FIRST EDITION

Leifer's INTRODUCTION TO Maternity and Pediatric Nursing in Canada

LISA KEENAN-LINDSAY, RN, MN, PNC(C)
Professor, School of Nursing
Seneca College of Applied Arts and Technology
Toronto, Ontario

US EDITOR
GLORIA LEIFER, RN, MA, CNE
Professor, Obstetric and Pediatric Nursing
Riverside City College
Riverside, California

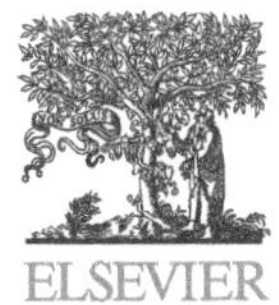

LEIFER'S INTRODUCTION TO MATERNITY AND PEDIATRIC NURSING IN CANADA, FIRST EDITION

ISBN: 978-1-77172-204-9

978-0-323-48397-1
(Softcover)

Notice

Practitioners and researchers must always rely on their own experience and knowledge in evaluating and using any information, methods, compounds, or experiments described herein. Because of rapid advances in the medical sciences, in particular, independent verification of diagnoses and drug dosages should be made. To the fullest extent of the law, no responsibility is assumed by Elsevier, authors, editors, or contributors for any injury and/or damage to persons or property as a matter of products liability, negligence, or otherwise, or from any use or operation of any methods, products, instructions, or ideas contained in the material herein.

Library of Congress Control Number: 2019909788

We are honoured to have received permission to reproduce the work, "Mother and Child", by Order of Canada award-winning Indigenous artist, Maxine Noel (Ioyan Mani), for this first Canadian edition, maternity and pediatric nursing text's cover.

Maxine has lent her voice and art to projects to improve the health and well-being of Indigenous women and girls; in projects related to maternal and infant health and, in collaboration with the NWAC in their work to raise awareness of the brutal dangers facing Indigenous women.

VP Education Content: Kevonne Holloway
Content Strategist, Canada Acquisitions: Roberta A. Spinosa-Millman
Director, Content Development Manager: Laurie Gower
Content Development Specialist: Sandy Matos
Publishing Services Manager: Julie Eddy
Project Manager: Abigail Bradberry
Design Direction: Renee Duenow

Printed in the United States of America

Last digit is the print number: 9 8 7 6 5 4 3 2

I would like to dedicate this book to the memory of both of my parents, Ruby Keenan (1932-2016) and Ross Keenan (1933-2018). My parents always inspired me and believed I could do anything I wanted. Their unwavering support throughout the years has made me the person I am today. As a perinatal nurse who usually cares for newborns and families at the beginning of life, it was an honour to care for both my parents during their final days. Love you Mom and Dad, you are never far from my thoughts.

Acknowledgements

I am grateful to the many patients and families I have cared for over the year. As a new nurse I worked at Sick Kids in Toronto which is where I learned to value the importance ensuring that care centred around the entire family and not just the child. This value has carried through in my care as a perinatal nurse. To the families I have cared for during birth, thank you for allowing me to be present at this most important time in your life and I hope I was able to assist in starting your family off in the right direction. It has been an honour to care for you.

To the many nurses I have met throughout my career from across the country, some of whom have contributed to this textbook, thank you for everything you have taught me. To the contributors of the textbook, thank you for understanding the value of accurate information for nursing students and working to provide this information. For those experts who I often refer to for questions that arise, thank you for your patience.

I would like to express my gratitude to my husband, John and my children, Katie, Emily and Jack for their encouragement and patience. Katie who is also my peer as a perinatal nurse, it is always a pleasure to discuss concerns and questions that would come up while working on this textbook with you. Your contributions have been invaluable. I would also like to acknowledge my new granddaughter, Hailey who has changed my life positively in so many ways and has taught me about the role of being a grandmother.

The group at Elsevier Inc. has been supportive of my vision for Canadian maternal-child textbooks. Thanks for believing in me and allowing me to provide this important resource for students. I embrace the challenge of ensuring that nursing students have the correct knowledge within the context of the Canadian health care system both in *Perry's Maternal Child Nursing Care in Canada,* for baccalaureate students and in this book, *Leifer's Introduction to Maternity and Pediatric Nursing in Canada,* for practical nursing students.

Thank you as well to Roberta Spinosa-Millman, Content Strategist at Elsevier Inc., Sandy Matos, Content Development Specialist for your continual support, guidance and the ability to keep me on track, and to my fantastic copy-editor Jerri Hurlbutt, who always makes everything so much clearer. This book would not have been completed without their support and hard work.

The role of the practical nurse is evolving in perinatal and pediatric nursing and it is vital that they have the most current knowledge to allow them to work effectively in a changing health care environment. It has been a pleasure to work with this team to develop this resource hat I hope will serve to educate and stimulate the appetite of the reader for continued education.

Finally, and most important, I would like to thank my many nursing students for helping me apply and redefine concepts of teaching and learning and for always keeping me on my toes.

Lisa Keenan-Lindsay

About the Author

Lisa J. Keenan-Lindsay graduated from the University of Toronto in 1983 with her BScN and returned to complete her MN in 2004. During her early career she worked in the area of pediatrics, mainly working in the pediatric intensive care unit at Sick Kids in Toronto. For the past 29 years, her work has focused on perinatal nursing, working in a variety of positions, including staff nurse in labour and birth and a prenatal clinic, educator for a maternal-newborn department, and a prenatal educator in the community. Currently Lisa is a professor of nursing at Seneca College and teaches perinatal nursing as well as other topics, to both baccalaureate and practical nursing students. She has been involved in many aspects of nursing education, including curriculum development, incorporation of simulation into the curriculum, and developing well written test questions. Lisa uses many active learning techniques in the classroom to enhance learning and critical thinking.

Lisa has been a member of the board of directors of the Canadian Association of Perinatal and Women's Health Nurses (CAPWHN) serving as President of CAPWHN in 2014 and 2015. Lisa has previously been involved with the Society of Obstetricians and Gynaecologists of Canada (SOGC) as an RN member for the Maternal-Fetal Medicine Committee and has co-authored many SOGC Clinical Practice Guidelines. Lisa has also been a Lamaze certified childbirth educator for many years. Lisa maintains her Perinatal Certification through the Canadian Nurses Association and is a member of the Perinatal Exam Committee. She is passionate about normalizing birth and works tirelessly at spreading the word in this endeavour.

CONTRIBUTORS AND REVIEWERS

CHAPTER CONTRIBUTORS

Jennifer Abbass-Dick, RN, BNSc, MN, IBCLC, PhD
Faculty of Health Science, Nursing
University of Ontario Institute of Technology
Oshawa, Ontario

Melanie Basso, RN, MSN, PNC(C)
Senior Practice Leader-Perinatal
BC Women's Hospital and Health Centre
Vancouver, British Columbia

Keri-Ann Berga, RN, BScN, MScN, IBCLC, PNC(C)
Assistant Professor
Department of Nursing Science, Faculty of Nursing
MacEwan University
Edmonton, Alberta

Jola Berkman, RN, BCur, BSc(med)Hons
Neonatal Outreach Coordinator for Perinatal Services of BC
Vancouver, British Columbia

Krystal Buchanan, PN, RN, BScN, MScN
Program Coordinator PN & PSW Programs, Orangeville Campus
Health, Wellness, and Sciences
Georgian College
Orangeville, Ontario

Martha Cope, RN, BA, MScN
Manager, Systemic Therapy & Oncology Nursing
Simcoe Muskoka Regional Cancer Program
Royal Victoria Regional Health Centre
Barrie, Ontario

Cheryl Dika, RN, MN, NP
Director, Curriculum Integrity and Faculty Development
Rady Faculty of Health Sciences College of Nursing
University of Manitoba
Winnipeg, Manitoba

Tanya Heuver, BScN, MN, Advanced Practice in Pediatrics
Assistant Professor
Department of Nursing Science
MacEwan University
Edmonton, Alberta

Kathleen Lindsay, RN, BScN
Registered Nurse
Labour and Delivery
St. Michael's Hospital
Toronto, Ontario

Andrea Logan, RN, MN, CPNP-PC, NP-Paediatrics
Registered Nurse
Emergency Department
The Hospital for Sick Children
Toronto, Ontario
Paediatric Nurse Practitioner
Simcoe Muskoka Paediatric Eating Disorder Program
Royal Victoria Regional Health Centre
Barrie, Ontario

Cheryl L. Pollard, PhD, RN, RPN
Associate Dean & Associate Professor
Faculty of Nursing
MacEwan University
Edmonton, Alberta

Cheryl A. Sams, RN, BScN, MSN
Professor Emerita
School of Health Sciences
Seneca College of Applied Arts and Technology
Toronto, Ontario

Angela Thable, BN, MN (NP)
Nurse Practitioner
Rady Faculty of Health Science College of Nursing
University of Manitoba
Winnipeg, Manitoba

Nancy Watts, RN, MN
Clinical Nurse Specialist
Perinatal
Mount Sinai Hospital
Toronto, Ontario

Ivanna Yau, MN, NP-Pediatrics
Pediatric Nurse Practitioner
Division of Neurology
Hospital for Sick Children
Toronto, Ontario

REVIEWERS

Tricia Anderson, RN, BScN, MN
Professor
St. Lawrence College
Kingston, Ontario

Krystal Buchanan, PN, RN, BScN, MScN
Program Coordinator PN & PSW Programs, Orangeville Campus
Health, Wellness, and Sciences
Georgian College
Orangeville, Ontario

Michelle A. Connell, RN, BScN, MEd
Nursing Professor
Ryerson, Centennial and George Brown Collaborative Nursing Degree Program
School of Community and Health Studies
Centennial College
Toronto, Ontario

Nancy Fleming, RN, HBScN, MAEd
Professor of Nursing
Confederation College & Lakehead University Collaborative BScN Program
Thunder Bay, Ontario

Joanna Gallacher, RN, MN
Professor
Durham College, Practical Nursing Program
Oshawa, Ontario

Erica Hurley, MN, BN, RN, CCNE
Nurse Educator
Western Regional School of Nursing
Memorial University of Newfoundland, Grenfell Campus
Corner Brook, Newfoundland and Labrador

Cindy Leclerc, RN, IBCLC
Saskatoon Health Region, Maternal Child Program
Saskatoon, Saskatchewan

Joan Paisley, RN, BN
Full Time Lab, Theory and Clinical Instructor
PN/PSW Program, Allied Health Program
New Brunswick Community College
Saint John, New Brunswick

Krista Patton, RN, BNSc, MN
Professor, School of Health Sciences
St. Lawrence College
Cornwall, Ontario

Rachael Wymer, RN, BScN, MSN
Nursing Faculty
Centennial College
Toronto, Ontario

To the Instructor

EDUCATION OF THE LICENSED/REGISTERED PRACTICAL NURSE

Depth with simplicity is the theme of this text, which is based on current Canadian health care practices and the need to adapt to advances in medicine and technology to maintain quality patient care. The role of the nurse is changing at every level, and the curriculum of educational programs for the practical nurse also must change to prepare graduates adequately for entry-level positions. Many practical nursing programs are considered "ladders" into a baccalaureate degree in nursing. This text contains the most accurate, current, and clinically relevant information within the scope of practice for the practical nurse, but with sufficient depth of knowledge and concepts essential to facilitate student success in the RN bridge program.

ABOUT THE TEXT

This combined maternity and pediatrics text highlights the ways in which infants and children differ from adults. Because of differences in anatomy, physiology, and psychology, techniques for caring for the infant, child, or pregnant woman may vary from those used for the adult medical-surgical patient. Principles of physiology and pathophysiology are presented in this text as a review to help students understand and identify normal and abnormal health.

This text provides comprehensive discussions of family-centred care, wellness, health promotion, illness prevention, and the growth and development of the child *and the parent*. **This information forms one continuum of knowledge that flows from conception to adulthood and is organized from simple to complex and health to illness.**

The normal process of growth and development—from conception to adulthood—is the core of perinatal and pediatric knowledge. Therefore, it is integrated as an essential feature of this text. The nurse must be able to provide parents with an awareness of the changing developmental needs of the growing fetus and child to promote healthy parenting.

The effects of illness and medication in the pregnant woman are influenced by the presence of a fetus; dosages are determined by the age and weight of the infant or young child, and illness or injury at a specific phase of growth and development may have an impact on the achievement of normal developmental tasks. Nothing is *standard* among these populations, and these are some of the unique challenges of perinatal and pediatric nursing.

The systems approach is maintained for the most part, in presenting physiological illness. **The organization of this text is designed to facilitate its use in a combined maternity and pediatric course, a maternity course followed by a separate pediatric course, or a medical-surgical course that integrates maternity and pediatric concepts.**

This edition encompasses the core aspects of evidence-informed maternal–child nursing in health and illness, incorporating updates in clinical care and technology. Practical nursing education includes tasks and technology used in acute-care hospitals. However, the modern trend of health care reform is moving the focus from the institution to the population. In addition, many parents use complementary or alternative therapies for themselves and their children. Chapter 21 discusses some common alternative or complementary therapies for which there is standard scientific evidence, as well as some readily available over-the-counter remedies. All nurses need a working knowledge of the actions, interactions, and safety of these interventions related to the child. An understanding of the trend toward active participation in one's own health care requires knowledge that can help the patient choose safe self-care practices.

The reader is encouraged to approach clinical problems using critical thinking rather than predetermined habit or memorization of fact. The strong base of knowledge provided by this text focuses on abilities (skills) and beginning concepts of critical thinking. Critical thinking is the basis of clinical decision making and is an essential part of nursing education at every level. Critical thinking questions are included in most chapters with answer guidelines available to the student on the Evolve website. Also, the three different types of care plan styles presented in this text (standard patient care plan, family care plan, and clinical pathway) are designed to assist readers in adapting to the style used in the area in which they practice. The unfolding case study can be used to challenge the student to apply concepts discussed in the text, using critical thinking that is enhanced by the open-ended questions relating to the presenting family in the chapter. Answers to the open-ended questions can be found in the student's resource materials provided online. Each chapter also offers online resources for students to use to enhance their evidence-based knowledge and critical thinking skills.

Positive communication skills are an essential part of caring nursing interventions. Cultural differences related to various perceptions of health and illness and traditional health practices are presented to enable the student nurse to begin developing cultural humility with the community served.

Clinical rotations, particularly in obstetrics and pediatrics, seem to be shortened each year because sites for hands-on clinical experiences are difficult to find. This text is designed to bridge the gap between the classroom and the clinical arena by presenting current facts, concepts, and principles that promote learning through comprehension rather than memorization. The inclusion of 38 detailed Skills—in addition to many photos and drawings of specific procedures—unique to obstetrics and pediatrics are designed to emphasize nursing actions and responsibilities. Each Skill includes several icons that symbolize common steps for *any* skill in *any* area of general medical-surgical nursing—checking the order, introducing yourself, identifying the patient, performing hand hygiene. It is essential for the student to understand the importance of these steps and to know when to perform each. Presented as a continuum of related images, these icons become engrained in the students' minds as steps that must be considered before performing any intervention. However, these icons also are standard and require critical thinking for students to determine the specific supplies and equipment they may need and when it is necessary to don personal protective equipment.

Every effort has been made to provide a readable text in a simplified format with an array of tables, figures and photographs and illustrations that allow a comprehensive understanding of techniques essential for effective perinatal and pediatric nursing care. It is hoped that the information presented in this text will help the practical nurse handle challenging clinical situations that require the use of a broad knowledge base and the ability to think critically, to prioritize, and to use specific clinical skills. This book, with its theme of *depth with simplicity,* is designed to prepare the practical nursing student for mobility in the profession as well as to enable the practical nurse to provide evidence-informed quality perinatal and pediatric nursing care to a diverse population in a rapidly changing world.

The first Canadian edition has been thoroughly revised with the most recent research and information, including Canadian guidelines from the Society of Obstetricians and Gynecologists of Canada (SOGC) and the Canadian Paediatric Society (CPS), the Breastfeeding Committee for Canada and the World Health Organization's Baby-Friendly Initiative (BFI), complementary and alternative therapies used in maternal–child care, nonpharmacological prevention and treatment of hypertension, updated immunization mandates, and preventing medication errors, among others.

HALLMARK FEATURES

The following are hallmark features of this book:

- Content that spans the **developmental continuum** is organized from **simple to complex** and from **health to illness,** making it easy to locate information.
- Focus is on **family-centred care, health promotion and illness prevention, women's health issues, and growth and development of child and parent.**
- **Perinatal content** includes exercise during pregnancy, routine screening tests done during pregnancy, nursing interventions and responsibilities for analgesia during childbirth, Canadian fetal health surveillance in labour information, current breastfeeding content, information related to Perinatal Mood Disorders (PMD), perinatal bereavement, and the understanding that the prenatal fetal environment impacts the health of the newborn as an adult.
- **Pictorial story of vaginal and cesarean births** includes photographs through birth, followed by delivery of placenta.
- Table 4.6 explains in detail the **physiological and psychosocial changes during trimesters** of pregnancy, signs and symptoms, and nursing interventions.
- **Cultural practices** as they relate to pregnancy and labour, maternal/infant care, and pediatric care are discussed.
- **Canada's Food Guide–2019 (Appendix C)** and the Public Health Agency of Canada guidelines on feeding children under 2 years of age have been incorporated into the chapters on nutrition to help promote healthy growth and development.
- **Pediatric content** includes pediatric language milestones and communication problems in pediatric growth and development, therapeutic play, and sickle cell crises.
- **Loss, death, and grief** and children's responses to death at various ages are presented in a new chapter on Chronic Conditions and Palliative Care: Caring for the Child and Family (Chapter 22).
- **Skills** unique to perinatal and pediatrics (with Performance Checklists for each on Evolve) cover a wide range of maternal and pediatric nursing interventions.
- **Nursing Care Plans** provide expected outcomes, interventions, and rationales for nursing interventions.
- **Unfolding Case Study** with open-ended critical thinking questions to assess application of content to practice as students follow one family through the conception and birth process.
- **Nursing Tips** throughout highlight pertinent information applicable in the clinical setting.
- **Pediatric laboratory values** have been included in Appendix B as a reference tool because they are not always standard content in lab books.

TEACHING AND LEARNING PACKAGE

FOR THE INSTRUCTOR

The comprehensive **Evolve Resources with TEACH Instructor Resource** include the following:

- Test Bank with approximately 1015 multiple-choice and alternate-format questions with correct answers and rationale
- TEACH Lesson Plans and TEACH PowerPoint slides with approximately 1860 slides
- Image Collection that contains all the illustrations and photographs in the textbook
- Open-Book Quizzes and Answer Keys for each chapter
- Suggestions for Working with ESL Students

FOR THE STUDENT

The Evolve **Student Resources** include the following assets and more:

- Answers and Rationales for end-of-chapter Review Questions and Unfolding Case Study questions
- Answer Guidelines for end-of-chapter Critical Thinking Questions
- Audio Glossary
- Calculators for instruction on how to determine body mass index (BMI), body surface area, fluid deficit, Glasgow coma score, IV dosages, and conversion of units
- Fluids and Electrolytes Tutorial
- Interactive Review Questions for the Certification Examination with immediate feedback, including answers and rationales
- Skills Performance Checklists for each Skill found in the textbook available for download
- Video clips

To the Student

READING AND REVIEW TOOLS

- **Objectives** introduce the chapter topics.
- **Key Terms** are listed. Difficult medical, nursing, or scientific terms are accompanied by simple phonetic pronunciations. Key Terms are considered essential to understanding chapter content and are in colour the first time they appear. Key Terms are briefly defined in the text, with complete definitions in the Glossary.
- Each chapter ends with a ***Get Ready for the Certification Exam!*** **section** that includes: (1) **Key Points** that reiterate the chapter objectives and serve as a useful review of concepts; (2) a list of **Additional Resources** including Online Resources; (3) a set of **Review Questions** with answers located on Evolve; and (4) **Critical Thinking Questions** for many chapters with answer guidelines located on Evolve.

CHAPTER FEATURES

Skills are presented in a logical format with defined *purpose*, relevant *illustrations*, and detailed and numbered nursing *steps*. Each Skill includes icons that serve as reminders to perform the basic steps applicable to *all* nursing interventions:

Check orders.

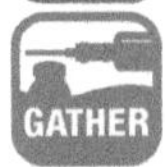

Gather necessary equipment and supplies.

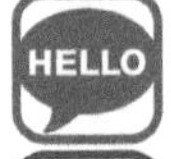

Introduce yourself.

Check patient's identification.

Provide privacy.

Explain the procedure/intervention.

Perform hand hygiene.

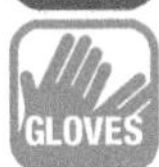

Don gloves (if applicable).

Not listing the exact supplies or equipment needed encourages you to think critically about what you might need to do or to gather according to hospital protocol before performing the specific Skill.

Nursing Care Plans, developed around specific case studies, include nursing diagnoses with an emphasis on patient goals and outcomes and questions to promote *critical thinking* and valuable sound *clinical decision-making skills.* An **Unfolding Case Study** uses open-ended questions to stimulate critical thinking in applying concepts discussed in the chapter that may relate to a specific family as they experience the various stages of pregnancy and birth.

Nursing Tips highlight pertinent information applicable in the clinical setting.

Safety Alerts and **Medication Safety Alerts** emphasize the importance of protecting patients, family, health care providers, and the public from accidents, medication errors, and the spread of disease.

Health Promotion boxes emphasize a healthy lifestyle, preventive behaviours, and screening tests to assist in the prevention of accidents and illness.

Medication tables provide quick access to information about commonly used medications related to perinatal or pediatric nursing care.

Cultural Considerations boxes explore select cultural preferences and how to address the needs of a culturally diverse patient and family when planning care.

Nutrition Considerations provide important nutrition information for the pregnant woman, infant, and growing child.

Patient Teaching boxes appear frequently in the text to help develop awareness of the vital role of patient/family teaching in health care today.

Communication boxes focus on communication strategies with real-life examples of nurse–patient dialogue.

Legal & Ethical Considerations present pertinent information about the legal issues and ethical dilemmas that may face the practicing nurse.

Home Care Considerations boxes discuss the issues facing patients and caregivers in the home setting.

Memory Joggers provide easy-to-remember mnemonics and acronyms for remembering specific information.

Table of Contents

APPENDICES

Overview of Perinatal and Pediatric Nursing in Canada

1

Lisa Keenan-Lindsay

http://evolve.elsevier.com/Canada/Leifer

Objectives

1. Define each key term listed.
2. Recall the history of perinatal and pediatric nursing care in Canada.
3. List the organizations concerned with setting standards for the care of maternity and pediatric patients.
4. Understand the legal responsibilities of the nurse to report certain diseases or conditions to the public health authorities.
5. Explain the role of the Public Health Agency of Canada.
6. Describe the impact of the social determinants of health on the health of Canadians.
7. Discuss how culture may influence the childbirth experience and care for the pediatric patient.
8. Define family as it relates to perinatal and pediatric nursing.
9. Explain how the Baby-Friendly Initiative supports breastfeeding.
10. Discuss why statistics are important and the common terms used in expressing the data.
11. List the five steps of the nursing process.
12. Define critical thinking.
13. Compare and contrast a nursing care plan with a clinical pathway.
14. Examine the importance of documentation as a nursing responsibility.
15. Describe the role of the community health nurse as a health care provider.
16. Describe the role of the Sustainable Development Goals and the impact on global health.

Key Terms

advanced practice nurses
advocate
clinical nurse specialist (CNS)
clinical pathways
critical thinking
cultural awareness
cultural competence
cultural humility
cultural safety
cultural sensitivity
culture
documentation
empowerment
evidence-informed practice
family care plan
midwives
Millennium Development Goals (MDGs)
morbidity
mortality
Personal Information Protection and Electronic Documents Act (PIPEDA)
primary care nurse practitioner
nursing care plan
nursing process
SBAR (or S-BAR) (ĔS-băr)
statistics

The word *obstetrics* is derived from the Latin term *obstetrix,* which means "stand by." It is the branch of medicine that pertains to the care of women during pregnancy, childbirth, and the postpartum period (puerperium). Perinatal nursing is the care given by the nurse to the expectant family before, during, and following birth.

A physician specializing in the care of women during pregnancy, labour, birth, and the postpartum period is an obstetrician. These physicians perform Caesarean births and treat women with known or suspected obstetrical problems as well as attend uncomplicated births. Many family physicians and registered midwives also provide assistance to women during the perinatal period and at birth. See further discussion regarding midwives later in chapter.

Pediatrics is defined as the branch of medicine that deals with the child's development and care and the diseases of childhood and their treatment. The word is derived from the Greek *pais, paidos,* meaning "child," and *iatreia,* "cure." Pediatric nursing is concerned with the protection, promotion, and optimization of health of children and their abilities, from newborn to young adulthood, focusing on the strengths of the child and family. Using a child- and family-centred care approach, pediatric nurses possess knowledge of psychomotor, psychosocial, and cognitive growth and development, as well as of the health problems and needs specific to people in this age group (Canadian Pediatric Nursing Standards Advisory Group, 2017).

THE HISTORY OF OBSTETRICAL AND PEDIATRIC CARE IN CANADA

The Indigenous people had their own traditional beliefs and practices related to pregnancy, childbirth, and health care. The early settlers to Canada also brought with them a wide variety of their own practices and beliefs about health care and the birth process.

In Canada, before the 1900s, most babies were born at home and a midwife or relative attended most births. Only very ill patients were cared for in hospitals. Maternal and child outcomes were poor in such institutions because of crowded conditions and unskilled nursing care. As a result, hospitals began to develop training programs for nurses. As the medical profession grew, physicians developed a closer relationship with hospitals. This, along with the advent of obstetrical instruments and anaesthesia, caused a shift toward hospital care during childbirth. By the 1950s, hospital practice in obstetrics was well established. By 1960, most births in Canada occurred in hospitals.

However, hospital care during that time did not embrace the family-centred approach. Often the father waited in a separate room during the labour and birth of his child. The mother was often sedated with "twilight sleep" and participated little during labour. After birth, the infant was not reunited with the parents for several hours, which resulted in a delay of parent–infant bonding. During the 1950s, the hospital stay for labour and birth was 1 week. Today, on average, a hospital stay is 1 to 2 days in uncomplicated cases, with routine follow-up of the newborn taking place within the first few days after discharge. For a summary of historical influences on pediatric and perinatal health care in Canada see Box 1.1.

Box 1.1 Historical Influences in Perinatal and Pediatric Health Care in Canada

The following is a chronological list of some of the important milestones in Canadian history related to improving perinatal and pediatric care:

- 1968 – The *Medical Care Act* was passed and universal health care was provided to all Canadians. This publically funded program divides costs between the federal and provincial governments. The pillars of the program are that it must be universal, publicly administered, portable, and comprehensive. Medications and dental care are covered in some provinces, although usually only for certain ages (e.g., older persons or children).
- 1971 – Canada adopted multiculturalism as an official policy that encompassed the value and dignity of all Canadians regardless of their racial, ethnic, language, or religious origins; the rights of Indigenous people; and the acknowledgement of two official languages (French and English).
- 1988 – Abortion was legalized in Canada.
- 1993 – The first midwifery education program was started, in Ontario.
- 2000 – The United Nations met and developed the Millennium Development Goals. These goals were developed to eradicate extreme poverty and hunger worldwide; achieve universal primary education; and promote gender equality and empower women, by the year 2015. The goals were revisited in 2015 and revised for future work.
- 2000 – The first Canadian Perinatal Certification exam was offered by the Canadian Nurses Association (CNA).
- 2000 – The ***Personal Information Protection and Electronic Documents Act (PIPEDA)*** was enacted, although it was amended in 2015. This legislation set standards to protect a person's privacy. Organizations must obtain an individual's consent when they collect, use, or disclose that individual's personal information. If an organization is going to use it for another purpose, they must obtain consent again (Office of the Privacy Commissioner of Canada, 2018). Some provinces have separate legislation covering patients' health information, but all legislation ensures that this information is kept private.
- 2001 – The Canadian Association of Midwives (CAM) was initiated.
- 2003 – The first Canadian Critical Care Pediatric certification exam was offered by the CNA.
- 2003 – The Canadian Patient Safety Institute (CPSI) was initiated and works with governments, health organizations, leaders, and health care providers to ensure patient safety and quality.
- 2004 – The Public Health Agency of Canada (PHAC) was formed to initially focus on population health and health promotion.
- 2005 – The Canadian Association of Neonatal Nurses (CANN) was formed.
- 2011 – The Canadian Association of Perinatal and Women's Health Nurses (CAPWHN) was formed, having previously been a section of the Association of Women's Health, Obstetric and Neonatal Nurses (AWHONN).
- 2012 – The Truth and Reconciliation Commission revealed the impact of the history of residential schools on the health and well-being of Indigenous Canadians and developed strategies for reconciliation. This report included recommendations for health care provider education.
- 2012 – The Breastfeeding Committee for Canada (BCC) developed the 10 indicators to achieve the Baby-Friendly Initiative.
- 2016 – The Canadian Association of Schools of Nursing published *Entry-to-Practice Competencies for Nursing Care of the Childbearing Family for Baccalaureate Programs in Nursing.*
- 2017 – The *Canadian Pediatric Nursing Standards* were published to guide and ensure consistent and high-quality nursing care for all Canadian children.
- 2018 – The first neonatal certification exam was offered by the Canadian Nurses Association
- 2018 – Perinatal nursing standards were published by CAPWHN.
- 2018 – The universal Pharmacare program is investigated by the federal government.

Source: Office of the Privacy Commissioner. (2018). *PIPEDA in brief.* Retrieved from https://www.priv.gc.ca/en/privacy-topics/privacy-laws-in-canada/the-personal-information-protection-and-electronic-documents-act-pipeda/pipeda_brief/.

Organizations concerned with setting standards for both perinatal and pediatric care were developed, starting in 1944. Obstetrical organizations include the Society of Obstetricians and Gynaecologists of Canada (SOGC), the Canadian Association of Midwives (CAM), and the Canadian Association of Perinatal and Women's Health Nurses (CAPWHN).

The Canadian Association of Pediatric Nurses (CAPN), the Canadian Association of Neonatal Nurses (CANN), and the Canadian Paediatric Society (CPS) have established a position of leadership in setting health standards for children. Children's Healthcare Canada supports pediatric health care organizations through education, research, and quality improvement initiatives to improve health service delivery for Canadian children and youth (Children's Healthcare Canada, 2019).

Legal and Ethical Considerations

The Canadian Nurses Association (CNA) develops standards of practice that serve as a guide to meet current challenges for both registered nurses and registered/licensed practical nurses. These standards are used when policies and procedures are established. Also, each province has its own regulatory body that determines the scope of practice for nurse practitioners, registered nurses, and practical nurses. Because these descriptions vary between provinces, nurses must stay informed about the laws in the province where they are employed.

Legal and Ethical Considerations

***Personal Information Protection and Electronic Documents Act* (PIPEDA)**

Health care personnel are expected to maintain strict confidentiality concerning all patient information. PIPEDA regulations mandate that the names and personal information of patients be kept in a secure and private place. Nurses and other health care personnel must maintain strict confidentiality of all patient information.

CURRENT ISSUES IN PERINATAL AND PEDIATRIC HEALTH CARE IN CANADA

HEALTH PROMOTION

Health promotion is key to improving the health of all Canadians. The role of the Public Health Agency of Canada (PHAC) is to empower Canadians to improve their own health. The PHAC works in partnership with federal, provincial, and community agencies, focusing on prevention of disease and injuries, promoting good physical and mental health, and providing information to support informed decision making regarding health throughout a person's life (Government of Canada, 2019).

Across Canada, disease prevention efforts are made at the national, provincial, and local levels. Municipal and regional health departments see to the inspection of the water, milk, and food supplies of communities and enforce the maintenance of proper sewage and garbage disposal. Epidemics are investigated and, when necessary, persons capable of transmitting diseases are isolated.

Preventing illness and disability is cost-effective; more important, it saves families from experiencing illness-related stress, disruptions, and financial burden. In addition, healthy children spend fewer days in the hospital.

Many conditions are currently treated in same-day surgery, ambulatory settings, or emergency departments. Rather than being separate entities, hospital and home care have become interdependent.

Legal and Ethical Considerations

Reportable Situations

The nurse has a legal responsibility to report certain diseases or conditions to the local public health authorities. A *reportable disease* is an illness that poses a health hazard to the public, such as a foodborne infection, tuberculosis, some sexually transmitted infections (STIs), or other communicable condition (see Chapters 2 and 32). Suspected child abuse must be reported immediately to protect the child from further harm. The nurse must have a basic understanding of legal and ethical responsibilities to provide meaningful support to the family.

SOCIAL DETERMINANTS OF HEALTH

The health of Canadians is dependent on many factors besides lifestyle and medical treatment. The primary factors that shape the health of Canadians are the living conditions they experience. These conditions have come to be known as the *social determinants of health* (Box 1.2). Social determinants influence a wide range of health vulnerabilities and capacities, health behaviours, and health management (Reading & Wein, 2009). Understanding the issues related to people's health can aid in determining the root causes of a problem and in developing strategies to address the problem, thus preventing health problems from occurring in the first place. This focus should assist in improving the health status of the whole society, while also considering the special needs and vulnerabilities of at-risk populations (Government of Canada, 2018b).

It is important to note that Indigenous people in Canada may be impacted by determinants of health that are different from those of non-Indigenous people. These determinants include circumstances and environments as well as social and political structures, systems, and institutions. See further discussion below regarding Indigenous Health.

CULTURE

Culture is a body of socially inherited characteristics that one generation hands down to the next. Culture consists of values, beliefs, and practices shared by members of the group. Culture becomes a patterned

Box 1.2 Social Determinants of Health

1. *Income and Social Status*—Health status improves at each step up the income and social hierarchy. High income determines living conditions such as safe housing and the ability to buy sufficient good food.
2. *Social Support Network*—Support from families, friends, and communities is associated with better health. Such social support networks can be important in helping people solve problems and deal with adversity, as well as in maintaining a sense of mastery and control over life circumstances.
3. *Education and Literacy*—Education contributes to health and prosperity by equipping people with knowledge and skills for problem solving, and it helps provide a sense of control and mastery over life circumstances. Education increases opportunities for job and income security and job satisfaction. And it improves people's ability to access and understand information to help keep them healthy.
4. *Employment and Working Conditions*—Unemployment, underemployment, and stressful or unsafe work are associated with poorer health.
5. *Social Environments*—Individuals within one's social environments (e.g., family, peers, community, and workplace) can add resources to an individual's repertoire of strategies to cope with changes and foster health.
6. *Physical Environments*—At certain levels of exposure, contaminants in air, water, food, and soil can cause a variety of adverse health effects, including cancer, birth defects, respiratory illness, and gastrointestinal ailments. In the built environment, factors related to housing, indoor air quality, and the design of communities and transportation systems can significantly influence physical and psychological well-being.
7. *Personal Health Practices and Coping Skills*—These are the actions by which individuals can prevent diseases and promote self-care, cope with challenges, develop self-reliance, solve problems, and make choices that enhance health.
8. *Healthy Child Development*—The effects of early experiences on brain development, school readiness, and health in later life can impact health. For example, a young person's development is greatly affected by their housing and neighbourhood, family income and level of parents' education, access to nutritious foods and physical recreation, genetic makeup, and access to dental and medical care.
9. *Biology and Genetic Endowment*—Genetic endowment provides an inherited predisposition to a wide range of individual responses that affect health status.
10. *Health Services*—Access to health services, particularly those designed to maintain and promote health, to prevent disease, and to restore health and function, contributes to population health.
11. *Gender*—Gender refers to the array of society-determined roles, personality traits, attitudes, behaviours, values, relative power, and influence that society ascribes to the two sexes on a differential basis.
12. *Culture*—Some persons or groups may face additional health risks due to a socioeconomic environment, which is largely determined by dominant cultural values that contribute to the perpetuation of conditions such as marginalization, stigmatization, loss or devaluation of language and culture, and lack of access to culturally appropriate health care and services.

Source: Public Health Agency of Canada. (2013). *What makes Canadians healthy or unhealthy?* Retrieved from https://www.canada.ca/en/public-health/services/health-promotion/population-health/what-determines-health/what-makes-canadians-healthy-unhealthy.html#social1

expression of thoughts and actions (called *traditions*), and these may affect the way patients respond to health care situations.

Canada is a culturally diverse nation. In caring for patients, nurses must develop **cultural awareness** and **cultural sensitivity** to practices and values that differ from their own. Only in this way can nurses develop the **cultural competence** that will enable them to adapt health care practices to meet the needs of patients from various cultures. **Cultural safety** goes beyond cultural awareness and sensitivity; it means understanding the power imbalances inherent in health care services and relationships and addressing these inequities in service delivery (Wiebe, van Gaalen, Langlois, et al., 2014). **Cultural humility** is the precursor to providing culturally competent care. Cultural humility is a process of self-reflection and discovery for building honest and trustworthy relationships (Yeager & Bauer-Wu, 2013). This lifelong process requires an understanding of one's own assumptions, biases, and values and how one's background and social environment have shaped one's experience (Yeager & Bauer-Wu, 2013). A key aspect of cultural humility is acknowledging that health care providers can never be "expert" or "competent" in another person's culture or history, but can instead demonstrate an openness to learning (CAPWHN, 2017).

The cultural background of the expectant family may influence their adaptation to the birth experience. Nursing Care Plan 1.1 lists nursing interventions for selected diagnoses that pertain to cultural diversity. One way that the nurse can gain important information about an individual's culture is to ask the patient or family what they consider normal practice. Data-collection questions for a pregnant woman might include the following:

- How does the woman view her pregnancy (as an illness, a vulnerable time, or a healthy time)?
- Is birth a public or private experience for her?
- In what position is she comfortable for giving birth (i.e., squatting, lithotomy, or some other position)?
- What type of help would she like before and after birth?
- What role does her immediate or extended family play in relation to the pregnancy and birth?

Nursing Care Plan 1.1 Care of Childbearing Families Related to Potential or Actual Stress Caused by Cultural Diversity

PATIENT DATA

A 22-year-old, $G_1T_0P_0A_0L_0$, is admitted to the labour room in active labour. Her partner is with her, and they do not speak English.

Selected Nursing Diagnosis Difficulty in verbal communication as a result of language barriers

Goals	Nursing Interventions	Rationales
The woman will have an opportunity to understand communication in her own language.	Arrange for a staff member interpreter or use an online translation app as needed.	An interpreter can provide support for the woman and help to lessen her anxieties. Poor communication can result in time delays, errors, and misinterpretation of intent. Use family members only when no other options are available.
	Clearly define instructions in woman's language of origin.	A common language is necessary for communication to take place.
	Provide written instructions in woman's language whenever possible.	Written instructions can be reviewed at a less stressful time by patient. In some cases it is necessary to determine if person can read.
	Explain the use and purpose of all instruments and equipment, along with the effects or possible effects on the mother and fetus.	Education of family lessens anxiety and provides family with a sense of control.
	Provide opportunities for clarification and questions.	Learning takes time; repetition of important material promotes learning. Nurse can determine woman's understanding of information and clarify misconceptions.

Selected Nursing Diagnosis Possible difficulty in family adaptation as a result of isolation, different customs, attitudes, or beliefs

Goals	Nursing Interventions	Rationales
Family members will state that they feel welcome and safe in the environment provided.	Encourage orientation visit to the maternity unit before birth.	Families who have clear, accurate information can better participate in the labour and birth process. Viewing the birthing unit before using it decreases anxiety about the unknown.
	Inform families about routines, visiting hours, and significant persons who can be present in labour and birth.	Families have different expectations of the health care system. They may hesitate to ask questions because of shyness or fear of "losing face."
	Determine and respect practices and values of family and incorporate them into nursing care plans as much as possible.	Clarification of culturally specific values and practices will prevent misunderstanding and conflict with the nurse's value system. Nursing care plans promote organization of care and communication among staff members.

Such information helps to promote understanding and individualizes patient care. It also increases the satisfaction of the patient and the nurse regarding the quality of care provided.

Cultural competence is also required for pediatric nursing care. Cultural beliefs may influence whether a family seeks help for a sick child and how the family perceives the recommended health care practices.

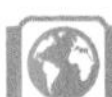
Cultural Considerations

Perception of Health and Illness

Cultural beliefs today, as in the past, affect how a family perceives health and illness and can affect the type of health care they may seek. Culturally sensitive nurses are aware of cultural diversity and incorporating this information into the plan for nursing care.

Impact of Immigration

Many people have immigrated to Canada from other countries, and some of these people may have difficulty accessing health care because of language difficulties or an inability to navigate the health care system. It is important to ensure that patients and families understand the health teaching that is provided to them; translators may need to aid in this process. It is also imperative that nurses consider the health beliefs of the person and family, as this may influence whether or not they follow through with suggested screenings and treatments.

Indigenous People

The health of Indigenous people in Canada declined after the colonization of Canada. There are many reasons for this decline, including a lack of support from settlers for Indigenous ways of healing. The health of Indigenous people has improved slightly over the past several decades, but Indigenous people continue to experience poorer health outcomes than those of non-Indigenous people as well as significant disparities related to health status (Health Canada, 2014). Indigenous health concerns include high infant and young-child mortality; high maternal morbidity and mortality; high levels of infectious disease (e.g., human immunodeficiency virus/acquired immunodeficiency syndrome [HIV/AIDS] and tuberculosis); malnutrition and stunted growth; shortened life expectancy; diseases and death associated with cigarette smoking; social problems, illnesses and death linked to misuse of alcohol and other drugs; accidents, poisonings, interpersonal violence, homicide, and suicide; obesity, diabetes, hypertension, cardiovascular, and chronic renal disease (lifestyle diseases); and diseases caused by environmental contamination (National Collaboration Centre for Aboriginal Health [NCCAH], 2013).

Some of these health disparities are due to lack of access to quality health care resulting from living in remote areas and the lack of Indigenous health care providers who understand the Indigenous traditions that are used to improve health and wellness. Many Indigenous people in Canada have lost their connection to their land, cultures, languages, and traditional ways of life, owing to colonial practices such as forced relocation and placement in residential schools. Residential schools first opened in Canada in the late 1800s; the last one closed in 1996. Often several generations of children experienced being removed from their families and communities, and this separation has had devastating effects on Indigenous people (NCCAH, 2013). The Truth and Reconciliation Commission (TRC) (2015) developed a call to action for Canadians to acknowledge the impact of the legacy of residential schools, as well as strategies for reconciliation that focus on mutual respect of all people. One recommendation of the TRC report is to include in the curriculum for all health care providers the findings of the commission.

Another issue related to the health of Indigenous people is the way health care is funded across the country. The complicated "patchwork" of policies, legislation, and agreements that delegate responsibility among federal, provincial, municipal, and Aboriginal governments in different ways in different parts of the country makes the equitable access to health care difficult for some Indigenous people (NCCAH, 2013).

Nurses need to acknowledge that an Indigenous approach to health care is often rooted in a holistic conception of well-being involving a healthy balance of four elements of wellness—physical, emotional, mental, and spiritual—and to incorporate these into the care provided.

LESBIAN, GAY, BISEXUAL, TRANSGENDER, QUEER, TWO-SPIRIT (LGBTQ2) HEALTH CONCERNS

Nurses need to be aware of health concerns of patients who identify as LGBTQ2, as it is known that LGBTQ2 people may have different health concerns than those of heterosexual persons and be at risk for certain health issues, including mental health, substance use, heart disease, smoking, cancer, and diet, weight, and body-image concerns (Ricca, Wahlskog, & Dewey Bergren, 2018). Some LGBTQ2 people are reluctant to access and use the health care system because they feel they may experience discrimination. Health care can be seen as heteronormative, which does not facilitate appropriate care for LGBTQ2 patients. Asking patients about their partners and not assuming heterosexuality is very important in this context. Offering an option for transgender or "other" is important when asking about gender, in order to be inclusive and supportive. Nurses also need to be supportive of children who identify as LGBTQ2; often the nurse is the first person the child will confide in.

In this text, LGBTQ2 concerns are integrated into the discussion when appropriate. Although the term *woman* is used mainly to describe patients who give birth, this may not always be the case for some patients. It is imperative that nurses be aware of this and provide care in a culturally safe manner for all patients.

FAMILY-CENTRED CARE

Family-centred care recognizes the importance of providing care for the individual and the family. Every family member is affected by the birth of a child; therefore, family involvement during pregnancy and birth is seen as integral for bonding and support. A child who is sick also impacts the whole family, and care must be provided within the context of the family.

In family-centred care, the strength and integrity of the family are placed at the core of planning and implementing health care. As caregivers and decision makers, family members are an integral part of both obstetrical and pediatric nursing. The philosophy, goals, culture, and health practices of the family contribute to their ability to accept and maintain control over the health care of family members. This control is called **empowerment**. The nurse's role in perinatal and pediatric family-centred care is to enter into a relationship or partnership with the family to achieve the goals of health for its members.

An important aspect of family-centred care is the definition of family. The Vanier Institute of the Family (2019) defines *family* as any combination of two or more persons who are bound together over time by ties of mutual consent, birth, and/or adoption or placement and who, together, provide some of the following:

- Physical maintenance and care of group members
- Socialization of children
- Social control of members
- Affective nurturance—love

The definition of family is broad to ensure that it encompasses all families and family experiences. It is a definition of family that focuses on relationships and roles—what families do, not what they look like (Vanier Institute, 2019). This definition encompasses the diversity of family structures in Canada.

Current maternity practice focuses on a high-quality family experience. *Childbearing is seen as a normal and*

Box 1.3 Family-Centred Maternity and Newborn Care Guidelines

Family-centred maternity and newborn care (FCMNC) is a process of providing safe, skilled, and individualized care. It responds to the physical, emotional, psychosocial, and spiritual needs of the woman, the newborn, and the family. FCMNC considers pregnancy and birth to be normal, healthy life events and recognizes the significance of family support, participation, and informed choice.

GUIDING PRINCIPLES

1. A family-centred approach to maternal and newborn care is optimal.
2. Pregnancy and birth are normal, healthy processes.
3. Early parent–infant attachment is critical for newborn and child development and the growth of healthy families.
4. Family-centred maternal and newborn care applies to all care environments.
5. Family-centred maternal and newborn care is informed by research evidence.
6. Family-centred maternal and newborn care requires a holistic approach.
7. Family-centred maternal and newborn care involves collaboration among care providers.
8. Culturally appropriate care is important in a multicultural society.
9. Indigenous peoples have distinctive needs during pregnancy and birth.
10. Care as close to home as possible is ideal.
11. Individualized maternal and newborn care is recommended.
12. Women and their families require knowledge about their care.
13. Women and their families play an integral role in decision making.
14. The attitudes and language of health care providers have an impact on a family's experience of maternal and newborn care.
15. Family-centred maternal and newborn care respects reproductive rights.
16. Family-centred maternal and newborn care functions within a system that requires ongoing evaluation.
17. Family-centred maternal and newborn care best practices from global settings may offer valuable options for Canadian consideration.

Source: Public Health Agency of Canada. (2017). *Family-centred maternity and newborn care in Canada: Underlying philosophy and principles*. Ottawa (ON): PHAC. Retrieved from https://www.canada.ca/content/dam/phac-aspc/documents/services/publications/healthy-living/maternity-newborn-care/maternity-newborn-care-guidelines-chapter-1-eng.pdf

healthy event. Parents are prepared for the changes that take place during pregnancy, labour, and birth. They are also prepared for changes in family dynamics after the birth. Treating each family according to their individual needs is considered paramount. The PHAC, along with experts across the country, has developed the *Family-Centred Maternity and Newborn Care Guidelines* (Government of Canada, 2018a). These guidelines are based on the principles listed in Box 1.3.

MIDWIFERY CARE

Throughout history, women have played an important role as birth attendants or midwives. In the 1940s public health nurses in rural Alberta provided midwifery care under legislation contained in the *Medical Profession Act.* The University of Alberta offered an Advanced Practical Obstetrics course to provide education for these nurses. In 1946, the CNA approved the practice of registered nurses as midwives in outlying areas where there were no physicians available. The practice of nurses who provided midwifery care usually depended on location and the availability of other health care providers. Throughout the years, changes have been made to midwifery care in different provinces depending on need.

In 1993, the first undergraduate program was started for a midwifery degree, in Ontario. This degree is separate from a nursing degree, and in 2001 the Canadian Association of Midwives (CAM) was established. Since that time other provinces have started midwifery education programs.

Presently the registered midwife (RM) is a regulated health provider who has graduated from an accredited midwife program and is nationally certified by CAM. Legislation regarding care provided by midwives is controlled by the individual provinces. The RM provides comprehensive prenatal, labour, and postnatal care for women who are considered low risk. Midwives assist women in giving birth either in the hospital or at home (see Chapter 6 for further discussion of settings for childbirth).

BABY-FRIENDLY INITIATIVE

In 1991, the World Health Organization (WHO) and UNICEF launched the Baby-Friendly Hospital Initiative in a global effort to implement practices that protect, promote, and support breastfeeding (WHO, 2019). The Baby-Friendly Initiative (BFI) was launched in Canada in 1998. The Breastfeeding Committee for Canada (BCC) plays an important leadership role overseeing the assessment and implementation of the BFI nationally, and also ensures that the standards and philosophy of the BFI are kept intact. The BCC has developed the BFI 10 Steps and WHO Code Outcome Indicators for Hospitals and Community Health Services, which set the international standards for the WHO/UNICEF global criteria within the Canadian context (Box 1.4). These 10 steps are the minimum standards that agencies must achieve in order to receive the BFI designation. There are presently 21 hospitals, 8 birthing centres, and 117 community centres designated

Box 1.4 10 Steps to Baby-Friendly Designation (BFI)

Step 1. Have a written breastfeeding policy that is routinely communicated to all health care providers and volunteers.
Step 2. Ensure that all health care providers have the knowledge and skills necessary to implement the breastfeeding policy.
Step 3. Inform pregnant women and their families about the importance and process of breastfeeding.
Step 4. Place babies in skin-to-skin contact with their mothers immediately following birth for at least an hour or until completion of the first feeding or as long as the mother wishes; encourage mothers to recognize when their babies are ready to feed, offering help as needed.
Step 5. Assist mothers in breastfeeding and maintaining lactation should they face challenges, including separation from their infants.
Step 6. Infants are not offered food or drink other than human milk for the first 6 months, unless *medically* indicated.
Step 7. Facilitate 24-hour rooming-in for all mothers; mothers and infants remain together.
Step 8. Encourage baby-led or cue-based breastfeeding. Encourage sustained breastfeeding beyond 6 months with appropriate introduction of complementary foods.
Step 9. Support mothers to feed and care for their breastfeeding babies without the use of artificial teats or pacifiers (dummies or soothers).
Step 10. Provide a seamless transition between the services provided by the hospital, community health services, and peer support programs.

Source: Breastfeeding Committee for Canada. (2017). *The BFI 10 steps and WHO code outcome indicators for hospitals and community health services.* Retrieved from http://breastfeedingcanada.ca/documents/Indicators%20-%20complete%20June%202017.pdf

as Baby-Friendly facilities in Canada (Government of Canada, 2018a). For further information on breastfeeding see Chapter 9.

STATISTICS

Statistics refers to the process of gathering and analyzing numerical data. Statistics concerning birth, illness (**morbidity**), and death (**mortality**) provide valuable information for determining or projecting the needs of a population or subgroup and for predicting trends. The Canadian Perinatal Surveillance System (CPSS) presents surveillance information on determinants of maternal, fetal, and infant health as well as maternal, fetal, and infant health outcomes. Examples of statistics that are collected include effect of maternal weight gain on pregnancy outcomes, maternal hypertension, rates of sudden infant death syndrome (SIDS), folic acid use among pregnant women, and Down syndrome rates. See Online Resources at the end of the chapter for more information on CPSS reports.

The *infant mortality rate* is the ratio of the number of deaths of infants younger than age 1 year during any given year to the number of live births occurring in the same year. The rate is usually expressed as the number of deaths per 1 000 live births. In Canada, the rate

Box 1.5 Common Vital Statistics Terms

birth rate: The number of live births per 1 000 population in 1 year
fertility rate: The number of births per 1 000 women ages 15 to 44 years in a given population
fetal mortality rate: The number of fetal deaths (fetuses weighing 500 g or more) per 1 000 live births per year
infant mortality rate: The number of deaths of infants under age 1 year per 1 000 live births per year
maternal mortality rate: The number of maternal deaths per 100 000 live births that occur as a direct result of pregnancy (includes the 42-day postpartum period)
neonatal mortality rate: The number of deaths of infants less than age 28 days per 1 000 live births per year
perinatal mortality rate: Includes both fetal and neonatal deaths per 1 000 live births per year

of infant mortality has remained stable and very low. In 2011, the rate of infant mortality was 5 deaths per 1 000 live births (PHAC, 2017). The infant death rate is highest in the first month and is referred to as the *neonatal mortality rate.* The infant mortality rate is considered to be one of the best means of determining the health of a country. To obtain accurate figures, all births and deaths must be registered. In Canada, each province requires this registration. See Online Resources at the end of the chapter for infant and mortality rates by province and territory.

Morbidity (*morbidus,* "sick") refers to the state of being diseased or sick. Morbidity rates show the incidence of disease in a specific population during a certain time frame. *Perinatology* is the study and support of the fetus and newborn. The term *perinatal mortality* designates fetal and neonatal deaths related to prenatal conditions and birth circumstances.

The infant mortality rate is highest among Indigenous people, often owing to poverty, lack of resources, and limited access to health care due to geography. Another factor contributing to the high infant mortality rate is the advances in technology that enable the live birth of very preterm newborns who subsequently die or have significant morbidity. Reducing infant morbidity rates can reduce the resulting incidence of disability, which can have an impact on the growth and development of children.

A nurse may use statistical data to become aware of reproductive trends, to determine populations at risk, to evaluate the quality of care, or to compare relevant information from province to province and country to country. Box 1.5 lists some frequently used terms in vital statistics.

Statistics show, for example, that although the rates of SIDS have decreased significantly since the early 1990s, this still remains the leading cause of death in infants under the age of 1 year. Unintentional injuries are the leading cause of childhood death and disability, and through the use of statistics, nurses can develop health promotion and prevention strategies to reduce these causes of death. The three leading causes of childhood injury-related deaths are motor vehicle collisions

(MVCs) (17%), drowning (15%), and threats to breathing (11%) (Yanchar, Warda, Fuselli, et al., 2012).

TECHNOLOGICAL ADVANCES

Technological advances have enabled many infants to survive who might otherwise have died (Fig. 1.1). High-risk prenatal clinics and the neonatal intensive care unit offer the 500 g preemie an opportunity to survive. Health care providers using such technological advances include pediatric cardiologists who treat children with heart problems. Pediatric surgeons provide much of the complex surgery needed by the newborn with a congenital defect. Many hospital laboratories are well equipped to test pediatric specimens. Chromosomal studies and biochemical screening have made identification of risks and family counselling more significant than ever. The field of perinatal biology has advanced to the forefront of pediatric medicine.

The interprofessional team works together to ensure the total well-being of the patient. Children with disabilities previously thought to be incompatible with life are provided with expert attention and care at specialized centres. After discharge, many of these children are cared for in their homes. The number of children with chronic disease and disability is growing. Some are dependent on sophisticated hospital equipment such as ventilators and home monitors. The required nursing care at home may call for the suctioning of a tracheostomy, central line care, and other highly technical skills. Parents must be educated and provided with continuous support. Although this type of care is cost-effective and best for the child and family, respite care is also extremely important, because 24-hour-a-day care can be extremely taxing for the family, both physically and psychologically.

Many children with chronic illness are living into adulthood, creating the need for more support services. Medically fragile and technology-dependent children may change the typical profile of chronically ill children. The nurse is often the initiator of support services to these patients through education and referral. Ideally, these services will assist the child to become as independent as possible, lead a productive life, and be integrated into society. It is expected that all children be given the same opportunities and access to education and resources. Full inclusion, signifying an expansion of mainstream policy, is being used more frequently today. The aim of early infant intervention programs for children with developmental disabilities is to reduce or minimize the effects of the disability. These services may be provided in a clinic or in the home. The need for in-home, family-centred pediatric care will continue to grow with the number of children with chronic illness who survive. See Chapter 22 for further discussion of caring for the child with a chronic illness.

Quality of life is particularly relevant. Organ transplants have saved many children; however, the complications, limited availability, and expense of these transplants create moral and ethical dilemmas. Older children with life-threatening conditions must be included in planning modified advance directives with their families and the medical team (see Chapter 22).

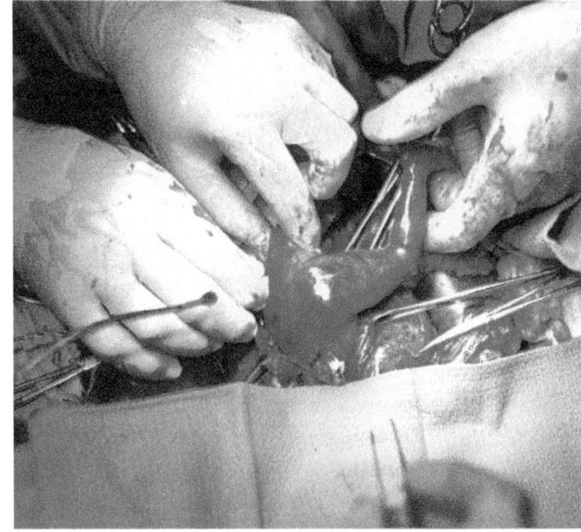

Fig. 1.1 Fetal surgery can be performed to repair a congenital defect before birth. (From Harrison, M. R., Globus, M. S., & Filly R. A. [Eds.]. [1991]. *The unborn patient: Prenatal diagnosis and treatment* [2nd ed.]. Philadelphia: Saunders.)

These developments, along with the explosion of information, an emphasis on individual nurses' accountability, new technology, and the use of computers in health care, make it especially imperative for nurses to maintain their knowledge and skills at the level necessary to provide safe care.

Technology and Teaching

Mobile applications (apps) for electronic devices have been developed to inform consumers about diet, exercise, and various general health issues. Mobile apps aid in teaching new parents the details of infant care and are popular with consumers. Health care technologists and health care providers are often involved in the development of information related to maternal–child care at the reading level of the consumer to supplement their individual patient teaching. For effective use, the nurse must be aware of the accuracy of the information provided in the app, the sources of the information, and the appropriateness to the individual patient or family. Research is ongoing, and nurses play a key role in the development of these apps for electronic devices. Use of these apps can result in an educated consumer with positive health behaviours and can help improve maternal–child care globally (Logsdon, 2017).

STANDARDS OF PRACTICE

The Canadian Association of Schools of Nursing (CASN) has developed entry-to-practice standards for nursing care for the childbearing family for the baccalaureate nursing student. These state the minimum standards that students should achieve prior to graduation (CASN, 2017).

CAPWHN has developed the Canadian Perinatal Nursing Standards, which aim to assist both novice and experienced nurses in performing their role as they provide care to childbearing women and their families within the context of their lives. The values and guiding principles of these standards include the following (CAPWHN, 2018):

- Caring
- Health and well-being
- Justice
- Informed decision-making
- Dignity
- Confidentiality
- Accountability

In 2017, standards were also developed for the practice of pediatric nurses. The standards serve as a framework for pediatric nursing delivery across all sectors and provide consistency in describing expertise and scope of practice of a pediatric nurse. The standards cover care in acute and community settings as well as the care for Indigenous and immigrant children. The aim of the standards is to ensure consistent and high-quality nursing care for all of Canada's children (Canadian Paediatric Nursing Standards Advisory Group, 2017).

Nursing Certification

The CNA offers a nationally recognized certification for registered nurses in specialty areas. The value of certification is that it demonstrates specialized knowledge and enhances professional credibility, and this is valued by employers. At the present time there are four certifications related to maternal–child nursing: community, perinatal, critical care pediatrics, and neonatal. The CNA is also developing certification exams for practical nurses.

INTERPROFESSIONAL NURSING CARE

As part of the health care team, nurses have many roles. For instance, electronic data entry and retrieval make it much easier to see the entries of other members of the health care team, enhancing collaborative care. The nurse is thus an important member of the interprofessional health care team!

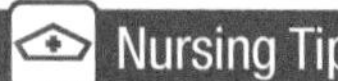

Nursing Tip

It is a nursing responsibility to collect data; it is vital for the nurse to initiate interventions for abnormal findings or refer patients for follow-up care and document findings and the follow-up provided.

Nursing Tip

Expanded nursing roles include the clinical nurse specialist, the pediatric nurse practitioner, and the primary care nurse practitioner.

Coordination of Care

The trend toward short hospital stays has resulted in the discharge of patients to home or the community who still require support, assistance, education, and follow-up care. The nurse participates on the health care team to help coordinate the care of the patient among the various providers of care to improve the quality of care; facilitate the transition from a pediatric care provider to an adult care provider; help the family access financial and local resources in the community to meet their identified needs; and avoid duplication of efforts. Care coordination is a vital aspect of the large health care team in decreasing the risk of fragmentation of care and ensuring that established goals are met. The nurse in the community may work with the local school system and family to meet the health care and educational needs of the child. The nurse can work with the family to teach parenting behaviours, understand the needs of the ill family member, utilize cultural awareness to assist in meeting these needs, and call on available resources within the community. Comprehensive care of the patient includes hospital care as well as follow-up care within the community. Nurses must be flexible and promote policies that make health care more available for all parents. Teaching must be integrated into care plans and individually tailored to the family's needs and their cultural and ethnic background.

The nurse must develop interprofessional values and communication skills in order to understand how different professionals have different roles and use different approaches to health care. *Trauma-informed care* involves power sharing, rather than a hierarchy of responsibilities, in providing health care (Sullivan, Murray, & Ake, 2015). Both the physical issues and the psychosocial aspects of care need to be addressed to help the child and family regain a sense of control over and empowerment in their own lives. For example, the nurse recognizes that the patient must be stabilized in order to treat the patient's illness; the nurse saves lives using the "ABCDE's" of care: *A*irway, *B*reathing and *C*irculation, *D*isability, and *E*xposure. However, because complete recovery requires a follow-up, *F*, to care, the "D-E-F" should include an additional focus on distress, emotional support, and family. The child's developmental age, prior experiences, and family cultural beliefs and practices are important to the responses to and recovery of the child. Talking to the decision maker of the family and respecting family wishes concerning support and referrals, rather than using a hierarchy of decision making by the health care team, means sharing the task of care to meet follow-up needs.

Another important aspect of trauma-informed care is to recognize the connections between violence, trauma, negative health outcomes, and behaviours. The goal is to create emotionally and physically safe environments and to ensure that members of the health care team do not retraumatize anyone who has had experience with trauma or violence (Government of Canada, 2018c).

Advanced Practice Nurses

The specialty of **primary care nurse practitioner** focuses on prevention of illness and maintenance of health rather than the treatment of illness. The primary care nurse practitioner provides ambulatory and primary care for patients often in clinics and offices.

The **clinical nurse specialist (CNS)** provides care in the hospital or community to specific specialty patients, such as perinatal, cardiac, neurological, or oncological care. CNSs conduct primary research and facilitate necessary changes in health care management of their patients. Often the nurse practitioner and the CNS are called **advanced practice nurses**, who are registered nurses (RN) with an advanced degree. Advanced practice nurses can specialize in perinatal, pediatric, or neonatal care.

An international board-certified lactation consultant (IBCLC) often works in perinatal and pediatric areas. The IBCLC assists women in having successful breastfeeding experiences. Some hospitals have an IBCLC on staff and some work in the community.

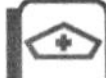 Nursing Tip

An important role of the nurse is that of being a patient advocate.

Nurses as Advocates

An **advocate** is a person who intercedes or pleads on behalf of another. Pediatric nurses are increasingly assuming the role of child advocate. Advocacy may be required for the child's physical and emotional health and may include other family members. Hospitalized children frequently cannot determine or express their needs. When nurses believe that the child's best interests are not being met, they must seek assistance. This usually involves taking the problem to the interdisciplinary team. Nurses must document their efforts to seek clarification and assistance.

Nurses also take on the role of advocating for the well-being of the childbearing woman, fetus, newborn, child, and family through practice, education, research, and leadership in a variety of care environments. It is also important for nurses to teach patients how to become their own advocates in relation to the care they require.

Community-Based Nursing

The community is now the major health care setting for patients, and the challenge is to provide safe, caring, cost-effective, high-quality care to mothers, children, and families. This challenge involves the nurse, who can advocate on behalf of patients and influence government, business, and the community to recognize the need for supporting preventive care of maternal–child patients to ensure a healthy population for the future. The nurse must work with the interprofessional health care team to identify needs within the community and create cost-effective approaches to comprehensive preventive and therapeutic care.

Involving schools, churches, health fairs, websites, and the media facilitates the role of the nurse as an educator within the community. Some nurses are branching out into the community as private practitioners, such as lactation consultants for new mothers. The nursing care plan is expanding to become a **family care plan**, because the nurse is providing care to the patient in the home. Growth and development of the family and family lifestyles are discussed in Chapter 13, and a sample family care plan is presented in Chapter 9. Creativity, problem solving, coordination of interdisciplinary caregivers, case management, assessment, and referral are just some of the essential skills required of a nurse providing community-based care to maternal–child and pediatric patients.

Preventive care is only one aspect of current and future home care and community-based nursing. Therapeutic care is also provided in the home setting, and the nurse must provide support for the family concerning care, monitoring, and the potential needs for professional referral. Specialized care such as fetal monitoring of high-risk pregnant women, apnea monitoring of high-risk newborns, diabetic glucose monitoring, heparin therapy, and total parenteral nutrition can be safely accomplished in the home setting, often supported by telephone or computer access to a nurse.

The future role of the nurse will involve providing health care in a variety of settings and working closely with the interprofessional health care team. The nurse will function as a caregiver, teacher, collaborator, advocate, manager, and researcher. Competence in care and accountability to the patient, family, community, and profession are core responsibilities of the nurse of today and tomorrow. Nurses play a key role in shaping the future picture of health care.

Nursing Tools

The nursing process

The **nursing process** refers to a series of steps describing the systematic problem-solving approach nurses use to identify, prevent, or treat actual or potential health problems. The steps of the nursing process include the following:

1. *Assessment:* Collection of patient data, both subjective and objective
2. *Diagnosis:* Analysis of data in terms of nursing needs of the individual patient or family that can be managed by nursing knowledge, skills, and actions or interventions with the development of a nursing diagnosis
3. *Planning:* Preparation of a plan of nursing care designed to achieve stated outcomes
4. *Implementation:* Carrying out of nursing interventions identified in the plan of care
5. *Evaluation:* Evaluation of outcome progress and redesigning of the plan, if necessary

The nursing process is a framework of action designed to meet the individual needs of patients. It is a problem-oriented and goal-directed process and involves the use of critical thinking, problem solving, and decision making. The nursing process is expressed in an individualized nursing care plan.

Nursing care plans

The **nursing care plan** is developed as a result of the nursing process. It is a written instrument of communication among staff members that focuses on individualized patient care. See Nursing Care Plan 1.1 for an example of a care plan. Other sample care plans of various types for maternity and pediatric nursing are provided throughout this text.

Clinical pathways

Clinical pathways, also known as *critical pathways, care maps,* or *multidisciplinary action plans,* are collaborative guidelines that define multidisciplinary care in terms of outcomes within a timeline. Fundamentally, the pathway is used to identify expected progress within a set timeline and benchmarks by which to recognize this progress. This expected progress of the patient becomes a standard of care; therefore, clinical pathways are based on research rather than on tradition. By setting specific recovery goals that the patient is expected to reach each day, deviations are readily identified. These deviations are called *variances.* If the patient's progress is slower than expected, the outcome (goal) is not achieved within the timeline and a negative variance occurs, and discharge from the hospital may be delayed. The use of clinical pathways improves the quality of care and reduces unnecessary hospitalization time. It promotes coordination of the entire health care team. Sample clinical pathways and multidisciplinary care plans are presented throughout this text.

Critical thinking

Nurses have job-specific knowledge and skills that they incorporate into their daily nursing practice by applying thought. *General thinking* involves random or memorized thoughts. An example of general thinking would be memorizing the steps of a clinical procedure or skill. **Critical thinking**, however, is a synthesis and analysis of all the information with the goal of developing purposeful, goal-directed thinking based on scientific evidence and previous knowledge rather than on assumption or memorization.

Nurses must consider factors that are specific to the individual patient or affected by the individual situation. For example, the cultural background of the patient or the age of the patient influences how effective a given intervention will be. If the problem is a protein deficiency and the nurse selects the intervention to teach the importance of meat in the diet, the intervention will be ineffective—that is, it will not have a positive outcome—if this patient is a vegetarian, because meat will not be eaten. Thus, critical thinking must enter the picture for optimum nursing care to be provided. Critical thinking entails applying creativity and ingenuity to solve a problem: combining basic standard principles with data specific to the patient.

Box 1.6 Process of Critical Thinking

1. Identify the problem.
2. Differentiate fact from assumption.
3. Check reliability and accuracy of data.
4. Determine relevant from irrelevant.
5. Identify possible conclusions or outcomes.
6. Set priorities and goals.
7. Evaluate response of patient.

Nursing Tip

Evidence-informed practice starts when the nurse uses the best evidence obtained from current, valid, published research. When the nurse combines that information with the critical thinking process, the nurse's experiences, and patients' needs, it is then possible to plan safe, effective nursing care for the patient.

The nursing process and critical thinking. The nursing process (assessment, diagnosis, planning, implementation, and evaluation) is a tool for effective critical thinking. When a nurse uses the nursing process in critical thinking, a clinical judgement can be made that is specific to the data collected and the clinical situation. In every clinical contact, a nurse must identify actual and potential problems and make decisions about a plan of action that will result in a positive patient outcome; know why the actions are appropriate; differentiate between those problems that the nurse can handle independently and those that necessitate contacting other members of the health care team; and prioritize those actions (Box 1.6).

Documentation

Documentation, or charting, has always been a legal responsibility of the nurse. Documentation—whether paper, electronic, audio, or visual—is used to monitor a client's progress and communicate with other care providers. It also reflects the nursing care that is provided to a client (College of Nurses of Ontario, 2008). When a medication is given or a treatment performed, it must be accurately documented on the patient's chart. Charting responsibilities also include head-to-toe assessment of the patient and a recording of both data pertinent to the diagnosis and the response to treatment.

Legal and Ethical Considerations

Documentation

Nurses must ensure that documentation is complete and accurate and presents a picture of the client, including nursing actions and client outcomes.

Electronic documentation has helped to decrease the number of medical errors caused by illegible handwriting and is now used by most hospitals. Electronic documentation is paperless, and a bar-coding system is often used to document medication administration at the patient's bedside. Security features are built in,

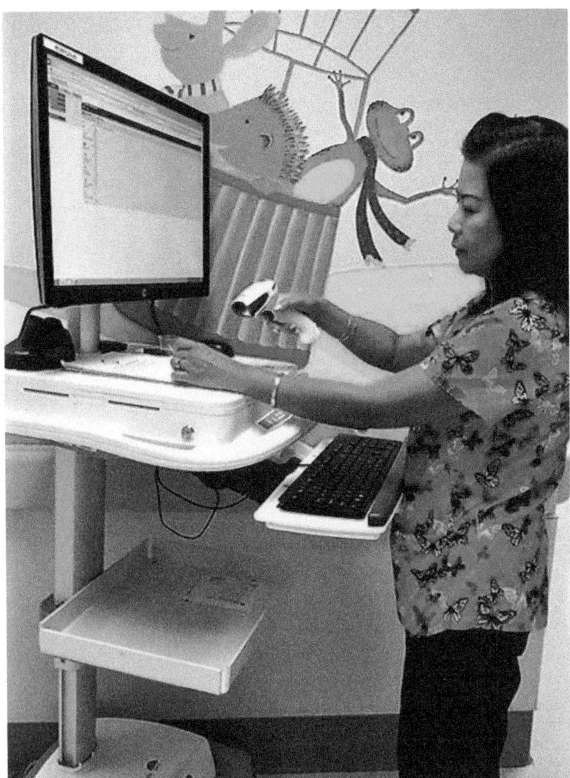

Fig. 1.2 The nurse uses a workstation on wheels (WOW), which contains the electronic health record system, to scan and confirm identity of the patient and the bar-coded medication she will be administering.

and integrated prompts encourage accurate and comprehensive documentation by requiring certain entries be made before the user can progress further through the system. The electronic documentation system can be on a separate computer in each patient room or can be accessed via a mobile unit, called a workstation on wheels (WOW) that can be wheeled by the nurse to each patient's room (Fig. 1.2). Critical ranges are programmed into the computer software system so the nurse is alerted to deviations from the norm as information is recorded. Using electronic documentation, all caregivers have simultaneous access to patient records on all patients at all times from various locations. For example, electronic tablets are used to document care given in both a community setting and hospital setting.

SBAR Communication

One technique of communication concerning the patient among the members of the health care team is the use of SBAR, a formal method of providing end-of-shift reports during the transition of care from one shift to the next, when sending the patient to different nursing unit, or when requesting assistance from another professional. Fig. 1.3 *A* shows a pocket SBAR that the nurse uses during shift report and can carry for quick reference and communication with the health care team and then use as a reference for the next shift report (Fig. 1.3 *B*). The SBAR process includes discussion of these elements:

- *Situation:* The status of the patient on the unit
- *Background:* The background or relevant history of the patient that may influence care
- *Assessment:* An analysis of the problem or continuing patient need based on assessments made or orders written
- *Recommendation:* What the current patient need is and the outcome goals

GLOBAL HEALTH

Sustainable Development Goals

In 2000, the member nations of the United Nations developed the Millennium Development Goals (MDGs), which were eight international goals that focused on improving the health and education of the global community. These goals included (United Nations, 2011):

1. To eradicate extreme poverty and hunger
2. To achieve universal primary education
3. To promote gender equality and empower women
4. To reduce child mortality
5. To improve maternal health
6. To combat HIV/AIDS, malaria, and other diseases
7. To ensure environmental sustainability
8. To develop a global partnership for development

The original plan was to meet the goals by 2015. While the goals were not completely met, the number of people living in extreme poverty declined by more than half; most girls are now in school and for longer periods; less children are dying before their fifth birthday; the maternal mortality rate has decreased; and rates of HIV/AIDS, tuberculosis, and malaria have decreased (United Nations, 2015). In 2015, the United Nations General Assembly endorsed the Sustainable Development Goals, an ambitious project for the next 15 years that has 17 goals to transform the world. The new goals include climate change and environmental protection (Fig. 1.4).

The CNA's position statement on global health and equity supports many of the Sustainable Development Goals and discusses the role of nurses in providing and advocating for appropriate care globally (CNA, 2009).

Interprofessional collaboration can advance health care to all, to make the world a better and healthier place. Communication, partnerships, and an understanding of how various health care beliefs of different cultures affect health care practices and delivery of care are essential within the local community as well as in various countries of the world. The graduate nurse, at all levels, must be aware of and participate in public health efforts to reduce disparities in global health. Nurses are leaders in the health care field, as well as innovators, mentors, and advocates, and can support efforts to increase education in other countries to understand major causes of illness and death and can share competencies needed to overcome disparities in global health care.

Nurses learn about various communicable diseases and need to understand how current travel practices contribute to the spread of these diseases. They also need to know the role of the nurse, as well as other professions, in preventing pandemics from occurring.

	Leifer's Pocket SBAR (Side 1)			
Situation	Pt. Name			
	Room:	Chip No.		
	Admit Date: Service:	Nurse ______ Dr. ______		
	Age:	Wt.: Mon/Thurs	Kg	Lbs.
Background	Allergy:			
	Dx:			
	Hx:	CPS	Fall Risk	
	Isolation:	Wounds	Drains	
	Diet:			
Assessment	IV:			
	O_2:	Pulse Ox:		
	Tx:			
	Labs:			
	Xray:			
	Procedures:			
	Pending:			

Recommendations				
0730	RR=	T=	HR=	BP=
0800	Morning care/Vitals Chart			
0900	Meds			
1000	Assess Chart			
1100	RR=	T=	HR=	BP=
1200	Lunch			
1300				
1400				
1500				
1600	RR=	T=	HR=	BP=
1700				
1800	I&O final			
Shift Report Summary:				
Leifer's Pocket SBAR (Side 2)				

A

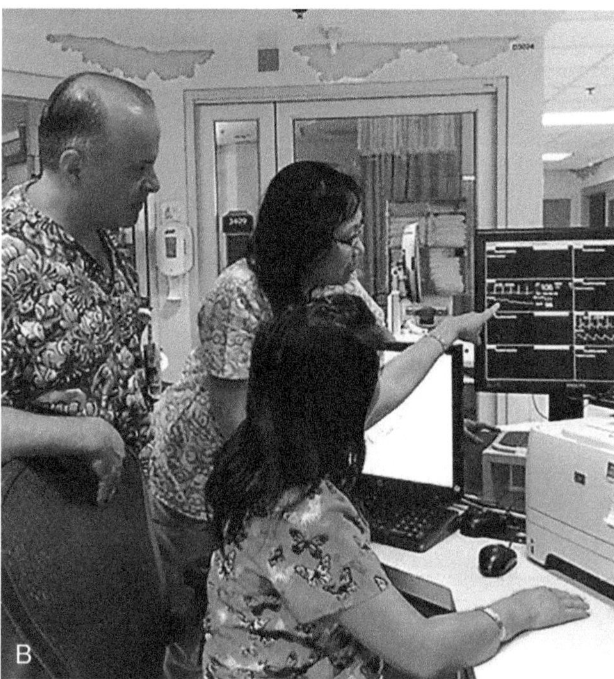

Fig. 1.3 **A,** Pocket SBAR. This pocket SBAR is a 7 × 12–cm card that can be carried in the pocket of the nurse's uniform. At the beginning of the shift the *S*: situation, *B*—background; *A*—assessments are completed. The *R*—recommend section becomes the plan of care for the patient with specific times noted for medications and treatments for the remainder of the shift. There is a space for a closing shift report to update new team members taking over the care, for a seamless transition of care. **B,** The nurse discusses the patient's vital signs during the end-of-shift report to the new nursing team.

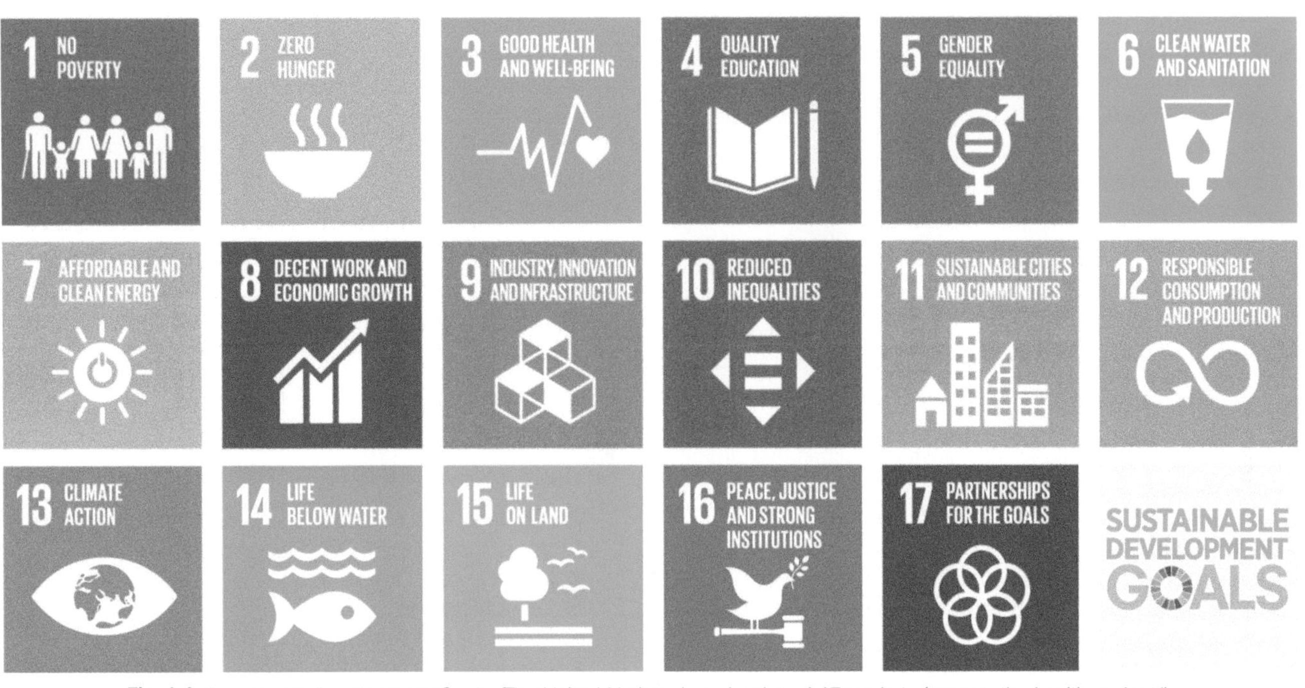

Fig. 1.4 Sustainable Development Goals. The United Nations has developed 17 goals to improve the health and well-being of the global community. (From United Nations. [2015]. *Sustainable Development Goals kick off with start of new year*. Retrieved from https://www.un.org/sustainabledevelopment/blog/2015/12/sustainable-development-goals-kick-off-with-start-of-new-year/.)

Get Ready for the Certification Examination!

Key Points

- The Public Health Agency of Canada focuses on health promotion and injury prevention.
- Nurses have legal and ethical responsibilities to report specific conditions to local public health agencies to protect the patient and the community.
- The health of Canadians is affected by the social determinants of health.
- Nurses must be aware of the impact of colonization on the health of Indigenous people.
- PIPEDA regulations mandate maintaining confidentiality concerning patient medical records and personal information.
- The culture of a society has a strong influence on family and child care.
- The nurse must understand the culture and tradition of the family and their influence on health practices.
- The educational focus for the childbearing family is that childbirth is a normal and healthy event.
- *Birth rate* refers to the number of live births per 1 000 population in 1 year.
- The nursing process consists of five steps: assessment, analysis, planning (with outcomes identification), implementation, and evaluation. It is an organized method in nursing practice and a means of communication among staff members.
- The nursing care plan is a written instrument of communication that uses the nursing process to formulate a plan of care for a specific patient. It uses nursing diagnoses and involves critical thinking and problem solving.
- Clinical pathways are collaborative guidelines that define multidisciplinary care in terms of outcomes within a timeline.
- Charting or documentation is the legal responsibility of the nurse and includes a head-to-toe assessment and data pertinent to the diagnosis and to the response of the patient to treatment.
- SBAR is a technique of communicating patient information among staff at the end of one shift and the beginning of the next, as well as communicating among healthcare professionals.
- Nurses at all levels have a responsibility to share knowledge to improve global health.
- The education and practice of all nurses must include a role in global health care.

Additional Learning Resources

evolve Go to your Evolve website (http://evolve.elsevier.com/Canada/Leifer) for the following learning resources:

- Answer Key for Critical Thinking Questions
- Answer Key for Textbook Review Questions
- Audio Glossary
- Fluids & Electrolytes tutorial
- Interactive Review Questions
- Skills Performance Checklists
- Video clips and more!

Online Resources

- Canadian Association of Perinatal and Women's Health Nursing (CAPWHN): http://www.capwhn.ca/en/capwhn/About_CAPWHN_p3185.html
- Canadian Paediatric Society: https://www.cps.ca/
- Canadian Perinatal Surveillance System (CPSS): https://www.canada.ca/en/public-health/services/injury-prevention/health-surveillance-epidemiology-division/maternal-infant-health.html
- Children's Healthcare Canada: https://www.childrenshealthcarecanada.ca/about/
- Government of Canada—*Family-Centred Maternity and Newborn Care: National Guidelines:* https://www.canada.ca/en/public-health/services/maternity-newborn-care-guidelines.html
- National Collaborating Centre for Aboriginal Health: *Health Inequalities and Social Determinants of Aboriginal Peoples' Health:* https://www.ccnsa-nccah.ca/docs/determinants/RPT-HealthInequalities-Reading-Wien-EN.pdf
- Society of Obstetricians and Gynaecologists of Canada (SOGC): https://www.sogc.org
- Statistics Canada—*Death and Mortality Rates by Age Group (and Province and Territory):* https://www150.statcan.gc.ca/t1/tbl1/en/tv.action?pid=1310071001
- World Health Organization: https://www.who.int

Review Questions

1. Which of the following are agencies that focus on global health and development? *(Select all that apply.)*
   a. World Health Organization
   b. United Nations
   c. Public Health Agency of Canada
   d. Canadian Nurses Association
2. The number of deaths of infants younger than age 28 days per 1 000 live births is termed which of the following?
   a. Infant death rate
   b. Neonatal birth rate
   c. Neonatal morbidity rate
   d. Neonatal mortality rate
3. An organization that sets standards of practice for nursing would be which of the following?
   a. Society of Obstetricians and Gynaecologists of Canada (SOGC)
   b. Canadian Nurses Association (CNA)
   c. Utilization review committee
   d. Canadian Paediatric Society (CPS)
4. The nurse is providing *evidenced-informed care* when the care provided does which of the following?
   a. Adheres to hospital procedure book guidelines
   b. Is based on protocols learned in nursing school

   c. Is provided on the basis of a request of the charge nurse or health care provider
   d. Is provided on the basis of what has been published in a professional journal or text
5. Which source would the nurse use to determine whether a specific nursing activity is within the scope of practice of a practical nurse?
   a. Nursing textbook
   b. Nursing procedure manual
   c. Head nurse or nurse manager
   d. Provincial nursing regulatory body
6. Nursing organizations that suggest standards of care in maternal–child nursing include which of the following? *(Select all that apply.)*
   a. CAPWHN
   b. CNA
   c. QSEN
   d. CPS

Critical Thinking Questions

1. What is culture, and how does it affect health care beliefs?
2. Describe two cultural practices that promote health.
3. What are the barriers to health care access in your community?

REFERENCES

Canadian Association of Perinatal and Women's Health Nursing (CAPWHN). (2017). *CAPWHN Position Statement on Cultural Safety/Humility*. Retrieved from: http://www.capwhn.ca/en/capwhn/CAPWHN_Position_Statement_on_Cultural_SafetyHumility_p4857.html.

Canadian Association of Perinatal and Women's Health Nursing (CAPWHN). (2018). *Perinatal Nursing Standards in Canada*. Retrieved from: http://www.capwhn.ca/uploads/documents//PERINATAL_NURSING_STANDARDS_IN_CANADA.pdf.

Canadian Association of Schools of Nursing. (2017). *Entry-to-Practice Competencies for Nursing Care of the Childbearing Family for Baccalaureate Programs in Nursing*. Retrieved from: https://www.casn.ca/wp-content/uploads/2016/09/FINAL-CHILDBEARING-FAMILY-COMPETENCIES-revised.pdf.

Canadian Nurses Association (CNA). (2009). *Position Statement: Global Health and Equity*. Retrieved from: https://www.cna-aiic.ca/-/media/cna/page-content/pdf-fr/ps106_global_health_equity_aug_2009_e.pdf#sthash.d1XSVQ3H.dpuf.

Canadian Paediatric Nursing Standards Advisory Group. (2017). *Canadian Paediatric Nursing Standards*. Retrieved from: https://ken.caphc.org/xwiki/bin/download/Other+Resources/Canadian+Paediatric+Nursing+Standards/FINAL-Paediatric%20Nursing%20Standards.pdf.

Children's Healthcare Canada. (2019). *About Children's Healthcare Canada*. Retrieved from: https://www.childrenshealthcarecanada.ca/about/.

College of Nurses of Ontario. (2008). *Practice Standard: Documentation (revised 2008)*. Toronto, ON: College of Nurses. Retrieved from: http://www.cno.org/globalassets/docs/prac/41001_documentation.pdf.

Government of Canada. (2018a). *Family-Centred Maternity and Newborn Care: National Guidelines*. Retrieved from: https://www.canada.ca/en/public-health/services/maternity-newborn-care-guidelines.html.

Government of Canada. (2018b). *Social Determinants of Health and Health Inequalities*. Retrieved from: https://www.canada.ca/en/public-health/services/health-promotion/population-health/what-determines-health.html.

Government of Canada. (2018c). *Trauma and Violence-Informed Approaches to Policy and Practice*. Retrieved from: https://www.canada.ca/en/public-health/services/publications/health-risks-safety/trauma-violence-informed-approaches-policy-practice.html#s3.

Government of Canada. (2019). *Public Health Agency of Canada*. Retrieved from: https://www.canada.ca/en/public-health.html.

Health Canada. (2014). *A Statistical Profile on the Health of First Nations in Canada: Determinants of Health, 2006 to 2010*. Retrieved from: https://www.canada.ca/en/health-canada/services/first-nations-inuit-health/reports-publications/aboriginal-health-research/statistical-profile-health-first-nations-canada-determinants-health-2006-2010-health-canada-2014.html.

Logsdon, M. C. (2017). Smart phone apps and maternal-child nursing. *Maternal Child Nursing (MCN)*, *42*(5), 247.

National Collaboration Centre for Aboriginal Health (NCCAH). (2013). *AnoverviewofAboriginalHealthinCanada*. Retrieved from: https://www.ccnsa-nccah.ca/docs/context/FS-OverviewAbororiginalHealth-EN.pdf.

Public Health Agency of Canada (PHAC). (2017). *Perinatal Health Indicators for Canada 2017*. Retrieved from: https://www.canada.ca/en/public-health/services/injury-prevention/health-surveillance-epidemiology-division/maternal-infant-health/perinatal-health-indicators-2017.html.

Reading, C. L., & Wein, F. (2009). *Health inequalities and social determinants of aboriginal peoples' health*. Prince George, BC: National Collaborating Centre for Aboriginal Health.

Ricca, P., Wahlskog, C., & Dewey Bergren, M. (2018). Enhancing cultural sensitivity in a community health care setting for LGBTQ patients. *Journal of Community Health Nursing*, *35*(4), 165–178. https://doi.org/10.1080/07370016.2018.1516420.

Sullivan, K. M., Murray, K. J., & Ake, G. S. (2015). Trauma-informed care for children in the child welfare system: An initial evaluation of a trauma-informed parenting workshop. *Child Maltreatment*, *21*(2), 147–155.

Truth and Reconciliation Commission of Canada (TRC). (2015). *Honouring the Truth, Reconciling for the Future: Summary of the Final Report of the Truth and Reconciliation Commission of Canada*. University of Manitoba: National Centre for Truth and Reconciliation. Retrieved from: http://nctr.ca/assets/reports/Final%20Reports/Executive_Summary_English_Web.pdf.

United Nations. (2011). *Millennium Development Goals: 2011 Progress Chart*. Retrieved from: http://www.un.org/millenniumgoals/pdf/%282011E%29_MDReport2011_ProgressChart.pdf.

United Nations. (2015). *The Millennium Development Goals Report 2015*. Retrieved from: http://www.un.org/millenniumgoals/2015_MDG_Report/pdf/MDG%202015%20PR%20Global.pdf.

Vanier Institute of the Family. (2019). *Definition of Family.* Retrieved from: https://vanierinstitute.ca/definition-family/.

Wiebe, P., van Gaalen, R., Langlois, K., et al. (2014). Towards culturally safe evidence informed decision making for First Nations and Inuit health policies and programs. *Pimatisiwin: A Journal of Aboriginal and Indigenous Community Health, 11*(1), 17–26. Retrieved from: http://www.arnbccommunitiesofpractice.ca/ahnn/wp-content/uploads/2014/10/Toward-Culturally-Safe-Evidence-Informed-Decision-Making.pdf.

World Health Organization (WHO). (2019). *Baby-Friendly Hospital Initiative.* Retrieved from: http://www.who.int/nutrition/topics/bfhi/en/.

Yanchar, N. L., Warda, L. J., Fuselli, P., et al. (2012). *Position Statement: Child and Youth Injury Prevention: A Public Health Approach.* Retrieved from: https://www.cps.ca/en/documents/position/child-and-youth-injury-prevention.

Yeager, K. A., & Bauer-Wu, S. (2013). Cultural humility: Essential foundation for clinical researchers. *Applied Nursing Research, 26*(4), 251–256. https://doi.org/10.1016/j.apnr.2013.06.008.

The Nurse's Role in Women's Health Care

2

Lisa Keenan-Lindsay

http://evolve.elsevier.com/Canada/Leifer

Objectives

1. Define each key term listed.
2. Explain aspects of preventive health care for women.
3. Explain the secondary prevention strategies for breast and cervical cancer.
4. Describe each menstrual disorder and its treatment.
5. Explain each gynecological infection in terms of cause, transmission, treatment, and care.
6. Describe the various methods of birth control, including indications, side effects, and contraindications of each.
7. Describe how to use natural family-planning methods for contraception or infertility management.
8. Explain the changes that occur during the perimenopausal period and after menopause.
9. Explain the medical and nursing care of women who are nearing or have completed menopause.

Key Terms

amenorrhea (ă-mĕn-ŏ-RĒ-ă)
climacteric (klī-MĂK-ŭr-ĭk)
coitus interruptus (KŌ-ĭ-tŭs ĭn-tŭr-RŬP-tŭs)
dysmenorrhea (dĭs-mĕn-ō-RĒ-ă)
dyspareunia (dĭs-pă-RŪ-nē-ă)
endometriosis (ĕn-dō-mē-trē-Ō-sĭs)
menopause (MĔN-ō-păwz)
menorrhagia (mĕn-ō-RĀ-zhă)
metrorrhagia (mĕ-trō-RĀ-zhă)
mittelschmerz (MĬT-ĕl-shmārts)
osteoporosis (ŏs-tē-ō-pă-RŌ-sĭs)
spermicides
spinnbarkeit (SPĬN-băhr-kīt)

Most women choose to be active participants in their health care and thus need information about their bodies, health promotion, self-care techniques, and choices concerning treatment options. Culturally competent communication is the key to empowering the woman to feel confident about her ability to care for herself and her family. In some cultures, women ask questions about their bodies and health care as these questions arise; in other cultures, women wait to be told what to do. To be an effective teacher about health behaviours, the nurse must understand the cultural practices, past experiences, and individual goals of the patient. The nurse offers support, knowledge, and caring behaviours that help the woman learn about screening tests or health concerns.

HEALTH PROMOTION

The goal of health promotion is the prevention or early identification of disease. The value of preventive health care is that some disabling conditions can be prevented or their severity lessened by specific measures, such as altering the diet or detecting the disorder early and at a more treatable stage. Health promotion includes primary, secondary, and tertiary prevention strategies. *Primary prevention* involves disease prevention through having a healthy lifestyle and decreasing exposure to environmental or other substances that increase the risk of disease. Examples of primary prevention are smoking cessation and immunization. *Secondary prevention* is the early detection of disease and trying to prevent the disease from developing further. Many screening tests are examples of secondary prevention. These tests are not diagnostic but can be used to identify whether additional testing is needed. Examples of screening tests that are common in women's health care include mammography to identify breast cancer and Pap tests for cervical cancer. Improving quality of life and managing symptoms of disease are examples of *tertiary prevention*. This may include learning to manage blood sugar levels and increase activity in someone with diabetes.

This chapter focuses on those disorders that are exclusive to or dominant in women.

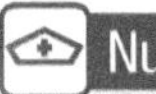
Nursing Tip

Encouraging women to practice preventive health care can help prevent some disorders or identify them early, when they are the most treatable.

BREAST CANCER

In Canada, breast cancer screening is recommended for women between the ages of 50 and 74 for women who have an average risk of developing breast cancer. Regular screening for breast cancer is recommended for this age group because about half of all new cases of breast cancer occur in women between 50 and 69 years of age. The most reliable way to find breast cancer early is screening mammography. Research has also shown that regular mammography can significantly lower the risk of women dying from breast cancer (Canadian Cancer Society, 2019c).

From an early age, women should be familiar with the appearance and feel of their breasts and report changes to a health care provider. However, routine breast self-examination (BSE) is no longer recommended as BSE does not save lives and leads to more unnecessary biopsies (Canadian Task Force on Preventative Health Care [CTFPHC], 2011). Women who wish to continue to perform BSE need to be given appropriate information that includes examination of breasts when they are not tender or swollen. Women who are breastfeeding should perform BSE when their breasts are empty. See Online Resources at the end of the chapter for how to do BSE. Clinical breast examination (CBE) by a qualified health care provider can be used to check for abnormalities, although research has not shown that CBE is an effective screening tool and is not recommended in women with a low risk for breast cancer (CTFPHC, 2011). All provinces and some territories have breast screening programs for women aged 50 to 69. These women receive letters telling them when they need to book appointments along with follow-up after the mammogram.

Women who have a higher risk for developing breast cancer (personal history of breast cancer, history of breast cancer in first-degree relative, known *BRCA1/BRCA2* mutation, or prior chest wall radiation) need more extensive breast cancer screening and will often start undergoing screening mammography earlier in consultation with their health care provider. The reader should consult a medical-surgical text for additional information about the diagnosis and treatment of breast cancer.

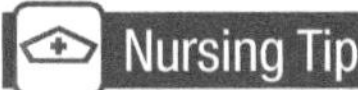
Nursing Tip

Preventive care for breast health involves screening mammography at the appropriate ages.

Mammography

Mammography involves very low-dose X-rays to visualize the breast tissue. Mammography can detect breast tumours very early—long before the woman or a professional can feel them. The breast is compressed firmly between two plates, which is briefly uncomfortable. Scheduling the mammogram after a menstrual period reduces the discomfort, because the breasts are less tender at that time. The CTFPHC currently recommends screening mammograms every 2 to 3 years for women age 50 to 74. Women who are aged 40 to 49 are not recommended for routine mammography (CTFPHC, 2011). If an abnormality is detected on the mammogram a diagnostic mammogram will be ordered by the women's primary health care provider.

VULVAR CANCER

Women should report any abnormalities of the vulva area to their health care provider. These abnormalities include itching; pain, tenderness, or discomfort; changes to the skin; and a lump or mass (Canadian Cancer Society, 2019b). They may indicate vulvar cancer. When found and treated early, the chances of successful treatment are better.

PELVIC EXAMINATION

The CTFPHC does not support routine pelvic exam screening (external inspection, internal speculum examination, bimanual examination, and rectovaginal examination) for noncervical cancer, pelvic inflammatory disease (PID), or other gynecological conditions in asymptomatic women (Tonelli, Connor Gorber, Moore, et al., 2016). The decision to perform routine pelvic examinations should be a shared decision between the woman and her health care provider (McNicholas & Peipert, 2017). Pelvic examinations are distinct from the Papanicolaou (Pap) test, which is used to screen for precancerous and cancerous lesions of the cervix. The current guidelines for routine Pap testing in women who are or have been sexually active are every 3 years from age 25 to 69 (CTFPHC, 2013). For women who are over the age of 70 who have been adequately screened (i.e., three successive negative Pap tests in the past 10 years), the recommendation is that routine screening may cease. For women aged 70 or over who have not been adequately screened, continued screening until three negative test results have been obtained is recommended (CTFPHC, 2013).

The pelvic examination should be scheduled between menstrual periods, and the woman should not douche or have sexual intercourse for at least 48 hours before the examination to avoid altering the Pap test. See a physical assessment text on how to complete a Pap test and pelvic examination.

Transmen who still have female reproductive organs also require routine Pap tests. This screening is often overlooked for the transman, and the nurse must provide education about the importance of the screening. This test can be extremely difficult for the man, thus a sensitive approach must be used.

MENSTRUAL DISORDERS

Menstrual cycle disorders can cause distress for many women. The nursing role in each depends on the disorder's cause and treatment. Common nursing roles involve explaining any recommended treatments (e.g., medications) and caring for the woman, including emotional support, before and after procedures.

AMENORRHEA

Amenorrhea is the absence of menstruation. It is normal before menarche, during pregnancy, and after menopause. Amenorrhea that is not normal may fall into one of two categories:

1. *Primary:* The absence of both menarche and secondary sexual characteristics by age 13 years or the absence of menses by age 16.5 years, regardless of normal growth and development.
2. *Secondary:* Cessation of menstruation for at least 6 months in a woman who previously had an established pattern of menstruation (Lobo, 2012).

Treatment of amenorrhea begins with a thorough history, physical examination, and laboratory examinations to identify the cause. Pregnancy testing is completed for any sexually active woman.

The specific treatment depends on the cause that is identified. For example, adolescents who are very thin or have a low percentage of body fat may experience amenorrhea, because fat is necessary for estrogen production. This group of women may include athletes but may also include patients who have eating disorders such as anorexia or bulimia. Therapy for the eating disorder may result in the resumption of normal periods. Other treatments are aimed at correcting the cause, which may be an endocrine imbalance.

ABNORMAL UTERINE BLEEDING

Abnormal uterine bleeding (AUB) may be defined as any variation from the normal menstrual cycle and includes changes in regularity and frequency of menses, in duration of flow, or in amount of blood loss, as well as bleeding that is not related to menses (Keenan-Lindsay, 2017b). **Metrorrhagia** (intermenstrual bleeding) is uterine bleeding that is usually normal in amount but occurs at irregular intervals. **Menorrhagia** refers to menstrual bleeding that is excessive in amount. The average woman loses about 35 mL of blood during normal menstruation. Blood loss greater than 80 mL/month is considered excessive and often results in anemia. Heavy menstrual bleeding is manifested by soaking through a menstrual pad or tampon within 1 hour, for several hours; passing clots the size of a quarter; and a gushing sensation, with menstrual blood often leaking through protection.

Common causes for any type of abnormal bleeding include the following:

- Bleeding disorders (e.g., von Willebrand disease)
- Pregnancy complications, such as an unidentified pregnancy that is ending in spontaneous abortion
- Lesions of the vagina, cervix, or uterus (benign or malignant)
- Breakthrough bleeding (BTB) that may occur in the woman taking oral contraceptives
- Endocrine disorders such as hypothyroidism
- Failure to ovulate or respond appropriately to hormones secreted with ovulation (dysfunctional uterine bleeding)

Treatment of AUB depends on the identified cause. Pregnancy complications and benign or malignant lesions are treated appropriately. BTB may be relieved by a change in the oral contraceptive used. Abnormal hormone secretion is treated with the appropriate medications. Surgical dilation and evacuation (D&E) may be necessary to remove intrauterine growths or aid in diagnosis. Hysterectomy may be performed for some disorders if the woman does not desire any or additional children. A technique called *laser ablation* can permanently remove the abnormally bleeding uterine lining without a hysterectomy. Menorrhagia can be treated with nonsteroidal anti-inflammatory drugs, (NSAIDs), oral contraceptives, the levonorgestrel-releasing intrauterine device (IUD), or tranexamic acid (an antifibrinolytic) (Singh, Best, Dunn, et al., 2013). NSAIDs reduce menstrual flow by 30 to 50% when taken daily during menstruation (Smith, 2018).

MENTRUAL CYCLE PAIN

Mittelschmerz

Mittelschmerz ("middle pain") is pain that many women experience around ovulation, near the middle of their menstrual cycle. Mild analgesics are usually sufficient to relieve this discomfort. The nurse can teach the woman that this discomfort is harmless.

Dysmenorrhea

Dysmenorrhea, painful menses or "cramps," affects many women. It occurs soon after the onset of menses and is spasmodic in nature. Discomfort is in the lower abdomen and may radiate to the lower back or down the legs. Some women also have diarrhea, nausea, and vomiting. It is most common in young women who have not been pregnant (nulliparas).

There are two types of dysmenorrhea: *primary,* which is associated with ovulatory cycles, and *secondary,* which develops usually after age 25 and is associated with a pathological condition.

Primary dysmenorrhea is a leading cause of short-term recurrent school absenteeism in adolescent girls. Characteristics include the following:

- Onset occurs shortly after menarche with heavy menstrual flow.
- Pain begins no more than a few hours before menstruation starts and lasts no more than 72 hours.
- Pelvic examination results are normal.

Prostaglandins from the endometrium (uterine lining) play an important role in dysmenorrhea. Some women produce excessive amounts of prostaglandins from the endometrium, and these substances are potent stimulants of painful uterine contractions. The following treatments may provide relief:

- Exercise

- Good nutrition—decreased salt and refined sugar consumption and increased water intake
- Prostaglandin-inhibitor drugs, primarily NSAIDs. Prostaglandin inhibitors are most effective if taken before the onset of menstruation and cramps.
- Oral contraceptives, which reduce the amount of prostaglandin secretion.
- Complementary and alternative health modalities (CAHM): heat application to the lower abdomen or back, massage, yoga, transcutaneous electrical nerve stimulation (TENS), as well as some herbal remedies

Secondary dysmenorrhea most commonly results from endometriosis, PID, uterine polyps, ovarian cysts, or fibroids. Treatment involves identifying and treating the cause. Some of the treatments for primary dysmenorrhea may be helpful.

ENDOMETRIOSIS

Endometriosis is the presence of tissue that resembles endometrium outside the uterus. This tissue responds to hormonal stimulation just as the uterine lining does. The lesions may cause pain, pressure, and inflammation to adjacent organs as they build up and slough during menstrual cycles.

Endometriosis causes pain in many women that is either sharp or dull. It is more constant than the spasmodic pain of dysmenorrhea. **Dyspareunia** (painful sexual intercourse) may be present. Endometriosis appears to cause infertility in some women.

Treatment of endometriosis may be either medical or surgical and depends on the severity of the symptoms and the reproductive goals of the woman. Combined hormonal contraceptives, ideally administered continuously, should be considered as first-line agents. Continuous use of oral contraceptive pills (OCPs) that have a low estrogen-to-progestin ratio can shrink endometrial tissue. Any low-dose OCPs can be used if taken for 15 weeks, followed by 1 week of withdrawal. This therapy is associated with minimal adverse effects and can be taken for extended periods (Leyland, Casper, LaBerge, et al., 2010). Medications such as danazol and agonists of gonadotropin-releasing hormone (GnRH) may be administered via nasal spray to reduce the buildup of tissue by inducing an artificial menopause. Lupron, given intramuscularly, is also effective. The woman may have hot flashes and vaginal dryness, similar to symptoms occurring at natural menopause. She is also at increased risk for other issues that occur after menopause, such as osteoporosis and serum lipid changes.

Surgical treatment includes the following:

- Hysterectomy with removal of the ovaries and all lesions if the woman does not desire any or another pregnancy
- Laser ablation (destruction) of the lesions if she wants to maintain fertility

Endometriosis has no effect on pregnancy once pregnancy has been achieved (Smith, 2018).

PREMENTRUAL DISORDERS

Premenstrual syndrome (PMS) and the more serious premenstrual dysphoric disorder (PMDD) are associated with abnormal serotonin response to normal changes in the estrogen levels during the menstrual cycle. A diagnosis of PMS is made when the following criteria are met (Taylor, Schuiling, & Sharp, 2013):

- Symptoms consistent with PMS occur in the period between ovulation and the onset of menses.
- A symptom-free period occurs in the week following the menstrual period.
- Symptoms are recurrent.
- Symptoms have a negative effect on some aspect of the woman's life.
- Other diagnoses that better explain the symptoms have been excluded.

PMDD is a more severe variant of PMS in which 3 to 8% of women have marked irritability, dysphoria, mood lability, anxiety, fatigue, appetite changes, and a sense of feeling overwhelmed (Lentz, 2012).

Treatment includes a diet rich in complex carbohydrates and fibre (to lengthen effects of the carbohydrate meal), stress management, and exercise. Medical management includes oral contraceptives (low-estrogen, progestin-dominant), diuretics during the luteal phase of the menstrual cycle (between ovulation and onset of menstruation), and NSAIDs.

Patient education concerning maintenance of a monthly calendar of symptoms, stress management, and dietary guidance are important concepts for the nurse to teach. Reduction of caffeine, simple sugars, and salty foods; regular exercise; and prevention of hypoglycemia are important lifestyle changes. Selective serotonin reuptake inhibitors (SSRIs) such as fluoxetine (Prozac) or sertraline (Zoloft), or short-acting antianxiety drugs such as alprazolam (Xanax) may be initiated 2 weeks before menses and discontinued when menses begins. CAHM therapies have been used to provide relief.

THE NORMAL VAGINA

At birth, the infant's vaginal epithelium is controlled by estrogen from the mother and is rich in glycogen, with a low pH of 3.7 to 6.3. When the maternal estrogen effect decreases, the vaginal epithelium atrophies, contains little glycogen, and the pH rises to 7. Estrogen influence returns at puberty, and glycogen increases. The interaction of glycogen and estrogen in the vaginal epithelium results in the growth of lactobacilli, which produce a bacteriostatic action. The pH falls to 3.5 to 4.5. The types of bacteria found in the vagina vary with the pH of the vagina. Factors that change the normal flora of the vagina and predispose to vaginal infection include the following:

- *Antibiotics:* Encourage yeast overgrowth
- *Douching:* Changes pH
- *Sexual intercourse:* Raises pH to 7 or higher for 8 hours after coitus

- *Uncontrolled diabetes mellitus:* Increases glucose that promotes organism growth

The normally acidic pH for the vagina is the first line of defense against vaginal infections. Normal vaginal secretions are made up of creamy white epithelial cells and mucus from the cervix, Skene glands, and Bartholin glands. The secretions prevent dryness and infection. At menopause, lowered estrogen causes vaginal dryness, and the pH may change, predisposing the woman to vaginal discomfort and infections. Other factors that can alter the pH of the vagina temporarily include the following:

- Deodorant soap
- Perfumed toilet tissue
- Spermicides
- Tampons
- Hot tubs and swimming pools
- Tight clothing made of synthetic fabrics

Health Promotion

Preventing Vaginal Infections

By promoting vaginal health, nurses can enhance the quality of life for the women they counsel. The promotion of vaginal health includes wearing cotton underwear, avoiding tight-fitting nylon or spandex pants, wiping front to back after toileting, and frequent hand hygiene. A healthy lifestyle, with a high-fibre, low-fat diet and exercise, strengthens the immune system and can prevent many infections. Douching increases the risk for vaginal infections. Women should not douche or use internal feminine hygiene products without first consulting their health care provider.

GYNECOLOGICAL INFECTIONS

Vaginal infections are a common reason for women to seek health care. Nurses play a key role in educating women about vaginal health and the prevention of sexually transmitted infections (STIs). Identifying high-risk behaviours and providing nonjudgemental, sensitive counselling and education should be part of every physical checkup. Education regarding safer sex practices provided in an individualized manner for each woman is an important aspect of primary prevention of STIs. Secondary prevention is the prompt treatment of the infection, which can also prevent further spread of the infection to others.

There are three classes of gynecological infections:

1. Toxic shock syndrome
2. Sexually transmitted infections
3. Pelvic inflammatory disease

TOXIC SHOCK SYNDROME

Toxic shock syndrome (TSS) is a rare and potentially fatal disorder. It is caused by strains of *Staphylococcus aureus* that produce toxins that can cause shock, coagulation defects, and tissue damage if they enter the bloodstream. TSS is associated with the trapping of bacteria within the reproductive tract for a prolonged period of time. Factors that increase the risk of TSS include the use of high-absorbency tampons for prolonged periods of time and the use of a diaphragm or cervical cap for contraception. Signs and symptoms of TSS include the following:

- Sudden spiking fever
- Flulike symptoms
- Hypotension
- Generalized rash that resembles sunburn
- Skin peeling from the palms and soles 1 to 2 weeks after the illness

The incidence of TSS has decreased, but nurses continue to play a role in prevention. The nurse's role is primarily one of education. The following teaching points should be included:

Tampon use:

- Perform hand hygiene before and after inserting a tampon.
- Change tampons at least every 4 hours.
- Do not use superabsorbent tampons.
- Use pads rather than tampons when sleeping, because tampons will likely remain in the vagina longer than 4 hours.

Diaphragm or cervical cap use:

- Perform hand hygiene before and after inserting the diaphragm or cervical cap.
- Do not use a diaphragm or cervical cap during the menstrual period or for 8 weeks after childbirth.
- Remove the diaphragm or cervical cap 6 to 8 hours after intercourse.

Treatment is supportive and includes hospitalization for vasopressor drugs, antimicrobial medication, and fluid replacement.

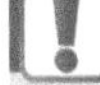

Safety Alert!

To prevent toxic shock syndrome, the woman should be taught to wash her hands well when using tampons or a diaphragm. The diaphragm should not be used during menstruation. Tampons should be changed every 4 hours and not used during sleep, which usually lasts longer than 4 hours.

SEXUALLY TRANSMITTED INFECTIONS

STIs are those that can be spread by sexual contact, although several of these infections have other modes of transmission as well. It is important that all sexual contacts of the infected person, even those persons who are asymptomatic, be completely treated to eradicate the infection. Table 2.1 provides specific information about STIs that the nurse may encounter. Chlamydia, gonorrhea, and infectious syphilis are reportable bacterial infections in Canada.

Nursing care related to STIs focuses primarily on patient education to prevent the spread of these infections. Such education includes the following:

- Teaching signs and symptoms that should be reported to the health care provider

Table 2.1 Sexually Transmitted Infections

INFECTION (CAUSATIVE ORGANISM)	SIGNS AND SYMPTOMS	DIAGNOSIS	PREGNANCY, FETAL, AND NEONATAL EFFECTS	TREATMENT	COMMENTS
Candidiasis (yeast) *(Candida albicans)*	Itching and burning on urination, inflammation of vulva and vagina, "cottage cheese" appearance to discharge	Signs and symptoms; speculum examination and potassium hydroxide preparation mixed with vaginal secretions—presence of buds and branches of yeast cells	Can infect newborn at birth	Fluconazole in a single dose can be prescribed. Fluconazole is contraindicated in pregnancy.	Medications are available OTC micomazole (Monistat) and clotrimazole (Canesten), but the woman should seek medical attention to diagnose her first infection or if she has persistent or recurrent infections.
Trichomoniasis *(Trichomonas vaginalis)*	Thin, foul-smelling, greenish yellow frothy, vaginal discharge, vulvar itching, edema, redness. Dysuria, and dyspareunia are often present.	Identification of the organism under microscope in a wet-mount	Associated with premature rupture of the membranes, preterm birth, and low birth weight	Metronidazole (Flagyl) 2 g in a single dose or 500 mg bid for 7 days.	Most infections are thought to be transmitted by sexual contact and the partner should also be treated. Abstaining from alcohol ingestion is recommended during and for 24 hours after treatment with metronidazole due to the risk of disulfuram (antabuse) reaction.
Bacterial vaginosis *(Gardnerella vaginalis)*	Thin, greyish white discharge that has a fishy odour	Microscopic evidence of clue cells (epithelial cells with bacteria clinging to their surface) and rapid detection tests	Associated with premature rupture of the membranes, chorioamnionitis, preterm labour, preterm birth and post-caesarean birth endometritis	Treatment with oral metronidazole is most effective.	See above for recommendations regarding metronidazole; treatment of partner is not recommended as sexual transmission is not proven.
Chlamydia *(Chlamydia trachomatis)*	Yellowish discharge, painful urination and postcoital bleeding Often asymptomatic in women, which delays treatment	Culture, rapid detection tests; DNA probe using urine specimen is noninvasive NAAT	Transmitted via birth canal Causes conjunctivitis and pneumonia in newborn	Azithromycin or doxycycline. Amoxicillin or erythromycin in pregnancy. Newborns have prophylactic eye care (see Chapter 6).	Reportable to a local health authority. All sexual partners who have had contact within 60 days before symptoms were evident need treatment. Untreated infection can ascend into fallopian tubes, causing scarring. Infertility or ectopic pregnancy may result. Can spread to newborn's eyes by contact with infected vaginal secretions.

Gonorrhea *(Neisseria gonorrhoeae)*	Purulent discharge, painful urination, dyspareunia, menstrual irregularities	Culture of organism, NAAT Noninvasive testing results are available within a few hours	Ophthalmia neonatorum, which can cause blindness; or systemic neonatal infection	Treatment with ceftriaxone plus zithromycin or cefixime plus azithromycin. Newborns have prophylactic eye care.	Can result in pelvic inflammatory disease with tubal scarring; all pregnant women should be screened at the first visit and those with positive screens or identified as at risk should be screened again at 36 weeks.
Syphilis *(Treponema pallidum)*	Three stages: *Primary:* Painless chancre on the genitalia, anus, or lips *Secondary:* 2 months after primary syphilis; enlargement of spleen and liver, headache, anorexia, generalized skin rash, wartlike growths on the vulva *Tertiary:* May occur many years after secondary syphilis and cause heart, blood vessel, nervous system damage	*Primary:* Examining material scraped from the chancre with darkfield microscopy to identify the spirochete organism; serological tests are not positive at this early stage *Secondary or tertiary:* Serological test (Venereal Disease Research Laboratory [VDRL] [less specific], and rapid plasma reagin (RPR) and fluorescent treponemal antibody absorption [FTA-ABS] [more specific])	Transmitted across placenta Causes congenital syphilis, stillbirth, spontaneous abortion It is recommended that all pregnant women be tested at the first prenatal visit and repeated at 28–32 weeks if high risk	Benzathine penicillin G; tetracycline, or erythromycin if allergic Tetracycline is not recommended during pregnancy.	Primary and secondary stages are the most contagious. Spread is through sexual contact or through the placenta from an infected mother.
Herpes genitalis (herpes simplex virus [HSV], types I and II)	Clusters of painful vesicles (blisters) on the vulva, perineum, and anal areas; fever, chills, malaise, and severe dysuria and may last 2–3 weeks Vesicles rupture in 1 to 7 days and heal in 12 days	By signs and symptoms; confirmed by viral culture antibody or DNA-based rapid test	Can cause spontaneous abortion, stillbirth Active genital infection necessitates Caesarean birth Causes neonatal central nervous system problems	No cure exists; acyclovir, famciclovir, or valacyclovir reduces symptoms. Treated with hygiene, sitz baths during pregnancy. Wearing loose clothing and cotton underwear is advised; oral analgesics to relieve pain.	HSV II usually causes genital lesions. The first episode is usually the most uncomfortable. The virus "hides" in the nerve cells and can re-emerge in later outbreaks that are as contagious as the first.

Continued

Table 2.1 Sexually Transmitted Infections—cont'd

INFECTION (CAUSATIVE ORGANISM)	SIGNS AND SYMPTOMS	DIAGNOSIS	PREGNANCY, FETAL, AND NEONATAL EFFECTS	TREATMENT	COMMENTS
Condylomata acuminata (human papillomavirus [HPV], genital warts)	Dry, wartlike growths on vagina, labia, cervix, and perineum	By typical appearance and location Over 40 subtypes can affect the genital tract HPV 6 and 11 cause warts HPV 16 and 18 cause most cervical concerns	Growth may obstruct birth canal	Removal with cryotherapy (cold), electrocautery, laser, or podophyllin applications are alternatives. Nurse should educate about application of local therapy.	Also, known as genital warts; associated with higher rates of cervical cancer. Women should have routine Papanicolaou (Pap) tests (see Pelvic Examination for screening guidelines); condom use can prevent transmission. The PHAC and NIAC recommends that males and females between 9–27 years of age receive the HPV vaccine series.
Human immunodeficiency virus ([HIV) Acquired immunodeficiency syndrome (AIDS)	Initially, no symptoms; later symptoms include weight loss, night sweats, fever and chills, fatigue, enlarged lymph nodes, skin rashes, diarrhea Late symptoms include immune suppression, opportunistic infections, and malignancies	Serology tests: positive enzyme-linked immunosorbent assay (ELISA), followed by positive Western blot test	Transmission can occur throughout the perinatal period. Women should be screened for HIV early in pregnancy so appropriate treatment can be instituted to decrease the rate of transmission to the newborn; Mother should be encouraged to formula feed	No cure is available yet. Antiretroviral treatment and close monitoring in pregnancy for complications are needed.	Transmitted through contact with nonintact skin or mucous membranes with infectious secretions, exposure to blood, and transmission from mother to fetus. Routine precautions reduce risk for caregivers. Condom use reduces risk for sexual transmission.

NAAT, Nucleic acid amplification test; *NAIC,* National Advisory Committee on Immunization; *OTC,* over the counter; *PHAC,* Public Health Agency of Canada.

Unnumbered Figure 1 from Grimes, D. E., & Grimes, R. M. (1994). *AIDS and HIV infection*. St. Louis: Mosby; unnumbered Figures 2 and 3 from Jarvis. C. (2000). *Physical examination and health assessment* (3rd ed.). Philadelphia: Saunders; unnumbered Figure 4 from Callen, J. P., Greer, K. E., Paller, A. S., & Swinyer, L. J. (2000). *Color atlas of dermatology* (2nd ed.). Philadelphia: Saunders.

Sources: Public Health Agency of Canada. (2013). *Canadian guidelines on sexually transmitted infections—Management and treatment of specific infections—Chlamydia*. Ottawa: Author. Retrieved from http://www.phac-aspc.gc.ca/std-mts/sti-its/cgsti-ldcits/section-5-2-eng.php; Public Health Agency of Canada. (2013). *Canadian guidelines on sexually transmitted infections—Management and treatment of specific syndromes—Vaginal discharge*. Retrieved from https://www.canada.ca/en/public-health/services/infectious-diseases/sexual-health-sexually-transmitted-infections/canadian-guidelines/sexually-transmitted-infections/canadian-guidelines-sexually-transmitted-infections-26.html; Public Health Agency of Canada. (2015). *Canadian guidelines on sexually transmitted infections: Management and treatment of specific infections—Human papillomavirus (HPV) infections*. Retrieved from https://www.canada.ca/en/public-health/services/infectious-diseases/sexual-health-sexually-transmitted-infections/canadian-guidelines/sexually-transmitted-infections/canadian-guidelines-sexually-transmitted-infections-33.html.

- Explaining diagnostic tests
- Teaching measures to prevent the spread of infection, such as the use of condoms
- Explaining treatment measures
- Emphasizing the importance of completing treatment and follow-up and of treating all sexual partners to eliminate the spread of infection

The incidence of STIs has increased during the past few decades and is a significant public health concern. Teaching STI prevention to women across the lifespan is important, because some viral STIs remain in the body for life and can include long-term complications.

Human papillomavirus (HPV) is the most common viral STI (also known as *condylomatata acuminate* or *vaginal warts*). It is estimated that 75% of Canadian adults will have at least one HPV infection in their lifetime, with the highest prevalence in women younger than 25 years (Public Health Agency of Canada [PHAC], 2019). There are more than 100 variations of HPV and of these 8 are associated with the development of malignant tumours. HPV types 16 and 18 are associated with serious cervical cancer.

The best prevention strategies for HPV is prophylactic vaccinations and the use of condoms. The PHAC and the National Advisory Committee on Immunization (NACI) recommend that a two-dose vaccination be given to females and males between the ages of 9 and 27, including women who have had previous Pap test abnormalities or cervical cancer, or individuals who have previously had genital warts. NACI also recommends that these vaccines be administered to individuals 27 years of age and older who are at ongoing risk of exposure to HPV (PHAC, 2019). All provinces and territories have publicly funded, school-based HPV vaccination programs for girls 9 to 13 years of age (grades 4 to 8), and some programs include vaccination of boys (Canadian Cancer Society, 2019a).

The use of condoms may not protect the woman if the male's lesion is on the scrotum or inguinal folds. It may take 3 to 6 months after infection to develop visible warts. Treatment includes cryotherapy, laser vaporization, electrodiathermy, and electrofulguration with a loop electrode excision procedure. Topical agents are used and lidocaine cream may be used 20 minutes before painful treatments.

Health Promotion

A two-dose series of vaccination for human papillomavirus (HPV) is recommended for all children and adults between 9 and 27 years of age. If women are at high risk of HPV exposure after age 27, they should also receive the vaccine.

Hepatitis B can be sexually transmitted if sexual practices include anal–oral sexual contact, digital rectal sexual intercourse, or multiple sex partners. Symptoms are nonspecific and include malaise, anorexia, nausea, and fatigue. Liver failure can develop. Hepatitis B vaccine can prevent the disease, and immunoglobulin can be administered if known exposure has occurred. All provinces and territories have either a universal school-based hepatitis B vaccination program aimed at children aged 9 to 13 or an infant vaccination program (PHAC, 2019).

The number of women newly diagnosed with human immunodeficiency virus (HIV) infection in Canada has held steady since 2011, although HIV continues to remain a worldwide health problem (Challacombe, 2019). Sexual contact and intravenous (IV) drug use are the most common risk behaviours for HIV infection. Patient education plays a key role in prevention, quality of life, and compassionate and knowledgeable referral. Early diagnosis, access to care, medications, and safer sex practices are improving outcomes and decreasing occurrence. HIV screening in pregnancy is strongly recommended for all women. It is important because many women in the early stages do not realize they are infected, and identification and treatment during pregnancy can prevent transmission to the fetus. Pre- and postscreening counselling must accompany all HIV testing. It is important to consider the older-person age group at risk, as well as opportunities for early detection and education for prevention that may be missed.

Prevention of STIs is the key role of the nurse. Teaching all age groups healthy behaviours such as safer sex practices and discussion of STI prevention is essential. Improving access to care and early detection are also important.

PELVIC INFLAMMATORY DISEASE

PID is an infection of the upper reproductive tract. Asymptomatic STIs are a common cause of PID. The cervix, uterine cavity, fallopian tubes, and pelvic cavity are often involved. Infertility may result.

The woman's symptoms vary according to the area affected. Fever (temperature >38.3°C), persistent pelvic pain, abnormal vaginal discharge, nausea and anorexia, and irregular vaginal bleeding are common. When examined, the abdomen and pelvic organs are often very tender. Laboratory tests can be used to identify common general signs of infection, such as elevated leukocytes and an elevated sedimentation rate. Cultures of the cervical canal are done to identify the infecting organism, which most commonly are *S. gonorrhoeae* or *C. trachomatis*. Urinalysis is usually done to identify infection of the urinary tract. The pelvic inflammation can result in scarring of the fallopian tubes, which can cause blockage and infertility or ectopic pregnancy.

Treatment includes antibiotics and patient education to prevent reinfection. Treatment may be administered on an inpatient or outpatient basis depending on the severity of the infection. Antimicrobials are begun promptly to treat the infection.

CONTRACEPTION AND FAMILY PLANNING

Family planning is influenced by many factors, including cultural practices and preference, religious beliefs, personal preferences, cost, knowledge of various methods, and the laws of human rights practiced in the country of residents. The nurse's role is to educate and guide the woman or couple concerning available choices, advantages, disadvantages, adverse effects, and long-term effects. The final decision rests with the individuals involved.

Contraception (birth control) may be part of the nurse's responsibility in family-planning clinics, in health care provider practices, or on the postpartum or gynecology units of an acute care hospital. In addition, family members and friends may turn to the nurse as a resource person who can answer their questions about contraception. The nurse can play a part in helping couples choose and correctly use contraceptive methods that enable them to have children at the appropriate time for the woman. Contraception does not always prevent pregnancy. An important consideration for patients is how likely the method is to fail. A contraceptive technique may fail because the method is ineffective or the user is using the method inappropriately.

NATURAL FAMILY PLANNING–FERTILITY AWARENESS

Natural family planning involves learning to identify the signs and symptoms associated with ovulation. The couple either abstains from intercourse or uses a barrier method during the period that is presumed to be fertile. The ovum is viable up to 24 hours after ovulation, and sperm are viable for up to 7 days in the fallopian tube, although most die within 24 hours.

Natural family planning methods are acceptable to most religions. They require no administration of systemic hormones or insertion of devices. They are not only reversible but also can be used to increase the odds of achieving pregnancy when the couple desires a child.

Natural family planning requires extensive assessment and charting of all the changes in the menstrual cycle. The woman must be highly motivated to track the many factors that identify ovulation. Both partners must be willing to abstain from intercourse for much of the woman's cycle if the method is used to prevent pregnancy. Couples must also be aware that the failure rate is approximately 24% (sexandu, 2019). Most women use a combination of the following methods for predicting when they are fertile to increase the predictive value over that of each method on its own.

Basal Body Temperature

The basal body temperature (BBT) is taken daily on awakening and before any activity (Fig. 2.1). This technique is based on the fact that there is a slight drop in basal temperature at ovulation (about 0.5°C) in some women although not all women. After ovulation the BBT increases slightly (0.4 to 0.8°C) and remains elevated until 2 to 4 days before menstruation. The fertile time is considered when the temperature drops, or the first elevation through 3 consecutive days of sustained temperature rise (Keenan-Lindsay, 2017a).

A *basal thermometer* is calibrated in tenths of a degree or an electronic digital format is used to detect these tiny changes. The woman charts each day's temperature to identify her temperature pattern. A rise in the BBT for the last 14 days of the cycle means that ovulation has probably occurred. Some electronic models have a memory to retain each day's temperature, and they display the pattern on a small screen.

Many factors can interfere with the accuracy of the BBT in predicting ovulation. Poor sleep, illness, jet lag, sleeping late, alcohol intake the evening before, or sleeping under an electric blanket or on a heated waterbed can make the BBT unreliable.

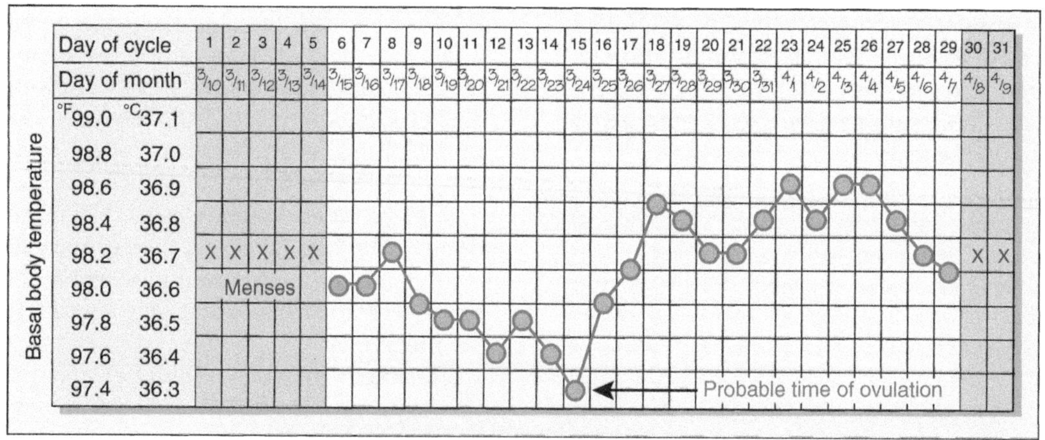

Fig. 2.1 Basal body temperature chart. By taking and recording her temperature, the woman can determine the probable time of ovulation.

Cervical Mucus Ovulation-Detection Method

The cervical mucus method of predicting ovulation requires that the woman notice the character and amount of cervical mucus changes during the menstrual cycle, because estrogen and progesterone influence the mucus-secreting glands of the cervix. Several days after menstruation, the cervical mucus is sticky, thick, and white. As ovulation nears, the mucus increases and becomes thin, slippery, and clear to aid the passage of sperm into the cervix. The slippery mucus can be stretched 6 cm or more and has the consistency of egg white (Fig. 2.2). The stretching characteristic of the mucus is called **spinnbarkeit**. After ovulation, the mucus disappears and the vagina feels drier. Factors that interfere with the accuracy of cervical mucus assessment include the use of antihistamines, vaginal infections, contraceptive foams or jellies, sexual arousal, and recent coitus. The noticeable changes in vaginal mucus before ovulation can aid in natural family planning and fertility awareness. This method can be used in women with irregular cycles.

Calendar or Rhythm Method

The woman charts her menstrual cycles on a calendar for several months. If the cycles are regular, she may be able to predict ovulation. The rhythm method is based on the fact that ovulation usually occurs about 14 days *before* the subsequent menstrual period. This would be about halfway through a 28-day cycle, but would be on day 18 of a 32-day cycle. A woman is fertile 5 days before and 1 day after ovulation and barrier methods of contraception can be used during this time to prevent pregnancy. This method is effective if the menstrual cycles are regular.

Breastfeeding: Lactational Amenorrhea Method

Breastfeeding is an effective although temporary method of birth control for up to 6 months postpartum in women if certain criteria are met. The woman must be exclusively (or nearly always) breastfeeding at least every 4 hours during the day and at least every 6 hours at night. The woman's period must also not have resumed and the infant must be less than 6 months of age. During the early life of an infant, frequent feeding ensures larger amounts of the hormone prolactin, which suppresses ovulation and the return of menstruation. The effectiveness of this method is 98% if all the criteria are met (Black, Guilbert, Costescu, et al., 2015b).

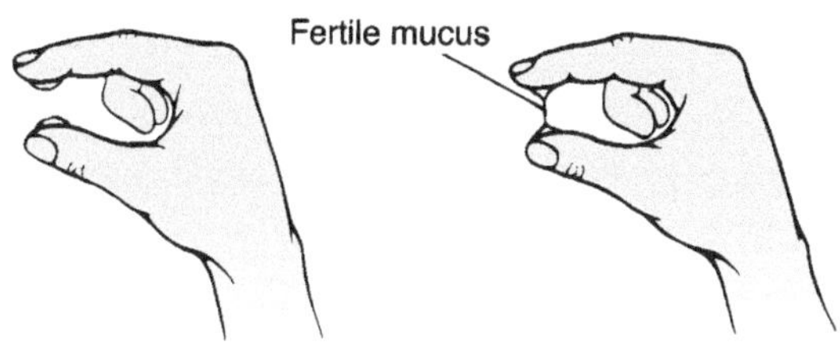

Fig. 2.2 Spinnbarkeit. The woman tests the capacity of her cervical mucus to stretch. This helps to determine the time of ovulation.

Coitus Interruptus

Withdrawal, or **coitus interruptus**, is withdrawal of the penis before ejaculation. It demands more self-control, which may be difficult for a man to achieve. Pre-ejaculatory secretions often contain sperm that can fertilize an ovum, and the failure rate is approximately 22% (Black, Guilbert, Costescu, et al., 2015a). Withdrawal also does not prevent STIs.

TEMPORARY CONTRACEPTION

Reversible contraception is defined as the temporary prevention of fertility.

Abstinence

Abstinence is 100% effective in preventing pregnancy and STIs. However, most couples believe that their sexual relationship adds to the quality of life. Therefore, abstinence is rarely an option the couple will consider.

Hormonal Contraceptives

Hormonal contraceptives include one or more of the following contraceptive effects:

- Prevent ovulation
- Make the cervical mucus thick and resistant to sperm penetration
- Make the uterine endometrium less hospitable if a fertilized ovum does arrive

Hormonal contraceptives do not protect either partner from STIs.

Oral contraceptives ("The Pill")

Oral contraceptives (OCs) are a popular, highly effective, and reversible method of birth control (Fig. 2.3). They contain either combined hormones (estrogen and progestin) or progestin alone ("minipill"). Progestin-only pills are recommended for breastfeeding mothers over the combined OC. A blood pressure assessment should be done prior to the woman receiving a prescription for an oral contraceptive.

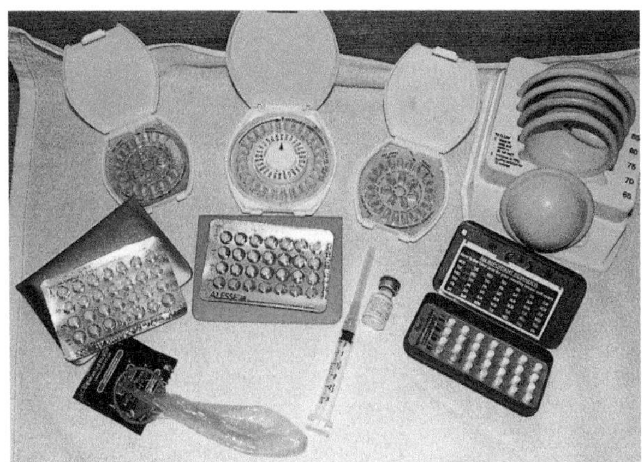

Fig. 2.3 Contraceptives. This photo shows common types of contraceptives: condoms, diaphragms, oral contraceptives, transdermal patch, and parenteral contraceptives.

Contraceptive regimens

Monthly contraception. Combination OCs are available in 21- or 28-pill packs. If the woman has a 21-pill pack, she takes one pill each day at the same time for 21 days, and then stops for 7 days. The woman who has a 28-day pack takes a pill each day; the last seven pills of the pack are inert (inactive) but help her maintain the habit of taking the pill each day. Menstruation occurs during the 7-day period when either no pills or inert pills are ingested.

Some pills are multiphasic in that their estrogen and progestin content changes during the cycle to mimic natural hormonal activity. If the woman takes multiphasic pills, it is very important that she take each pill in order. Taking the pills at the same time each day is important, regardless of the type of OC, to maintain a stable blood level of the hormones. It is most important that the medication-free interval not be extended beyond 7 days.

Extended-dose contraception. Extended-dose contraception is also known as *induced amenorrhea.* Research has shown that there are no specific health benefits to monthly menstruation. The woman can take an OC with no breaks. There has been no noted evidence of adverse effects with the extended-dose regimen, and it has a lower failure rate as compared to conventional (monthly) administration. Women should be made aware that there is often bleeding or spotting in the first 3 months but after that bleeding is minimal (Black, Guilbert, Costescu, et al., 2016).

Adverse effects and contraindications. Common adverse effects of OCs include nausea, headache, breast tenderness, weight gain, and spotting between periods or amenorrhea. These effects generally decrease within a few months and are seen less frequently with low-dose OCs.

Women with the following disorders should not take OCs or should take them with caution:

- Thromboembolic disorders (blood clots)
- Cerebrovascular accident or heart disease
- Estrogen-dependent cancer or breast cancer
- A smoking pattern of more than 15 cigarettes a day for women older than 35 years (women who are older than 35 years and who smoke should take progestin-only contraception)
- Impaired liver function
- A confirmed or possible pregnancy
- Undiagnosed vaginal bleeding
- Lactation less than 6 weeks

Safety Alert!

Smoking increases the chance of experiencing complications related to combined oral contraceptives, particularly in women older than 35 years.

The first episode of menstrual bleeding after a miscarriage or abortion is usually preceded by ovulation, and therefore contraception should begin immediately to prevent pregnancy. However, after a term birth there is a high risk of thromboembolism; therefore, the contraceptive is usually started 3 to 4 weeks postpartum, if the woman is not breastfeeding.

The use of combination OCs also may decrease breastmilk production, so OC use may be contraindicated in the breastfeeding woman until lactation is well established. The progestin-only OC (minipill) is a better option for breastfeeding women.

Memory Jogger

The mnemonic *ACHES* can help a woman recall the warning signs to report when taking OCs:

- **A**bdominal pain (severe)
- **C**hest pain, dyspnea, bloody sputum
- **H**eadache (severe), weakness, or numbness of the extremities
- **E**ye problems (blurring, double vision, vision loss)
- **S**evere leg pain or swelling, speech disturbance

Extended-dose oral contraceptives have been used successfully to minimize the bloating, fluid retention, and symptoms of PMDD usually associated with oral contraceptives.

Some medications decrease the effectiveness of OCs, including the following:

- Some anticonvulsants
- Some antiretrovirals, rifampin and griseofulvin

Nursing care. The woman needs thorough teaching if the contraceptive pill is to be a satisfactory method for her. Teaching should be done in her own language and should be supplemented by written materials if she is able to read. Teaching points should include the following:

- How to take the specific medication
- What to do if a dose is missed or if she decides to stop using it and does not want to become pregnant (see *Stay on Schedule* resource in Online Resources for information regarding this)
- Common adverse effects and signs and symptoms that should be promptly reported
- Backup contraceptive methods, such as barrier methods (discussed later in this chapter)
- Supplemental barrier methods of contraception to use, in addition to OCs, that also reduce the risk of STIs

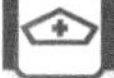

Nursing Tip

The more birth control pills a woman misses, the greater her risk that pregnancy will occur.

Injectable contraception

Depot medroxyprogesterone acetate (DMPA; Depo-Provera) is an injectable form of slow-release progestin. Its contraceptive action is similar to that of the minipill. It provides 3 months of highly effective contraception; therefore, it must be administered every 12 to 13 weeks. Fertility returns about 6 to 10 months after stopping the injections (sexandu, 2019).

Adverse effects and contraindications. The adverse effects and contraindications of hormone injections are similar to those of OCs. Menstrual irregularities, breakthrough bleeding, and amenorrhea are common concerns and are often the reason that women stop taking the drug. There is no STI protection with this method. The failure rate for women with typical use is 6%, although with perfect use it is 99% effective.

Nursing care. The woman should be taught about the adverse effects and problems to report. It should be emphasized that she must return for continued injections if she wants to maintain a constant hormone level, thus preventing pregnancy. A backup contraceptive method should be taught for use if she decides to stop the injections or is delayed in returning for subsequent injections. Women with seizure disorders can use this method of contraception without fear of interaction with their antiseizure medication and it may decrease the number of seizures in these women (sexandu, 2019). Women with coagulation problems or with sickle cell anemia benefit from this type of contraception, which suppresses ovulation and reduces blood loss.

Intrauterine contraception

An intrauterine device (IUD) is a reversible method of birth control that requires a prescription and a health care provider to insert it. They are effective (99% or greater) and reversible, and no specific actions are required related to intercourse. Health care providers are encouraged to consider IUDs as the first line of contraception for all women whether or not they have given birth, owing to the low risk of adverse effects and the high rates of effectiveness (Black et al., 2016). Depending on the device, the IUD can remain in for 3 to 10 years before needing to be replaced (Sexandu. 2019). The copper IUD is a small, T-shaped, copper-containing plastic device that does not contain hormones and is effective for up to 5 years. The main mechanism of the copper IUD is as a spermicide and it prevents a fertilized ovum from implanting in the endometrium. The levonorgestrel-releasing intrauterine system (Mirena, Kyleena, or Jaydess) has a small cylinder that contains progestin or levonorgestrel that is diffused into the uterus each day. The action is local in the uterine cavity, and blood levels do not increase. This type of IUD thickens cervical mucus (making it difficult for sperm to move into the uterus), inhibits sperm movement in the uterus, and thins the lining of the uterus, and the Mirena can sometimes prevent ovulation. On removal of the IUD, fertility rapidly returns. The IUD does not protect against STIs.

Adverse effects and contraindications. Cramping and bleeding are likely to occur with insertion. Insertion should not be attempted during menses. Increased menstruation and dysmenorrhea may occur, and these are common reasons that a woman decides to have the IUD removed. The woman who has heavier periods may need iron supplementation.

Nursing care. The woman is taught about adverse effects and how to take iron supplements if they are prescribed. The woman will need to feel for the fine plastic strings (tail) that protrude from the vagina and are connected to the IUD to verify that it is in place. She should check the tail weekly for the first 4 weeks after insertion, then monthly. The woman is taught to report if she cannot feel the tail that protrudes into the vagina, or if it is longer or shorter than previously. The nurse can teach her the signs of infection (fever, pain, change in vaginal discharge).

Transdermal patch

A transdermal patch contains hormones (norelgestromin/ethinyl-estradiol) and is applied to the skin once a week for 3 weeks, followed by a 1-week patch-free interval to allow for menstruation to occur. The patch provides safe and effective contraception similar to that of OCs. The transdermal patch may be less effective in women with a weight of greater than 90 kg (Black, Guilbert, Costescu, et al., 2017).

Vaginal ring

A flexible, one-size vaginal ring (NuvaRing) that releases estrogen and progestin locally instead of systemically is a highly effective method if used properly. The ring is worn in the vagina for 3 weeks and is removed for 1 week to allow for withdrawal bleeding. The vaginal ring may reduce menstrual flow and cramps.

Barrier Methods

Barrier methods work by blocking the entrance of semen into the woman's cervix. **Spermicides** (sperm-killing chemicals) play a part in some of these methods. They help the woman avoid the use of systemic hormones. Some barrier methods offer some protection against STIs by providing a barrier to contact.

Some barrier methods must be applied just before intercourse (condoms, spermicidal foams, and suppositories), whereas others can be inserted a few hours earlier (diaphragm, cervical cap). Spermicidal foams and suppositories are messy and may drip from the vagina. These methods are not suitable for people who are uncomfortable with touching their bodies. They are often used as a backup method for contraception.

Barrier methods are inexpensive per use. The diaphragm and cervical cap require a fitting and prescription, which adds to their initial cost. Other barrier methods are over-the-counter purchases. These methods are often chosen as backup methods or when the woman is lactating, or if she cannot tolerate OCs or an IUD.

Diaphragm and cervical cap

Diaphragms and cervical caps are rubber domes that fit over the cervix and are used with spermicides to kill sperm that pass the mechanical barrier. A health care provider fits the diaphragm and cervical cap.

The woman must learn how to insert and remove the diaphragm or cervical cap and to verify proper placement. User misplacement, especially of the small cervical cap, is a common reason for unintended pregnancy. The typical failure rate is approximately 12%.

Before insertion of a diaphragm, the woman should check either device for weak spots or pinholes by holding it up to the light (Skill 2.1). Spermicidal jelly or cream is applied to the ring and the centre of the diaphragm before inserting it and positioning it over the cervix. It may be inserted 2 hours before intercourse, and it should remain in place for at least 6 hours after intercourse, but not more than 24 hours to prevent pressure on local tissue. More spermicidal jelly or cream must be inserted into the vagina if the couple repeats coitus within 6 hours. The diaphragm must be refitted after each birth or after a weight loss or gain of 20%. The cap must be checked yearly and after birth or gynecological surgery. Women who have an allergy to latex or spermicides are not good candidates for the diaphragm or cervical cap.

Vaginal sponge

A vaginal sponge is a soft concave sponge that contains a spermicide and is moistened thoroughly in water and inserted by the woman with the cupped side against the cervix. A loop facilitates removal after use. It can be left in place for up to 24 hours after intercourse, then discarded. The sponge absorbs and traps sperm as well as vaginal secretions and can cause vaginal dryness and subsequent vaginal irritation. Changes in the shape of the cervix may occur after giving birth, which can affect the proper fitting and effectiveness of the sponge in preventing pregnancy. The failure rate of the vaginal sponge is fairly high and it is less effective in women who have previously given birth. The sponge does not protect against STIs.

Nursing care. The health care provider who fits the device will provide much of the teaching on insertion, verification of placement, and removal. The nurse often reinforces the teaching, especially about the use and reapplication of spermicide for repeat intercourse. The nurse should teach the woman about signs of uterine infection (pain, foul-smelling drainage, or fever) and of sensitivity to the product (irritation or itching).

Male condom

Male condoms are sheaths of thin latex, polyurethane, or natural membrane ("skins") worn on the penis during intercourse. Condoms collect semen before, during, and after ejaculation. They come in various styles, such as ribbed, lubricated, and coloured. They are single-use, low-cost items that are widely available from vending machines, drugstores, and family-planning clinics. Latex condoms provide some protection from STIs. Natural membrane condoms do not prevent the passage of viruses. See Skill 2.2 for the correct use of the condom.

To prevent condom breakage, water-soluble lubricants should be used if the condom or vagina is dry. Unlike other, oil-based lubricants, water-soluble lubricants do not damage the latex or cause breakage. The penis should be withdrawn from the vagina immediately if the man feels that the condom is breaking or is becoming dislodged. The condom is removed and a new one is applied. Condoms are not reused, because even a pinhole can lead to pregnancy or permit the entry of viruses, including HIV.

The nurse should educate patients on how to prevent common condom mistakes, including the following:

- Allowing the penis to lose erection while still in the vagina
- Opening the condom package with the teeth or a sharp object, which can tear the condom
- Unrolling the condom before applying it to the penis
- Using out-of-date condoms
- Using baby oil, cold cream, vegetable oil, or petroleum jelly to lubricate the condom
- Reusing the condom
- Storing condoms in the wallet (heat destroys spermicide)
- Not leaving space between the tip of the penis and the condom to provide a reservoir for ejaculate

Side effects and contraindications. Side effects of and contraindications to condom use are rare. Either of the partners may be allergic to latex, in which case a polyurethane condom can often be used successfully. The failure rate for condoms is 18%.

Female condom

Female condoms are essentially used for the same purpose as male condoms—to prevent pregnancy and to protect the woman from STIs (Fig. 2.4). The female condom has two flexible rings, one that fits into the vagina and one that remains outside, connected by a polyurethane sheath. Female condoms are prelubricated, single-use items that are available over the counter. They allow the woman control over her exposure to infections without having to rely on the cooperation of her partner. Its failure rate in pregnancy prevention is 5% if used perfectly (sexandu, 2019) and 21% with typical use. It is slightly more expensive than a male condom and some people find it is noisier during intercourse.

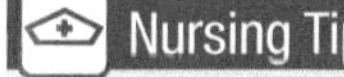

Nursing Tip

It is important to educate adolescents about contraception, reproductive health, and the importance of safer sex.

Spermicides

Spermicidal foam, cream, jelly, film, and suppository capsules are over-the-counter contraceptives. They are inserted into the vagina before intercourse to neutralize vaginal secretions, destroy sperm, and block entrance to the uterus. Each product has specific directions for use. Vaginal films and suppositories must melt before

Skill 2.1 Teaching How to Use a Diaphragm

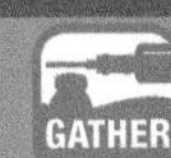

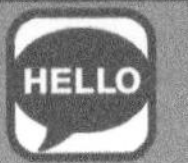

PRIVACY

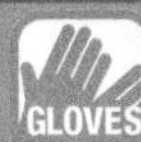

PURPOSE

To learn to use a diaphragm for contraception

NOTE: A diaphragm can be inserted up to 2 hours before intercourse. Insertion and removal skills increase with practice.

STEPS

1. Apply spermicidal cream or gel inside at centre and around the rim of the diaphragm. This aids the insertion and offers a more complete seal.

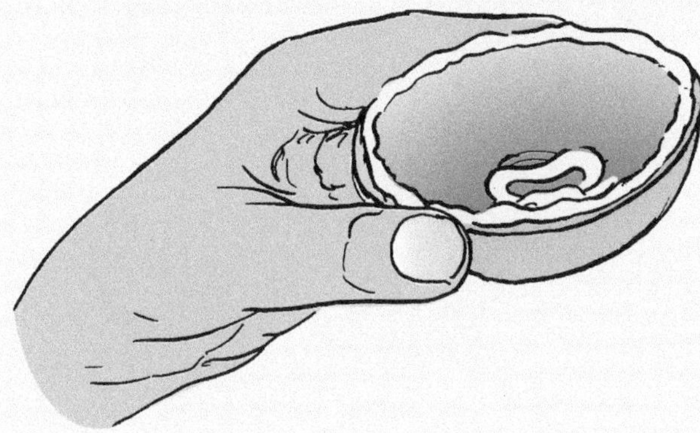

2. Hold diaphragm between your thumb and finger and compress diaphragm. Use fingers of other hand to spread the labia (lips of the vagina).
3. Begin to insert diaphragm into vagina with spermicide toward the cervix. Squatting or placing one foot on a chair makes insertion (and removal) easier.
4. Insert diaphragm into vagina. Direct it inward and downward behind and below the cervix.

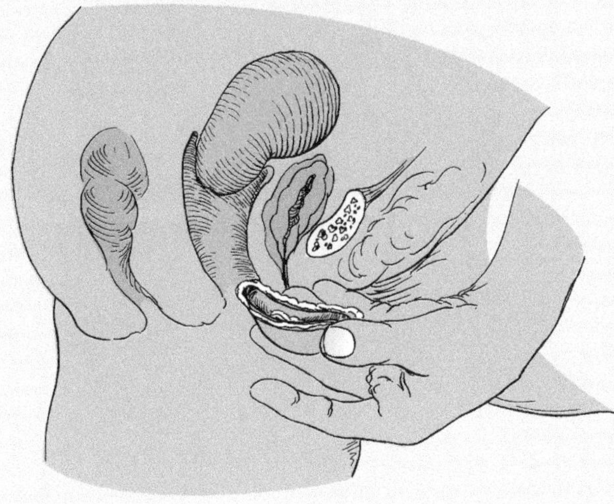

5. Tuck the front of the rim of diaphragm behind the pubic bone.

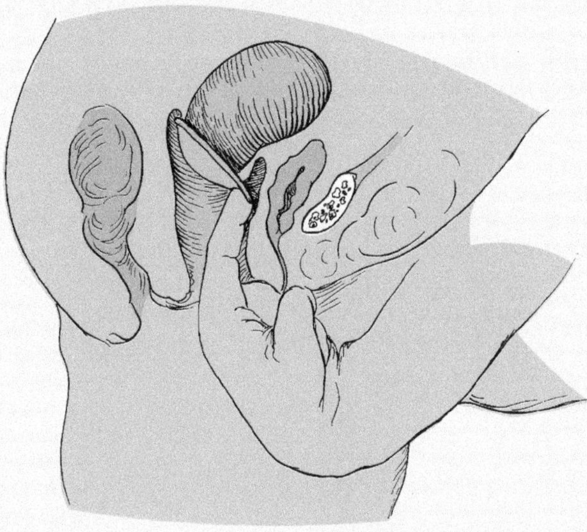

6. Feel your cervix through the centre of the diaphragm.
7. Leave diaphragm in place at least 6 hours after intercourse.
8. To remove diaphragm, assume squatting position and bear down. Hook a finger over the top rim to break suction, and pull diaphragm down and out.

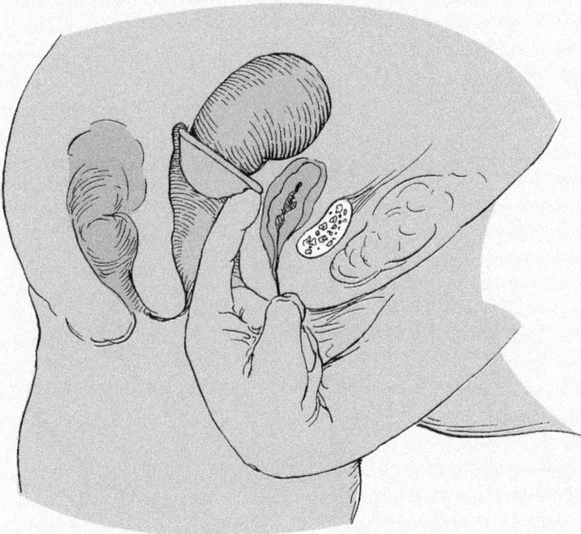

9. Wash diaphragm with mild soap and dry well after each use.
10. Dust diaphragm with cornstarch. Scented talc or baby powder can weaken the rubber.
11. Inspect diaphragm regularly for small holes by holding it up to light.

Skill 2.2 Teaching How to Use the Male Condom

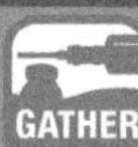

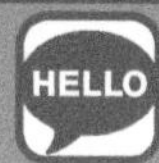

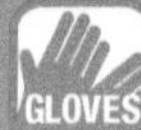

PURPOSE

To learn to use a condom for contraception

STEPS

1. Use a new condom each time you have intercourse.
2. Check the expiration date on packages, because condoms deteriorate over time.
3. Apply the condom before you have any contact with the woman's vagina, because there are sperm in the secretions before you ejaculate.
4. Squeeze the air from the tip when placing the condom over the end of your penis. Leave 1 cm of space at the tip to allow sperm to collect and to prevent breakage.

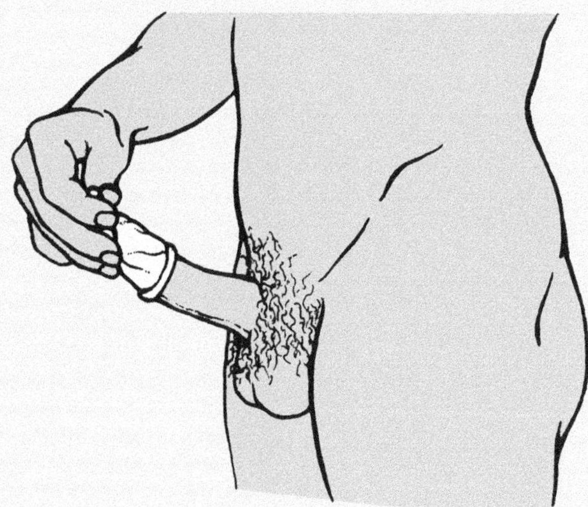

5. Hold the tip while you unroll the condom over the erect penis.

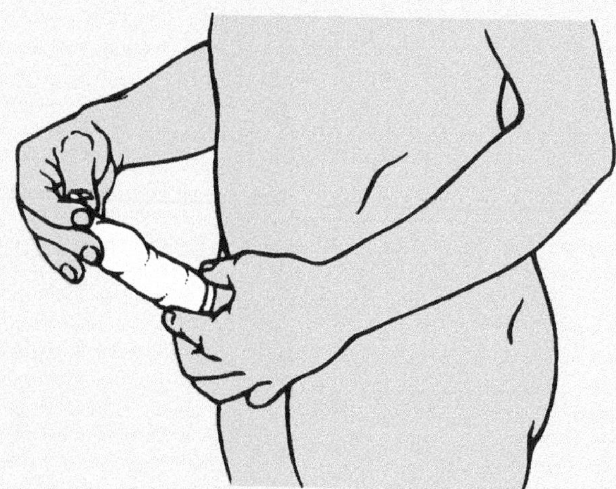

6. Do not use petroleum jelly, grease, or oil as lubricants because they can cause the condom to break. Instead, use a water-soluble lubricant such as K-Y Jelly.
7. Hold on to the condom at the base of the penis to prevent spillage as you withdraw from the vagina.

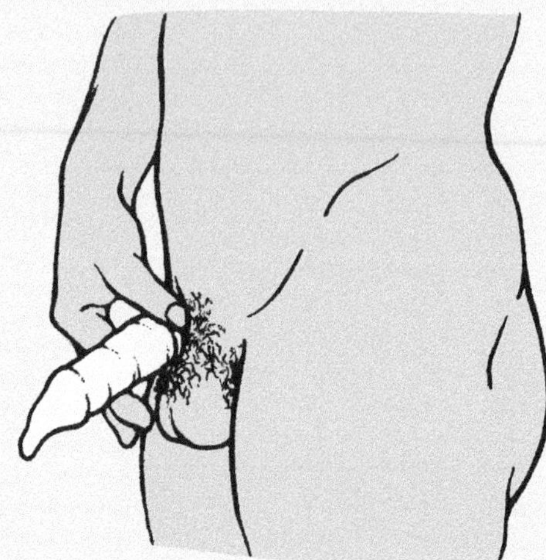

8. Remove the condom carefully to be sure that no semen spills from it.
9. Place the condom in the trash or in some safe disposal.

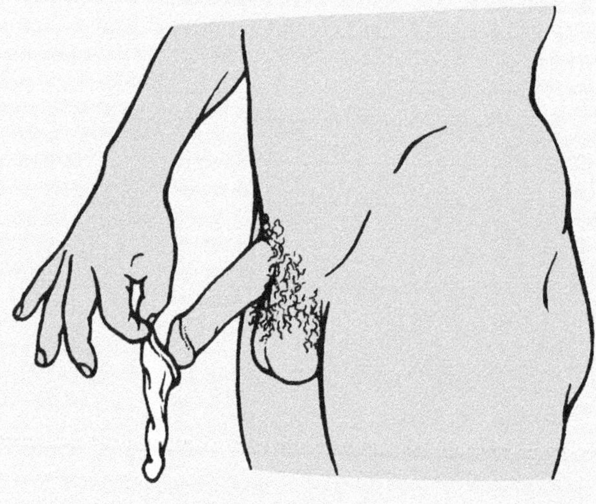

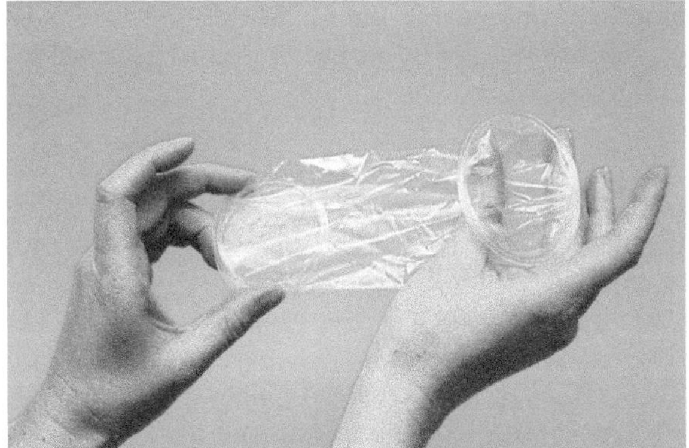

Fig. 2.4 Female condom. (From Grimes, D. E., & Grimes, R. M. [1994]. *AIDS and HIV infection.* St. Louis: Mosby.)

they are effective, which takes about 15 minutes. Most spermicides are effective for no more than 1 hour. Reapplication is needed for repeated coitus. The woman should not douche for at least 6 to 8 hours after intercourse. Vaginal spermicides are the least effective method of birth control with high failure rates (18 to 28%). Spermicides should be used with another barrier form of contraception (diaphragm or condom).

Adverse effects and contraindications. Spermicides can cause local irritation in the vagina or on the penis. The irritation can cause tiny cracks that provide portals of entry for infection.

EMERGENCY CONTRACEPTION

Emergency contraception (EC) is a method of preventing pregnancy after unprotected sexual intercourse. It can be used if contraceptives fail (such as a condom that tears), in cases of sexual assault, or in other situations as needed. It is not to be used as a regular method of birth control but rather as an occasional method. There are two options for EC available in Canada: hormonal methods or the postcoital insertion of a copper IUD.

The one-step EC Plan B contains the progestin levonorgestrel in a one-dose pill "morning after" regime that is available in pharmacies without a prescription. It is most effective if used within 72 hours of unprotected intercourse, but may be effective if used within 120 hours after unprotected sexual intercourse.

Placement of a copper IUD within 5 days of unprotected intercourse is the most effective method of EC and also has the advantage of providing long-term contraception at a low cost (Black et al., 2015a).

The woman should be referred for counselling and follow-up care after use of EC.

PERMANENT CONTRACEPTION

Sterilization

Sterilization is a permanent method of birth control that is almost 100% effective in preventing pregnancy. Although the procedures may be reversed in some cases, reversal is expensive and not always successful. Therefore, patients should think carefully about this decision and should consider it permanent.

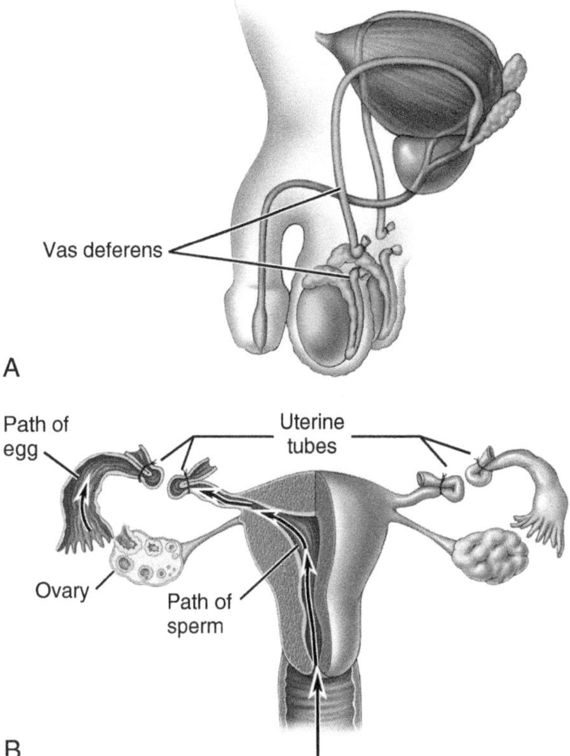

Fig. 2.5 Surgical methods of birth control. **A,** Vasectomy, the cutting and ligation (tying off) of the vas deferens. **B,** Tubal ligation, the ligation of the fallopian tubes. (From Herlihy, B. [2014]. *The human body in health and illness* [5th ed.]. St. Louis: Saunders.)

Advantages

The advantages of sterilization relate to the fact that the person can consider the risk of pregnancy to be near zero. Minimal anxiety about becoming pregnant may help the individual to enjoy the sexual relationship more.

Disadvantages

A major disadvantage of sterilization is the same as its primary advantage: permanence. Divorce, marriage, death of a child, or a change in attitude toward having children may make the person regret their decision. The procedures require surgery, and, although the risks are small, they are the same as for other surgical procedures: hemorrhage, infection, injury to other organs, and anaesthesia complications.

Male sterilization

Male sterilization, or *vasectomy,* is performed by making a cut in each side of the scrotum and cutting each vas deferens, the tube through which the sperm travel (see Fig. 2.5, *A*). Because sperm are already present in the system distal to the area of ligation, sterility is not immediate. Another method of birth control must be implemented until all sperm have left the system, usually about 1 to 3 months. The man should return to his health care provider for analysis of his semen to verify that it no longer contains sperm. Many men need information about the anatomy and physiology of their sex organs. They need reassurance that they will still have erections and ejaculations and that intercourse will remain pleasurable.

The surgery takes about 20 minutes and is performed on an outpatient basis with a local anaesthetic. There is some pain, bruising, and swelling after the surgery. Rest, a mild analgesic, and the application of an ice pack are comfort measures. As in other surgeries, the man should report the following:

- Bleeding or substantial bruising
- Separation of the suture line, drainage, or increasing pain

Female sterilization

Tubal ligation. Tubal ligation involves blocking or ligating the fallopian tubes (Fig. 2.5, *B*). This can be accomplished by using electrocautery or clips. Tubal ligation is easy to perform during the immediate postpartum period, because the fundus, to which the tubes are attached, is large and near the surface. Female permanent contraception may be performed abdominally, laparoscopically, or by *minilaparotomy,* in which an incision is made near the umbilicus in the immediate postpartum period or just above the symphysis pubis at other times. In a minilapartomy, the physician makes a tiny incision, brings each tube through it, and ligates and cuts the tube.

The discomfort after the minilaparotomy or laparoscopy is usually easily relieved with oral analgesia. Some women experience nausea from the anaesthesia. Even though this is not considered major surgery, the woman requires 1 or 2 days to recuperate. She should report signs of bleeding or infection, as with the male vasectomy.

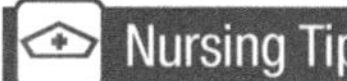

Nursing Tip

When discussing sexual issues with a couple, the nurse should use the word *partner* until the couple indicates a preference for an alternative term.

MENOPAUSE

The definition of **menopause** is the cessation of menstrual periods for a 12-month period due to changes in estrogen production. The **climacteric** (change of life) is also known as the *perimenopausal period,* which extends for 2 to 8 years before menstruation ceases. The average age for menopause is 51.4 years with a range from 35 to 60 years (Keenan-Lindsay, 2017b). In the 2- to 8-year period before this time, the ova slowly degenerate and menstrual cycles are often anovulatory and irregular. Estrogen production by the ovaries decreases. Pregnancy can occur during the climacteric, and the woman should be encouraged to continue any birth control that she has used in the past. Decreasing estrogen in the woman increases her risk for osteoporosis, arteriosclerosis, and increases in cholesterol levels in the blood. Menopause may be induced at any age by surgery, pelvic irradiation, or extreme stress.

PHYSICAL CHANGES

The decrease in estrogen specifically causes the following:

- Changes in the menstrual cycle
- Vasomotor instability (hot flashes)
- Decreased moisture and elasticity of vagina that can cause dyspareunia (painful intercourse)

Other symptoms such as mood swings and irritability are also experienced. Hot flashes are a well-known phenomenon. The woman suddenly feels a burning or hot sensation of her skin followed by perspiration. Hot flashes often occur during the night, and some women have several sleep interruptions because of them. They are more likely to occur when menopause is artificial, such as through oophorectomy (removal of the ovaries), rather than when it occurs naturally. The woman may also notice chills, palpitations, dizziness, and tingling of the skin as part of the vasomotor instability.

The reproductive organs are estrogen dependent, leading to changes as the estrogen level declines. The uterus shrinks, and the ovaries atrophy. The sacral ligaments relax, and pelvic muscles weaken, which can result in pelvic floor dysfunction. The cervix becomes pale and shrinks. The vagina becomes shorter, narrower, and less elastic. There is less lubrication. Some women notice a change in *libido* (sexual desire) at this time. Coitus may be uncomfortable because of vaginal dryness. Urinary incontinence may be a problem, because the muscles controlling urine flow atrophy. The breasts atrophy.

Loss of estrogen secretion also means an end to its protective effect on the woman's cardiovascular and skeletal systems. Estrogen increases the amount of high-density lipoproteins, which carry cholesterol from body cells to the liver for excretion. The incidence of heart disease rises after menopause, because low-density lipoproteins, which carry cholesterol into body cells (including blood vessels), increase.

Estrogen assists the deposition of calcium in the bones to strengthen them. Loss of bone mass accelerates as estrogen levels fall, resulting in **osteoporosis**. Osteoporosis is a leading cause of vertebral, hip, and other fractures in postmenopausal women, because the bones become very fragile. Both males and females lose bone mass as they age. Females, who have a lower bone mass to begin with because they are smaller, lose more in proportion to the total amount as they age. In addition, women generally live longer than men, so the loss continues longer. Therefore, problems such as hip fractures related to age affect many more women than men. The bones may be so fragile that a fracture occurs and causes a fall, rather than the fracture being the result of a fall.

PSYCHOLOGICAL AND CULTURAL VARIATIONS

Women from different cultures experience menopause differently. How society views aging, the role of the female, and femininity itself have a bearing. In countries in which age is revered, menopause is practically a "nonevent." In North America, with its emphasis on youth, sex appeal, and physical beauty, menopause can threaten the woman's feelings of health and self-worth. A positive aspect of menopause is that it is a time of liberation from monthly periods, cramps, and the fear of unwanted pregnancy. It can be the beginning of a satisfying postreproductive life.

MANAGEMENT OF SYMPTOMS

Menopause is a stage of health within the health–illness continuum in a woman's life. It is not approached as a disease or illness but rather as a unique stage of life and as a normal, healthy process. Partnership-building communication with the health care team can help the woman cope with lifestyle changes that may be necessary to maintain health. The nurse can help educate the woman to understand the changes that are occurring and develop coping mechanisms to promote comfort in handling minor discomforts. Vaginal dryness can be relieved by the use of lubricants, Kegel exercises can counter genital atrophy, and maintaining good hydration and techniques to prevent urinary tract infections can promote general well-being. Exercise, an increase in the dietary intake of calcium and magnesium, and a high-fibre, low-fat diet rich in antioxidants are essential. Limiting intake of alcohol, nicotine, and caffeine may also decrease menopause symptoms and improve the lifestyle of the woman.

Hormone therapy (HT) is sometimes used to manage moderate to severe menopause symptoms. It is recommended that health care providers prescribe HT at the lowest dose required, and for the least duration necessary, to treat troubling menopause symptoms. Current research confirms that HT is both a safe and effective way to treat symptoms of menopause (Reid, Abramson, Blake, et al., 2014). HT helps restore balance in a woman's body after her ovaries have stopped producing estrogen and progestin. An HT program may involve the use of estrogen alone (estrogen therapy, or ET), or estrogen and progestin in combination (EPT). Today, HT decisions are based on the individual patient, with the benefits and risks clearly identified. Nurses should counsel their patients who are taking HT to have regular follow-up care and to report any signs of complications, such as headache, vision changes, signs of thrombophlebitis, or cardiac symptoms.

Contraindications for HT include estrogen-dependent breast cancer, endometrial cancer, thromboembolic disease, a history of malignant melanoma, chronic liver disease, severe hypertriglyceridemia, gallbladder disease, and seizure disorders. Although women who are *BRCA-1* gene carriers have a 60 to 80% chance of developing breast cancer, prophylactic surgery before menopause lowers the risk of developing cancer. Women should have breast cancer surveillance as advised by their health care provider.

Table 2.2 Popular Herbs Used in Menopause and for Other Reproductive Concerns

HERB	USES AND CONTRAINDICATIONS
Black cohosh (*Cimicifuga racemosa*)	Diminishes hot flashes by reducing luteinizing hormone (LH); reduces joint pain, hot flashes, and other menopausal discomforts
Sage (*Salvia officinalis*)	Contains phytosterols and bioflavonoids; effective for night sweats and hot flashes and has been used to decrease breastmilk production
Dong quai (*Angelica sinensis*)	Contains phytoestrogens; contraindicated for use in presence of midcycle spotting and fibroids
Chasteberry (*Vitex agnus-castus*)	Reduces hot flashes and dizziness caused by high levels of follicle-stimulating hormone (FSH); balances hormonal fluctuations when combined with other herbs
Motherwort (*Leonurus cardiaca*)	Relieves hot flashes and moodiness; reduces anxiety and insomnia

Data from Heber, D. (2007). *PDR for herbal medicines* (4th ed.). Montvale, NJ: Medical Economics; Rakel, D. (2018). *Integrative medicine* (4th ed.). Philadelphia: Elsevier.

Complementary and Alternative Health Modalities

The use of CAHM therapy during menopause has become very popular. See Table 2.2 for discussion of some herbs that are used for menopause and other reproductive concerns for women.

Homeopathy, acupuncture, and relaxation techniques can also be helpful. See Chapter 33 for more information concerning CAHM therapies.

Therapy for Osteoporosis

Osteoporosis occurs when the loss of calcium from the bones is faster than its deposition in the bones. Signs of osteoporosis include a loss of height, the development of a dowager's hump (a dorsal kyphosis and cervical lordosis), curvature of the upper spine, and increased susceptibility to hip and spinal fractures. Calcium intake from food sources such as dairy products, dark green leafy vegetables, soybeans, wheat bread, and/or calcium and vitamin D supplements can prevent complications of osteoporosis. A daily intake of 1 200 mg calcium is needed for the woman over age 50 and 600 IU of vitamin D per day is needed to absorb calcium from the gastrointestinal tract (Health Canada, 2019). Weight-bearing exercises such as walking, hiking, stair climbing, and dancing are advisable to strengthen the musculoskeletal system. High-impact exercises should be avoided. To assess risk for osteoporosis, bone mineral density (BMD) testing is recommended for postmenopausal women older than 65 years. Bisphosphonates may be prescribed to increased bone mineral density and to prevent potential fractures. Esophageal and gastric irritation are common adverse effects of bisphosphonates, and the woman should be instructed to drink 250 mL of plain water and to sit upright for 30 minutes after taking the medication and before eating a meal. Parathyroid hormones and calcitonin show promise in reducing the risk of fractures and possibly increasing bone formation. Denosumab (Prolia) is a bone metabolism regulator that may be prescribed to reduce bone loss.

NURSING CARE OF THE MENOPAUSAL WOMAN

Nursing Care Plan 2.1 offers further nursing interventions in addition to those discussed here. The woman's knowledge of the changes surrounding menopause is assessed. If she is near the age for the climacteric to begin, any symptoms are identified. Treatments or tests that the woman will have, such as bone density studies, are clarified. The nurse must determine the woman's understanding of the risks and benefits of HT when helping her to decide about the therapy, with written information provided to reinforce verbal teaching.

The woman is taught the signs and symptoms that she should report, such as vaginal bleeding that recurs after the cessation of menstrual periods. She should also report signs of vaginal irritation or signs of urinary tract infection, because these are more common with atrophy of vaginal tissues.

The woman is also taught how to take prescribed medications properly. For example, the nurse must teach the woman that calcium is best absorbed if she also takes vitamin D. Taking foods or other medications before allowing at least 30 minutes (preferably 1 hour) for alendronate to be absorbed will negate the benefit of that dose. Lying down after taking a bisphosphonate can cause severe esophageal irritation.

The woman should be informed of medication-related adverse effects to report. She should contact her health care provider if she has headaches visual disturbances, signs of thrombophlebitis, heaviness in her legs, chest pain, or breast lumps because these symptoms may indicate adverse effects associated with HT. Basic education concerning the use of CAHM and their adverse effects and interactions should be included in the teaching plan.

The woman should be taught about the value of weight-bearing exercise in slowing bone loss. She must be helped to identify suitable exercises that she enjoys and cautioned about the high-impact ones that she should avoid. Because even minor falls can result in disabling fractures in women who have osteoporosis, the nurse should teach the woman ways to make her environment safer. Safety needs may be as simple as making sure there are adequate lights with handy switches and that loose cords and obstructions are secured outside of walking paths. Nonskid bath and shower floors and convenient grab bars reduce the risk of falls when bathing.

The nurse should identify the woman's perception of her menopausal status with consideration of cultural factors, sexuality concerns, access to care, and use of self-medication. Teaching the woman about available support groups in the community and the physiology of menopause can increase adherence to preventive health measures.

Unfolding Case Study

Tess is a 22-year-old woman who comes to the clinic with her partner, Luis, for information on contraception so she will not become pregnant until they are ready.

QUESTIONS

1. What can the nurse teach Tess about the contraceptive options that are available for her?
2. What other options for temporary birth control are available for Tess?
3. What can the nurse teach Tess about possible adverse effects of contraceptives that she should report to her health care provider?

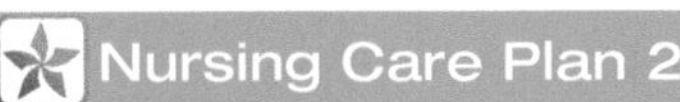

Nursing Care Plan 2.1 The Woman Experiencing Perimenopausal Symptoms

PATIENT DATA

A 52-year-old woman comes to the clinic and tells the nurse that she is experiencing a lot of discomfort relating to her beginning menopause. She states she is having hot flashes and does not enjoy having sex anymore, among other "embarrassing" symptoms.

Selected Nursing Diagnosis Discomfort as a result of vasomotor symptoms (hot flashes)

Goals	Nursing Interventions	Rationales
The woman will verbalize measures to increase her comfort during vasomotor symptoms.	Suggest that she wear layered cotton clothes.	This allows the woman to take off or put on clothes during hot flashes or chills; cotton allows easier passage of air than synthetic fabric.
	Counsel her to limit caffeine consumption (coffee, tea, colas, chocolate).	Hot flashes often occur at night; caffeine is a stimulant and will contribute to insomnia and perspiration.
	Explain that stress exacerbates the condition; explore activities that she finds relaxing.	Stress affects virtually every system of the body, including the endocrine and cardiovascular systems, worsening the hot flashes.
	Suggest she discuss hormone therapy (HT) with her health care provider.	HT is effective at relieving vasomotor symptoms when given at the lowest dose and for the shortest period of time possible, but the individual patient must evaluate its benefits and risks.
	Teach her that complementary and alternative health modalities may reduce vasomotor symptoms.	Some women should not take or choose not to take HT, and these measures provide an alternative.

Selected Nursing Diagnosis Painful intercourse as a result of vaginal dryness

Goals	Nursing Interventions	Rationales
The woman will state measures to reduce vaginal dryness. The woman will express no discomfort with intercourse.	Teach the woman to use water-soluble lubricant before intercourse.	Thinning of vaginal walls and drying of secretions can lead to discomfort during intercourse unless additional lubrication is used; oil-based lubricants can promote bacterial growth.
	Teach which products are available without a prescription to provide relief for vaginal dryness for several days.	These products lubricate the vagina for a longer time, reducing tissue trauma.
	If estrogen vaginal cream is prescribed, teach that it should be inserted at bedtime.	Topical applications of estrogen reduce vaginal atrophy; applying at bedtime reduces loss and increases absorption.

Selected Nursing Diagnosis Stress urinary incontinence and infection as a result of genital atrophy

Goals	Nursing Interventions	Rationales
The woman will restate measures to promote urinary tract health.	Teach Kegel exercises: Contract muscles as if to stop urine flow. Repeat 10 times. Do the cycle of 10 Kegel exercises five times each day. Do not actually stop urine flow while urinating.	Kegel exercises increase muscle tone around the urinary meatus and the vagina. Repeatedly stopping the stream of urine could cause retention that could lead to infection.
	Drink at least eight glasses of water each day. Caffeine-containing drinks should not be included in the target amount of fluid.	Adequate intake of liquid dilutes urine and promotes regular emptying, both of which discourage bacterial growth. Caffeine acts as a diuretic, which reverses some of the benefits of the fluid ingested.
	Urinate regularly; do not allow the bladder to become overly distended.	Prevents the stasis of urine that promotes the growth of bacteria.
	Wipe from front to back after toileting.	Prevents bringing anal organisms to the urinary meatus or vagina, where they could cause infection.

Get Ready for the Certification Examination!

Key Points

- Health promotion involves primary, secondary, and tertiary health prevention strategies.
- Routine mammograms can help in diagnosing breast cancer early and reducing the morbidity from breast cancer.
- Amenorrhea can be caused by a lack of body fat, and often changing eating habits may result in resumption of a normal period.
- Several self-help measures can relieve some symptoms of premenstrual syndrome.
- Prevention of toxic shock syndrome involves not allowing microorganisms the time to grow in the woman's reproductive tract.
- Sexually transmitted infections (STIs) must be adequately treated in all sexual contacts to stop the transmission and to prevent resistance to antibiotics.
- Contraception is an individual choice. The role of the nurse is to educate the woman about the risks and benefits of contraceptive methods.
- Fertility awareness methods can be used both to prevent pregnancy and to increase the chance of achieving it.
- Contraceptive choices include temporary contraception, such as barrier methods or hormones, or permanent contraception, such as sterilization or vasectomy.
- Emergency contraception, Plan B, is a progestin-only medication taken within 72 hours of unprotected sexual intercourse and is available without a prescription.
- Condoms (male and female) offer the best protection from STIs.
- Common menopausal symptoms, such as hot flashes and vaginal dryness, stem from the cessation of ovulation and the decrease in hormonal activity, particularly that of estrogen and progesterone.
- Prevention of osteoporosis begins with adequate calcium and vitamin D intake during youth to achieve maximum bone mass. Reducing risk for osteoporosis after menopause is best accomplished by adequate calcium and vitamin D intake combined with exercise.
- Complementary and alternative health modalities for menopause symptoms are available for women.

Additional Learning Resources

evolve Go to your Evolve website (http://evolve.elsevier.com/Canada/Leifer) for the following learning resources:

- Answer Key for Critical Thinking Questions
- Answer Key for Textbook Review Questions
- Audio Glossary
- Fluids & Electrolytes tutorial
- Interactive Review Questions
- Skills Performance Checklists
- Video clips and more!

Online Resources

- CATIE—Canada's source for HIV and hepatitis C information: https://www.catie.ca/en/home
- HealthLinkBC—*Breast Self-Examination:* https://www.healthlinkbc.ca/health-topics/hw3791
- Menopause & U: http://www.menopauseandu.ca/
- Osteoporosis Canada: https://osteoporosis.ca/
- Sex & U—A resource for sexual and reproductive health: https://www.sexandu.ca/
- Society of Obstetricians and Gynaecologists of Canada: https://sogc.org/
- Stay on Schedule—A guide to taking contraception after a missed or extended dose: https://www.sexandu.ca/sos/

Review Questions

1. What would be the best method to screen for breast cancer in low-risk women?
   a. Monthly breast self-examination
   b. Yearly clinical breast examination by a health care provider
   c. Mammograms every 2-3 years after the age of 50
   d. Magnetic resonance imaging scan every 3 years after age 40
2. Which factors change the normal flora of the vagina and predispose to vaginal infection? *(Select all that apply.)*
   a. use of antibiotics.
   b. douching.
   c. sexual intercourse.
   d. daily baths.
3. What is a reliable temporary (reversible) birth control method? *(Select all that apply.)*
   a. Douching
   b. Breastfeeding
   c. Transdermal patch
   d. Vasectomy
   e. IUD
4. In order to relieve or reduce symptoms of premenstrual dysphoric disorder, what should a nurse teach a woman to do?
   a. Avoid simple sugars and caffeine consumption.
   b. Use oral contraceptive medication.
   c. Avoid physical exercise.
   d. Limit water intake to 1 000 mL/day.
5. A nurse should teach the woman who is experiencing menopause which of the following? *(Select all that apply.)*
   a. Calcium is best absorbed when vitamin D intake is adequate.
   b. Weight-bearing exercise is important.
   c. Lying down and resting after each meal is important.
   d. An increased intake of vitamin C will enhance calcium absorption.
   e. Limiting alcohol intake will help decrease symptoms.

Critical Thinking Question

1. A woman, age 52 years, requests help in controlling her anxiety level. She reports hot flashes, night sweats, sleep pattern disturbances, and mood swings. She is afraid her partner will leave her, and she wants medication to "calm her down." Based on her age and history, what is the best response of the nurse?

REFERENCES

Black, A., Guilbert, E., et al. (2015a). SOGC clinical practice guideline: Canadian contraception consensus (Part 1 of 4). *Journal of Obstetrics and Gynecology of Canada, 37*(10), S1–S28.

Black, A., Guilbert, E., et al. (2015b). SOGC clinical practice guideline: Canadian contraception consensus (Part 2 of 4). *Journal of Obstetrics and Gynecology of Canada, 37*(11), S1–S39.

Black, A., Guilbert, E., et al. (2016). SOGC clinical practice guideline: Canadian contraception consensus (Part 3 of 4). *Journal of Obstetrics and Gynecology of Canada, 38*(2), 182–222.

Black, A., Guilbert, E., et al. (2017). SOGC clinical practice guideline: Canadian contraception consensus (Part 4 of 4). *Journal of Obstetrics and Gynecology of Canada, 39*(4), 229–268.

Canadian Cancer Society. (2019a). *All About HPV Vaccines.* Retrieved from: http://www.cancer.ca/en/prevention-and-screening/reduce-cancer-risk/make-informed-decisions/get-vaccinated/all-about-hpv-vaccines/?region=on.

Canadian Cancer Society. (2019b). *Finding Vulvar Cancer Early.* Retrieved from: http://www.cancer.ca/en/cancer-information/cancer-type/vulvar/finding-cancer-early/?region=on.

Canadian Cancer Society. (2019c). *Screening for Breast Cancer.* Retrieved from:http://www.cancer.ca/en/cancer-information/cancer-type/breast/screening/?region=on.

Canadian Task Force on Preventative Health Care (CTFPHC). (2011). Recommendations on screening for breast cancer in average-risk women aged 40–74 years. *Canadian Medical Association Journal, 183*(17), 1991–2001. https://doi.org/10.1503/cmaj.110334.

Canadian Task Force on Preventative Health (CTFPH). (2013). Recommendations on screening for cervical cancer. *Canadian Medical Association Journal, 185*(1), 35–45.

Challacombe, L. (2019). *The Epidemiology of HIV in Females.* Retrieved from: http://www.catie.ca/fact-sheets/epidemiology/epidemiology-hiv-women.

Health Canada. (2019). *Vitamin D and Calcium: Updated Dietary Reference Intakes.* Retrieved from: https://www.canada.ca/en/health-canada/services/food-nutrition/healthy-eating/vitamins-minerals/vitamin-calcium-updated-dietary-reference-intakes-nutrition.html#a7.

Keenan-Lindsay, L. (2017a). Infertility, contraception and abortion. In S. Perry, M. Hockenberry, D. Lowdermilk, et al. (Eds.), *Maternal child nursing care in canada* (2nd ed.). St. Louis: Mosby.

Keenan-Lindsay, L. (2017b). Reproductive health. In S. Perry, M. Hockenberry, D. Lowdermilk, et al. (Eds.), *Maternal child nursing care in canada* (2nd ed.). St. Louis: Mosby.

Lentz, G. M. (2012). Primary and secondary dysmenorrheal, premenstrual syndrome, and premenstrual dysphoric disorder. In G. M. Lentz, R. A. Lobo, D. M. Gershenson, et al. (Eds.), *Comprehensive gynecology* (6th ed.). Philadelphia: Mosby.

Leyland, N., Casper, R., Laberge, P., et al. (2010). SOGC clinical practice guideline: Endometriosis: Diagnosis and management. *Journal of Obstetrics and Gynaecology Canada, 32*(7, Suppl. 2), S1–S32.

Lobo, R. A. (2012). Primary and secondary amenorrhea and precocious puberty. In G. M. Lentz, R. A. Lobo, D. M. Gershenson, et al. (Eds.), *Comprehensive gynecology* (6th ed.). Philadelphia: Mosby.

McNicholas, C., & Peipert, J. (2017). Is it time to abandon the routine pelvic examination in asymptomatic non-pregnant women? *Journal of American Medical Association, 317*, 910–911. https://doi.org/10.1001/jama.2017.0899.

Public Health Agency of Canada (PHAC). (2019). *Canadian Guidelines on Sexually Transmitted Infections.* Retrieved from: https://www.canada.ca/en/public-health/services/infectious-diseases/sexual-health-sexually-transmitted-infections/canadian-guidelines/sexually-transmitted-infections.html.

Reid, R., Abramson, B., Blake, J., et al. (2014). SOGC clinical practice guideline: Managing menopause. *Journal of Obstetrics and Gynecology of Canada, 36* (9, eSuppl. A), S1–S80.

Sexandu. (2019). *Contraception.* Retrieved from: https://www.sexandu.ca/contraception/.

Singh, S., Best, C., Dunn, S., et al. (2013). SOGC clinical practice guideline: Abnormal uterine bleeding in pre-menopausal women. *Journal of Obstetrics and Gynaecology Canada, 35* (5 eSuppl.), S1–S28.

Smith, R. (2018). *Netter's obstetrics and gynecology* (3rd ed.). Philadelphia: Elsevier.

Taylor, D., Schuiling, K., & Sharp, B. (2013). Menstrual cycle pain and discomforts. In K. Schuiling, & F. Likis (Eds.), *Women's gynecologic health* (2nd ed.). Burlington. MA: Jones & Bartlett.

Tonelli, M., Connor Gorber, S., Moore, A., & Thombs, B. D. (2016). Recommendations on routine pelvic examination. *Canadian Family Physician, 62*(3), 211–214.

3 Fetal Development

http://evolve.elsevier.com/Canada/Leifer

Lisa Keenan-Lindsay

Objectives

1. Define each key term listed.
2. Describe the process of gametogenesis in human reproduction.
3. Explain human fertilization and implantation.
4. Describe embryonic development.
5. Describe fetal development and the maturation of body systems.
6. Describe the development and functions of the amniotic fluid, placenta, and umbilical cord.
7. Compare fetal circulation to circulation after birth.
8. Explain the similarities and differences in the two types of twins.

Key Terms

age of viability
amniotic sac (ăm-nē-Ŏ-tĭk SĂK)
autosomes
chorion (KŌ-rē-ŏn)
decidua (dĕ-SĬD-yū-ă)
diploid (DĬP-loid)
dizygotic (DZ) (dī-zī-GŎT-ĭk)
fertilization
gametogenesis (găm-ĕ-tō-JĔN-ĕ-ĭs)
germ layers
haploid (HĂP-loid)
monozygotic (MZ) (mŏn-ō-zī-GŎT-ĭk)
oogenesis (ō-ō-JĔN-ĕ-sĭs)
placenta (plă-SĔN-tă)
spermatogenesis (spŭr-mă-tō-JĔN-ĕ-sĭs)
teratogens (TĔR-ă-tō-jĕnz)
Wharton's jelly

The human body contains many millions of cells at birth, but life begins with a single cell created by the fusion of a sperm with an ovum. Deoxyribonucleic acid (DNA) programs a genetic code into the nucleus of the cell; the nucleus controls the development and function of the cell. Defects in the DNA code can result in inherited disorders. The genes and chromosomes contained within the DNA determine the uniqueness of the traits and features of the developing person.

Normal human chromosomes begin in pairs, one supplied by the female and the other by a male. Each body cell contains 46 chromosomes, made up of 22 pairs of **autosomes** (body chromosomes) and 1 pair of sex chromosomes that determine the sex of the fetus. Cell division then occurs, which is the basis of human growth and regeneration.

Biological development is not isolated. It is influenced by the external environment, such as maternal drug use (**teratogens** that cause damage to growing cells, including some prescribed medications), maternal undernutrition, or smoking by the mother, and it is known that sounds such as music are heard by the fetus and are recognized by the newborn. All these factors influence prenatal growth and development. The experience of the fetus during prenatal life influences the healthy outcome of the newborn and also influences susceptibility to diseases that may occur when the fetus reaches adulthood. Preconception as well as early prenatal care is essential to the optimum outcome of the pregnancy (see Chapter 4).

It is also important to consider the health of the parents prior to conception as this establishes the foundation for their new child's health throughout the child's life. The goals for preconception care are to improve the health status of women and men before conception and to reduce those behaviours and individual and environmental factors that could contribute to poor maternal and child health outcomes (Government of Canada, 2018).

CELL DIVISION AND GAMETOGENESIS

The division of a cell begins in its nucleus, which contains the gene-bearing chromosomes. The two types of cell division are mitosis and meiosis. *Mitosis* is a continuous process by which the body grows and develops and dead body cells are replaced. In this type of cell division, *each daughter cell contains the same number* of chromosomes as the parent cell. The 46 chromosomes in a body cell are called the **diploid** number of chromosomes. The process of mitosis in the sperm is called **spermatogenesis**, and in the ovum it is called **oogenesis**.

Meiosis is a different type of cell division, in which the reproductive cells undergo two sequential divisions. During meiosis, the number of chromosomes in each cell is reduced by half, to 23 chromosomes per cell, each including only one sex chromosome. This is called the **haploid** number of chromosomes. This process is completed in the sperm before it travels toward the fallopian tube and in the ovum if it is fertilized after ovulation. At the moment of **fertilization** (when the sperm and the ovum unite), the new cell contains 23 chromosomes from the sperm and 23 chromosomes from the ovum, thus returning to the diploid number of chromosomes (46); traits are therefore inherited from both the female and male partner. The formation of gametes by this type of cell division is called **gametogenesis** (Fig. 3.1).

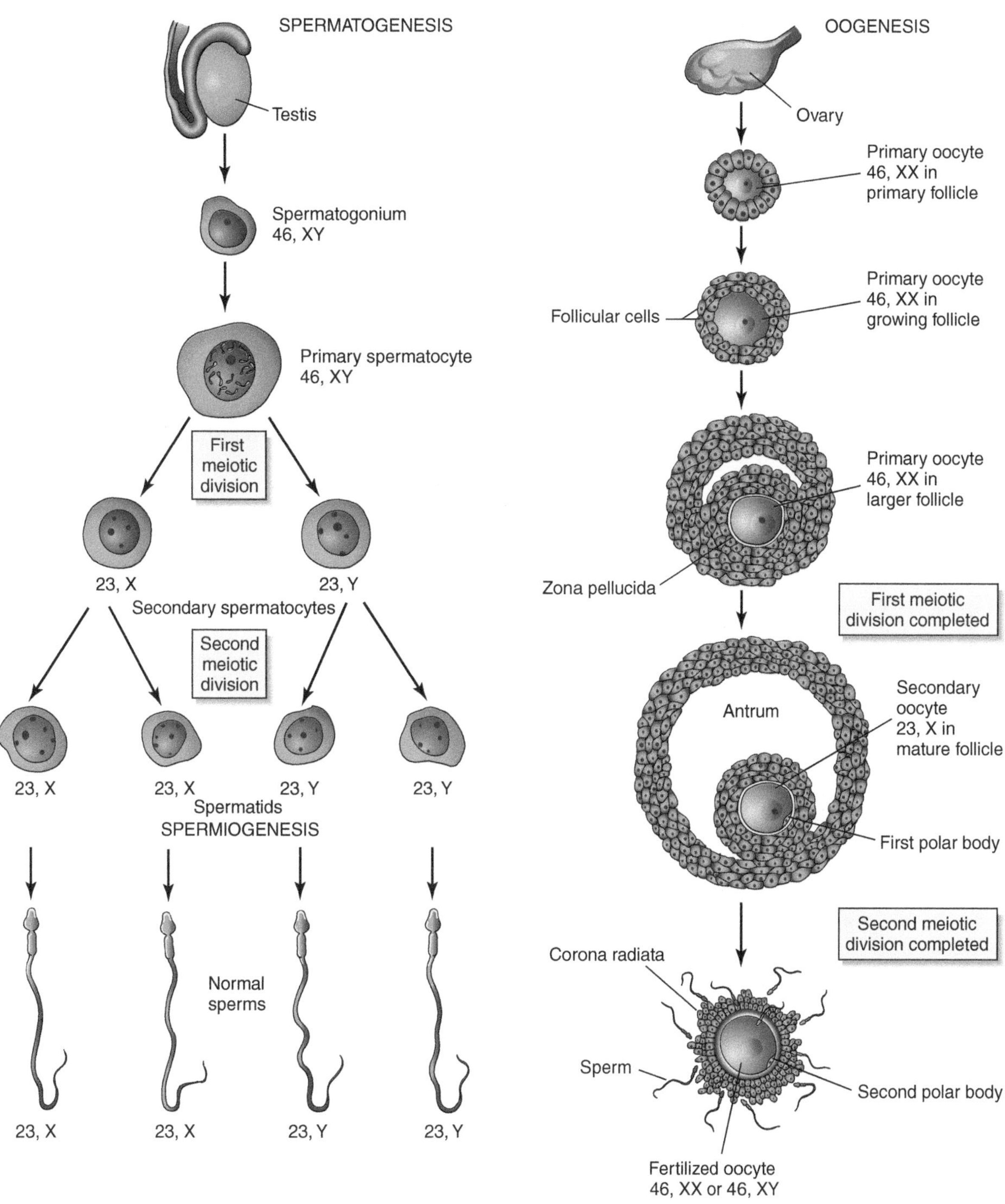

Fig. 3.1 Normal gametogenesis. Four sperm develop from one spermatocyte, each with 23 chromosomes—including one sex chromosome, either an X or a Y. In oogenesis, one ovum develops with 23 chromosomes—including one sex chromosome, always an X. An XY combination produces a boy, and an XX combination produces a girl. (From Moore, K. L., Persaud, T. V. N., & Torchia, M.G. [2016]. *The developing human: Clinically oriented embryology* [10th ed.]. Philadelphia: Saunders.)

FERTILIZATION

Fertilization occurs when a sperm penetrates an ovum and unites with it, restoring the total number of chromosomes to 46. It normally occurs in the outer third of the fallopian tube, near the ovary (Fig. 3.2). The sperm pass through the cervix and the uterus and into the fallopian tubes by means of the flagellar (whiplike) activity of their tails and can reach the fallopian tubes within 5 minutes after sexual intercourse, although the average transit time is 4 to 6 hours. As soon as fertilization occurs, a chemical change in the membrane around the fertilized ovum prevents penetration by another sperm.

The time during which fertilization can occur is brief because of the short lifespan of mature gametes. The ovum is estimated to survive for up to 24 hours after ovulation. The sperm remains capable of fertilizing the ovum for up to 7 days after being ejaculated into the area of the cervix, although this usually occurs within the first 24 hours.

Nursing Tip

During sexual counselling, the nurse should emphasize that the survival time of sperm ejaculated into the area of the cervix may be up to 7 days and that pregnancy can occur with intercourse as long as 5 days before ovulation.

SEX DETERMINATION

The sex of human offspring is determined at fertilization. The ovum always contributes an X chromosome (gamete), whereas the sperm can carry an X or a Y chromosome (gamete). When a sperm carrying the X chromosome fertilizes the X-bearing ovum, a female child (XX) results. When a Y-bearing sperm fertilizes the ovum, a male child (XY) is produced (Fig. 3.3).

Because sperm can carry either an X or a Y chromosome, the male partner determines the sex of the child. However, the pH of the female reproductive tract and the estrogen levels of the woman's body affect the survival rate of the X- and Y-bearing sperm, as well as the speed of their movement through the cervix and the fallopian tubes. Thus, the female physiology has some influence on which sperm fertilizes the mature ovum.

By 6 to 7 weeks' gestation, the male embryo differentiates under the influence of the Y chromosome and by 8 weeks' gestation, testosterone secretion begins. Female gonadal development occurs in the presence of estrogen and the absence of testosterone, and by 6 to 8 weeks' gestation, two female gonads develop into ovaries, which will produce the life's supply of ova during fetal life (Moktar, Rodway, & Huether, 2017).

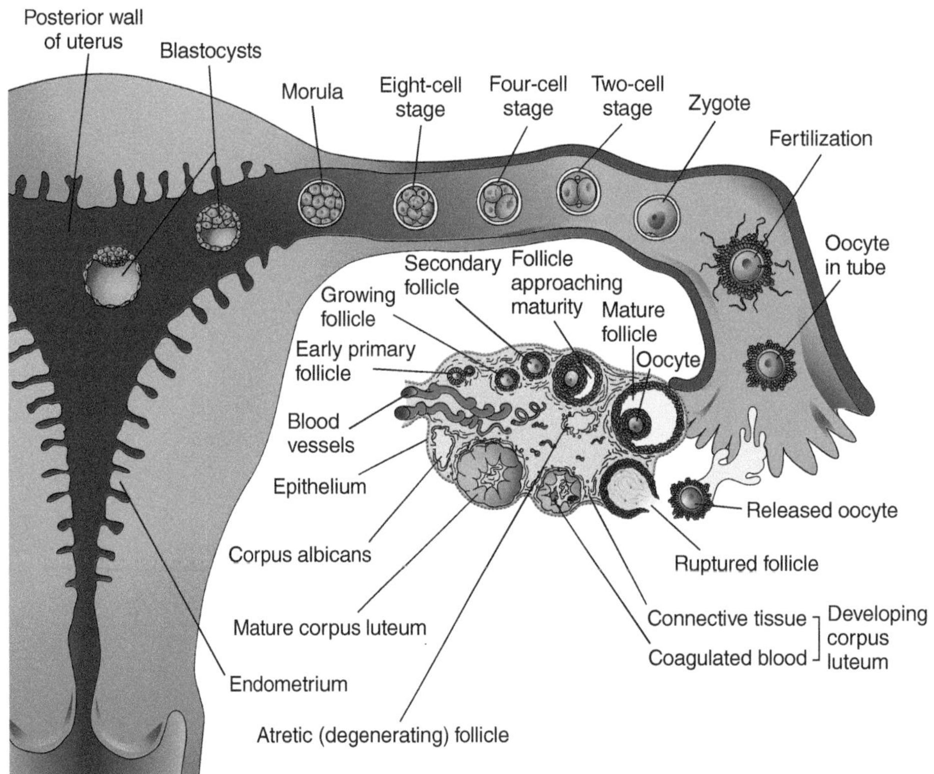

Fig. 3.2 Ovulation and fertilization. Ovulation occurs; the egg is caught by the fimbriae (fingerlike projections of the fallopian tube) and is guided into the fallopian tube where fertilization occurs. The zygote continues to multiply (but not grow in size) as it passes through the fallopian tube and implants into the posterior wall of the uterus. (From Moore, K. L., Persaud, T. V. N., & Torchia, M. G. [2016]. *The developing human: clinically oriented embryology* [10th ed.]. Philadelphia: Saunders.)

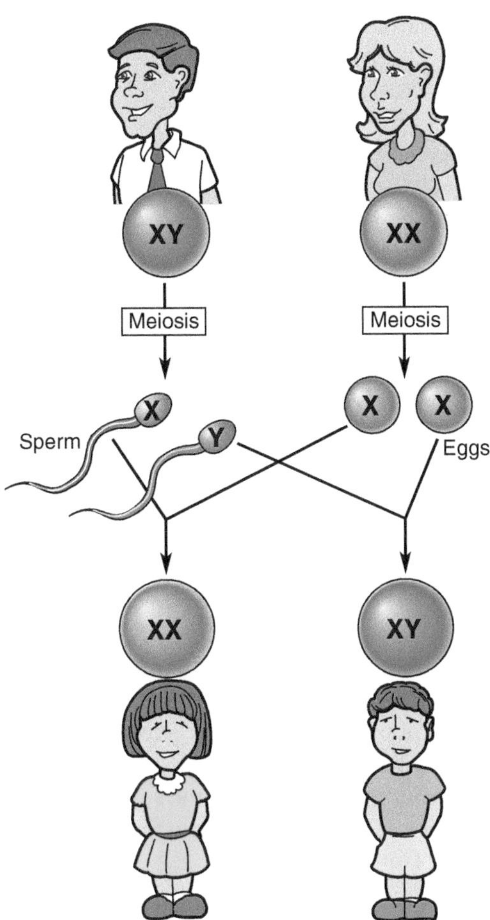

Fig. 3.3 Sex determination. If an X chromosome from the male unites with an X chromosome from the female, the child will be a female (XX). If a Y chromosome from the male unites with an X chromosome from the female, the child will be a male (XY). (From Herlihy, B., & Maebius, N. K. [2014]. *The human body in health and illness* [5th ed.] Philadelphia: Saunders.)

> **Nursing Tip**
>
> The sex of an offspring is influenced by both maternal and paternal factors, although the male partner contributes the actual sex chromosome.

INHERITANCE

Each gene (a segment of the DNA chain) is coded for inheritance. The coded information carried by the DNA in the gene is responsible for individual traits, such as eye and hair colour, facial features, and body shape. Genes carry instructions for *dominant* and *recessive* traits. Dominant traits overpower recessive traits and are passed on to the offspring. If only one parent carries a dominant trait, an average of 50% of the offspring will have (and thus display) that dominant trait. If *each* parent carries a recessive trait, there is a higher chance that one of the offspring will display that trait.

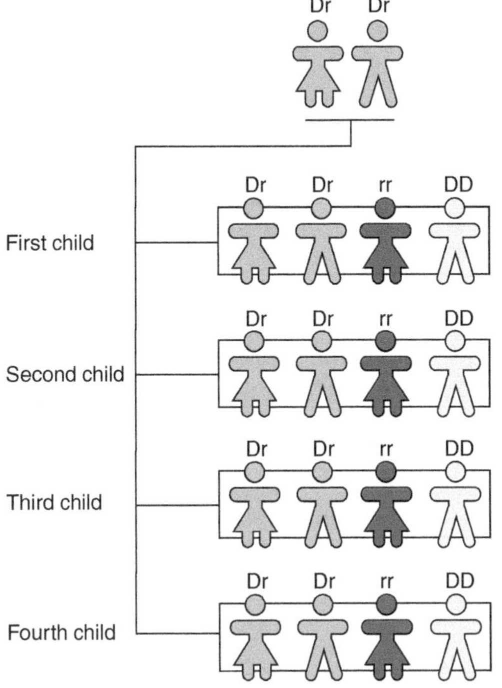

Fig. 3.4 Recessive inheritance. This figure shows how a disorder carried as a recessive trait can be passed along to an offspring when each parent is a carrier of that recessive trait. *D* represents a dominant gene; *r* represents a recessive gene.

Knowledge of inheritance enables the nurse to offer relevant information and suggest to potential parents appropriate referrals related to reproductive decision making, if required. Most genes are paired, with only one of the pair passing on to the fertilized egg from the mother and one from the male partner. An alteration or defect in just one gene of the pair can cause a disorder in the developing fetus that is labelled as a *dominant disorder.* When a single defective gene is passed on to the fetus and the other gene is normal, the newborn has a 50% chance of developing the disorder. Therefore, it is important for the nurse to inform the parents that each pregnancy has a 50% chance of resulting in an affected child; giving birth to one child with a genetic disorder does not necessarily increase the chance of the next child having that genetic defect. Examples of dominant disorders are Huntington disease, Marfan syndrome, neurofibromatosis, and achondroplasia (dwarfism). Recessive disorders are those in which both genes of a pair must be abnormal in order for the disorder to be passed on to the fetus. The transmission of a recessive disorder is shown in Fig. 3.4. Examples of recessive disorders include Tay-Sachs disease, sickle cell anemia, and cystic fibrosis. Genetic testing can be used to diagnose disorders, predict risk of future disorders, and assist in reproductive decisions. The nurse must understand the trends and changes in genetic testing and assist clients in finding the resources that are available to meet the individual needs of the parents or parents-to-be.

TUBAL TRANSPORT OF THE ZYGOTE

The *zygote* is the cell formed by the union of the sperm and the ovum, and it is transported through the fallopian tube and into the uterus. During transport through the fallopian tube, the zygote undergoes rapid mitotic division, or cleavage. Cleavage begins with two cells, which subdivide into four and then eight cells to form the *blastomere*. The size of the zygote does not increase; rather, the individual cells become smaller as they divide and eventually form a solid ball called the *morula* (see Fig. 3.2).

The morula enters the uterus on the third day and floats there for another 2 to 4 days. The cells form a cavity, and two distinct layers evolve. The inner layer is a solid mass of cells called the *blastocyst* (see Fig. 3.2), which develops into the embryo and the embryonic membranes. The outer layer of cells, called the *trophoblast*, develops into an embryonic membrane, the chorion. Occasionally the zygote does not move through the fallopian tube and instead becomes implanted in the lining of the tube, resulting in a tubal ectopic pregnancy (see Chapter 5).

IMPLANTATION OF THE ZYGOTE

The zygote usually implants in the upper section of the posterior uterine wall. The cells burrow into the prepared lining of the uterus, called the endometrium. The endometrium is now called the **decidua**; the area under the blastocyst is called the *decidua basalis* and gives rise to the maternal part of the placenta (Fig. 3.5).

DEVELOPMENT

CELL DIFFERENTIATION

During the week between fertilization and implantation, the cells within a zygote are identical to one another. After implantation, the cells begin to differentiate and develop special functions. The chorion, the amnion, the yolk sac, and the primary germ layers appear.

Chorion

The **chorion** develops from the trophoblast (outer layer of embryonic cells) and envelops the amnion, embryo, and yolk sac. It is a thick membrane with fingerlike projections called *villi* on its outermost surface. The villi immediately below the embryo extend into the decidua basalis on the uterine wall and form the embryonic or fetal portion of the placenta (see Fig. 3.5).

Amnion

The *amnion* is the second membrane; it is a thin structure that envelops and protects the embryo. It forms the boundaries of the amniotic cavity, and its outer aspect meets the inner aspect of the chorion.

The chorion and the amnion together form an **amniotic sac** filled with fluid (bag of waters) that permits the embryo to float freely. The volume of amniotic fluid steadily increases from about 30 mL at 10 weeks of pregnancy to 350 mL at 20 weeks. The volume of fluid is about 700 to 1 000 mL at term. In the latter part of pregnancy, the fetus may swallow up to 400 mL of amniotic fluid per day and normally excretes urine into the fluid. The following are functions of amniotic fluid:

- Maintains a constant body temperature
- Prevents the amniotic sac from adhering to the fetal skin facilitating symmetrical growth
- Acts as a barrier to infection
- Allows buoyancy and fetal movement
- Acts as a cushion to protect the fetus and the umbilical cord from injury

Yolk Sac

On the ninth day after fertilization, a cavity called the *yolk sac* forms in the blastocyst. It functions only during embryonic life and initiates the production of red blood cells. This function continues for about 6 weeks until the embryonic liver takes over. The umbilical cord then encompasses the yolk sac, and the yolk sac degenerates.

Germ Layers

After implantation, the zygote in the blastocyst stage transforms its embryonic disc into three primary **germ layers** known as ectoderm, mesoderm, and endoderm. Each germ layer develops into a different part of the growing embryo. The specific body parts that develop from each layer are listed in Box 3.1.

PRENATAL DEVELOPMENTAL MILESTONES

Table 3.1 follows the developmental milestones during intrauterine development. Three basic stages characterize prenatal development: zygote, embryo, and fetus. The zygote continues to grow and develop as it passes through the fallopian tube and implants into the wall of the uterus. The second to the eighth week of development is known as the *embryonic stage*; the developing infant is called an *embryo*. From the ninth week of development until birth, the developing infant

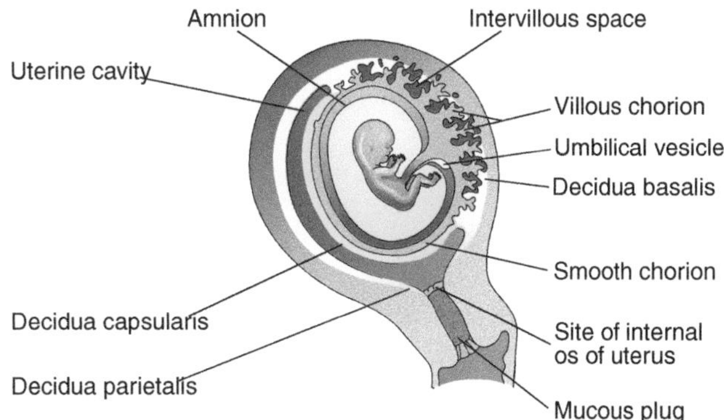

Fig. 3.5 The pregnant uterus at 8 weeks showing the relationship of the fetal membranes to the decidua of the uterus and the embryo. (From Moore, K. L., Persaud, T. V. N., & Torchia, M. G. [2008]. *Before we are born: Essentials of embryology and birth defects* [7th ed.]. Philadelphia: Saunders.)

Box 3.1 Body Parts That Develop From the Primary Germ Layers

ECTODERM
Outer layer of skin
Oil glands and hair follicles of skin
Nails and hair
External sense organs
Mucous membrane of mouth and anus

MESODERM
True skin
Skeleton
Bone and cartilage
Connective tissue
Muscles
Blood and blood vessels
Kidneys and gonads

ENDODERM
Lining of trachea, pharynx, and bronchi
Lining of digestive tract
Lining of bladder and urethra

is called a *fetus*. By the second week after fertilization, the ectoderm, the endoderm, and the amnion begin to develop.

By the third week the mesoderm and neural tube form, and the primitive heart begins to pump. It is at this time that some women first realize they have "missed" their menstrual period and suspect they are pregnant (therefore, the fetus is affected by maternal influences even before the pregnancy becomes known).

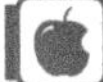 Nutrition Considerations

FOLIC ACID AND NEURAL TUBE DEFECTS

It is now known that folic acid supplements can prevent most neural tube defects such as spina bifida. However, in an unplanned pregnancy, it is possible for a neural tube defect to occur before the mother confirms her pregnancy state. Early prenatal care with good nutrition and folic acid supplements prior to pregnancy are desirable so that the embryo is protected in the very first days and weeks of development. See Chapter 4 for further discussion.

By 8 weeks' gestation the ovaries or testes are present, the beginnings of all systems have developed, and there is movement in the extremities. The fetal period begins at the ninth week, and by the tenth week the external genitalia may be visible to ultrasonography. At the end of the fourth week, maternal–fetal circulation is established. At this time, the placenta attaches to the uterine wall. Failure of adequate attachment of the placenta to the uterine wall can result in spontaneous abortion (miscarriage). An abnormal attachment to the uterine wall can result in placenta accreta or placenta previa, which will present as a serious complication at birth (see Chapter 8). At the fourteenth week, the fetus moves in response to external stimuli. By 22 weeks' gestation the lungs have matured functionally enough for the fetus to survive outside the uterus (**age of viability**), but special care in the neonatal intensive care unit (NICU) would be required. By 28 weeks, the eyes open and the fetal position in the uterus becomes more stable. The fetus is considered to be term if more than 37 weeks' gestation.

The development of the fetus (see Table 3.1) can be correlated with the psychological and physical changes in the mother that occur prenatally.

Table 3.1 Embryonic and Fetal Development

AGE	LENGTH AND WEIGHT	DEVELOPMENT
Week 3 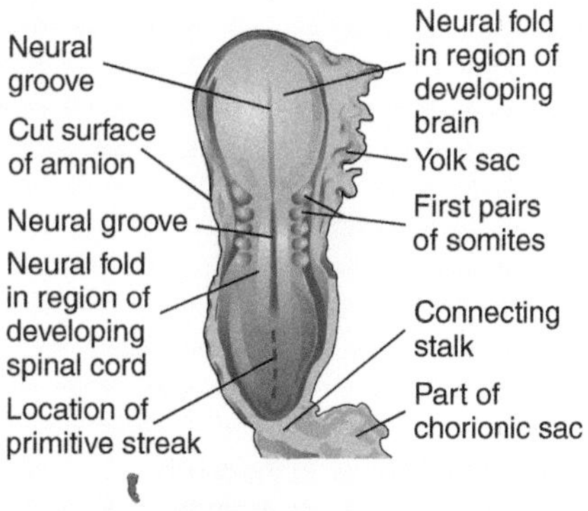 Actual size 2.5 mm	1.5–2.5 mm	*Cardiovascular:* Single tubular heart is formed. *Nervous:* Neural tube forms; primitive spinal cord and brain appear.
Week 4 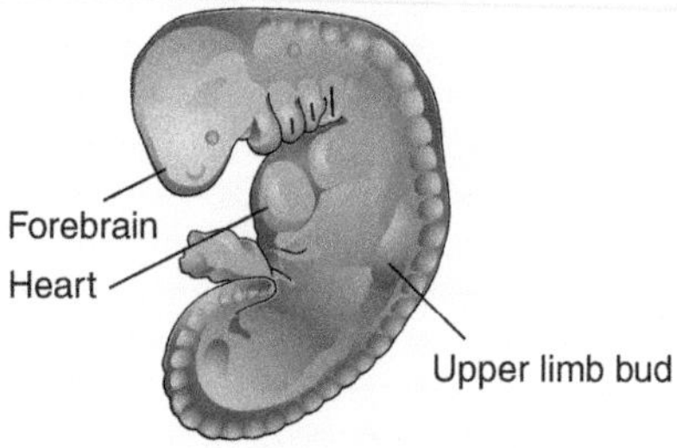	3.5–4 mm	*Gastrointestinal (GI):* Esophagus and trachea separate; stomach forms. *Nervous:* Neural tube closes; forebrain forms. *Musculoskeletal:* Upper and lower limb buds appear. *Senses:* Ears and eyes begin to form.
Week 6 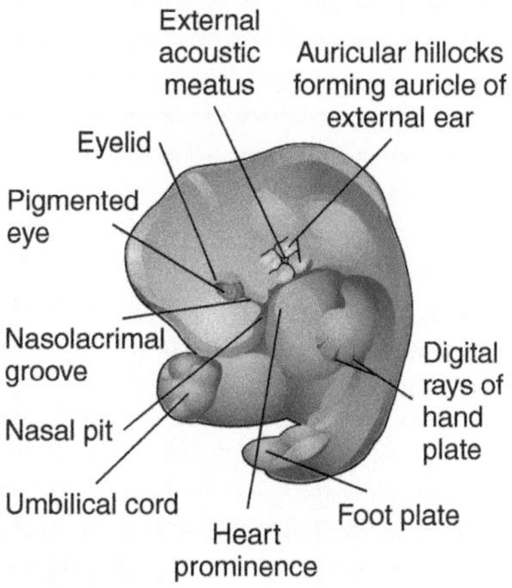 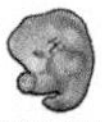 Actual size 11.0 mm	11–13 mm	*Senses:* Auditory canal forms; eye is obvious. *Cardiovascular:* Heart has all four chambers. *GI:* Nasal cavity and upper lip form.
Week 8 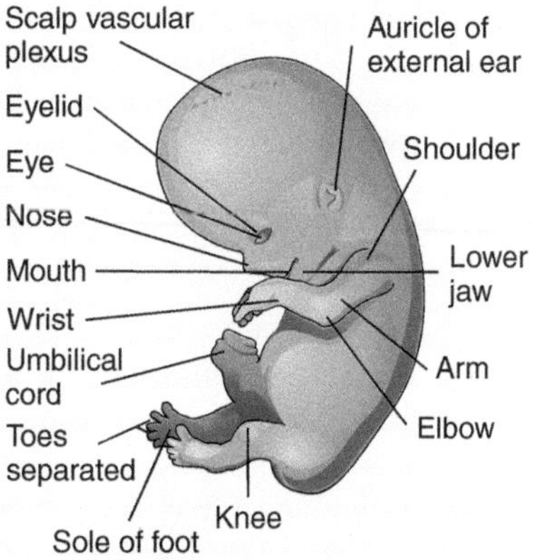 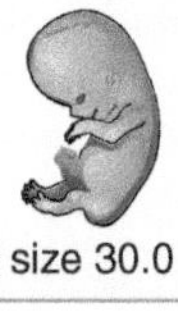 Actual size 30.0 mm	30 mm crown–rump 6 g	Embryo has distinct human appearance. Purposeful movements occur. Tail has disappeared. Sex organs form. Beginnings of most external and internal structures are formed. Embryo enters fetal period.

Table 3.1 Embryonic and Fetal Development—cont'd

AGE	LENGTH AND WEIGHT	DEVELOPMENT
Week 17 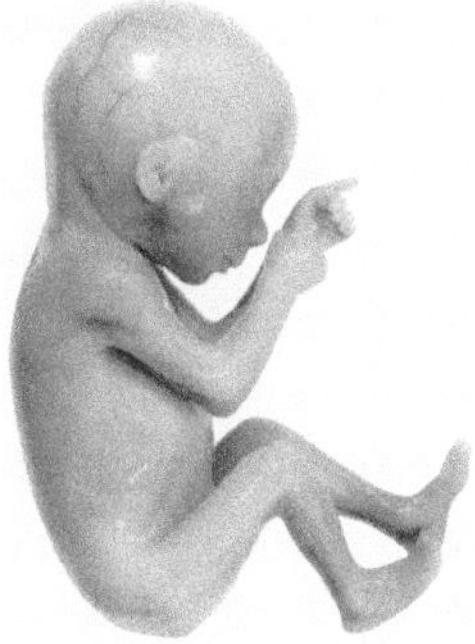	150 mm crown–rump 260 g	Genitalia and leg movements are visible on ultrasound and may be felt by the mother (quickening). Bones are ossified. Eye movements occur. Fetus sucks and swallows amniotic fluid. Ovaries contain ova. No subcutaneous fat is present. Thin skin allows blood vessels of scalp to be visible.
Week 25 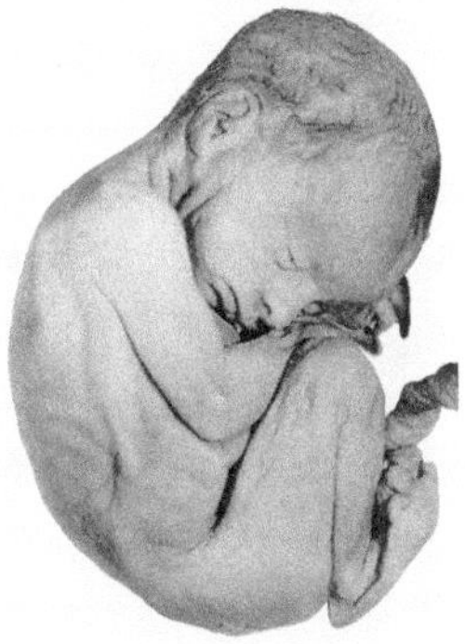	28 cm (11.2 in) crown–heel 780 g (1 lb 10 oz)	Wrinkled skin, lean body results from lack of subcutaneous fat. Eyes are open. Fetus is now viable. Mother feels stronger movement. Fetus has schedule of sleeping and moving. Vernix caseosa is present on skin. Lanugo covers body. Brown fat is formed. Lungs begin to secrete surfactant. Fingernails are present. Respiratory movements begin.
Week 29 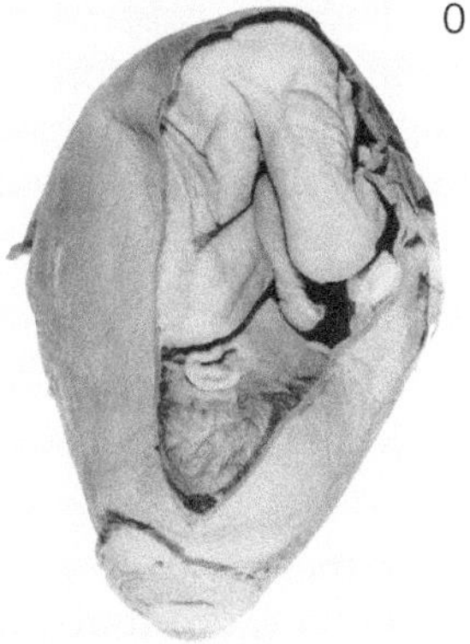 0	38 cm (15 in) crown–heel 1260 g (2 lb 10 oz)	Fetus assumes stable (cephalic) position in utero. Central nervous system is functioning. Skin is less wrinkled because of the presence of subcutaneous fat. Spleen stops forming blood cells, and bone marrow starts to form blood cells. Increased surfactant is present in lungs.
Week 36 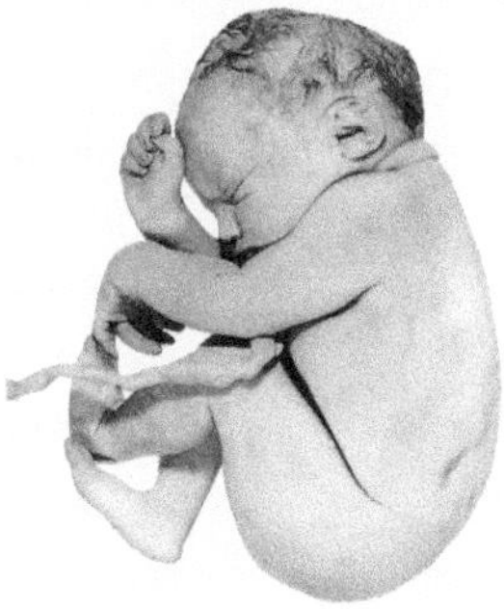 1	48 cm (19 in) crown–heel 2500 g (5 lb 12 oz)	Subcutaneous fat is present. Skin is pink and smooth. Grasp reflex is present. Circumferences of head and abdomen are equal. Surge in lung surfactant production occurs.

Note: Full term is considered to be greater than 37 weeks' gestation. The crown–heel length is 45–55 cm, and the weight is 2 500–4 000 g.
Figures from Moore, K. L., Persaud, T. V. N., & Torchia, M. G. (2016). *The developing human: Clinically oriented embryology* (10th ed.). Philadelphia: Saunders.

ACCESSORY STRUCTURES OF PREGNANCY

The placenta, the umbilical cord, and the fetal circulation support the fetus as it completes prenatal life and prepares for birth.

PLACENTA

The placenta (afterbirth) is a temporary organ for fetal respiration, nutrition, and excretion. It also functions as an endocrine gland. The placenta forms when the chorionic villi of the embryo extend into the blood-filled spaces of the mother's decidua basalis. The maternal part of the placenta arises from the decidua basalis and has a beefy, red appearance. The fetal side of the placenta develops from the chorionic villi and the chorionic blood vessels. The amnion covers the fetal side and the umbilical cord and gives them a greyish, shiny appearance at term.

The placenta plays an important role in fetal development as it provides adequate blood flow to the fetus. Examples of factors that decrease blood flow through the placenta include maternal hypertension and cocaine use. Stress, undernutrition, exposure to steroids during pregnancy, and chronic hypoxia can cause a small placenta (see Chapter 8).

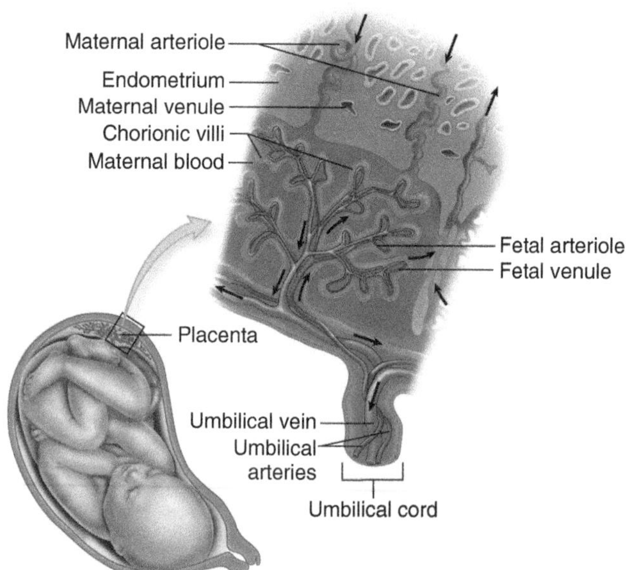

Fig. 3.6 Maternal–fetal circulation showing the relationship of the fetus and the placenta in the uterus. Close placement of the fetal blood supply to the maternal blood in the placenta is shown. The maternal blood in the lacuna permits the diffusion of nutrients and other substances; some harmful substances are prevented from passing through by a thin placental barrier. No mixing of fetal or maternal blood occurs. (From Patton, K. T., & Thibodeau, G. A. [2016]. *Anatomy & physiology* [9th ed.]. St. Louis: Mosby.)

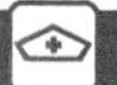 **Nursing Tip**

The placenta is much larger than the developing infant during early pregnancy, but the fetus grows faster. At term, the placenta weighs about one-sixth the weight of the infant. Placenta size can be an important indicator of nutritional or environmental problems in the newborn that may require follow-up care.

Placental Transfer

A thin membrane separates the maternal and fetal blood, and the two blood supplies do not normally mix. However, separation of the placenta at birth may allow some fetal blood to enter the maternal circulation, which can cause problems in subsequent pregnancies if the blood types are not compatible (see Chapter 5).

Fetal deoxygenated blood and waste products leave the fetus through the two umbilical arteries and enter the placenta through the branch of a main stem villus, which extends into the intervillus space (lacuna). Oxygenated, nutrient-rich blood from the mother spurts into the intervillus space from the spiral arteries in the decidua (Fig. 3.6; see Fig. 3.5). The fetal blood releases carbon dioxide and waste products and takes in oxygen and nutrients before returning to the fetus through the umbilical vein.

The thin placental membrane provides some protection but is not a barrier to most substances ingested by the mother. Many harmful substances such as medications (therapeutic and recreational), nicotine, and viral infectious agents are transferred to the fetus. Some drugs can cause neonatal opioid withdrawal syndrome [NOWS] (also known as *neonatal abstinence syndrome*) or congenital anomalies. Viruses can also cause congenital anomalies or fetal infections.

Placental Hormones

Four hormones are produced by the placenta: progesterone, estrogen, human chorionic gonadotropin (hCG), and human placental lactogen (hPL).

Progesterone

Progesterone is first produced by the corpus luteum and later by the placenta. It has the following functions during pregnancy:

- Maintains uterine lining for implantation of the zygote
- Reduces uterine contractions to prevent spontaneous abortion or preterm labour
- Prepares the alveoli of the breasts for lactation
- Stimulates maternal metabolism
- Stimulates testes to produce testosterone, which aids the male fetus in developing the reproductive tract

Estrogen

Estrogen has three important functions during pregnancy:

- Stimulates uterine growth
- Increases the blood flow to uterine vessels
- Stimulates a proliferation of breast glandular tissue to prepare for lactation

The effects of estrogen not directly related to pregnancy include the following:

- Increased skin pigmentation (such as the "mask of pregnancy")
- Vascular changes in the skin and the mucous membranes of the nose and mouth
- Increased salivation

Human chorionic gonadotropin

hCG is the hormone that preserves the function of the corpus luteum to continue the production of estrogen and progesterone necessary to sustain pregnancy. hCG is detectable in maternal blood as soon as implantation occurs—usually 7 to 9 days after fertilization—and is the basis for most pregnancy tests.

Human placental lactogen

hPL is also known as human chorionic somatomammotropin (hCS). hPL causes decreased insulin sensitivity and utilization of glucose by the mother, making more glucose available to the fetus to meet growth needs.

UMBILICAL CORD

The umbilical cord develops with the placenta and fetal blood vessels and is the lifeline between mother and fetus. Two arteries carry blood away from the fetus, and one vein returns blood to the fetus. Wharton's jelly covers and cushions the cord vessels and keeps the three vessels separated. The vessels are coiled within the cord to allow movement and stretching without restricting circulation. The normal length of the cord is about 55 cm (22 inches). The umbilical cord usually protrudes from the centre of the placenta.

Memory Jogger

An easy way to remember the number and type of umbilical cord vessels is the mnemonic *AVA:* **A**rtery, **V**ein, **A**rtery.

FETAL CIRCULATION

After the fourth week of gestation, circulation of blood through the placenta to the fetus is well established (see Fig. 3.6). Because the fetus does not breathe and the liver does not have to process most waste products, several physiological diversions in the fetal circulatory route are needed. There are three fetal circulatory shunts:

1. *Ductus venosus:* diverts some blood away from the liver as it returns from the placenta
2. *Foramen ovale:* diverts most blood from the right atrium directly to the left atrium, rather than circulating it to the lungs
3. *Ductus arteriosus:* diverts most blood from the pulmonary artery into the aorta

CIRCULATION BEFORE BIRTH

Oxygenated blood enters the fetal body through the umbilical vein. About half of the blood goes to the liver through the portal sinus, with the remainder entering the inferior vena cava through the *ductus venosus* (Fig. 3.7, *A*). Blood in the inferior vena cava enters the right atrium, where most of it passes directly into the left atrium through the *foramen ovale.* A small amount of blood is pumped to the lungs by the right ventricle. The rest of the blood from the right ventricle joins that from the left ventricle through the *ductus arteriosus.* After circulating through the fetal body, blood containing waste products is returned to the placenta through the umbilical arteries.

CIRCULATION AFTER BIRTH

Fetal shunts are not needed after birth when the infant breathes and blood is circulated to the lungs. The foramen ovale closes, because pressure in the right side of the heart falls as the lungs become fully inflated and there is now little resistance to blood flow. The infant's blood oxygen level rises, causing the ductus arteriosus to constrict. The ductus venosus closes when the flow from the umbilical cord stops (Fig. 3.7, *B*).

Closure of Fetal Circulatory Shunts

The foramen ovale closes functionally (temporarily) within 2 hours after birth and permanently by age 3 months. The ductus arteriosus closes functionally within 15 hours and permanently in about 3 weeks. The ductus venosus closes functionally when the cord is cut and permanently in about 1 week. After permanent closure, the ductus arteriosus and the ductus venosus become ligaments.

Because the foramen ovale and ductus arteriosus are initially closed functionally, some conditions may cause one or the other to reopen after birth. A condition that impedes full lung expansion (e.g., respiratory distress syndrome) can increase resistance to blood flow from the heart to the lungs, causing the foramen ovale to reopen. Similar conditions often reduce the blood oxygen levels and can cause the ductus arteriosus to remain open. See Chapter 26 for further discussion of newborn congenital cardiac problems.

FETAL LUNG PREPARATION FOR BIRTH

Fluid in the fetal lung maintains lung expansion and allows for lung growth. Lung fluid decreases during labour to provide for the transition to extrauterine breathing of air. Several hormones increase in the fetus during the labour process that decrease lung fluid production and increase lung fluid resorption to prepare the lung to accept air. In Caesarean births or precipitous (quick) labour, this process is limited and thought to be the cause of "wet lung" in the newborn (Ross & Erwin, 2017).

IMPAIRED PRENATAL DEVELOPMENT AND SUBSEQUENT ILLNESS

Research has shown that undernutrition in utero can result in permanent changes in fetal structure, physiology, and metabolism and can influence the development of conditions such as heart disease and stroke in adult life (see Health Promotion box). Other factors that influence health in later life can be exposure to toxins in utero or factors that occur in the first 3 years of growth and development after birth.

Health Promotion

Some social determinants of health, including social risk, economic risk, low income, or low literacy, can increase the risk for some poor pregnancy outcomes (e.g., preterm birth, stillbirth, small-for-gestational-age infant). Dietary counselling is associated with improved infant birth weight and reduced risk of some poor pregnancy outcomes. The Canada Prenatal Nutrition Program funds community groups to develop or enhance programs for vulnerable pregnant women with the aims of reducing the incidence of unhealthy birth weights, improving the health of infants and mothers, and encouraging breastfeeding (O'Connor, Blake, Bell, et al., 2016).

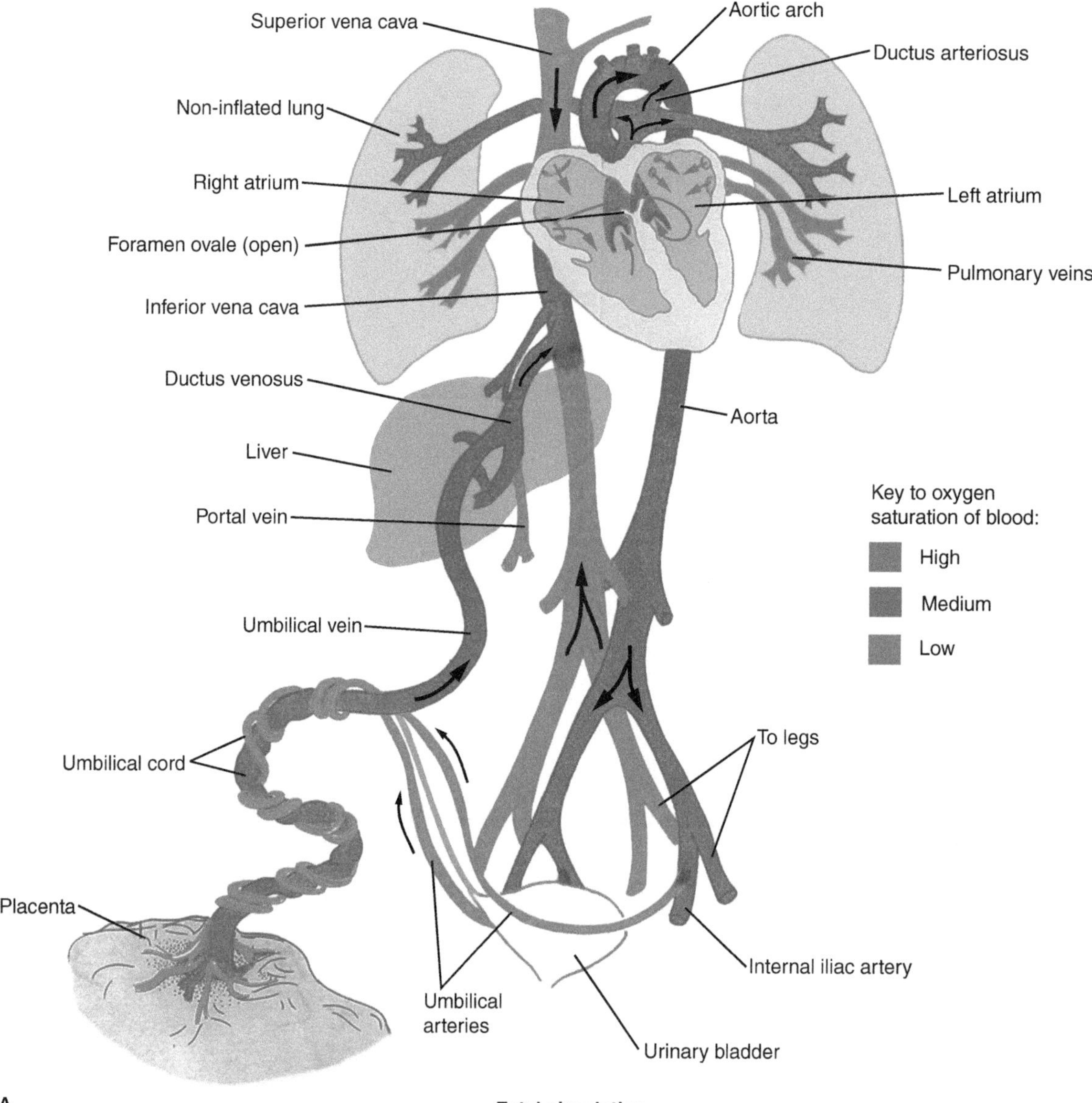

Fig. 3.7 **A,** Fetal circulation. Three shunts allow most blood from the placenta to bypass the fetal lungs and liver; they are the ductus venosus, ductus arteriosus, and foramen ovale.

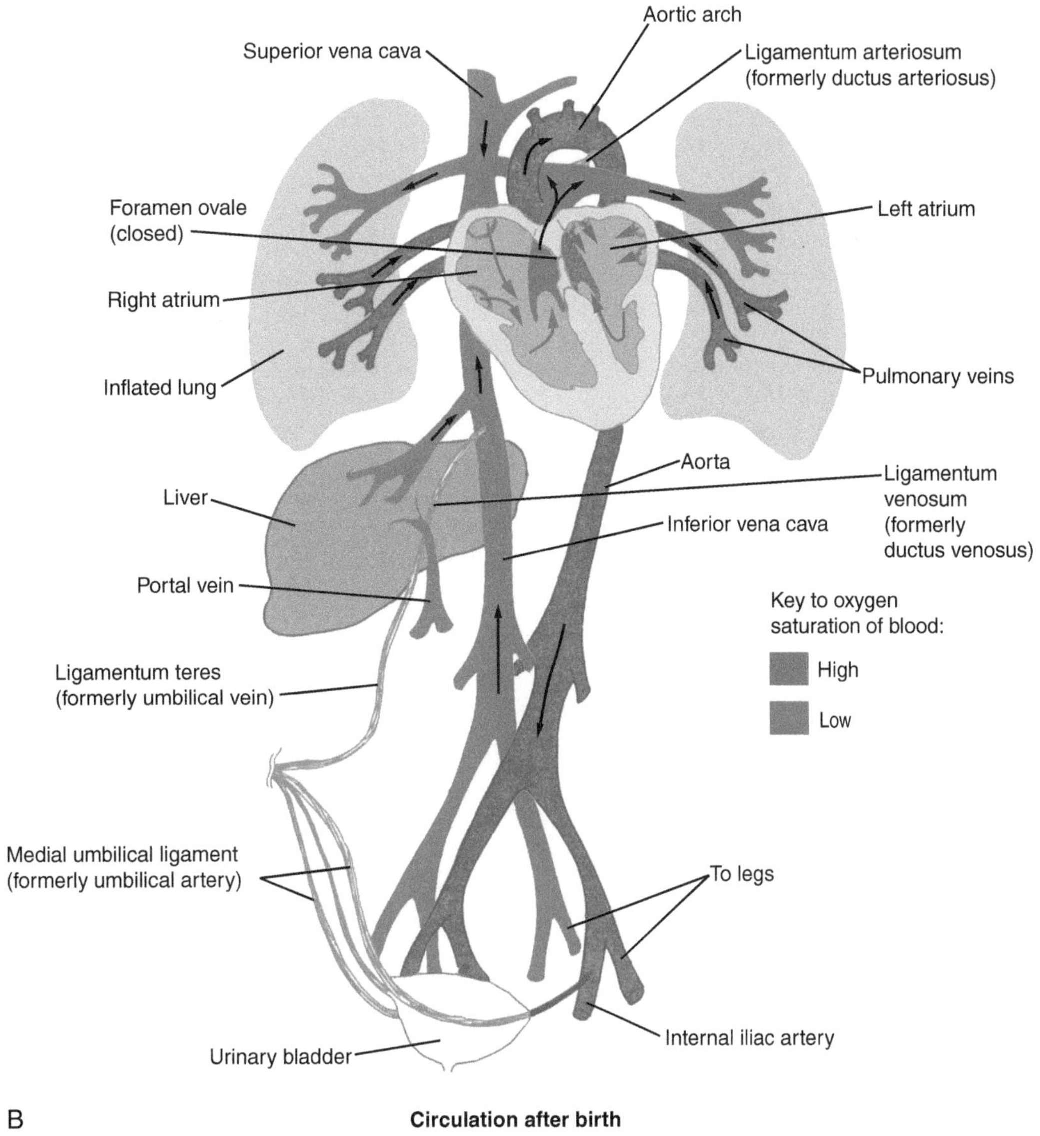

Fig. 3.7, cont'd B, Circulation after birth. Note that the fetal shunts have closed. The umbilical vessels (ductus venosus and ductus arteriosus) will be converted to ligaments. (From McKinney, E. S., James, R. S., Murray, S. S., Nelson, K. A., & Ashwill, J. W. [2017]. *Maternal-child nursing* (5th ed.). St. Louis: Saunders.)

During the first 3 months of fetal life, the fetus is most susceptible to external influences such as undernutrition. However, different organs and tissues undergo rapid development at specific times during gestational life and are therefore sensitive to undernourishment or viral and toxic influences during these periods.

Infants with intrauterine growth restriction may have a reduced number of cells in their organs and can thus be predisposed to the development of specific diseases later in life. For example, a reduced number of pancreatic beta cells can impair insulin secretion and result in a health problem in the adult. Obesity, inactivity, and other factors during the lifespan influence the timing and severity of adult-onset diseases.

It is also possible that in utero changes in vascular or renal structures or in hormonal systems resulting from in utero malnourishment can influence the development of hypertension later in life. Studies have also shown that impaired fetal liver growth in late gestation can permanently impair lipid metabolism and predispose the person to increased cholesterol levels in adult life (Ross & Desai, 2017).

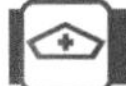
Nursing Tip

The best assessment of fetal growth takes weight, length of gestation, placental size, and newborn head circumference into consideration.

MULTIFETAL PREGNANCY

Twins occur once in every 43 pregnancies in North America (Benirschke, 2014). The rates of multiple births has increased owing to the increase in fertility treatments. When hormones are given to assist with ovulation, twinning and other multifetal births (triplets, quadruplets, and quintuplets) are more likely to occur.

Monozygotic (MZ) twins (Fig. 3.8, *A*), often called identical twins, are genetically identical, are of the same sex, and look alike, because they develop from a single fertilized ovum. Physical differences between monozygotic twins are caused by prenatal environmental factors involving variations in the blood supply from the placenta. Most monozygotic twins begin to develop at the end of the first week after fertilization. The result is two identical embryos, each with its own amnion but with a common chorion and placenta and some common placental vessels. If the embryonic disc does not divide completely, various types of conjoined (formerly called Siamese) twins may form. They are named according to the regions that are joined (e.g., *thoracopagus* indicates an anterior connection of the thoracic regions). Conjoined twins have a single amnion.

Dizygotic (DZ) twins (Fig. 3.8, *B*), also called *fraternal twins*, may or may not be of the same sex, and they develop from two separate ova fertilized by two separate sperm. Dizygotic twins always have two amnions, two chorions, and two placentas, although their chorions and placentas sometimes fuse. Dizygotic twin pregnancies tend to repeat in families, and the incidence increases with maternal age. The twins are about as much alike as any other siblings.

Many twin or higher multiples are born prematurely, because the uterus becomes overly distended. The placenta may not be able to supply sufficient nutrition to both fetuses, with the result that one or both twins is smaller than average.

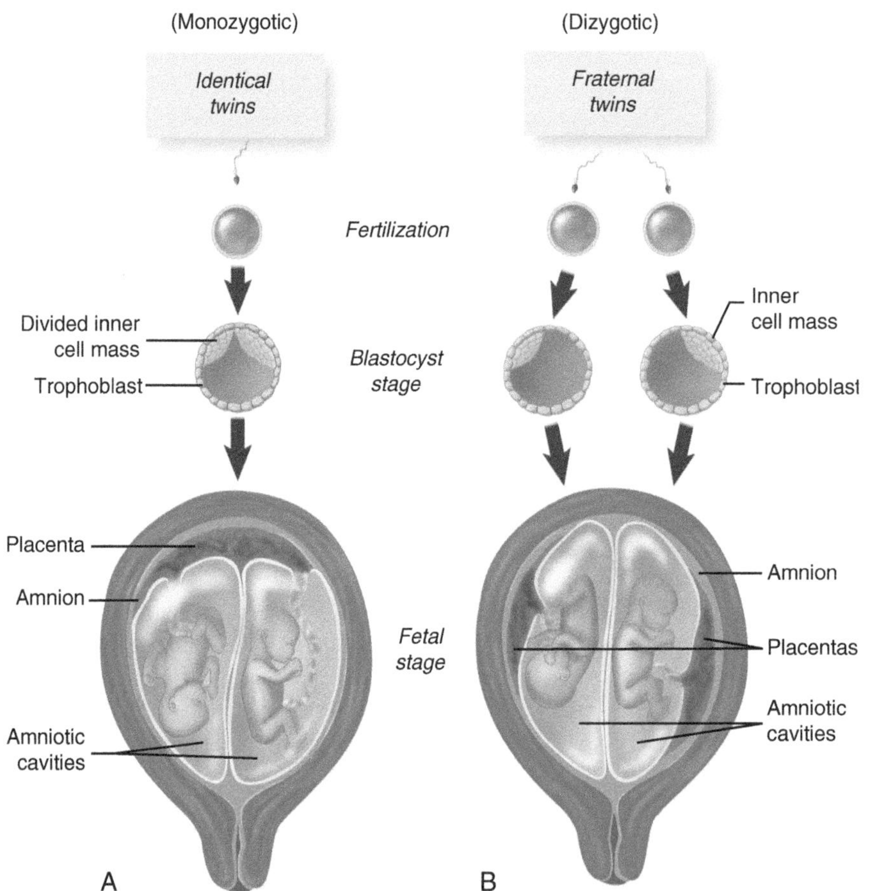

Fig. 3.8 Multiple births. **A,** Identical (monozygotic) twins develop when the embryonic tissue from a single egg splits to form two individuals. The twins share the placenta. **B,** Fraternal (dizygotic) twins develop when two different ova are fertilized at the same time by two different sperm, producing separate zygotes. Each twin has its own placenta, amnion, and chorion. (From Thibodeau, G. A., & Patton, K. T. [2016]. *Anatomy & physiology* [9th ed.]. St. Louis: Mosby.)

Get Ready for the Certification Examination!

Key Points

- The uniqueness of each individual results from the blending of genes on the 46 chromosomes contained in each body cell and the environment of the embryo and fetus during development.
- Gametogenesis in the male is called spermatogenesis. Each mature sperm has 22 autosomes, plus either an X or a Y sex chromosome, for a total of 23. Gametogenesis in the female is called oogenesis. It begins at ovulation and is not completed until fertilization occurs. The mature ovum has 22 autosomes plus the X sex chromosome, for a total of 23. At conception, the total number of chromosomes is restored to 46.
- When the ovum is fertilized by an X-bearing sperm, a female offspring results; when it is fertilized by a Y-bearing sperm, the child will be male.
- After fertilization in the fallopian tube, the zygote enters the uterus, where implantation is complete by 7 days after fertilization. If the zygote fails to move through the tube, implantation occurs there, and a tubal ectopic pregnancy results.
- When implantation occurs in the uterine lining, the cells of the zygote differentiate and develop into the following structures: chorion, amnion, yolk sac, and primary germ layers. The chorion develops into the embryonic or fetal portion of the placenta; the amnion encloses the embryo and the amniotic fluid; the primary germ layers develop into different parts of the growing fetus; and the yolk sac, which functions only during embryonic life, begins to form red blood cells.
- The three germ layers of the embryo are the ectoderm, the mesoderm, and the endoderm. All structures of the individual develop from these layers.
- All body systems are formed and functioning in a simple way by the end of the eighth week.
- The accessory structures of pregnancy are the placenta and the umbilical cord. These along with the fetal circulation continuously support the fetus throughout prenatal life in preparation for birth.
- The amniotic fluid maintains a constant body temperature around the fetus, allows free floating and symmetrical growth, protects against infection, and acts as a cushion to protect the fetus and the umbilical cord.
- The placenta is an organ for fetal respiration, nutrition, and excretion. It is also a temporary endocrine gland that produces progesterone, estrogen, human chorionic gonadotropin (hCG), and human placental lactogen (hPL).
- The umbilical cord contains two arteries that carry blood *away* from the fetus and one vein that carries blood *to* the fetus.
- Fetal circulation transports oxygen and nutrients to the fetus and disposes of carbon dioxide and other waste products from the fetus. The temporary fetal circulatory structures are the *foramen ovale,* the *ductus arteriosus*, and the *ductus venosus.* They divert most blood from the fetal liver and lungs, because these organs do not fully function during prenatal life.
- *Monozygotic twins* develop from a single ovum and are identical. *Dizygotic twins* develop from two separate ova and two separate sperm and have a separate amnion and placenta.

Additional Learning Resources

evolve Go to your Evolve website (http://evolve.elsevier.com/Canada/Leifer) for the following learning resources:

- Answer Key for Critical Thinking Questions
- Answer Key for Textbook Review Questions
- Audio Glossary
- Fluids & Electrolytes tutorial
- Interactive Review Questions
- Skills Performance Checklists
- Video clips and more!

Online Resources

- Female reproductive system: https://www.nlm.nih.gov/medlineplus/femalereproductivesystem.html
- Fetal circulatory system: http://www.indiana.edu/~anat550/cvanim/fetcirc/fetcirc.html
- Government of Canada, *Family-Centred Maternity and Newborn Care in Canada: National Guidelines* (Chapter 2, Preconception Care): https://www.canada.ca/en/public-health/services/publications/healthy-living/maternity-newborn-care-guidelines-chapter-2.html
- Government of Canada, *Genetic Testing and Screening:* https://www.canada.ca/en/public-health/services/fertility/genetic-testing-screening.html
- The Visible Embryo: http://www.visembryo.com/

Review Questions

1. What determines a child's sex?
   - **a.** The dominance of either the X or the Y chromosome.
   - **b.** The number of X chromosomes in the ovum.
   - **c.** The ovum, which contributes either an X or a Y chromosome.
   - **d.** The sperm, which contains either an X or a Y chromosome.
2. A woman who wants to become pregnant should avoid all medications unless they are prescribed by a health care provider who knows she is pregnant, due to which reason?
   - **a.** The placenta allows many medications to cross into the fetus.
   - **b.** Medications often have adverse effects when taken during pregnancy.
   - **c.** Fetal growth is likely to be slowed by many medications.
   - **d.** The pregnancy is likely to be prolonged by some medications.

3. When a couple has unprotected sexual intercourse 3 days before the woman ovulates, the risk of the woman becoming pregnant is:
   a. limited, because the ova only lives for 24 hours.
   b. possible, because the sperm survive for up to 7 days.
   c. unknown.
   d. very low, because that is not the woman's "fertile period."
4. The purpose of the foramen ovale is to:
   a. increase fetal blood flow to the lungs.
   b. limit blood flow to the liver.
   c. raise the oxygen content of fetal blood.
   d. reduce blood flow to the lungs.
5. Why are twins often born early?
   a. The uterus becomes overdistended.
   b. The placenta becomes distended.
   c. The woman's body cannot tolerate the weight.
   d. The fetuses become too large to be born vaginally.
6. The nurse is responsible for examining the umbilical cord of the newborn infant. The nurse knows which of the following? *(Select all that apply.)*
   a. The umbilical cord has two veins and one artery.
   b. The umbilical cord has two arteries and one vein.
   c. The umbilical cord has two arteries and two veins.
   d. Umbilical arteries carry blood *away* from the fetus.
   e. Umbilical arteries carry blood *to* the fetus.

Critical Thinking Questions

1. A patient discusses her family-planning decisions. She states that she will come to the clinic for prenatal care and will begin to take prenatal vitamins as soon as she knows she is pregnant. What would be the best response from the nurse?
2. A patient in the thirty-second week of gestation states that she wants to give birth to her fetus now, because she feels so "big and uncomfortable." She states that she knows the baby has been fully formed since the first trimester and does not mind if it is a little small at birth. What would be the best response from the nurse?

REFERENCES

Benirschke, K. (2014). Multiple gestation. The biology of twinning. In R. K. Creasy, R. Resnik, J. D. Iams, et al. (Eds.), *Creasy & Resnik's Maternal-Fetal Medicine: Principles and Practice* (7th ed.). Philadelphia: Saunders.

Government of Canada. (2018). *Preconception care. Family-centred maternity and newborn care: national guidelines*. Retrieved from: https://www.canada.ca/en/public-health/services/publications/healthy-living/maternity-newborn-care-guidelines-chapter-2.html.

Moktar, A., Rodway, W., & Huether, S. (2017). Structure and function of the reproductive system. In S. Huether & K. McCance (Eds.), *Understanding pathophysiology* (6th ed.). St. Louis: Elsevier.

O'Connor, D. L., Blake, J., Bell, R., et al. (2016). SOGC clinical practice guideline: Canadian consensus on female nutrition: Adolescence, reproduction, menopause, and beyond. *Journal of Obstetrics and Gynaecology Canada*, *38*(6), 508–554.

Ross, M. G., & Desai, M. (2017). Developmental origins of adult health and disease. In S. Gabbe, J. Niebyl, J. Simpson, et al. (Eds.), *Obstetrics: Normal and problem pregnancies* (7th ed.). Philadelphia: Elsevier.

Ross, M. G., & Erwin, M. G. (2017). Fetal development and physiology. In S. Gabbe, J. Niebyl, J. Simpson, et al. (Eds.), *Obstetrics: Normal and problem pregnancies* (7th ed.). Philadelphia: Elsevier.

Prenatal Care and Adaptations to Pregnancy

4

Lisa Keenan-Lindsay

http://evolve.elsevier.com/Canada/Leifer

Objectives

1. Define each key term listed.
2. List the goals of prenatal care.
3. Discuss prenatal care for a normal pregnancy.
4. Explain the nurse's role in prenatal care.
5. Calculate the expected date of birth and the duration of pregnancy.
6. Differentiate between the presumptive, probable, and positive signs of pregnancy.
7. Describe the physiological changes that occur during pregnancy.
8. Identify the effects of medication ingestion on pregnancy and lactation.
9. Identify nutritional needs for pregnancy and lactation.
10. Discuss the importance of exercise in pregnancy.
11. Describe patient education related to travel and common discomforts of pregnancy.
12. Review immunization administration during pregnancy.
13. State three herbal products contraindicated in pregnancy.
14. Discuss nursing support for emotional changes that occur in a family during pregnancy.
15. Identify special needs of the pregnant adolescent, the lone parent, and the older couple.
16. Apply the nursing process to develop a culturally appropriate plan for care during pregnancy.
17. Explain the role of the prenatal environment in the long-term health of a person.

Key Terms

abortion
alternative therapy
antepartum
aortocaval compression (a-ŏr-tō-KĀ-văl kŏm-PRĔSH-ŭn)
Braxton Hicks contractions
Chadwick sign
chloasma
colostrum (kŏ-LŌS-trŭm)
complementary therapy
estimated date of birth (EDB)
gestational age
Goodell sign
gravida (GRĂV-ĭ-dă)
Hegar sign
intrapartum
lactation (lăk-TĀ-shŭn)
last menstrual period (LMP)
lightening
McDonald sign
multigravida
multipara (mŭl-TĬP-ă-ră)
Nägele's rule (NĀ-gĕ-lēz rūl)
parity
postpartum
primigravida (prĭ-mĭ-GRĂV-ĭ-dă)
primipara (prĭ-MĬP-ă-ră)
pseudoanemia (sū-dō-ă-NĒ-mē-ă)
quickening
supine hypotension
trimesters

Pregnancy is a temporary, normal physiological process that affects the woman physically and emotionally. All systems of her body adapt to support the developing fetus. There are three phases of the childbearing period: **antepartum** or prenatal (pregnancy—before birth), **intrapartum** (during birth), and **postpartum** (after birth). The focus of nursing care during pregnancy is to teach the mother how to maintain good health or, in the case of a mother with a condition that places her or her fetus at risk, to improve her health as much as possible to promote a healthy outcome for both mother and fetus. Good prenatal care can also help prevent adult-onset diseases in the infant. This chapter reviews prenatal care, the physiological and psychological changes of pregnancy, and nursing care to meet the needs of women and families.

PRECONCEPTION CARE

During pregnancy, maternal diet, exercise, smoking, stress, drugs, and environmental pollutants can affect the adult health of the developing fetus. Thus the goal of prenatal care is no longer limited to the outcome of a healthy mother and newborn but has been expanded to the prevention of adult disease in the newborn infant. Ideally, health care for childbearing begins before conception (Afshar & Han, 2017). Preconception care identifies risk factors that may be changed before conception, to reduce their negative impact on the outcome of pregnancy. For example, the woman may be counselled and provided resources to improve her nutritional state before pregnancy, or she may receive immunizations to prevent infections that would be harmful to the developing fetus. An adequate folic acid intake before conception can reduce the incidence of congenital anomalies. Although some risk factors cannot be eliminated, such as pre-existing diabetes, preconception care helps the woman to begin pregnancy in the best possible state of health.

Preconception care involves a discussion of pregnancy intention, access to care, use of folic acid, smoking cessation, sexually transmitted infections (STIs), recreational and prescription drug use, and mental health issues. Education related to healthy weight, glycemic control, and use of *teratogenic* (causing developmental malformations) medications should be provided, and family history and any chronic illness should be discussed.

PRENATAL CARE

Prenatal care is a primary example of primary prevention.

Early and regular prenatal care is the best way to promote a healthy outcome for both mother and child. Obstetricians, family practice physicians, registered midwives (RMs), and nurse practitioners provide prenatal care. The nurse assists the health care provider in evaluating the expectant family's physical, psychological, and social needs and can provide teaching about women's self-care. The major goals of prenatal care include the following:

- Promote the health of the mother, fetus, newborn, and family.
- Ensure a safe birth for mother and child by promoting good health habits and reducing risk factors.
- Teach health habits that may be continued after pregnancy.
- Educate regarding self-care for pregnancy.
- Develop a partnership with parents and family to provide continuous and coordinated health care.
- Provide physical care.
- Prepare parents for the responsibilities of parenthood.

To achieve these goals, health care providers must do more than offer physical care. All health care providers must work as an interprofessional team to create an environment that allows for respectful cultural and individual differences while also being supportive of the entire family.

Nursing Tip

The major roles of the nurse during prenatal care include collecting data from the pregnant woman, identifying and re-evaluating risk factors, educating in self-care, providing nutrition counselling, and promoting the woman and family's adaptation to pregnancy.

Legal and Ethical Considerations

Documenting abnormal data such as high blood pressure *must* be followed by documentation of intervention or referral for follow-up care.

DEFINITION OF TERMS

The following terms are used to describe a woman's obstetrical history:

- ***Gravida:*** Any pregnancy, regardless of duration; also, the number of pregnancies, including the one in progress, if applicable.
- *Nulligravida:* A woman who has never been pregnant.
- ***Primigravida:*** A woman who is pregnant for the first time.
- ***Multigravida:*** A woman who has been pregnant before, regardless of the duration of the pregnancy.
- ***Parity:*** The number of pregnancies that have reached 20 weeks' gestation, regardless of the number of fetuses born and regardless of whether those children are now living.
- ***Primipara:*** A woman who has given birth to her first child (past the point of viability), regardless of whether the child was alive at birth or is now living. The term is also used informally to describe a woman before the birth of her first child.
- ***Multipara:*** A woman who has given birth to two or more children (past the point of viability), regardless of whether the children were alive at birth or are presently alive. The term is also used informally to describe a woman before the birth of her second child.
- *Nullipara:* A woman who has not given birth to a child who reached the point of viability (22 weeks' gestation).
- ***Abortion:*** Premature termination of pregnancy, either spontaneous or induced.
- ***Gestational age:*** Prenatal age of the developing fetus calculated from the first day of the woman's last menstrual period.
- *Age of viability:* A fetus that has reached the stage (usually at 22 weeks' gestation) where it is capable of living outside of the uterus.

Box 4.1 GTPAL System to Describe Parity

G Number of all pregnancies (including current one)
T Number of *term* infants born (infants born after at least 37 weeks of gestation)
P Number of *preterm* infants born (infants born after 20 weeks or before 37 weeks of gestation)
A Number of pregnancies *aborted before 20 weeks of gestation* (spontaneously or induced)
L Number of children now *living*

EXAMPLE

Katie Field is pregnant for the fourth time. She has had one child at 34 weeks' gestation, one at 39 weeks' gestation, and one miscarriage at 12 weeks' gestation.

G/P	GRAVIDA	TERM	PRETERM	ABORTION	LIVING
G_4P_2	4	1	1	1	2

The GTPAL system (Box 4.1) is a standardized way to describe a woman's detailed obstetrical history on her prenatal record.

Some centres use the G/P system for obstetrical history. In this system the word *gravida* indicates the number of pregnancies. The word *para* indicates the outcome of the pregnancies. The gravida number increases by 1 each time a woman is pregnant, whereas the para number increases *only* when a woman has a pregnancy that lasts 20 weeks of gestation (see example in Box 4.1). This system does not provide enough information about the woman's history so its use should be limited.

DETERMINING THE ESTIMATED DATE OF BIRTH

The average duration of a term pregnancy is 40 weeks (280 days) after the first day of the **last menstrual period (LMP)**. **Nägele's rule** is used to determine the **estimated date of birth (EDB)**. To calculate the EDB, one identifies the first day of the last menstrual period, adds 7 days, and counts forward 9 months or alternatively counts backward 3 months and then adds 7 days (Box 4.2). The year is updated, if applicable. The EDB is an *estimated* date, and many births occur before or after this date. Nägele's rule assumes a 28-day menstrual cycle so it is not accurate for women with irregular periods.

In order to determine as accurate a due date as possible the Society of Obstetricians and Gynaecologists of Canada (SOGC) recommends the following:

- Ultrasound is the most accurate method to determine EDB when performed accurately and done prior to 23 weeks' gestation.
- Ideally, every pregnant woman should be offered a first-trimester dating ultrasound; however, if the availability of obstetrical ultrasound is limited, it is reasonable to use a second-trimester scan to assess gestational age; first-trimester crown–rump length is the best parameter for determining gestational age and should be used whenever appropriate.
- If more than one first-trimester ultrasound is done, the earliest scan after 7 weeks' gestation should be used for the EDB (Butt, Lim, & Diagnostic Imaging Committee, 2014).

Box 4.2 Nägele's Rule to Determine the Estimated Date of Birth (EDB)

1. Determine first day of the last menstrual period (LMP).
2. Add 7 days.
3. Count forward 9 months.
4. Correct the year if necessary.

EXAMPLE

1. First day of last normal menstrual period: January 27
2. Add 7 days: February 3
3. Count forward 9 months: November 3 is the EDB

Pregnancy is divided into three 13-week stages called **trimesters**. Predictable changes occur in the woman and the fetus in each trimester. Understanding these developments helps to better provide anticipatory guidance and identify deviations from the expected pattern of development.

PRENATAL VISITS

Prenatal care should begin if not before conception then as soon as a woman suspects that she is pregnant. A complete history and physical examination will help identify problems that may affect the woman or her fetus. The history should include the following:

- *Obstetrical history:* Number and outcomes of past pregnancies; concerns for the mother or infant
- *Menstrual history:* Usual frequency of menstrual cycles and duration of flow; first day of the LMP; any "spotting" since the LMP
- *Contraceptive history:* Type used; whether an oral contraceptive was taken before the woman realized she might be pregnant; whether an intrauterine device is still in place
- *Medical and surgical history:* Infections such as hepatitis or pyelonephritis; surgical procedures; trauma that involved the pelvis or reproductive organs
- *Family history of the woman and her partner:* To identify genetic or other factors that may pose a risk for the pregnancy
- *Health history of the woman and her partner:* To identify risk factors (e.g., genetic defects or the use of alcohol, drugs, or tobacco) and possible blood incompatibility between the mother and the fetus
- *Psychosocial history of the woman and her partner:* To identify any concerns related to lifestyle, ability to access resources and support; significant cultural practices or health beliefs that may affect the pregnancy

The woman has a complete physical examination on her first visit. The aim is to evaluate her general health, determine her baseline weight and vital signs, evaluate her nutritional status, and identify current physical or social problems. A pelvic examination may be performed to evaluate the size and condition of the pelvis and reproductive organs, and to assess for signs of pregnancy.

Health Promotion

Optimal prenatal care includes "teachable moments" to introduce knowledge and lifelong skills in self-care and wellness that includes continuing health care screening, immunizations, and regular follow-up of all risk factors throughout life for each member of the family.

As discussed earlier, the woman's EDB is calculated on the basis of the LMP. An ultrasound examination may be done at this visit or at a later visit to confirm the EDB. An assessment for risk factors that may affect the pregnancy is performed during the first visit and is updated at subsequent visits.

Several routine laboratory tests are performed during the first or second prenatal visit. Others are done at specific times during pregnancy and may be repeated at certain intervals. Several tests are done for all pregnant women; others are based on the presence of various risk factors. Table 4.1 lists prenatal laboratory tests. To prevent unnecessary fears or stress, it is important that the nurse explain that most tests are used to establish a baseline normal for comparison throughout pregnancy.

In Canada, the SOGC recommends that all women be offered the option of a prenatal screening test in the first trimester. This screening may include blood work along with an ultrasound for nuchal translucency between 11 and 14 weeks, if available. Nuchal translucency is an ultrasound that measures the thickness of the fluid under the skin at the back of the neck of the fetus. If this area is thicker than normal, it can be an early sign of Down syndrome, trisomy 18, or heart problems. If ultrasound for nuchal translucency is not available the women should be offered first- and second-trimester serum screening. The option of noninvasive prenatal testing (NIPT) is also available and involves obtaining blood from the mother. NIPT is a screening test that presently is not covered by any provincial health insurance plans in Canada, so the woman must pay for it herself, although some provinces fund this screening for women who have some high-risk criteria. If the test is positive, further invasive testing is required before any decisions can be made related to the continuation of the pregnancy (Audibert, De Bie, Johnson, et al., 2017). All women should also receive an ultrasound at 18 to 22 weeks to assess for fetal anatomy and placental location.

! Safety Alert!

Early and regular prenatal care is important for reducing morbidity and mortality for mothers and newborns.

The present recommended schedule for prenatal visits in an uncomplicated pregnancy is as follows:

- Conception to 28 weeks—every 4 weeks
- 29 to 36 weeks—every 2 weeks
- 37 weeks to birth—weekly

The pregnant woman is seen more often if complications arise. Routine assessments made at each prenatal visit include the following:

- Review of known risk factors and assessment for new ones.
- Vital signs: The woman's blood pressure should be taken in the same arm and in the same position (horizontal and at heart level) each time for accurate comparison with her baseline value.
- Weight to determine if the pattern of gain is normal: Low prepregnancy weight or inadequate gains are risk factors for preterm birth, a low-birth-weight infant, and other issues.
- Urinalysis for protein and ketones.
- Blood glucose screening between 24 and 28 weeks of gestation (or earlier if high risk for gestational diabetes): Additional testing is done if the result of this screening test is abnormal.
- STI testing may also be performed at 36 weeks of gestation if the woman is considered high risk for contracting an STI.
- Fundal height to determine if the fetus is growing as expected and the volume of amniotic fluid is appropriate (Fig. 4.1).
- Leopold manoeuvres to assess the presentation and position of the fetus by abdominal palpation.
- Fetal heart rate: Assessed during the end of the first trimester with a Doppler transducer. Beating of the fetal heart can be seen on ultrasound examination as early as 8 weeks after the LMP.
- Fetal movement counting ("kick counts"): Low-risk women should be aware of any changes in movement; for high-risk women fetal movement counting should be done daily after 26 to 32 weeks (see Chapter 5).
- Review of emotional health and psychological well-being.
- Discomforts or problems that have arisen since the last visit.

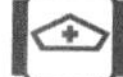
Nursing Tip

The nurse listens to concerns and answers questions from the expectant family during each prenatal visit. This is a prime time for teaching good health habits because most women are highly motivated to improve their health.

The nurse establishes rapport with the expectant family by conveying interest in their needs, listening to their concerns, and directing them to appropriate resources. The health care team must create a culturally safe environment and incorporate as many cultural and health beliefs as possible into care. For example, Muslim laws of modesty dictate that a woman be covered (hair, body, arms, and legs) when in the presence of an unrelated male, thus a female health care provider is often preferred. An Asian woman may nod her head when the nurse teaches her, leading the nurse to believe that she understands and will use the teaching. However, the woman may be showing respect to the nurse, rather than agreement with what is being taught. Eye contact may be expected during conversations, but in some cultures this may be seen as confrontational.

GROUP PRENATAL CARE

Group prenatal care is an alternative model of providing prenatal care and is often called *Centering Pregnancy* care. Instead of individual prenatal appointments, a

Table 4.1 **Routine Prenatal Tests***

TEST	PURPOSE
First Trimester (Routine)	
Blood type, Rh factor, and antibody screen	Determines risk for maternal–fetal blood incompatibility
Hemoglobin, hematocrit, WBC, differential	Detects anemia, infection, or cell abnormalities
VDRL	Identifies untreated syphilis
Rubella, varicella, and parvovirus B19 titre	Determines immunity to rubella, chicken pox, and parvovirus
Tuberculin skin screening (depending on woman's history)	Screening test for exposure to tuberculosis
Hepatitis B screen	Identifies carriers of hepatitis B
Human immunodeficiency virus (HIV) screen	Detects HIV infection (with patient consent following pre- and postcounselling)
Urinalysis and culture	Detects infection, renal disease, hypertension disease of pregnancy, or diabetes
Papanicolaou (Pap) test	Screens for cervical cancer, herpes simplex type 2, and human papillomavirus (HPV) (if not done within 3 years before conception)
Vaginal culture	Detects sexually transmitted infections (STIs) such as gonorrhea, *Chlamydia,* or HPV
First-Trimester Screening (FTS)	
Ultrasound at 11 to 14 weeks including nuchal translucency (NT)	Determines accurate dating, identification of twins, early detection of major structural abnormalities, screening for Down syndrome, and aneuploidy screening
Maternal serum biochemical markers (pregnancy-associated plasma protein-A [PAPP-A] and free beta-human chorionic gonadotropin [β-hCG])	Screens for Down syndrome and trisomy 18
First Trimester (If Indicated)	
Hemoglobin electrophoresis	Identifies presence of hemoglobinopathies (e.g., sickle cell anemia or β-thalassemia)
Second Trimester (Routine)	
1-hour glucose tolerance: sample drawn 1 hour after 50 g of liquid glucose is ingested	Routine test done at 28 weeks of gestation to identify gestational diabetes; done earlier if there are risk factors
2-hour glucose tolerance (if required)	Screens for diabetes in women with an elevated 1-hour glucose screen
Ultrasound—between 18 and 22 weeks	Fetal anatomy scan as well as to detect fetal anomalies (open neural tube defects) and placenta location
Second Trimester (If Indicated)	
Amniocentesis	Performed at 16–20 weeks of gestation when screening test is positive for a genetic condition
Third Trimester (Routine)	
Group B streptococcus (GBS) (vaginal and rectal swab)	Performed at 36–37 weeks. If woman tests positive she is treated during labour to prevent GBS sepsis in the newborn. Treated with penicillin G every 4 hours until birth or if the woman is allergic to penicillin cefazolin or clindamycin, every 8 hours until birth, or vancomycin every 12 hours until birth
Third Trimester (If Indicated)	
Biophysical profile	Ultrasound for fetal well-being, performed when problem is suspected. Assesses fetal breathing movements, fetal movements, fetal tone, and amniotic fluid volume (AFV). Score of 2 for each part of assessment for a total score of 8. Any score less than 8 requires further assessment.
Ultrasound	In tandem with amniocentesis, determines fetal lung maturity (lecithin and sphingomyelin ratio)—rarely done
Transvaginal ultrasound	To assess cervical length as a predictor for preterm labour
Doppler blood flow	To assess placental function and sufficiency
Cervical fibronectin assay	Determines risk of preterm labour when risk factors are present

EDB, Estimated date of birth; *VDRL*, Venereal Disease Research Laboratory (test); *WBC,* white blood cell.
*Additional optional prenatal diagnostic tests are described in Table 5.1.
Sources: Audibert, F., De Bie, I., Johnson, J., et al. (2017). No. 348 Joint SOGC-CCMG guideline: Update on prenatal screening for fetal aneuploidy, fetal anomalies, and adverse pregnancy outcomes. *Journal of Obstetricians and Gynaecologists of Canada, 39*(9), 805–817. https://doi.org/10.1016/j.jogc.2017.01.032; Green, P., Argylan, A., Mutal, F, et al. (2017). Implementation of universal cervical length screening is associated with reduction in the rate of spontaneous preterm deliveries in low risk cohorts. *American Journal of Obstetrics & Gynecology, 216*(1), S10; Money, D., Allen, V. M., & Infectious Diseases Committee. (2013). SOGC clinical practice guideline: The prevention of early-onset neonatal group B streptococcal disease. *Journal of Obstetrics and Gynaecology Canada, 35*(10), e1–e1; Pandipati, S., Combs, C., & Fishman, A. (2017). Transabdominal ultrasound for cervix length screening—or not. *American Journal of Obstetrics & Gynecology, 216*(6), 621–622.

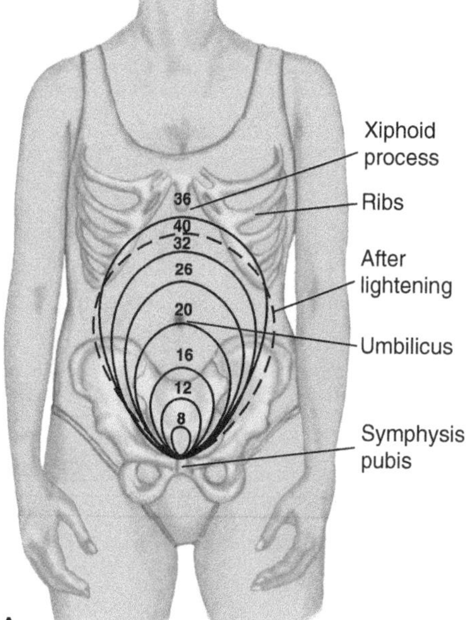

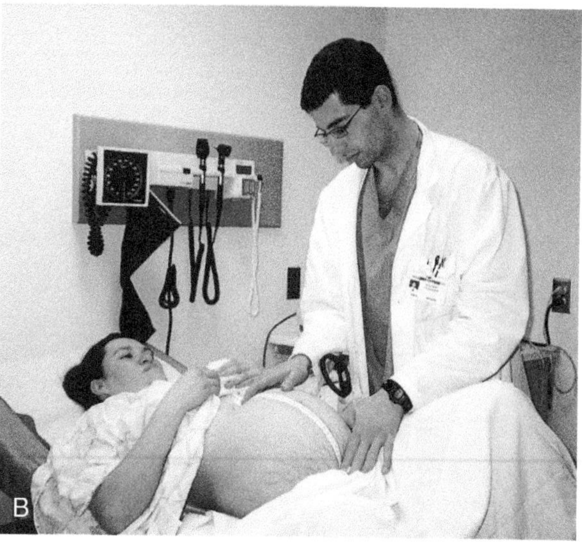

Fig. 4.1 Height of fundus during gestation. **A,** The numbers represent the weeks of gestation, and the circles represent the height of the fundus expected at that stage of gestation. **Note:** The fortieth week is represented by a dotted line to indicate lightening has occurred. **B,** A healthcare provider measures the height of the fundus during a clinic visit. (**A** from Murray, S. S., McKinney, E. S., & Gorrie, T. M. [1998]. *Foundations of maternal-newborn nursing* [2nd ed.]. Philadelphia: Saunders. **B** courtesy Pat Spier, RN-C.)

facilitator meets with a group of 8 to 12 women with a similar due date, monthly until the last few weeks of pregnancy (Thielen, 2012). This type of care has proven to be effective, as the women become responsible for some of their own care and there is an atmosphere of mutual education and support (Thielen, 2012). Benefits of group prenatal care include improved birth outcomes, improved patient satisfaction, and higher breastfeeding initiation rates (Herrman, Rogers, & Ehrenthahl, 2012).

SIGNS OF PREGNANCY

The signs of pregnancy are divided into three general groups: *presumptive, probable,* and *positive,* depending on how likely they are to be caused by factors other than pregnancy (Box 4.3).

PRESUMPTIVE SIGNS OF PREGNANCY

The presumptive indications of pregnancy are those from which a definite diagnosis of pregnancy cannot be made. These are subjective signs that are felt by the woman and are signs and symptoms that are common during pregnancy but can often be caused by other conditions.

Amenorrhea, the cessation of menses, in a healthy and sexually active woman is often the first sign of pregnancy. However, strenuous exercise, changes in metabolism and endocrine dysfunction, chronic disease, certain medications, anorexia nervosa, early menopause, or serious psychological disturbances may also be the cause.

Box 4.3 Signs of Pregnancy

PRESUMPTIVE
Amenorrhea
Nausea
Breast tenderness
Fatigue
Urinary frequency
Quickening

PROBABLE
Goodell sign
Chadwick sign
Hegar sign
McDonald sign
Abdominal enlargement
Braxton Hicks contractions
Ballottement
Positive pregnancy test (serum or urine)

POSITIVE
Audible fetal heartbeat
Fetal movement felt by examiner
Ultrasound visualization of fetus

Nausea and sometimes *vomiting* occur in 50 to 75% of all pregnancies and may be the result of an increase of human chorionic gonadotropin (hCG) levels in early pregnancy and are not associated with unfavourable outcomes for mother or infant (Stotland, Bodnar, & Abrams, 2014). "Morning sickness" describes the symptoms, but they may occur at any time of day. Distaste for certain foods or their odours may be the main symptom. The nausea begins between the first

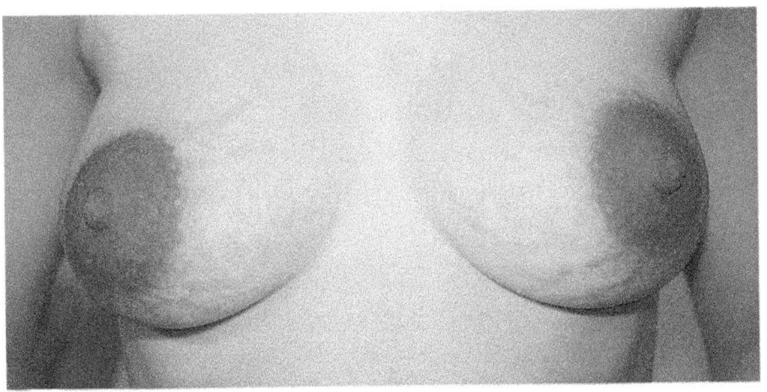

Fig. 4.2 Striae and pigmentation of breasts. Note the darkened pigmentation of areolae and the pink-white lines at the base of the breasts that are caused by stretching of the elastic tissue as the breasts enlarge. Pigmentation will disappear after pregnancy, and striae will fade into silvery strands. (From Swartz, M. H. [2014]. *Textbook of physical diagnosis: History and examination* [7th ed.], Philadelphia: Saunders.)

and second missed period and usually improves by the end of the twentieth week. By screening the woman for nausea and vomiting during prenatal visits, the nurse can offer interventions and supportive care that can increase the quality of the pregnancy experience (see discussion later in chapter, Discomforts in Pregnancy). Emotional problems or gastrointestinal upsets may also cause nausea and vomiting. When diet and lifestyle changes do not relieve morning sickness, medication may be prescribed by the healthcare provider. Pyridoxine/doxylamine (Diclectin) is a delayed-release tablet that is administered at bedtime. An adverse effect may be drowsiness.

Breast changes include tenderness and tingling as hormones from the placenta stimulate growth of the ductal system in preparation for breastfeeding. Similar breast changes also occur premenstrually in many women. *Striae* are pink to brown lines that may develop as the breasts enlarge (Fig. 4.2).

Fatigue and *drowsiness* are early symptoms of pregnancy. It is believed that fatigue is caused by increased metabolic needs of the woman and fetus. In an otherwise healthy young woman, it is a significant sign of pregnancy. However, illness, stress, or sudden changes in lifestyle may also cause fatigue.

Frequency and *urgency of urination* are common in the early months of pregnancy. The enlarging uterus, along with the increased blood supply to the pelvic area, exerts pressure on the bladder. Urinary frequency occurs in the first trimester until the uterus expands and becomes an abdominal organ in the second trimester. The pregnant woman experiences frequency of urination again in the third trimester when the presenting part descends in the pelvis in preparation for birth. Causes of urinary disturbances other than pregnancy are urinary tract infections and pelvic masses.

Quickening, or fetal movement felt by the mother, is first perceived at 16 to 20 weeks of gestation as a faint fluttering in the lower abdomen in primiparous women. Women who have previously given birth often report quickening as early as 14 weeks. Abdominal gas, normal bowel activity, and false pregnancy (pseudocyesis) are other possible causes of this fluttering in the lower abdomen.

PROBABLE SIGNS OF PREGNANCY

The probable indications of pregnancy provide stronger evidence of pregnancy and are mainly objective signs that can be observed by an examiner. However, these also may be caused by other conditions.

Goodell sign is the softening of the cervix and the vagina caused by increased vascular congestion. **Chadwick sign** is the purplish or bluish discoloration of the cervix and vaginal mucosa caused by increased vascular congestion. Hormonal imbalance or infection may also cause both Goodell and Chadwick signs. **Hegar sign** is a softening of the lower uterine segment. Because of the softening, it is easy to flex the body of the uterus against the cervix, which is known as **McDonald sign**.

Abdominal and uterine enlargement occurs rather irregularly at the onset of pregnancy. By the end of the twelfth week, the uterine fundus may be felt just above the symphysis pubis, and it extends to the umbilicus between the twentieth and twenty-second weeks (see Fig. 4.1). Uterine or abdominal tumours may also cause enlargement.

Braxton Hicks contractions, also known as *prelabour contractions*, are irregular, painless uterine contractions that begin in the second trimester. These contractions give the sensation of the abdomen being hard and tense. They may become progressively more noticeable as term approaches and are more pronounced in multiparas. They may become strong enough to be mistaken for true labour. Uterine fibroids (benign tumours) may also cause these contractions.

Ballottement is a manoeuvre by which the fetal part is displaced by a light tap of the examining finger on the cervix, and then the part rebounds quickly. Uterine or cervical polyps (small tumours) may cause the sensation of ballottement on the examiner's finger.

Fetal outline may be identified by palpation after the twenty-fourth week. It is possible to mistake a tumour for a fetus.

Pregnancy tests use maternal urine or blood to determine the presence of hCG, a hormone produced by the chorionic villi of the placenta. Home pregnancy tests based on the presence of hCG in the urine are capable of greater than 97% accuracy, but the instructions must be followed *precisely* to obtain this accuracy. A highly reliable pregnancy test is the *radioimmunoassay* (RIA). The RIA is a blood test that accurately identifies pregnancy as early as 1 week after ovulation. Pregnancy tests of all types are probable indicators, because several factors may interfere with their accuracy: medications such as antianxiety or anticonvulsant drugs, blood in the urine, malignant tumours, or premature menopause.

POSITIVE SIGNS OF PREGNANCY

Only a developing fetus causes positive signs of pregnancy. They include demonstration of fetal heart activity, fetal movements felt by an examiner, and visualization of the fetus with ultrasound.

Fetal heartbeat may be detected as early as 10 weeks of pregnancy by using a Doppler device. When assessing the fetal heartbeat, the woman's pulse rate must be assessed at the same time to be certain that the fetal heart is what is actually heard. The fetal heart rate at term ranges between 110 and 160 beats/min. The rate is higher in early gestation and slows as term approaches.

Additional sounds that may be heard while assessing the fetal heartbeat are the uterine and funic souffles. *Uterine souffle* is a soft, blowing sound heard over the uterus during auscultation. The sound is synchronous with the mother's pulse and is caused by blood entering the dilated arteries of the uterus. The *funic souffle* is a soft, swishing sound heard as the blood passes through the umbilical cord vessels.

A trained examiner can feel fetal movements in the second trimester. The examiner must distinguish fetal activity because, to a prospective mother, normal intestinal movements can appear similar to the faint fetal movements typical of early pregnancy. Fetal movements can be seen with ultrasonography.

Identification of the embryo or fetus by means of ultrasonography of the gestational sac is possible as early as 4 to 5 weeks of gestation, with 100% reliability. This noninvasive method is the earliest positive sign of a pregnancy. An ultrasound is often routinely performed between 11 and 14 weeks of gestation (Fig. 4.3).

PHYSIOLOGICAL CHANGES IN PREGNANCY

The woman's body undergoes dramatic changes as her metabolic demands change and she provides a nurturing environment for the fetus. Most of these changes reverse shortly after birth.

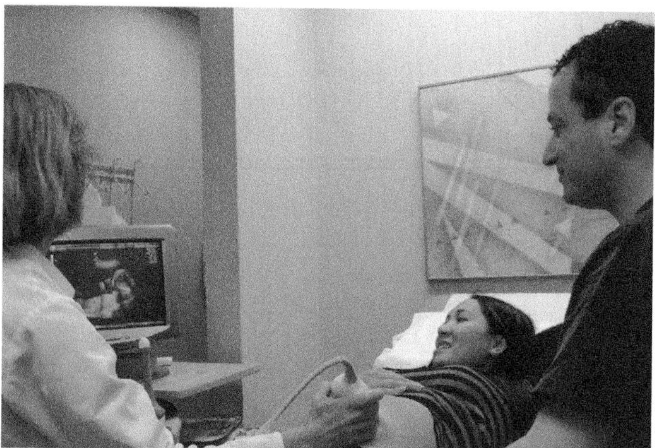

Fig. 4.3 The pregnant woman's family may be present during an ultrasound.

ENDOCRINE SYSTEM

Hormones are essential to maintain pregnancy, and the dramatic increase in hormones during pregnancy affects all body systems. Most hormones are produced by the corpus luteum initially and later by the placenta. The most striking change in the endocrine system during pregnancy is the addition of the placenta as a temporary endocrine organ that produces large amounts of estrogen and progesterone to maintain the pregnancy (as well as hCG and human chorionic somatomammotropin). Table 4.2 further discusses pregnancy hormones.

REPRODUCTIVE SYSTEM

Uterus

The uterus undergoes the most obvious changes in pregnancy. Before pregnancy, the uterus is a small, muscular, pear-shaped pelvic organ that weighs about 60 g, measures 7.5 cm long × 5 cm wide × 1 to 2.5 cm, and has a capacity of about 10 mL. The uterus expands gradually during pregnancy by increasing both the number of myometrial (muscle) cells during the first trimester and the size of individual cells during the second and third trimesters. The uterus becomes a temporary abdominal organ at the end of the first trimester. At term, the uterus reaches the woman's xiphoid process and weighs about 1 000 g. Its capacity is about 5 000 mL, enough to house the term fetus, the placenta, and amniotic fluid.

Cervix

Soon after conception, the cervix changes in colour and consistency. Chadwick and Goodell signs appear. The glands of the cervical mucosa increase in number and activity. Secretion of thick mucus leads to the formation of a *mucous plug* that seals the cervical canal. The mucous plug prevents the ascent of vaginal organisms into the uterus. With the beginning of cervical thinning *(effacement)* and opening *(dilation)* near the onset of labour, the plug is loosened and expelled.

Ovaries

The ovaries do not produce ova (eggs) during pregnancy. The *corpus luteum* (empty graafian follicle) remains on the ovary and produces progesterone to maintain the *decidua* (uterine lining) during the first 6 to 7 weeks of the pregnancy until the placenta can perform this function.

Vagina

The vaginal blood supply increases, causing the bluish colour of Chadwick sign. The vaginal mucosa thickens, and rugae (ridges) become prominent. The connective tissue softens to prepare for distention as the child is born. *Leukorrhea* (vaginal secretions) increase during pregnancy. In addition, the vaginal pH becomes more acidic to protect the vagina and uterus from pathogenic microorganisms. However, the vaginal secretions

Table 4.2 **Hormones Essential in Pregnancy**

HORMONE	SOURCE AND SIGNIFICANCE
Estrogen	Produced by corpus luteum until 14 weeks and then by the placenta Responsible for enlargement of uterus, breasts, and genitals Promotes fat deposit changes Stimulates melanocyte-stimulating hormone in hyperpigmentation of skin Promotes vascular changes Relaxes pelvic ligaments Alters sodium and water retention Decreases ability of pancreas to process insulin
Progesterone	Produced by corpus luteum and ovary until 14 weeks and then by the placenta Maintains endometrium for implantation Inhibits uterine contractility, preventing miscarriage Promotes development of secretory ducts of breasts for lactation Stimulates sodium secretion Reduces smooth muscle tone (causing constipation, heartburn, varicosities)
Thyroxine (T_4)	Influences thyroid gland size and activity and increases heart rate Increases basal metabolic rate during pregnancy
Human chorionic gonadotropin (hCG)	Produced early in pregnancy by fertilized ovum and chorionic villi Stimulates progesterone and estrogen by corpus luteum to maintain pregnancy until placenta takes over Used in pregnancy tests to determine pregnancy
Human chorionic somatomammotropin (previously called human placental lactogen [hPL])	Produced by placenta Affects glucose and protein metabolism Has a diabetogenic effect—allows increased glucose to stimulate pancreas and increase insulin level Contributes to breast development
Melanocyte-stimulating hormone (MSH)	Produced by anterior pituitary gland Causes pigmentation of skin to darken, resulting in brown patches on face (chloasma [melasma gravidarum]), dark line on abdomen (linea nigra), darkening of moles and freckles, and darkening of nipples and areolae
Relaxin	Produced by corpus luteum and placenta Remodels collagen, causing connective tissue of symphysis pubis to be more movable and cervix to soften Inhibits uterine activity
Prolactin	Prepares breasts for lactation
Oxytocin	Produced by posterior pituitary gland Stimulates uterine contraction Is inhibited by progesterone during pregnancy After birth, helps keep uterus contracted Stimulates milk ejection reflex during breastfeeding

also have higher levels of glycogen, a substance that promotes the growth of *Candida albicans*, the organism that causes yeast infections.

A common cause of vaginal discharge is *bacterial vaginosis* (BV), in which there is a decrease in normal lactobacilli and an increase in bacteroids and other anaerobic microorganisms. There may be a profuse, thin, milky-white vaginal discharge that has a fishy odour, but often there are no other clinical symptoms. Bacterial vaginosis has been associated with premature rupture of the membranes, chorioamnionitis, preterm labour, and post-Caesarean endometritis (Public Health Agency of Canada [PHAC], 2013). Pregnant women should be treated to relieve vaginal symptoms and the signs of infection.

Breasts

Hormone-induced breast changes occur early in pregnancy. High levels of estrogen and progesterone prepare the breasts for **lactation**. The areolae of the breasts usually become deeply pigmented, and sebaceous glands in the nipples (tubercles of Montgomery) become prominent. The tubercles secrete a substance that lubricates the nipples.

In the last few months of pregnancy, a thin yellow fluid called **colostrum** may be expressed from the breasts. This "premilk" is high in protein, fat-soluble vitamins, and minerals, but it is low in calories, fat, and sugar. Colostrum contains the mother's antibodies to diseases and is secreted for the first 2 to 3 days after birth in the breastfeeding woman.

RESPIRATORY SYSTEM

The pregnant woman breathes more deeply, but her respiratory rate may increases only slightly. These changes increase oxygen and carbon dioxide exchange, because she moves more air in and out with each breath. Oxygen consumption increases by 20 to 40% during pregnancy. The expanding uterus exerts upward pressure on her diaphragm, causing it to rise about 4 cm. To compensate, the rib cage flares, increasing the circumference of the chest about 6 cm. Dyspnea may occur until the fetus descends into the pelvis (**lightening**), relieving upward pressure on the diaphragm.

Increased estrogen levels during pregnancy cause edema or swelling of the mucous membranes of the nose, pharynx, mouth, and trachea. The woman may have nasal stuffiness and epistaxis (nosebleeds). A similar process occurs in the ears, causing a sense of fullness or earaches.

CARDIOVASCULAR SYSTEM

The growing uterus displaces the heart upward and to the left. The blood volume gradually increases *(hypervolemia)* to about 40 to 50% greater (1 500 mL) than that of the prepregnant state by 32 to 34 weeks of gestation, at which time it levels off or declines slightly. This increase provides added blood for these purposes:

- Exchange of nutrients, oxygen, and waste products within the placenta
- Needs of expanded maternal tissue
- Reserve for blood loss at birth

Cardiac output increases by 30 to 50%, because more blood is pumped from the heart with each contraction, the pulse rate increases by 10 to 15 beats/min, and the basal metabolic rate (BMR) may increase 10 to 20% during pregnancy.

Blood pressure does not increase with the higher blood volume because resistance to blood flow through the vessels decreases. A blood pressure of 140/90 mm Hg or a significant elevation above the woman's baseline measurement calls for attention. **Supine hypotension**, also called **aortocaval compression**, may occur if the woman lies on her back (Fig. 4.4). The supine position allows the heavy uterus to compress the inferior vena cava, reducing the amount of blood returned to her heart. Circulation to the placenta may also be reduced by increased pressure on the woman's aorta, resulting in fetal hypoxia. Symptoms of supine hypotension include faintness, lightheadedness, dizziness, and agitation. Displacing the uterus to one side by turning the patient to a lateral position (preferably to the left) is all that is needed to relieve the pressure. If the woman must remain flat for any reason, a small towel roll placed under one hip will also help to prevent supine hypotension.

Orthostatic hypotension may occur whenever a woman rises from a recumbent position, resulting in faintness or lightheadedness. Cardiac output decreases because venous return from the lower body suddenly drops. *Palpitations* (sudden increase in heart rate) may occur from increases in thoracic pressure, particularly if the woman moves suddenly.

Although both plasma (fluid) and red blood cells (erythrocytes) increase during pregnancy, they do not increase by the same amount. The fluid part of the blood increases more than the erythrocyte component. This leads to a *dilutional anemia* or **pseudoanemia** (false anemia). As a result, the normal prepregnant hematocrit level of 0.37 to 0.47 may fall to 0.33. Although this is not true anemia, the hematocrit count is re-evaluated to determine patient status and needs. The white blood cell (leukocyte) count also increases about 8% (mostly neutrophils) during the second and third trimesters and returns to prepregnant levels by the sixth day postpartum (Table 4.3).

There are increased levels of clotting factors VII, VIII, and X and plasma fibrinogen during the second and third trimesters of pregnancy. This hypercoagulability state helps prevent excessive bleeding after birth when the placenta separates from the uterine wall. However, these changes increase the possibility of thrombophlebitis or thromboembolism during pregnancy and are the reason that the pregnant patient requires careful assessment for this risk and specific teaching to prevent the venous stasis that can lead to thrombophlebitis. The risk for a thromboembolism increases after labour,

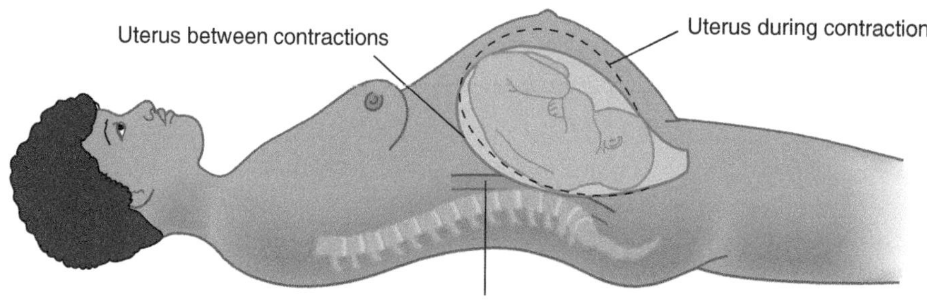

Fig. 4.4 Supine hypotension. When a pregnant woman lies on her back (supine), the weight of the uterus with its fetal contents presses on the vena cava and the abdominal aorta. Placing a wedge pillow under the woman's hip helps to relieve compression of these vessels. (From Matteson, P. S. [2001]. *Women's health during the childbearing years: A community-based approach*. St. Louis: Mosby.)

thus prevention strategies need to be put in place for high-risk women (see Chapter 10).

Venous pressure may increase in the femoral veins as the size and weight of the uterus increase, resulting in varicose veins in the legs of some women. Pregnant women should be encouraged to exercise during pregnancy. The effects of exercise on the cardiovascular system that already has an increased blood volume, increased cardiac output, and increased coagulability during pregnancy must be reviewed before an exercise plan is implemented.

GASTROINTESTINAL SYSTEM

The growing uterus displaces the stomach and intestines toward the back and sides of the abdomen (Fig. 4.5). Increased salivary secretion (ptyalism) sometimes affects taste and smell. The mouth tissues may become tender and bleed more easily because of increased blood vessel development caused by high estrogen levels. Contrary to popular belief, teeth are not affected by pregnancy, although poor dental hygiene can lead to dental caries, which may be a risk for preterm birth, low birth weight, and pre-eclampsia (Russell & Mayberry, 2008).

The demands of the growing fetus increase the woman's appetite and thirst. The acidity of gastric secretions is decreased; emptying of the stomach and motility (movement) of the intestines are slower. Women often feel bloated and may experience constipation and hemorrhoids. *Pyrosis* (heartburn) is caused by relaxation of the cardiac sphincter of the stomach, which permits reflux (backward flow) of the acid secretions into the lower esophagus.

Glucose metabolism is altered because of increased insulin resistance during pregnancy. This allows more glucose use by the fetus but also places the woman at risk for the development of gestational diabetes mellitus (GDM). Progesterone and estrogen relax the muscle tone of the gallbladder, resulting in the retention of bile salts, and this can lead to increased risk of cholelithiasis (gallstones).

URINARY SYSTEM

The urinary system excretes waste products for both the mother and the fetus during pregnancy. The glomerular filtration rate of the kidneys increases. The renal tubules increase the reabsorption of substances that the body needs to conserve, but the tubules may not be

Table 4.3 Normal Blood Values in Nonpregnant and Pregnant Women

VALUE	NONPREGNANT	PREGNANT
Hemoglobin (g/L)	120–160	>110
Hematocrit	0.37–0.47	>0.33
Red blood cells (×10^{12}/L)	4.2–5.4	5–6.25
White blood cells (×10^{9}/L) (increase during labour and up to 6 days postpartum)	5–10	5–15
Fibrinogen (g/L)	2–5	Levels increase late in pregnancy

Source: Blackburn, S. (2013). *Maternal, fetal and neonatal physiology: A clinical perspective* (4th ed.). Philadelphia: Saunders.

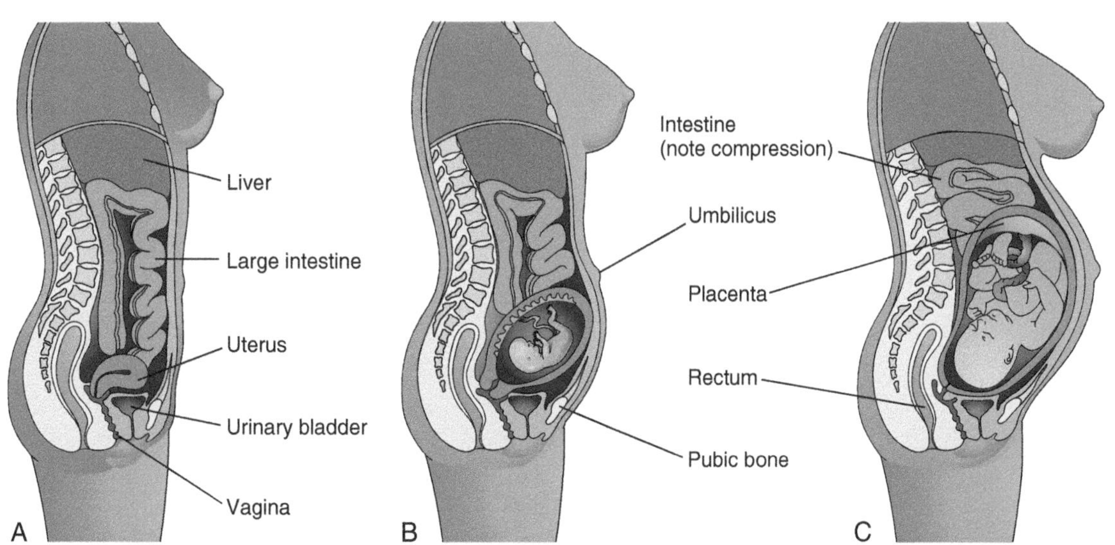

Fig. 4.5 Compression of abdominal contents as the uterus enlarges. The nonpregnant state **(A)** shows the relationship of the uterus to the abdominal contents. As the uterus enlarges at 20 weeks of gestation **(B)** and 30 weeks of gestation **(C)**, the abdominal contents are displaced and compressed. (From Moore, K. L., Persaud, T. V. N., & Torchia, M. G. [2016]. *The developing human: Clinically oriented embryology* [10th ed.]. Philadelphia: Saunders.)

able to keep up with the high load of some substances filtered by the glomeruli (e.g., glucose). Therefore, glycosuria and proteinuria are more common during pregnancy. Water is retained because it is needed for increased blood volume and for dissolving nutrients that are provided for the fetus.

The relaxing effects of progesterone cause the renal pelvis and ureters to lose tone, resulting in decreased peristalsis to the bladder. The diameter of the ureters and the bladder capacity increase because of the relaxing effects of progesterone, causing urine stasis. The combination of urine stasis and nutrient-rich urine makes the pregnant woman more susceptible to urinary tract infection. Consuming at least eight glasses of water each day reduces the risk for urinary tract infection. Although the bladder can hold up to 1 500 mL of urine, the pressure of the enlarging uterus causes increasing frequency of urination, especially in the first and third trimesters. Changes in the renal system may take 6 to 12 weeks after birth to return to the prepregnant state.

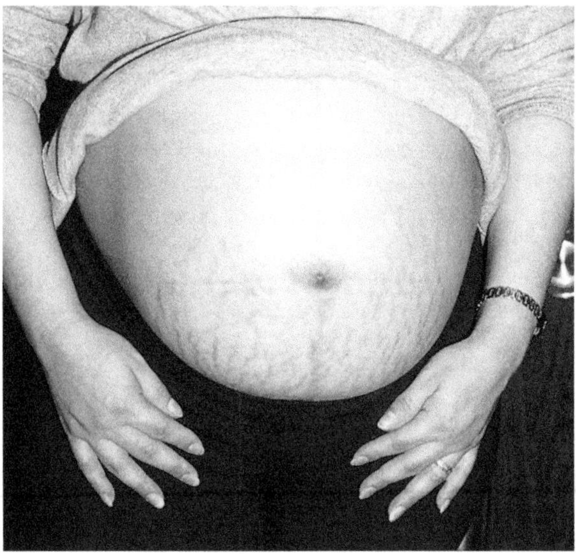

Fig. 4.6 Abdominal striae are pinkish white or purple-grey lines that may occur in pregnancy. They may be found on the breasts, abdomen, and thighs. The dark line at the midline is the linea nigra, an area of increased pigmentation most noticeable in dark-skinned women.

Fluid and Electrolyte Balance

The increased glomerular filtration rate in the kidneys increases sodium filtration by 50%, but the increase in the tubular resorption rate results in 99% reabsorption of the sodium. Because of the need for increased maternal intravascular and extracellular fluid volume, additional sodium is needed to expand fluid volume and maintain an isotonic state. As efficient as the renal system is, it can be overstressed by excessive dietary sodium intake or restriction or by the use of diuretics (Keenan-Lindsay, 2017a).

In pregnancy, blood is slightly more alkaline than in the nonpregnant state, and this mild alkalemia is enhanced by the hyperventilation that often occurs during pregnancy. This status does not affect a normal pregnancy.

INTEGUMENTARY AND SKELETAL SYSTEMS

The high levels of hormones produced during pregnancy cause a variety of temporary changes in the integument (skin) of the pregnant woman. The sweat and sebaceous glands of the skin become more active to dissipate heat from the woman and fetus. Small red elevations of skin with lines radiating from the centre, called *spider nevi,* may occur. The palms of the hands may become deeper red. Most skin changes are reversed shortly after giving birth. Mild pruritus is a common discomfort of pregnancy that has no known physiological reason.

Abdominal striae (stretch marks) are fine, pinkish white or purplish-grey lines that some women develop when the elastic tissue of the skin has been stretched to its capacity (Fig. 4.6). Increased amounts of estrogen cause a rise in adrenal gland activity. This change, in addition to the stretching, is believed to cause breakdown and atrophy of the underlying connective tissue in the skin. Striae are seen on the breasts, thighs, abdomen, and buttocks. After pregnancy, the striae lose their bright colour, and they become thin, silvery lines. Striae may occur with skin stretching from any cause, such as weight gain.

Pigmentation changes that occur include increased pigmentation of the face (**chloasma**, or "mask of pregnancy"), breasts (darkening of the areolae), and abdomen (*linea nigra,* a line extending in the midline of the abdomen from just above the umbilicus to the symphysis pubis) (see Fig. 4.6).

The woman's posture changes as her child grows within the uterus. The anterior part of her body becomes heavier with the expanding uterus, and the lordotic curve in her lumbar spine becomes more pronounced. The woman often experiences low backaches, and, in the last few months of pregnancy, rounding of the shoulders may occur along with aching in the cervical spine and upper extremities.

The pelvic joints relax with hormonal changes during late pregnancy and entry of the fetal presenting part into the pelvic brim in the last trimester. A woman often has a "waddling" gait in the last few weeks of pregnancy because of a slight separation of the symphysis pubis.

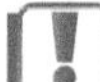

Safety Alert!

A change in the centre of gravity and joint instability because of the softening of the ligaments predispose the pregnant woman to problems with balance. Interventions concerning safety should be part of prenatal education.

THE EFFECT OF PREGNANCY AND LACTATION ON MEDICATION METABOLISM

The physiological changes in pregnancy affect the metabolism of medications administered to the mother. Subtherapeutic drug levels may occur because of the increased plasma volume, cardiac output, and glomerular filtration that occur during pregnancy. A decreased gastric emptying time during pregnancy changes absorption of medications and can delay onset of action. Parenteral medication may be absorbed more rapidly because of increased blood flow and may have a faster onset of action than in the nonpregnant state. The increased levels of estrogen and progesterone may alter hepatic (liver) function, resulting in medication accumulation in the body.

Medications can cross the placenta and have an impact on fetal development, especially in the first trimester, and have increased absorption levels in the developing fetus in the third trimester. The mother should be instructed to check with her healthcare provider before taking over-the-counter medications. Taking ibuprofen in the third trimester can cause early closure of the ductus arteriosus, resulting in fetal distress.

Medications can pass into breastmilk by diffusion and be can be ingested by the newborn during breastfeeding. If the lactating mother must take certain medication, they should be administered after the infant breastfeeds, if possible, to minimize passage to the infant. All women of childbearing age should be counselled about the risk of ingesting medications during pregnancy and lactation.

PREGNANCY CONSIDERATIONS

NUTRITION

Good nutrition is vital to good health and essential for normal growth and development. It is also essential for establishing and maintaining a healthy pregnancy and giving birth to a healthy child. Good nutritional habits begun before conception and continued during pregnancy promote adaptation to maternal and fetal needs. Health Canada has developed prenatal nutrition guidelines that provide women with the needed information to ensure adequate prenatal nutrition. Pregnant and lactating women should be encouraged to follow *Canada's Food Guide* (see Appendix C) (see Online Resources at the end of this chapter).

 Nutrition Considerations

MATERNAL DIET AND FETAL HEALTH

There is a high correlation between maternal diet and fetal health. To ensure that nutritional deficiencies do not occur during the critical first weeks of pregnancy, the nurse can teach women of childbearing age the value of eating well-balanced meals so they can start pregnancy in a good nutritional state.

A healthy, balanced, nutrient-dense diet is at the core of *Canada's Food Guide*. It recommends the following foods in the diet (Government of Canada, 2019a):

- Eat plenty of vegetables and fruit. Choose dark green and orange vegetables each day. Examples might include spinach or broccoli, and squash or carrots.
- Choose whole-grain foods like bread, rice, and pasta.
- Dairy products like yogurt and cheese contribute to healthy bones for mother and baby. Women who do not drink milk should drink fortified soy beverages.
- Choose lean meats, dried peas, beans, tofu, and lentils. Have cooked fish each week that is low in mercury.

Pregnant women require more nutrition and should eat a little more food every day, especially during the second and third trimesters. One extra snack is often enough to cover the nutritional needs of the pregnant woman (Government of Canada, 2019b). The *Food Guide* also focuses on reading nutrition labels to assist in choosing foods that are lower in fat, sodium, and sugar. Refer to Table 13.5 for culturally diverse food patterns.

During pregnancy and lactation, an adequate dietary intake of docosahexaenoic acid–omega 3 fatty acid (DHA) is essential for optimal brain development of the fetus and infant. Dietary sources are preferred; Government of Canada (2009) recommends that pregnant women eat 150 g of cooked fish each week. The types of fish that generally have low levels of contaminants, such as salmon, trout, herring, haddock, canned light tuna, pollock (Boston bluefish), sole, flounder, anchovy, char, hake, mullet, smelt, Atlantic mackerel, and lake white fish, should be chosen (Government of Canada 2009). High levels of mercury can be harmful to the developing fetus's brain. Fish oil supplements in pregnancy may be associated with a decrease in asthma and wheezing in offspring (Ramsden, 2016).

Nursing Care Plan 4.1 lists some common nursing diagnoses and suggested interventions related to nutrition during pregnancy and lactation.

RECOMMENDED DIETARY ALLOWANCES AND RECOMMENDED DIETARY INTAKES

In Canada, the Food and Nutrition Board of the Institute of Medicine (IOM) in partnership with Health Canada developed recommended dietary allowances (RDAs) of nutrient intake required to maintain optimal health. In the past, RDAs reflected the fact that nutrients were primarily supplied by foods, in particular, nonfortified ones. Research by the Food and Nutrition Board showed an increasing use of dietary supplements and fortified foods, resulting in the need to describe upper limits of intake levels to prevent toxicity. Adverse responses (toxicity) can occur if the combination of intake in the form of supplements and food, whether fortified or not, exceeds the present upper limits of safety. When scientific evidence is insufficient to determine RDA, an

Nursing Care Plan 4.1 Nutrition During Pregnancy and Lactation

PATIENT DATA

Mrs. Switzer is seen in the clinic. She is 35 years old, in the first trimester of her first pregnancy, and appears interested in learning how to "start a healthy diet" in order to have a healthy pregnancy outcome.

Selected Nursing Diagnosis Need for education concerning the importance of nutrition in pregnancy and lactation

Goals	Nursing Interventions	Rationales
Patient will verbalize the importance of good nutrition during pregnancy and lactation.	Determine age, parity, present weight, body mass index (BMI), prepregnant nutritional status, food preferences and dislikes, food intolerances, and general health of pregnant patient.	Many factors influence nutritional status of the patient during pregnancy and lactation; nutrition teaching must be individualized to best meet her pregnancy nutritional needs. Teaching regarding appropriate weight gain depends on prepregnancy BMI.
	Determine socioeconomic and cultural factors that may influence food choices. Make recommendations to fit specific needs. Consult with a dietitian if patient's nutritional needs are complex.	Socioeconomic and cultural factors affect the patient's food choices. These factors must be considered to increase the chance that a patient will be able to follow dietary recommendations. The assessment may identify the need for referral to programs such as the Canadian Prenatal Nutrition Program.
	Review specific nutritional needs and food sources for optimal outcome of pregnancy and successful lactation.	If patient understands specific nutritional needs of pregnancy and food sources, she is more likely to choose foods that meet these needs.
	Provide written information in patient's primary language regarding nutrition and food preparation. Modify information to incorporate cultural practices or food dislikes or intolerances.	Written information reinforces verbal teaching and helps patient to recall forgotten information. Recommendations must fit within a patient's individual needs to increase the chance that she will follow them.
	Encourage her to ask questions, and provide appropriate answers.	Encouraging the patient's questions allows the nurse to identify and correct areas of inadequate knowledge or misunderstanding.
Patient will implement good nutrition during pregnancy and lactation, as evidenced by a 24-hour food diary.	Teach patient the purpose of and how to maintain a 24-hour food diary. Teach patient to eat normally and to write down everything she eats and drinks, including approximate amounts, for 1 day.	A 24-hour food diary helps the nurse to evaluate a patient's usual diet and her likes and dislikes, as well as how to improve her diet. It may help identify the need for a dietitian referral.
	Review 24-hour intake from the diary and make appropriate recommendations for improvement. Refer patient to a dietitian if nutritional assessment shows complex needs.	Analysis of usual meals and snacks enables the nurse to identify adequate and inadequate intake of specific nutrients. The 24-hour diary allows the nurse to reinforce areas of adequate intake and concentrate on areas of deficient nutrients.
	Teach patient about *Canada's Food Guide* and how to read nutrition labels.	Choices on the *Canada's Food Guide* provide essential nutrients on a daily basis. Reading of labels helps the patient to select more nutritious items from those that are available.
Patient will demonstrate a gradual weight gain appropriate for her pregnancy (11.5–16 kg for women with a normal BMI).	Maintain a chart to show patient's actual weight at each visit.	Weight chart identifies both the amount and pattern of weight gain and can be used to identify inadequate or excessive gain.
	Review progress of weight with patient at each visit and compare it with the recommended amount of gain for that point in pregnancy.	Reviewing the patient's weight identifies whether the patient's weight gain is normal and whether additional teaching or exploration of needs is required.

CRITICAL THINKING QUESTIONS

1. Mrs. Switzer says she is eager to complete the clinic appointment because she wants to "light up a cigarette." What is your major concern about her smoking? What interventions would be appropriate?
2. Mrs. Switzer states that her dietary pattern is heavily influenced by her perceived "food cravings," which have occurred increasingly in the past month. What would be your approach to this concern?

adequate intake is likely provided by an adequate diet. Consuming dietary supplements of trace elements can result in toxicity if upper limits of intake are consistently exceeded.

Health Canada has published RDAs focusing on specific nutrients (see Additional Learning Resources). Future nutrient recommendations will be expressed as dietary reference intakes (DRIs). *DRI* is an umbrella term that includes the RDA, adequate intakes (AI), and tolerable upper levels of intake. The RDA will be retained for any nutrient for which revision to the new DRI has not been made.

Safety Alert!

Avoid exceeding recommended doses of vitamins and minerals, because a balance is needed for health. For example, excess intake of vitamin C can inhibit the absorption of vitamin B_{12}.

RECOMMENDED WEIGHT GAIN

In the past, a woman's weight gain was restricted during pregnancy, but evidence shows that low maternal weight gain is associated with complications such as preterm labour and intrauterine growth restriction (IUGR), and recommendations for weight gain during pregnancy have gradually increased. Guidelines for weight gain during pregnancy are based on the woman's prepregnant weight and body mass index (BMI). (The BMI considers the height and weight of the individual.) A BMI calculator is available online (see Additional Learning Resources). Women with a BMI of 18.5 to 24.9 are considered as having a healthy weight; women with a BMI of less than 18.5 are considered underweight; women with a BMI of 25 to 25.9 are considered overweight; and women with a BMI greater than 30 are considered obese. A pregnancy weight gain calculator is available online (see Additional Learning Resources). Current Government of Canada (2014) recommended weight gains during pregnancy with a *single* fetus are as follows:

- Normal-weight women (BMI 18.5–24.9): 11.5 to 16 kg (25 to 35 lb)
- Underweight women (BMI <18.5): 12.5 to 18 kg (28 to 40 lb)
- Overweight women (BMI 25–29.9): 7 to 11.5 kg (15 to 25 lb)
- Obese women (BMI ≥30): 5 to 9 kg (11 to 20 lb)

Women carrying *twins* should gain more weight:

- Normal-weight women: 17 to 25 kg (37 to 54 lb)
- Overweight women: 14 to 23 kg (31 to 50 lb)
- Obese women: 11 to 19 kg (25 to 42 lb)

Pregnant adolescents should gain in the upper part of the range currently recommended for adult women as they are not only nourishing a fetus but also require extra nutrients for their own growth.

The pattern of weight gain is also important. The general recommendation is that women who have a normal BMI gain up 1 to 2 kg during the first trimester and approximately 0.4 kg per week during the rest of pregnancy. Nausea and vomiting and some transient food dislikes often limit weight gain or cause weight loss during the first trimester, but the weight is usually regained when the gastrointestinal upsets subside.

Women often want to know why they should gain so much weight when their infant weighs only 3 to 4 kg. The nurse can use the distribution of weight gain during pregnancy shown in Fig. 4.7 to teach women about all the factors that contribute to weight gain.

Nutritional Requirements During Pregnancy

Four nutrients are especially important in pregnancy: protein, calcium, iron, and folic acid.

Protein

Added protein is needed for metabolism and to support the growth and repair of maternal and fetal tissues. An intake of 71 g/day is recommended during pregnancy, which is an increase of 25 g over the nonpregnant diet. The best sources of protein are meat, fish, poultry, and dairy products.

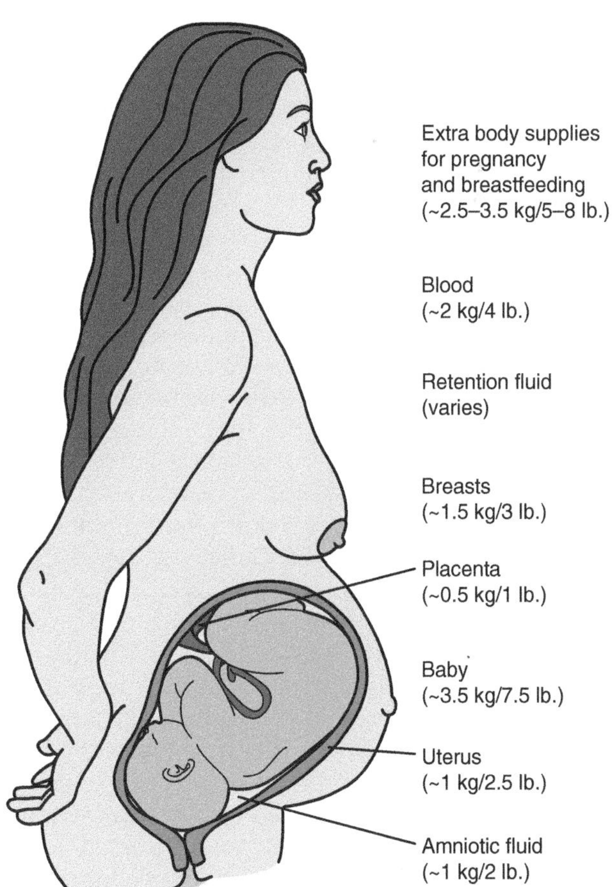

Fig. 4.7 Example of distribution of weight gain for a woman with a normal body mass index (BMI). (From https://www.healthyfamiliesbc.ca/home/articles/weight-gain-during-pregnancy-trimester.)

Examples of complementary plant protein combinations are corn and beans, lentils and rice, and peanut butter and bread. Plant proteins are also complemented with animal proteins, such as in grilled cheese sandwiches, cereal with milk, and chili made of meat and beans. The complementary foods must be eaten together, because all the amino acids necessary for building tissues (essential amino acids) must be present at the same time.

Information about nonmeat sources of protein should be provided to women who are vegetarians to ensure that their protein needs are met. The information can also help reduce the family's food budget, because many plant protein sources are less expensive than animal sources. Raw meat and raw eggs can be contaminated and their consumption should be avoided during pregnancy and lactation.

Calcium

Calcium requirements during pregnancy are the same as for nonpregnant women. The DRI of calcium for all women under 19 is 1 300 mg and for women over 19 is 1 000 mg. This requirement is the same in pregnancy. Dairy products are the single most plentiful source of this nutrient. Other sources of calcium include enriched cereals, legumes, nuts, dried fruits, broccoli, green leafy vegetables, and canned salmon and sardines that contain bones. Calcium supplements are necessary for women who do not drink milk (or do not eat sufficient amounts of equivalent products). Calcium supplements should be taken separately from iron supplements for best absorption. An adequate intake of vitamin D is required to enhance calcium absorption.

Iron

Pregnancy causes a heavy demand for iron, because the fetus must store an adequate supply to meet its needs in the first 3 to 6 months after birth. In addition, the pregnant woman increases her production of erythrocytes. The DRI is 15 mg/day for nonpregnant adult women and 27 mg/day for pregnant women. Women who have a known iron deficiency may need more.

It is difficult to obtain this much iron from the diet alone, thus Government of Canada (2019b) recommends that all pregnant women take a multivitamin that has 16 to 20 mg of iron. A resource on iron-rich foods is available from the Dietitians of Canada (see Additional Learning Resources). Iron supplements may need to be started in the second trimester after morning sickness decreases, as some women find the iron difficult to tolerate. Taking the iron on an empty stomach improves absorption, but many women find it difficult to tolerate it without food. It should not be taken with coffee or tea or with high-calcium foods such as milk, as these foods decrease the absorption of calcium. Vitamin C (ascorbic acid) may enhance iron absorption (Mahan, & Raymond, 2017).

Iron comes in two forms, *heme* (found in red and organ meats) and *nonheme* (found in plant products). The body absorbs heme iron best. Nonheme plant foods that are high in iron include molasses, whole grains, iron-fortified cereals and breads, dried fruits, and dark green, leafy vegetables.

Folic acid

Folic acid or folate is a water-soluble B vitamin essential for the formation and maturation of both red and white blood cells in bone marrow. This vitamin can also reduce the incidence of neural tube defects (NTD) such as spina bifida and anencephaly *when taken before conception and during early pregnancy,* because the neural tube begins to close within the first month of gestation. Women who are considering pregnancy should consume 0.4 mg per day of folic acid in a multivitamin and should continue taking this amount throughout the pregnancy. Women who are at high risk to have a fetus with an NTD (e.g., diabetes, epilepsy, obesity, or a family history of NTD) should take 1.0 mg of folic acid before pregnancy and for the first 3 months of the pregnancy, at which time this amount can be decreased to 0.4 mg (Wilson & Genetics Committee, 2015). Food sources of folic acid are liver, lean beef, kidney and lima beans, dried beans, potatoes, whole-wheat bread, peanuts, and fresh, dark green, leafy vegetables.

Vitamins and minerals

Health Canada has established DRIs of specific vitamins. Although adequate intake of vitamins is essential during pregnancy, and supplements in the form of prenatal vitamins are routinely prescribed, excess intake of some vitamins can result in problems. For example, excess vitamin A can cause fetal anomalies and cardiac defects, and intake should not exceed 3 000 mcg/day. Vitamin D is important to enhance the absorption of calcium. Vitamin D needs sunlight to be metabolized properly. Vitamin D deficiency is more common in women who are overweight, if they live at a northern latitude (north of 37°N), or who have darker pigmented skin (Keenan-Lindsay, 2017b). Thus, Indigenous women are at risk of vitamin D deficiency and must be adequately counselled regarding this. Vitamin B_6 (pyridoxine) is often prescribed to reduce the nausea of pregnancy, but excess intake can cause numbness and muscle weakness. An adequate intake of zinc is required during pregnancy, especially in vegetarian and vegan diets, because whole grains decrease zinc absorption. Water-soluble vitamins are not stored in the body, so daily intake is important.

Most vitamins essential during pregnancy are part of the prenatal vitamin supplement that pregnant women take. Women should be referred for counselling from a registered dietitian if they have multiple gestations, an eating disorder, or a restricted diet such as vegan or vegetarian.

 Nutrition Considerations

Vitamin B_6 and ginger may be recommended to relieve the common discomfort of nausea during pregnancy.

Fluids

The pregnant woman should drink three litres of fluid each day, most of which should be water. Caffeinated drinks and drinks high in sugar should be limited. Caffeine acts as a diuretic, which counteracts some of the benefit of fluid intake. The woman should limit her daily caffeine consumption to 300 mg of caffeine daily (two cups of coffee or equivalent) (Government of Canada, 2017). Women at risk for insufficient amniotic fluid (oligohydramnios) have had successful outcomes by increasing their daily fluid intake (Gilbert, 2017).

Sodium

Sodium intake is essential for maintaining normal sodium levels in plasma, bone, brain, and muscle because both tissue and fluid expand during the prenatal period. Sodium should not be restricted during pregnancy, but foods high in sodium, such as lunchmeats and chips, or using additional salt at mealtime should be avoided during pregnancy.

Diuretics to rid the body of excess fluids are not recommended for the healthy pregnant woman because they reduce fluids necessary for the fetus. The added fluid during pregnancy supports the mother's increased blood volume.

Food Safety

Foodborne illness (food poisoning) is a serious problem in pregnant women because they have a weaker immune system to fight off the infection. Some infections, such as listeria, can travel to the placenta and can effect the growing fetus. If contacted in the first 3 months of pregnancy there is an increased risk of miscarriage and if later in pregnancy, the risk of preterm birth or stillbirth increases. Box 4.4 lists foods that should be avoided to decrease the risk of a foodborne illness. Also see *Safe Food Handling for Pregnant Women,* in Additional Learning Resources at the end of this chapter.

Box 4.4 Food to be Avoided During Pregnancy to Decrease Risk of Foodborne Illness

- Hot dogs straight from the package (cook first)
- Non-dried deli meats, such as bologna, roast beef, and turkey breast
- Raw or lightly cooked eggs, or egg products that contain raw eggs, including some salad dressings, cookie dough, cake batter, sauces, and drinks (like homemade eggnog)
- Raw or undercooked meat or poultry
- Raw seafood, such as sushi
- Raw oysters, clams, and mussels
- Refrigerated smoked seafood
- Raw or unpasteurized dairy products
- Unpasteurized and pasteurized soft cheeses, such as Brie and Camembert
- Unpasteurized and pasteurized semi-soft cheeses, such as Havarti
- All unpasteurized and pasteurized blue-veined cheeses
- Raw sprouts, such as alfalfa, clover, radish, and mung beans
- Refrigerated pâtés and meat spreads
- Unpasteurized fruit juice and cider

Source: Government of Canada. (2019). Food safety for pregnant women. Retrieved from https://www.canada.ca/en/health-canada/services/food-safety-vulnerable-populations/food-safety-pregnant-women.html

Special Nutrition Considerations

Pregnant adolescent

Inadequate weight gain and nutrient deficits are more likely to occur in the pregnant adolescent. The girl's continuing growth plus the growth of the fetus may make it difficult for her to meet her nutritional needs. In addition, a body image in which she sees herself as overweight at a time when appearance is a high priority, combined with peer pressure to eat "junk" foods, places the pregnant adolescent at special risk. The nurse and teen need to collaborate in order to help her find nutritious foods that allow her to fit in eating with her friends.

Even a moderate positive change in diet helps, and the nurse should give the teen positive reinforcement for her efforts. Fast foods with poor nutritional content may be the adolescent's foods of choice. However, the nurse can point out to the adolescent that many fast-food restaurants offer salads, chicken, tacos, baked potatoes, and pizza. These foods provide many important nutrients and still allow her to socialize with her peers at mealtimes.

Education regarding nutrition is necessary early in prenatal care to ensure a healthy mother and child. The younger and smaller teenage adolescent will need additional food in order to meet her own growth needs and those of the developing fetus. Their weight gain should be at the high end of the range for someone of a similar BMI.

Many communities offer programs for adolescents that provide social support, education about prenatal care, and nutritional advice. Adolescents often respond well to these peer groups. The nurse can refer these young women to programs such as the Canadian Prenatal Nutrition Program, which is a community-based program that provides support to improve the health and well-being of pregnant women, new mothers, and babies facing challenging life circumstances. The federal government also supports a program for Indigenous women living on reserves, called the Aboriginal Head Start on Reserve Program. The goal of this program is to support early intervention strategies to address the learning and developmental needs of young children living in Indigenous communities. One of the components of this program is ensuring adequate healthy nutrition.

Vegetarian or vegan diets

Women who follow vegetarian or vegan diets should focus on protein-rich foods, such as soy milk, tofu, tempeh, and beans, and they should supplement the diet with prenatal vitamins to meet the dietary needs of pregnancy. A vegan diet may require supplements of vitamin B_{12}, calcium, vitamin D, iron, and zinc because sources in plant foods may not be adequate. A registered dietitian may need to be consulted.

Pica

The craving for and ingestion of nonfood substances such as clay, dirt, starch, raw flour, and cracked ice is called *pica*. Ingestion of small amounts of these substances may be harmless, but frequent ingestion in large amounts may cause significant health problems. Starch can interfere with iron absorption and thus cause anemia, and large amounts of clay may cause fecal impaction. Any other nonfood substance ingested in large quantities may be harmful, because the necessary nutrients for healthy fetal development will not be available as the woman is too full to eat healthy food.

Pica is a difficult habit to break, and the nurse often becomes aware of the practice when discussing nutrition, food cravings, and myths with the pregnant woman. The nurse should educate the pregnant woman in a nonjudgemental way about the importance of good nutrition so the pica habit can be eliminated or at least decreased.

Lactose intolerance

Intolerance to lactose is caused by a deficiency of lactase, the enzyme that digests the sugar in milk. Some women cannot digest milk or milk products, which increases their risk for calcium deficiency. Indigenous people, Latin Americans, and persons of African, Middle Eastern, and Asian descent have a higher incidence of lactose intolerance than White people. Signs and symptoms of lactose intolerance include abdominal distention, flatulence, nausea, vomiting, and loose stools after ingestion of dairy products. In such cases, a daily calcium supplement can be taken.

Substitutes for dairy products are listed in the section on calcium. Lactose-intolerant women may tolerate cultured or fermented milk products such as aged cheese, buttermilk, and yogurt. The enzyme lactase (LactAid) is available in tablet form or as a liquid to add to milk.

Cultural preferences

People of varied cultures believe that specific foods include a dominant trait that affects the "humoral balance" in the body when ingested. Classification of food as "hot" or "cold" has nothing to do with the actual temperature. Examples of hot foods include peanuts, mangoes, ice cream, tea, cereal grains, and hard liquor. Examples of cold foods include milk, green leafy vegetables, freshwater fish, chicken, bananas, and citrus fruits. In this belief framework, several health problems are classified as hot or cold, requiring a cold or hot food for balance.

To support the nutritional needs of patients from various cultures, teachings must include an understanding these cultural beliefs and practices.

Gestational diabetes mellitus

GDM is first diagnosed during pregnancy (see Chapter 5). Women with GDM should be taught that food intake should be evenly distributed during the day among three meals and three snacks to maintain adequate and stable blood glucose levels. Pregnant diabetic women are susceptible to hypoglycemia (low blood glucose level) during the night, because the fetus continues to use glucose while the mother sleeps. It is suggested that the final bedtime snack be one of protein and a complex carbohydrate to provide more blood glucose stability. Referral to a registered dietitian may be required to provide appropriate dietary counselling for the pregnant woman with GDM. Glycemic control during the first and second trimesters is most important in preventing complications such as macrosomia (abnormally large newborn). Women with uncontrolled diabetes and high fasting blood glucose levels in the last trimester have an increased risk of stillbirth. See Chapter 5 for additional information concerning GDM.

EXERCISE DURING PREGNANCY

There is evidence that exercising during normal pregnancy is beneficial and has been associated with fewer newborn complications (e.g., large for gestational age). Many maternal health benefits are associated with exercise, including the following (Mottola, Davenport, Ruchat, et al., 2019):

- Decreased risk of pre-eclampsia
- Decreased gestational hypertension
- Decreased gestational diabetes
- Decreased rates of Caesarean birth
- Decreased rates of instrumental births
- Decreased urinary incontinence
- Improved mood and decreased depression
- Decreased severity of depressive symptoms
- Decreased total gestational weight gain
- Improved blood glucose
- Reduced feelings of stress
- Enhanced sleep
- Enhanced postpartum recovery
- Increased energy levels
- Reduced constipation
- Decreased back pain

The SOGC and the Canadian Society for Exercise Physiology (CSEP) recommend that pregnant women take part in 150 minutes of moderate-intensity physical activity per week and that it should be accumulated over a minimum of 3 days per week; however, being active every day is encouraged (Mottola et al., 2019). Pregnant women should incorporate a variety of aerobic and resistance training activities to achieve greater benefits.

Adding yoga, gentle stretching, or both may also be beneficial (Mottola et al., 2019). For pregnant women not currently meeting these guidelines, a progressive adjustment toward these goals is recommended (Mottola et al., 2019). Women who partake in vigorous exercise can continue this as long as they are able to tolerate the exercise. A guidepost for women indicating they are not overdoing it is being able to carry on a conversation throughout the activity. Range of motion (ROM) should not extend beyond prepregnancy abilities, as joint instability caused by hormonal changes may result in injury if the woman engages in deep flexion or extension of joints (Fig. 4.8). Women who are active in high-impact aerobics and running may need to consider decreasing these activities as the pregnancy progresses if they are no longer able to tolerate them. Activities to avoid include horseback riding, downhill skiing, ice hockey, gymnastics, or Olympic lifts (Mottola et al., 2019).

Women should be assessed using the PARmed-X for PREGNANCY, which is a guideline for health screening before participation in a prenatal fitness class or other exercise (see Online Resources at the end of the chapter). Practising safety measures is advisable because of the changes in the body's centre of gravity as the uterus enlarges. Women should be encouraged to start with a warm-up and end with a cool-down period. Liquid and caloric intake should be adjusted to meet the needs of pregnancy as well as the demands of exercise. Women who have complications or medical conditions such as hypertension or multiple gestations should consult a health care provider before engaging in any exercise program during pregnancy.

In healthy women, water aerobics can relieve edema because the hydrostatic pressure forces fluid into the circulation, stimulating glomerular filtration and excretion of water.

Elevated Body Temperature

Exercise can elevate the maternal temperature and result in decreased fetal circulation and cardiac function. Maternal body temperature should not exceed 38°C (100.4°F), which means that use of hot tubs and saunas should be avoided during pregnancy. Maternal heat exposure during the first trimester of pregnancy has been associated with NTDs and miscarriage. Exercise-related increases in body temperature are somewhat more easily tolerated because of the normal physiology of pregnancy as it pertains to increased peripheral blood flow, thermal inertia from weight gain, and peripheral venous pooling. Women should be instructed to drink lots of water before, during, and after physical activity to avoid overheating and dehydration. They should also refrain from being active outdoors on overly hot or humid days.

SUBSTANCE USE DURING PREGNANCY

Smoking

Smoking during pregnancy may increase the risk of vaginal bleeding, premature birth, placental abruption, placenta previa, and spontaneous abortion in the mother. The impact on the fetus includes increased perinatal mortality and lower birth weight. Exposure of the fetus to second-hand smoke may increase the risk of sudden infant death syndrome (SIDS), asthma, upper and lower respiratory tract illness, allergies, colic, and possible child behaviour issues including hyperactivity and aggression (Pregnets, 2012). Studies have shown a relationship between maternal smoking and psychiatric disorders in the offspring, such as schizophrenia and attenion-deficit/hperactivity disorder (ADHD) (Niemela, Sourander, Surcel, et al., 2016). Smoking during pregnancy also may affect the developing eggs of the female fetus, which in turn

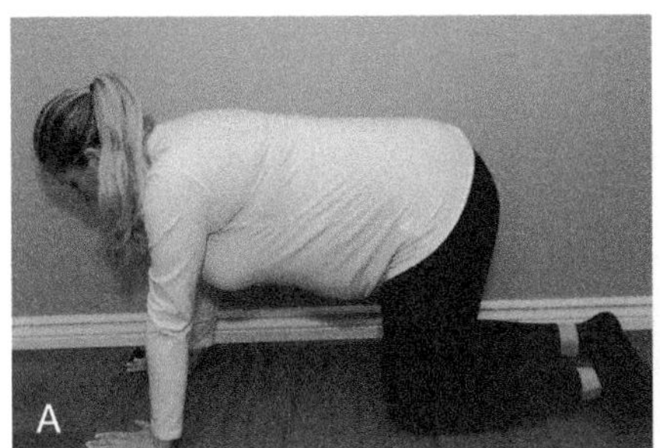

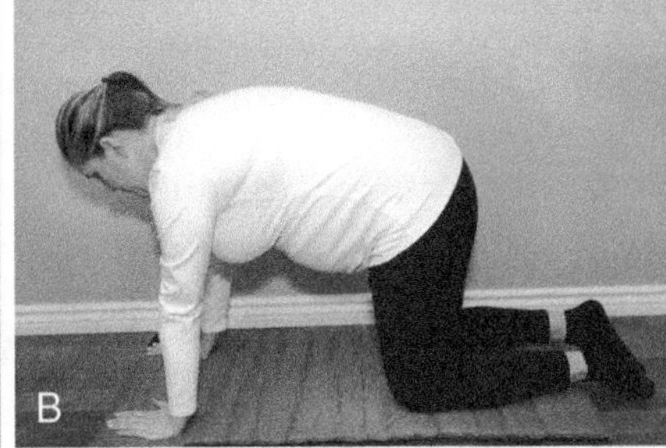

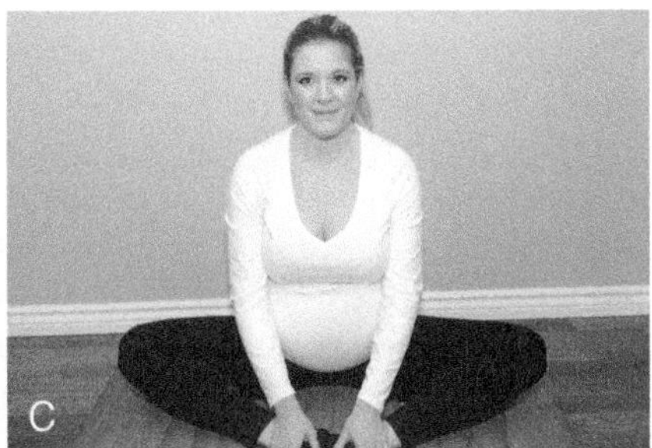

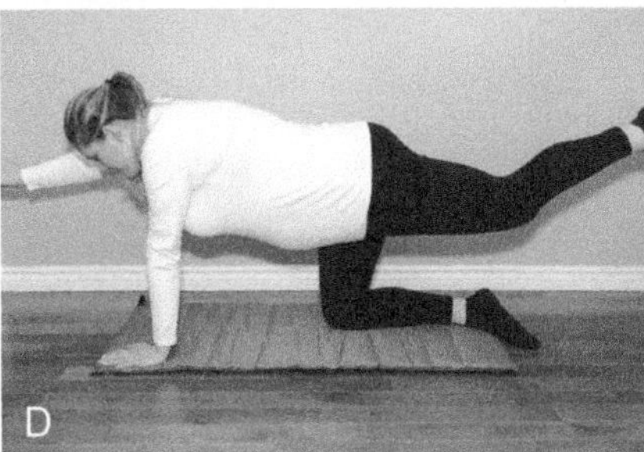

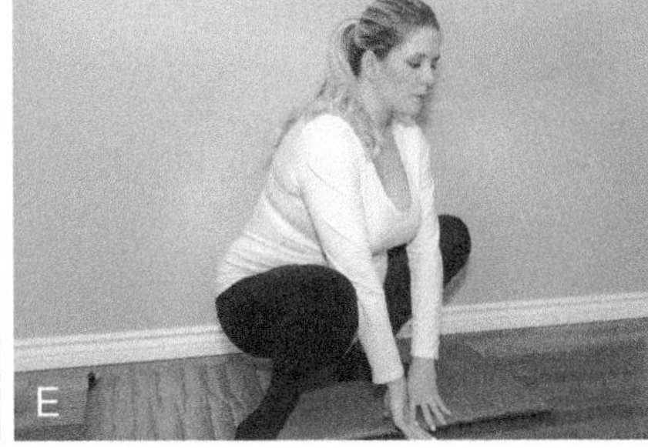

Fig. 4.8 Exercises during pregnancy. **A** and **B,** The pelvic tilt. **C,** Tailor sitting position. **D,** Proper stretch position. **E,** Proper squat position. (Courtesy of Sandy Matos)

will affect the grandchildren of the smoker (Halliday, 2017).

Pregnant women who smoke should be counselled regarding smoking cessation. Pregnancy and postpartum are opportune times to promote smoking cessation interventions, as women are often motivated to do so at these times. The use of a brief intervention such as the 4A's—*Ask*, *Advise*, *Assist*, and *Arrange*—has been shown to be effective in reducing tobacco consumption (Registered Nurses Association of Ontario [RNAO], 2017). The RNAO (2017) recommends treating or referring all pregnant or postpartum women at every encounter for intensive behavioural counselling for tobacco harm reduction, cessation, and relapse prevention, in conjunction with nicotine replacement therapy, on a case-by-case basis. Counselling should have an individualized, woman-centred approach that emphasizes the benefits of harm reduction or cessation for the woman and her fetus. Pharmacotherapy interventions (e.g., nicotine replacement therapy) should be considered in consultation with the primary health care provider (RNAO, 2017).

Cannabis

Cannabis use during pregnancy may also impact the neurodevelopment of the fetus, beyond the adverse health effects related to maternal and fetal exposure to smoking. The adverse effects caused by cannabis exposure can be lifelong; it is recommended that women who are pregnant or contemplating pregnancy abstain from cannabis use (Government of Canada, 2019d; SOGC, 2017). The use of marijuana during pregnancy is also associated with preterm birth (Leemaqz, Dekker, McCowan, et al., 2016).

Alcohol

Drinking alcohol during pregnancy can result in fetal alcohol spectrum disorder (FASD) in the newborn. *FASD* is a nondiagnostic term that describes a range of disabilities (physical, social, mental/emotional) that may affect people whose birth mothers drank alcohol while they were pregnant. Given the risk of FASD, the PHAC and the SOGC recommend that women not drink any alcohol during pregnancy, because it is not known what the safe limit is (Carson, Cox, Crane, et al., 2010; Government of Canada, 2019c). All pregnant women should be screened for alcohol consumption. Ideally, at-risk drinking should be identified before pregnancy, allowing for change in behaviour. Health care providers should create a safe environment for women to report alcohol consumption (Carson et al., 2010).

TRAVEL DURING PREGNANCY

Many women choose to maintain a normal lifestyle and travel during a normal pregnancy. For women with no risk factors, air travel is generally safe for the pregnant woman, up to 36 weeks' gestation. Because of the increased levels of clotting factors and plasma fibrinogen that normally occur during pregnancy, the woman should be counselled to avoid long periods of sitting, because there is an increased risk of developing thromboembolism (American College of Obstetrics and Gynecology [ACOG], 2018). She should also avoid locations that pose a high risk for exposure to infectious diseases.

Guidance concerning hand hygiene and dietary precautions to prevent diarrhea are essential. The woman should be advised to wear comfortable shoes and long-sleeved clothing and use mosquito nets around the bed in insect-prone areas. Insect repellants that contain the chemical abbreviated as *DEET* are usually safe after the first trimester. Sunblock should be applied as appropriate.

If a woman is travelling in a car she also needs to be encouraged to take frequent breaks to get out and walk. The wearing of seatbelts is important as any collision in a car can increase the risk of a *placental abruption* (placental separation), which can cause fetal death. Seat belts need to be placed low across the hip bones and the shoulder strap placed above the uterus.

IMMUNIZATIONS DURING PREGNANCY

Live-virus vaccines are contraindicated during pregnancy because of possible adverse effects on the fetus. Vaccines contraindicated during pregnancy include human papillomavirus (HPV), measles, mumps, and rubella (MMR), chicken pox, and the Sabin (oral) poliomyelitis vaccine (no longer used in the Canada). A woman is advised to avoid pregnancy for at least 1 month following an MMR immunization.

Vaccines consisting of killed viruses that may be administered during pregnancy include tetanus, diphtheria, recombinant hepatitis B, rabies vaccines, and most influenza vaccines (Watts, 2017). The influenza vaccine is recommended for pregnant women as there is higher risk of complications from the flu when pregnant (Government of Canada, 2018). If the pregnant woman is exposed to varicella, the varicella immune globulin can be given, ideally within 4 days, but up to 10 days of exposure (Centers for Disease Control and Prevention [CDC], 2018). Whooping cough (Tdap) vaccine is recommended after 26 weeks of gestation and has a protective effect on the fetus and newborn infant (Government of Canada, 2019a). Vaccines in vials with natural rubber tops should not be administered to women who are allergic to latex.

COMPLEMENTARY AND ALTERNATIVE HEALTH MODALITIES (CAHM) DURING PREGNANCY

Complementary therapy refers to non-Western medical therapy that is used *with* traditional or conventional (Western medical) therapy. An example would be the treatment of hypertension with medication *plus* relaxation or biofeedback techniques. **Alternative therapy** refers to unconventional or nontraditional therapy that

Table 4.4 **Common Herbs Contraindicated in Pregnancy and Lactation**

HERB	USE	CONTRAINDICATION
Aloe vera	Treats constipation Aids wound healing	Causes engorgement of pelvic vessels that can result in increased bleeding and spontaneous abortion; avoid use during pregnancy.
Garlic, ginkgo biloba	Decreases cholesterol Prevents motion sickness Lessens depression	Avoid use in pregnancy; do not use with other antiplatelet medications. Inhibits platelet activity and may cause bleeding.
St. John's wort	Lessens depression	Avoid exposure to sun. Increases tone of uterus. Use with caution in pregnancy. Interacts with alcohol, cold and flu medications, chocolate, aged cheese, beer, oral contraceptives, and SSRI drugs.
Angelica (dong quai)	Used for gynecological disorders, menstrual discomfort, and post-menopausal symptoms	Avoid use during pregnancy and breastfeeding because of uterine stimulation. Prolongs prothrombin time and causes poor glycemic control in diabetics.
Chamomile	Prevents urinary tract infections, gastrointestinal spasms; used for sedation	Avoid use in pregnancy. May cause abortion and teratogenic effects in fetus.
Feverfew	Used for migraine headache and menstrual problems	Avoid use during pregnancy and lactation. Can cause withdrawal symptoms.
Flax (flaxseed)	Used for bowel concerns	Contraindicated during pregnancy; potential for toxicity. Must be refrigerated.
Ginseng	Aids resistance to stress Used to increase stamina	Avoid use during pregnancy and lactation. May be toxic. CNS effects increase when used with coffee or tea. Interacts with St. John's wort and MAOIs.
Kava	Reduces anxiety and stress	Avoid use during pregnancy and lactation. May cause nutritional deficiencies or blood dyscrasias. May be toxic to the liver and cause CNS depression.
Ma huang (ephedra)	Used as CNS stimulant	Avoid use during pregnancy. Can cause cardiac dysrhythmia, urinary retention, and uterine contractions.
Nettle	Used as diuretic	Diuresis can cause electrolyte imbalance.
Saw palmetto	To improve urinary flow	Affects androgen activity and can harm fetus. Increases dyspepsia.

CNS, Central nervous system; MAOIs, monoamine oxidase inhibitors; SSRI, selective serotonin reuptake inhibitor.
Data from Rakel, D. (2018). *Integrative medicine* (4th ed.). Philadelphia: Elsevier; Skidmore-Roth, L. (2010). *Mosby's handbook of herbs & natural supplements* (4th ed.). St. Louis: Elsevier; Tsai, H., Lin, H., & Pickard, A. (2016). Evaluation of documented interactions and contraindications associated with herbs and dietary supplements in a systematic literature review. *International Journal of Clinical Practice, 66,* 1056–1058; Carlo, W. A., & Ambalavana, N. (2016). Maternal medication and toxin exposure and the fetus. In R. M. Kliegman, B. F. Stanton, J. St. Geme, et al. (Eds.), *Nelson textbook of pediatrics* (20th ed.). Philadelphia: Elsevier.

replaces conventional or traditional therapy. Women may view complementary and alternative health modalities and herbal remedies as "natural remedies" and therefore may not be aware of the possible dangers to themselves or their growing fetus. The woman may have been using herbal products before becoming pregnant, and the question of whether or not to continue during pregnancy, labour, and birth must be discussed with the health care provider. Table 4.4 lists commonly used herbs that are contraindicated for use during pregnancy.

In general, herbs that promote menstruation are contraindicated for use in pregnancy. Tannic acid and bran decrease the absorption of iron from foods, and thus tea with meals should be avoided during pregnancy in a woman with anemia. Health Canada has recommendations regarding use of herbal tea during pregnancy (Box 4.5).

Box 4.5 **Herbal Teas During Pregnancy**

Teas that are safe to consume in moderation (2–3 cups per day): citrus peel, ginger, lemon balm, orange peel, rose hip

Teas that are contraindicated during pregnancy: chamomile, aloe, coltsfoot, juniper berries, pennyroyal, buckthorn bark, comfrey, Labrador tea, sassafras, duck roots, lobelia and senna leaves

Sources: Government of Canada. (2017). Health Canada is advising Canadians about safe levels of caffeine consumption. Retrieved from: http://healthycanadians.gc.ca/recall-alert-rappel-avis/hc-sc/2017/63362a-eng.php ; Perth District Health Unit (n.d.). *Herbal teas and products*. Retrieved from http://www.pdhu.on.ca/health-topics/healthy-eating/pregnancy/herbal-teas/

COMMON DISCOMFORTS IN PREGNANCY

Various discomforts occur during normal pregnancy as a result of physiological changes. The nurse should teach the woman measures to relieve these discomforts (Table 4.5). The nurse should also explain signs

Table 4.5 Common Discomforts of Pregnancy

DISCOMFORT	INFLUENCING FACTORS	SELF-CARE MEASURES
First Trimester		
Nausea with or without vomiting ("morning sickness")	Cause is unknown, may be related to elevation in hormones, decrease in gastric motility, fatigue, emotional factors; usually does not last beyond 16 weeks If vomiting persists and the woman is unable to tolerate any food or fluid may lead to hyperemesis gravidarum	Avoid an empty stomach. Eat dry crackers or toast ½ to 1 hour before rising in the morning. Eat small, frequent meals. Avoid drinking fluids with meals (drink between meals). Ensure adequate fluid intake (2 L/day) Avoid greasy, odourous, spicy, or gas-forming foods. Increase vitamin B_6. Use ginger. Use acupressure wrist bands. Reduce strong odours (sniff lemons or limes or get fresh air). Medication may be ordered by healthcare provider if above methods fail.
Breast tenderness	Increased vascular supply and hypertrophy of breast tissue caused by estrogen and progesterone Results in tingling, fullness, and tenderness	Wear a supportive bra (to alleviate tingling and tenderness). Avoid applying soap on the nipples (to prevent cracking).
Urinary frequency	Pressure of growing uterus on bladder in both first and third trimesters Progesterone relaxes smooth muscles of bladder	Void when urge is felt (to prevent urinary stasis); increase fluid intake during day. Practice Kegel exercises.
Nasal stuffiness, epistaxis	Caused by edema of nasal tissues as a result of the high level of estrogen	Use saline nasal drops or room humidifiers.
Vaginal discharge (leukorrhea) (often noted throughout pregnancy)	Increased production of mucus by endocervical glands in response to elevated estrogen levels and increased blood supply to the pelvic area, causing white, viscid vaginal discharge	Wear cotton underwear. Avoid tight undergarments and pantyhose. Keep the perineal area clean and dry. Avoid douching. Wipe the perineal area from front to back after toileting. Contact healthcare provider if there is a change in colour, odour, or character of discharge.
Fatigue	Unexplained, but may be due to hormonal changes in early pregnancy; more prominent in early months of pregnancy	Try to get 8–10 hours of sleep. Take naps during the day if possible. Use relaxation techniques, meditation, or change of scenery. Eat a healthy diet.
Second and Third Trimesters		
Heartburn (pyrosis or acid indigestion)	Increased production of progesterone, causing relaxation of esophageal sphincter Regurgitation or backflow of gastric contents into the esophagus, causing burning sensation behind the sternum, burping, and sour tastes in mouth	Sit up for 30 minutes after eating a meal. Avoid gas-forming and greasy foods. Avoid overeating. Drink hot herbal tea. Primary healthcare provider may order antacids.
Constipation and flatulence (gas)	Increased levels of progesterone, causing bowel sluggishness with decreased water absorption (results in hardened stool) Pressure of enlarging uterus on intestine Diet, lack of exercise, and decreased fluids Iron supplements contributing to hardening of stools	Increase fluid intake (a minimum of 8 glasses of water per day) and roughage in diet. Exercise to stimulate peristalsis. Establish regular schedule for bowel movement. Do not take mineral oil or enemas. Consult healthcare provider about taking a stool softener.

Table 4.5 Common Discomforts of Pregnancy—cont'd

DISCOMFORT	INFLUENCING FACTORS	SELF-CARE MEASURES
Hemorrhoids	Varicosities (distended veins) of rectum caused by vascular enlargement of pelvis, straining from constipation, and descent of fetal head into pelvis May disappear after birth, when pressure is relieved	Use anaesthetic ointment, cool witch hazel pads, or warm sitz baths. Increase fibre in diet, and have regular bowel habits to avoid constipation.
Backache	Result of the spine's adaptation to posture changes as the uterus enlarges Enlarging uterus altering centre of gravity, resulting in lordosis (exaggeration of lumbosacral curve) and muscle strain	Maintain correct posture with head up and shoulders back; use good body mechanics. Avoid exaggerating lumbar curve. Squat rather than bending over when picking up objects (bend at knees, not waist). Wear low-heeled shoes to help maintain better posture. Do exercises such as tailor sitting (cross-legged), shoulder circling, and pelvic rocking. Rest; applying localized heat or ice may help. Physiotherapy, acupuncture, and massage may help.
Round ligament pain	Abdominal ligaments stretched by enlarging uterus, causing pain in lower abdomen after sudden movements	Avoid jerky or quick movements. Relieve cramping by bringing knees to chest; heat may help. Use good body mechanics.
Leg cramps	Pressure of uterus on nerves supplying lower extremities to legs Pointing toes when stretching legs Imbalance in the calcium/phosphorus ratio	Dorsiflex foot and straighten leg with downward pressure on knee or stand with feet flat on floor when cramps occur Evaluate diet and calcium intake.
Headache	Emotional tension and fatigue Increased circulatory blood volume and heart rate causing dilation and distention of cerebral vessels	Obtain emotional support. Practice relaxation exercises. Eat regular meals. Apply heat or cold Take over-the-counter analgesics (check with health-care provider). If headaches continue and become worse, report to healthcare provider (potential pre-eclampsia).
Varicose veins	Relaxation of smooth muscle in walls of veins caused by elevated progesterone Pressure of enlarging uterus causing pressure on veins, resulting in development of varicosities in vulva, rectum, and legs	Avoid lengthy standing or sitting, constrictive clothing, and bearing down during bowel movements. Walk frequently. Rest with legs elevated. Wear support stockings; avoid tight knee-highs. Exercise (to stimulate venous return). Relieve hemorrhoid swelling with warm sitz baths, local application of astringent compresses, or analgesic ointment.
Edema of feet and ankles	Circulatory congestion of lower extremities made worse with long standing or sitting	Elevate legs when sitting. Increase rest periods. Drink adequate fluid (natural diuretic). Avoid wearing constrictive clothing and prolonged standing or sitting.
Faintness and dizziness	Vasomotor instability or postural hypotension Standing for long periods with venous stasis in lower extremities	Avoid sudden changes in position, prolonged standing, and warm, crowded areas. Move slowly from rest position. Avoid hypoglycemia by eating 4–5 small meals daily. Lie on side when resting to avoid supine hypotension (pressure of uterus on vena cava). If symptoms do not lessen, report to healthcare provider.
Dyspnea	Later in pregnancy, caused by uterus rising into abdomen and pressing on diaphragm	Sleep with several pillows under head. Use deep chest breathing before going to sleep. Use proper posture while sitting or standing. Avoid exertion.

of problems that can be confused with the normal discomforts of pregnancy. Providing information written in the woman's primary language gives her a reference if she has questions later.

PSYCHOSOCIAL ADAPTATIONS TO PREGNANCY

Pregnancy creates a variety of confusing feelings for all members of the family, whether or not the pregnancy was planned. Early in the pregnancy, both parents may feel ambivalence about the pregnancy and being a parent. First-time parents may be anxious about how the infant will affect their relationship as a couple. Parents who already have a child may wonder how they can stretch their energies, love, and finances to another infant and how the infant will affect their older child or children. The nurse who provides prenatal care can help families work through this phase in their lives. Identifying and providing support for psychosocial concerns is essential to the positive outcome of pregnancy.

Identifying barriers to accessing care is a primary nursing responsibility. Financial problems, knowledge deficit concerning community resources, lack of transportation, and the need for day care for other children or older parents are examples of concerns that can be referred to a social service worker. Frequent housing relocation may indicate intimate partner violence or legal or financial difficulties that may need attention to ensure the woman is able to attend regular prenatal care. Nutritional needs should also be discussed. Tobacco and substance use should be assessed. Stress in the life of the mother should be reviewed, and appropriate referrals to mental health providers or educational programs should be made to reduce the levels of stress that can affect pregnancy outcome.

Impact on the Mother

In 1984, researcher Reva Rubin noted four maternal tasks that the woman accomplishes during pregnancy as she becomes a mother:

1. Seeking safe passage for herself and her fetus. This involves both obtaining health care by a professional and adhering to important cultural practices.
2. Securing acceptance of herself as a mother and for her fetus. Will her partner accept the infant? Does her partner or family have strong preferences for a child of a particular sex? Will the child be accepted even if he or she does not fit the ideal?
3. Learning to give of self and to receive the care and concern of others. The woman will never again be the same carefree woman she was before her infant's arrival. She depends on others in ways she has not experienced before.
4. Committing herself to the child as she progresses through pregnancy. Much of the emotional work of pregnancy involves protecting and nurturing the fetus.

Pregnancy is more than a physical event in a woman's life. During the months of pregnancy, she first accepts the fetus as part of herself and gradually moves to acceptance of the child as an independent person. She evolves from being a pregnant woman to being a mother. The woman's responses change as pregnancy progresses. These changes will be discussed here within the framework of the three trimesters of pregnancy.

First trimester

The woman may have difficulty believing that she is pregnant during early pregnancy because she may not feel different. If a home pregnancy test was positive, the woman often feels "more pregnant" after a professional confirms it. An early ultrasound can help the woman see the reality of the developing fetus within her. Women (and their partners) often show off their ultrasound photos just as they will show their infant pictures later.

Most women have conflicting feelings about being pregnant *(ambivalence)* during the early weeks. Many pregnancies are unplanned. The parents may have wanted to wait longer so they could achieve career or educational goals or to have longer spacing between children. Women who have planned their pregnancy or even worked hard to overcome infertility also feel ambivalence. They wonder if they have done the right thing and at the right time. Moreover, women often feel that they should not have these conflicting feelings. The nurse can help the woman to express these feelings of ambivalence and reassure her that they are normal.

The woman focuses on herself during this time. She feels many new physical sensations, but none of them seem related to a child. These physical changes and the higher hormone levels cause her emotions to be more unstable *(labile)*. The nurse can reassure the woman and her partner (who is often confused by her moods) about the cause of these fluctuations and that they are for the most part normal. Excessive anxiety is not normal and may need further assessment.

Second trimester

The fetus becomes real to the woman during the second trimester. Her weight increases, and the uterus becomes obvious as it ascends into the abdomen. If she has not already heard the fetal heartbeat or seen it beating on an ultrasound, the woman usually will have an opportunity to hear it early in the second trimester. She feels fetal movement, and this is a powerful aid in helping her to distinguish the fetus as a separate person from herself.

The second trimester is a more stable time of pregnancy during which most women have resolved many of their earlier feelings of ambivalence and begin to take on the role of an expectant mother. The woman becomes totally involved with her developing child and her changing body image *(narcissism)*. She often devotes a great deal of time to selecting just the right foods and the best environment to promote her health and that of her infant. She welcomes the solicitous concern of others when they caution her not to pick up a heavy package or work too hard. She begins to devote herself to the project of nurturing her fetus. The nurse can take advantage of her heightened interest in healthful living to teach good nutrition and other habits that can benefit the woman and her family long after the child is born.

The woman "tries on" the role of mother by learning what infants are like. She wants to hear stories of what she and her partner were like when they were infants. She often fantasizes about how her child will look and behave or what sex the child will be. The woman who previously has had a child undergoes a similar transition as she imagines what this specific child will be like and how the child will compare to any siblings.

The body changes resulting from pregnancy become evident during the second trimester. The woman may welcome them as a sign to all that her fetus is well protected and thriving (Fig. 4.9). However, these same changes may be unwelcome to some women, because they can be perceived as unattractive and can cause discomfort.

The body changes may alter her sexual relationship with her partner as well. Both partners may fear harming the developing fetus. Her increasing size, discomforts, and the other changes of pregnancy may make one or both partners have less interest in intercourse. The nurse can assure them that these changes are temporary and can help them explore other expressions of love and caring. The nurse can also discuss different positions for intercourse that may be more comfortable for the woman. Sexual interest is often decreased in the first trimester due to fatigue and breast discomfort and during the third trimester due to the discomfort. Sexual desire often increases in the second trimester.

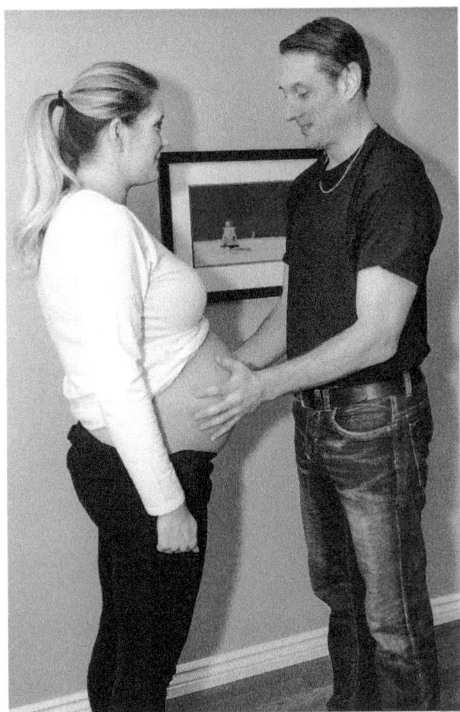

Fig. 4.9 The body changes during pregnancy are evident, and the woman may welcome them as a sign to all that her pregnancy is real and her fetus is thriving. (Courtesy of Sandy Matos)

Third trimester

As her body changes even more dramatically, the woman may alternate between feeling "absolutely beautiful and productive" and feeling "as big as a house and totally unloved" by her partner. These mood swings reflect her sense of increased vulnerability. She becomes introspective about the challenge of labour that is ahead and its outcome. Her moods may again be more labile.

The woman begins to separate herself from the pregnancy and to commit herself to the care of an infant. She and her partner begin making concrete preparations for the infant's arrival. They buy clothes and equipment the infant will need. Many take childbirth preparation classes. The woman's thinking gradually shifts from "I am pregnant" to "I am going to be a mother."

The minor discomforts of pregnancy become tiresome during the last weeks before birth, and the woman may feel that the pregnancy will never end. With the understanding and support of her family and health care providers, she can develop inner strength to accomplish the tasks of birth.

Impact on the Partner

Responses of partners vary widely. Some want to be fully involved in the physical and emotional aspects of pregnancy. Others prefer a management role, helping the woman adhere to recommendations of her health care provider. Some partners want to "be there" for the woman, but prefer not to take an active role during pregnancy or birth. Cultural values influence the role of partners, because pregnancy and birth are viewed exclusively as women's work in some cultures. The nurse should not assume that a partner is disinterested if they take a less active role in pregnancy and birth.

Partners go through phases similar to those of expectant mothers. Pregnancy is considered the beginning of a separate developmental stage called "growth and development of a parent" (see Table 13.4). Partners who do not anticipate changes specific to the normal event of pregnancy may be confused or concerned by new feelings or behaviours and the changes that occur in family dynamics.

For partners, the announcement phase begins when pregnancy is confirmed. Initially they may also have difficulty perceiving the fetus as real. Ambivalence and self-questioning about their readiness for parenthood are typical. Partners who attend prenatal appointments with the woman can see the fetus on ultrasound or hear the fetal heartbeat, making the child seem more like a real person. Acceptance of the pregnancy results in strengthening of the family support system and expansion of the social network. Rejection of the pregnancy may result in lack of communication and resentment.

The second phase of the partner's response is the adjustment phase. The partner may revise financial plans, become involved in planning the child's room or furniture, and actively listen to the fetal heartbeat and feel fetal movement (Fig. 4.10). Lack of adjustment may result in an increase in outside interests or the development of various symptoms in a struggle to regain the attention they may feel they have lost to the fetus.

The third phase of the partner's response is the focus phase, where active plans for participation in the labour process, birth, and change in lifestyle result in the partner "feeling like a parent." The nurse's role is to help the partner achieve positive outcomes in each phase.

The partner is often asked to provide emotional support to the pregnant woman while struggling themselves with the issue of parenthood. Too often, the partner receives the message that their only job is to support the pregnant woman rather than to be a parent who is also important and who has needs. The nurse should explore the partner's feelings and encourage them during prenatal appointments, childbirth preparation classes, and labour and birth. Both parents are trying to learn the role of being a parent.

Documenting the health history of the partner is also important because health concerns such as genetic disorders or chronic illness, or lifestyle practices such as substance or tobacco use can adversely affect the health of the mother, infant, and family. The father's blood type and Rh are also important when the mother is Rh negative.

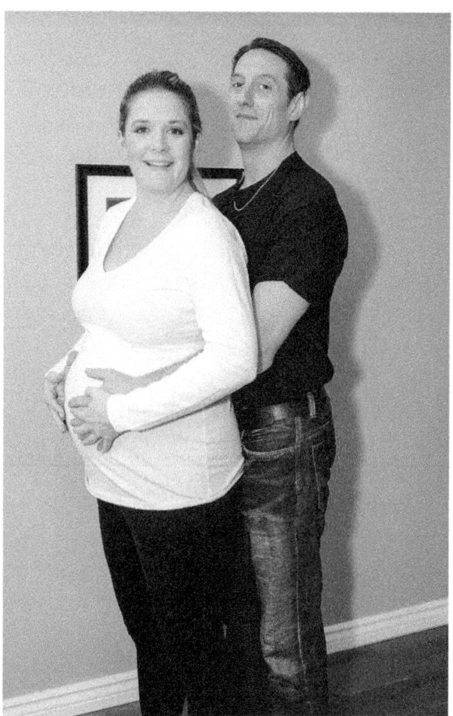

Fig. 4.10 The father begins to develop a relationship with the fetus as he hears the fetal heartbeat and feels fetal movement. (Courtesy of Sandy Matos)

Impact on the Pregnant Adolescent

Pregnant adolescents often have to struggle with feelings they find difficult to express. They may be fraught with conflict about how to handle the pregnancy. Initially, they must face the anxiety of breaking the news to their parents and to the father of the child. Denial of the pregnancy until late in gestation is not uncommon. There may be financial problems, shame, guilt, relationship problems with the infant's father, and feelings of low self-esteem. Alcoholism and substance use may also be a part of the complex picture.

The nurse must assess the teen's developmental and educational level and her support system to best provide care for her. A critical variable is the girl's age. Young adolescents may have difficulty considering the needs of others, such as the fetus. The very young adolescent is at increased risk for poor pregnancy outcomes; however, when prenatal care is initiated early and consistently the very young adolescent (and her newborn) is at no greater risk than older pregnant women (Watts, 2017). The nurse can help the adolescent girl to complete the developmental tasks of adolescence while assuming the new role of motherhood. Ideally, separate prenatal classes tailored to their needs help adolescent girls learn to care for themselves and assume the role of mother.

The nurse must consider the girl's developmental level and the priorities typical of her age, such as the importance of her peer group, focus on appearance, and possible difficulty considering the needs of others. The pregnant adolescent must cope with two of life's most stress-laden transitions simultaneously: adolescence and parenthood.

Impact on the Older Couple

Women who become pregnant for the first time after age 35 years are described as "elderly primips" or of "advanced maternal age," because they are at a later stage in their childbearing cycle, and they may face special problems during pregnancy and labour. Many factors contribute to the trend of postponing pregnancy until after age 35 years:

- Effective birth control alternatives
- Increasing career options for women
- High cost of living (delays childbearing until financial status is secure)
- Development of fertilization techniques to enable later pregnancy

The "older couple" usually adjusts readily to pregnancy, because they are often well educated, have achieved life experiences that enable them to cope with the realities of parenthood, and are ready for the lifestyle change. Although the older couple may adjust to the process of pregnancy and parenthood, they may find themselves "different" from their peers, and this can result in impaired social interaction. Concerns of the older parent relate to age and energy level as the child grows, confronting the issues of their own mortality, and child care requirements. Meeting financial needs of a college-age child at retirement is a special issue that may require discussion and planning. Some older mothers may be labelled "high-risk"; however, the pregnancy should be treated as normal unless problems are identified.

Advances in maternal care and birthing practices have decreased the risk of unfavourable pregnancy outcomes, although special problems do exist. Delayed childbearing (maternal age ≥35) is associated with increased obstetrical and perinatal complications, including increased risk of spontaneous abortion, ectopic pregnancy, placenta previa, pregestational diabetes, eclampsia, gestational hypertension, Caesarean birth, and induction of labour (Johnson, Tough, & SOGC Genetics Committee, 2012). There also may be an increased risk for multiple pregnancy if fertility drugs were used, which increase fetal risk. The greater risk of a congenital anomaly may result in special tests being offered during pregnancy (e.g., chorionic villi sampling, amniocentesis).

Impact on the Lone Mother

Whether an adolescent or a mature woman, the lone mother has special emotional needs. Some lone mothers can turn to their parents, siblings, or close friends for support. Women who do not have emotional support from significant others will have more difficulty completing the tasks of pregnancy. Their uncertainty in day-to-day living competes with mastering the emotional tasks of pregnancy.

Some lone mothers may have conceived by in vitro fertilization because of a strong desire to have a child. These women often are nearing the end of their childbearing years and perceive a "now or never" view of motherhood. Single women who plan pregnancies often prepare for the financial and lifestyle changes. Achieving social acceptance is not as difficult today as it was many years ago when single motherhood was taboo and was considered a distinct disgrace to the maternal family. The nurse should maintain a nonjudgemental attitude and assist the lone mother to successfully achieve the psychological tasks of pregnancy.

Impact on the Lone Father

The lone father may take an active interest in and financial responsibility for the child. The couple may plan marriage eventually, but it is often delayed. A lone father may provide emotional support for the mother during the pregnancy and birth. He often has strong feelings of surprise and accomplishment when he becomes aware of his partner's pregnancy. He may want to participate in plans for the child and take part in infant care after birth. However, the woman sometimes rejects his participation.

Impact on Grandparents

Prospective grandparents have different reactions to a woman's pregnancy as well. They may eagerly anticipate the announcement that a grandchild is on the way, or they may feel that they are not ready for the role of grandparent, which they equate with being old. The first grandchild often causes the most excitement in grandparents. Their reaction may be more subdued if they have several grandchildren, which may hurt the excited pregnant couple.

Grandparents have different ideas of how they will be involved with their grandchildren. Distance from the younger family dictates the degree of involvement for some. They may want to be involved fully in the plans for the infant and to help with child care, and they often travel a great distance to be there for the big event. Other grandparents want less involvement, because they welcome the freedom of a childless life again. Many grandparents are in their 40s and 50s, a time when their own career demands and care of their aging parents compete with their ability to be involved with grandchildren.

If grandparents and the expectant couple have similar views of their roles, little conflict is likely. However, disappointment and conflict may occur if the pregnant couple and the grandparents have significantly different expectations of their role and involvement. The nurse can help the young couple understand their parents' reactions and help them to negotiate solutions to conflicts that are satisfactory to both generations.

Impact on Siblings

Preparation for the arrival of a new baby in the family should start before the arrival of the newborn and before the sibling feels the change that a new family member brings (Fig. 4.11). All siblings will be affected

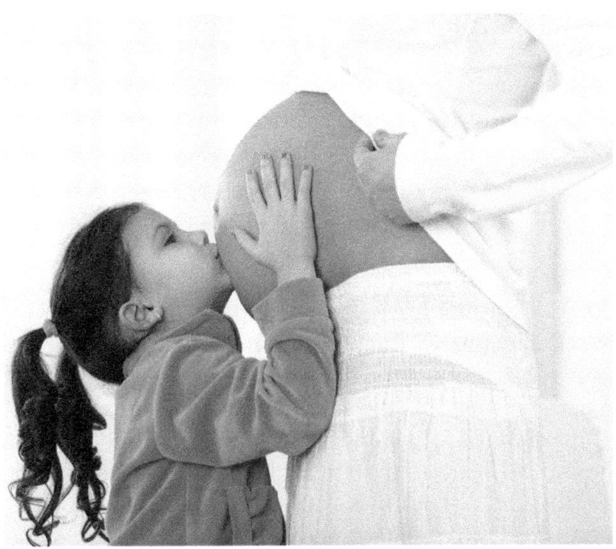

Fig. 4.11 A sibling begins to anticipate the birth of her brother. (Source: iStock.com/fotostorm)

by the arrival of a new baby into the family. Young children may lack resources to cope with their feelings of being displaced, and some behaviour changes may be expected. It is important to teach parents that regression to previous behaviours is a normal reaction that should not be punished. It is best to ignore negative behaviours and reward positive ones. Special time and efforts are needed to make siblings feel that they are loved as they were before.

THE INFLUENCE OF PRENATAL CARE ON THE ADULT HEALTH OF THE NEWBORN

Many newborns who survive today may not have survived just a few years ago. Early prenatal care, fetal surgery, use of prenatal glucocorticoids, technology, and neonatal intensive care have all played a role in increasing the positive outcome of pregnancy. Today, there is an increasing awareness of the "developmental origins of adult disease" (Ross & Desai, 2017). What happens to the fetus in utero affects the health of the newborn at birth as well as throughout their adult life. Prevention of many adult diseases may thus start in utero. *Epigenetics* is a genetic process that switches genes on and off in response to external or environmental factors. This "gestational programming" occurs during pregnancy and may be influenced by nutrition; hormones; the intrauterine environment, which includes maternal stress; environmental toxins; and medications, all of which permanently alter the physiology and gene expression in the offspring and may have significant effects on the health of the newborn and through to adult life (Ross & Desai, 2017). The role of maternal nutrition is known because of the impact of prenatal supplementation of folic acid, which has decreased the occurrence of NTDs in the newborn. There is also evidence that the risks of obesity in metabolic syndrome can be markedly influenced by early life events, particularly prenatal and newborn growth and environmental exposures (Ross & Desai, 2017). Research has shown that there is a relationship between birth weight and adult obesity, cardiovascular disease, and insulin resistance, with increasing risks for both low–birth weight and high–birth weight newborns (Ross & Desai, 2017). Therefore, prevention of low and high birth weight in utero is essential to reduce cardiovascular disease and strokes in adults.

The exposure of the fetus to multiple courses of glucocorticoid medications during pregnancy has shown a relationship to the development of cardiovascular and renal problems in adulthood and has a possible negative effect on the learning, cognitive, emotional, and behavioural problems in the older child (Ross & Desai, 2017). Thus maternal glucocorticoid use should be directed only at those infants most likely to benefit and those most likely to be born preterm (Ross & Desai, 2017). Caesarean birth has been associated with the development of obesity in the older child and subsequently into adulthood, possibly owing to the altered exposure to normal microbiota in the gut, which play a role in preventing obesity and its many complications (Yuan, Gaskins, Blaine, et al., 2016).

This knowledge of the impact of various prenatal exposures can lead to interventions initiated during pregnancy and at birth that can prevent specific adult-onset diseases later in life. A healthy diet and regular exercise during pregnancy improve insulin sensitivity, and the combination is more effective than reduction of calorie intake to prevent maternal obesity, which is associated with adult-onset cardiovascular disease.

Skin-to-skin contact immediately after any birth may enhance the gut microbes in the newborn as the infant is able to pick up the healthy maternal microbes and ingest them. Improvement of the fetal environment in utero may prevent long-term negative consequences in the developing fetus, in turn resulting in a reduction of noncommunicable diseases in adults in both developed and undeveloped countries and thus having a positive, long-term effect on global health. Thus, the focus of perinatal care must not only be the healthy outcome of mother and fetus at birth but also include efforts to reduce the long-term negative consequences of the prenatal environment that can impact prevention or reduction of adult-onset diseases for generations to come.

THE ROLE OF MICROBIOMES IN PREGNANCY

Recent research has revealed that the *microbiome* (the normal microbes in the individual's own body) also plays a role in maintaining pregnancy, preparation for labour, and the microbiome that is passed on to the newborn. For example, these microbiomes contribute to development of the acidic vaginal changes that occur during pregnancy that protect the woman from vaginal infections and may play a role in preventing preterm births. Research has shown that the microbes in the oral cavity of the mother are spread by the blood to the placenta and has explained the relationship between periodontal (dental) disease and preterm birth as being due to the influence of placental functions (Antony, Racusin, Aagaard, et al., 2017). The microbiomes in the breastmilk of mothers as well as on the mother's skin also contribute to the establishment of a gut microbiome in the newborn infant after birth and are important in the health of the infant as it grows and develops (Pannaraj, Li, Cerini, et al., 2017).

NURSING CARE DURING PREGNANCY

Table 4.6 describes the physiological and psychological changes that occur during pregnancy, the related signs and symptoms noted in the mother, and some suggested nursing interventions or teaching points that are appropriate to that phase. The rationales for a nursing care plan can be based on the information within this table. Teaching for the prenatal patient should include the risks of smoking and of alcohol and illicit drug use, as well as the advantages of breastfeeding and good nutrition during pregnancy.

Table 4.6 Physiological and Psychological Changes in Pregnancy, Nursing Interventions, and Teaching—cont'd

MATERNAL CHANGES	SIGNS AND SYMPTOMS	NURSING INTERVENTIONS AND TEACHING
Third Trimester		
Weight gain typically approaches 9–11 kg.	Patient tires easily.	Teach patient about the need for rest periods and organization of work.
Colostrum forms.	Colostrum may leak from breasts.	Teach patient care of nipples. Introduce nipple pads. Avoid nipple stimulation to prevent preterm labour if woman is at risk for preterm labour.
Maximum increase in cardiac output (increase in stroke volume) occurs.	Patient tires easily.	Teach patient of need for rest periods.
Edema of hands and wrists is possible.	Risk for carpal tunnel syndrome increases.	Teach patient warning signs of hypertensive disorder of pregnancy and assess water retention.
Uterus increases in size.	Pressure on stomach occurs. Pressure on diaphragm occurs. Venous congestion increases.	Discuss how to cope with decrease in appetite and shortness of breath. Teach patient how to avoid constipation and leg varicosities.
Awareness of Braxton Hicks contractions increases.	Fetal head may engage (uterus drops) (lightening).	Teach patient signs of labour and when to come to hospital. Offer tour of labour and birth unit.
Hormone levels increase.	Woman becomes self-centred and worries how she will manage labour.	Review labour management learned in prenatal classes. Discuss sibling care and support system.

PRENATAL EDUCATION

Prenatal education is an interactive process that requires input from the patient concerning individual needs and assessment of outcome: a healthy mother, child, and family unit. A plan for prenatal education is based on the desired outcome and includes the development of positive attitudes and perceptions, achievement of knowledge of facts, and learning of skills to cope with pregnancy, labour, and the transition into parenthood. Examples include the *perception* that pregnancy is a normal process that is enhanced by good nutrition and a healthy lifestyle; the *knowledge* to select the proper diet; and the learning of *skills* to perform exercises, breathing, and relaxation techniques to prepare the woman for labour.

Prenatal education should progress according to the nursing process, as follows:

- *Assess* the history and cultural needs.
- *Diagnose* the knowledge deficit.
- *Plan* the goals and priorities.
- *Outcomes identification* clarifies expected outcomes.
- *Teach* (implement) the facts and rationales.
- *Evaluate* the knowledge gained and the goals achieved.

Collecting data to assess cultural needs can be individualized to the patient. Teaching can occur in formal childbirth education classes or informally during a clinic visit. Every contact a nurse has with a pregnant patient is an opportunity for teaching.

Unfolding Case Study

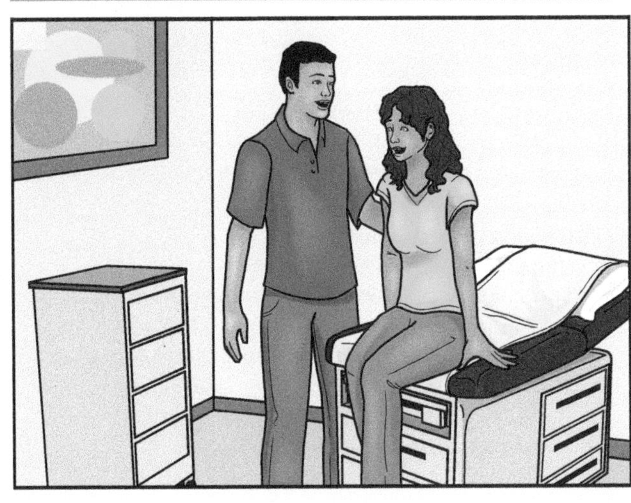

Tess is a 22-year-old woman who comes to the clinic with her partner, Luis, for a prenatal checkup on May 10, 2019. This is her first pregnancy, and they are both very excited about starting a family. Her physical exam is within normal limits, but she states she has nausea in the mornings. Her LMP was March 1, 2019.

QUESTIONS

1. What is Tess's GTPAL?
2. When is her expected date of birth?
3. How many weeks pregnant is she today?
4. What advice would the nurse give Tess concerning her symptoms of nausea?
5. Describe the probable signs of pregnancy that the health care provider will assess for during this first visit.
6. Tess says that she and her partner, Luis, want to take a last vacation together before starting their family responsibilities. They plan to leave on a 2-week trip to Europe starting November 30. What teaching should the nurse provide?

Get Ready for the Certification Exam!

Key Points

- Early and regular prenatal care promotes the healthiest possible outcome for mother and infant.
- The woman's estimated date of birth is calculated from her last menstrual period.
- The length of a pregnancy is 40 weeks after the last menstrual period. The expected date of birth can be determined by using Nägele's rule, although a first-trimester ultrasound is more accurate.
- Specific laboratory screening tests are performed during pregnancy to ensure a positive outcome for both mother and infant.
- Obstetrical ultrasound has been incorporated into routine care.
- Presumptive signs of pregnancy often have other causes. Probable signs more strongly suggest pregnancy but can still be caused by other conditions. Positive signs have no other cause except pregnancy. The three positive signs of pregnancy include detection of a fetal heartbeat, recognition of fetal movements by a trained examiner, and visualization of the embryo or fetus on ultrasound.
- The optimal weight gain during pregnancy for a woman with a normal body mass index is 11.5 to 16 kg (25 to 35 lb).
- The uterus undergoes the most obvious changes in pregnancy: It increases in weight from approximately 60 g to 1 000 g; it increases in capacity from about 10 mL to 5 000 mL. Pregnancy affects all body systems.
- The mother's blood volume is about 40 to 50% greater than her prepregnant volume to enable perfusion of the placenta and extramaternal tissues. Her blood pressure does not increase, because resistance to blood flow in her arteries decreases. The fluid portion of her blood increases more than the cellular portion, resulting in a pseudoanemia.
- The common discomforts of pregnancy occur as a result of hormonal, physiological, and anatomical changes normally occurring during pregnancy. The nurse should teach relief measures and explain abnormal signs to report to the health care provider.
- Supine hypotension, also known as aortocaval compression, may occur if the pregnant woman lies flat on her back. Turning to one side or placing a small pillow under one hip can help relieve this hypotension.
- To provide for the growth of the fetus and maternal tissues, the mother needs an extra snack per day. Important nutrients that must be increased are protein, iron, and folic acid.
- Adequate folic acid intake before conception of 0.4 mg/day can reduce the incidence of neural tube defects (NTD) such as anencephaly or spina bifida in the newborn in the low-risk woman. If the risk for an NTD is increased, women should take 1.0 mg/day before conception and for the first 3 months of pregnancy.
- Adequate vitamin intake is essential for optimum fetal development. However, excess vitamin intake can be toxic.
- Live-virus vaccines are contraindicated during pregnancy.
- The physiological changes during pregnancy influence the metabolism of ingested medications.
- Medications and herbal remedies ingested during pregnancy can affect fetal development.
- Partners should be included in prenatal care to the extent they and the woman desire.
- The health history of the partner is important, because genetics, illness, or lifestyle practices may affect the health of all members of the family.
- Adaptation to pregnancy occurs in the mother, the partner, and other family members. Prenatal care involves physical and psychological aspects and should be family centred.
- The intrauterine environment of the fetus can influence the adult health of the newborn.
- Normal microbes living in the individual mother's body play a role in maintaining pregnancy, preparing for labour, and establishing a microbiome in the gut of the newborn.
- Childbirth education includes formal classes and informal counselling. Education may include appropriate nutrition, healthy lifestyle, breathing and relaxation techniques for labour, the birth process, newborn care, safety issues, and parenting skills.

Additional Learning Resources

evolve Go to your Evolve website (http://evolve.elsevier.com/Canada/Leifer) for the following learning resources:

- Answer Key for Critical Thinking Questions
- Answer Key for Textbook Review Questions
- Audio Glossary
- Fluids & Electrolytes tutorial
- Interactive Review Questions
- Skills Performance Checklists
- Video clips and more!

Online Resources

- *Body Mass Index (BMI) Calculator:* https://www.diabetes.ca/diabetes-and-you/healthy-living-resources/weight-management/body-mass-index-bmi-calculator
- Canada's Food Guide: https://www.canada.ca/en/health-canada/services/canada-food-guides.html
- Dietitians of Canada—*How to Get More Iron:* http://www.unlockfood.ca/en/Articles/Vitamins-and-Minerals/How-To-Get-More-Iron.aspx?aliaspath=%2fen%2fArticles%2fNutrients-(vitamins-and-minerals)%2fHow-to-get-more-iron

- Government of Canada—*Healthy Eating and Pregnancy:* https://www.canada.ca/en/public-health/services/pregnancy/healthy-eating-pregnancy.html
- Health Canada—*Dietary Reference Intake Tables:* https://www.canada.ca/en/health-canada/services/food-nutrition/healthy-eating/dietary-reference-intakes/tables.html
- Health Canada—*Eating Well with Canada's Food Guide—First Nations, Inuit and Métis:* https://www.canada.ca/en/health-canada/services/food-nutrition/reports-publications/eating-well-canada-food-guide-first-nations-inuit-metis.html
- Health Canada—*Pregnancy Weight Gain Calculator:* http://www.hc-sc.gc.ca/fn-an/nutrition/prenatal/bmi/index-eng.php
- Health Canada: *Safe Food Handling for Pregnant Women:* http://healthycanadians.gc.ca/alt/pdf/eating-nutrition/healthy-eating-saine-alimentation/safety-salubrite/vulnerable-populations/pregnant-enceintes-eng.pdf
- Lamaze International: https://www.lamaze.org
- *PARmed-X for PREGNANCY:* http://www.csep.ca/cmfiles/publications/parq/parmed-xpreg.pdf
- Pregnets: *Smoking Cessation for Pregnant and Post-partum Women: A Toolkit for Healthcare Providers:* www.pregnets.org/dl/Toolkit.pdf
- SOGC—*Pregnancy Info:* https://www.pregnancyinfo.ca/

Review Questions

1. A woman arrives in the clinic for her prenatal visit. She states that she is currently 28 weeks pregnant with twins; has a 5-year-old son who was born at 39 weeks' gestation; and a 3-year-old daughter born at 34 weeks' gestation; and her last pregnancy terminated at 16 weeks' gestation. The nurse will interpret her obstetrical history as:
   a. $G_4\ T_2\ P_2\ A_1\ L_4$.
   b. $G_3\ T_2\ P_0\ A_1\ L_2$.
   c. $G_3\ T_1\ P_1\ A_1\ L_2$.
   d. $G_4\ T_1\ P_1\ A_1\ L_2$.
2. Exercise during pregnancy should be practiced to achieve which of the following goals?
   a. Improving obstetrical outcomes.
   b. Minimizing weight gain.
   c. Achieving weight loss.
   d. Improving physical fitness.
3. During a prenatal examination at 30 weeks of gestation, a woman is lying on her back on the examining table. She suddenly states she feels dizzy and feels faint. The most appropriate response of the nurse would be to:
   a. reassure the woman and take measures to reduce her anxiety level.
   b. offer the woman some orange juice or other rapidly absorbed form of glucose.
   c. place a pillow under the woman's head.
   d. turn the woman onto her side.
4. A woman being seen for her first prenatal care appointment has a positive home pregnancy test, and her chart shows her obstetrical history to be G4T3P0A1L2. The nurse would anticipate that:
   a. minimal prenatal teaching will be required because this is her fourth pregnancy.
   b. the woman will need help in planning the care of her other children at home during her labour and birth.
   c. the woman should experience minimal anxiety because she is familiar with the progress of pregnancy.
   d. this pregnancy will be considered high risk, and measures to reduce anxiety will be needed.
5. A woman's LMP was on April 1, 2019. She has been keeping her prenatal clinic appointments regularly but states she needs to alter the dates of a future appointment because she and her partner are going on an ocean cruise vacation for the New Year's celebration from December 30 through January 7, 2020. The best response of the nurse would be:
   a. "Prenatal visits can never be altered. Every visit is important."
   b. "Be sure to take antinausea medication when going on an ocean cruise."
   c. "Perhaps you might consider rescheduling your vacation earlier rather than the New Year's dates."
   d. "I will reschedule your clinic appointment to accommodate your vacation plans."
6. A nurse is explaining probable signs of pregnancy with a group of women. Probable signs of pregnancy include which of the following? (*Select all that apply.*)
   a. Fetal heart beat
   b. Abdominal enlargement
   c. Amenorrhea
   d. Braxton Hicks contractions
   e. Hegar sign

Critical Thinking Questions

1. A 35-year-old primipara woman in her twentieth week of pregnancy states that she does not want to drink the liquid glucose for the routine blood glucose screen because it does not taste good. She states that she is not a diabetic and does not think the test is necessary for her. What is the best response by the nurse?
2. A woman entering her second trimester of pregnancy states that she is noticing increasing stretch marks on her abdomen. She is afraid these marks will remain prominent after pregnancy, and she wants to go on a low-calorie diet to prevent her abdomen from becoming too large. What information should the nurse include in her teaching plan for this patient?

REFERENCES

Afshar, Y., & Han, S. (2017). Trimester zero: Pregnancy wellness begins before positive pregnancy test. *Contemporary Ob/Gyn, 62*(3), 28–34.

American College of Obstetrics and Gynecology. (2018). *Air travel during pregnancy*. Retrieved from: https://www.acog.org/Clinical-Guidance-and-Publications/Committee-Opinions/Committee-on-Obstetric-Practice/Air-Travel-During-Pregnancy.

Antony, K., Racusin, D., Aagaard, K., et al. (2017). Maternal physiology. In S. F. Gabbe, J. R. Niebyl, & J. L. Simpson (Eds.), *Obstetrics: Normal and problem pregnancies* (7th ed.). Philadelphia: Saunders.

Audibert, F., De Bie, I., Johnson, J., et al. (2017). No. 348-Joint SOGC-CCMG guideline: Update on prenatal screening for fetal aneuploidy, fetal anomalies, and adverse pregnancy outcomes. *Journal of Obstetricians and Gynecologists of Canada, 39*(9), 805–817.

Butt, K., Lim, K., & Diagnostic Imaging Committee. (2014). SOGC clinical practice guideline: Determination of gestational age by ultrasound. *Journal of Obstetricians and Gynecologists of Canada, 36*(2), 171–181.

Carson, G., Cox, L. V., Crane, J., et al. (2010). SOGC clinical practice guideline: Alcohol use and pregnancy: Consensus clinical guideline. *Journal of Obstetricians and Gynecologists of Canada, 32*(8), s1–s31.

Centers for Disease Control and Prevention (CDC). (2018). *Managing people at high risk for varicella*. Retrieved from: https://www.cdc.gov/chickenpox/hcp/persons-risk.html.

Gilbert, W. M. (2017). Amniotic fluid disorders. In S. F. Gabbe, J. R. Niebyl, & J. L. Simpson (Eds.), *Obstetrics: Normal and problem pregnancies* (7th ed.). Philadelphia: Saunders.

Government of Canada. (2017). *Health Canada is advising Canadians about safe levels of caffeine consumption*. Retrieved from: http://healthycanadians.gc.ca/recall-alert-rappel-avis/hc-sc/2017/63362a-eng.php.

Government of Canada. (2018). *Canadian immunization guide chapter on influenza and statement on seasonal influenza vaccine for 2017–2018*. Retrieved from: https://www.canada.ca/en/public-health/services/publications/healthy-living/canadian-immunization-guide-statement-seasonal-influenza-vaccine-2017-2018.html.

Government of Canada. (2019a). *Canadian immunization guide: Immunization in pregnancy and breastfeeding*. Retrieved from: https://www.canada.ca/en/public-health/services/publications/healthy-living/canadian-immunization-guide-part-3-vaccination-specific-populations/page-4-immunization-pregnancy-breastfeeding.html.

Government of Canada. (2019b). *Healthy eating and pregnancy*. Retrieved from: https://www.canada.ca/en/public-health/services/pregnancy/healthy-eating-pregnancy.html.

Government of Canada. (2019c). *The sensible guide to a healthy pregnancy: Alcohol and pregnancy*. Retrieved from: https://www.canada.ca/en/public-health/services/health-promotion/healthy-pregnancy/healthy-pregnancy-guide.html#a3.

Government of Canada. (2019d). *Thinking of using cannabis before or during pregnancy*. Retrieved from: https://www.canada.ca/en/health-canada/services/drugs-medication/cannabis/health-effects/before-during-pregnancy.html.

Halliday, A. (2017). *Smoking during pregnancy may affect eggs in the ovary of the developing fetus*. NYU Bristol News Release 4/27/17 and presented at International Meeting for Autism Research 2017.

Government of Canada. (2009). *Prenatal nutrition guidelines for health professionals—Fish and omega-3 fatty acids*. Retrieved from: https://www.canada.ca/en/health-canada/services/food-nutrition/reports-publications/nutrition-healthy-eating/prenatal-nutrition-guidelines-health-professionals-fish-omega-3-fatty-acids-2009.html.

Government of Canada. (2014). *Prenatal nutrition guidelines for health professionals: Gestational weight gain*. Retrieved from: https://www.canada.ca/en/health-canada/services/food-nutrition/healthy-eating/prenatal-nutrition/eating-well-being-active-towards-healthy-weight-gain-pregnancy-2010.html.

Herrman, J. W., Rogers, S., & Ehrenthal, D. B. (2012). Women's perceptions of centering pregnancy: A focus group study. *MCN: The American Journal of Maternal/Child Nursing, 37*(1), 19–26.

Johnson, J., Tough, S., & SOGC Genetics Committee. (2012). Delayed child-bearing. *Journal of Obstetrics & Gynaecology Canada, 34*(1), 80–93.

Keenan-Lindsay, L. (2017a). Anatomy and physiology of pregnancy. In S. Perry, M. Hockenberry, D. Lowdermilk, et al. (Eds.), *Maternal child nursing care in Canada* (2nd ed.). Toronto, ON: Elsevier.

Keenan-Lindsay, L. (2017b). Maternal and fetal nutrition. In S. Perry, M. Hockenberry, D. Lowdermilk, et al. (Eds.), *Maternal child nursing care in Canada* (2nd ed.). Toronto, ON: Elsevier.

Leemaqz, S., Dekker, G., McCowan, L., et al. (2016). Maternal marijuana use has independent effects on risk for spontaneous birth but not for other common pregnancy complications. *Reproductive Toxicology, 62*, 77–86. https://doi.org/10.1016/j.reprotox.2016.04.021.

Mahan, L. K., & Raymond, J. (2017). *Krause's food and the nutrition care process* (14th ed.). St. Louis: Elsevier.

Mottola, M. F., Davenport, M. H., Ruchat, S., et al. (2019). Canadian guideline for physical activity throughout pregnancy. *British Journal of Sports Medicine, 52*, 1339–1346.

Niemela, S., Sourander, A., Surcel, H. M., et al. (2016). Prenatal nicotine exposure and risk of schizophrenia among offspring in national birth cohort. *American Journal of Psychiatry, 173*(8), 799–806.

Pannaraj, P. S., Li, F., Cerini, C., et al. (2017). Association between breast milk bacterial communities and establishment and development of the infant gut microbiome. *Journal of the American Medical Association Pediatrics, 171*(7), 647–654. https://doi.org/10.1001/jamapediatrics.2017.0378.

Pregnets. (2012). *Smoking cessation for pregnant and postpartum women: A toolkit for healthcare providers*. Retrieved from: http://www.pregnets.org/dl/Toolkit.pdf.

Public Health Agency of Canada (PHAC). (2013). *Canadian guidelines on sexually transmitted infection—Management and treatment of specific syndromes: Vaginal discharge*. Retrieved from: https://www.canada.ca/en/public-health/services/infectious-diseases/sexual-health-sexually-transmitted-infections/canadian-guidelines/sexually-transmitted-infections/canadian-guidelines-sexually-transmitted-infections-26.html.

Ramsden, C. (2016). Breathing easier with fish oil: A new approach to preventing asthma? *New England Journal of Medicine, 375*, 2596.

Registered Nurses Association of Ontario (RNAO). (2017). *Integrating tobacco interventions into daily practice* (3rd ed.). Toronto, ON: Author.

Ross, M. G., & Desai, M. (2017). Developmental origins of adult health and disease. In S. G. Gabbe, J. R. Niebyl, J. L. Simpson, et al. (Eds.), *Obstetrics: Normal and problem pregnancies* (7th ed.). Philadelphia: Saunders.

Russell, S., & Mayberry, L. (2008). Pregnancy and oral health. *American Journal of Maternal Child Nursing, 33*(1), 32–37.

Society of Obstetricians and Gynaecologists of Canada (SOGC). (2017). *SOGC position statement: Marijuana use during pregnancy*. Retrieved from: https://sogc.org/files/letSOGCstatementCannabisUse.pdf.

Stotland, N. E., Bodnar, L. M., & Abrams, B. (2014). Maternal nutrition. In R. Resnik, R. Creasy, J. Iams, et al. (Eds.), *Creasy and Resnik's maternal-fetal medicine: Principles and practice* (7th ed.). Philadelphia: Saunders.

Thielen, K. (2012). Exploring the group prenatal care model: A critical review of the literature. *Journal of Perinatal Education, 21*(4), 209–218. https://doi.org/10.1891/1058-1243.21.4.209.

Watts, N. (2017). Nursing care during pregnancy. In S. Perry, M. Hockenberry, D. Lowdermilk, et al. (Eds.), *Maternal child nursing care in Canada* (2nd ed.). Toronto, ON: Elsevier.

Wilson, R. D., & Genetics Committee. (2015). Pre-conception folic acid and multivitamin supplementation for the primary and secondary prevention of neural tube defects and other folic acid–sensitive congenital anomalies. *Journal of Obstetrics & Gynaecology Canada, 37*(6), 534–549.

Yuan, C., Gaskins, A. J., Blaine, A. I., et al. (2016). Cesarean birth and risk of offspring obesity in childhood, adolescence and early adulthood. *Journal of American Medical Association Pediatrics, 170*(11), e162385.

Nursing Care of Women With Complications During Pregnancy

5

Nancy Watts

http://evolve.elsevier.com/Canada/Leifer

Objectives

1. Define each key term listed.
2. Explain the purpose of fetal diagnostic tests offered during pregnancy.
3. Identify health promotion strategies during pregnancy to decrease risks for antepartum complications.
4. Describe possible prenatal complications, their treatment options, and associated nursing care.
5. Discuss the nursing care and management of pregnancies complicated by concurrent medical conditions.
6. Describe environmental hazards that may adversely affect the outcome of pregnancy.
7. Describe care for the pregnant trauma victim.
8. Describe psychosocial nursing interventions for a woman with a high-risk pregnancy and her family.

Key Terms

abortion
age of viability
cerclage (sĕr-KLĂHZH)
disseminated intravascular coagulation (DIC)
eclampsia (ĕ-KLĂMP-sē-ă)
gestational diabetes mellitus (GDM)
hemolytic disease of the newborn
hydramnios (hī-DRĂM-nē-ŏs)
incompetent cervix (ĭn-KŎM-pă-tănt SŬR-vĭkz)
isoimmunization (ī-sō-ĭm-myū-nĭ-ZĀ-shŭn)
pre-eclampsia (prē-ĕ-KLĂMP-sē-ă)
preterm labour
products of conception (POC)
teratogen (TĔR-ă-tō-jĕn)
tonic-clonic seizures

Many women have pregnancies that are free of complications. Some, however, have complications that threaten their well-being and that of their babies. Many problems can be anticipated in the course of prenatal care and made less severe or possibly prevented. Others occur acutely and without warning.

Women who have no prenatal care or begin care late in pregnancy may have complications that are more severe because they were not identified earlier. Danger signs that should be taught to every pregnant woman and reinforced at each prenatal visit are listed in the Patient Teaching box. The woman should be taught to notify her healthcare provider if any of these danger signs occur. A *high-risk pregnancy* is defined as one in which the health of the mother or fetus is in jeopardy.

The causes of high-risk pregnancies usually include the following characteristics:

- They relate to the pregnancy itself.
- They occur because the woman has a medical condition or injury that complicates the pregnancy.
- They result from environmental hazards that affect the mother or her fetus.
- They arise from maternal behaviours or lifestyles that have a negative effect on the mother or fetus.

Early and consistent assessment for risk factors during prenatal visits and developing a plan for ongoing care are essential for a positive outcome for the mother and fetus.

Nursing Tip

The nurse should teach the woman to report promptly any danger signs that occur during pregnancy.

Patient Teaching

Danger Signs in Pregnancy

The nurse should teach the woman to report any of the following signs if they occur during pregnancy and to seek treatment promptly:

- A sudden gush of fluid from the vagina prior to 37 weeks' gestation
- Vaginal bleeding
- Abdominal pain
- Decreased or absent fetal movements ("kick count") (after 26–28 weeks)
- Persistent vomiting
- Epigastric pain
- Significant edema of face and hands
- Severe, persistent headache
- Blurred vision or dizziness
- Chills with fever greater than 38.0°C (100.4°F)
- Painful urination or reduced urine output
- Feeling something is "just not right"

ASSESSMENT OF FETAL HEALTH

Technical advances have enabled the management of high-risk pregnancies so that the health of both the mother and the fetus is optimized through either a termination of the pregnancy or the family being offered information and support for continuing the pregnancy if that is their desire. Various tests can be used prenatally to assess the well-being of the fetus. Nursing responsibilities during the assessment of fetal health include preparing the patient, explaining the reason for the test, and clarifying and interpreting the results in collaboration with other healthcare providers. The nurse can provide the psychosocial support that can allay or reduce parental anxiety. Fig. 5.1 shows an amniocentesis and Table 5.1 reviews common diagnostic tests used to assess the status of the fetus. Fetal assessment techniques used during labour are discussed in Chapter 6.

The future of fetal assessment, particularly for rural and northern, less populated areas, is in the ability to transmit images to health care centres where specialists can review and provide advice to those nearby. This process may facilitate keeping the woman and family together rather than forcing her to travel long distances to obtain testing. Telemedicine, a growing field, is a specialized technology used in "virtual prenatal care." Noninvasive prenatal assessment technologies, reviewed in Table 5.1, aid in reducing risks to the fetus and increase the accuracy of assessments and intervention for a positive birth outcome. Such technologies continue to be researched and developed.

PREGNANCY-RELATED COMPLICATIONS

HYPEREMESIS GRAVIDARUM

Nausea and vomiting are the most common conditions in pregnancy, affecting 50 to 80% of women (Campbell, Rowe, Azzam et al., 2016). Dietary suggestions may be helpful in relieving symptoms, as well as complementary medicine such as acupressure, mindfulness-based cognitive therapy, and ginger supplements (Campbell et al., 2016). While mild nausea and vomiting are common during pregnancy (discussed in Chapter 4), women with hyperemesis gravidarum have excessive nausea and vomiting that can significantly interfere with food intake and fluid balance as well as work, family, and every aspect of these women's lives. Fetal growth may be restricted, resulting in a low-birth-weight infant. Dehydration impairs perfusion of the placenta, reducing the delivery of blood oxygen and nutrients to the fetus. Hyperemesis gravidarum is present in 0.5 to 2% of women, usually between 10 and 20 weeks of pregnancy (Fletcher, Waterman, Nelson, et al., 2015).

Manifestations

Hyperemesis gravidarum differs from "morning sickness" of pregnancy in one or more of the following ways:

- Persistent nausea and vomiting, often with complete inability to retain food and fluids
- Significant weight loss (more than 5% of prepregnant weight)
- Dehydration as evidenced by a dry tongue and mucous membranes, decreased turgor (elasticity) of the skin, decreased urinary volume with increased concentration, and a high serum hematocrit level
- Electrolyte and acid–base imbalances
- Ketonuria
- Psychological factors such as unusual stress, emotional immaturity, passivity, or ambivalence about the pregnancy

Most cases resolve by 20 weeks of pregnancy, but in more severe cases (10–45%) affected women continue to have severe nausea and vomiting until giving birth (Fletcher et al., 2015).

Treatment

The healthcare provider should rule out other causes for the excessive nausea and vomiting, such as gastroenteritis or liver, gallbladder, or pancreatic disorders, before making this diagnosis. The medical treatment for hyperemesis gravidarum is to correct dehydration and electrolyte or acid–base imbalances with oral or intravenous (IV) fluids. Antiemetic drugs such as doxylamine/pyridoxine (Diclectin) can be prescribed (Campbell et al., 2016). Other medications given include metoclopramide (Reglan) and phenothiazines. Ondansetron (Zofran) can be used in pregnancy when other antiemetics do not work (Campbell et al., 2016). Severe cases necessitate hospitalization and total parenteral nutrition. The condition is self-limiting in most women, although it is quite distressing to the woman and her family.

Nursing Care

Nursing care focuses on patient teaching because most care occurs in the home. The woman should be taught how to reduce factors that trigger nausea and vomiting, such as avoiding food odours.

Accurate intake and output and daily weight records are kept to assess fluid balance. Frequent, small amounts of food and fluid keep the stomach from becoming too full, which can trigger vomiting and decrease gastric distention. Easily digested carbohydrates, such as crackers or baked potatoes, are tolerated best. Foods with strong odours should be eliminated from the diet if possible. Sitting upright after meals reduces gastric reflux (backflow) into the esophagus.

The nurse needs to be aware of the effect of this diagnosis on the woman and her family, offer support and encouragement, and collaborate with them

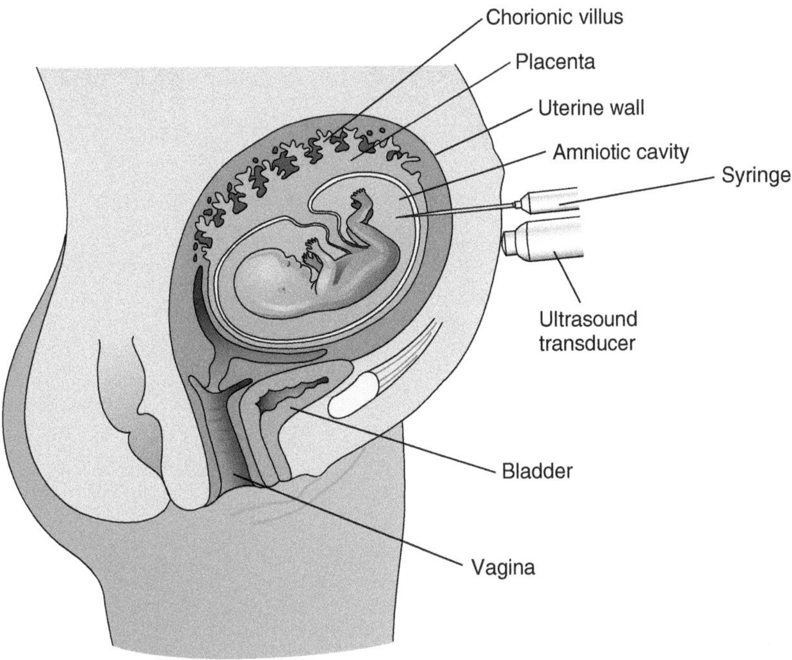

Fig. 5.1 Amniocentesis. An ultrasound transducer on the abdomen ensures needle placement away from the body of the fetus and the placenta. A needle is inserted into the amniotic cavity, and a sample of amniotic fluid is collected for laboratory examination and fetal assessment. (From Moore K. L., Persaud, T. V. N., & Torchia, M. G. [2016]. *The developing human: Clinically oriented embryology* [10th ed.]. Philadelphia: Saunders.)

Table 5.1 Fetal Diagnostic Tests

TEST	DESCRIPTION	USE(S) DURING PREGNANCY
Ultrasound examination	High-frequency sound waves are used to visualize structures within the body; the examination may use a transvaginal probe or an abdominal transducer. Abdominal ultrasound during early pregnancy requires a full bladder for proper visualization (have the woman drink 1–2 litres of water before the examination). A transvaginal ultrasound requires an empty bladder. A targeted comprehensive ultrasound detects specific anomalies. A first-trimester combined screen of ultrasound for nuchal translucency and a maternal blood test detects chromosomal anomalies at 11 to 14 weeks. A transvaginal ultrasound in the third trimester is used to determine cervix length to detect risk of preterm birth if there is a history of preterm birth. A first-trimester ultrasound can determine the gestational age (estimated date of birth [EDB]).	Visualize a gestational sac in early pregnancy to confirm the pregnancy. Identify the site of implantation (uterine or ectopic). Verify fetal viability or death. Identify a multifetal pregnancy, such as twins or triplets. Diagnose some fetal structural abnormalities. Guide procedures, such as chorionic villus sampling, amniocentesis, or percutaneous umbilical blood sampling. Locate the placenta. Determine the amount of amniotic fluid. Observe fetal movements. Determine EDB. Between 7 and 14 weeks the crown–rump length can indicate fetal age. After 12 weeks, the biparietal diameter of the fetus and the femur length provide an accurate estimation of fetal age.
Amniotic fluid volume (AFV)	This ultrasound scan measures the amniotic fluid pockets in all four quadrants surrounding the mother's umbilicus and produces an amniotic fluid index (AFI).	From 5 to 19 cm is considered normal; <5 cm is known as *oligohydramnios* (insufficient amniotic fluid) and is associated with growth restriction and decreased placental function (occasionally also with fetal renal abnormalities). A measurement >30 cm is *polyhydramnios* (excess amniotic fluid) and is associated with neural tube defects, gastrointestinal obstruction, and fetal hydrops.

Continued

Table 5.1 **Fetal Diagnostic Tests—cont'd**

TEST	DESCRIPTION	USE(S) DURING PREGNANCY
Magnetic resonance imaging (MRI)	This imaging technique provides a noninvasive radiological view of fetal structures, including the placenta.	Used when there is high suspicion of an anomaly.
Kick count/Fetal movement counting	Maternal awareness and understanding of fetal movement for all women beginning at 26–28 weeks is important to ensure fetal health. Decreased placental perfusion and fetal acidosis are associated with decreased movements. Counting movements daily is encouraged for women at high risk for complications (e.g., hypertension and cardiac conditions) (Liston, Sawchuck, & Young, 2018).	While lying on her side, 1 hour after a meal (usually an active time for fetal movement), the pregnant woman counts fetal movements (minimum of 6 in 2 hours). A daily fetal movement record is kept for women at high risk for adverse perinatal outcomes. The sleep cycle of the fetus should be considered when selecting a time to evaluate fetal movement.
Doppler ultrasound blood flow assessment	This assessment uses high-frequency sound waves to study the flow of blood through vessels. Colour doppler can detect the speed and direction of blood flow within fetal vessels (i.e., the umbilical artery).	Determine adequacy of blood flow through the placenta and umbilical cord vessels in women in whom it is likely to be impaired (such as those at risk for having a fetus with intrauterine growth restriction) (Liston et al., 2018).
First-trimester screening (FTS)	This test is done at 11–13 weeks of pregnancy and includes a nuchal translucency ultrasound combined with a single blood test. This blood test provides results sooner. If the patient does not present until 14–15 weeks in pregnancy, there is still an option for serum screening, but the nuchal translucency cannot be considered.	Identify high levels of two pregnancy-specific substances, pregnancy-associated plasma protein-A (PAPP-A) and human chorionic gonadotropin (hCG), which are associated with open defects, such as spina bifida (open spine), anencephaly (incomplete development of the skull and brain), or gastroschisis (open abdominal cavity). Identify low levels, which are associated with chromosome abnormalities or gestational trophoblastic disease (hydatidiform mole).
Chorionic villus sampling (CVS)	Sampling consists of obtaining a small part of the developing placenta to analyze fetal cells at 10 to 12 weeks of gestation.	Identify chromosome abnormalities or other defects that can be determined by analysis of cells. Results of chromosome studies are available 24 to 48 hours later. Cannot be used to determine spina bifida or anencephaly (see FTS). Higher rate of spontaneous abortion after procedure than after amniocentesis. Reports of limb reduction defects in newborns. Rh_0(D) immune globulin is given to the Rh-negative woman.
Cell free DNA (noninvasive prenatal testing [NIPT])	This is a test of maternal blood.	Screening test to identify chromosomal anomalies. If woman screens positive, further testing must be done (Liston et al., 2018). Maternal use of anticoagulants or aspirin can decrease availability of cell free DNA in maternal circulation (Nitsche, Barnard, Conran, et al., 2017).
Amniocentesis	This procedure consists of insertion of a thin needle through the abdominal and uterine walls (guided by ultrasound) to obtain a sample of amniotic fluid, which contains cast-off fetal cells and various other fetal products (see Fig. 5.1). Standard genetic amniocentesis is done at 15–17 weeks of gestation.	*Early pregnancy:* Identify chromosome abnormalities and biochemical disorders (such as Tay-Sachs disease). *Late pregnancy:* Identify severity of maternal–fetal blood incompatibility and assess fetal lung maturity. Rh_0(D) immune globulin is given to the Rh-negative woman.

Table 5.1 **Fetal Diagnostic Tests—cont'd**

TEST	DESCRIPTION	USE(S) DURING PREGNANCY
Non–stress test (NST)	The test comprises evaluation with an electronic fetal monitor of the fetal heart rate (FHR). Two accelerations of at least 15 beats/min lasting 15 seconds in a 20-minute period and usual fetal movement patterns is considered normal in a fetus greater than 32 weeks. If the test is normal, it should be classified and documented. If atypical or abnormal, a health care-provider should review the test results.	Identify fetal compromise in conditions associated with decreased placental function, such as hypertension, diabetes mellitus, or post-term gestation. Adequate accelerations of the FHR are normal, demonstrating that the placenta is functioning properly and the fetus is well oxygenated.
Contraction stress test (CST)	This test is an evaluation of the FHR response to mild uterine contractions, by using an electronic fetal monitor; contractions may be induced by a low dose of oxytocin given as an intravenous infusion. The woman must have at least three contractions at least 40 seconds in duration in a 10-minute period for interpretation of the CST. This test must be done in a setting that can accommodate an emergency Caesarean birth if needed. It should not be performed if vaginal birth is contraindicated (Liston et al., 2018).	Purposes are the same as for the NST; the CST may be done if the NST results are atypical or abnormal (the FHR does not accelerate). Normal CST results mean there are normal characteristics in the fetal monitor strip such as baseline and variability and the fetus can probably tolerate labour.
Biophysical profile (BPP)	This profile consists of a group of five fetal assessments: FHR and reactivity (the NST), and four assessments done by ultrasound: fetal breathing movements, fetal body movements, fetal tone e.g., (closure of the hand), and the volume of amniotic fluid (AFI). Some centres omit the NST, and others assess only the NST and AFI.	Identify reduced fetal oxygenation in conditions associated with decreased placental function, but with greater precision than the NST alone. As fetal hypoxia gradually increases, FHR changes occur first, followed by cessation of fetal breathing movement, gross body movements, and finally loss of fetal tone. AFV is reduced when placental function is decreased (shows pockets of low or absent amniotic fluid).
Percutaneous umbilical blood sampling (PUBS)	Procedure serves to obtain a fetal blood sample from a placental vessel or from the umbilical cord; this may be used to give a blood transfusion to an anemic fetus.	Identify fetal conditions that can be diagnosed only with a blood sample. Blood transfusion may be necessary for fetal anemia caused by maternal–fetal blood incompatibility, placenta previa, or placental abruption.
Tests of fetal lung maturity	This test uses a sample of amniotic fluid (obtained by amniocentesis) to determine substances that indicate fetal lungs are mature enough to adapt to extrauterine life.	Evaluate whether the fetus is likely to have respiratory complications in adapting to extrauterine life. May be done to determine whether the fetal lungs are mature before performing an elective Caesarean birth or inducing labour if the gestational age is questionable. Also used to evaluate whether the fetus should be born immediately or allowed to mature further when the membranes rupture and the gestation is at <37 weeks or if the gestation is questionable.
Lecithin/sphingomyelin (L/S) ratio	A 2:1 ratio indicates fetal lung maturity (3:1 ratio desirable for diabetic mother); fluid is usually obtained by amniocentesis.	

Data from Liston, R., Sawchuck, D., Young, D., et al. (2018). No. 197a-Fetal health surveillance: Antepartum consensus guideline. *Journal of Obstetrics and Gynaecology Canada, 40*(4), e251–e271; Nitsche, J., Barnard, A., Conrad, S., & Onslow, M. (2017). Effect of maternal heparin/aspirin on the amount of cell free DNA in maternal circulation. *American Journal of Obstetricians and Gynecologists, 216*(1), S20, Supplement.

to determine helpful strategies. Women with this diagnosis have described their fears regarding leaving the comfort of their home because they may become nauseated or have to vomit; their inability to care for themselves or their families; and their concerns about the inability to work. While in the past, stress and depression were thought to be the cause of hyperemesis gravidarum, it is now understood to be multifactorial, and many emotional responses are recognized as coming from the condition rather than being the cause (Dean, Bannigan, & Marsden, 2018). The nurse should provide support by listening to the woman's feelings about pregnancy, child-rearing, and living with constant nausea. Involving other resources, during a hospital admission or as an outpatient in the clinic, such as social work or mental health counselors may be helpful if done in collaboration with the patient. If the patient is in the hospital the nurse can help her explore how she can continue to communicate with her family. The nurse may also help her use community resources for hydration and medication.

BLEEDING DISORDER OF EARLY PREGNANCY

Several bleeding disorders can complicate early pregnancy, such as spontaneous abortion (miscarriage) (Fig. 5.2), ectopic pregnancy (Fig. 5.3), or hydatidiform mole (Fig. 5.4). Maternal blood loss can decrease the oxygen-carrying capacity of the blood, resulting in fetal hypoxia, and places the fetus at risk.

Abortion

Abortion is the spontaneous (miscarriage) or intentional termination or interruption of a pregnancy before 20 weeks of gestation. Up to 10% of pregnancies end in spontaneous loss within the first trimester and up to 30% by 20 weeks (Sapra, Joseph, Gallea, et al., 2017). Abortion is the second most common reproductive health procedure experienced by 31% of Canadian women (Costescu, Guillbert, Bernardin, et al., 2016). Table 5.2 differentiates the various types of abortions.

Treatment

When a *threatened* abortion occurs, efforts are made to keep the fetus in utero until the **age of viability**. In recurrent pregnancy loss, causes are investigated that could include genetic, immunological, anatomical, endocrine, or infectious factors. **Cerclage**, or suturing of an **incompetent cervix** that opens when the growing fetus presses against it, is successful in many cases. A low human chorionic gonadotropin (hCG) level by 8 weeks of gestation may be an ominous sign about the health of the pregnancy. While bleeding is a significant predictor of loss, the absence of nausea and vomiting associated with the pregnancy is also more likely to be associated with a possible miscarriage (Sapra et al., 2017).

Termination of pregnancy after 20 weeks of gestation may be done, usually in cases of fetal abnormalities that are incompatible with life or severe health risk

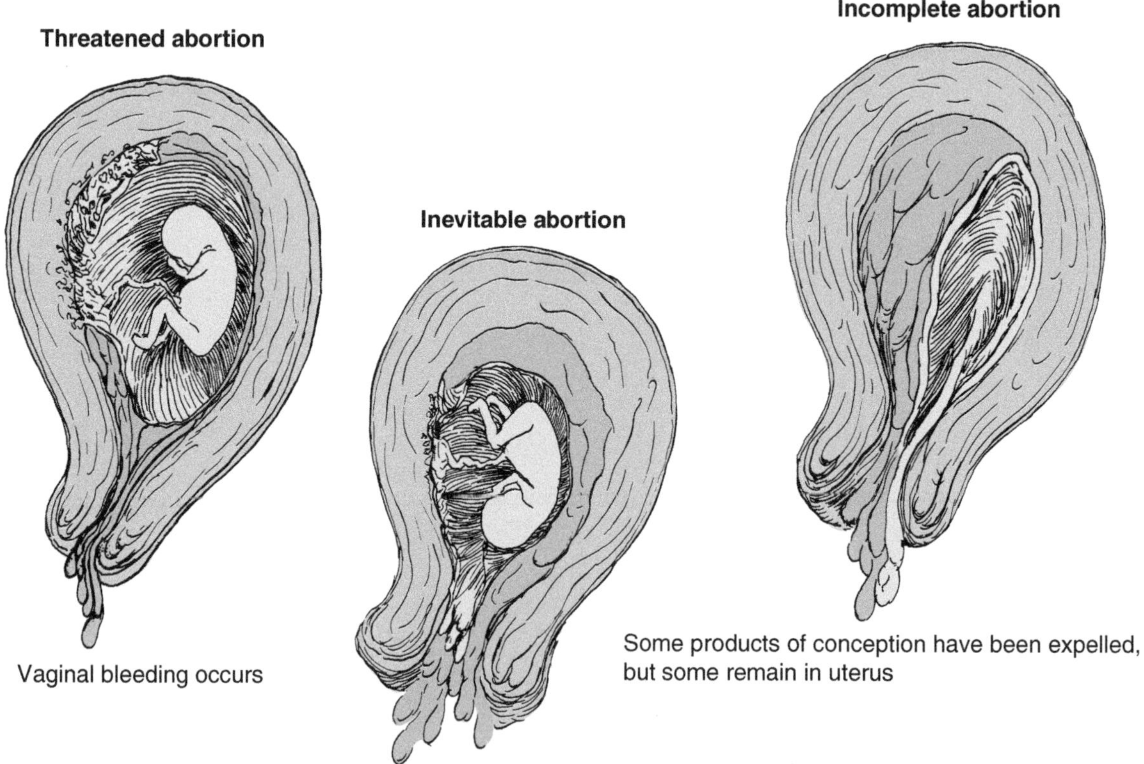
Threatened abortion
Vaginal bleeding occurs
Inevitable abortion
Membranes rupture and cervix dilates
Incomplete abortion
Some products of conception have been expelled, but some remain in uterus

Fig. 5.2 Three types of spontaneous abortion.

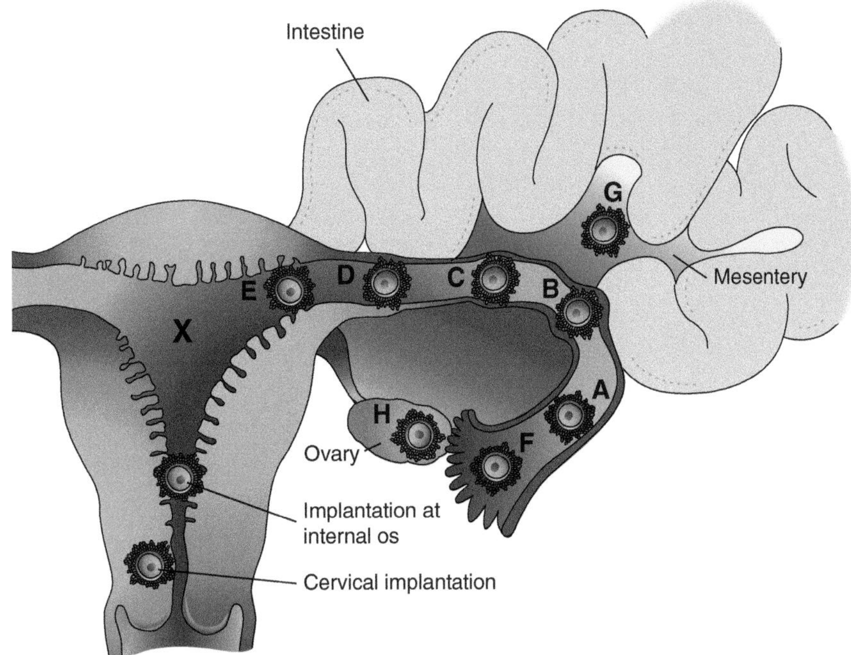

Fig. 5.3 The ovary *(H)*, uterus, and fallopian tubes, illustrating various abnormal implantation sites. *A* to *F* are tubal pregnancies (the most common); *G* is an abdominal pregnancy; and *X* indicates the wall of the uterus where normal implantation should occur. (From Moore K. L., Persaud, T. V. N., Torchia, & M. G. [2016]. *The developing human: Clinically oriented embryology* [10th ed.]. Philadelphia: Saunders.)

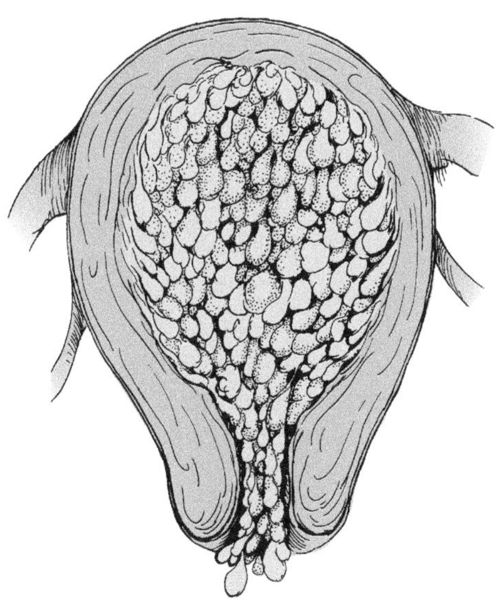

Fig. 5.4 A hydatidiform mole (gestational trophoblastic disease).

to the mother. In all cases of pregnancy loss, counselling of the parent(s) is essential. Even when the woman elects to terminate pregnancy, there are emotional responses that need to be recognized and addressed. The nurse's recognition that this may have been a very difficult decision to make is important to the care provided during this time. In Canada, termination or interruption of pregnancy can be done surgically with a dilatation and evacuation (D&E) procedure or medically with a combination of two medications, mifepristone and misoprostol. They are given 24 hours apart and, depending on gestational age, may be dispensed after seeing a healthcare provider, or the woman may be hospitalized (Costescu et al., 2016).

Oxytocin controls blood loss before and after curettage, much as the medications do after term birth. Rh_0(D) immune globulin (300 mcg) is given to Rh-negative women after any abortion to prevent development of antibodies that might harm a fetus during a subsequent pregnancy.

Nursing care

Physical care. The nurse documents the amount and character of bleeding and saves anything that looks like clots or tissue for evaluation by a pathologist during a spontaneous abortion. A pad count with an estimate of saturation (e.g., 50%, 75%) or weighing pads is the most accurate method to determine blood loss. The woman with threatened abortion who remains at home is taught to report increased bleeding or passage of tissue.

The nurse should check the hospitalized woman's bleeding and vital signs to identify excessive blood loss that may result in hypovolemic shock if the blood loss continues (Box 5.1). She should not eat (remain NPO) if she has active bleeding, to prevent aspiration if anesthesia is required for D&E treatment. Laboratory tests, such as a hemoglobin level and hematocrit, will be ordered.

After vacuum aspiration or curettage, the amount of vaginal bleeding is observed. The blood pressure, pulse, and respirations are checked every 15 minutes

Table 5.2 Types of Abortions

TYPE	DESCRIPTION	TREATMENT OR INTERVENTION
Spontaneous (Nonintentional) Abortion: Unintentional Termination of Pregnancy Before Viability (22 Weeks of Gestation)		
Threatened abortion (Fig. 5.2, A)	Cramping and backache with light spotting; cervix is closed, and no tissue is passed	Ultrasound is used to determine if fetus is living; limited activity is prescribed; avoid coitus.
Inevitable abortion (Fig. 5.2, B)	Increased bleeding, cramping; cervix dilates	Patient is placed on limited activity and monitored; awaits natural evacuation of uterus. Save peripads.
Incomplete abortion (Fig. 5.2, C)	Bleeding, cramping, dilation of cervix, passage of tissue	Uterus may be emptied of remaining tissue by dilation and evacuation (D&E) or vacuum extraction. Save peripads.
Complete abortion	Passage of all products of conception (POC); cervix closes; bleeding stops	Patient is monitored, and emotional support is given. Give Rh_0(D) immune globulin if indicated.
Missed abortion	Fetus dies in utero but is not expelled; uterine growth stops; sepsis can occur	If fetus is not expelled, uterus is evacuated by D&E.
Recurrent abortion	Two or more consecutive spontaneous abortions (habitual abortion), usually caused by incompetent cervix or progesterone levels inadequate to maintain pregnancy	Incompetent cervix may be treated with cerclage, a reinforcement of the cervix with a surgical suture; the patient is then monitored for early signs of labour and the cerclage removed to prevent injury.
Induced Abortion: Intentional Termination of Pregnancy Before Age of Viability		
Abortion	Intentional termination of pregnancy for reasons related to fetal diagnosis or diagnoses or to maternal choice	Induced abortion is legal in Canada when performed by a qualified healthcare provider. Supportive counselling must be part of the plan of care. May involve a D&E procedure, mini-suction, hypertonic saline, or vacuum curettage. Medical abortions are also done using methotrexate or Mifegymiso, which is a combination of mifepristone and misoprostol.

Box 5.1 Signs and Symptoms of Hypovolemic Shock

- Rising, weak pulse (tachycardia)
- Rising respiratory rate (tachypnea)
- Shallow, irregular respirations; air hunger (oxygen saturation less than 95%)
- Decreasing blood pressure (hypotension)
- Decreased (usually less than 30 mL/hr) or absent urine output
- Pale skin or mucous membranes
- Cold, clammy skin
- Faintness
- Thirst

for 1 hour, then every 30 minutes until discharge from the postanaesthesia care unit. The woman's temperature is checked on admission to the recovery area and every 4 hours until discharge, to monitor for infection.

Most women are discharged directly from the recovery unit to their home after the procedure. Guidelines for self-care at home include the following:

- Assess ongoing bleeding and report if it increases.
- Do not use tampons, which may cause infection.
- Take temperature every 8 hours for 3 days. Report signs of infection (temperature of 38°C [100.4°F] or higher; foul odour or brownish vaginal discharge).
- Take an oral iron supplement if prescribed.
- Sexual activity may be resumed as recommended by the healthcare provider (usually after the bleeding has stopped).
- Return to the healthcare provider at the recommended time for a checkup and contraception information. Seek help sooner if challenged with sleeping, eating, or depressed mood.
- Pregnancy can occur before the first menstrual period returns after the abortion procedure.

Emotional care. The emotional distress spontaneous abortion causes a woman and her family is often underestimated. Even if the pregnancy was not planned or suspected, they often grieve for what might have been. Their grief may last longer and be deeper than they or other people expected. The nurse needs to listen to the woman and acknowledge the grief she and her partner feel. The Communication box gives examples of effective and ineffective techniques for communicating with the family experiencing pregnancy loss. Spiritual support of the family's choice as well as community support groups may help the family work through the grief of any pregnancy loss. Supporting both the woman and her partner is critical to their grief and their ongoing relationship. Offering resources, for example, community bereavement groups, to both is helpful in ongoing healing. Nursing Care Plan 5.1 suggests interventions for families experiencing early pregnancy loss.

 Nursing Care Plan 5.1 **The Family Experiencing Early Pregnancy Loss**

PATIENT DATA

A woman is admitted at 18 weeks of gestation and within a few hours gives birth to a fetus that is 400 g and has no heart rate at the time of miscarriage. The woman asks what she has done wrong to cause this loss.

Selected Nursing Diagnosis Grief as a result of loss of anticipated infant

Goals	Nursing Interventions	Rationales
The woman and family will express grief to significant others within the next 2 weeks.	Promote expression of grief by providing privacy, eliminating time restrictions, encouraging support persons of choice to visit, and recognizing individualized grief expressions and cultural differences.	Grief is an individual process, and people react to it in different ways; these measures encourage the woman and family to express grief and begin resolving it.
The woman and family will complete each stage of the grieving process within individual time frames.	Use the four stages of grief as a basis for nursing interventions: • *Stage 1:* Shock and disbelief at loss; characterized by numbness, apathy, and impaired decision making • *Stage 2:* Seeking answers for why loss happened; characterized by crying, tears, guilt, loss of appetite, insomnia, and blame placing • *Stage 3:* Disorganization; characterized by feelings of purposelessness and malaise; gradual resumption of normal activities • *Stage 4:* Reorganization; characterized by sad memories but return of daily functioning Knowledge of normal stages of grieving helps the nurse identify whether it is progressing normally or if there is dysfunctional grieving in any family member. Stages help the nurse better interpret patients' behaviour—for example, blame placing is a normal part of grieving and is not necessarily directed at the nurse or caregivers. This allows the nurse to reassure the patient that feelings are normal, without diminishing the intensity of the feelings. Use open communication techniques: • Quiet presence • Expression of sympathy ("I'm sorry this happened.") • Open-ended statements ("This must be really sad or hard for you.") • Reflection of patient's expressed feelings ("You feel guilty because you didn't eat healthy?")	
	Reinforce explanations given by the healthcare provider or others (e.g., what the problem was, why it occurred); use simple language.	Grieving people often do not hear or understand explanations the first time they are given because their concentration is impaired.

CRITICAL THINKING QUESTIONS

1. What steps should the nurse take to assist the woman in coping with the loss of her pregnancy?
2. How should questions be formulated to foster communication with the patient?
3. This patient and family may be in the hospital for only a short time and will just be starting to move through the stages of grief. What information will the nurse give to the patient and family to help them understand their grief process over the next weeks and months? What resources would the nurse most appropriately suggest?

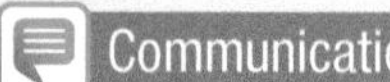

Communication

The Family Experiencing Pregnancy Loss

EXAMPLES OF EFFECTIVE STRATEGIES

Keep the family together.
Wait quietly with the family: "Be there."
Say, "I'm sorry," or "I'm here if you need to talk."
Touch (This may not be appreciated by some people or in some cultures.)
Refer to spontaneous abortion as "miscarriage."
Provide mementos, as appropriate (lock of hair, photograph, footprint), if the family would like these; save keepsakes for later retrieval if the family does not want them immediately.
Alert other hospital personnel to the family's loss, to prevent hurtful comments or questions.
Allow the family to see the fetus if they wish; prepare them for the appearance of the fetus.
Reduce the number of staff with whom the family must interact.
Summon a hospital chaplain if women or family wishes.
Make referrals to support groups in the area.

EXAMPLES OF INEFFECTIVE STRATEGIES

Giving selective or no information
Separating family members
Discouraging expressions of sadness; for example, expecting the partner to be strong for the woman's sake
Avoiding interaction with the family and talking about their loss
Acting uncomfortable with the family's expressions of grief
Encouraging the family not to cry
Minimizing the importance of the pregnancy by comments such as "You're young—you can always have more children"; "At least you didn't lose a real baby"; "It was for the best; the baby was abnormal"; or "You have another healthy child at home."
Saying, "I know how you feel." Self-disclosure of a similar experience must be used carefully and only if it is likely to be therapeutic to the patient.

Ectopic Pregnancy

Ectopic pregnancy occurs when the fertilized ovum (*zygote*) is implanted outside the uterine cavity (see Fig. 5.3). Of all ectopic pregnancies, 95% occur in the fallopian tube (*tubal pregnancy*). An obstruction or other abnormality of the tube prevents the zygote from being transported into the uterus. Scarring from a previous pelvic infection or abnormality of the fallopian tubes or inhibition of normal tubal motion to propel the zygote into the uterus may result from the following:

- Hormonal abnormalities
- Inflammation
- Infection
- Adhesions
- Congenital defects
- Endometriosis (uterine lining occurring outside the uterus)

A woman who has had a previous tubal pregnancy or a failed tubal ligation is also more likely to have an ectopic pregnancy.

A zygote that is implanted in a fallopian tube cannot survive for long because the blood supply and size of the tube are inadequate. The zygote or embryo may die and be resorbed by the woman's body, or the tube may rupture with bleeding into the abdominal cavity, creating a surgical emergency.

Manifestations

The woman has a history of a missed menstrual period and often describes symptoms of lower abdominal pain, sometimes accompanied by light vaginal bleeding. If the tube ruptures, she may have sudden severe lower abdominal pain, vaginal bleeding, and signs of hypovolemic shock (see Box 5.1). The amount of vaginal bleeding may be minimal, because most blood is lost into the abdomen rather than externally through the vagina. Shoulder pain is a symptom that often accompanies bleeding into the abdomen (referred pain).

Treatment

A sensitive pregnancy test for hCG is done to determine if the woman is pregnant. Transvaginal ultrasound examination determines whether the embryo is growing within the uterine cavity. Culdocentesis (puncture of the upper posterior vaginal wall with removal of peritoneal fluid) may occasionally be performed to identify blood in the woman's pelvis, which suggests tubal rupture. A laparoscopic examination may be done to view the damaged tube with an endoscope (lighted instrument for viewing internal organs).

The surgeon attempts to preserve the tube if the woman wants other children, but this is not always possible. The priority medical treatment is to control blood loss. Blood transfusion may be required for massive hemorrhage. One of the following three courses of treatment is chosen, depending on the gestation and the amount of damage to the fallopian tube:

1. No action is taken if the woman's body is resorbing the pregnancy.
2. Medical therapy with methotrexate (if the tube is not ruptured) inhibits cell division in the embryo and allows it to be resorbed.
3. Surgery to remove the **products of conception (POC)** from the tube is performed if damage is minimal; severe damage requires removal of the entire tube and, occasionally, the uterus.

Nursing care

Nursing care includes observing for hypovolemic shock as in spontaneous abortion. Vaginal bleeding is assessed, although most lost blood may remain in the abdomen. The nurse should report increasing pain, particularly shoulder pain, to the healthcare provider.

If the woman has surgery, preoperative and postoperative care is similar to that for other abdominal surgeries, including the following:

- Measurement of vital signs to identify hypovolemic shock and of temperature to identify infection

- Assessment of lung and bowel sounds
- IV fluid; blood replacement may be ordered if the loss was substantial
- Antibiotics as ordered
- Pain assessment and options such as patient-controlled analgesia (PCA) after surgery
- NPO status preoperatively; oral intake usually resumes after surgery, beginning with ice chips and then clear liquids or full diet may be resumed immediately depending on the health care provider's orders
- Indwelling Foley catheter as ordered. Urine output is a significant indicator of fluid balance and will fall or stop if the woman hemorrhages; minimum acceptable urine output is 30 mL/hr
- Bed rest before surgery; progressive ambulation postoperatively. The nurse should have adequate assistance when the woman first ambulates, because she is more likely to experience orthostatic hypotension if she lost a significant amount of blood.

In addition to physical preoperative and postoperative care, the nurse provides emotional support because the woman and her family may experience grieving similar to that accompanying spontaneous abortion. Loss of a fallopian tube threatens future fertility and is another source of grief. However, future pregnancies are possible if the remaining fallopian tube is normal.

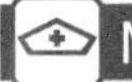 **Nursing Tip**

Supporting and encouraging the grieving process in families who have undergone a pregnancy loss, such as a spontaneous abortion or ectopic pregnancy, help them to resolve their grief.

Hydatidiform Mole

Hydatidiform mole (*gestational trophoblastic disease*; also known as a *molar pregnancy*) occurs when the chorionic villi (fringelike structures that form the placenta) increase abnormally and develop vesicles (small sacs) that resemble tiny grapes (see Fig. 5.4). The mole may be complete, with no fetus present, or partial, in which only part of the placenta has the characteristic vesicles. Hydatidiform mole may cause hemorrhage, clotting abnormalities, hypertension, and, potentially, later development of cancer (choriocarcinoma). Chromosome abnormalities are found in many cases of hydatidiform mole. It is more likely to occur in women at the age extremes of reproductive life. A woman who has had one molar pregnancy has a 1% chance of having another molar pregnancy in the future (Eagles, Sebire, Short, et al., 2015).

Manifestations

Signs associated with hydatidiform mole appear early in pregnancy and can include the following:

- Bleeding, which may range from spotting to profuse hemorrhage and may be of a brown colour; cramping may be present
- Rapid uterine growth and a uterine size that is larger than expected for the gestation
- Failure to detect fetal heart activity
- Signs of hyperemesis gravidarum (see discussion earlier in chapter)
- Unusually early development of gestational hypertension (see discussion later in chapter)
- Higher than expected levels of hCG
- A distinctive "snowstorm" pattern on ultrasound but no evidence of a developing fetus in the uterus

Treatment

A transvaginal ultrasound verifies the diagnosis. The uterus is evacuated by vacuum aspiration and D&E. The level of hCG is tested and retested until it is undetectable, and the levels are followed for at least 1 year. Persistent or rising levels suggest that vesicles remain or that malignant change has occurred. The woman should delay conceiving until follow-up care is complete, because a new pregnancy would confuse tests for hCG. $Rh_o(D)$ immune globulin is prescribed for the Rh-negative woman.

Nursing care

The nurse observes for bleeding and shock; care is similar to that given in spontaneous abortion and ectopic pregnancy. If the woman also experiences hyperemesis or pre-eclampsia, the nurse needs to incorporate care related to those conditions as well. The woman has also lost a pregnancy, so the nurse should provide care related to grieving, similar to that for a spontaneous abortion. The need to delay another pregnancy may be a concern if the woman is nearing the end of her reproductive life and wants a child; therefore, the need for follow-up examinations is reinforced. The woman is encouraged and taught how to use contraception (see Chapter 2).

BLEEDING DISORDERS OF LATE PREGNANCY

Placenta previa and placental abruption often cause bleeding in late pregnancy (Table 5.3).

Placenta Previa

Placenta previa occurs when the placenta develops in the lower part of the uterus rather than the upper. There are three degrees of placenta previa, depending on the location of the placenta in relation to the cervix (Fig. 5.5, *A*, Table 5.3).

A low-lying placenta is implanted near the cervix but does not cover any of the opening. This variation is not a true placenta previa and may or may not be accompanied by bleeding. The low-lying placenta may be discovered during a routine ultrasound examination in early pregnancy. It also may be diagnosed during

Table 5.3 Comparison of Placenta Previa and Placental Abruption

	PLACENTA PREVIA	PLACENTAL ABRUPTION
Description	Abnormal implantation of the placenta in the lower uterus *Low lying:* Approaches, but does not reach, the cervical opening (within 2 to 3 cm) *Partial:* Partially covers the cervical opening *Total:* Completely covers the cervical opening	Premature separation of the normally implanted placenta *Partial:* Detachment of part of the placenta *Marginal:* Detachment at the edge of the placenta *Central:* Detachment of the centre surface of the placenta; edges stay attached *Total:* Complete detachment of the placenta
Bleeding	Obvious vaginal bleeding, usually bright; may be profuse	Visible dark vaginal bleeding or concealed bleeding within the uterus; enlargement of uterus suggests that blood is accumulating within the cavity
Pain	None, other than from normal uterine contractions if in labour	Gradual or abrupt onset of pain and uterine tenderness; possibly low back pain
Uterine consistency	Uterus is soft; no abnormal contractions or irritability	Uterus is firm and boardlike; may be irritable, with frequent, brief contractions
Fetus	Fetus may be in an abnormal presentation, such as breech or transverse lie (see Chapter 8)	Fetal presentation usually normal
Blood clotting	Normal	Often accompanied by impaired blood clotting
Postpartum complications	*Infection:* Placental site is near the nonsterile vagina *Hemorrhage:* Lower uterine segment does not contract as effectively to compress bleeding vessels Signs of neonatal compromise if maternal shock or extensive placental detachment occur Fetal or neonatal anemia may occur because of blood loss	*Infection:* Bleeding into uterine muscle fibres predisposes to bacterial invasion *Hemorrhage:* Bleeding into uterine muscle fibres damages them, inhibiting uterine contraction after birth Signs of neonatal compromise, depending on amount and location of placental surface that is disrupted Fetal or neonatal anemia may occur because of blood loss

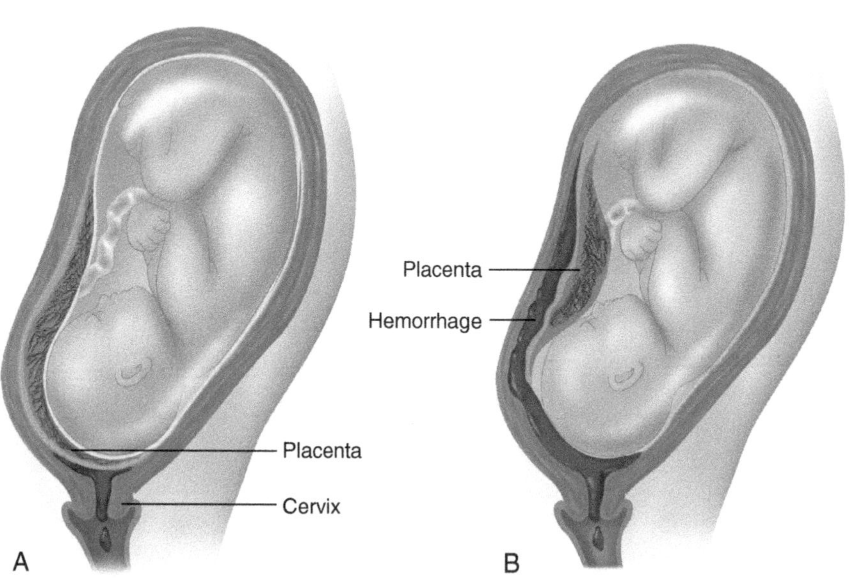

Fig. 5.5 Placenta previa and placental abruption. **A,** Placenta previa. The placenta *(purple shading)* is implanted low in the uterus. Detachment of the placenta from the uterine wall occurs as the cervix dilates, resulting in bleeding. **B,** Placental abruption. The placenta *(purple)* is implanted normally in the uterus but separates from the uterine wall. If the fetal head is engaged, bleeding *(red lining)* may accumulate in the uterus instead of being expelled externally. (From Patton, K. T., & Thibodeau, G. A. [2015]. *Anatomy & physiology* [9th ed.]. St. Louis: Mosby.)

late pregnancy because the woman has signs similar to those of a true placenta previa.

Manifestations

Painless vaginal bleeding, usually bright red, is the main characteristic of placenta previa. The woman's risk of hemorrhage increases as term approaches and the cervix begins to efface (thin) and dilate (open). These normal prelabour changes disrupt the placental attachment. The fetus may be in an abnormal presentation (e.g., breech or transverse lie) because the placenta occupies the lower uterus, which often prevents the fetus from assuming the normal head-down presentation.

The fetus or newborn may have anemia or hypovolemic shock because some of the blood lost may be fetal blood. Fetal hypoxia may occur if a large disruption of the placental surface reduces the transfer of oxygen and nutrients.

The woman with placenta previa is more likely than others to experience an infection or hemorrhage after birth for the following reasons:

- Infection is more likely to occur because vaginal organisms can easily reach the placental site, which is a good growth medium for microorganisms.
- Postpartum hemorrhage may occur because the lower segment of the uterus, where the placenta was attached, has fewer muscle fibres than the upper uterus. The resulting weak contraction of the lower uterus does not compress the open blood vessels at the placental site as effectively as would the upper segment of the uterus.

Treatment

Medical care depends on the length of gestation and the amount of bleeding. The goal is to maintain the pregnancy until the fetal lungs are mature enough that respiratory distress is less likely. Birth will be considered if bleeding is sufficient to jeopardize the mother or fetus, regardless of gestational age.

If the woman is bleeding she should lie on her side or have a pillow under one hip to avoid supine hypotension. If bleeding is extensive or the gestation is near term, a Caesarean section is performed for partial or total placenta previa. The woman with a low-lying placenta or marginal placenta previa may be able to give birth vaginally unless the blood loss is excessive.

Nursing care

The priorities of nursing care include monitoring the fetal heart and the character of contractions. Documenting and reporting vaginal blood loss and signs and symptoms of shock are important. Vital signs are taken every 15 minutes if the woman is actively bleeding, and oxygen is often given to increase the amount delivered to the fetus. Vaginal examination is not done because it may precipitate bleeding if the placental attachment is disrupted. The fetal heart rate is monitored continuously. If required, the nurse implements care for a Caesarean birth (see Chapter 8). The parents of the infant are often fearful for their child, particularly if a preterm birth is required. Supportive care should be provided.

Nursing Tip

If placenta previa is suspected, the surgeon will perform a sterile speculum examination with preparations for both vaginal and Caesarean birth (a double setup) in place.

Placental Abruption

A placental abruption is the premature separation of a placenta that is normally implanted. Predisposing factors include the following:

- Hypertension
- Cocaine use (which causes vasoconstriction)
- Tobacco and inadequate nutrition (e.g., folate deficiency)
- Trauma to the abdomen, such as with intimate partner violence or motor vehicle collision
- Previous history of placental abruption

Placental abruption may be partial or total (Fig. 5.5, *B*); it may be marginal (separating at the edges) or central (separating in the middle). Bleeding may be visible or concealed behind the partially attached placenta.

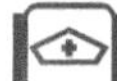
Nursing Tip

Pain that is felt between contractions is an important symptom that distinguishes placental abruption from placenta previa.

Manifestations

Bleeding accompanied by abdominal or low back pain is the typical characteristic of placental abruption. Unlike the bleeding in placenta previa, most or all of the bleeding may be concealed behind the placenta. Obvious dark-red vaginal bleeding occurs when blood leaks past the edge of the placenta. The woman's uterus is tender and unusually firm (boardlike) because blood leaks into its muscle fibres. Frequent, cramplike uterine contractions often occur (uterine irritability).

The fetus may or may not be compromised, depending on how much placental surface is disrupted. As in placenta previa, some of the blood lost may be fetal, and the fetus or newborn may have anemia or hypovolemic shock.

Disseminated intravascular coagulation (DIC) is a complex disorder that may complicate placental abruption. The large blood clot that forms behind the placenta consumes clotting factors, which leaves the rest of the mother's body deficient in these factors. Clot formation and anticoagulation (destruction of clots) occur simultaneously throughout the body in the woman with DIC. She may bleed from her mouth, nose, incisions, or venipuncture sites because the clotting factors are depleted.

Postpartum hemorrhage may also occur, because the injured uterine muscle does not contract effectively to control blood loss. Infection is more likely to occur, because the damaged tissue is susceptible to microbial invasion.

Treatment

The treatment of choice, immediate Caesarean birth, is performed because of the risk for maternal shock, clotting disorders, and fetal death. Blood and clotting factor replacement may be needed because of DIC. The mother's clotting action quickly returns to normal after birth because the source of the clotting abnormality is removed.

Nursing care

Preparation for Caesarean birth and close monitoring of vital signs and fetal heart are essential. Signs of shock and bleeding from the nose, the gums, or other unexpected sites should be promptly reported. Rapid increase in the size of the uterus suggests that blood is accumulating within it. The uterus is usually very tender and hard. Nursing care after birth is similar to that with placenta previa.

The fetus sometimes dies before birth. See Nursing Care Plan 5.1 and Chapter 9 for nursing care related to fetal death (stillbirth) and support of the grieving family. Many therapeutic communication techniques outlined in the Communication box earlier in the chapter are appropriate. The care of a pregnant woman with excessive bleeding is summarized in Box 5.2.

HYPERTENSIVE DISORDERS DURING PREGNANCY (HDP)

Hypertension may exist before pregnancy; this is known as *pre-existing (chronic) hypertension.* Pre-existing hypertension is also defined as hypertension that develops prior to 20 weeks' gestation. When hypertension develops as a complication during pregnancy it is known as *gestational hypertension* (GH). GH is a transient form of hypertension that occurs after 20 weeks' gestation during pregnancy but can become chronic hypertension later in life. Rates of pre-existing hypertension and GH are increasing (Raio, Bollo, & Baumann, 2015). At the same time, the maternal mortality rate in Canada is at 11/100 000 births (Public Health Agency of Canada [PHAC], 2013), with 10% of these related to hypertension.

Increased blood pressure causes vasospasm, which impedes blood flow to the mother's organs and placenta. Severe HDP can also affect the central nervous system, eyes, urinary tract, liver, gastrointestinal system, and blood clotting function. Table 5.4 summarizes laboratory tests that aid in diagnosis of an HDP.

Proteinuria develops as reduced blood flow damages the kidneys. This damage allows protein to leak into the urine. A clean-catch (midstream) or catheterized urine specimen is used to check for proteinuria because vaginal secretions might lead to a false-positive result. The primary health care provider may choose a 24-hour urine collection for protein or a protein/creatinine ratio test for more information.

Pre-eclampsia

The term **pre-eclampsia** is usually defined as an increase in blood pressure that occurs after 20 weeks' gestation with proteinuria (protein in the urine) in a woman who had a normal blood pressure before pregnancy or a woman with pre-existing hypertension (Magee, Pels, Helewa, et al., 2014). While proteinuria has been a classic symptom of pre-eclampsia, it may also be hypertension combined with systemic involvement such as thrombocytopenia, renal insufficiency, elevated liver enzymes or epigastric pain, or cerebral symptoms such as a sudden acute headache (Magee et al., 2014; Raio et al., 2015).

Box 5.2 Care of the Pregnant Woman With Excessive Bleeding

Document blood loss (by weighing peripads, if possible).
Closely monitor vital signs, including intake and output.
Observe for:
- Pain
- Uterine rigidity or tenderness

Verify that orders for blood typing and cross-match have been implemented.
Monitor intravenous infusion and give fluid bolus.
Prepare for surgery, if indicated.
Monitor fetal heart rate and contractions.
Monitor laboratory results, including coagulation studies.
Administer oxygen by mask.
Prepare for newborn resuscitation.

Table 5.4 Laboratory Tests for Patients With Hypertensive Disorder of Pregnancy (HDP)

TEST	RATIONALE
Hemoglobin and hematocrit	Detects hemoconcentration for indication of severity of HDP
Platelets	Thrombocytopenia suggests pre-eclampsia
Urine for protein	Proteinuria confirms pre-eclampsia
Serum creatinine	Elevated creatinine and oliguria suggest pre-eclampsia
Serum uric acid	Elevated uric acid suggests pre-eclampsia
Serum transaminase	Elevated transaminase confirms liver involvement in pre-eclampsia

Data from Gabbe, S. F., Niebyl, J. R., & Simpson, J. L., et al. (Eds.). (2017). *Obstetrics: Normal and problem pregnancies* (7th ed.). Philadelphia: Saunders.

Risk factors for development of pre-eclampsia include the following:

- Pregnancy at extremes of maternal age (adolescents or women >40 years)
- Obesity, pre-existing hypertension
- Diagnosis of pre-eclampsia in a previous pregnancy
- Diabetes or renal disease
- Nulliparity, or pregnancy with a new partner
- Multiple gestation
- Pre-existing autoimmune diseases such as antiphospholipid antibody syndrome

Nonsevere pre-eclampsia is defined as the following:

- Blood pressure (BP) reading of ≥140/90 mm Hg × two readings 15 minutes apart
- Presence of proteinuria 1+
- Presence of one or more adverse conditions (e.g., possible headache, visual problems, epigastric pain, elevated creatinine, low platelets)

Severe pre-eclampsia is defined as the following:

- BP reading ≥160/110 mm Hg on two separate readings 15 minutes apart
- Presence of proteinuria: a urine dipstick results of 2+ to 3+ or greater on two separate urine specimens
- Presence of one or more severe complications (e.g., severe headache; blurred vision, photophobia, blind spots on fundoscopy, elevated creatinine, platelets <50 × 10^9/L, hepatic dysfunction, decreased placental function which can result in an intrauterine growth-restricted [IUGR] fetus) (Magee et al., 2014).

Pre-eclampsia progresses to **eclampsia** when convulsions occur. Convulsions due to eclampsia can occur antepartum, intrapartum, or postpartum (one sometimes hears the term *toxemia,* an old term for pre-eclampsia).

Manifestations of severe pre-eclampsia

Other signs and symptoms occur with severe pre-eclampsia. All are related to decreased blood flow and edema of the organs involved.

Central nervous system. A severe, unrelenting headache may occur because of brain edema and small cerebral hemorrhages. The severe headache often precedes a convulsion. Deep tendon reflexes become hyperactive because of central nervous system irritability.

Eyes. Visual disturbances such as blurred or double vision or "spots before the eyes" occur because of arterial spasm and edema surrounding the retina. Visual disturbances often precede a convulsion.

Urinary tract. Decreased blood flow to the kidneys reduces urine production (oliguria) and worsens hypertension.

Respiratory system. Pulmonary edema (accumulation of fluid in the lungs) may occur with severe pre-eclampsia.

Gastrointestinal system and liver. Epigastric pain or nausea occurs because of liver edema, ischemia, and necrosis and often precedes a convulsion. Liver enzyme levels are elevated because of reduced circulation and small hemorrhages.

Blood clotting. HELLP syndrome is a variant of GH that involves **h**emolysis (breakage of erythrocytes), **el**evated **l**iver enzymes, and low **p**latelets. Hemolysis occurs as erythrocytes break up when passing through small blood vessels damaged by the hypertension. Obstruction of hepatic blood flow causes the liver enzyme levels to become elevated. Low platelet levels occur when the platelets gather at the site of blood vessel damage, reducing the number available in the general circulation. Low platelet levels cause abnormal blood clotting. Right upper quadrant (RUQ) or epigastric pain, nausea, vomiting, and malaise may signal that HELLP is developing. Liver enzyme laboratory reports should be monitored. HELLP syndrome can also develop postpartum, thus all patients with hypertension should be closely monitored during the postpartum period. The patient with severe HELLP syndrome may be monitored in the critical care unit and given magnesium sulphate to prevent convulsions and antihypertensive medications. The need regarding whether the woman should give birth is evaluated. The woman is monitored closely for bleeding.

Postpartum, the mother is evaluated for fluid intake and output, laboratory values, and pulse oximetry for at least 48 hours. Most patients improve after the birth.

Effects on the fetus

Pre-eclampsia reduces maternal blood and nutrition flow through the placenta and decreases the oxygen available to the fetus. Fetal hypoxia may result in meconium (first stool) passage into the amniotic fluid. The fetus may have IUGR and at birth will be small for gestational age. Fetal death or stillbirth is a higher risk with pre-eclampsia. In women with pre-existing or GH, administration of magnesium sulphate should be considered for fetal neuroprotection if imminent preterm birth will occur (at ≤31 + 6 weeks) (Magee et al., 2014).

Eclampsia

Progression to eclampsia occurs when the woman has one or more generalized **tonic-clonic seizures**. Facial muscle twitching is followed by generalized contraction of all muscles (tonic phase), then alternate contraction and relaxation of the muscles (clonic phase). An eclamptic seizure may result in cerebral hemorrhage, placental abruption, fetal compromise, or death of the mother or fetus. Magnesium sulphate is administered to control seizures. Close fetal monitoring is essential as well as monitoring of uterine contractions. Measures to prevent aspiration are the responsibility of the nurse. Birth may be expedited.

Prevention

Correction of some risk factors reduces the risk for pre-eclampsia. For example, improving the woman's diet may prevent pre-eclampsia and promote normal fetal growth. Other risk factors, such as family history, cannot be changed. Early and regular prenatal care enables prompt diagnosis of pre-eclampsia so it can be more effectively managed. Calcium supplementation is recommended for women with low dietary intake of calcium (<600 mg/day). The following recommendations may also be beneficial to decrease the risk of pre-eclampsia: abstention from alcohol for prevention of fetal alcohol effects, exercise to maintain or enhance fitness, periconceptual use of a folate-containing multivitamin for prevention of neural tube defects, and smoking cessation for prevention of low-birth-weight and preterm birth (Magee et al., 2014). Low-dose aspirin, started between 12 and 14 weeks' gestation, has anticoagulant and anti-inflammatory properties that aid in the prevention of pre-eclampsia for patients with a high risk of developing eclampsia (Fantasia, 2018).

Management and treatment of hypertension during pregnancy

Antihypertensives may not be given to women with mild hypertension, but frequent prenatal visits and fetal monitoring are scheduled. Treatment of hypertension is similar, whether the woman has pre-existing hypertension or GH. Initial therapy in pregnancy can be with one of the following antihypertensives: methyldopa, labetalol, other beta blockers (acebutolol, metoprolol, pindolol, and propranolol), and calcium channel blockers (nifedipine). If a woman is admitted to the hospital for hypertension, initial antihypertensive therapy should be with nifedipine short-acting capsules, parenteral hydralazine, or parenteral labetalol (Magee et al., 2014). Angiotensin-converting enzyme inhibitors and angiotensin receptor blockers should not be used during pregnancy (Magee et al., 2014).

Treatment of pre-eclampsia depends on the severity of the hypertension and on the gestational age of the fetus. Treatment focuses on (1) maintaining blood flow to the woman's vital organs and the placenta and (2) preventing convulsions. Birth is the cure for pre-eclampsia. If the fetus is mature, pregnancy is ended by labour induction or Caesarean birth. If pre-eclampsia is severe, the fetus is often in greater danger from being in the uterus than from being born prematurely.

Inpatient care should be provided for women with severe hypertension or severe pre-eclampsia. Home care can be considered for women with nonsevere pre-eclampsia or nonsevere pre-existing or GH (Magee et al., 2014).

The pregnant patient who develops pre-eclampsia requires frequent fetal evaluations, including ultrasounds, nonstress tests, and possibly early birth at 36 to 37 weeks' gestation. The patient should be instructed to report symptoms such as headaches or visual changes and the nurse monitors laboratory tests for abnormal results.

Safety Alert!

When taking the blood pressure (BP) of a woman with a hypertensive disorder during pregnancy, the BP should be measured with the woman in the sitting position with her arm at the level of her heart. An appropriately sized cuff (i.e., length 1.5 times the circumference of the arm) should be used. Korotkoff phase V should be used to designate diastolic blood pressure. If BP is consistently higher in one arm, the arm with the higher values should be used for all BP measurements. The BP can be measured using a mercury sphygmomanometer, a calibrated aneroid device, or an automated BP machine that has been validated for use in pre-eclampsia (Magee et al., 2014).

Because HDP are closely related to the development of complications such as placental abruption, fetal growth restriction, pre-eclampsia, prematurity, and stillbirth, special care of the pregnant woman with hypertension is essential. The Society of Obstetricians and Gynaecologists of Canada (SOGC) recommends BP screening and assessment for proteinuria at each health care visit during pregnancy to detect HDP (Magee et al., 2014).

Conservative treatment, whether at home or in the hospital, includes the following:

- Activity restriction to allow blood that would be circulated to skeletal muscles to be conserved for circulation to the mother's vital organs and the placenta. The woman should remain on reduced activity with frequent rest periods lying on her side to improve blood flow to the placenta. Complete bed rest is not recommended because of risk factors of being immobilized.
- Maternal assessment of fetal activity ("kick counts") (see Chapter 4). She should seek medical assessment if there is a decrease in movements or if none occur during a 3-hour period (if greater than 26 to 28 weeks' gestation) (see Table 5.1).
- BP monitoring two to four times per day in the same arm and in the same position. A family member must be taught the technique if the woman can safely remain at home.
- Checking urine for protein with a dipstick using a first-voided, clean-catch specimen, as needed (Magee et al., 2014; Sperling & Gassett, 2017).

Home Care Considerations

Hypertension in Pregnancy

Patient teaching for home care should include the following:

- Activity as tolerated, with frequent rest periods
- Recommendation to discontinue smoking and alcohol use
- Primary management is without medications, because blood pressure normally falls in the first two trimesters of pregnancy
- Blood pressure measurement two to four times per day (preferably at the same time each day)
- Urine dipstick for protein, as needed
- Monitor fetal movements and uterine activity
- Encourage a balanced diet with sufficient protein and fluids to replace loss
- Teach signs and symptoms of problems to report
- Encourage side lying during rest periods

Diuretics and sodium restriction are not prescribed for pre-eclampsia. The woman's diet should have adequate calories and protein (see Chapter 4 for prenatal dietary guidelines). See Table 5.1 for fetal assessment tests that may be done.

Several medications may also be used to treat HDP, as described in the sections above. *Magnesium sulphate* is an anticonvulsant administered to prevent seizures. It also may slightly reduce the BP, but its main purpose is as an anticonvulsant. It is usually given by IV infusion (controlled with an infusion pump). Administration continues for at least 12 to 24 hours after birth because the woman remains at risk for seizures. Steroids may be given to aid in fetal lung maturity if labour induction is planned.

The kidneys excrete magnesium. Decreased urine output (less than 30 mL/hr) may result in serum levels of magnesium reaching toxic levels. Excess magnesium first causes loss of the deep tendon reflexes, which is followed by depression of respirations; if levels continue to rise, collapse and death can occur. Close monitoring of the respiratory rate and sedation scale is essential in women who receive magnesium sulphate. Calcium gluconate reverses the effects of magnesium and should be available for immediate use when a woman receives magnesium sulphate.

Nursing care

Nursing care focuses on (1) assisting women in obtaining prenatal care, (2) helping them cope with therapy, (3) caring for acutely ill women, and (4) administering medications.

Promoting prenatal care.

Nurses can promote awareness of how prenatal care allows risk identification and early intervention if complications arise. The nurse should develop a therapeutic relationship with the woman and family, tailoring the information to the identified learning needs and conditions present, which will encourage regular attendance of prenatal care (Logsdon, Davis, Myers, et al., 2018). Providing clear information about warning signs and symptoms and where to go if they occur is critical to maternal and fetal health. The woman with gestational or pre-existing hypertension will need to come more often for assessment and possibly for evaluation of therapy and presence of complications, so spending time with this woman and her family is important.

Helping to cope with therapy. The nurse can help the woman understand the importance of reduced activity and frequent rest periods and to plan ways to manage them. Activity diverts blood from the placenta, reducing the infant's oxygen supply, so the nurse must impress upon the woman how important rest is to her child's well-being. Positioning the patient on her side during rest helps to improve blood flow to the placenta and more effectively provides oxygen and nutrients to the fetus. See the discussion of preterm labour (Chapter 8) for more information about care related to limited activity.

Caring for the acutely ill woman. The acutely ill woman requires intensive nursing care directed by an interdisciplinary team including anesthesiology, obstetrical staff, and one-to-one nursing care by a registered nurse. A quiet, low-light environment reduces the risk of pre-eclampsia becoming eclampsia (seizure). The woman should remain on bed rest, on her side, often the left side, to promote maximum fetal oxygenation. Side rails should be padded and raised to prevent injury if a seizure occurs. Stimulation such as loud noises or bumping of the bed should be avoided. Visitors are usually limited to one or two support persons. Suction equipment to assist with respiratory effort needs to be available for immediate use.

If a seizure occurs, the nursing focus is to prevent injury and restore oxygenation to the mother and fetus. If the woman is not already on her side, the nurse should try to turn her before the seizure begins. The nurse should not forcibly hold the woman's body but protect her from injury caused by striking hard surfaces.

Breathing can stop during a seizure. An oral airway, inserted *after* the seizure, facilitates breathing and suctioning of secretions. Aspiration of secretions can occur during a seizure, so the healthcare provider may order chest radiographs and arterial blood gas measurements. Oxygen by face mask improves fetal oxygenation. The woman is reoriented to the environment when she regains consciousness. Labour may progress rapidly after a seizure, often while the woman is still drowsy, and the fetus must be monitored continuously (see Chapter 6 for signs of impending birth).

Providing postpartum care. Pre-eclampsia is of concern for the prenatal patient and the fetus and continues to be a threat in the postpartum period. Women with pre-existing hypertension are at risk for pulmonary edema, renal failure, and eclampsia. Close monitoring for 48 to 72 hours after birth is essential. Women requiring antihypertensive medications postpartum who are breastfeeding can be given nifedipine XL, labetalol, methyldopa, captopril, and enalapril (Magee et al., 2014). Other antihypertensive drugs may have adverse effects on the breastfeeding infant. Diuretics decrease milk production and are generally not administered. Women should be taught to seek care after discharge if they have symptoms of blurred vision or headache that is increasing in severity, as this may continue to be a concern in the first week postpartum.

BLOOD INCOMPATIBILITY BETWEEN THE PREGNANT WOMAN AND THE FETUS

The placenta allows maternal and fetal blood to be close enough to exchange oxygen and waste products without actually mixing (see Fig. 3.6). However, small leaks that allow fetal blood to enter the mother's circulation may occur during pregnancy or when the placenta detaches at birth. No problem occurs if the maternal and fetal blood types are compatible. However, if the maternal and fetal blood factors differ, problems can arise.

Rh and ABO Incompatibility

People either have the Rh blood factor on their erythrocytes or they do not. If they have the factor, they are Rh positive; if not, they are Rh negative. An Rh-positive person can receive Rh-negative blood with no untoward effects (if all other factors are compatible) because in Rh-negative blood this factor is absent. However, the reverse is not true—Rh incompatibility between the woman and fetus can occur if the woman is Rh negative and the fetus is Rh positive.

A person with Rh-negative blood is not born with antibodies against the Rh factor. However, exposure to Rh-positive blood causes the person to make antibodies to destroy Rh-positive erythrocytes. The antibodies remain ready to destroy any future Rh-positive erythrocytes that enter the circulation (sensitization).

If fetal Rh-positive blood leaks into the Rh-negative mother's circulation, her body may respond by making antibodies to destroy the Rh-positive erythrocytes. This process is called **isoimmunization**. Because this leakage usually occurs at birth, the first Rh-positive child is rarely seriously affected. However, the woman's blood levels of antibodies increase rapidly each time she is exposed to more Rh-positive blood (in subsequent pregnancies with Rh-positive fetuses). Antibodies against Rh-positive blood cross the placenta and destroy the fetal Rh-positive erythrocytes before the infant is born, which can cause hemolytic disease of the newborn. A similar response occurs with ABO incompatibility when the mother is type O and the infant's blood type is type A or type B, but the response is rarely life-threatening in the newborn, although the newborn may develop jaundice after birth and should be monitored.

Manifestations

The woman has no obvious effects if her body produces anti-Rh antibodies. Rising antibody titres in laboratory tests evidence increased levels of these antibodies in her blood. Noninvasive DNA testing of maternal plasma can also determine fetal Rh status. When these maternal anti-Rh antibodies cross the placenta and destroy fetal erythrocytes, **hemolytic disease of the newborn** (erythroblastosis fetalis) results (Fig. 5.6). The effect on the newborn is discussed in Chapter 12.

Prevention, treatment, and nursing care

The primary management to prevent the manufacture of anti-Rh antibodies is by giving Rh_0(D) immune globulin to the Rh-negative woman at 28 weeks of gestation and within 72 hours after birth of an Rh-positive infant or after a miscarriage or abortion. It is also given after amniocentesis and to women who experience bleeding during pregnancy, because fetal blood may leak into the mother's circulation at these times. Rh_0(D) immune globulin has greatly decreased the incidence of infants with Rh-incompatibility problems.

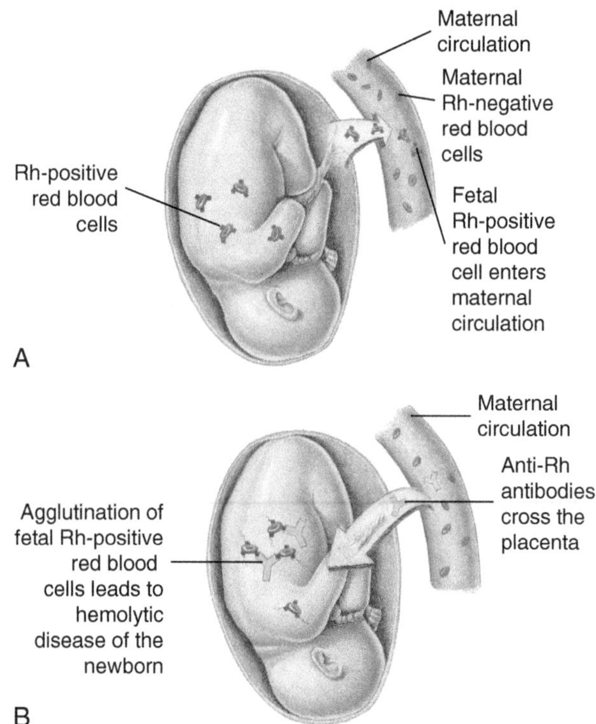

Fig. 5.6 Hemolytic disease of the newborn. **A,** A few fetal Rh-positive red blood cells enter the circulation of the Rh-negative mother during pregnancy or at birth, causing the mother to produce antibodies against Rh-positive blood cells. **B,** The Rh-positive antibodies from the maternal circulation cross the placenta, enter the fetal circulation, and destroy fetal Rh-positive blood cells. (From Patton, K. T., & Thibodeau, G. A. [2015]. *Anatomy & physiology* [9th ed.]. St. Louis: Mosby.)

However, some women are still sensitized, usually because they did not receive Rh_0(D) immune globulin after childbirth or abortion. Rh_0(D) immune globulin will not be effective if sensitization has already occurred.

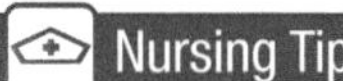

Nursing Tip

Most cases of Rh incompatibility between an Rh-negative mother and an Rh-positive fetus can be prevented with the administration of Rh_0(D) immune globulin if incompatibility is indicated.

The woman who is sensitized to destroy Rh-positive blood cells is carefully monitored during pregnancy to determine if too many fetal erythrocytes are being destroyed. Several fetal assessment tests may be used, including the Coombs' test, amniocentesis, or percutaneous umbilical blood sampling (see Table 5.1). A Doppler ultrasound to detect increased blood flow in the middle cerebral artery of the fetus detects fetal anemia that can occur due to Rh incompatibility.

An intrauterine transfusion may be performed for the severely anemic fetus. The Rh factor should be documented on the chart and the healthcare provider notified if the woman is Rh negative. See Chapter 12 for the effect of Rh and ABO incompatibility on the newborn.

PREGNANCY COMPLICATED BY MEDICAL CONDITIONS

Health problems that are present before pregnancy can influence the outcome of a pregnancy and necessitate special management. Health problems discussed in this section include diabetes mellitus, heart disease, anemia, and infections.

DIABETES MELLITUS

Diabetes mellitus (DM) can be classified according to whether it preceded pregnancy or had its onset during pregnancy. Types of DM include the following (Feig, Berger, Donovan, et al., 2018):

- *Type 1 diabetes mellitus:* Usually caused by an autoimmune destruction of the beta cells of the pancreas resulting in an insulin deficiency
- *Type 2 diabetes mellitus:* Usually caused by insulin resistance; usually has a strong genetic predisposition and is associated with obesity
- *Pregestational diabetes mellitus:* Type 1 or 2 diabetes that existed before pregnancy occurred
- **Gestational diabetes mellitus (GDM)**: Glucose intolerance with onset during pregnancy. In true GDM, glucose usually returns to normal by 6 weeks postpartum, although women with GDM have increased risk of developing type 2 diabetes later in life (Berger, Gagnon, Sermer, et al., 2016).

Effect of Pregnancy on Glucose Metabolism

Pregnancy affects a woman's metabolism (whether or not she has DM) as there are additional requirements, that is, the need for glucose to be available to the growing fetus. Hormones (estrogen and progesterone), an enzyme (insulinase) produced by the placenta, and increased prolactin levels have two effects:

- Increased resistance of cells to insulin
- Increased speed of insulin breakdown

Most women respond to these changes by secreting extra insulin to maintain normal carbohydrate metabolism while still providing plenty of glucose for the fetus. If the woman cannot increase her insulin production, she will have periods of *hyperglycemia* (increased blood glucose levels) as glucose accumulates in the blood. Because the fetus continuously draws glucose from the mother, maternal *hypoglycemia* (low blood glucose) can occur between meals and during the night. There is also a normally increased tissue resistance to maternal insulin action in the second and third trimesters, and the fetus is then at risk for organ damage resulting from hyperglycemia. The newborn is at risk for hypoglycemia because it leaves the high insulin environment that was present in utero and enters a lower insulin environment, thus close monitoring of the newborn is required after birth.

Pre-existing Diabetes Mellitus

Women who are diabetic before pregnancy may need to alter management of their condition. Preconception planning is encouraged for these women to ensure that they understand the risks of pregnancy and plan for changes that can occur throughout (Berger et al., 2016). The time of major risk for congenital anomalies to occur from maternal hyperglycemia is during the embryonic period of development in the first trimester. Therefore, women who are diabetic *before* pregnancy have a greater risk of having a newborn with a congenital anomaly than a woman who develops gestational diabetes, which is usually manifested after the first trimester. With careful management, most diabetic women can have successful pregnancies and healthy babies. Nevertheless, there are many potential complications of diabetes (Box 5.3).

Box 5.3 Effects of Diabetes in Pregnancy

MATERNAL EFFECTS

Spontaneous abortion
Gestational hypertension
Preterm labour and premature rupture of the membranes
Hydramnios (excessive amniotic fluid; also called *polyhydramnios*)
Infections:
- Vaginitis
- Urinary tract infection

Complications of macrosomia:
- Birth canal injuries
- Caesarean birth

Ketoacidosis

FETAL AND NEWBORN EFFECTS

Congenital abnormalities
Macrosomia
Intrauterine growth restriction
Birth injury
Delayed lung maturation; respiratory distress syndrome
Neonatal hypoglycemia
Neonatal hypocalcemia
Neonatal hyperbilirubinemia and jaundice
Neonatal polycythemia (excess erythrocytes) caused by hypoxia
Perinatal death

Gestational Diabetes Mellitus

GDM is common, affecting up to 3 to 20% of women, depending on their risk factors (Feig et al., 2018), The following factors in a woman's history are associated with high risk for GDM (Feig et al., 2018):

- Body mass index (BMI) ≥30 kg/m^2
- History of macrosomic infant (>4 000 g or about 9 lb [Fig. 5.7])
- Maternal age greater than 35 years
- Previous unexplained stillbirth or infant having congenital abnormalities
- History of GDM in a previous pregnancy
- Family history of DM
- Using corticosteroid medication
- Glucose challenge test (50 g glucose) results: 7.8 to 11.0 mmol/L

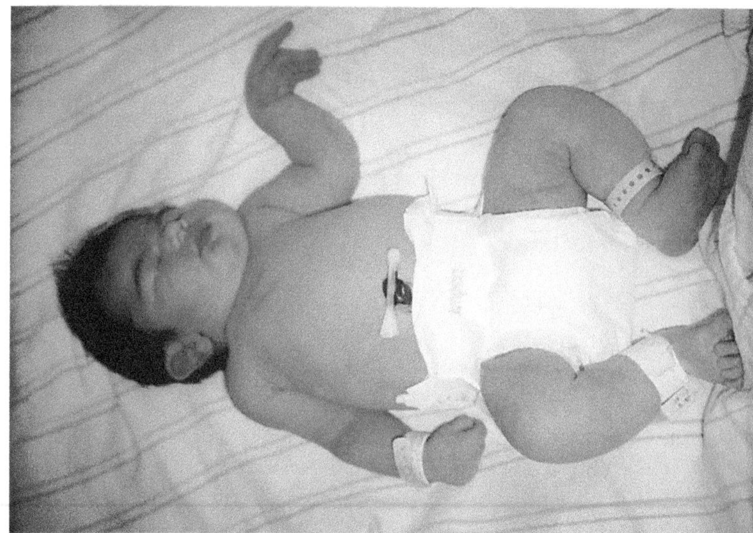

Fig. 5.7 Macrosomic infant. A newborn with macrosomia caused by maternal diabetes mellitus during pregnancy. This infant weighed 5 kg (11 lb) at birth. Newborns with macrosomia often have respiratory and other problems. (From Zitelli, B. J., & Davis, H. W. [Eds.]. [2017]. *Atlas of pediatric physical diagnosis* [7th ed.]. St. Louis: Mosby.)

Identification of GDM

If the woman does not have pre-existing diabetes, a prenatal screening test to identify GDM is often routinely performed between 24 and 28 weeks of gestation but may be done earlier if risk factors are present. In the prenatal screening test for GDM, the woman drinks 50 g of an oral glucose solution (fasting is not necessary) (Berger et al., 2016) and a blood sample is taken 1 hour later and analyzed for glucose. If the blood glucose level is 7.8 mmol/L or higher, a more complex, 3-hour glucose tolerance test is done (an initial fasting, then at 1 hour and 2 hours). One abnormal result in the 3-hour glucose tolerance tests is diagnostic for GDM (Berger et al., 2016).

Treatment of GDM

Diet modifications. The woman is counselled to avoid single large meals with high amounts of simple carbohydrates. Advice on meal planning for women with GDM should emphasize a healthy diet during pregnancy, with a minimum of 175 g/day of carbohydrate distributed over three moderate-sized meals and two or more snacks (one of which should be at bedtime), as well as replacing high-glycemic index foods with low-glycemic index ones (Feig et al., 2018). The timing and content of meals and snacks may require adjustment to prevent early-morning hypoglycemia. A bedtime snack is important to minimize the risk of hypoglycemia. Dietary guidance in collaboration with a registered dietitian is important.

Monitoring of blood glucose levels. To ensure a successful pregnancy, the woman must try to keep her blood glucose levels as close to normal as possible. She should be taught the signs and symptoms of both hypoglycemia and hyperglycemia (Table 5.5). The pregnant diabetic woman needs to monitor her blood glucose levels as directed by the healthcare provider; blood glucose self-monitoring is discussed in Chapter 31. Glycated hemoglobin ($HgbA_{1C}$) is performed every 3 months to provide an indication of long-term (4- to 6-week) glucose control, and lower values can indicate successful glucose management of the pregnant diabetic. $HgbA_{1C}$ monitoring cannot be used as a guide to adjust daily insulin needs during pregnancy, but levels may warn of a risk for fetal anomalies.

Monitoring of ketones. During pregnancy, the woman may check her urine for ketones as part of her diabetic care. She would be given instructions about when to contact her diabetic clinic nurse or other healthcare provider if she was concerned, particularly when combining ketone levels with hypoglycemic values.

Insulin administration. Oral hypoglycemic drugs have been used to treat GDM with some success, although further research is needed (Feig et al., 2018). Glyburide, which does not cross the placenta, is considered superior to metformin, which does cross the placenta but has not been shown to be teratogenic to the fetus. However, because both oral agents often require supplemental injectable insulin to maintain adequate glucose control, injectable insulin is the preferred medication to lower blood glucose levels during pregnancy. GDM may be controlled by diet and exercise alone, or the woman may require insulin injections. The dose and frequency of insulin injections are tailored to a woman's individual needs. Insulin is often administered on a sliding scale, in which the woman varies her dose of insulin based on each blood glucose level.

The insulin regimen of a diabetic woman is different during pregnancy than in the nonpregnant state. Typically, the insulin dosage may have to be reduced to avoid hypoglycemia in the first trimester, when nausea decreases appetite and physical activity may be reduced. In the second trimester, increasing placental hormones increases insulin resistance, and the dosage of insulin may have to be increased. Insulin requirements may drop again at 38 weeks of gestation. GDM resolves promptly after birth, when the insulin-antagonistic (diabetogenic) effects of pregnancy cease.

Table 5.5 **Comparison of Hypoglycemia and Hyperglycemia in the Diabetic Woman**

HYPOGLYCEMIA	HYPERGLYCEMIA
Cause	
Excess insulin, excess exercise, and/or inadequate food intake	Inadequate insulin, increased insulin resistance of placenta, reduced activity, and/or excessive food intake; more likely if the woman has an infection, because this increases her need for insulin
Blood Glucose Level	
Below normal (usually <3.3 mmol/L if diet controlled or <3.7 if on insulin)	Above normal (>6.7 mmol/L)
Urine	
Urine glucose absent	Glycosuria (glucose in the urine); possibly ketonuria (ketones in the urine)
Behavioural and Physiological Manifestations	
Hunger; trembling; weakness; faintness; lethargy; headache; irritability; sweating; pale, cool, moist skin; blurred vision; loss of consciousness	Fatigue; headache; flushed, hot skin; dry mouth; thirst; dehydration; frequent urination; weight loss; nausea and vomiting; rapid, deep respirations (Kussmaul's respirations); acetone odour to the breath; depressed reflexes
Corrective Measures	
Drink a glass of milk or juice; eat a piece of fruit or two crackers; recurrent hypoglycemia necessitates adjustment of insulin or food intake	Evaluate food intake; emphasize importance of patient being honest if she "cheats," to prevent inappropriately adjusting insulin dose; identify and treat infections; insulin dose often adjusted throughout pregnancy to maintain normal glucose levels

! Safety Alert!

Insulin is a high-risk medication. In many institutions, before administering insulin to an antepartum, intrapartum, or postpartum woman, two identifiers for the medication dosage and patient are required, particularly if given intravenously. When a woman is diagnosed with DM and she requires insulin, education and teaching are required to assist her in safely injecting herself, drawing up the appropriate dose or using a device such as a pen in which the dose is programmed, and learning to do capillary sampling. The nurse also needs to help her understand what the blood glucose values mean and how to seek help if needed.

Aspart insulin and lispro are fast-acting insulins that are highly effective if given before meals. Long-acting insulin such as glargine is also effective and has no adverse effects (Feig et al., 2018). The use of an insulin pump has proved to be of great value for glucose control in pregnant patients with DM and reduces hypoglycemic events. (See Chapter 31 for the discussion of insulin administration and insulin pumps.)

Exercise. A pregnant woman with pre-existing diabetes may have vascular damage, and exercise may then result in ischemia (decreased circulation) to the placenta and in hypoxia (decreased oxygen) to the fetus. The healthcare provider should prescribe the level of exercise, and blood glucose levels should be monitored closely. In GDM, however, exercise can help control blood glucose levels, and diet and exercise can minimize the need for insulin. The woman with GDM should be counselled that exercise after meals is preferred, because glucose levels are higher at that time. Hypoglycemia can occur if the woman exercises when the effects of the last insulin dose are at their peak. Hyperglycemia can occur if the woman exercises when the effects of the last dose of insulin have decreased. Therefore, blood glucose levels should be monitored before, during, and after exercise, and a readily absorbed glucose source should be on hand for the woman to manage any hypoglycemia (see Table 5.5).

Fetal assessments. Assessments (see Table 5.1) may help identify fetal growth and the placenta's ability to provide oxygen and nutrients. Ultrasound examinations are used to identify IUGR, macrosomia, excess amniotic fluid (polyhydramnios) in the woman with poorly controlled diabetes, or decreased amniotic fluid (oligohydramnios) in placental failure.

Diabetes can affect the blood vessels that supply the placenta, impairing the transport of oxygen and nutrients to the fetus and the removal of fetal wastes. The non–stress test and the biophysical profile provide information about how the placenta is functioning. Tests of fetal lung maturity may be done if early birth is considered.

Care during labour. Labour is work (exercise) that affects the amount of insulin and glucose needed. Some women receive an IV infusion of a dextrose solution plus regular insulin as needed. Regular insulin is the *only* type given intravenously. Blood glucose levels are assessed hourly, and the insulin dose is adjusted accordingly. Because macrosomia (large fetal size) is a common complication of any type of DM, close monitoring of the progress of labour is essential, and Caesarean birth may be required. (See Chapter 8 for care of a woman requiring Caesarean section.)

Care of the newborn. Infant complications after birth may include hypoglycemia, respiratory distress, and injury caused by macrosomia. Some infants experience growth restriction because the placenta functions poorly. Neonatal nurses and a neonatologist (a physician specializing in care of newborns) are often present at the birth. (See Chapter 12 for a discussion of these neonatal concerns.)

Nursing care

Nursing care of the pregnant woman with DM involves helping her to learn to care for herself and providing emotional care to meet the demands imposed by this complication. Care during labour primarily involves careful monitoring for signs of fetal distress and the progress of labour.

Teaching self-care. Most women with pre-existing diabetes already know how to check their blood glucose level and administer insulin. They should be taught why diabetes management changes during pregnancy. The woman with newly diagnosed GDM must be taught these self-care skills.

The woman is taught how to select appropriate foods for three meals and snacks throughout the day. A woman is more likely to maintain the diet if her caregivers are sensitive to her food preferences and cultural needs and she has input into creating the diet. A dietitian can determine foods to meet her needs and wishes. Frequent meetings with an interdisciplinary team throughout pregnancy, including the dietitian, endocrinologist, and nurse, may assist with support and encouragement in these care requirements.

The woman who takes insulin may experience episodes of hypoglycemia or hyperglycemia (see Table 5.5). The woman must be taught how to recognize and respond to each condition, and family members should be included in the teaching. Maintaining glycemic control during pregnancy is essential to prevent later complications such as macrosomia or stillbirth. Follow-up care is important, as patients with GDM have an increased risk of developing type 2 DM 5 to 10 years after giving birth.

Providing emotional support. Pregnant women with diabetes often find that living with the glucose monitoring, diet control, and frequent insulin administration can be challenging. The expectant mother is already anxious about the outcome for herself and her child, and this change adds to these concerns. Therapeutic communication can help her to express her frustrations and fears. For example, to elicit her feelings about her condition the nurse might say, "Many women find that all the changes they have to make are demanding. How has it been for you?" It may help to emphasize that the close management is usually temporary, especially if she has GDM. Knowing that the woman is at risk of later developing type 2 diabetes, the nurse may also want to point out that the nutritional counselling and diet she is following are good practices to continue while breastfeeding and for her family's health as well as her own.

A woman who is actively involved in her own care is more likely to maintain the prescribed therapy. Referral to a diabetes management centre is often helpful.

Encouraging breastfeeding. Studies have shown that newborns who have been exclusively breastfed have a lower incidence of developing diabetes later in life. Women with pre-existing diabetes should be encouraged to breastfeed immediately after birth and for at least 4 months postpartum, as this may contribute to the reduction of neonatal hypoglycemia, limit offspring obesity, and prevent development of diabetes (Feig et al., 2018). Blood glucose levels of newborns are monitored closely in the first 24 hours of life. Breastfeeding uses glucose reserves in the mother, thus glucose monitoring of the mother after breastfeeding is important. Taking in fluids or food before or during breastfeeding may be necessary.

Postpartum contraception. The preferred method of postpartum contraception for the woman with DM is one of the barrier methods, an intrauterine device (IUD), or progestin-only oral contraceptives (see Chapter 2) (Feig et al., 2018). The adverse effects of combined oral contraceptive use, such as the development of blood clots and cardiac problems, may be increased in women with DM. Carbohydrate metabolism may be affected by the progestin in the combined oral contraceptive, and an increased resistance to insulin may occur. Combined oral contraceptives thus should not be first-line recommendations.

HEART DISEASE

Heart disease affects a small percentage of pregnant women—1 to 4% of pregnancies (Elkayam, Golland, Petronella, et al., 2016). This number is increasing, as the number of women with congenital heart disease is increasing as well as those with other complications and advanced maternal age in pregnancy. During a normal pregnancy, an increase in heart rate, blood volume, and cardiac output places a physiological strain on the heart that may not be tolerated in a woman with pre-existing heart disease. Cardiac failure can occur prenatally, during labour, or in the postpartum period.

Manifestations

Increased levels of clotting factors predispose a woman to *thrombosis* (formation of clots in the veins). If her heart cannot meet these increased demands of pregnancy, heart failure (HF) results, and the fetus suffers from reduced placental blood flow. Box 5.4 lists signs and symptoms of HF.

During labour, each contraction temporarily shifts 300 to 500 mL of blood from the uterus and placenta into the woman's circulation, possibly overloading her weakened heart. Excess interstitial fluid rapidly returns to the circulation after birth, predisposing the woman to circulatory overload during the postpartum

Box 5.4 Signs of Heart Failure During Pregnancy

- Orthopnea (having to sit upright to breathe more easily)
- Persistent cough, often with expectoration of mucus that may be blood-tinged
- Moist lung sounds because of fluid within lungs
- Difficulty breathing on exertion
- Palpitations
- Fatigue or fainting on exertion
- Severe pitting edema of the lower extremities or generalized edema
- Changes in fetal heart rate indicating hypoxia or growth restriction if placental blood flow is reduced

period. She remains at an increased risk for HF after birth until her circulating blood volume returns to normal levels in the postpartum period; therefore, close monitoring is required.

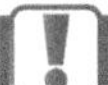 **Safety Alert!**

The nurse should observe the woman with heart disease for signs of heart failure, which can occur before, during, or after birth.

Treatment

The pregnant woman with heart disease is usually under the care of both a cardiologist and an obstetrician. She needs more frequent antepartum visits to determine how her heart is coping with the increased demands of pregnancy. Excessive weight gain must be avoided, because it adds to the demands on her heart. Preventing anemia with adequate diet and supplemental iron prevents a compensatory rise in the heart rate, which would add to the strain on the woman's heart. The priority of care is to limit physical activity to decrease the demands made on the heart. The limitation of activity can range from frequent rest periods to more limited activity depending on the degree of heart impairment. A woman on prolonged bed rest for any reason has a greater risk for forming venous thrombi (blood clots) and should be monitored for 12 weeks after birth. She is also at risk for obstetrical complications such as preterm labour and her fetus at risk for IUGR, so it is important to assess her pregnancy closely.

Medication therapy may include low-molecular-weight heparin to prevent clot formation, as heparin does not cross the placenta. Anticoagulants such as warfarin (Coumadin) may cause fetal anomalies and are not given during pregnancy. Beta-adrenergic blocking drugs used to treat hypertension and dysrhythmias can cause fetal *bradycardia* (slow heartbeat), respiratory depression, and hypoglycemia. Lasix (furosemide) may be used to treat chronic HF, but thiazide diuretics can cause harmful effects on the fetus, especially if administered in the third trimester. Digitalis and most antiarrhythmic drugs may be used to treat a pregnant woman, but they should be used with caution.

Box 5.5 Normal Blood Values of Significance for the Woman With a Heart Defect

LABORATORY TESTS	NORMAL VALUES
Partial thromboplastin time (PTT)	10–13 seconds
Activated partial thromboplastin time (aPTT)	30–40 seconds
Platelets	150–400 × 10^9/L

A vaginal birth is preferred over Caesarean birth because it carries less risk for infection or respiratory complications that would further tax the impaired heart. Forceps or a vacuum extractor may be used to decrease the need for maternal pushing in the second stage. An early epidural may also be planned for decreased stress in labour. Each cardiac condition will be evaluated separately to determine an individual plan of care by the interdisciplinary team.

Nursing Care

A woman with heart disease may already be familiar with its management. She should be taught about any necessary changes, such as the change from warfarin anticoagulants to subcutaneous heparin, and should be instructed in how to inject the medication. Laboratory tests include partial thromboplastin time (PTT), activated partial thromboplastin time (aPTT), and platelet counts. Box 5.5 specifies the normal values. She should promptly report signs of excess anticoagulation, such as bruising without reason, petechiae (tiny red spots on the skin), nosebleeds, or bleeding from the gums when brushing her teeth.

The woman is taught signs that may indicate HF so she can promptly report them. The nurse can help her to identify how she can balance activity with rest to minimize the demands on her heart. She should avoid exercise in extreme temperatures. She should be taught to stop an activity if she experiences dyspnea, chest pain, or tachycardia.

The woman may need help to plan her diet so that she has enough calories to meet her needs during pregnancy while not gaining too much weight. She should be taught about foods that are high in iron and folic acid to prevent anemia. She should avoid foods high in sodium, such as smoked meats and potato chips. Patients receiving heparin therapy should avoid foods high in vitamin K.

Stress can also increase demands on the heart. The nurse should discuss stressors in the woman's life and help her to identify ways to reduce or cope with them. During hospitalization, the healthcare provider should be notified if the pulse exceeds 100 beats/min or respirations are greater than 25 breaths/min at rest. Signs of *dyspnea* (difficulty in breathing), coughing, and abnormal breath sounds should be recorded and reported. Postpartum bradycardia should be reported to the healthcare provider, because the heart may fail as a result of the increased blood volume and diaphoresis that occur after birth.

ANEMIA

Anemia is the reduced ability of the blood to carry oxygen to the cells. Hemoglobin levels that are lower than 105 g/L in the second trimester and that are below 110 g/L in the first and third trimesters indicate anemia during pregnancy (Kilpatrick, 2014). Four anemias are significant during pregnancy: two nutritional anemias (iron-deficiency anemia and folic acid–deficiency anemia), and two anemias resulting from genetic disorders (sickle cell disease and thalassemia).

Nutritional Anemias

Most women with anemia have vague symptoms, if any. The anemic woman may fatigue easily and have little energy. Her skin and mucous membranes are pale. Shortness of breath, palpitations, and a rapid pulse may occur with severe anemia. The woman who develops anemia gradually has fewer symptoms than the woman who becomes anemic abruptly, such as through blood loss.

Iron-deficiency anemia

Pregnant women need additional iron for their own increased blood volume, for transfer to the fetus, and for a cushion against the blood loss expected at birth. The RBCs are small (microcytic) and pale (hypochromic) in iron-deficiency anemia. The tannic acid in tea and bran may decrease absorption of iron from foods eaten at the same meal.

Prevention. Iron supplements are commonly used to meet the needs of pregnancy and maintain iron stores. Vitamin C enhances the absorption of iron. Iron should not be taken with milk or antacids, because calcium impairs absorption.

Treatment. The woman with iron-deficiency anemia needs extra iron to correct the anemia and replenish her stores. She is treated with oral doses of *elemental iron* and continues this therapy for about 3 months after the anemia has been corrected.

Folic acid–deficiency anemia

Folic acid (also called *folate* or *folacin*) deficiency is characterized by large, immature RBCs (megaloblastic anemia). Iron-deficiency anemia is often present at the same time. Anticonvulsants, oral contraceptives, sulfa drugs, and alcohol can decrease the absorption of folate from food.

Prevention. Folic acid is essential for normal growth and development of the fetus. Folic acid deficiency has been associated with neural tube defects in the newborn. A daily supplement of 0.4 mg ensures adequate folic acid and is now recommended for all women of childbearing age (Wilson & Genetics Committee, 2015).

Treatment. Treatment of folate deficiency is with folic acid supplementation, as diet alone cannot provide the folic acid needed. The preventive dosage of supplementary folic acid may be higher for women who have previously had a child who had a neural tube defect (see Chapter 4 for further discussion).

Genetic Anemias

Sickle cell disease

Unlike those with nutritional anemias, people with sickle cell disease have abnormal hemoglobin that causes their erythrocytes to become distorted into a sickle (crescent) shape during episodes of hypoxia or acidosis. It is an autosomal recessive disorder, meaning that the affected person receives an abnormal gene from each parent. The abnormally shaped blood cells do not flow smoothly, and they clog small blood vessels. The sickle cells are destroyed more rapidly, resulting in chronic anemia. (See Chapter 27 for further discussion of sickle cell disease.)

Pregnancy may cause a sickle cell crisis, with onset of increased pain often in the joints, accompanied by massive erythrocyte destruction and occlusion of blood vessels. The main risk to the fetus is occlusion of vessels that supply the placenta, leading to preterm birth, growth restriction, and fetal death.

The woman should have frequent evaluation and treatment for anemia during prenatal care. Fetal evaluations concentrate on fetal growth and placental function. Oxygen, warm blankets or the use of an underbody warmer, and fluids are provided continuously during labour to prevent sickle cell crisis. Genetic counselling should be offered. An early epidural is encouraged, to decrease stress and promote pain relief in labour.

Thalassemia

Thalassemia is a genetic trait that causes an abnormality in one of two chains of hemoglobin, the alpha (α) or beta (β) chain. The β-chain variety is most often encountered in North America. The person can inherit an abnormal gene from each parent, causing β-thalassemia major, or Cooley's anemia. If only one abnormal gene is inherited, the person will have β-thalassemia minor.

The woman with β-thalassemia minor usually has few problems other than mild anemia, and the fetus does not appear to be affected. However, administration of iron supplements may cause iron overload in a woman with β-thalassemia because the body absorbs and stores iron in higher-than-usual amounts.

Nursing Care for Anemias During Pregnancy

The woman is taught which foods are high in iron and folic acid to help her prevent or treat anemia. She is taught how to take the supplements in a way that they are optimally effective. For example, the nurse should explain that although milk is good to drink during pregnancy, it should not be taken at the same time as the iron supplement, or the iron will not be absorbed as easily. Taking iron supplements on an empty stomach and eating with foods high in vitamin C enhance absorption.

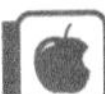

Nutrition Considerations

Foods Recommended in Pregnancy

FOODS HIGH IN IRON

Meats, chicken, fish, liver, legumes, green leafy vegetables, whole or enriched grain products, nuts, molasses, tofu, eggs, dried fruits

FOODS HIGH IN FOLIC ACID

Green leafy vegetables, asparagus, green beans, fruits, whole grains, liver, legumes, yeast

FOODS HIGH IN VITAMIN C (ENHANCES ABSORPTION OF IRON)

Citrus fruits and juices, strawberries, cantaloupe, cabbage, green and red peppers, tomatoes, potatoes, green leafy vegetables

To prevent or correct nutritional anemias, such as iron and folic acid deficiencies, the nurse should teach all women appropriate food sources for those nutrients.

The woman is taught that when she takes iron, her stools may be dark green to black and that mild gastrointestinal discomfort may occur. She should contact her primary healthcare provider if these side effects trouble her; another iron preparation may be better tolerated. She should not take antacids with iron.

The woman with sickle cell disease requires close medical and nursing care. She should be taught to prevent dehydration and activities that cause hypoxia. The woman with β-thalassemia is taught to avoid situations in which exposure to infection is more likely (e.g., crowds during flu season) and to report any symptoms of infection promptly. (See Chapter 27 for a discussion of sickle cell anemia and thalassemia.)

OBESITY, BARIATRIC SURGERY, AND PREGNANCY

The obese woman who is pregnant has a high risk for developing complications during pregnancy, such as gestational diabetes, hypertension, cardiac problems, pre-eclampsia, and respiratory problems. The obese patient is often placed in a high-risk category for prenatal care to receive special assessments, guidance, and close follow-up care. Ultrasounds may be scheduled over several visits as they may need to be focused on specific areas of the fetus only, given the challenges of body size of the mother. Planning during pregnancy for labour and birth is important to ensure that the facility has the right equipment for labour or a Caesarean birth. Working with an interdisciplinary team is ideal to ensure that obese women who are pregnant receive sensitive, compassionate care that addresses all of their needs.

When childbearing-age women undergo gastric bypass surgery, they are cautioned to delay pregnancy for 1 to 2 years, to avoid weight loss during pregnancy. However, the reduced absorption in the stomach and small bowel may result in a deficiency of essential nutrients during pregnancy. In this instance, nutritional guidance from a registered dietitian during pregnancy is essential. In some patients who have had bariatric surgery, consumption of simple sugars can lead to a condition known as "dumping syndrome," which is manifested by nausea, vomiting, cramping, and diarrhea. Blood glucose levels should be monitored. Abdominal symptoms during pregnancy should be monitored closely to determine whether they are related to the gastric bypass surgery. Internal intestinal herniation can occur, and abdominal pain, nausea, and vomiting in the third trimester in a patient with a history of bariatric surgery should be managed promptly (Bryant, 2016). When bariatric surgery via gastric band placement is undertaken, the band can be adjusted during pregnancy to allow adequate nutrient intake during pregnancy.

INFECTIONS

The mnemonic *TORCH* has been used to describe infections that can be devastating for the fetus or newborn. The letters stand for the first letters of four infections or infectious agents: **to**xoplasmosis, **r**ubella, **c**ytomegalovirus, and **h**erpes simplex virus; the **O** is sometimes used to designate "**o**ther" infections. However, there are many more infections that can be devastating for the mother, fetus, or newborn. Some of these are damaging any time they are acquired, whereas others are relatively harmless except when acquired during pregnancy. See Chapter 4, Table 4.1, for routine prenatal laboratory testing.

Viral Infections

Viral infections often have no effective therapy and may have serious consequences for the mother, fetus or newborn, or both. However, immunizations can prevent some of these infections. An infant born to a mother with an active viral infection, such as rubeola or varicella, must be placed on airborne and contact isolation.

Cytomegalovirus

Cytomegalovirus (CMV) infection is a herpes infection and can be sexually transmitted as well as transmitted in other ways. The infection is often asymptomatic in the mother. CMV immunoglobulin can be given to the symptomatic mother during pregnancy (Schleiss, 2016). An infected infant may have some of the following serious problems:

- Developmental delays
- Seizures
- Blindness
- Deafness
- Dental abnormalities
- Petechiae (often called a "blueberry muffin" rash)

Treatment and nursing care. Primary prevention via hand hygiene is essential. Therapeutic pregnancy termination may be offered if CMV infection is discovered during early pregnancy. Ganciclovir and valganciclovir are antiviral drugs that hold promise in improving the developmental outcome in newborns (Britt, 2016).

Rubella

Rubella is a mild viral disease with a low fever and rash. However, its effects on the developing fetus can be destructive. Rubella occurring in very early pregnancy can disrupt the formation of major body systems, whereas rubella acquired later is more likely to damage organs that are already formed. Some effects of rubella on the embryo or fetus include the following:

- Microcephaly (small head size)
- Developmental delays
- Congenital cataracts
- Deafness
- Cardiac defects
- IUGR

Treatment and nursing care. Immunization against rubella infection has been available for some time, but some women of childbearing age are still susceptible. When a woman of childbearing age is immunized, she should not get pregnant for at least 1 month after the immunization. The vaccine is offered during the postpartum period to nonimmune women. It is *not* given during pregnancy, because it is a live attenuated (weakened) form of the virus.

Nursing Tip

Rubella is a cause of birth defects that is almost completely preventable by immunization before childbearing age. The nurse should check each postpartum woman's chart for rubella immunity and notify the healthcare provider if the woman is not immune. Information should also be given to the postpartum woman who receives the vaccine about possible adverse effects, such as rash in 10 days to 2 weeks.

Herpes virus

There are two types of herpes viruses. Type 1 is more likely to cause fever blisters or cold sores. Type 2 is more likely to cause genital herpes. After the primary infection occurs, the virus becomes dormant in the nerves and may be reactivated later as a recurrent (secondary) infection. Initial infection during the first half of pregnancy may cause spontaneous abortion. The infant is infected in one of the following ways:

- The virus ascends into the uterus after the membranes rupture.
- The infant has direct contact with infectious lesions during vaginal birth.

Neonatal herpes infection can be either localized or disseminated (widespread). Disseminated neonatal infection has a high mortality rate, and survivors may have neurological complications.

Treatment and nursing care. Avoiding contact with the lesions can prevent neonatal herpes infection. If the woman has active genital herpes lesions when the membranes rupture or labour begins, a Caesarean birth may be required to prevent fetal contact during birth or the development of an ascending infection. Caesarean birth is not necessary if there are no active genital lesions. The mother and infant do not need to be isolated as long as direct contact with lesions is prevented. Breastfeeding is safe if there are no lesions on the breasts. Antiviral drugs such as acyclovir may be given orally during pregnancy to reduce the occurrence of active lesions at the time of birth (PHAC, 2016). Infected newborns may receive acyclovir and are followed closely after birth.

Hepatitis B

Blood, saliva, vaginal secretions, semen, and breastmilk can carry the virus that causes hepatitis B infection; the infection can also cross the placenta. The woman may be asymptomatic or acutely ill with chronic low-grade fever, anorexia, nausea, and vomiting. Some individuals become chronic carriers of the virus. The fetus may be infected transplacentally or by contact at birth with blood or vaginal secretions. The infant may become a chronic carrier and a continuing source of infection. Box 5.6 lists those who are at greater risk of having hepatitis B infection.

Treatment and nursing care. All women should be screened for hepatitis B during the course of prenatal care, and the screening should be repeated during the third trimester for women in high-risk groups. Infants born to women who are positive for hepatitis B should receive a single dose of hepatitis B immune globulin (for temporary immunity right after birth) followed by hepatitis B vaccine (for long-term immunity). Both should be given within the first 12 hours of life. Immunization during pregnancy is not contraindicated. If possible, injections should be delayed until after the infant's first bath, so that blood and other potentially infectious secretions are removed

Box 5.6 Persons at Higher Risk for Hepatitis B Infection

- Intravenous drug users
- Persons with multiple sexual partners
- Persons with repeated infection with sexually transmitted infections
- Health care workers with occupational exposure to blood products and needle-sticks
- Hemodialysis patients
- Recipients of multiple blood transfusions or other blood products
- Household contact with hepatitis carrier or hemodialysis patient
- Persons arriving from countries where there is a higher incidence of the disease

to avoid introducing them under the skin. Because healthcare staff have occupational exposure to blood and other infectious secretions, they should be immunized against hepatitis B. Some provinces provide hepatitis B vaccine to all newborns at birth and at 1 to 2 months and 6 to 18 months, but some provinces do this when the child is in grade 8. Please refer to the provincial schedule for immunizations and Chapter 32 for more information.

Zika virus infection

Zika virus is spread by the bite of an *Aedes* mosquito and can also be spread by sexual contact (PHAC, 2019). Currently, there is no preventive vaccination or treatment for the infection. Criteria for testing for Zika infection include history of travel to high-risk areas, unprotected sexual contact with a partner from a high-risk area within 6 months, or evidence of exposure (Epps, Rac, Dunn, et al., 2017). Acquiring the infection during the first trimester and subsequent transmission to the fetus may lead to the development of congenital Zika syndrome, which includes the following severe birth defects (Government of Canada, 2018a):

- Hearing loss
- Club foot and contracted limbs
- Incomplete brain development, including abnormally small heads (microcephaly)
- Abnormal development of the eyes, including visual problems
- Other neurological abnormalities, including:
  - Irritability
  - Seizures
  - Spasticity

The mosquito bite results in an infection that has mild and nonspecific signs and symptoms in the mother, such as a rash and headache. Prevention involves eliminating breeding sources for the mosquito, wearing long-sleeved shirts and pants, and use of plant-derived insect repellants containing DEET, picaridin, oil of lemon, eucalyptus, or para-menthane-diol (PMD). Oil of eucalyptus and PMD should not be used on children younger than 3 years of age, and any insect repellant is contraindicated for infants under 2 months of age (Government of Canada, 2018a). The use of window screens and mosquito netting is advised in affected areas. Sexual transmission of the virus can be prevented by use of condoms (Government of Canada, 2018a). Pregnant women should be assessed for Zika virus exposure and be offered preventive education (Society of Obstetricians and Gynaecologists of Canada [SOGC], 2016).

Pertussis

Bordetella pertussis is a respiratory pathogen that is most critical for infants less than 6 months of age. As a result, pregnant women are being encouraged to obtain a single dose of Tdap (tetanus, diphtheria, and acellular pertussis) (Costillo & Poliquin, 2018; Government of Canada, 2015). The timing of this vaccination is between 26 and 32 weeks in pregnancy, with the intention of increasing antibodies in preparation for birth.

Sexually Transmitted Infections

Sexually transmitted infections (STIs) are those for which a common mode of transmission is sexual intercourse, although several can also be transmitted in other ways. Herpes virus has already been discussed. Other infections that are typically transmitted sexually are syphilis, gonorrhea, chlamydia, trichomoniasis, condylomata acuminata (genital warts), and human immunodeficiency virus (HIV).

Changes in the vaginal secretions that occur during pregnancy can increase the risk of developing a vaginal infection. The high estrogen levels present during pregnancy thicken the vaginal mucosa and increase secretions that have a high glycogen content. This makes the woman susceptible to yeast infections and infections by other microorganisms. Later in pregnancy the pH of the vagina decreases, resulting in a protective effect.

All sexual contacts of persons infected with a disease that can be sexually transmitted should be informed and treated; otherwise the cycle of infection and reinfection will continue. Consistent use of a latex condom, including the female condom, helps to reduce the sexual spread of STIs. STIs and vaginal infections are discussed in detail in Chapter 2.

Human immunodeficiency virus

Human immunodeficiency virus (HIV) is the causative organism of acquired immunodeficiency syndrome (AIDS). The virus eventually affects the immune system, making the person susceptible to infections that eventually can result in death. There is no known immunization or curative treatment, but control of opportunistic infections has increased life expectancy. See Chapter 2 and a medical-surgical text for further discussion of HIV/AIDS and its treatment.

The incidence of HIV infection has declined overall, although in 2016 the rate increased slightly. The incidence of women newly diagnosed with AIDS accounts for 23.4% of the overall total for 2016 (Bourgeois, Edmunds, Awan, et al., 2017). HIV infection is acquired in one of the following four ways:

1. Unprotected (through condom nonuse, breakage, or slippage) sexual contact (anal, vaginal, or oral) with an infected person
2. Sharing a needle with an infected person
3. Mucous membrane exposure to infected body fluids
4. Perinatal exposure (infants)

The infant may be infected in one of the following three ways:

1. Transplacentally
2. Through contact with infected maternal secretions at birth
3. Through breastmilk

Box 5.7 High-Risk Factors for Human Immunodeficiency Virus (HIV)

- Intravenous problematic substance use and needle sharing
- Multiple sexual partners
- Sex trade worker
- History of sexually transmitted infections
- Immigration from geographical areas where infection is endemic
- Sexual partner in a high-risk group
- Sexual partner with HIV infection

If a woman is identified with an HIV infection and adequately treated throughout the pregnancy and if she does not breastfeed, the chance of transmitting the virus to her newborn is less 1% (Money, Tullock, Boucoiran, et al., 2014). The key to prevention of HIV infection in newborns is universal screening of all pregnant women. All pregnant women should be offered HIV testing, with appropriate pre- and post-test counselling, as part of their routine prenatal care in each pregnancy. This testing should be repeated in each trimester in women who are recognized to be at high and ongoing risk for HIV infection (Money et al., 2014).

Nursing care. Counselling should be provided to all women concerning behaviours that place them at risk for contracting HIV (Box 5.7). Pregnant women with AIDS are more susceptible to infection, and the fetus may develop an impaired immune system that increases the risk of opportunistic infections after birth. It is recommended that mothers who live in developed countries, who are HIV positive, not breastfeed.

The fetus and the woman are monitored closely during the antepartum period. All infants born to HIV-positive women are presumed to be HIV positive, and routine precautions are initiated for both the mother and the infant. The infant may receive medication therapy with zidovudine starting 6 to 12 hours after birth and continuing during the first 6 weeks of life. The nurse should help the mother cope with the anxiety that is almost certain to occur about whether the newborn is infected. Community resources can help the family with the care of the child at home. During the hospital stay, it is important to keep the information regarding the HIV status confidential, as some women may not have shared this information with all of their family or friends. Women should be taught about the risks of sharing needles, the importance of using condoms, and the need to avoid oral sex.

Safety Alert!

The nurse should wear protective equipment, such as gloves, with *every* potential exposure to a patient's body secretions. This practice protects the nurse from direct exposure to many pathogenic organisms.

Nonviral Infections

Toxoplasmosis

Toxoplasmosis is caused by *Toxoplasma gondii*, a parasite that may be acquired by contact with cat feces or raw meat and transmitted through the placenta. The woman is usually asymptomatic or has mild symptoms. Congenital toxoplasmosis includes the following possible signs in the newborn:

- Low birth weight
- Enlarged liver and spleen
- Jaundice
- Anemia
- Inflammation of eye structures
- Neurological damage

Treatment and nursing care. Treatment of the mother reduces the risk of congenital infection. Pyrimethamine (Daraprim) and sulfadiazine are used after the first trimester and leucovorin after 18-weeks' gestation. Spiramycin (Rovamycine), although controversial, is typically well tolerated. Treatment of infants involves pyrimethamine, sulfadiazine, and leucovorin for 1 year, which may reduce the severity of the congenital effects of the disease (McLeod, VanTubbergen, & Boyer, 2016). Nurses can teach women the following measures to reduce the likelihood of acquiring the infection:

- Cook all meat thoroughly.
- Wash hands and all kitchen surfaces after handling raw meat.
- Avoid touching the mucous membranes of the eyes or mouth while handling raw meat.
- Avoid uncooked eggs and unpasteurized milk.
- Wash fresh fruits and vegetables well.
- Avoid materials contaminated with cat feces, such as litter boxes, sand boxes, and garden soil.

Group B streptococcus infection

Group B streptococcus (GBS) is a leading cause of perinatal infections that result in a high neonatal mortality rate. The organism can be found in the woman's rectum, vagina, cervix, urine, throat, or skin. Although she is colonized with the organism, the woman is usually asymptomatic, but the infant may be infected through contact at birth with vaginal secretions. The risk is greater if the woman has a long labour or premature rupture of membranes. GBS is a significant cause of maternal postpartum infection (endometritis, or infection of the uterine interior), especially after Caesarean birth. Symptoms include an elevated temperature within 12 hours after birth, rapid heart rate (tachycardia), and abdominal distention. Diagnosis of GBS is confirmed by vaginal and rectal culture.

GBS infection can be deadly for the infant. A newborn may have either early-onset (before 7 days) or late-onset (after 7 days) GBS infection.

Prevention and treatment. A culture of the woman's rectum and lower vagina for the presence of GBS is routinely taken at 35 to 37 weeks of gestation. If results are not known, the woman is ordered antibiotics based on her risk factors, such as previous history of GBS infection, prolonged rupture of the membranes (>18 hours), or fever above 37.7°C (100°F) during labour, to prevent GBS infection. Any GBS-positive urine culture during pregnancy is considered a cause for antibiotic treatment during labour, and the newborn may be treated with antibiotics at birth (Jefferies & Canadian Paediatric Society, Fetus and Newborn Committee, 2017). Regular assessment of the newborn after birth up to 24 to 48 hours is also part of the intervention if a woman is determined to be GBS positive during pregnancy.

Tuberculosis

There are about 1 600 new cases of tuberculosis (TB) each year, and about 90% of these cases affect two main populations: 70% of cases occur among foreign-born individuals, and 20% of cases occur among Canadian-born Indigenous peoples (Government of Canada, 2018b). Drug-resistant strains of the bacterium continue to emerge (Centers for Disease Control and Prevention [CDC], 2017). Pregnant women are screened for pulmonary TB by either a tuberculin skin test or a serum interferon gamma release assay (IGRA), more commonly known as a QuantiFERON-TB Gold (QFT-G) or T-spot test, as would be the case for any other patient (refer to a medical-surgical nursing text). If the screening test is positive, the woman should have a chest radiograph (X-ray film) with the pregnant abdomen shielded by a lead apron. If required, sputum cultures that are positive for the bacterium confirm the diagnosis.

The adult with TB experiences fatigue, weakness, loss of appetite and weight, fever, and night sweats. The newborn may acquire the disease by contact with an untreated mother after birth.

Treatment and nursing care. The local public health department is notified of positive cultures and/or chest radiograph results, and isoniazid and rifampin are usually prescribed for 9 months. Pregnant women who are taking isoniazid should usually take pyridoxine to reduce the risk of peripheral neuritis. Ethambutol may be prescribed if drug-resistant TB is suspected. If the mother has active pulmonary TB, the infant must be kept in a separate area away from the mother. The local health department must be notified, and the discharge plan of the mother and infant must be approved before they are allowed to leave the hospital. The infant may receive preventive therapy with isoniazid for 3 months after birth. The health care staff, including nurses, must teach the family how the organism is transmitted and the importance of continuing the antitubercular medications consistently for the full course of therapy. Incompletely treated TB is a significant cause in the development of medication-resistant organisms. Modern antitubercular drugs usually render the sputum culture negative within 2 weeks; thus, home care is the protocol, with health department follow up.

Urinary Tract Infections

Urinary tract infections (UTIs) are common in females because of the short urethra and the ease of contamination of the urethra from the rectum. Bacteriuria involving GBS was discussed above in the section on GBS.

The urinary tract is normally self-cleaning; acidic urine inhibits the growth of microorganisms and flushes them out of the body with each voiding. Pregnancy alters this self-cleaning action, because pressure on urinary structures keeps the bladder from emptying completely and because the ureters dilate and lose motility under the relaxing effects of the hormone progesterone. Urine that is retained in the bladder becomes more alkaline, providing a favourable environment for the growth of microorganisms.

Some women have excessive microorganisms in their urine but no symptoms (asymptomatic bacteriuria). The asymptomatic infection may eventually cause cystitis (bladder infection) or pyelonephritis (kidney infection). The woman with cystitis has the following signs and symptoms:

- Burning with urination
- Increased frequency and urgency of urination
- A normal or slightly elevated temperature

If not treated, cystitis can ascend in the urinary tract and cause pyelonephritis. Pyelonephritis is a particularly serious infection in pregnancy and is accompanied by these signs and symptoms:

- High fever
- Chills
- Flank pain or tenderness
- Nausea and vomiting

Maternal hypertension, chronic renal disease, and preterm birth may occur with pyelonephritis during pregnancy. The high maternal fever is dangerous for the fetus because it increases the fetal metabolic rate, which in turn increases fetal oxygen needs to levels that the mother cannot readily supply.

Treatment

UTIs are treated with short-term oral antibiotics. Asymptomatic bacteriuria is treated with oral antibiotics for 10 days. Pyelonephritis is treated with multiple antibiotics, initially administered intravenously. Cystitis in pregnant women is treated with a full 7 days of antibiotic therapy.

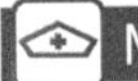
Nursing Tip

The nurse should teach all females measures to reduce their risk for urinary tract infections.

Nursing care

All females should be taught how to reduce the introduction of rectal microorganisms into the bladder. For example, a front-to-back direction should be used when wiping after urination or a bowel movement, when doing perineal cleansing, or when applying and removing perineal pads. The nurse can begin teaching during the woman's prenatal visits and reinforce the teaching during the postpartum stay. The mother should be taught how to clean and diaper an infant girl to avoid fecal contamination of her urethra.

Adequate fluid intake promotes frequent voiding. Drinking at least eight glasses of liquid per day and excluding caffeine-containing beverages help to flush urine through the urinary tract regularly. Cranberry juice may make the urine more acidic and therefore less conducive to the growth of infectious organisms.

Sexual intercourse mildly irritates the bladder and urethra, which can promote a UTI. Urinating before intercourse reduces irritation; urinating afterward flushes urine from the bladder. Using water-soluble lubricant during intercourse can also reduce periurethral irritation.

Pregnant women should be taught the signs and symptoms of cystitis and pyelonephritis so that they will know what to watch for and to seek treatment at once.

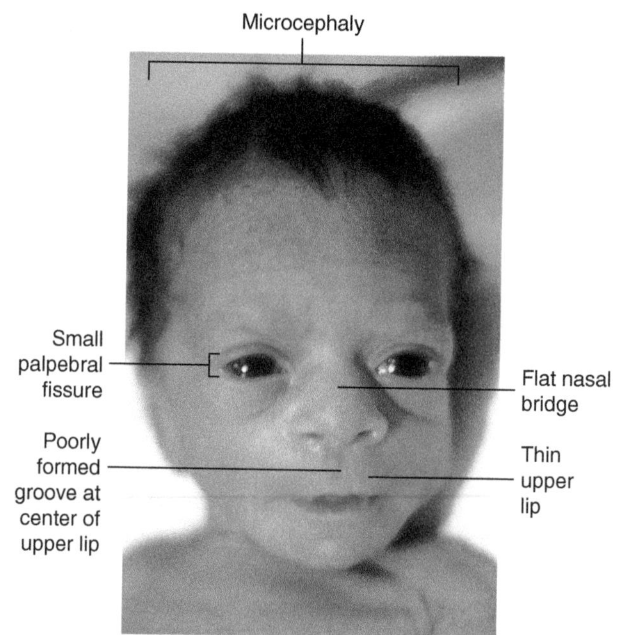

Fig. 5.8 Fetal alcohol spectrum disorder (FASD). The facial features of an infant with FASD include short palpebral (eye) fissures; a flat nasal bridge; a thin, flat upper lip; a poorly formed groove at the center of the upper lip; and a small head (microcephaly). (From Clark, D. A. [2000]. *Atlas of neonatology: A companion to Avery's diseases of the newborn* [7th ed.]. Philadelphia: Saunders.)

ENVIRONMENTAL HAZARDS DURING PREGNANCY

A **teratogen** is a substance that causes an adverse effect on the developing embryo or fetus. Some birth defects are caused by a combination of genetic and environmental factors. The specific anomaly that develops depends on the time of exposure to the environmental teratogen in relation to the stage of development of the embryo. In the first weeks of life, the vital organs are developing, and exposure to an environmental teratogen may cause miscarriage. Exposure to a teratogen in later pregnancy might result in growth restriction. The four main teratogens of concern during pregnancy are drugs, chemicals, infectious agents, and radiation.

SUBSTANCE USE

The use of illicit or recreational drugs during pregnancy has an adverse effect on both the mother and the fetus. The most common substances used during pregnancy are tobacco and alcohol (Finnegan, 2013), with rates of about 10% among childbearing women. Cannabis is the most commonly used illicit substance used by pregnant women (Finnegan, 2013). Multiple drugs may be used together, and other factors such as inadequate nutrition and prenatal care may also combine to decrease the overall health of a woman and her fetus.

For pregnant women dealing with issues related to medication or illicit substance use, MotherToBaby is a resource on the risks and safety of all medication use during pregnancy. This information is available to healthcare providers and laypeople; see the Online Resources section at the end of the chapter. A woman with persistent pain or conditions requiring opioid medications in pregnancy needs support to enable her to meet her needs. It is important for this patient to review her options with her healthcare providers during this time, particularly if she wishes to breastfeed after birth. It will be important for her to know that her infant will be assessed and scored for neonatal opioid withdrawal syndrome (NOWS), also often known as *neonatal abstinence syndrome (NAS)*, after birth and to know the comfort measures she can carry out to decrease withdrawal symptoms (see Chapter 12 for further discussion of NOWS).

It is well established that several (prescribed and recreational) substances are harmful to the developing fetus (Fig. 5.8). The fetus of the woman who uses substances or takes prescription medications such as opioids for chronic pain is exposed to higher levels of the substance for a longer time because the substances become concentrated in the amniotic fluid and the fetus ingests the fluid. Many environmental substances are most harmful to the fetus early in pregnancy, perhaps before the woman realizes she is pregnant. Table 5.6 reviews some substances that are harmful to the fetus.

Nursing Tip

When asking questions about substance use during pregnancy, the nurse should focus on how the information will help nurses and other healthcare providers provide the safest and most appropriate care to the pregnant woman and her infant. All women should be asked about past and current alcohol, nicotine, marijuana, and illicit and prescribed medication use with open-ended questions in a nonthreatening manner (Ordean, Wong, Graves, et al., 2017).

Treatment and Nursing Care

Care focuses on identifying a woman's substance use early in the pregnancy, educating her about the

Table 5.6 Substances Harmful to the Fetus

SUBSTANCE	EFFECTS
Alcohol	Alcohol is commonly used by women of childbearing age. Fetal alcohol spectrum disorder (FASD) is well documented (see Fig. 5.8) and includes growth restriction, developmental delays, and facial abnormalities. No "safe" level of alcohol ingestion during pregnancy is known; therefore, the Society of Obstetricians and Gynaecologists of Canada (SOGC) recommends that women abstain from alcohol during pregnancy because of the unknown risks (Senikas, Kluka, Wood, et al., 2010).
Cocaine	Cocaine is a powerful central nervous system stimulant that causes vasoconstriction that may precipitate preterm labour. It can cause hypertension, seizures, and stroke in the mother; fetal anomalies such as genitourinary malformations, intrauterine growth restriction (IUGR), and placental abruption; and behavioural problems in the child long term.
Marijuana	Cannabis may now be the most commonly used substance during pregnancy. Effects of cannabis during pregnancy may cause preterm labour, low birth weight, offspring with lower IQ scores, and impulsivity and hyperactivity in childhood (SOGC, 2018). Initial effects on the newborn are related to decreased self-quieting ability, fine tremors, and sleep pattern changes. It passes into breastmilk easily. The woman who is using marijuana is encouraged to quit, based on the effects related to judgement and decision making while using this substance as a new parent.
Tobacco	Smoking can cause fetal growth restriction, placental previa, and placental abruption, as well as spontaneous abortion. Nicotine causes vasoconstriction that reduces blood flow to the placenta. Childhood asthma, behavioural problems, and attention-deficit/hyperactivity disorder (ADHD) have been connected long term to smoking during pregnancy.
Heroin	The heroin-addicted woman may also be exposed to human immunodeficiency virus (HIV) because the drug is taken intravenously and may include needle sharing and other high-risk behaviours. Withdrawal syndrome (agitation, cramps, diarrhea, rhinorrhea [runny nose]) occurs if the drug is stopped suddenly. Neonatal opioid withdrawal syndrome occurs within 24 hours of birth (high-pitched cry, tremors, seizures, and disrupted sleep–wake cycles). Serious maternal and fetal effects occur.
Amphetamines	These are often associated with maternal malnutrition and tachycardia. Their use can cause fetal anomalies, IUGR, and neonatal opioid withdrawal syndrome symptoms (NOWS) in the newborn, or can cause fetal death. This type of drug enters breastmilk and is dangerous to the infant.
Anticoagulants	Warfarin (Coumadin) can cross the placenta and cause spontaneous abortion, growth restriction, central nervous system problems, and facial defects (fetal warfarin syndrome). Heparin and enoxaparin (Lovenox) do not cross the placenta and are the medications of choice when an anticoagulant is required.
Antibiotics	Tetracycline (Sumycin) exposure can cause yellowing of the deciduous teeth and hyperplasia of the enamel. To prevent tooth discoloration, tetracycline is not advised for children under 7 years. Medications such as streptomycin and kanamycin are associated with damage to the eighth cranial nerve and hearing loss in the newborn. Amoxicillin is safe, but the addition of clavulanate (Augmentin) can cause necrotizing enterocolitis (NEC) in the newborn. Sulfonamides increase the risk of hyperbilirubinemia in the newborn. Cephalosporins are considered generally safe.
Anticonvulsants	Phenytoin (Dilantin) can cause craniofacial abnormalities and developmental delays in the newborn. The risk of medication and the benefits of seizure control during pregnancy should be evaluated. Pregnant women who must take valproic acid (Depakene) or carbamazepine (Tegretol) should have fetal assessments for skeletal anomalies and neural tube defects. Most anticonvulsants increase the risk for fetal anomalies; folic acid supplementation is recommended (1 mg vs. 0.4 mg).
Isotretinoin (Accutane) and vitamin A derivatives	Isotretinoin and etretinate are used for skin disorders (mainly acne); they are clearly associated with fetal anomalies and are contraindicated for use in pregnancy. Birth control is advised for a minimum of 3 months after isotretinoin therapy.
Antiasthmatic	Cromolyn sodium is considered safe during pregnancy. Isoproterenol and metaproterenol aerosols are considered safe, but oral or intravenous use may decrease uterine blood flow.
Cough medicine	Any cough medicine containing iodide can cause a goiter in the fetus that could affect respirations in the newborn and thus should be avoided.
Decongestants	Topical nasal sprays, rather than systemic medication, are considered preferable during pregnancy.

Continued

Table 5.6 Substances Harmful to the Fetus—cont'd

SUBSTANCE	EFFECTS
Angiotensin-converting enzyme (ACE) inhibitors (captopril, enalapril)	ACE inhibitors can cause fetal kidney anomalies, growth restriction, and oligohydramnios (decreased amniotic fluid). Enalapril (Vasotce) and captopril (Capoten) in the second trimester can cause craniofacial anomalies. The medication valsartan can cause lung problems in the newborn and oligohydramnios in the mother.
Folic acid antagonists (methotrexate, amethopterin)	Folic acid antagonists cause spontaneous abortion and serious fetal anomalies. Use of cyclosporine evidenced no anomalies but premature birth can occur. Chloroquine for malaria prevention is considered generally safe.
Lithium	Lithium is associated with development of congenital heart disease. It can also be toxic to the thyroid and kidneys of the fetus. Discontinuation during pregnancy may not be in the best interest of maternal health.

Data from Niebyl, J., Weber, R., & Briggs, G. (2017). Drugs and environmental agents in pregnancy and lactation: Tetralogy and epidemiology. In S. F. Gabbe, J. R. Niebyl, & J. L. Simpson, et al. (Eds.), *Obstetrics: Normal and problem pregnancies* (7th ed.). Philadelphia: Saunders; Smith, R. (2018). *Netter's obstetrics and gynecology* (3rd ed.). Philadelphia: Elsevier; Senikas, V., Kluka, S., Wood, R., et al. (2010). SOGC clinical practice guideline: Alcohol use and pregnancy consensus clinical guideline. *Journal of Obstetrics and Gynaecology Canada, 32*(8), Suppl. 3; Society of Obstetricians & Gynaecologists of Canada. (2018). The SOGC urges Canadians to avoid cannabis use during pregnancy and breastfeeding. Retrieved from: https://sogc.org/files/Cannabis%20campaign_web.pdf.

effects of substance use, and encouraging her to reduce or eliminate use. Appropriate referrals should be made.

A partnership should be created with the woman, and a plan for treatment should be developed. Dietary support, monitoring of the woman's weight gain, and fetal assessment promote better pregnancy outcomes. Flexibility in patient scheduling and allowing late arrival for appointments are critical to developing rapport with this woman (Ordean et al., 2017). Pregnancy is the ideal time for the woman to make a change, as the motivation of the infant's health as well as her own may be higher than at any other time in her life. Harm reduction may be a consideration, such as substituting methadone therapy for opioid use.

In the case of therapeutic medications, the woman's need for the medication is weighed against the potential for fetal harm it may cause and the fetal or maternal harm that may occur if the woman is not treated. In general, the healthcare provider will choose the least teratogenic medication that is effective and prescribe it at the lowest effective dosage.

Educating females about the effect of medications on a developing fetus is best done before pregnancy. Women should be taught to try to eliminate the use of any recreational substances before becoming pregnant. Women should be encouraged to tell their healthcare provider if they think they are pregnant (or are trying to conceive) before having a nonemergency X-ray, being prescribed a medication, or taking herbal or food supplements.

A trusting, therapeutic nurse–patient relationship makes it more likely that a woman will be truthful about the use of substances, both legal and illicit. The nurse who collects data must use a nonjudgemental approach and treat the issue as a health problem rather than a moral problem. The nurse should support the woman who is trying to reduce her drug use. The nurse should also praise her efforts to improve her overall health and to have a successful pregnancy.

In the context of substance and medication use, a multidisciplinary approach is needed to plan for the care of a mother and her newborn that includes referral to community agencies after discharge or child protective services, if needed. Medications that are contraindicated for use in women who are breastfeeding are identified in various drug references; these references should be used as a guide in counselling mothers concerning breastfeeding.

TRAUMA DURING PREGNANCY

Trauma during pregnancy is the leading cause of nonobstetrical maternal mortality, with 20% of maternal deaths caused by such injuries (Jain, Chari, Maslovitz, et al., 2015). The incidence of trauma during pregnancy may continue to rise because women are increasingly employed at some jobs that entail greater risk of injury. There is also a trend toward more violence in society. Although pregnant women usually are more careful to protect themselves from harm, increased stress from pregnancy may lead to injury both inside and outside of the home. Falls, motor vehicle collisions, and intimate partner violence are the leading causes of trauma in pregnancy.

Falls are not uncommon, because of the woman's altered sense of balance (approximately 25% of women describe a fall during pregnancy). The pregnant woman needs to be especially careful in winter weather with snow and ice, in circumstances where water on surfaces makes them slippery, and when taking any medications that may increase her drowsiness.

A pregnant woman needs to wear a seat belt every time she is in a car, both as a driver and as a passenger. The lap portion of the belt is placed low, just below her protruding abdomen. The pregnant woman and her fetus are more likely to suffer severe injury or death because of not being restrained during a crash than they are to be injured by the restraint itself. Air bags are a supplemental restraint and are intended for use in addition to seat belts.

Physical trauma is usually blunt trauma (falls or blows to the body) but may be penetrating trauma (knife or gunshot wounds). Physical abuse against women is a significant cause of trauma. Intimate partner violence occurs in all ethnic groups and all social strata. It often begins or becomes worse during pregnancy. The abuser is usually her male partner, although it may also be a female partner.

Women abused during pregnancy are more likely to have miscarriages, stillbirths, and low-birth-weight babies. They often enter prenatal care late, if at all. The risk of homicide escalates during pregnancy.

Abuse during pregnancy, as at other times, may take many forms. It is not always physical abuse; many women are abused emotionally. Emotional abuse makes leaving the relationship especially difficult, because it lowers the woman's self-esteem and isolates her from sources of help. The time of greatest danger to the abused woman occurs when she leaves her abuser.

MANIFESTATIONS OF INTIMATE PARTNER VIOLENCE

In addition to having late or erratic prenatal care, the abused woman may have bruises or lacerations in various stages of healing. An X-ray may show old fractures. The woman tends to minimize injury or "forget" its severity. She may assume responsibility for the trauma, as evidenced by remarks such as "If I had only kept the children quiet, he wouldn't have gotten so mad." Her abuser is often particularly attentive after the abusive episode.

TREATMENT AND NURSING CARE OF THE PREGNANT WOMAN EXPERIENCING TRAUMA

Nurses must be aware that any woman may be in a current abusive relationship or have experienced abuse in the past. Therapeutic, nonjudgemental communication helps establish a trusting nurse–patient relationship. Emotional abuse often supplements physical abuse, making the woman feel that she is "stupid" or "no good" and that she is "lucky that he loves her, because no one else would ever love her." She usually feels that she has no choice but to stay in the abusive relationship. She may assume part of the blame, believing that her abuser will stop hurting her if she tries harder.

Women should be assessed for abuse in privacy. The nurse determines whether there are factors that increase the risk for severe injuries or homicide, such as drug use by the abuser, a gun in the house, previous use of a weapon, or violent behaviour by the abuser outside the home. The nurse also needs to determine whether children in the family are being hurt. It is vital that the abuser not discover that the woman has reported the abuse or that she intends to leave, as this can escalate the abuse.

Safety Alert!

If a woman confides that she is being abused during pregnancy, this information must be kept absolutely confidential. Her life may be in danger if her abuser learns that she has told anyone. She should be referred to local shelters, but the decision to leave her abuser is hers alone.

Nurses can refer a woman to shelters and other services if she wishes to leave the abuser. However, the decision about whether to end the relationship rests with the woman. Abuse of children must be reported to appropriate authorities.

In addition to a routine comprehensive assessment, the pregnant woman who has any type of trauma should have fetal monitoring for at least 4 hours. If the woman has any adverse factors such as abdominal pain, uterine tenderness, or atypical fetal heart rate and is greater than 23 weeks' gestation, she should be observed for a minimum of 24 hours, based on the risk for internal bleeding. If any vaginal bleeding is noted, no vaginal examination should be performed and an immediate ultrasound should be done as soon as possible (Jain et al., 2015). The nurse should understand the changes in anatomy and physiology that normally occur during pregnancy and should ensure that the pregnant woman is not positioned on her back, to prevent supine hypotension (see Chapter 4).

Nursing care for the acutely injured pregnant woman supplements medical management: The focus is on stabilizing the mother's condition when life-threatening injuries occur. In major trauma, the assessment, stabilization, and care of the pregnant women is the first priority. Then, if the fetus is viable (≥22 weeks), fetal heart rate auscultation and fetal monitoring can be initiated and an obstetrical consultation obtained as soon as feasible (Jain et al., 2015). An assessment of vital signs and urine output reflects blood circulation to the kidneys. Modifications in the technique of performing cardiopulmonary resuscitation (CPR) on a pregnant woman are described in Box 5.8.

Safety Alert!

The pregnant woman with trauma should not be placed in a supine position. A rolled towel can be placed under her right hip to displace the uterus to the left, to avoid compromising fetal oxygenation.

Pelvic fractures can cause injuries to the uterus that can result in fatal bleeding due to the increased blood flow during pregnancy. Until 14 weeks' gestation, the uterus is protected by pelvic bones. Maternal hypovolemia can cause fetal loss; therefore, any initial treatment of the mother after an injury must include maintenance of blood volume. In the third trimester of pregnancy, the fetus is better able to cope with a decrease in fetal oxygen delivery (Brown, 2017). If

Box 5.8 Modification of Standard Cardiopulmonary Resuscitation (CPR) for Pregnant Women

- A minimum of four responders is recommended (adult, neonatal, airway management, chest compressions).
- Displace uterus laterally by placing a wedge or rolled blanket under right hip (prevents supine hypotension.
- If defibrillation is used, place the paddles one rib interspace higher than usual (because of the normal heart displacement caused by the enlarged term uterus).
- Chest compressions may be administered in the centre of the chest in the lower portion of the sternum. Do NOT use abdominal thrusts.
- Determine resting uterine tone after CPR of a pregnant woman.
- Provide hemodynamic monitoring for the woman after CPR.
- Maintain continuous electronic fetal monitoring of the fetus.

Kikuchi, J., & Deering, S. (2018). Cardiac arrest in pregnancy. *Seminars in Perinatology, 42*, 33–38.

the mother suffers shock as a result of her injury, her blood will be recirculated away from her uterus to her vital organs, which could result in fetal death. Close fetal heart monitoring and documentation of contractions are essential nursing functions after trauma to a pregnant woman. Maternal vital signs should be recorded and reported. Blunt abdominal trauma could result in placental abruption, which could occur up to 48 hours after the injury; thus pregnant women experiencing trauma should be observed closely for several hours.

Because of the increased coagulability of the pregnant woman, the aftermath of trauma can result in a high risk for blood-clotting problems such as thrombophlebitis and DIC.

The use of tocolytics to delay labour may be contraindicated in some types of trauma, such as burns. Magnesium sulphate is a vasodilator and also may be contraindicated for use in some types of trauma and shock. Electrical shock injuries can be more serious to the fetus even though the mother does not seem to be seriously injured, because amniotic fluid offers low resistance to the passage of the electrical current to the fetus. In general, it is important for the nurse to understand and correlate the physiology of pregnancy to help the mother and fetus who are victims of trauma.

Safety Alert!

Even minor motor vehicle accidents can cause increased abdominal pressure on the pregnant abdomen via flexion of the body or seat belt pressure and can result in stretching or tearing of vessels within the uterus. Therefore, every pregnant woman in the emergency room who has experienced trauma should receive close uterine and fetal monitoring.

EFFECTS OF A HIGH-RISK PREGNANCY ON THE FAMILY

Normal pregnancy can be experienced as a crisis because it is a time of significant change and growth. The woman with a complicated pregnancy has stressors even beyond those of normal pregnancy. Women who are hospitalized may wait in anticipation for long periods of time during their pregnancy with fear and anxiety, which may be experienced as pain related to inactivity (Schlegel, Whalen, & Williamsen, 2016). Her family may also be affected by the pregnancy and the impending birth.

A variety of complementary therapies, such as relaxation therapy, massage, acupuncture, and other anxiety-reducing activities, have been used with success in women with high-risk pregnancy (Schlegel et al., 2016). Many new noninvasive technologies have been developed to detect problem pregnancies and to enable early diagnosis and treatment, including intrauterine surgery. The most important complication prevention methods are early preconception care, prenatal care, and surveillance.

DISRUPTION OF USUAL ROLES

The woman who experiences a difficult pregnancy must often remain on limited activity at home or in the hospital, sometimes for several weeks. Others must assume her usual roles in the family, in addition to their own obligations. Finding caregivers for young children in the family may be difficult if extended family lives far away. Placing the children in day care may not be an option if financial problems exist.

Nurses can help families adjust to these disruptions by identifying sources of support to help maintain reasonably normal household function.

DELAYED ATTACHEMENT TO THE INFANT

Pregnancy normally involves gradual acceptance of and emotional attachment to the fetus, especially after the woman feels fetal movement. Partners feel a similar attachment, although usually at a slower pace. The woman who has a high-risk pregnancy often halts planning for the child and may withdraw emotionally to protect herself from pain and loss if the outcome is poor. Maternal anxiety may also influence her attitude toward positive parenting and put her at higher risk for postpartum mood disorders after birth (Schlegel et al., 2016). Partners may also experience challenges with perinatal anxiety and with attachment to their infant (Dollberg, Rozenfeld, & Kupfermincz, 2016). Assessment of coping with the high-risk pregnancy should happen regularly with both parents, and resources should be provided, if possible, to help the couple become parents to this infant postpartum.

Unfolding Case Study

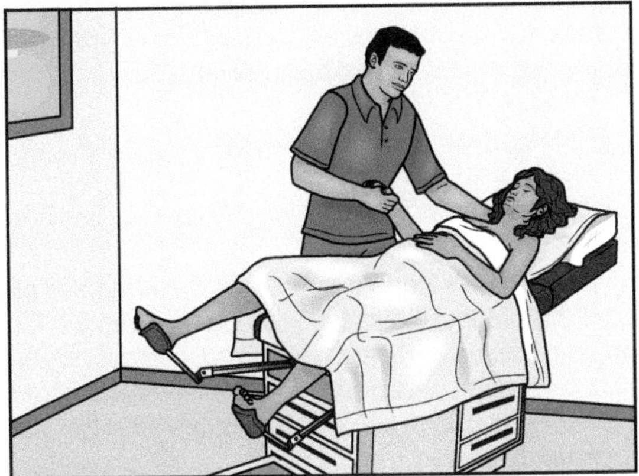

Tess and her partner, Luis, were introduced to the reader in Chapter 2 and will be followed throughout the maternity section of this text.

Tess becomes pregnant and her obstetrical history is $G_1T_0P_0A_0L_0$. She is now 10 weeks pregnant. She visits the prenatal clinic before her scheduled appointment and has symptoms of spotting and worsening of her nausea with some vomiting. An examination shows that her cervix is closed and Chadwick sign is positive, but no fetal heart tones are heard.

QUESTIONS

1. What is the significance of a positive Chadwick sign?
2. What are the causes of bleeding early in pregnancy?
3. What data concerning history will the nurse obtain from Tess?
4. When would nausea and vomiting during pregnancy not be considered a normal occurrence?
5. How is excessive nausea and vomiting during pregnancy treated?
6. What is the significance of the fact that the healthcare provider cannot hear fetal heart tones at this visit?

Get Ready for the Certification Examination!

Key Points

- A routine, noninvasive ultrasound examination can be used to confirm pregnancy, detect some anomalies, and possibly identify the sex of the fetus.
- Hyperemesis gravidarum is persistent nausea and vomiting of pregnancy and often interferes with nutrition and fluid balance.
- The most common reason for early spontaneous abortion is abnormality of the developing fetus or the placenta.
- An abortion is the termination of pregnancy before 20 weeks' gestation.
- If a woman has a tubal rupture from an ectopic pregnancy, the nurse should observe for shock.
- Because of hemorrhage into the abdomen in the case of a tubal rupture, vaginal blood loss may be minimal, even though intra-abdominal blood loss can be massive.
- The woman who has gestational trophoblastic disease (hydatidiform mole) should have follow-up medical care for 1 year to detect the possible development of choriocarcinoma. She should not become pregnant during this time.
- Placenta previa is the abnormal implantation of the placenta in the lower part of the uterus.
- Placental abruption is the premature separation of the placenta that is normally implanted.
- A blood pressure of 140/90 mm Hg or above is considered hypertension in the pregnant patient.
- The main manifestations of pre-eclampsia are hypertension and proteinuria.
- Patients at risk for pre-eclampsia should be given low-dose aspirin.
- Eclampsia occurs when the woman has a seizure.
- Positioning the mother on her left side during bed rest helps improve blood flow to the placenta and prevents pressure on the vena cava.
- Rh_o(D) immune globulin can be administered to an Rh-negative mother to prevent blood incompatibilities between the mother and an Rh-positive fetus (hemolytic disease of the newborn).
- Gestational diabetes mellitus (GDM) first occurs during pregnancy and resolves after pregnancy. The newborn may be excessively large (macrosomia), and the mother may develop DM later in life. Control of blood glucose level is essential to protect the fetus.
- Nutrition counselling and ongoing dietary management of the woman with GDM are essential for a positive outcome for the mother and fetus.
- TORCH diseases of pregnancy include **to**xoplasmosis, **r**ubella, **c**ytomegalovirus, and **h**erpes, with the **o** also denoting **o**thers.
- Pregnant women should be assessed for Zika virus exposure.
- Urinary tract infections are more common during pregnancy because compression and dilation of the ureters result in urine stasis.
- Preterm labour is more likely to occur if a woman has pyelonephritis.
- Prescribed medications, recreational substances, and alcohol consumed by the mother can cross the placenta and adversely affect the developing fetus.
- The nurse must be prepared to recognize the effects of adverse environmental factors on the patient and fetus.
- The nurse must consider the physiological changes that occur during pregnancy to understand and care for the pregnant trauma victim. Both the mother and the fetus must be monitored closely.

Additional Learning Resources

evolve Go to your Evolve website (http://evolve.elsevier.com/Canada/Leifer) for the following learning resources:

- Answer Key for Critical Thinking Questions
- Answer Key for Textbook Review Questions
- Audio Glossary
- Glossary
- Fluids & Electrolytes tutorial
- Interactive Review Questions
- Skills Performance Checklists
- Video clips and more!

Online Resources

- California Maternal Quality Care Collaborative—*Cardiovascular Disease (CVD) Signs and Symptoms:* https://www.cmqcc.org/resource/cvd-signs-and-symptoms-infographic-english-pdf
- Diabetes Canada—*Living with Gestational Diabetes:* http://www.diabetes.ca/diabetes-and-you/living-with-gestational-diabetes
- Health Canada, *Physical Activity and Pregnancy:* https://www.canada.ca/en/public-health/services/health-promotion/healthy-pregnancy/healthy-pregnancy-guide.html
- HIV and hepatitis C information: https://www.catie.ca/en/home
- MotherToBaby: http://www.mothertobaby.org/

Review Questions

1. A woman has an incomplete abortion followed by vacuum aspiration. She is now in the recovery room with her partner and is crying softly. Select the most appropriate nursing action.
   a. Leave the couple alone, except for necessary recovery-room care.
   b. Tell the couple that most abortions are for the best, because the infant would have been abnormal.
   c. Tell the couple that spontaneous abortion is very common and does not mean that they cannot have other children.
   d. Express your regret at their loss and remain nearby if they want to talk about it.
2. A woman with a diagnosis of pre-eclampsia receives magnesium sulphate intravenously. Which of the following nursing interventions are priorities when caring for a patient who has received magnesium sulphate? *(Select all that apply.)*
   a. Monitor uterine tone.
   b. Monitor urine output.
   c. Keep patient NPO.
   d. Monitor respiratory rate.
3. It is important to emphasize to a woman who has gestational trophoblastic disease (hydatidiform mole) that she should continue to receive follow-up medical care after initial treatment, because of which of the following?
   a. Choriocarcinoma sometimes occurs after the initial treatment.
   b. She has lower levels of immune factors and is vulnerable to infection.
   c. Anemia complicates most cases of hydatidiform mole.
   d. Permanent elevation of her blood pressure is more likely.
4. What is the primary difference between the symptoms of placenta previa and placental abruption?
   a. Fetal presentation
   b. Presence of pain
   c. Abnormal blood clotting
   d. Presence of bleeding
5. During a prenatal clinic visit, a nurse provides interventions to a woman who is a victim of intimate partner violence. The nurse's interventions should focus on which of the following?
   a. Persuading her to leave her abusive partner
   b. Informing her of her safety options
   c. Convincing her to notify the police
   d. Placing her in a shelter for abused women
6. If a pregnant woman is admitted to the emergency room in shock after an accident, the nurse would help relieve the effect of shock by doing which of the following? *(Select all that apply.)*
   a. Placing her in Trendelenburg position
   b. Placing her flat in bed in a supine position
   c. Placing a small pillow under the right hip of the woman
   d. Closely observing and documenting fetal heart rate and contractions

REFERENCES

Berger, H., Gagnon, R., Sermer, M., et al. (2016). SOGC clinical practice guideline: Diabetes in pregnancy. *Journal of Obstetrics and Gynaecology Canada, 38*(7), 667–679.

Bourgeois, A. C., Edmunds, M., Awan, A., et al. (2017). HIV in Canada—Surveillance report, 2016. *Canada Communicable Disease Report, 43*(12), 248–256. Retrieved from: https://www.canada.ca/content/dam/phac-aspc/documents/services/reports-publications/canada-communicable-disease-report-ccdr/monthly-issue/2017-43/ccdr-volume-43-12-december-7-2017/ccdr-43-12-ar01-eng.pdf.

Britt, W. (2016). Cytomegalovirus. In R. M. Kliegman, B. F. Stanton, J. W. St. Geme, et al. (Eds.), *Nelson textbook of pediatrics* (20th ed.). Philadelphia: Saunders.

Brown, H. (2017). Trauma and related surgery in pregnancy. In S. F. Gabbe, J. R. Niebyl, J. L. Simpson, et al. (Eds.), *Obstetrics: Normal and problem pregnancies* (7th ed.). Philadelphia: Saunders.

Bryant, A. (2016). Pregnancy associated internal hernia after gastric bypass. *New England Journal of Medicine, 21*(7), 52.

Campbell, K., Rowe, H., Azzam, H., et al. (2016). SOGC clinical practice guideline: The management of nausea and vomiting of pregnancy. *Journal of Obstetrics and Gynaecology Canada, 38*(12), 1127–1137.

Centers for Disease Control and Prevention (CDC). (2017). Tuberculosis—United States, 2016. *MMWR Morbidity and Mortality Weekly Report, 66*(11), 289–294.

Costescu, D., Bernardin, E., Black, J., et al. (2016). SOGC clinical practice guideline: Medical abortion. *Journal of Obstetrics and Gynaecology Canada, 38*(4), 366–389.

Costillo, E., & Poliquin, V. (2018). SOCG clinical practice guideline: No. 357: Immunization in pregnancy. *Journal of Obstetrics and Gynaecology, 40*(4), 478–489.

Dean, C., Bannigan, K., & Marsden, J. (2018). Reviewing the effect of hyperemesis gravidarum on women's lives and mental health. *British Journal of Midwifery, 26*(2), 109–119.

Dollberg, D., Rozenfeld, T., & Kupfermincz, M. (2016). Early parental adaptation, prenatal distress, and high risk pregnancy. *Journal of Pediatric Psychology, 41*(8).

Eagles, N., Sebire, N., Short, D., et al. (2015). Risk of recurrent molar pregnancies following complete and partial hydatidiform moles. *Human Reproduction, 30*(9), 2055–2063.

Elkayam, U., Goland, S., Petronella, P., et al. (2016). High-risk cardiac disease in pregnancy: Part 1. *Journal of the American College of Cardiology, 68*(4), 396.

Epps, C., Rac, M., Dunn, J., et al. (2017). Testing for Zika virus in pregnancy: Key concepts to deal with an emerging epidemic. *American Journal of Obstetrics & Gynecology, 216*(3), 209–225.

Fantasia, H. (2018). Low-dose aspirin for the prevention of preeclampsia. *Nursing for Women's Health, 22*(1), 87–92.

Feig, D., Berger, H., Donovan, D., et al. (2018). 2018 clinical practice guidelines: Diabetes and pregnancy. *Canadian Journal of Diabetes, 42*, 5255–5285.

Finnegan, L. (2013). *Substance use in Canada: Licit and illicit drug use during pregnancy: Maternal, neonatal and early childhood consequences*. Ottawa: Canadian Centre on Substance Use. Retrieved from: http://www.ccdus.ca/Resource%20Library/CCSA-Drug-Use-during-Pregnancy-Report-2013-en.pdf.

Fletcher, S., Waterman, H., Nelson, L., et al. (2015). Holistic assessment of women with hyperemesis gravidarum: A randomised controlled trial. *International Journal of Nursing Studies, 52*, 1669–1679.

Government of Canada. (2015). *Update on pertussis vaccination in pregnancy*. Retrieved from: https://www.canada.ca/en/public-health/services/publications/healthy-living/update-pertussis-vaccination-pregnancy.html.

Government of Canada. (2018a). *Prevention of Zika*. Retrieved from: https://www.canada.ca/en/public-health/services/diseases/zika-virus/prevention-zika-virus.html.

Government of Canada. (2018b). *Surveillance of tuberculosis (TB)*. Retrieved from: https://www.canada.ca/en/public-health/services/diseases/tuberculosis-tb/surveillance-tuberculosis-tb.html.

Jain, V., Chari, R., Maslovitz, S., et al. (2015). SOGC clinical practice guideline: Guidelines for the management of a pregnant trauma patient. *Journal of Obstetrics and Gynaecology Canada, 37*(6), 553–571.

Jefferies, A., & Canadian Paediatric Society, Fetus and Newborn Committee (2017). *Position statement: Management of term infants at increased risk for early onset bacterial sepsis*. Retrieved from: https://www.cps.ca/en/documents/position/management-infant-sepsis. Revised 2018.

Kilpatrick, S. J. (2014). Anemia and pregnancy. In R. Resnick, R. K. Creasy, J. Iams, et al. (Eds.), *Creasy & Resnik's maternal–fetal medicine: Principles and practice* (7th ed.). Philadelphia: Saunders.

Logsdon, M., Davis, D., Myers, J., et al. (2018). Do new mothers understand the risk factors for maternal mortality? MCN. *The American Journal of Maternal/Child Nursing*. 43(4), 201–205. https://doi.org/10.1097/NMC.0000000000000434.

Magee, L. A., Pels, A., Helewa, M., et al. (2014). Diagnosis, evaluation, and management of the hypertensive disorders of pregnancy. *Pregnancy and Hypertension, 4*(2), 105–145.

Mcleod, R., VanTubbergen, C., & Boyer, K. M. (2016). Toxoplasmosis (Toxoplasma gondii). In R. M. Kliegman, B. F. Stanton, J. W. St. Geme, et al. (Eds.), *Nelson textbook of pediatrics* (20th ed.). Philadelphia: Saunders.

Money, D., Tullock, K., Boucoiran, I., et al. (2014). SOGC clinical practice guideline: Guidelines for the care of pregnant women living with HIV and interventions to reduce perinatal transmission. *Journal of Obstetrics and Gynaecology Canada, 36*(8e, Suppl. A), S1–S46.

Ordean, A., Wong, S., Graves, L., et al. (2017). Substance use in pregnancy. *Journal of Obstetrics and Gynaecology Canada, 39*(10), 922–937e2.

Public Health Agency of Canada (PHAC). (2013). *Maternal mortality in Canada*. Retrieved from: https://www.med.uottawa.ca/sim/data/assets/documents/Mortality-EN-Final-PDF.pdf.

Public Health Agency of Canada (PHAC). (2016). *Canadian guidelines on sexually transmitted infections—Management and treatment of specific infections—Genital herpes simplex virus (HSV) infections*. Retrieved from: http://www.phac-aspc.gc.ca/std-mts/sti-its/cgsti-ldcits/section-5-4-eng.php.

Public Health Agency of Canada (PHAC). (2019). *Zika virus prevention and treatment recommendations*. Retrieved from: https://www.canada.ca/en/public-health/services/publications/diseases-conditions/zika-virus-prevention-treatment-recommendations.html?&_ga=2.54234080.930114984.1525962085-440366529.1516216001#a9.

Raio, L., Bolla, D., & Baumann, M. (2015). Hypertension in pregnancy. *Current Opinion in Cardiology, 30*, 411–415.

Sapra, K., Joseph, K., Galea, S., et al. (2017). Signs and symptoms of early pregnancy loss: A systematic review. *Reproductive Sciences, 24*(4), 502–513.

Schlegel, M., Whalen, J., & Williamsen, P. (2016). Integrative therapies for women with a high risk pregnancy. *MCN, The American Journal of Maternal Child Nursing, 41*(6)356–362.

Schleiss, M. (2016). Principles of antiviral therapy. In R. M. Kliegman, B. F. Stanton, J. W. St. Geme, et al. (Eds.), *Nelson textbook of pediatrics* (20th ed.). Philadelphia: Saunders.

Society of Obstetricians and Gynaecologists of Canada (SOGC). (2016). *SOGC recommendation on ZIKA virus exposure for clinicians caring for pregnant women and those who intend to get pregnant*. Retrieved from: https://www.cfpc.ca/uploadedFiles/Resources/_PDFs/Recommendation%20on%20Zika%20Virus.pdf.

Society of Obstetricians and Gynecologists of Canada (SOGC). (2018). No. 197a Fetal Health Surveillance: Antepartum consensus guideline. *Journal of Obstetrics and Gynaecology Canada, 40*(4), e251–e271.

Sperling, J. D., & Gassett, D. (2017). Screening for preeclampsia and USPTF recommendations. *Journal of the American Medical Association, 425*(317), 1629.

Wilson, R. D., & Genetics Committee. (2015). Pre-conception folic acid and multivitamin supplementation for the primary and secondary prevention of neural tube defects and other folic acid-sensitive congenital anomalies. *Journal of Obstetrics and Gynaecology Canada, 37*(6), 534–549.

Nursing Care of the Mother and Infant During Labour and Birth

6

Katie Lindsay and Lisa Keenan-Lindsay

http://evolve.elsevier.com/Canada/Leifer

Objectives

1. Define each key term listed.
2. Compare the advantages and disadvantages for each type of childbearing setting: hospital, freestanding birth centre, and home.
3. Describe the five *Ps* of the birth process: **p**owers, **p**assage, **p**assenger, **p**osition, and **p**syche.
4. Describe how the five *Ps* of labour interrelate to result in the birth of an infant.
5. Explain the normal processes of childbirth: premonitory signs, mechanisms of birth, and stages and phases of labour.
6. Explain how prelabour differs from true labour.
7. Determine appropriate nursing care for the intrapartum patient, including the woman in prolonged prelabour and the woman having a vaginal birth after Caesarean (VBAC).
8. Explain common nursing responsibilities during labour and birth.
9. Describe the care of the newborn immediately after birth.

Key Terms

absent variability
accelerations
acrocyanosis (ăk-rō-sī-ă-NŌ-sĭs)
amnioinfusion (ăm-nē-ō-ĭn-FYŪ-zhŭn)
amniotomy (ăm-nēŎT-ō-mē)
baseline fetal heart rate
bloody show
cold stress
coping
crowning
dilate
doula (DŪ-lă)
early decelerations
efface (ĕ-FĀS)
fetal bradycardia
fetal tachycardia
fontanelle (FŎN-tă-nĕl)
late decelerations
Leopold manoeuvre
lie
marked variability
moderate variability
microbiata
microbiome
minimal variability
moulding
neutral thermal environment
nitrazine test
nuchal cord (NŪ-kăl kŏrd)
ophthalmia neonatorum (ŏf-THĂL-mē-ă nē-ō-nă-TŎR-ăm)
periodic changes
prolonged decelerations
station
sutures
tachysystole
trial of labour after Caesarean (TOLAC)
uteroplacental insufficiency (yū-tăr-ō-plă-SĔN-tăl ĭn-sŭ-FĬSH-ăn-sē)
vaginal birth after Caesarean (VBAC)
variability
variable decelerations

Childbirth is a normal physiological process that involves caring for the health of the mother and a fetus. The nursing care is unique because every nursing intervention involves the welfare of two patients and the use of skills from medical-surgical and pediatric nursing, psychosocial and communication skills, and specific skills involved in obstetrical care. In addition, labour and birth are often a family affair, with partners, grandparents, siblings, and others closely involved. Each family participant often remembers the details of this experience for a long time.

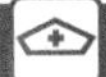

Nursing Tip

The overall aim of caring for women during labour and birth is to engender a positive experience for her and her family while maintaining her and her baby's health, preventing complications, and responding to emergencies (Public Health Agency of Canada [PHAC], 2018).

The privacy and rights of the mother must be protected, the policies and procedures of the institution must be considered, and the nurse must be familiar with the scope of practice set out by the provincial regulatory board of nursing. This chapter provides information concerning the birth process and the nursing responsibilities during labour and birth.

Communication throughout labour and birth needs to be ongoing and responsive to the woman's needs. It is imperative that all members of the health care team establish rapport with the woman and ask her about her wishes and expectations for labour and birth. Women must be treated with respect, supported to make informed choice throughout labour and birth, and encouraged to actively participate in their care decisions (Public Health Agency of Canada [PHAC], 2018).

CULTURAL INFLUENCE ON BIRTH PRACTICES

The needs of the woman giving birth may be influenced by her cultural background, which may be very different from that of the nurse but must be understood and respected. Patient and cultural preferences require flexibility on the part of the nurse. Women of many cultures prefer the presence of a support person at all times during labour and birth, and that can include the woman's partner or family as well as professional staff. It is important to consider that it is not appropriate for the father to attend the birth in some cultures, and this practice must be respected. Nurses should not make assumptions about patient and family behaviours, such as assuming the father is uninvolved because he does not attend the birth, as this could be related to a cultural practice.

While some cultural groups may have specific beliefs and act certain ways during childbirth, it is important to remember that not everyone who is from a certain cultural group will have the same beliefs. Nurses must engage in culturally competent practice, which involves knowing about cultural practices, but also understanding the individual beliefs of each woman.

FEMALE GENITAL MUTILATION

In some cultures, female genital mutilation (FGM) is a routine practice, involving the stitching of the inner layers of the labia minor or majora, the removal of the clitoris or other parts of the genitalia, or both for cultural or nontherapeutic reasons (World Health Organization [WHO], 2014). The practice of FGM is recognized internationally as a harmful practice and a violation of girls' and women's rights to life, physical integrity, and health (Perron, Senikas, Burnett, et al., 2013). The practice of FGM can interfere with the birthing process as it may cause obstructed labour and is associated with an increased risk of vaginal/vulvar lacerations, although it is not an indication for a Caesarean birth (Perron et al., 2013). It is important to provide dignity and respect to these vulnerable women who have undergone FGM and not to stigmatize them. Some women may feel that FGM is culturally necessary but may also feel emotionally horrified by their experience. Nurses and other health care providers need to be aware of these complexities and respond appropriately (Scamell & Ghumman, 2019). Prior to birth, women must be educated that repairing the previous infibulation will be declined on medical grounds because repetitive cutting and suturing of the vulva is likely to increase scar tissue, thus causing or perpetuating painful intercourse (dyspareunia) or voiding difficulties. Any incision that is made will be repaired. Women also need good pain relief measures following the birth due to possible increase in pain.

CARING FOR THE LGBTQ2 PATIENT

Nurses will encounter patients in relation to childbirth who identify as lesbian, gay, bisexual, transgender, queer, or two-spirited (LGBTQ2). Increasingly, lesbian and gay couples are becoming parents, through either artificial insemination or surrogacy. To provide compassionate and respectful care to these patients it is important to develop a therapeutic relationship with them. It is also important to ask them about their plans for birth and what names the parents will be called (e.g., both *mother*) and to then use the appropriate names. Like heterosexual couples, gay couples also need opportunities to bond and provide skin-to-skin contact with their newborn.

Transmen may also become pregnant if the reproductive organs are still present. This requires them to stop taking the hormones they take to minimize their feminine characteristics, which can be distressing for some men, as they worry they will lose their gender identity. The important aspect of caring for a transman is to recognize possible concerns with gender identity. Transmen sometimes have difficulty coping with labour as they do not perceive themselves as being of the sex who would be able to give birth to a baby. The parent may also want to nurse the infant if the breasts are still intact; extra support is needed in this situation. Referring to the process as *chest feeding* rather than *breastfeeding* may be more appropriate. Privacy and respect are paramount to providing excellent care. The transman should be asked what he wants to be referred to (e.g., *dad*) and his wishes should be honoured.

Gender nonconforming (GNC) is defined as not subscribing to being either male or female (Wolfe-Roubatis, & Spatz, 2015). Persons who are GNC may also make the decision to have a baby. It is important to ask the patient how they would like to be referred to. The patient's preferred pronoun and gender identity must be documented (Wolfe-Roubatis & Spatz, 2015).

SETTINGS FOR CHILDBIRTH

Depending on facilities available in the area and the risks for complications, a woman can choose among three settings in which to give birth to her child. Most women in Canada give birth in the hospital, although others may choose freestanding birth facilities or their own home, with a registered midwife in attendance. Registered midwives in Canada are educated through a 4-year university program and are regulated by the Canadian Association of Midwives. Midwives assist low-risk women to give birth at home, in birth centres, or in hospitals. Not all provinces and territories presently have legislation regarding the practice of midwives, although most do. Midwives usually provide all the prenatal, labour, and postpartum care to women. In some locations, nurses may assist the midwife for the birth.

HOSPITALS

The woman who chooses a hospital birth may give birth in a setting in which she labours, gives birth, and recovers in separate rooms. After the recovery period, she is transferred to the postpartum unit. A more common setting for hospital maternity care is the birthing room, often called a *labour, birth, and recovery (LBR)* room. The woman labours, gives birth, and recovers, all in the same room. She is then transferred to the postpartum unit for continuing care. The appearance of the birthing room is more homelike than institutional (Fig. 6.1). The birthing beds have receptacles for various fittings, such as a "squat bar," which facilitates squatting during second-stage labour.

Another hospital birth setting is single-room maternity care, often called a *labour, birth, recovery, and postpartum (LBRP)* room. It is similar to the LBR room, but the mother and infant remain in the same room until discharge. An advantage of hospital-based birth settings is the ability to provide family-centred care for the woman who has a complicated pregnancy.

FREESTANDING BIRTH CENTRES

Some communities have birth centres that are separate from hospitals where registered midwives usually attend the births. Women who are cared for by registered midwives are seen throughout the pregnancy by the same group of midwives and they also care for them in labour. Advantages of freestanding birth centres include a homelike setting for the low-risk woman.

HOME

Women who are at low obstetrical risk may make the decision to give birth at home. In Canada, home births are usually attended by registered midwives.

Advantages of a home birth include the following:

- Control over persons who will or will not be present for the labour and birth, including children and other family members
- No risk of acquiring pathogens from other patients
- A low-technology birth, which is important to some families
- Lower rates of interventions

Research has shown that low-risk women who have home births attended by midwives in a jurisdiction where home birth is well integrated into the health care system is not associated with a difference in serious adverse newborn outcomes but rather associated with fewer intrapartum interventions (Hutton, Cappelletti, Reitsma, et al., 2015). The Society of Obstetricians and Gynaecologists of Canada (SOGC) stresses the importance of choice for women and their families in the birthing process and recognizes that women will continue to choose the setting in which they will give birth (SOGC, 2009).

COMPONENTS OF THE BIRTH PROCESS

Five interrelated components, often called the "five Ps," make up the process of labour and birth: the *p*owers, the *p*assageway, the *p*assenger, maternal *p*osition, and the *p*syche. These factors can impact the progress of labour, either positively or negatively, and are discussed in detail in the sections that follow.

THE POWERS

The *powers* of labour are forces that cause the cervix to open and that push the fetus downward through the birth canal. The two powers are the uterine contractions and the mother's pushing efforts.

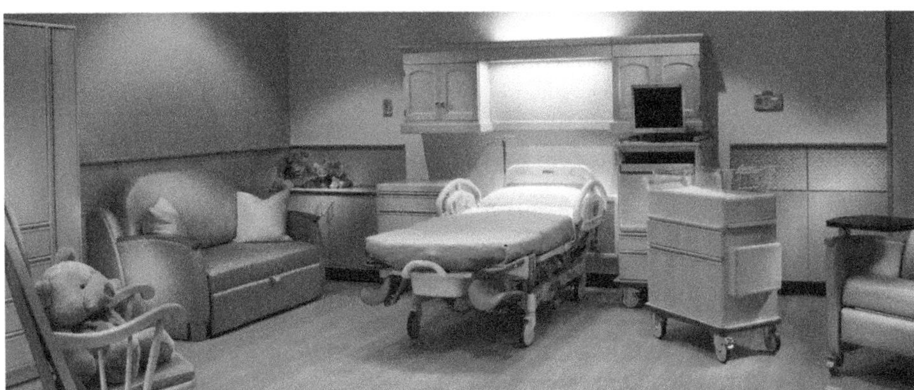

Fig. 6.1 Typical labour, birth, and recovery (LBR) room. Homelike furnishings can be quickly adapted if needed during labour. (Courtesy Hill-Rom Services, Batesville, IN.)

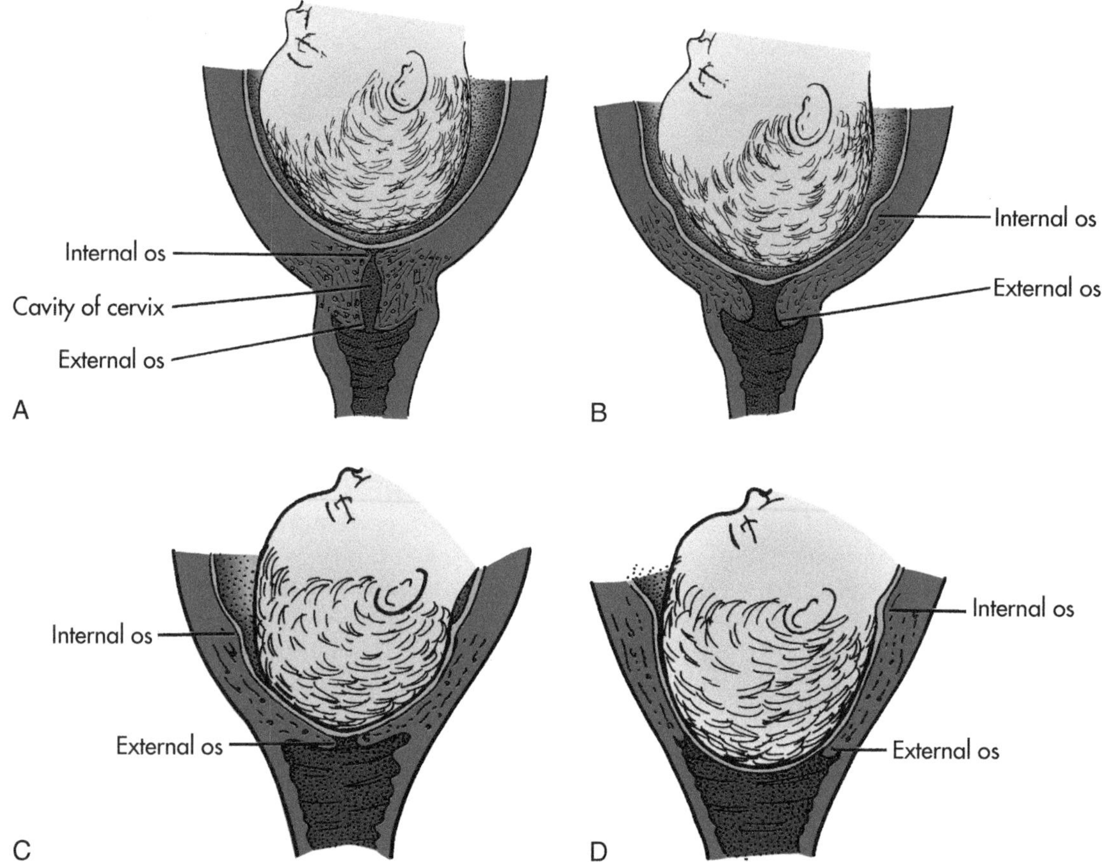

Fig. 6.2 Cervical effacement and dilation. **A,** No effacement, no dilation. **B,** Early effacement and dilation. **C,** Complete effacement, some dilation. **D,** Complete dilation and effacement. (From Lowdermilk, D. L., Perry, S. E., Cashion, K., et al. [2016]. *Maternity & women's health care* [11th ed.]. St. Louis: Elsevier.)

Uterine Contractions

Uterine contractions are the primary powers of labour during the first stage of labour (from onset until full dilation of the cervix). Uterine contractions are involuntary smooth muscle contractions; the woman cannot consciously cause them to stop or start. However, their intensity and effectiveness are influenced by a number of factors, such as walking, maternal position, medications, and maternal anxiety.

Effect of contractions on the cervix

Contractions cause the cervix to **efface** (thin) and **dilate** (open) to allow the fetus to descend in the birth canal (Fig. 6.2). Before labour begins, the cervix is a tubular structure about 2 to 3.8 cm long. Contractions simultaneously push the fetus downward as they pull the cervix upward (an action similar to pushing a ball out of a balloon). This causes the cervix to become thinner and shorter. Effacement is determined by a vaginal examination and is described as a percentage of the original cervical length or in length in centimetres. When the cervix is 100% effaced, it feels like a thin, slick membrane over the fetus.

Dilation of the cervix is also determined during a vaginal examination. Dilation is described in centimetres, with full dilation being 10 cm (Fig. 6.3). Both dilation and effacement are estimated by touch rather than being precisely measured.

Phases of contractions

Each contraction has the following three phases (Fig. 6.4):

1. *Increment:* The period of increasing strength
2. *Peak,* or *acme:* The period of greatest strength
3. *Decrement:* The period of decreasing strength

Contractions are described by their frequency, duration, and intensity.

Frequency

Frequency is the elapsed time from the beginning of one contraction until the beginning of the next contraction. Frequency is described in minutes and fractions of minutes, such as "contractions every 4½ minutes." If contractions occur more often than every 2 minutes, they are too close together and may reduce fetal oxygen supply and should be reported.

Duration

Duration is the elapsed time from the beginning of a contraction until the end of the same contraction. Duration is described as the average number of seconds for which contractions last, such as "duration of 45 to 50 seconds." Persistent contraction durations longer than 90 seconds may reduce fetal oxygen supply and should be reported.

Intensity

Intensity is the approximate strength of the contraction. In most cases, intensity is described in words such as "mild," "moderate," or "strong," which are defined as follows:

- *Mild contractions:* Fundus is easily indented with the fingertips; the fundus of the uterus feels similar to the tip of the nose.
- *Moderate contractions:* Fundus can be indented with the fingertips but with more difficulty; the fundus of the uterus feels similar to the chin.
- *Strong contractions:* Fundus cannot be readily indented with the fingertips; the fundus of the uterus feels similar to the forehead. The resting tone is the tone of the uterus between contractions and is described as soft or firm. Resting tone should be soft; if it is firm there is not enough time between contractions for the fetus to recover from the previous contraction.

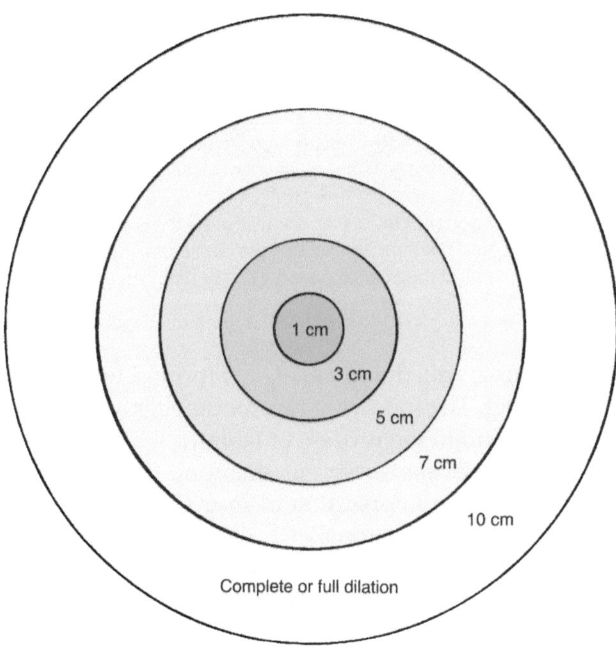

Fig. 6.3 Cervical dilation in centimetres. Full dilation is 10 cm (1 cm is approximately one finger's width).

Safety Alert!

Report to the primary health care provider any contractions that occur more frequently than every 2 minutes, last longer than 90 seconds, or when resting tone is and the interval between contractions is less than 60 seconds.

Maternal Pushing

When the woman's cervix is fully dilated, she adds voluntary pushing to involuntary uterine contractions. The combined powers of uterine contractions and voluntary maternal pushing in the second stage of labour propel the fetus downward through the pelvis. Most women feel a strong urge to push or bear down when the cervix is fully dilated and the fetus begins to descend. However, factors such as maternal exhaustion or sometimes epidural analgesia (see Chapter 7) may reduce or eliminate the natural urge to push. Some women feel a premature urge to push before the cervix is fully dilated, because the fetus pushes against the rectum or because of the occiput-posterior position of the fetus. Women should be assisted to try not to push at this time because it may contribute to swelling of the cervix, tearing of maternal soft tissues, and maternal exhaustion. The practice of "labouring down" is discussed below.

THE PASSAGEWAY

The *passageway* consists of the mother's bony pelvis and the soft tissues (cervix, muscles, ligaments, and fascia) of her pelvis and perineum.

Types of Pelves

There are four basic types of pelves (Fig. 6.5). Most women have a combination of pelvic characteristics rather than having one pure type. Each type of pelvis has implications for labour and birth:

- The *gynecoid* pelvis is the classic female pelvis, with rounded anterior and posterior segments. This type is most favourable for vaginal birth.

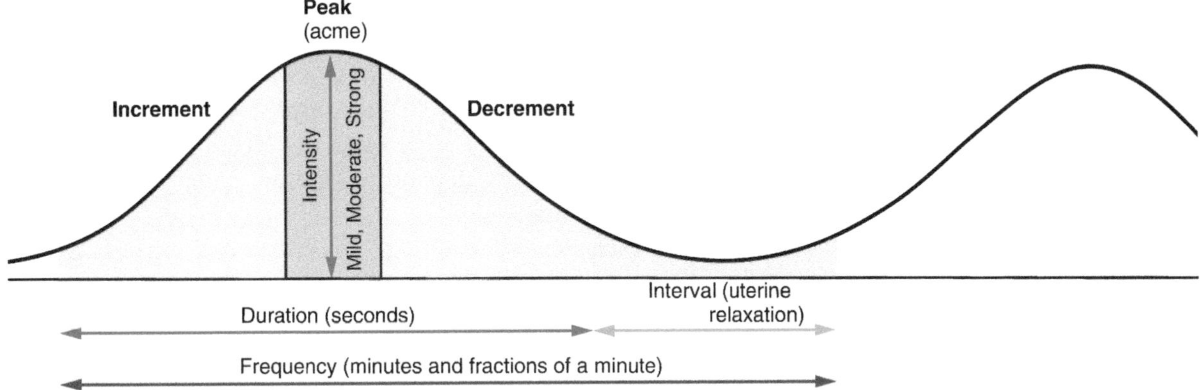

Fig. 6.4 Contraction cycle. Each contraction can be likened to a bell shape, with an increment, peak (acme), and decrement. The frequency of contractions is the average time from the beginning of one to the beginning of the next. The duration is the average time from the beginning to the end of one contraction.

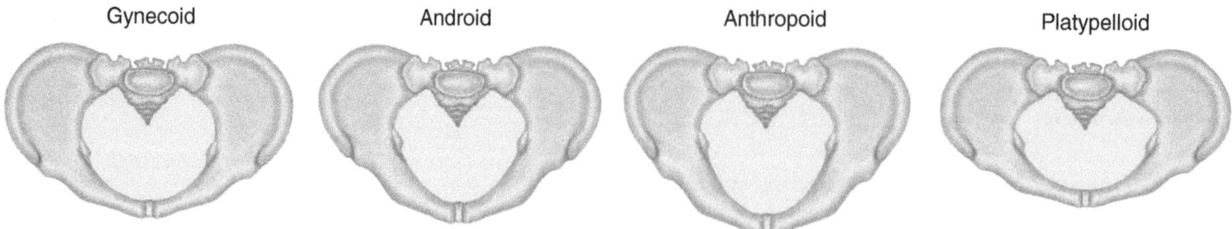

Fig. 6.5 Four types of pelves. The gynecoid pelvis is the typical female pelvis and is optimum for passage of the fetal head. (From Murray, S. S., McKinney, E. S., & Gorrie, T. M. [2002]. *Foundations of maternal–newborn nursing* [3rd ed.]. Philadelphia: Saunders.)

- The *android* pelvis has a wedge-shaped inlet with a narrow anterior segment; it is typical of the male anatomy.
- The *anthropoid* pelvis has an anteroposterior diameter that equals or exceeds its transverse diameter. The shape is a long, narrow oval. Women with this type of pelvis can usually give birth vaginally, but their infant is more likely to be born in the occiput posterior (back of the fetal head toward the mother's sacrum) position.
- The *platypelloid* pelvis has a shortened anteroposterior diameter and a flat, transverse oval shape. This type is unfavourable for vaginal birth.

Bony Pelvis

The pelvis is divided into two major parts: (1) the false pelvis (upper, flaring part) and (2) the true pelvis (lower part). The true pelvis, which is directly involved in childbirth, is further divided into the inlet at the top, the midpelvis in the middle, and the outlet near the perineum. It is shaped somewhat like a curved cylinder or a wide, curved funnel. The maternal bony pelvis must be adequate to allow the fetal head to pass through or cephalopelvic disproportion (CPD) will occur, and a Caesarean birth may be indicated (Fig. 6.6 and Fig. 6.7, B).

Soft Tissues

In general, women who have had previous vaginal births have quicker labours than those of women having their first births, because their soft tissues yield more readily to the forces of contractions and pushing efforts. This advantage is not present if the woman's previous births were Caesarean. Soft tissue may not yield as readily in older mothers, women who have long gaps between children, or after cervical procedures that have caused scarring.

THE PASSENGER

The *passenger* is the fetus along with the placenta (afterbirth) and amniotic membranes. The fetus usually enters the pelvis head first (cephalic presentation), and the structure of the fetal head impacts the process of labour.

The Fetus

Fetal head

The fetal head is composed of several bones separated by strong connective tissue called sutures (Fig. 6.7).

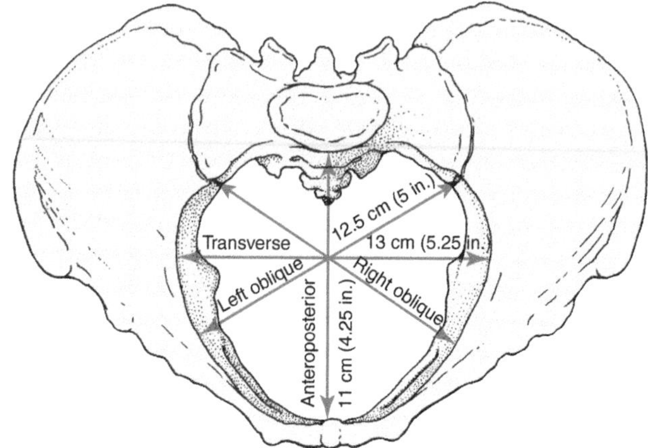

Fig. 6.6 Four important pelvic inlet diameters are the anteroposterior, the transverse, and the right and left oblique diameters. (Modified from *Stedman's illustrated medical dictionary* (1990). (25th ed.). Baltimore: Williams & Wilkins.)

A wider area, called a fontanelle, is formed where the sutures meet. The following two fontanelles are important in relation to the process of labour:

1. The *anterior fontanelle,* a diamond-shaped area formed by the intersection of four sutures (frontal, sagittal, and two coronal)
2. The *posterior fontanelle,* a tiny triangular depression formed by the intersection of three sutures (one sagittal and two lambdoid)

The sutures and fontanelles of the fetal head allow it to change shape as it passes through the pelvis (moulding). They are important landmarks in determining how the fetus is oriented within the mother's pelvis during birth.

The main transverse diameter of the fetal head is the biparietal diameter, which is measured between the points of the two parietal bones on each side of the head. The anteroposterior diameter of the fetal head can vary depending on how much the head is flexed or extended.

Fetal lie

Lie describes how the fetus is oriented to the mother's spine (Fig. 6.8). The most common orientation is the *longitudinal* lie, in which the fetus is positioned parallel to the mother's spine. The fetus in a *transverse* lie is at right angles to the mother's spine. The transverse lie may also be called a *shoulder presentation.* In an *oblique* lie, the fetus is between a longitudinal lie and

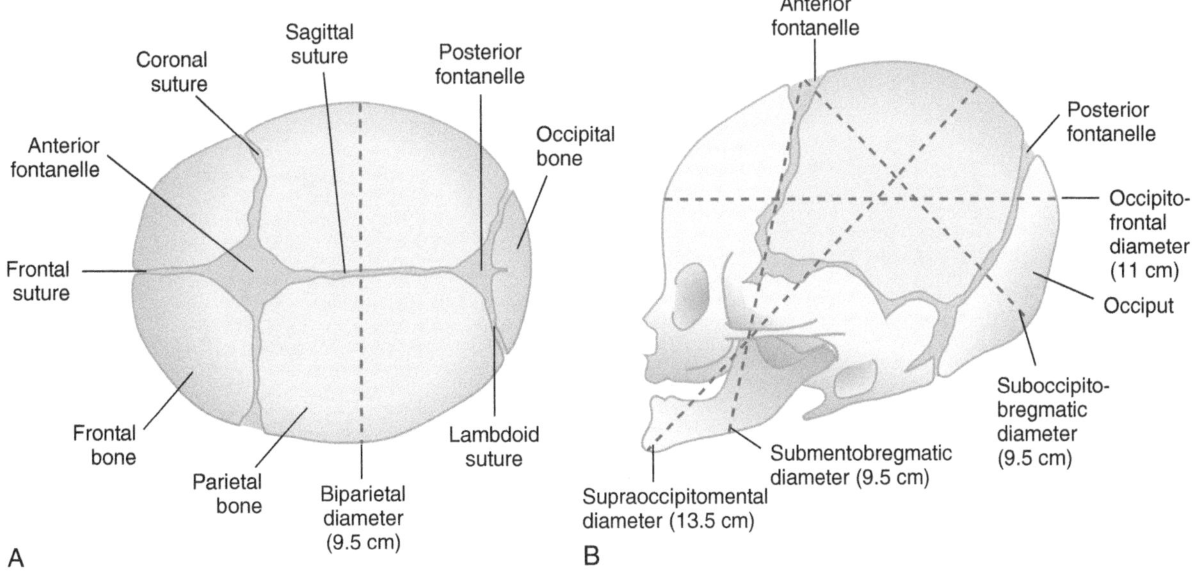

Fig. 6.7 The fetal skull, showing sutures, fontanelles, and important measurements. **A,** Superior view. Note that the anterior fontanelle has a diamond shape; the posterior fontanelle is triangular. The biparietal diameter is an important fetal skull measurement. **B,** Lateral view. The measurements of the fetal skull are important to determine if cephalopelvic disproportion will be a problem. The mechanisms of labour allow the fetal head to rotate so that the smallest diameter of the head passes through the pelvis as it descends. (From Matteson, P. S. [2001]. *Women's health during the childbearing years: A community-based approach*. St. Louis: Mosby.)

a transverse lie.

Fetal attitude

The fetal attitude is normally one of flexion, with the head flexed forward and the arms and the legs flexed. The flexed fetus is compact and ovoid and most efficiently occupies the space in the mother's uterus and pelvis. Extension of the head, the arms, and/or the legs sometimes occurs, and labour may be prolonged.

Fetal presentation

Presentation refers to the fetal part that enters the pelvis first. Cephalic presentation is the most common type. Any of the following four variations of cephalic presentations can occur, depending on the extent to which the fetal head is flexed (Fig. 6.9):

1. *Vertex presentation:* The fetal head is fully flexed. This is the most favourable cephalic variation, because the smallest possible diameter of the head enters the pelvis. It occurs in about 96% of births.
2. *Sinciput (military) presentation:* The fetal head is neither flexed nor extended.
3. *Brow presentation:* The fetal head is partly extended. The longest diameter of the fetal head is presenting. This presentation is unstable and tends to convert to either a vertex or a face presentation.
4. *Face presentation:* The head is fully extended and the face presents.

The next most common presentation is the breech, which can have the following three variations (see Fig. 6.9, *E* to *G*):

1. *Frank breech:* The fetal legs are flexed at the hips and extend toward the shoulders; this is the most common type of breech presentation. The buttocks present at the cervix.
2. *Full or complete breech:* A reversal of the cephalic presentation, with flexion of the head and extremities. Both feet and the buttocks present at the cervix.
3. *Footling breech:* One or both feet are present first at the cervix.

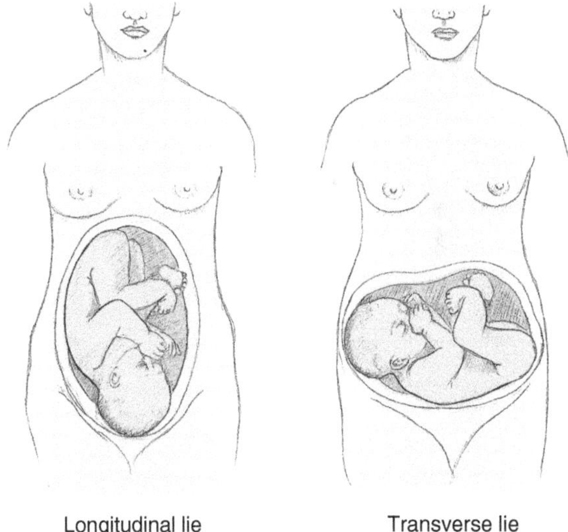

Fig. 6.8 Lie. In the longitudinal lie, the fetus is parallel to the mother's spine. In the transverse lie, the fetus is at right angles to the mother's spine. The shoulder presents at the cervix.

Many women with a fetus in the breech presentation have a Caesarean birth because the head, which is the largest single fetal part, is the last to be born and may not pass through the pelvis easily as flexion of the fetal head cannot occur (see Fig. 8.6). After the fetal

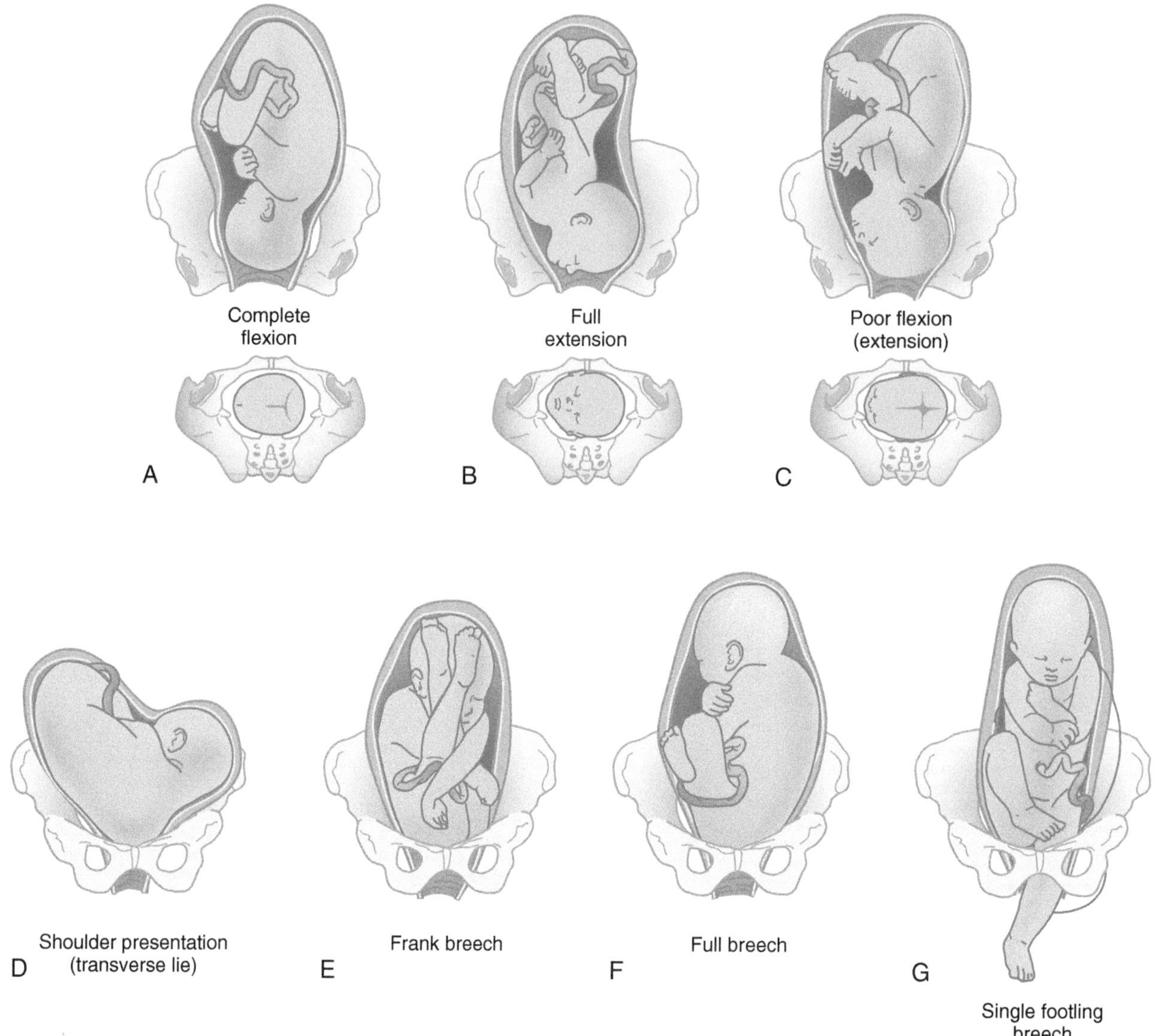

Fig. 6.9 Fetal presentations. **A,** Cephalic vertex. **B,** Cephalic face. **C,** Cephalic brow. **D,** Shoulder. **E,** Frank breech. **F,** Full or complete breech. **G,** Footling breech (can be single or double). The vertex presentation in which the fetal chin is flexed on the chest is the most common and favourable for a vaginal birth because it allows the smallest diameter of the head to go through the bony pelvis of the mother. Note how the anterior and posterior fontanelles can be used to determine fetal presentation and position in the pelvis. (From Matteson, P. S. [2001]. *Women's health during the childbearing years: A community-based approach*. St. Louis: Mosby.)

body is born, the head must be born quickly so that the fetus can breathe; at this point, part of the umbilical cord is outside the mother's body and the remaining part is subject to compression by the fetal head against the bony pelvis. Although many women with a breech presentation give birth by Caesarean, vaginal birth is recommended for some women and can be as safe as elective Caesarean birth. The SOGC states that planned vaginal birth is reasonable in selected women with a term singleton breech fetus. With careful labour management, these women have similar outcomes to those in women who have planned Caesarean birth, and long-term neurological outcomes in the infants do not differ by planned mode of birth, even in the presence of serious short-term newborn morbidity (Kotaska, Menticoglou, Gagnon, et al., 2009).

When the fetus is in a transverse lie, the fetal shoulder enters the pelvis first. A fetus in this orientation must be born by Caesarean section because it cannot safely pass through the pelvis.

Fetal position

Position refers to how a reference point on the fetal presenting part is oriented within the mother's pelvis. The term *occiput* is used to describe how the head is oriented if the fetus is in a cephalic vertex presentation. The term *sacrum* is used to describe how a fetus in a breech presentation is oriented within the pelvis. The shoulder and back are reference points if the fetus is in a shoulder presentation.

The maternal pelvis is divided into four imaginary quadrants: right and left anterior and right and left posterior. If the fetal occiput is in the left front quadrant of the mother's pelvis, it is described as *left occiput anterior.* If the sacrum of a fetus in a breech presentation is in the mother's right posterior pelvis, it is described as *right sacrum posterior.*

Abbreviations describe the fetal presentation and position within the pelvis (Box 6.1). Three letters are used for most abbreviations:

1. *First letter:* Right or left side of the woman's pelvis. This letter is omitted if the fetal reference point is directly anterior or posterior, such as occiput anterior (OA).
2. *Second letter:* Fetal reference point (occiput for vertex presentations; mentum [chin] for face presentations; and sacrum for breech presentations).
3. *Third letter:* Front or back of the mother's pelvis (anterior or posterior). Transverse (T) denotes a fetal position that is neither anterior nor posterior.

Fig. 6.10 shows various fetal presentations and positions.

Box 6.1 Classifications of Fetal Presentations and Positions

CEPHALIC PRESENTATIONS

Vertex Presentations

1. LOA—left occiput anterior
2. ROA—right occiput anterior
3. ROT—right occiput transverse
4. LOT—left occiput transverse
5. OA—occiput anterior
6. OP—occiput posterior

Face Presentations

1. LMA—left mentum anterior
2. RMA—right mentum anterior
3. LMP—left mentum posterior
4. RMP—right mentum posterior

BREECH PRESENTATIONS

1. LSA—left sacrum anterior
2. RSA—right sacrum anterior
3. LSP—left sacrum posterior
4. RSP—right sacrum posterior

Abbreviations that designate brow, military, and shoulder presentations are not included here because they occur infrequently.

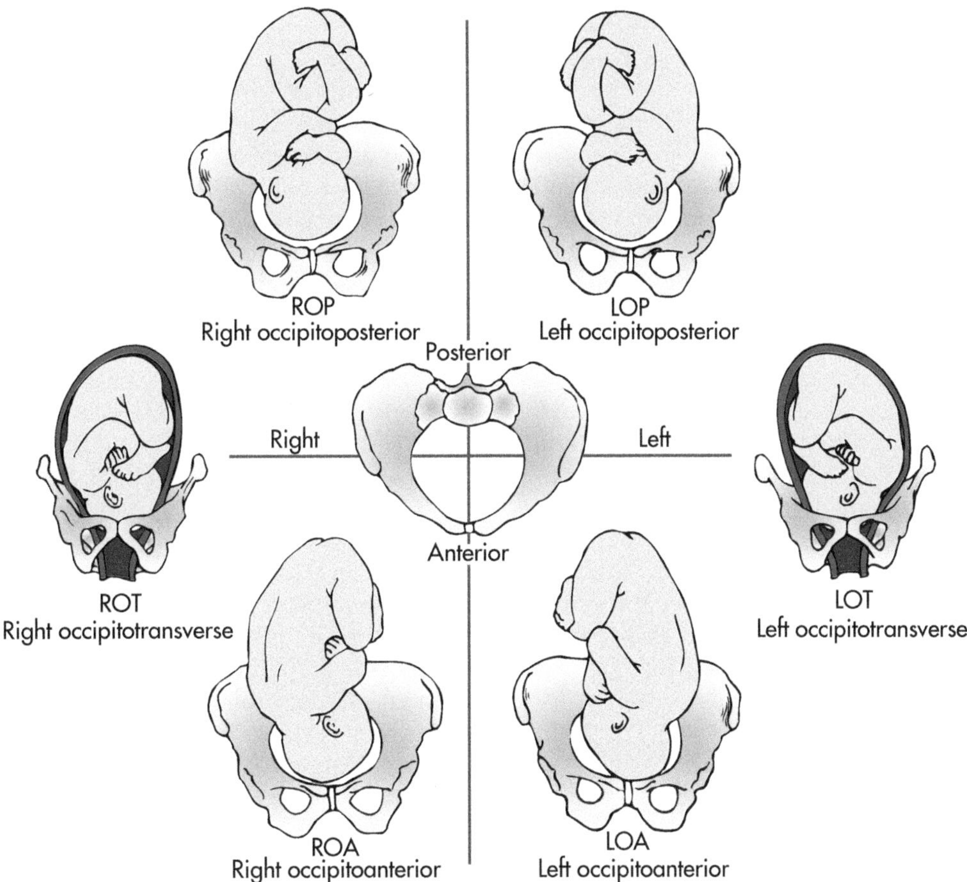

Lie: Longitudinal or vertical
Presentation: Vertex
Reference point: Occiput
Attitude: General flexion

Fig. 6.10 Fetal position. The right occipitoanterior *(ROA)* or left occipitoanterior *(LOA)* is most favourable for normal labour. When the occiput faces the posterior section of the woman's pelvis, a longer, "back labour" birth process is anticipated. (From Matteson, P. S. [2001]. *Women's health during the childbearing years: A community-based approach.* St. Louis: Mosby.)

POSITION OF THE LABOURING WOMAN

Maternal position has a significant impact on the progress of labour. Women who are in upright positions (walking, squatting, sitting, or kneeling) often have shorter labours as gravity and the force of contractions work to facilitate effacement and dilatation and also promote the descent of the fetus. Changing positions can also enhance pain relief so women should be encouraged to find a position that is comfortable for them. Women should also be encouraged to change positions frequently to facilitate the process of labour. The supine position is not beneficial for labour, as blood flow to the uterus and fetus is decreased and supine hypotension may result.

THE PSYCHE

Childbirth is more than a physical process; it involves the woman's entire being. Women remember and describe births in emotional terms, like those they use to describe marriages, anniversaries, religious events, or even deaths. Families often have great expectations about the *birth experience,* and the nurse can promote a positive childbearing experience by incorporating as many of the family's birth expectations as possible. For example, in some cultures the woman's position during birth may be upright or squatting rather than recumbent; if her cultural preferences are not respected, this may affect the way the woman copes during the labour and birth process.

A woman's *perception* of the process and her mental state can influence the course of her labour. For example, the woman who is relaxed and positive during labour may be better able to manage the discomfort and work with the physiological processes. By contrast, marked anxiety can increase her perception of pain and reduce her tolerance of it. Anxiety and fear also cause the secretion of stress compounds from the adrenal glands. These compounds, called *catecholamines,* inhibit uterine contractions and divert blood flow from the placenta.

A woman's cultural and individual values influence how she views and copes with childbirth, as does her preparation. Women who take childbirth education classes have a better understanding of what to expect during labour and birth, which can have a positive impact on the birth experience.

Nursing Tip

Nurses must provide emotional support to the labouring woman to decrease her anxiety and fear. Excessive anxiety or fear can cause greater pain, inhibit the progress of labour, and reduce blood flow to the placenta and fetus.

PROCESS OF CHILDBIRTH

The specific event that triggers the onset of labour remains unknown. Many factors play a part in initiating labour, which is an interaction of the mother and fetus. These factors include stretching of the uterine muscles, hormonal changes, placental aging, and increased sensitivity to oxytocin. Labour normally begins when the fetus is mature enough to adjust easily to life outside the uterus, yet still small enough to fit through the mother's pelvis. This point is usually reached at 40 weeks' gestation, or approximately 280 days after the woman's last menstrual period.

SIGNS OF IMPENDING LABOUR

Signs and symptoms that labour is about to start may occur from a few hours to a few weeks before the actual onset of labour.

Braxton Hicks Contractions

Braxton Hicks contractions are irregular contractions that begin during early pregnancy and may intensify as full term approaches. They can often become regular and somewhat uncomfortable, leading many women to believe that labour has started (see discussion of true and prelabour later in this chapter). Braxton Hicks contractions play a part in preparing the cervix to dilate and in adjusting the fetal position within the uterus.

Lightening

Lightening (or "dropping") is when the fetus settles into the true pelvis and the fundus no longer presses on the diaphragm. The woman may feel an increased urge to void but is able to breathe better. She may also feel increased pelvic pressure. In first-time mothers this may occur 2 to 4 weeks prior to the birth, whereas in multiparous women lightening may not occur until during labour.

Backache

Prior to the onset of labour some women may experience backache. This pain is different from the back pain she may have experienced during pregnancy. It is often intermittent and not relieved by methods she used for backache during pregnancy.

Cervical Changes

As the time for birth approaches, the cervix undergoes changes in preparation for labour. It softens ("ripens"), effaces, and may dilate slightly.

Vaginal Discharge

Women who are pregnant have increased vaginal discharge, but as labour nears, the discharge may increase. Also, as the cervix begins to soften, the mucous plug that has sealed the uterus during pregnancy is dislodged from the cervix, tearing small capillaries in the process. **Bloody show** is thick mucus mixed with pink or dark brown blood. It may begin a few days before labour, or a woman may not have bloody show until labour is underway. A woman occasionally has a small amount of blood-tinged discharge if she has had a recent vaginal examination or intercourse.

Energy Spurt

Many women have a sudden burst of energy shortly before the onset of labour ("nesting"). The nurse should teach women to conserve their strength, even if they feel unusually energetic.

Weight Loss

Occasionally a woman may notice that she loses 0.5 to 1.5 kg shortly before labour begins. Hormonal changes cause her to excrete extra body water.

Flu-like Symptoms

Some women experience flu-like symptoms before the onset of labour. This may involve diarrhea, nausea, vomiting, and indigestion. It is important for a mother to determine if she is actually sick and requires further follow up.

Rupture of the Membranes

The amniotic sac (bag of waters) sometimes ruptures before labour begins. Infection is more likely if many hours elapse between rupture of the membranes and birth, because the amniotic sac seals the uterine cavity against organisms from the vagina. There is also a slightly increased chance that the umbilical cord may slip down and become compressed between the mother's pelvis and the fetal presenting part. This is more common in multiparous women. Women are usually encouraged to go to the birth facility for assessment when their membranes rupture, even if they have no other signs of labour. Often they will be sent home to wait until labour starts after the assessment.

MECHANISMS OF LABOUR

As the fetus descends into the pelvis, it undergoes several positional changes so that it adapts optimally to the changing pelvic shape and size. Many of these mechanisms, also called *cardinal movements,* occur simultaneously (Fig. 6.11).

Descent

Descent is required for all other mechanisms of labour to occur and for the infant to be born. Descent occurs as each mechanism of labour comes into play. **Station** describes the level of the presenting part (usually the head) in the pelvis. Station is estimated in centimetres from the level of the ischial spines in the mother's pelvis (at 0 [zero] station). Minus stations are above the ischial spines, and plus stations are below the ischial spines (Fig. 6.12). As the fetus descends, the minus numbers decrease (e.g., −2, −1) and the plus numbers increase (e.g., +1, +2).

Engagement

Engagement occurs when the presenting part (usually the biparietal diameter of the fetal head) passes the pelvic inlet; the head is said to be engaged.

Flexion

The fetal head should be flexed to pass most easily through the pelvis. As labour progresses, uterine contractions increase the amount of fetal head flexion until the fetal chin is on the chest.

Internal Rotation

When the fetus enters the pelvis head first, the head is usually oriented so the occiput is toward the mother's right or left side. As the fetus is pushed downward by contractions, the curved, cylindrical shape of the pelvis causes the fetal head to turn until the occiput is directly under the symphysis pubis (occiput anterior [OA]).

Extension

As the fetal head passes under the mother's symphysis pubis, it must change from flexion to extension so it can properly negotiate the curve. To do this, the fetal neck stops under the symphysis, which acts as a pivot. The head swings anteriorly as it extends with each maternal push until it is born.

Restitution and External Rotation

When the head is born in extension, the shoulders are crosswise in the pelvis and the head is somewhat twisted in relation to the shoulders. The head spontaneously turns to one side as it realigns with the shoulders (restitution). The shoulders then rotate within the pelvis until their transverse diameter is aligned with the mother's anteroposterior pelvis. The head turns farther to the side as the shoulders rotate within the pelvis.

Expulsion

The anterior shoulder and then the posterior shoulder are born, quickly followed by the rest of the body.

ADMISSION TO THE BIRTHING UNIT

Nursing care includes admission assessments, collection of data, and the initiation of necessary procedures. Some women have prelabour and are discharged after a short observation period.

During late pregnancy the woman should be instructed in when to go to the hospital or birth centre. There is no *exact* time, but the general guidelines are as follows:

- *Contractions:* The woman should go to the hospital when the contractions have a pattern of increasing frequency, duration, and intensity. The woman having her first child is usually advised to enter the facility when contractions have been regular (every 4 to 5 minutes) for 1 hour and the contractions last approximately 60 seconds. Women having second or later children should go sooner, when regular contractions are approximately 5 to 7 minutes apart for a period of 1 hour. All women should be instructed

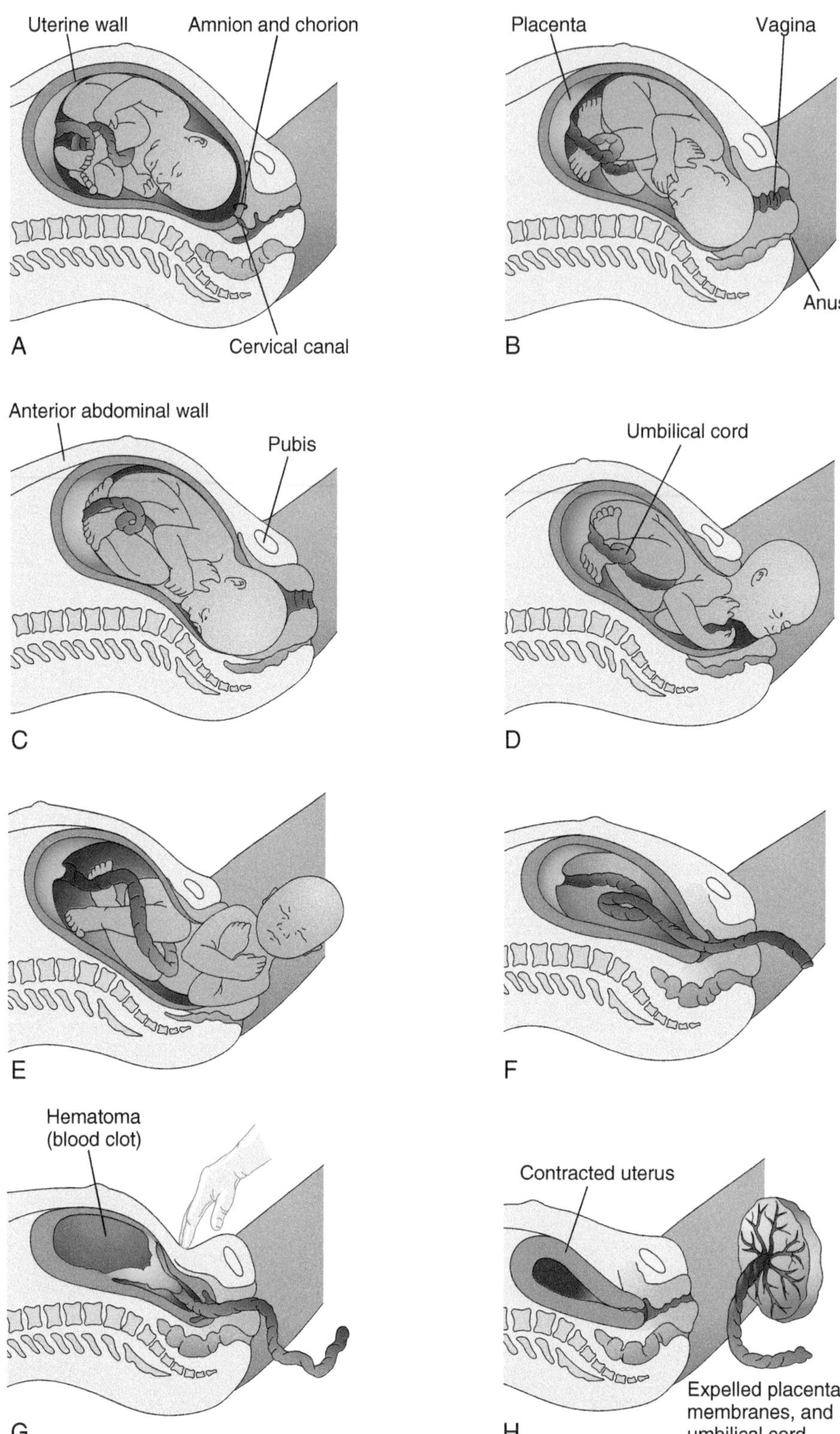

Fig. 6.11 Mechanisms of labour are also called cardinal movements (A-E). The positional changes allow the fetus to fit through the pelvis with the least resistance. **A,** Descent, engagement, and flexion. **B,** Internal rotation. **C,** Beginning extension. **D,** Birth of the head by complete extension. **E,** External rotation, birth of shoulders and body. **F,** Separation of placenta begins. **G,** Complete separation of placenta from uterine wall. **H,** Placenta is expelled and uterus contracts. (From Moore, K. L., Persaud, T. V. N., & Torchia, M. G. [2016]. *The developing human: Clinically oriented embryology* [10th ed.] Philadelphia: Saunders.)

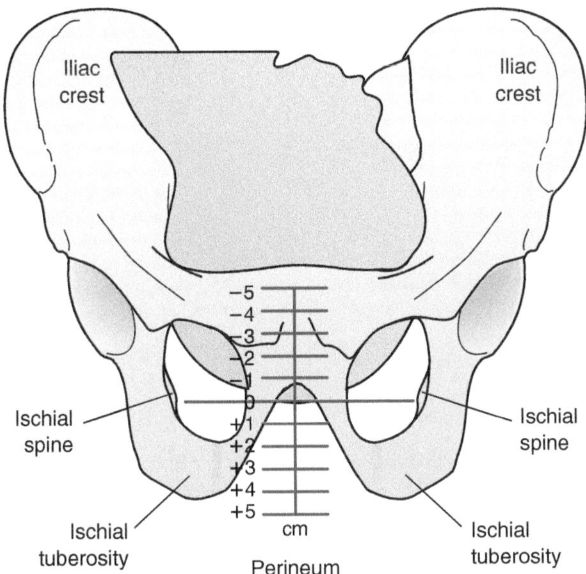

Fig. 6.12 Station. The station describes the level of the presenting part in relation to the ischial spines of the mother's pelvis. The "minus" stations are above the ischial spines, and the "plus" stations are below the ischial spines. (From Matteson, P. S. [2001]. *Women's health during the childbearing years: A community-based approach*. St. Louis: Mosby.)

to go to the hospital when they cannot cope anymore at home regardless of the timing of the contractions.

- *Ruptured membranes:* Most women are instructed to go to the birthing facility if her membranes rupture or if she thinks they may have ruptured. If the amniotic fluid is clear and the woman is group B streptococcus (GBS) negative, she may be instructed to stay home until labour begins or to come to the hospital after a specified amount of time.
- *Bleeding other than bloody show:* Bloody show is a mixture of blood and thick mucus. Active bleeding is free flowing, bright red, and not mixed with thick mucus.
- *Decreased fetal movement:* The woman should be evaluated if the fetus is moving less than usual. Many fetuses become quiet shortly before labour, but decreased fetal activity can also be a sign of fetal compromise.
- *Any other concern:* Because these guidelines cannot cover every situation, the woman should contact her health care provider or go to the birth facility for evaluation if she has any other concerns, including severe pain that she is unable to cope with.

ADMISSION DATA COLLECTION AND PROCEDURES

When a woman is admitted, the nurse establishes a therapeutic relationship by welcoming her and her family members. The nurse continues developing the therapeutic relationship during labour by determining the woman's expectations about birth and helping her to achieve them. Some women have a written birth plan that they have discussed with their healthcare provider, and this should be facilitated as much as possible by the nurse. The woman's partner and other family members she wants to be part of her care are included. From the first encounter, the nurse needs to convey confidence in the woman's ability to cope with labour and give birth to her child.

The three major assessments performed promptly on admission are (1) fetal condition, (2) maternal condition, and (3) impending (nearness to) birth.

If the maternal and fetal conditions are normal, and if birth is not imminent, other data can be gathered in a more leisurely way. Most birth facilities use computerized documentation to guide admission assessments. Women who have had prenatal care should have a prenatal record on file for retrieval of that information. Examples of the assessment data needed are as follows:

- Basic information should be obtained—the woman's reason for coming to the facility, the name of her healthcare provider, medical and obstetrical history, GBS status, allergies, food intake, any recent illness, and medication use (including illicit substances).
- The woman's plans for birth should be determined.
- The status of labour should be evaluated. The registered nurse (RN), registered midwife (RM), or physician does a vaginal examination to determine cervical effacement and dilation as well as fetal presentation, position, and station. Contractions are assessed for frequency, duration, and intensity by palpation.
- A woman's general condition should be evaluated by performing a brief physical examination. Any abdominal scars should be further explored. Baseline vital signs should be obtained.

Birth Plans

A birth plan is a tool for a woman to articulate her preferences and hopes for childbirth, to build trust with her care team, and to receive necessary information. Birth plans should be developed collaboratively during prenatal care to assist families and the healthcare team discuss their respective expectations. When a woman is admitted into the facility where she will give birth, it is important that the nurse ask about her birth plan and discuss her expectations and wishes. It is the role of the nurse to advocate for the woman and to provide nursing care that will help the woman and family achieve their wishes. Research has shown that a woman's satisfaction with her birth experience is positively affected when more of the requests on her birth plan are accommodated (PHAC, 2018). See the Additional Learning Resources section at the end of this chapter for an example of a birth plan template.

Fetal Condition

The fetal heart rate (FHR) is assessed with a handheld Doppler transducer or an external fetal monitor. When the amniotic membranes are ruptured, the colour, amount, and odour of the fluid are assessed, and the FHR is recorded.

Previously, all women who were admitted to the labour unit had an electronic fetal monitor strip done for a minimum of a 20-minute assessment. The SOGC does not support this practice for low-risk, healthy women. The fetus can be assessed with intermittent auscultation. If the woman is considered high risk, then an admission electronic fetal monitor strip should be done (Liston, Sawchuck, Young, et al., 2018).

Determining fetal position and presentation

The nurse can determine the fetal position and presentation by performing abdominal palpations called **Leopold manoeuvre** (Fig. 6.13). Leopold manoeuvre is also helpful in locating the fetal back, which is the best location for hearing the FHR, and thus determining optimal placement of the fetal monitor sensor.

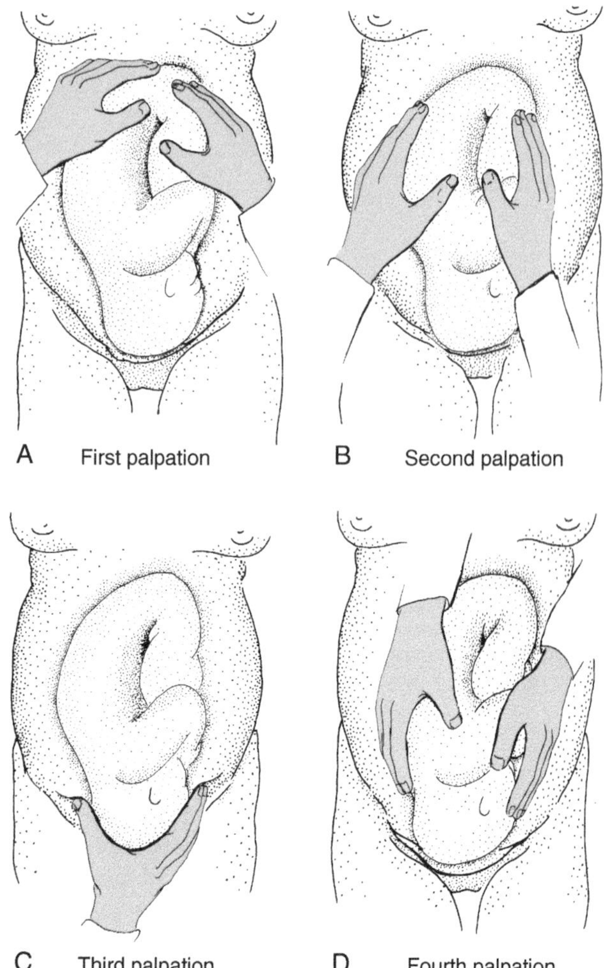

Fig. 6.13 Leopold manoeuvre. **A,** Presentation. Hands are placed on either side of the maternal abdomen to palpate the uterine fundus to determine if a round, hard object is felt at the fundus (the fetal head, indicating a breech presentation) or a soft, irregular contour (the fetal buttocks, indicating a vertex presentation). **B,** Position. Hands are placed on either side of the maternal abdomen. Support one side of the abdomen while palpating the other side. Palpating a hard, smooth contour indicates location of the fetal back, whereas feeling soft, irregular objects indicates the small parts or extremities. **C,** Confirm presentation. The suprapubic area is palpated to determine that the vertex or head is presenting. Feeling a hard, round area that does not move may indicate that the head is engaged. **D,** Attitude. Attitude of the fetal head is determined by palpating the maternal abdomen with fingers pointing toward the maternal feet. The hand is moved downward toward the symphysis pubis. Feeling a hard, round object on the same side as the fetal back indicates the fetus is in extension. Feeling the hard, round object opposite the fetal back indicates the head is in flexion.

Maternal Condition

The mother's temperature, pulse, respirations, and blood pressure are assessed for signs of infection or hypertension. The woman's contractions are also assessed; when they began, how far apart they are, how long they last are important questions to ask the woman. It is also important to assess how the woman is coping with labour. Is she anxious, able to manage the pain, or does she need assistance to help her cope?

Permission and Consent Forms

The mother gives consent, usually verbally, for her care and the care of her infant during labour, birth, and the postbirth period. Permission for routine care is covered with this consent; for other nonroutine care, written consent must be obtained. The health-care provider and the nurse must witness all signatures and confirm that proper information was given to the patient.

Laboratory Tests

A blood sample for blood group and type as well as in some institutions, a complete blood count (CBC) is taken on admission. A clean-catch urine specimen may be obtained for determination of hydration status, presence of infection, and presence of protein. The woman who did not have prenatal care will undergo prenatal screening, which includes tests discussed in Table 4.1. If the GBS or human immunodeficiency virus (HIV) status is unknown, a rapid test may be done, if available (see Table 4.1).

If the woman is GBS positive, administration of intravenous (IV) antibiotics is recommended after rupture of membranes or when labour starts, to reduce risk of transmission of GBS to the newborn. If GBS status is unknown, then risk factors are taken into consideration for a treatment plan for the newborn.

NURSING CARE OF THE WOMAN IN PRELABOUR

Prelabour (prodromal) contractions, sometimes called *false labour*, help prepare the woman's body and the fetus for true labour. True labour is characterized by changes in the cervix (effacement and dilation), which is the key distinction between true labour and prelabour. Table 6.1 lists characteristics of true labour and of prelabour.

The woman may be observed briefly, but is usually sent home with teaching about what to expect and

Table 6.1 Comparison of Prelabour and True Labour

PRELABOUR (PRODROMAL LABOUR)	TRUE LABOUR
Contractions are irregular or do not increase in frequency, duration, and intensity.	Contractions gradually develop a regular pattern and become more frequent, longer, and more intense.
Walking tends to relieve or decrease contractions.	Contractions become stronger and more effective with walking.
Discomfort is felt in the abdomen and groin.	Discomfort is felt in the lower back and the lower abdomen; it often feels like menstrual cramps at first.
Bloody show is usually not present.	Bloody show is often present.
There is no change in effacement or dilation of the cervix.	Progressive effacement and dilation of the cervix occur.

when she should return to the hospital. The woman is encouraged to walk, because if she is in true labour, walking often helps to intensify the contractions and bring about cervical effacement and dilation.

The woman in prelabour is often frustrated and needs generous reassurance that her symptoms will eventually change to true labour. No one stays pregnant forever, although it may feel that way to a woman who has had several false alarms and is tired of being pregnant. Guidelines for coming to the facility should be reinforced before she leaves.

! Safety Alert!

Encourage the woman in prelabour to return to the facility when she thinks she should. It is better to have another "trial run" than to wait at home until she is in advanced labour.

If the woman's membranes are ruptured, she may be admitted even if labour has not begun, because of the risk for infection, although some women are given a choice to wait 24 hours to see if labour will begin on its own. Women who are GBS positive will be induced shortly after membranes rupture if they are not yet in labour (see Chapter 8).

NURSING CARE DURING LABOUR

After admission to the labour unit, nursing care consists of the following elements:

- Monitoring the fetus
- Monitoring the labouring woman
- Providing supportive care to the labouring woman to help her cope

STAGES AND PHASES OF LABOUR

There are four stages of labour, and women giving birth display common physical and behavioural characteristics in each of the four stages of labour. The four stages of labour are as follows:

- First stage (0–10 cm)
  - Latent (early) (0–3 cm)
  - Active (4–10 cm)
- Second stage (10 cm to birth of infant)
- Third stage: Delivery of placenta
- Fourth stage: 1–2 hours following birth

Those who receive an epidural analgesic during labour may not exhibit the behaviours and sensations associated with each stage and phase. The nurse must also realize that women are individuals and that each responds to labour in her own way. Table 6.2 summarizes the stages and phases of labour, the related behavioural changes, and the nursing care responsibilities.

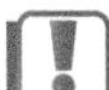

Safety Alert!

If a woman suddenly loses the ability to focus or listen, becomes irritable, or is shaking or vomiting, suspect that she has progressed to the late active phase of labour.

FETAL HEALTH SURVEILLANCE

Intrapartum care of the fetus includes assessment of FHR patterns and the amniotic fluid. In addition, several observations of the mother's status, such as vital signs and contraction pattern, are closely related to fetal well-being, because they influence fetal oxygen supply.

Fetal Heart Rate

The goal of fetal monitoring is to enable early detection of fetal hypoxia, which can have many causes, and to allow prompt interventions that will avoid fetal injury. FHR can be assessed by intermittent auscultation using a Doppler transducer or by continuous electronic fetal monitoring (EFM). (See Skill 6.1 for the procedure for assessing FHR.) FHR monitoring requires additional training.

Intermittent auscultation should be the fetal monitoring method of choice for healthy term women in spontaneous labour in the absence of risk factors (Liston et al., 2018). EFM should be used for women at increased risk for poor perinatal outcome as continuous EFM has been associated with increased intervention and Caesarean birth rates. No matter what type of fetal health surveillance is used, one-to-one labour support from a nurse or midwife is recommended because supportive care has the potential to enhance outcomes (Liston et al., 2018).

Intermittent auscultation

Intermittent auscultation allows the mother greater freedom of movement, which is helpful during labour. Intermittent auscultation does not automatically record the results, so the nurse must provide careful documentation. Intermittent auscultation of the FHR should be performed as noted in Skill 6.1 and Box 6.2.

Table 6.2 Stages of Labour and Role of the Nurse

CHARACTERISTICS	PATIENT BEHAVIOURS	NURSING INTERVENTIONS
First Stage—Dilation and Effacement		
Latent (Early) Phase		
Cervix dilation is 0–3 cm.	Happy, excited	May be sent home and will need education regarding when to return. Establish positive relationships.
Amniotic membranes may be intact.	Alert	Encourage alternating ambulation and rest.
There may be bloody show.	Talkative	Review breathing and relaxation techniques with woman and partner.
Contractions: 5 to 30 minutes apart	Welcomes diversions	Assess fetal heart rate.
• *Duration:* 30–45 seconds	Thirsty	Time contractions.
• *Intensity:* mild to moderate	May be at home	Document colour of vaginal discharge.
	Rests or sleeps if possible	Assess for distended bladder. Provide opportunity to void.
		Assist into comfortable positions.
		Provide mother ice chips and fluids.
		Assess vital signs every 2–4 hours.
		Woman may take shower or bath.
		Teach what to expect as labour progresses.
Active Phase (Approximately 2–8 Hours)		
Cervix dilation is 4–10 cm.	Apprehensive	Help partner implement coping strategies learned in prenatal classes (breathing, relaxation).
Amniotic membranes may rupture.	Anxious	Continue maternal and fetal assessments. Report colour, odour, and amount of vaginal discharge; report if meconium is seen.
Effacement of cervix occurs.	Introverted	Reassure woman.
Contractions: 2–5 minutes apart	Less social	Praise progress.
• *Duration:* 40–90 seconds	Focused on breathing	Provide back massage.
• *Intensity:* moderate to strong	Perspires	Facilitate position changes (avoid lying flat on back).
	Facial flushing	Provide ice chips to moisten mouth.
	May request pain relief	Continue to provide supportive care and determine what pain relief the woman wants.
	Fears losing control	
	Irritable	Watch for bladder distension.
	Rejects support person	Encourage voiding.
	Tremor of legs	Woman may shower or use tub (hydrotherapy).
	Restless	Provide general comfort measures.
		Provide firm coaching of breathing and relaxation techniques, focusing.
		Support coach.
		Keep woman and support person informed as to progress with each contraction.
		Accept negative comments from woman.
		Maintain a positive approach.
Second Stage—Pushing of Fetus (30 Minutes to 2 Hours or More)		
Cervix dilation is 10 cm.	Bulging perineum	Assist woman to assume position that helps her push.
Contractions: every 2–3 minutes	Mother may pass stool	Assist with open glottis pushing technique and coping strategies.
• *Duration:* 60–80 seconds	Uncontrollable urge to push	Support coach.
• *Intensity:* strong	States "baby is coming"	Maintain communication with healthcare provider.
	Exhaustion after each contraction	Monitor contractions and fetal heart rate every 5 minutes.

Table 6.2 **Stages of Labour and Role of the Nurse—cont'd**

CHARACTERISTICS	PATIENT BEHAVIOURS	NURSING INTERVENTIONS
Second stage ends with birth of infant.	Excitement concerning imminent birth	Assess perineum and vaginal discharge.
		Report bulging or crowning.
		Observe for bladder distension.
		Prepare instruments for birth.
		Prepare infant resuscitation equipment.
		Provide feedback to woman and partner.
Third Stage—Expulsion of Placenta		
Duration: 5–30 minutes	Elation	Observe and document blood loss.
Contractions: intermittent	Relief	Document delivery of placenta.
• *Intensity:* mild to moderate	Tremors	Examine placenta to determine if all of it was expelled (retained placenta causes hemorrhage because it prevents the uterus from contracting).
Umbilical cord is cut.	Increased physical energy	Monitor mother's vital signs every 15 minutes.
Signs of placental separation include the following:	Curiosity about infant	Assess vaginal discharge.
	Desire to breastfeed infant	Assess uterus to determine location and firmness.
• Lengthening of cord	Pain is minimal as placenta is expelled	Administer oxytocin to mother as ordered.
• Uterine fundus rises and becomes firm		Obtain cord blood if needed.
• Fresh blood expelled from vagina		Note parent–infant interaction.
Placenta is expelled by Schultze mechanism (shiny fetal side first) or by Duncan's mechanism (dull, rough maternal side first) (see Fig. 6.25).		Dry newborn and place skin-to-skin with mother (or partner).
Uterus contracts to size of a grapefruit.		Assess and provide immediate newborn care.
Laceration or episiotomy is sutured by healthcare provider.		Perform Apgar evaluation.
		Apply proper identification to mother, infant, and partner.
Fourth Stage—Recovery (1–2 Hours After Birth)		
Uterus remains midline, firmly contracted at or slightly below umbilicus level.	A get-acquainted period between woman, partner, and infant	Maintain skin-to-skin contact and encourage breastfeeding within the first hour.
Lochia rubra saturates perineal pad (no more than one pad per hour).	Mother breastfeeds infant	Assess fundus and massage to maintain firm contraction (a fundus that is displaced to the side indicates a full bladder is pressing against it).
Cramping may occur.		Assess lochia (no more than one saturated pad per hour).
Woman may have shaking chills that may be a thermoregulation response.		Assess woman's vital signs every 15 minutes.
		Assess maternal voiding.
		Monitor heart rate and temperature of newborn.
		Provide warmth to newborn.
		Assess newborn for anomalies.
		Enhance bonding between parent and infant.
		Change mother's gown and underpads.

Skill 6.1 How to Perform Fetal Health Surveillance

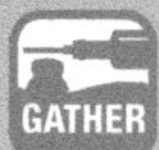

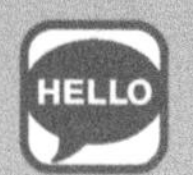

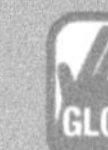

PURPOSE

To assess and document the fetal heart rate (FHR)

STEPS

1. Determine the best location for assessing FHR by performing Leopold manoeuvre (see Fig. 6.13).
2. The clearest fetal heart sounds will most likely be found over the fetal back (see Fig. 6.14).
3. Assess the mother's pulse while doing intermittent auscultation to make sure that the FHR and maternal pulse are different.
4. Assess fetal heart rate using one of the following methods:

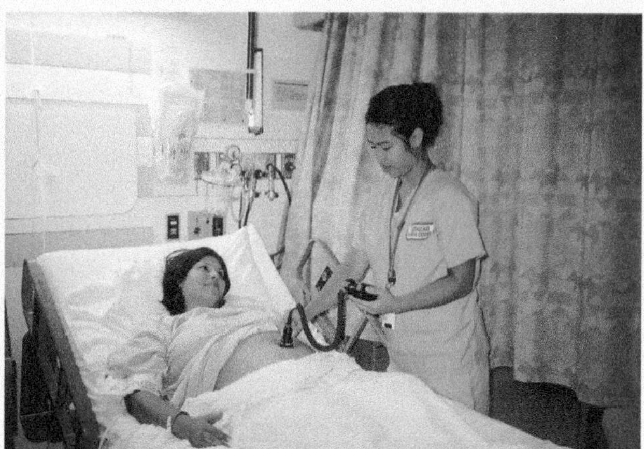

Fetoscope

a. Place the head attachment (if there is one) over your head and earpieces in your ears.
b. Place bell in the approximate area of the fetal back and press firmly while listening for muffled fetal heart sounds. When they are heard, count rate for 1 minute.
c. Assess rate after a contraction.

Doppler Transducer

a. Place water-soluble gel on the head of the handheld transducer.
b. Position earpieces in your ears, or connect transducer to a speaker.
c. Turn switch on and place transducer head over approximate area of the fetal back.
d. Count as instructed with fetoscope. If earpieces are used, let the parents hear the fetal heartbeat.

Continuous External Fetal Monitor

This is used to monitor the FHR continuously.

a. Put water-soluble gel on transducer and apply as instructed for Doppler transducer.
b. Belts, a wide band of stockinette, or an adhesive ring is used to secure the transducer for external fetal monitoring.
c. The rate is calculated by the monitor and displayed on an electronic panel and changes as FHR changes.
d. A second belt goes over the fundus of the uterus to monitor uterine contractions. The belt should not be placed too tight and the transducer should be moved every 30 to 60 minutes to decrease skin pressure.

5. See Table 6.3 for interpretation of FHR findings.
6. Document the rate. The guidelines for a normal FHR at term are as follows:
   - Lower limit of 110 beats/min
   - Upper limit of 160 beats/min

Box 6.2 How Often to Assess and Document Fetal Heart Rate

Use these guidelines for assessing and documenting the fetal heart rate (FHR) when the woman has intermittent or routine auscultation or continuous electronic fetal monitoring.

Assessment and documentation should occur:

1. Every hour in the latent phase (every 15 minutes if oxytocin is infusing)
2. Every 15 to 30 minutes in the active phase
3. Every 5 minutes in the second stage

Intermittent auscultation should be used for low-risk women, with no risk factors identified.

ROUTINE AUSCULTATION

This should be done:

1. When membranes rupture (spontaneously or artificially)
2. Before and after medication or anaesthesia administration or a change in medication
3. At the time of peak action of analgesic medications
4. After a vaginal examination
5. After catheterization
6. If uterine contractions are abnormal or excessive

CONTINUOUS ELECTRONIC FETAL MONITORING

This is recommended for women who have increased risk for adverse outcomes.

Modified from Liston, R., Sawchuck, D. Young, D., et al. (2018). No. 197b Fetal health surveillance: Intrapartum consensus guideline. *Journal of Obstetrics and Gynaecology Canada*, 40(4), e298–e322

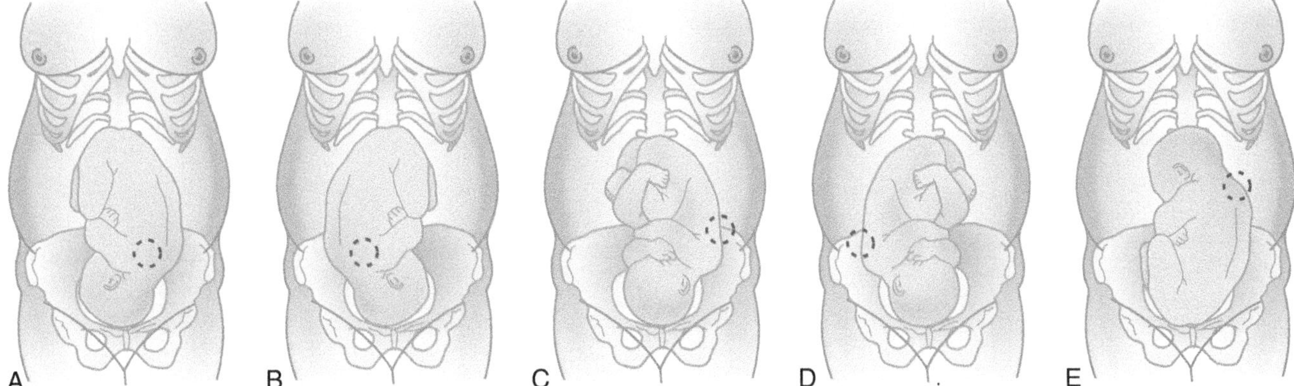

Fig. 6.14 **A–E,** Determining placement of fetoscope or sensor to assess fetal heart rate. Approximate the location of the strongest fetal heart sound when the fetus is in various positions and presentations. The fetal heart sounds are heard best in the lower abdomen in a cephalic (vertex) presentation and higher on the abdomen when the fetus is in a breech presentation **(E)**. **A,** Left occipitoanterior (LOA); **B,** right occipitoanterior (ROA); **C,** left occipitoposterior (LOP); **D,** right occipitoposterior (ROP); **E,** left sacrum anterior (LSA). (From Matteson, P. S. [2001]. *Women's health during the child-bearing years: A community based approach*. St. Louis: Mosby.)

Fig. 6.14 shows the approximate locations of the fetal heart sounds according to various presentations and positions of the fetus.

Continuous electronic fetal monitoring

Continuous EFM provides information about the FHR and uterine contraction patterns. This information is continuously recorded. The permanent recording becomes part of the mother's chart. Some monitors make use of telemetry (like a cordless telephone), so the woman is able to walk while a transmitter sends the data back to the monitor to be recorded at the nurses' station.

The recommendation is that continuous EFM be used only for high-risk pregnancies, although it continues to be used in low-risk women as well. Some of the reasons for the high use of EFM are the following (Rivard & Morin, 2017):

- Lack of nursing staff to provide one-to-one supportive care
- Caregiver skill and comfort with intermittent auscultation
- False belief that EFM will prevent all bad outcomes
- False caregiver belief that an EFM record will prevent medical legal actions

> **Safety Alert!**
>
> Fetal heart rate monitoring should be done every 15 to 30 minutes in the active phase of the first stage of labour and every 5 minutes in the second stage.

EFM can also be performed with *internal* devices. Internal devices require that the membranes be ruptured and the cervix dilated 1 to 2 cm for device insertion. Internal devices are disposable, thus reducing transmission of infection. A small spiral electrode applied to the fetal presenting part allows internal FHR monitoring. Two types of devices are used for internal contraction monitoring. One uses a fluid-filled catheter connected to a pressure-sensitive device on the monitor. The other uses a solid catheter with an electronic pressure sensor in its tip.

Evaluating fetal heart rate patterns. The FHR is recorded on the upper grid of the paper strip and is expressed as beats per minute (beats/min, or bpm); the uterine contraction pattern is recorded on the lower grid. Both grids must be evaluated together for accurate interpretation of FHR patterns. The contractions are assessed for frequency and duration. The FHR is evaluated for baseline rate, variability, and periodic and episodic changes. *Episodic changes* are those changes in the FHR that are *not* associated with uterine contractions. **Periodic changes** *are* associated with uterine contractions.

- **Baseline fetal heart rate** is the average FHR that occurs during a 10-minute period and does not include any accelerations, decelerations, or periods of marked variability. The baseline FHR should be 110 to 160 beats/min, and it should be present for at least a 2-minute period within a 10-minute window.
- **Fetal bradycardia** occurs when the FHR is below 110 beats/min for 10 minutes or longer. Causes of fetal bradycardia can be fetal cardiac anomalies, hypoxia, maternal hypoglycemia, maternal hypotension, maternal hypothermia, prolonged umbilical cord compression, or viral infections. The significance of bradycardia depends on the reason why it has occurred, along with whether it is accompanied by a loss of baseline variability or by late decelerations.
- **Fetal tachycardia** is a baseline FHR greater than 160 beats/min that lasts for more than 10 minutes. Common causes are maternal infection, fever, medication administration, or maternal dehydration, although it can also be a sign of fetal hypoxemia. When fetal tachycardia occurs along with loss of baseline variability or with late decelerations, intervention is required.

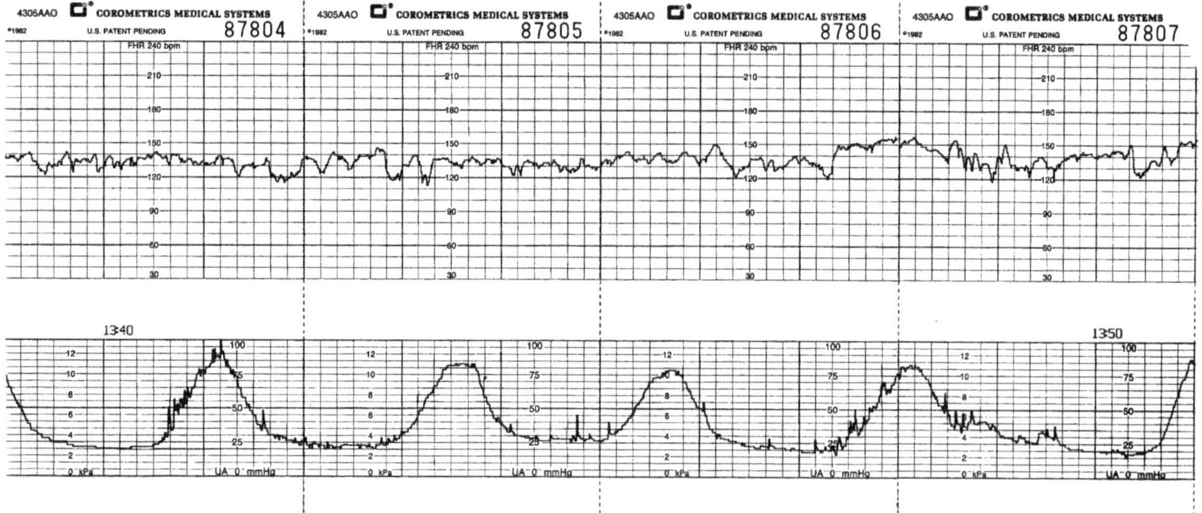

Fig. 6.15 Recording of the fetal heart rate (FHR) in the upper grid and the uterine contractions in the lower grid. Note the sawtooth appearance of the FHR tracing that is a result of the constant changes in the rate (variability). **Note:** The space between each dark black line on the strip represents 1 minute. The small squares, or the space between each light black line, represents 10 seconds. (Courtesy Corometrics Medical Systems, Wallingford, CN. Redrawn with permission.)

- **Variability** describes fluctuation or constant changes in the baseline FHR above and below the baseline, excluding accelerations and decelerations in a 10-minute window (Fig. 6.15). Variability causes a recording of the FHR to have a sawtooth appearance.
- **Absent variability** is a 0 to 2 beats/min change from baseline for a 10-minute period and is typically caused by uteroplacental insufficiency but can also be caused by maternal hypotension, cord compression, and fetal hypoxia. See Table 6.3 for nursing interventions related to this.
- **Minimal variability** is FHR changes of less than 6 beats/min and is often due to medications administered to the mother, maternal smoking, or fetal sleep. If minimal variability lasts for 40 to 80 minutes, it is considered atypical, but if it lasts longer than 80 minutes, it is considered an abnormal finding and the primary healthcare provider should be notified.
- **Moderate variability** is defined as changes of 6 beats/min to 25 beats/min from the baseline FHR. It is considered normal because it indicates good oxygenation of the central nervous system (CNS) and fetal well-being.
- **Marked variability** occurs when there are more than 25 beats/min of fluctuation over the FHR baseline; the significance of marked variability is uncertain. It may be due to a normal variation or decreased fetal oxygenation (Miller, Miller, & Tucker, 2013).

See Table 6.3 for interpretation and interventions of fetal monitor findings.

Accelerations. **Accelerations** are temporary, abrupt rate increases of at least 15 beats/min above the baseline FHR that last 15 seconds but less than 2 minutes from onset to return to baseline in a fetus greater than 32 weeks' gestation. This pattern suggests a fetus that is well oxygenated. Accelerations can be episodic or periodic. Accelerations may occur with fetal movement and are the basis for interpretation of the non–stress test (NST) (see Chapter 5 for further discussion). An acceleration that lasts 2 to 10 minutes is considered a prolonged acceleration. An acceleration that lasts longer than 10 minutes may be considered a baseline FHR change.

Decelerations

Early decelerations. **Early decelerations** are temporary, gradual FHR decreases during contractions; the FHR always returns to the baseline rate by the end of the contraction. The peak of deceleration occurs at the same time as the peak of the contraction. This shows a U-shaped pattern that begins early with the uterine contraction and ends near the end of the uterine contraction. They are usually caused by compression of the fetal head, although sometimes they may be due to CPD, especially if seen early in labour. They are normally felt to be a good sign, as evidence that the CNS is responding in a normal way, although if seen early in labour the woman needs to be assessed for labour progress.

Variable decelerations. **Variable decelerations** are abrupt decreases of at least 15 beats/min below baseline, lasting 15 seconds to 2 minutes in the full-term fetus. These decreases begin and end abruptly; on the monitor they are V-, W-, or U-shaped (Fig. 6.16). They do not always exhibit a consistent pattern in relation to contractions. Variable decelerations suggest that the umbilical cord is being compressed, sometimes because it is around the fetal neck (**nuchal cord**) or because there is inadequate amniotic fluid to cushion the cord. It is not associated with fetal hypoxia but is associated with fetal respiratory acidosis. Variable decelerations are further classified as:

Table 6.3 Fetal Heart Rate Interpretation System and Nursing Care

CATEGORY	FETAL HEART RATE (FHR) TRACINGS	NURSING RESPONSIBILITIES
Normal	Normal baseline rate (110–160 beats/min) Variability • 6–25 beats/min (moderate) • <5 beats/min for <40 min Decelerations • None or occasional uncomplicated variables or early decelerations Accelerations • Spontaneous accelerations present	Provide routine labour care.
Atypical	Baseline FHR • 100–110 beats/min • >160 beats/min for >30 min to <80 min • Rising baseline Variability • ≤5 beats/min for 40–80 min Decelerations • Repetitive ≥3 uncomplicated variable decelerations • Occasional late decelerations • Single prolonged deceleration >2 min but <3 min Accelerations • Absence of accelerations with fetal scalp stimulation	Provide vigilant assessment, especially when more than one symptom is present. Attempt to correct the cause of fetal compromise, provide intrauterine resuscitation (change maternal position, increase IV rate, decrease oxytocin, administer oxygen), or do further fetal evaluation.
Abnormal	Baseline FHR • <100 beats/min • >160 beats/min for >80 min • Erratic baseline Variability • ≤5 beats/min for >80 min Decelerations • Repetitive (≥3) complicated variable decelerations • Late decelerations >50% of contractions • Single prolonged decelerations >3 min but <10 min Accelerations • Usually absent	Prompt interventions are indicated: intrauterine resuscitation and/or prompt birth (vaginal or Caesarean) unless there is normal fetal scalp pH.

From Liston, R., Sawchuck, D. Young, D., et al. (2018). No. 197b Fetal health surveillance: Intrapartum consensus guideline. *Journal of Obstetrics and Gynaecology Canada, 40*(4), e298–e322.

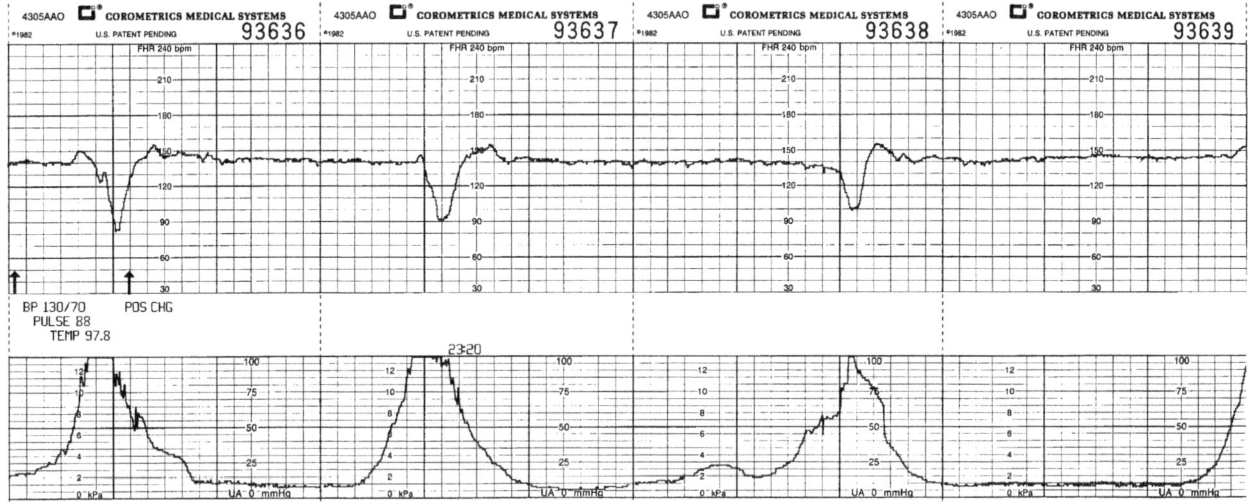

Fig. 6.16 Variable decelerations, showing their typically abrupt onset and offset. They are caused by umbilical cord compression. The first response to this pattern is to reposition the mother to relieve pressure on the cord. (Courtesy Corometrics Medical Systems, Wallingford, CN. Redrawn with permission.)

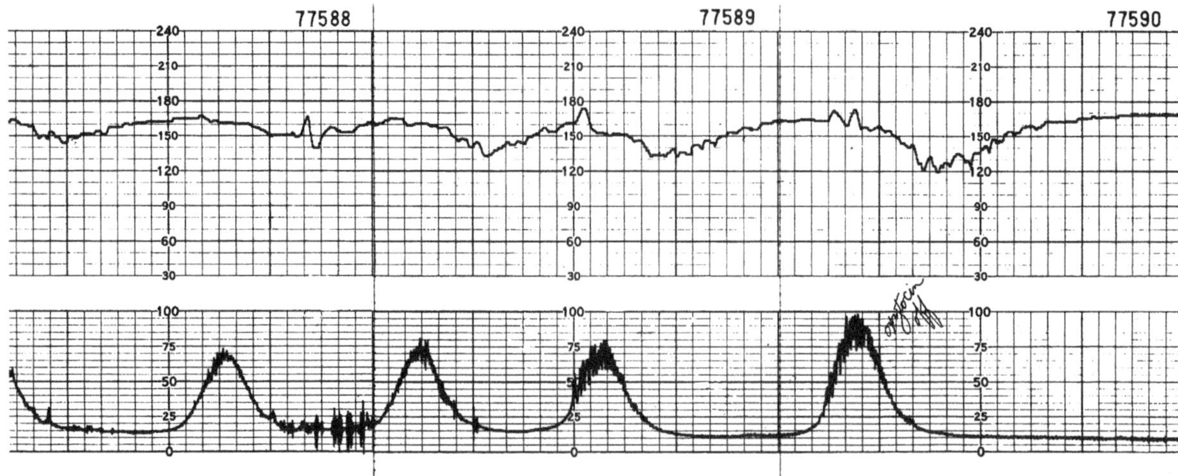

Fig. 6.17 Late decelerations, showing their pattern of slowing, which persists after the contraction ends. The usual cause is reduced blood flow from the placenta (uteroplacental insufficiency). Measures to correct this include repositioning the woman, increasing nonmedicated intravenous fluid, giving oxygen, and stopping administration of oxytocin if it is being given. (Courtesy Corometrics Medical Systems, Wallingford, CN. Redrawn with permission.)

Uncomplicated: Deceleration that have acceleration at the beginning or end of contraction. Usually they are not clinically significant unless present with other abnormal FHR signs.

Complicated: Deceleration to 70 beats/min for more than 60 seconds, slow return to baseline. If repetitive (>3) they are considered abnormal.

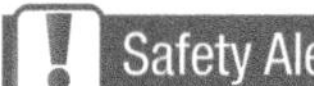

Safety Alert!

Report any questionable fetal heart rate or contraction pattern to the healthcare provider for complete evaluation.

Late decelerations. Late decelerations of the FHR look similar to early decelerations, except that they begin *after* the beginning of the contraction and do not return to the baseline FHR until *after the contraction ends* (Fig. 6.17). Late decelerations suggest that the placenta is not delivering enough oxygen to the fetus (uteroplacental insufficiency), and this could be due to chronic conditions in the mother or placental conditions. Late decelerations that are accompanied by decreased variability and absent accelerations are abnormal and require immediate intervention by the health care provider.

Prolonged decelerations. Prolonged decelerations are abrupt FHR decreases of at least 15 beats/min from baseline that last longer than 2 minutes but less than 10 minutes. These are caused by an interruption of oxygen supply to the fetus, possibly due to cord compression or prolapse, maternal supine hypotension, or regional anaesthesia. A prolonged deceleration that lasts longer than 10 minutes may be considered a change in the baseline rate (Liston et al., 2018).

Sinusoidal pattern. *Sinusoidal pattern* is a specific FHR pattern that has a smooth, wavelike appearance or undulating pattern with a wave frequency of 3 to 5 waves per minute and persists for 20 minutes or longer. It may be caused by fetal response to medication provided to the mother in labour, such as opioids, or occur in a fetus who is anemic (Miller et al., 2013).

Nursing response to monitor patterns

The significance of and, thus, nursing response to FHR changes depend on the pattern or category identified (see Table 6.3). For example, accelerations and early decelerations are normal and thus necessitate no intervention other than continued assessment. Repositioning the woman is usually the first corrective response to a pattern of variable decelerations. Changing the mother's position can relieve pressure on the umbilical cord and can improve blood flow through it. The woman is turned to her side. Other positions, such as the knee–chest or a slight Trendelenburg (head-down) position may be tried if the side-lying position does not restore the pattern to a normal one.

Any abnormal FHR or atypical FHR that does not respond to a position change should be promptly reported to the obstetrical healthcare provider.

The purpose of FHR monitoring is to assess the adequacy of oxygenation and uterine activity during labour, to avoid hypoxic injury to the fetus. FHR patterns are not diagnostic, as they have many possible causes, but instead they are used to detect possible identifiable complications that may be causing interruptions in fetal oxygen supply. Atypical and abnormal FHR patterns often require an improvement in fetal oxygenation (see Table 6.3). These include the following nursing interventions:

- *Position changes* can relieve the pressure on the fetal umbilical cord (knee–chest position) or pressure on the inferior vena cava (left-lateral position).
- *Increase in IV fluids* increases the circulating volume and enhances uteroplacental perfusion. The nurse should observe for fluid volume overload and pulmonary edema.

Skill 6.2 Testing for Presence of Amniotic Fluid (Nitrazine Paper Test)

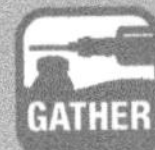

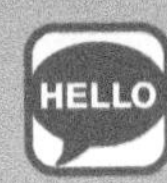

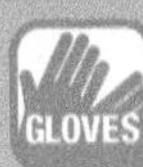

PURPOSE

To determine the presence of amniotic fluid in vaginal secretions

STEPS

1. Place a piece of nitrazine paper into fluid from vagina.
2. Read the colour on the strip of paper.
   a. A blue-green or deep-blue colour of nitrazine paper indicates the fluid is alkaline and most likely amniotic fluid.
   b. A yellow to yellow-green colour of the strip paper indicates the fluid is acidic and is most likely urine.
3. Document and report results; offer and provide pericare; remove gloves and perform hand hygiene.
4. Document presence of bloody show, which may alter accuracy of the results.

- *Decrease oxytocin* if labour is being augmented.
- *Correct any hypotension,* which may be caused by dehydration or be a response to the epidural analgesic.
- *Administration of oxygen* via face mask at 6 L/min may be used, although it is not always effective, as healthy labouring women already have high levels of circulating oxygen.
- **Amnioinfusion**—instilling of a saline infusion by catheter into the uterine cavity to restore amniotic fluid volume in order to relieve umbilical cord compression that can interrupt fetal oxygenation (see Chapter 8). This is done by the obstetrical healthcare provider.
- *Altered pushing and breathing techniques in the second stage of labour:*
  1. Changing from Valsalva (holding the breath and pushing) to open glottis pushing
  2. Fewer pushing efforts during contractions
  3. Pushing with every other contraction
  4. Pushing only with the urge to push

If the above corrective measures do not improve the FHR tracing, more aggressive interventions are required. These may include fetal scalp blood pH or fetal stimulation, which may be done by the obstetrical healthcare provider to assess the fetal status and urgency for birth for a positive outcome. The SOGC recommends that after the birth, umbilical arterial and venous gases be assessed to determine if further care is required (Liston et al., 2018). Umbilical artery gases reflect the status of the fetus, and venous gases reflect how well the placenta functions (Miller et al., 2013).

Inspection of Amniotic Fluid

The membranes may rupture spontaneously, or the healthcare provider may rupture them artificially in a procedure called an **amniotomy**. The colour, odour, and amount of fluid are recorded. The normal colour of amniotic fluid is clear, possibly with flecks of white vernix (fetal skin protectant) or slightly pink from the changes in the cervix. The amount of amniotic fluid is usually estimated as scant (only a trickle), moderate (about 500 mL), or large (about 1 000 mL or more). Green-stained fluid may indicate the fetus has passed meconium (the first stool) before birth, a situation associated with fetal compromise that can cause respiratory problems at birth. Cloudy or yellow amniotic fluid with an offensive odour may indicate an infection and should be reported immediately.

The FHR should be assessed for at least 1 full minute after the membranes rupture and must be documented. Marked slowing of the rate or variable decelerations suggests that the fetal umbilical cord may have descended with the fluid gush and is being compressed.

A **nitrazine test** or fern test may be performed if it is not clear whether the mother's membranes have ruptured. Nitrazine paper is a pH paper; alkaline amniotic fluid turns it dark blue-green or dark blue. Commercial high-tech strips are available, such as AmniSure, the use of which involves swabbing vaginal secretions and inserting the swab into a vial to determine the pH of the vaginal fluid. In the fern test, a sample of amniotic fluid is spread on a microscope slide and allowed to dry. It is then viewed under the microscope; the crystals in the fluid look like tiny fern leaves (Skill 6.2).

ASSESSMENT OF THE LABOURING WOMAN

Intrapartum care of the woman includes assessing her vital signs, contractions, progress of labour, intake and output, and responses to labour. The physiological changes that occur during labour are listed in Table 6.4.

Impending Birth

The nurse continually observes the woman for behaviours that suggest she is about to give birth, including the following:

- Making grunting sounds
- Bearing down with contractions
- Stating "The baby's coming"

Table 6.4 Physiological Changes in Labour and Nursing Interventions

SYSTEM	PHYSIOLOGY	CLINICAL SYMPTOMS	NURSING INTERVENTIONS
Cardiovascular	Uterine contractions release 400 mL of blood into vascular system, causing increase in cardiac output.	BP increases by 10 mm Hg; pulse rate increases slightly.	Assess BP between contractions.
	Ascending vena cava and descending aorta are compressed by weight of the uterus.	Supine hypotension can occur.	Have woman avoid lying on her back. Encourage left side-lying position.
	Holding the breath and forceful pushing increase intrathoracic pressure and reduce venous return and can cause fetal hypoxia.	Forceful rather than spontaneous pushing (Valsalva manoeuvre) causes redness of face, increase in BP, and slowing of pulse rate.	Encourage open-glottis pushing and discourage forceful pushing during the second stage.
	White blood cell (WBC) count increases.	Increase in WBC count is not related to infection.	Correct interpretation of laboratory results intrapartum and postpartum is important.
Respiratory	Increased physical activity of labour increases oxygen consumption. Anxiety can also increase oxygen consumption.	Respiratory rate increases.	Encourage relaxation between contractions.
	Paced breathing techniques can prevent development of respiratory alkalosis.	Tingling of the hands and feet, dizziness, or numbness may indicate hyperventilation, which can cause respiratory alkalosis.	Coach the labouring woman in breathing techniques.
Renal (kidneys)	Breakdown in muscle tissue resulting from work of labour can cause proteinuria.	Palpate above symphysis pubis to detect a full bladder.	Encourage voiding every 2 hours; catheterize if bladder is distended and if the woman is unable to void.
	A full bladder can be obstructed by a full uterus and the fetal head.	Spontaneous voiding may occur during contractions.	Do not confuse spontaneous urination with rupture of bag of waters. Nitrazine paper can show whether fluid discharge is urine or amniotic fluid.
Musculoskeletal	Muscle activity increases during labour. Increased joint laxity can cause backaches.	Observe for diaphoresis, fatigue, and increased temperature.	Encourage rest between contractions; use comfort measures for diaphoresis and positioning for back and joint pain.
Neurological	Euphoria changes to self-centredness as labour progresses. Amnesia during the second stage is common, and fatigue and elation occur in the third and fourth stages. Endorphins produce natural, general sedation, whereas ischemia of perineal tissues by pressure of presenting part causes a decrease in perception of perineal pain.	Behaviour of patient may change during each stage of labour.	Provide support; allow sleep whenever possible; provide for safety and privacy.

Continued

Table 6.4 Physiological Changes in Labour and Nursing Interventions—cont'd

SYSTEM	PHYSIOLOGY	CLINICAL SYMPTOMS	NURSING INTERVENTIONS
Gastrointestinal (GI)	Mouth breathing during labour dries the lips and tongue; GI motility is decreased during labour.	Dry lips and mouth may be noted. Nausea and vomiting of undigested food may occur.	Assess for signs of dehydration. Use ice chips to moisten the lips or tongue during active labour. Allow the woman to eat and drink as desired if not at risk for general anaesthetic. Rectal pressure and urge to defecate may indicate imminent birth.
Endocrine	Estrogen increases and progesterone decreases. Metabolism increases during labour; work of labour may decrease glucose levels.	Close monitoring of the mother with diabetes (including blood glucose levels) during labour is essential.	Encourage rest whenever possible between contractions.
Blood	The increased blood volume during pregnancy enables a 500-mL blood loss during birth without problems unless the woman is anemic.	Decrease in BP should be reported.	Monitor vital signs during labour and birth.
	Increased levels of fibrinogen and other clotting factors during pregnancy decrease the risk for hemorrhage during birth but increase risk for thrombosis.	If possible, avoid prolonged use of stirrups to support her legs during birth.	

BP, Blood pressure.

- Bulging of the perineum or the fetal presenting part becoming visible at the vaginal opening

If it appears that birth is imminent, the nurse must not leave the woman but summon help or use the call bell. The nurse's priority is to prevent injury to the mother and infant. The nurse should don gloves and assist with the birth until help arrives (Skill 6.3).

Nursing Tip

It is unlikely that a practical nurse will be called on to help a woman give birth to an infant during a precipitous birth, but the process should be reviewed in case this does occur.

Vital Signs

The temperature is checked every 4 hours, or every 2 hours if it is elevated or if the membranes have ruptured (frequency varies among facilities). A temperature of 38°C (100.4°F) or higher should be reported. If the temperature is elevated, the amniotic fluid is assessed for signs of infection. Blood cultures may be drawn to accurately treat an infection. IV antibiotics may be given to a woman who has a fever because of the risk that the infant will acquire an infection. The pulse, blood pressure, and respirations are assessed every 30 to 60 minutes. Maternal hypotension (particularly if the systolic pressure is below 90 mm Hg) or hypertension (greater than 140/90 mm Hg) can reduce blood flow to the placenta.

Contractions

Contractions can be assessed by palpation or by continuous EFM. When palpation is used to evaluate contractions, the fingertips are placed lightly on her uterine fundus (Fig. 6.18; see Skill 6.4). Normal contractions are fewer than five in a 10-minute period (Table 6.5).

Progress of Labour

A vaginal examination is done periodically to determine how labour is progressing. The cervix is evaluated for effacement and dilation. The descent of the fetus is determined in relation to the ischial spines (station) (see Fig. 6.12). There is no set interval for doing vaginal examinations. The observant nurse watches for physical and behavioural changes associated with the progression of labour to reduce the number of vaginal examinations needed. Vaginal examinations should be limited to prevent infection, especially if the membranes are ruptured. They also can be uncomfortable for the woman.

Intake and Output

Women in labour do not usually need strict measurement of intake and output, but the time and approximate amount of each urination are recorded. The woman may not sense a full bladder, so she should be checked every 1 or 2 hours for a bulge above the symphysis pubis. A full bladder is a source of vague discomfort and can impede fetal descent. It often causes

Skill 6.3 Assisting With an Emergency Birth

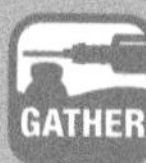

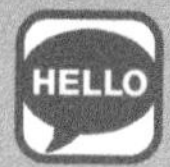

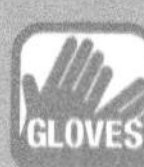

PURPOSE

To prioritize care and prevent injury to the mother and child

STEPS

1. Obtain an instrument tray (an emergency birth tray if available).
2. Do not leave the woman if she exhibits any signs of imminent birth, such as grunting, bearing down, perineal bulging, or a statement that the baby is coming. Summon help with the call bell and try to remain calm.
3. Put on gloves and a cover gown. Use of either clean or sterile gloves is acceptable because no invasive procedures will be done. Gloves and a cover gown are used primarily to protect the nurse from exposure to body fluids while supporting the infant during the birth.
4. Support the infant's head and body as it emerges. Wipe secretions from the infant's face.
5. Feel around the infant's neck for presence of the umbilical cord (nuchal cord). If the cord is around the infant's neck, it may be long enough to slip over the infant's head or it may be clamped with two clamps and cut.
6. Control delivery of the head to prevent laceration of the perineum, but do not hold the head back.
7. Clamp and cut the cord.
8. Dry infant quickly, ensure the airway is clear, place skin-to-skin with the mother, and cover with a warm blanket to maintain infant's temperature.
9. Observe infant's colour and respirations. The cry should be vigorous and the colour pink (bluish hands and feet are normal). Rub the back and stimulate as needed.
10. Observe for placental detachment and bleeding. After the placenta detaches, observe for a firm fundus. If fundus is not firm, massage it. The infant can suckle at the mother's breast to promote release of oxytocin, which stimulates uterine contraction.
11. Document events as they occurred and include the sex of the infant, time of birth, and expulsion of the placenta.

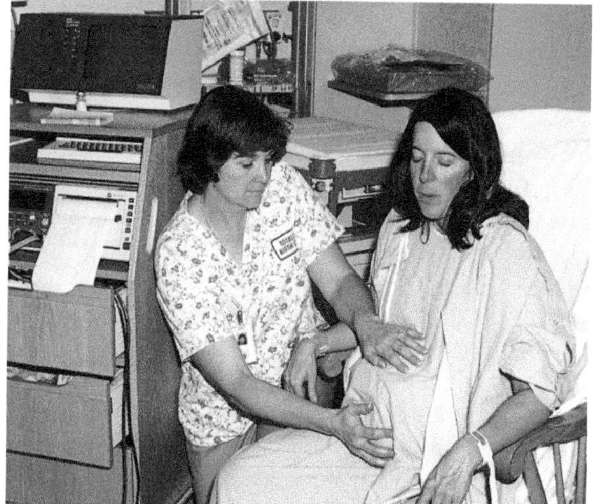

Fig. 6.18 The nurse helps the mother maintain control and use breathing techniques during active labour. Assessment of strength of contractions is done using the fingertips. (Courtesy Pat Spier, RN-C.)

discomfort that persists after an epidural block has been initiated.

Policies about oral intake vary among birth facilities, although the SOGC states that women who are at low risk of requiring general anaesthesia should have the choice to eat or drink as desired or tolerated in labour (Lee, Dy, Azzam, et al., 2016). Ice chips or popsicles may be offered to keep the mouth moistened. Routine IVs are not usually started. They would be initiated in women who are having labour induced or augmented, are receiving antibiotics, have epidural analgesia, have a fetus with an abnormal FHR, or are vomiting and unable to keep oral fluids in place.

Response to Labour

The nurse assesses the woman's response to labour, including her use of breathing and relaxation techniques, and supports the woman to cope during labour. Nonverbal behaviours that suggest difficulty coping with labour include a tense body posture and thrashing in bed. The healthcare provider should be notified if the woman requests added pain relief, such as epidural analgesia.

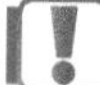

Safety Alert!

Signs suggesting rapid progress of labour need to be promptly addressed. Bloody show may increase markedly, and the perineum may bulge as the fetal head stretches it. The practical nurse should summon an RN with the call bell if bloody show or perineal bulging increases or if the woman exhibits behaviours typical of imminent birth (listed earlier in this chapter). Do not leave the woman if birth is imminent!

Skill 6.4 Determining Contractions by Palpation

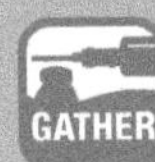

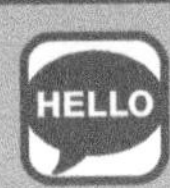

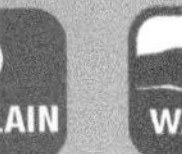

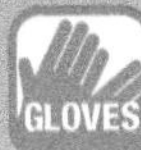

PURPOSE

To provide intermittent assessment of uterine contractions

STEPS

1. Place fingertips of one hand lightly on the upper uterus. Keep fingers relatively still, but move them occasionally so that mild contractions can be felt.
2. Palpate at least three to five contractions for an accurate estimate of their average characteristics.
3. Note the time when each contraction begins and ends.
   a. Calculate the *frequency* by counting the elapsed time from the beginning of one contraction to the beginning of the next.
   b. Calculate the *duration* by determining the number of seconds from the beginning to the end of each contraction.
4. Estimate the *intensity* by trying to indent uterus at the contraction's peak. If it is easily indented (like the tip of the nose), the contraction is mild; if it is harder to indent (like the chin), it is moderate; if it is nearly impossible to indent (like the forehead), it is firm.
5. Chart average frequency (in minutes and fractions), duration (in seconds), and intensity.
6. Report contractions more frequent than every 2 minutes or lasting longer than 90 seconds or intervals of relaxation shorter than 60 seconds.

Table 6.5 Describing Uterine Activity

UTERINE ACTIVITY	DESCRIPTION
Normal	Five or less contractions within 10 minutes averaged over a 30-minute period
Tachysystole (increased uterine activity)	More than five contractions within 10 minutes averaged over 30 minutes • Tachysystole should always be qualified by presence or absence of associated FHR changes. • Tachysystole may occur in both spontaneous and stimulated labour.

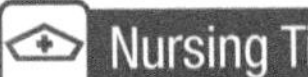

Nursing Tip

If a labouring woman says her baby is coming, believe her.

HELPING THE WOMAN COPE WITH LABOUR

Coping is a dynamic process in which emotions and stress affect and influence each other; coping changes the relationship between the individual and the environment. The nurse must understand the physiology of the normal process of labour to recognize abnormalities. The nurse collects, records, and interprets data during labour, such as FHR responses to uterine contractions (see discussion of electronic fetal monitoring earlier in chapter), maternal physical responses (e.g., vital signs and duration of contractions), and psychological responses (e.g., anxiety and tension). The nurse also needs to maintain open communication with the healthcare provider and provide general hygiene and comfort measures for the mother according to the needs presented. In addition to consistent assessment of the fetal and maternal conditions, the nurse helps the woman to cope with labour by comforting, positioning, teaching, and encouraging her (Fig. 6.19). Another aspect of intrapartum nursing is care of the woman's partner and family.

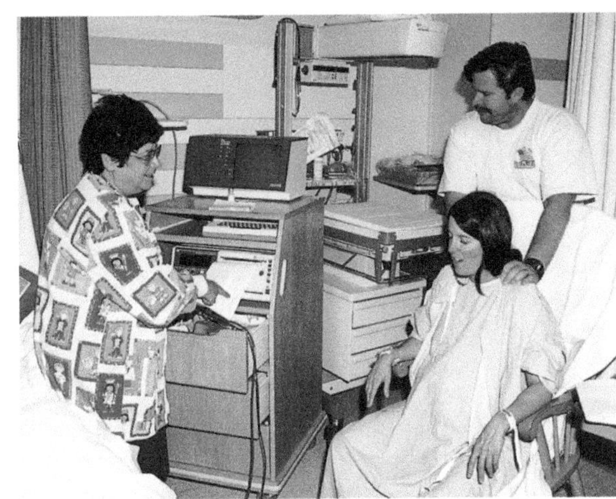

Fig. 6.19 The nurse teaches the woman and her partner about electronic fetal monitoring to reduce anxiety and promote the woman's comfort during labor. Electronic fetal monitoring is only one method used to evaluate fetal well-being during labour.

Childbirth is a normal and natural process, but today, with modern medicine and technology, few women in the hospital setting give birth without some intervention. The World Health Organization (WHO) has developed new recommendations to establish global care standards for healthy pregnant women during labour and to reduce unnecessary medical interventions (WHO, 2019). The guideline recognizes that every labour and childbirth is unique and that the duration of the active first stage of labour varies from one woman to another.

Labour Support

The nurse should provide continuous labour support in a hands-on, in-person manner rather than rely on monitors viewed from outside the labour room. The environment of the labour room can be controlled by having the woman listen to familiar music brought from home, which can produce a calming effect. Her maintaining an upright position during labour can shorten the first stage (Lee et al., 2016). Positions of comfort for the labouring woman include sitting upright on a rocking chair or birthing ball, which uses the natural force of gravity to promote fetal descent. The lateral Sims position encourages rest and helps prevent pressure on the sacrum.

In addition to controlling the environment, nonpharmacological pain-relief techniques such as touch, effleurage, massage, back pressure, application of heat or cold, and various relaxation techniques are effective means of labour support. Hydrotherapy is an effective method for managing pain. Nonpharmacological pain relief methods are further discussed in Chapter 7. Walking or resting during labour is based on the woman's preference for comfort (Selby, Valencia, Garcia, et al., 2012). During labour, the nurse should encourage the woman to assume positions that favour fetal rotation and descent. Emotional support, encouragement, communication concerning progress, and promoting positive thoughts are also essential. Providing support for women during active labour and birth significantly increases families' satisfaction with the birth experience, reduces the use of medications and interventions, and enhances the positive attitude women need to care for their babies (PHAC, 2018).

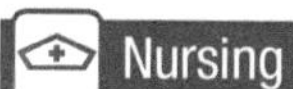 Nursing Tip

Regular changes of position may make the labouring woman more comfortable and promote the normal processes of labour.

Back Labour

A common cause of a longer labour is a fetus that remains in a persistent occiput posterior (OP) position (left [LOP] or right [ROP]). The fetal occiput occupies either the left or the right posterior quadrant of the mother's pelvis. In most women, the fetal head rotates in a clockwise or counterclockwise direction until the occiput is in one of the anterior quadrants of the pelvis (left [LOA] or right [ROA]). Intense and poorly relieved back and leg pain characterize labour when the fetus is in the OP position. Women with a small or average-sized pelvis may have difficulty giving birth to infants who remain in a persistent OP position. The obstetrical healthcare provider may try to manually rotate the infant using their hand while the woman is pushing. If this is not successful, they may attempt using forceps to rotate the fetal head into an occiput anterior position.

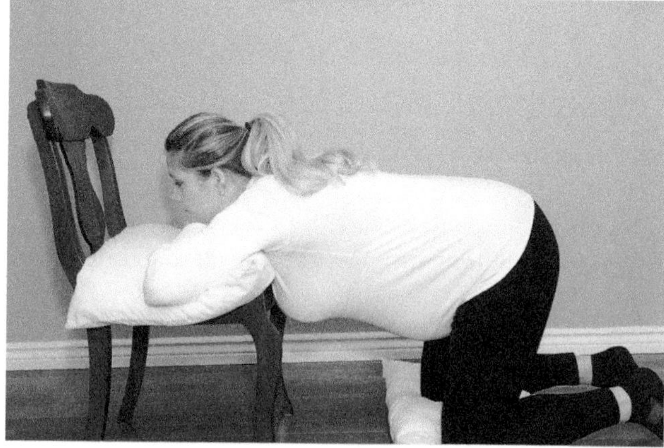

Fig. 6.20 The hands-and-knees position can help the fetus rotate from an occiput posterior to an occiput anterior position. Gravity causes the fetus to float downward toward the pool of amniotic fluid. This position can be practiced before labour. (Courtesy of Sandy Matos)

Good positions to relieve the pain of back labour include the following:

- Sitting, kneeling, or standing while leaning forward
- Rocking the pelvis back and forth while on hands and knees (Fig. 6.20) to encourage rotation
- Side-lying (on the left side for an ROP position, on the right side for an LOP position)
- Squatting (for second-stage labour) increases the diameter of the pelvis, facilitating fetal rotation and descent
- Lunging by placing one foot in a chair with the foot and knee pointed to that side; lunging sideways repeatedly during a contraction for 5 seconds at a time. Lunging helps the femur press on the ischium to increase pelvic space and facilitates rotation of the fetus that is in OP position.

Teaching

Teaching the labouring woman and her partner is an ongoing task of the nurse. Even women who attended childbirth classes may find that the measures they learned need adaptation. Positions or breathing techniques different from those learned in class can be tried. A woman should usually try a change in technique or position for two or three contractions before abandoning it.

Many women are discouraged when their cervix is about 5 cm dilated, because it has taken many hours to reach that point. They think they are only halfway through labour (full dilation is 10 cm); however, a 5-cm dilation signifies that about two thirds of the labour is completed, because the rate of progress increases. Labouring women often need support and reassurance to overcome their discouragement at this point.

Providing Encouragement

Encouragement is a powerful tool for intrapartum nursing care, because it helps the woman to summon

Table 4.6 Physiological and Psychological Changes in Pregnancy, Nursing Interventions, and Teaching

MATERNAL CHANGES	SIGNS AND SYMPTOMS	NURSING INTERVENTIONS AND TEACHING
First Trimester		
Fertilization occurs. Increased progesterone levels result in amenorrhea. Sodium (Na) retention increases. Nitrogen (N) stores decrease.	Pregnancy test is positive.	Teach patient about nutritional needs and folic acid requirements. Encourage patient to seek early prenatal care. Assess attitude toward this pregnancy and how it affects family.
Blood volume increases. Levels of relaxin hormone increase. Levels of human chorionic gonadotropin (hCG) hormone increase.	Fainting is possible. Morning nausea can occur. Relaxation of gastrointestinal (GI) muscles can cause "heartburn." Sensitivity to odours increases.	Teach patient how to rise slowly from prone position. Teach patient how to cope with nausea without medication (see Table 4.5).
Pituitary gland releases melanin-stimulating hormone.	Pigmentation deepens on face (chloasma) and on abdomen (linea nigra).	Discuss body changes and assure patient that pigmentation will fade after puerperium.
Fetus grows. Uterus begins to enlarge.	Abdomen enlarges at end of first trimester when uterus rises out of pelvis. Small weight gain occurs. Enlarged uterus presses on bladder.	Teach methods to minimize fetal problems: • Avoid high temperatures around abdomen (baths and spas). • Discuss effects of medications and herbs on fetal development (see Table 4.4).
		Discuss impact of frequency of urination on lifestyle and activities. Facilitate communication with partner concerning sexual relationships during pregnancy. Discuss nutritional needs.
For partners, announcement phase begins when pregnancy is confirmed, followed by adjustment phase and, finally, focus phase in third trimester and during labour, when "feeling like a parent" develops.	Parents adjust to reality of pregnancy.	Review partner's role as well as mother's responses. Refer to community agencies as needed. Assess for misinformation and knowledge deficit. Help parents identify concerns. Answer questions. Discuss relevant topics, such as care of siblings and role of grandparents.
Second Trimester		
Corpus luteum is absorbed, and placenta takes over fetal support (between third and fourth months).	Blood volume increases in placental bed.	Teach patient how to manage symptoms of increased congestion.
Broad ligament stretches as uterus enlarges.	Occasional pain in groin area occurs.	Teach patient Kegel exercises to strengthen pelvic muscles.
Vascularity of pelvis increases.	Sexual pleasure and desire increase. White discharge may occur.	Discuss modifications of positions for sexual comfort and pleasure. Teach patient to avoid routine douches. Teach patient perineal skin hygiene.
Blood volume and vasomotor lability increase.	Orthostatic hypotension can occur.	Teach patient to change positions slowly and to avoid warm, crowded areas.
Cardiac output increases.	Physiological anemia may occur.	Iron supplements may be prescribed for anemia. Teach patient how to prevent constipation, and teach about change in stool colour during iron therapy.
Renal threshold decreases.	Gestational diabetes may occur.	Test glucose tolerance test in second trimester to rule out gestational diabetes.
Uterus rises out of pelvis. Estrogen relaxes sacroiliac joint.	Body's centre of gravity changes.	Teach patient proper shoe and heel height to prevent falling. Teach placement of automobile restraints across hips rather than across abdomen. Teach patient to try to avoid lying supine in bed after fourth month of pregnancy to prevent supine hypotension. Teach posture and pelvic rocking exercises.

Continued

Table 4.6 Physiological and Psychological Changes in Pregnancy, Nursing Interventions, and Teaching—cont'd

MATERNAL CHANGES	SIGNS AND SYMPTOMS	NURSING INTERVENTIONS AND TEACHING
	Pressure on bladder and rectum increases.	Instruct patient to anticipate urinary frequency during long trips. Teach patient Kegel exercises to strengthen pelvic floor.
Enlarging uterus compresses nerves supplying lower extremities.	Leg muscle spasms occur, especially when reclining.	Teach patient how to dorsiflex the foot to help relieve spasms. Massage foot.
Late in second trimester cardiac reserve begins to decrease and respiratory effort to increase.	Exercise levels may need to be decreased.	Teach patient that inability to converse without taking frequent breaths is a sign of physiological stress. Teach patient to stop exercising if numbness, pain, or dizziness occurs.
Hormonal influence on emotions	Mood swings occur.	Prepare spouse or significant other and family for mood swings, and labile emotions.
Levels of relaxin hormone increase.	Sphincter of stomach relaxes, and gastrointestinal motility is slowed.	Teach patient how to prevent constipation. Instruct patient to increase fluid intake and avoid gas-forming foods.
Increase in estrogen levels causes increased excretory function of skin.	Skin itches.	Teach patient to wear loose clothing, shower frequently, and use mild soaps and oils for comfort.
Anterior pituitary secretes melanin-stimulating hormone.	Skin pigmentation deepens.	Prepare patient to anticipate development of spider nevi and skin pigmentation. Reassure patient that most fade after puerperium.
Estrogen levels increase.	Increased estrogen levels develop increased vascularity of oral tissues, resulting in gingivitis and stuffy nose. Estrogen levels develop network of increased arterioles.	Teach proper oral hygiene techniques. Edema can occur. Assess blood pressure, and report proteinuria.
Pituitary gland secretes prolactin.	Breasts enlarge.	Avoid soaps, ointments, and alcohol that dry skin. Teach patient not to stimulate nipples by massage or exercise, because doing so may increase risk for preterm labour in some women.
As breast size increases, drooping of shoulders causes traction on brachial plexus.	Fingers tingle.	Teach patient proper posture. Encourage use of a supportive maternity bra.
Placental barrier allows certain elements and organisms to pass through to fetus.	Some medications can pass through placental barrier and cause fetal defects.	Counsel patient about risks of smoking and about smoking cessation strategies. Teach patients that exposure to toxic substances must be avoided in the workplace.
Travel becomes more difficult.	Because of placental permeability, travelling to countries that have endemic diseases can have negative effect on fetus; active, live viral immunization should be avoided. Lowered oxygen levels can cause fetal hypoxia.	Counsel patient about travel options. Most commercial airlines have cabin pressure controlled at or below 1 500-m (5 000-ft) level and therefore do not pose risk to fetus.
Increased levels of platelets occur.	Women are prone to thrombophlebitis if they are inactive for long periods.	Encourage patient to keep hydrated because of low cabin humidity in airplanes and to move around to help prevent thrombophlebitis.
Fetal growth continues.	Mother feels signs of life; fetus moves and kicks.	Teach nutrition that fosters fetal growth without adding extra "empty" calories. Encourage patient to attend child care and parenting classes.

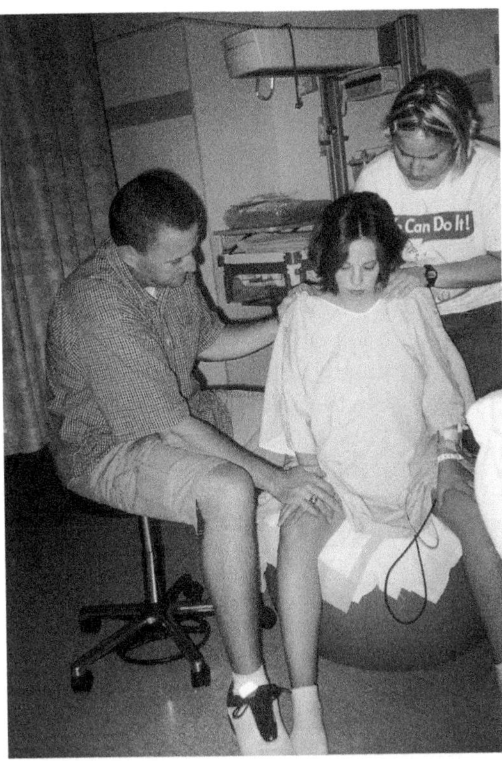

Fig. 6.21 The doula. The labouring woman sits on a birthing ball as her partner provides encouragement and the doula massages her shoulders. (Courtesy Pat Spier, RN-C.)

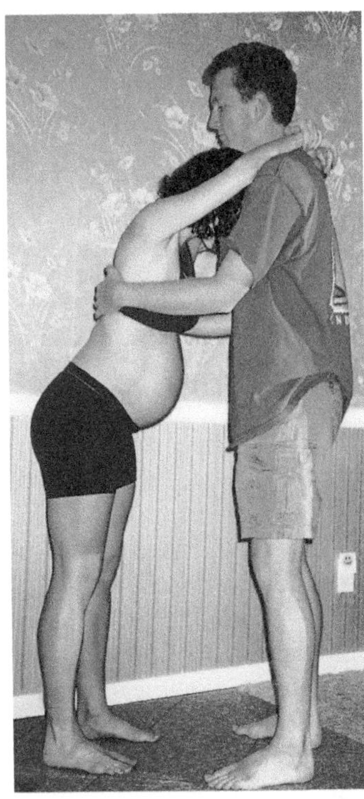

Fig. 6.22 Standing and walking during early labour and leaning on the partner during contractions use gravity to aid in fetal descent, reduce back pain, and stimulate contractions. Maintaining an upright position can shorten the first stage of labour.

inner strength and gives her courage to continue. After each vaginal examination, she is told of the progress in cervical change or fetal descent. She needs to hear praise as she successfully uses techniques to cope with labour. Her partner needs encouragement as well, because supporting a woman in labour is a demanding job. Some women may use a **doula**, a person whose only job is to support and encourage the woman in the task of giving birth (Fig. 6.21). Doulas do not perform any clinical tasks, diagnose medical conditions, offer personal opinions, or give medical advice; they provide support for women who choose a hospital or out-of-hospital birth with either a physician or a midwife (PHAC, 2018). Research on the use of doulas has shown the importance of having a nonclinical person present just to support the woman and her partner. Compared to women without doula support, women who have a doula have a higher rate of spontaneous vaginal births, shorter duration of labour, and fewer Caesarean births or instrumental vaginal births. Their use of any analgesia is less, their newborns have higher 5-minute Apgar scores, and they have more positive feelings about the childbirth experience (Bohren, Hofmeyr, Sakala, et al., 2017). Couples have stated that they feel their relationship with their partner and their baby is better because of the supportive, continuous presence of a doula (PHAC, 2018). The doula is considered a member of the healthcare team, and nurses and doulas can work alongside each other to provide the best support for the labouring family.

As a source of support and encouragement for the labouring woman and her partner, the nurse's caring presence cannot be overlooked. Just being present helps, even if no specific care is given, because they see the nurse as a support.

Supporting the Partner

Partners vary considerably in their degree of involvement during labour and how comfortable they are with that process. The labour partner is most often the infant's father but may be the woman's partner, mother, or friend. Some partners take a leading role in helping the woman cope with labour (Fig. 6.22). Others are willing to assist if they are shown how, but they will not take the initiative. Still other couples are content with the partner's encouragement and support but do not expect that person to have an active role. The partner should be permitted to provide the type of support comfortable for the couple. The nurse does not take the partner's place but remains available as needed. The partner should be encouraged to take a break and periodically eat a snack or meal. Many partners are reluctant to leave the woman's bedside, but they may faint during the birth if they have not eaten. A chair or stool near the bed allows the partner to sit down as much as possible.

 Patient Teaching

Teaching the Partner What to Expect

The partner should be taught the following:
- How labour pains affect the woman's behaviour and attitude
- How to adapt responses to the woman's behaviour
- What to expect in their own emotional responses as the woman becomes introverted or negative
- Effects of epidural analgesia

VAGINAL BIRTH AFTER CAESAREAN

Many women may be appropriate candidates for a **trial of labour after a Caesarean section (TOLAC)** and for **vaginal birth after Caesarean (VBAC)**. See Chapter 8 for more information about Caesarean births. The healthcare provider should discuss the potential benefits and risks of a TOLAC versus a repeat Caesarean section, and documentation of the counselling and plan of care should be included in the medical record.

Nursing care for women who plan to have a VBAC is similar to that for women who have had no Caesarean births. The main concern is that the uterine scar will rupture (see Chapter 8), which can disrupt the placental blood flow and cause hemorrhage. Observation for signs of uterine rupture should be part of the nursing care for all labouring women, regardless of whether they have had a previous Caesarean birth. The signs of rupture include severe pain in the lower abdomen and an abnormal FHR.

Women having a VBAC may need more support than other labouring women. They are often anxious about their ability to cope with labour's demands and to give birth vaginally, especially if they have never done so. If their Caesarean birth occurred during rather than before labour, they may become anxious when they reach the same point in the current labour. The nurse must provide empathy and support to help the woman cross this psychological barrier. However, the nurse cannot promise the woman that a repeat Caesarean birth will not be needed, because one may be required for many reasons. It is essential that an obstetrician and the surgical team be available during all stages of labour for this woman.

WATER BIRTH

Some women may choose to labour and give birth in water. These women are often cared for by a registered midwife and may give birth at a birthing centre or at home. Relaxing in a birth pool can be comforting and helpful in managing contractions. The use of water for labour pain (hydrotherapy) is discussed in Chapter 7. Presently, there are very few studies investigating the safety of water birth. There is not enough information to make conclusions about the safety of giving birth to a baby under water. Women who decide to have a water birth must ensure that the tub, hoses, and water are all very clean.

NURSING CARE DURING THE SECOND STAGE OF LABOUR

When the cervix is fully dilated, the second stage of labour begins, and the nurse teaches and supports effective pushing techniques. If the woman is pushing effectively and the fetus is tolerating labour well, the nurse should not interfere with her efforts. The woman takes a deep breath and exhales at the beginning of a contraction. She then takes another deep breath and pushes with her abdominal muscles while exhaling. Prolonged breath holding while pushing can impair fetal blood circulation (Valsalva manoeuvre). The woman should push for a maximum of 6 seconds at a time. If she is in a semi-sitting position in bed, she may find pulling back on her knees, with her hands behind her thighs, or using the handholds on the bed more comfortable.

The nurse may need to help the woman to avoid pushing before her cervix is 10 cm or fully dilated. She can be taught to blow out in short puffs when the urge to push is strong before the cervix is fully dilated. Pushing before full dilation can cause maternal exhaustion, possible swelling of the cervix, and fetal hypoxia, thus slowing labour progress rather than speeding it up.

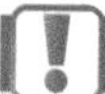 Safety Alert!

Closed glottis pushing decreases fetal oxygenation and should be avoided.

Labouring down is a term that describes an intervention during the second stage of labour that allows passive fetal decent before active pushing is encouraged, usually when an epidural is in place. Women are encouraged to rest until they have a strong urge to push. This may increase the length of the second stage of labour (Yee, Bailit, Reddy, et al., 2017).

The woman who is pushing needs to be encouraged to change position frequently if she is not making good progress. The "towel-pull" involves the woman pulling on a towel that is secured to the foot of the bed during contractions, which uses the abdominal muscles and aids in expulsion efforts.

There is no exact time when the nurse should be ready for the woman to actually give birth. In general, the woman having her first child is usually close to giving birth when about 3 to 4 cm of the fetal head is visible (**crowning**) at the vaginal opening. The multiparous woman is usually close when her cervix is fully dilated but before crowning has occurred. If the woman must be transferred to a delivery room rather than giving birth in an LBR room, she should be moved early enough to avoid a last-minute rush. The primary healthcare provider should be called at this point if not already present.

The nurse should observe the appropriate infection-control measures when caring for a woman during birth. Water-repellent gowns, eye shields, and gloves should be worn in the birthing area, and the newborn infant is handled with gloves until after the first bath.

If the woman does not have full sensation or movement of the legs because of an epidural anaesthetic, padded stirrups may be used, and the woman should be observed closely for excess pressure behind the knees, which can cause thrombophlebitis (blood clot).

A woman can give birth in many different positions. The "traditional" position—semi-sitting and using foot supports—improves access to her perineum but may not be the most comfortable for her or the best one for pushing out the infant. She may give birth in a side-lying position, squatting, standing, or in other positions.

Nursing Tip

Support the woman's partner so that they can be as helpful as possible during labour. Encourage the partner or support person to support the mother's head or leg during pushing.

EPISIOTOMY AND LACERATIONS

Episiotomy is the surgical enlargement of the vaginal opening during birth. The healthcare provider performs and repairs an episiotomy. A *laceration* is a tear of the tissues that results in a jagged wound. Lacerations of the perineum and episiotomy incisions are treated similarly.

Perineal lacerations and often episiotomies are described by the amount of tissue involved:

- *First degree:* Involves the superficial vaginal mucosa or perineal skin
- *Second degree:* Involves the vaginal mucosa, perineal skin, and deeper tissues of the perineum
- *Third degree:* Same as second degree, plus involves the anal sphincter
- *Fourth degree:* Extends through the anal sphincter into the rectal mucosa

Women with third- and fourth-degree lacerations are often prescribed stool softeners to prevent discomfort that can occur with constipation after birth. They may also require more pain-relief measures during the postpartum period.

The research does not support episiotomy being done routinely during vaginal birth but it may be used with specific indications when problems occur during the expulsion stage of labour, such as abnormal FHR (Lee et al., 2016). Perineal massage before labour may decrease the need for an episiotomy during birth.

An episiotomy is either (Fig. 6.23):

- *Midline (median),* extending directly from the lower vaginal border toward the anus, or
- *Mediolateral,* extending from the lower vaginal border toward the mother's right or left

The mediolateral incision causes greater scarring during healing and may cause painful sexual intercourse and is very rarely used. A laceration that extends a median episiotomy is more likely to involve the rectal sphincter than one that extends the mediolateral episiotomy.

The main complication from an episiotomy is postpartum pain. Women who have first- and second-degree lacerations have less pain than one who has an episiotomy. As in other incisions, infection is a risk in an episiotomy or laceration. An additional risk is extension of the episiotomy with a laceration into or through the rectal sphincter (third or fourth degree), which can cause prolonged perineal discomfort and stress incontinence.

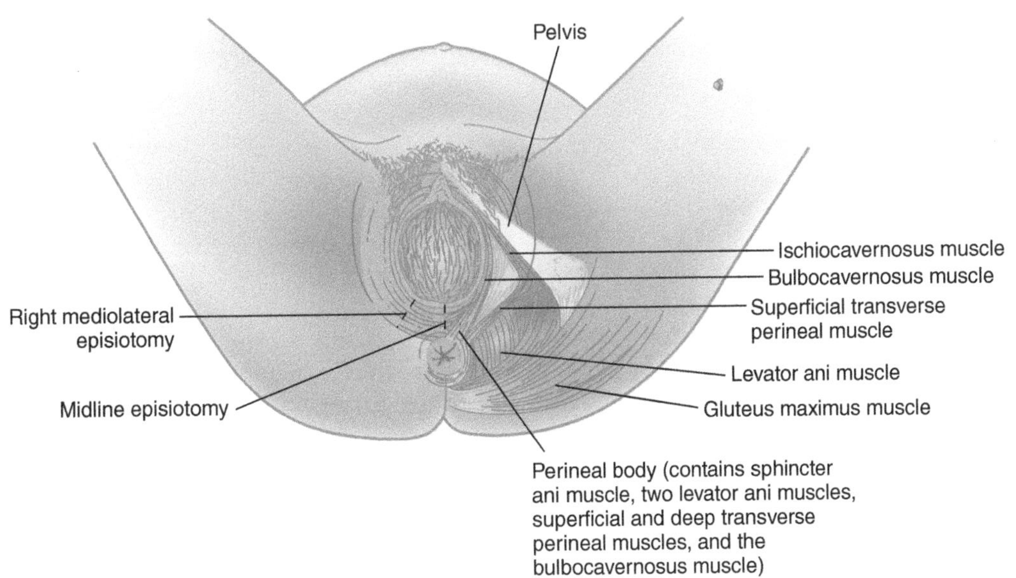

Fig. 6.23 Episiotomies. The two common types of episiotomies are midline (median) and mediolateral. (From Matteson, P. S. [2001]. *Women's health during the childbearing years: A community-based approach*. St. Louis: Mosby.)

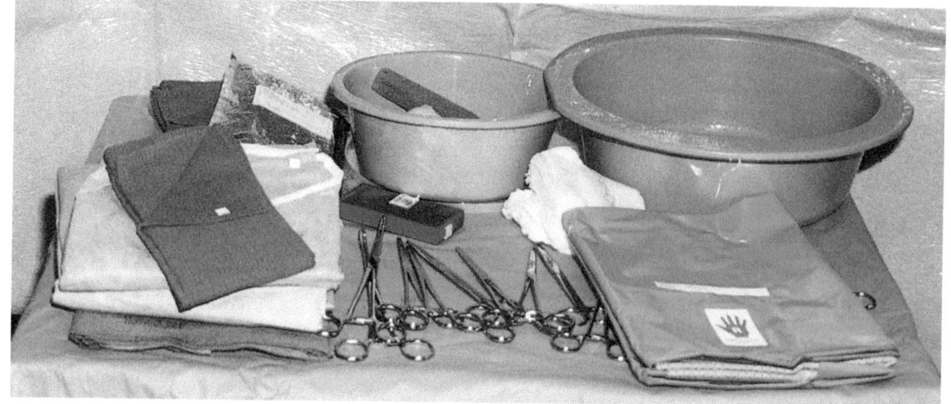

Fig. 6.24 The table contains the sterile instruments that the healthcare provider will use for the birth. The table not opened until it is ready for use in order to maintain sterility.

Table 6.6 Apgar Scoring System

SIGN	0	1	2
Heart rate	Absent	<100 beats/min	≥100 beats/min
Respiratory effort	No spontaneous respirations	Slow; weak cry	Spontaneous, with a strong, lusty cry
Muscle tone	Limp	Minimal flexion of extremities; sluggish movement	Active spontaneous motion; flexed body posture
Reflex irritability	No response to suction or stimulation	Minimal response (grimace) to stimulation	Prompt response to stimulation, with cry or active movement with a backrub
Colour	Blue or pale	Body pink, extremities blue	Completely pink (light skin) or absence of cyanosis (dark skin)

Note: The nurse evaluates each sign in the Apgar system and totals the score at 1 and 5 minutes after birth to assess the condition of the infant. A score of 8 to 10 requires no action other than continued observation and support of the infant's adaptation. A score of 4 to 7 means the infant needs gentle stimulation such as rubbing the back; the possibility of opioid-induced respiratory depression should also be considered. Scores less than 3 mean that the infant needs active resuscitation.

NURSING RESPONSIBILITIES

The nurse needs to be prepared to do the following at the birth:

- Prepare the instruments needed for the birth and infant equipment (Fig. 6.24).
- Administer medications to the mother or infant.
- Provide initial care to the infant, such as drying the skin, and placing the infant skin-to-skin with the mother or partner.
- Assess the infant's Apgar score (Table 6.6).
- Assess the infant for obvious abnormalities.
- Make a note if the infant has a stool or urinates.
- Identify the mother and infant with like-numbered identification bands (the partner or other support person usually receives a band as well).
- Promote parent–infant bonding and initial breastfeeding by encouraging parents to hold and explore the infant (observe for eye contact, fingertip or palm touch of the infant, and talking to the infant, all of which are associated with initial bonding; these observations continue throughout the postpartum period).
- Examine the placenta to be sure it is intact (Fig. 6.25). The primary healthcare provider will examine the placenta and cord for any abnormalities. These may be correlated with fetal anomalies.
- The obstetrical healthcare provider will examine the maternal perineum for lacerations or bleeding.

Fig. 6.26 shows the entire process of an infant being born in the vertex presentation in a spontaneous vaginal birth.

NURSING CARE IMMEDIATELY AFTER BIRTH

THE THIRD AND FOURTH STAGES OF LABOUR

The third stage of labour is the expulsion of the placenta. The nurse examines the placenta and monitors the woman's vital signs (see Table 6.2). The fourth stage of labour is the first 1 to 2 hours after birth when the mother and newborn become physiologically stable. Nursing care during the fourth stage of labour includes the following general care:

- Identifying and preventing hemorrhage
- Administering oxytocin as needed to contract the uterus
- Evaluating and intervening for pain
- Observing bladder function and urine output
- Evaluating recovery from anaesthesia
- Initiating skin-to-skin contact and breastfeeding
- Providing initial care to the newborn infant

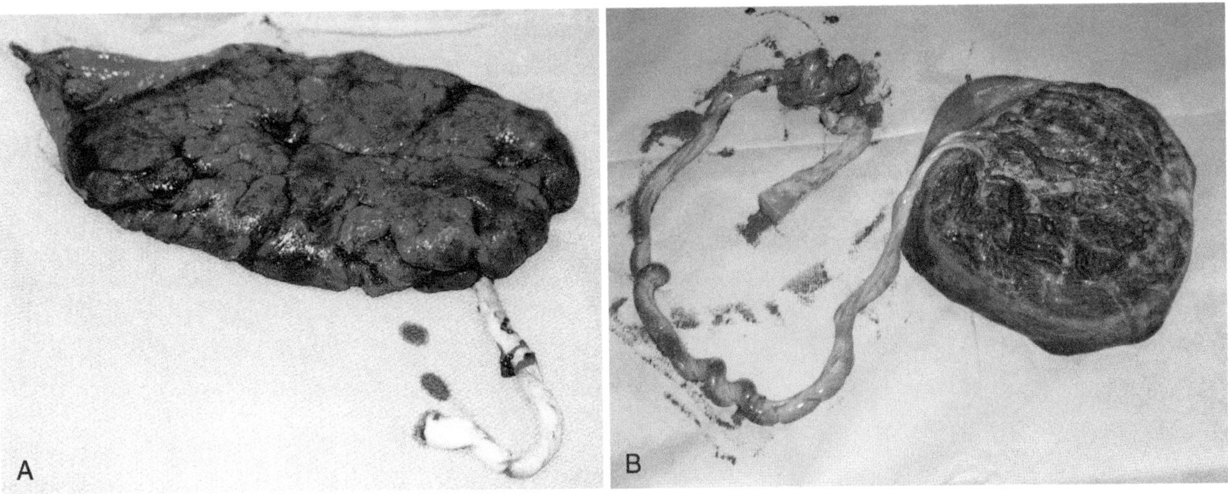

Fig. 6.25 The placenta after delivery. **A,** Duncan's delivery: The maternal side of the placenta, which is dull and rough, is delivered first. **B,** Schultze delivery: The fetal side of the placenta, which is shiny and smooth, is delivered first. (Courtesy Pat Spier, RN-C.)

- Promoting bonding and attachment between the infant and family

CARE OF THE MOTHER

Facility protocols will vary, but a common schedule for assessing the mother during the fourth stage is every 15 minutes for 1 hour, every 30 minutes during the second hour, and hourly until transfer to the postpartum unit. After transfer to the postpartum unit, applicable routine assessments are made every 4 to 8 hours. The following should be included at each maternal assessment during the fourth stage:

- Vital signs (temperature may be taken hourly if normal)
- Skin colour
- Location and firmness of the uterine fundus (see Chapter 9)
- Amount and colour of lochia (see Chapter 9)
- Presence and location of pain
- IV infusion and medications
- Fullness of the bladder or urine output from a catheter
- Condition of the perineum for vaginal birth
- Condition of dressing for Caesarean birth
- Level of sensation and ability to move lower extremities if an epidural or spinal block was used

Observing for Hemorrhage

The uterine fundus is assessed for firmness, height in relation to the umbilicus, and position (midline or deviated to one side). Refer to Chapter 9 for assessment of the fundus. Vaginal bleeding should be dark red (lochia rubra). No more than one pad should be saturated in an hour, and the woman should not pass large clots. A continuous trickle of bright red blood suggests a bleeding laceration. The blood pressure, pulse rate, and respirations are checked to identify a rising pulse rate or falling blood pressure, which suggests shock (see Chapter 10 for further discussion). An oral temperature is taken and reported if it is 38°C (100.4°F) or higher or if the woman has a higher risk for infection.

Observing for Bladder Distention

The bladder is assessed for distention, which may occur soon after birth. The woman may not feel the urge to urinate because of the effects of the anaesthetic, perineal trauma, and loss of fetal pressure against the bladder. If her bladder is full, the uterus will be higher than expected and often displaced to one side. A full bladder inhibits uterine contraction and can lead to hemorrhage. Catheterization may be needed if the woman cannot urinate.

Promoting Comfort

Many women have a shaking chill after birth yet deny that they are cold. A warm blanket over the woman can make her feel more comfortable until the chill subsides. The warm blanket also maintains the infant's warmth while parents get acquainted.

Nursing care for an episiotomy or laceration begins during the fourth stage of labour. Cold packs should be applied to the perineum for the first 24 hours to reduce pain, bruising, and edema. After 24 hours of cold applications, warmth in the form of heat packs or sitz baths increases blood circulation, enhancing comfort and healing. Mild oral analgesics are usually sufficient for pain management. See Chapter 9 for postpartum nursing care of the woman with an episiotomy or laceration.

The infant stays with the mother or parents during recovery if there were no complications.

CARE OF THE NEWBORN IMMEDIATELY AFTER BIRTH

The priority care of the newborn involves promoting respiratory function and maintaining the temperature.

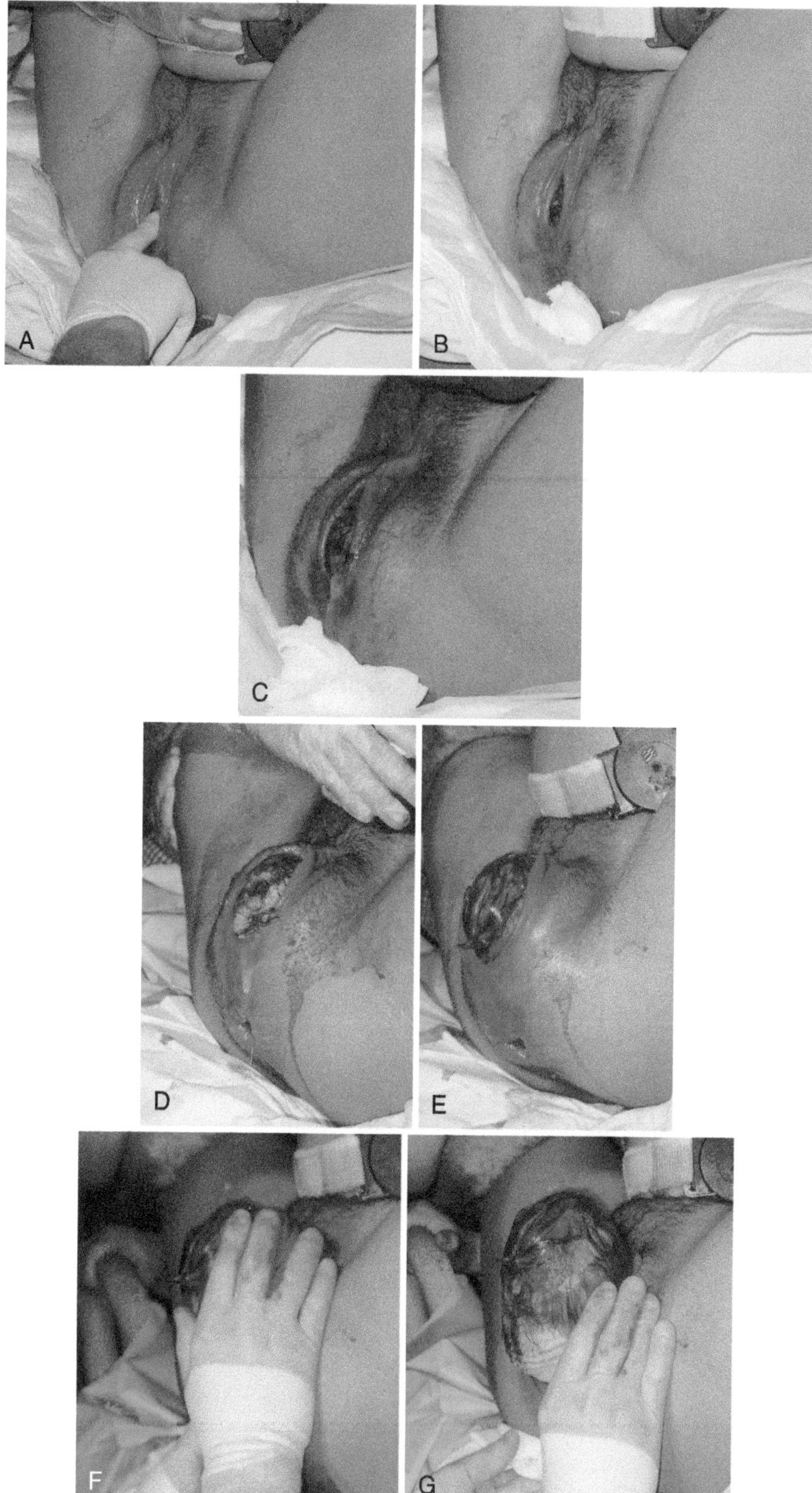

Fig. 6.26 Vaginal birth of a fetus in vertex presentation. **A,** The healthcare provider palpates the fontanelle of the fetus to confirm the position of the head. **B,** A portion of the fetal head is visible during a contraction. This is called *crowning*. **C,** The perineum bulges, and more of the fetal head is visible as the woman bears down. Amniotic fluid drips from the vaginal orifice. **D,** The perineum has been cleansed with an antimicrobial solution as the fetal head begins extension. Note the distention of the perineum and anus. **E,** The head is about to be born through the process of extension. Note the thinning, redness, and distention of the perineal area. **F,** The healthcare provider supports the perineum as the head emerges. **G,** The healthcare provider checks for cord around the neck.

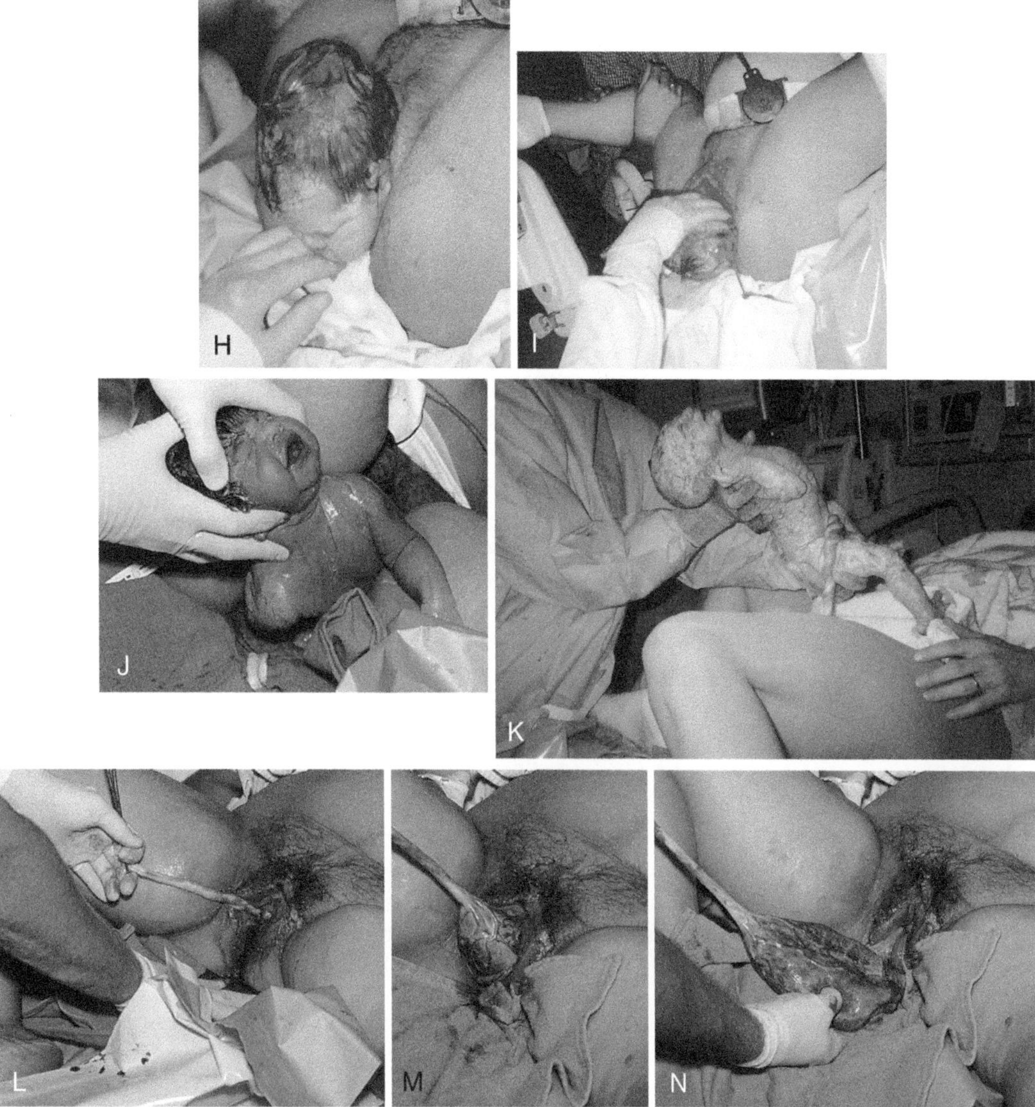

Fig. 6.26, cont'd **H,** The perineum is covered as the head is born. **I,** The healthcare provider exerts gentle pressure on the head to release the anterior shoulder from under the symphysis pubis. **J,** The posterior shoulder and chest are delivered. **K,** The newborn infant, covered with thick white vernix, is lifted onto the abdomen of the mother, where his cord is cut after a 60-second delay. **L–N,** Delivery of placenta. (**A** to **I** courtesy Pat Spier, RN-C; **J, L, M,** and **N** courtesy Michael S. Clement, MD, Mesa, AZ. In Lowdermilk, D. L., Perry, S. E., Cashion, M. C., & Alden, K. R. [2016]. *Maternity and women's health care* [11th ed.]. St. Louis: Mosby.)

See Chapter 11 for care of the newborn. Initial care of the newborn includes the following:

- Maintaining cardiorespiratory function
- Maintaining thermoregulation
- Encouraging bonding and breastfeeding
- Observing and documenting for urination and passage of meconium
- Identifying the mother, the father or partner, and the newborn
- Performing and documenting a brief assessment for major anomalies
- Administering medications

The infant will be covered in blood, vernix, and amniotic fluid at birth. All caregivers should wear gloves when handling the newborn until after the first bath to protect themselves from body fluids. The first hour after birth is critical and sometimes called the *golden hour*. Important aspects of care during the first hour after birth include delayed cord clamping, skin-to-skin contact for at least an hour or until the newborn breastfeeds, performance of newborn assessments on the maternal abdomen, delaying nonurgent tasks (e.g., weighing the newborn) for at least 60 minutes, and early initiation of breastfeeding. Care provided during the golden hour contributes to improved neonatal thermoregulation, decreased stress levels in a woman and her newborn, and improved mother–newborn bonding. Implementation of these actions is further associated with increased rates and duration of breastfeeding (Neczypor & Holley, 2017).

Delayed cord clamping for 1 to 3 minutes has some advantages for the healthy term infant, such as higher

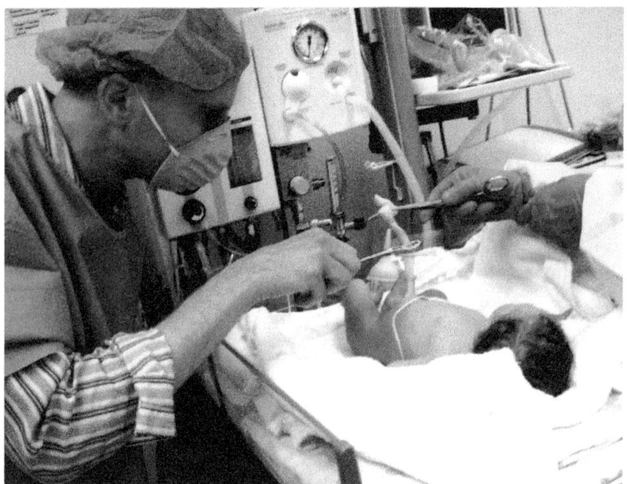

Fig. 6.27 The nurse assists the father in cutting the umbilical cord to a proper length after the umbilical clamp has been applied.

birth weight, early hemoglobin concentration, and increased iron reserves up to 6 months after birth. These need to be balanced against a small, additional risk of jaundice in newborns that requires phototherapy (Garofalo & Abenhaim, 2012; McDonald, Middleton, Dowswell, et al., 2013).

Performing Apgar Scoring

Dr. Virginia Apgar devised a system for evaluating the infant's condition and response to resuscitation that is provided at birth (see Table 6.6). Five factors are evaluated at 1 minute and 5 minutes after birth:

1. Heart rate
2. Respiratory effort
3. Muscle tone
4. Reflex response to suction or gentle stimulation
5. Skin colour

The Apgar score is not a predictor of future intelligence or abilities and disabilities. It was meant to identify only the infant's condition and how the newborn is adapting to the extrauterine environment. Equipment, medications, and personnel must be readily available for resuscitation at any birth, because the need cannot always be anticipated. If the Apgar score is not 7 or more at 5 minutes, the score will be repeated at 10 minutes.

Maintaining Cardiorespiratory Function

Physiological changes in the cardiopulmonary circulation in the newborn are discussed in Chapter 11. Respiratory support immediately after birth includes the following:

- The face, nose, and mouth are gently wiped to remove mucus and excess amniotic fluid.
- A cord clamp is applied by the healthcare provider in the first 1 to 3 minutes after birth (Fig. 6.27).
- At birth, if the infant is stable, it should be placed on the mother's chest.

Spontaneous breathing usually begins within a few seconds after birth. The infant's colour at birth may be cyanotic (blue) but quickly turns pink (often except for the hands and feet). As the infant cries, the skin colour will be pink. **Acrocyanosis** is the bluish colour of hands and feet of the newborn that is normal and is caused by sluggish peripheral circulation.

Some signs of respiratory distress that require administration of oxygen via face mask and that should be immediately reported include the following:

- Persistent cyanosis (other than the hands and feet)
- Grunting respirations: a noise heard without a stethoscope as the infant exhales
- Flaring of the nostrils
- Retractions (indrawing): under the sternum or between the ribs
- Sustained respiratory rate higher than 60 breaths/min
- Sustained heart rate greater than 160 beats/min or less than 110 beats/min

Maintaining Thermoregulation

A critical factor in the transition of the newborn is maintaining a **neutral thermal environment** in which heat loss is minimal and oxygen consumption needs are lowest. *Hypothermia* (low body temperature) can cause *hypoglycemia* (low blood glucose level), because the infant's body uses glucose to generate heat. Hypoglycemia is associated with the development of neurological problems in the newborn. Hypothermia can also cause **cold stress**, in which the increased metabolic rate required to generate body heat causes increased respiratory rate and oxygen consumption. If the infant cannot supply the increased demand for oxygen, hypoxia will result and cause further problems.

Essential nursing interventions to maintain a neutral thermal environment include the following:

- *Drying the infant* with a towel prevents heat loss caused by evaporation of amniotic fluid on the skin.
- *Placing the infant skin-to-skin with the mother (or partner)* (see Skill 12.2) or breastfeeding can also prevent heat loss.
- *Placing a hat on the infant's head* after the head is dried. The head is the largest body surface area in the newborn, and significant heat loss can occur if the moist head is left open to room air.
- *Wrapping the infant* in warm blankets if the mother or partner is unable to place the infant skin-to-skin.

If the infant is unable to stabilize body temperature the best place for it to be is skin-to-skin with the mother. The first bath is delayed a minimum of 8 to 12 hours and until the infant's temperature is stabilized at 36.5°C to 37°C. The WHO recommends delaying the first bath until after 24 hours (WHO, 2015).

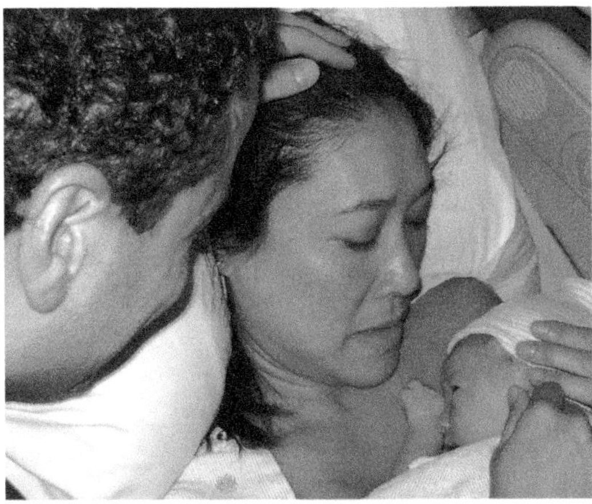

Fig. 6.28 The mother and father bond with the newborn infant in the labour, birth, and recovery room.

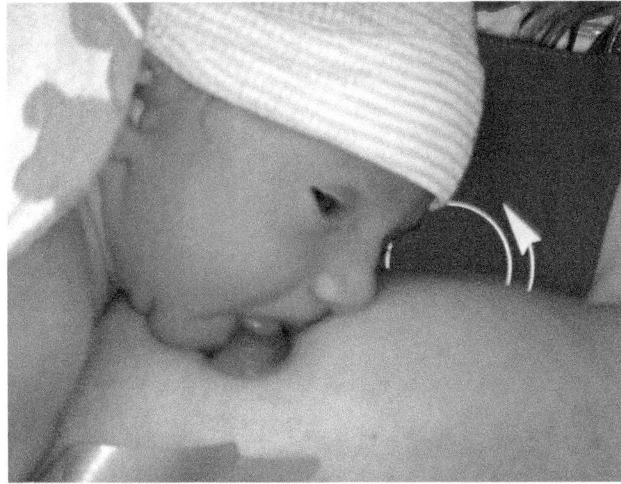

Fig. 6.29 The naked infant placed on the bare chest of the mother will move toward the breast and breastfeed. Studies show this is beneficial to infant neurodevelopment and behaviour and parent–infant bonding as well as improved breastfeeding success. (From Leifer, G. [2012]. *Maternity nursing* [11th ed.]. St. Louis: Saunders.)

Promoting Maternal–Infant Bonding and Initiating Breastfeeding

Every attempt should be made to facilitate maternal–infant contact. As long as the infant is stable, the newborn should be placed skin-to-skin with the mother or partner (Fig. 6.28). The infant is alert in the first hour of life; therefore, this is the best time to initiate breastfeeding and bonding.

One of the focuses of the Baby-Friendly Initiative (BFI) is promotion of early and uninterrupted skin-to-skin contact between a mother and infant as soon as possible after birth and initiation of breastfeeding within the first hour (Fig. 6.29). Skin-to-skin contact between mother and infant shortly after birth helps to initiate early breastfeeding and increases the likelihood of exclusive breastfeeding for the first 1 to 4 months of life as well as the overall duration of breastfeeding. Infants placed in early skin-to-skin contact with their mother also appear to interact more with their mothers and cry less (WHO, 2017). The Baby-Friendly Initiative and breastfeeding are discussed in Chapter 9.

Identifying the Infant

Wristbands with preprinted numbers are placed on the mother, the infant, and often the partner or other support person in the birthing room as the primary means of identifying the infant. The nurse should check to be sure that all numbers in the set are identical. Other identifying information is completed, such as mother's name, the birth attendant's name, the date and time of birth, the sex of the infant, and usually the mother's hospital identification number. The bands are applied relatively snugly on the infant's wrist and ankle with only a finger's width of slack, because infants lose weight after birth.

The nurse must check the preprinted identification band numbers to see that they match every time an infant newborn assessment is done. The nurse should either look at the numbers to see that they are identical or have the mother read her own band number while looking at the infant's band. Often, the identification band is embedded with a security chip compatible with the hospital's security system or another security band is placed on the infant.

Observing Urinary Function and Passage of Meconium

Newborns may not urinate for as long as 24 hours after birth. If the infant voids in the LBR room, it must be documented on the chart. Meconium, the first stool of the newborn, should be passed before 24 hours and occasionally occurs during labour. Whenever meconium is passed it should also be documented in the chart. Passing meconium and voiding help determine the status of the gastrointestinal and genitourinary systems.

Administering Medication

Eye care

Most provinces have legislation requiring that all newborn infants receive erythromycin eye ointment to prevent ophthalmia neonatorum, which is caused by *Neisseria gonorrhoeae* or *Chlamydia trachomatis.* The recent statement from the Canadian Paediatric Society (CPS) does not support the administration of erythromycin eye ointment, owing to the lack of research to support its use (Moore, MacDonald, & CPS Infectious Diseases and Immunization Committee, 2015), although it presently is still used in most provinces and territories. Ontario has recently changed the legislation regarding mandatory prophylactic eye treatment and allows parents to opt out of the treatment if a written request is made to their healthcare provider and if the parents

Skill 6.5 Administering Eye Ointment to the Newborn

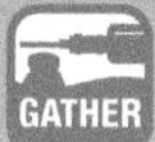

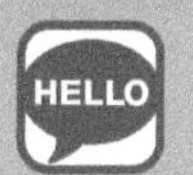

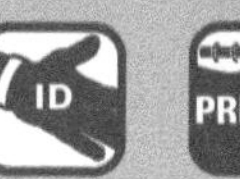

PRIVACY
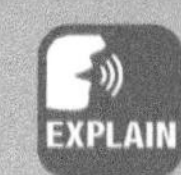

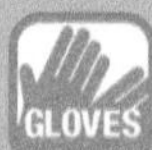

PURPOSE

To protect against ophthalmia neonatorum in the newborn

STEP

1. Apply an antimicrobial ointment to the lower conjunctival sac of the newborn's eyes.

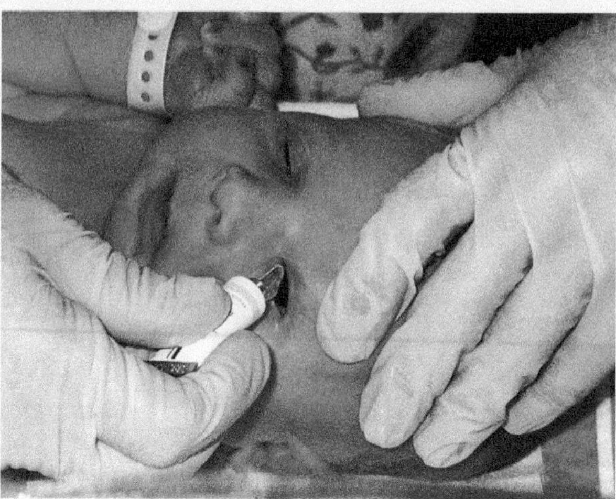

Photo courtesy Pat Spier, RN-C.

have made an informed decision and the newborn is not at risk for ophthalmia neonatorum (Ontario Ministry of Health and Long-Term Care, 2018). If parents in other provinces or territories refuse this medication for their child, protocols must be in place in institutions on how to proceed in this situation. Eye care is administered from a single-dose tube within 2 hours after birth (so that the infant and mother can bond in that first hour) (Skill 6.5).

Vitamin K (AquaMEPHYTON)

Newborns need vitamin K to assist in blood clotting. Vitamin K is naturally produced from intestinal flora, which is absent in the newborn. One single dose of vitamin K is injected into the vastus lateralis muscle (thigh) intramuscularly within 6 hours after birth (Skill 6.6). Vitamin K can be administered orally if the parents refuse an intramuscular injection for their newborn. This method of administration requires follow-up as more than one dose is required. It is not a common method of administering Vitamin K.

A detailed assessment for anomalies and gestational age is completed either in the labour room or on admission to the maternal–child unit. See discussion in Chapter 11.

CORD BLOOD BANKING

Blood from the placenta and umbilical cord had traditionally been treated as a waste product and discarded. However, cord blood, like bone marrow, contains regenerative stem cells that can be stored and used for transplant to replace diseased cells or to treat many malignant or genetic diseases in children and adults; these cells are less likely to cause a potentially fatal rejection response. Cord blood contains hematopoietic stem cells that have a distinct advantage over bone marrow or peripheral stem cells for use in treatment of multiple diseases such as immune, genetic, or neurological disorders (Armson, Allan, & Casper, 2015). Private and public cord blood banks have been established in Canada. Private blood banks serve the needs of one family, for a collection and maintenance fee. Public cord blood banks are free to donors and are run by the Canadian Blood Services, although not all hospitals have access to this service. Public banks can be used by anyone who needs stem cell treatment.

The cord blood is collected immediately after the birth of the infant and after the cord has been clamped and cut. The healthcare provider or nurse usually performs collection with appropriate equipment to prevent contamination, and the cord blood bank is notified in advance. The collection of umbilical cord blood must not adversely affect the health of the mother or newborn and should not interfere with delayed cord clamping (Armson et al., 2015). Healthcare providers should inform pregnant women and their partners of the benefits of delayed cord clamping and of its impact on cord blood collection and banking (Armson et al., 2015).

The blood must be transported within 48 hours of collection for cryopreservation. The registry provides the parents with containers for storage of the cord blood until it is picked up by the registry.

Skill 6.6 Administering Intramuscular Injections to the Newborn

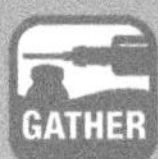

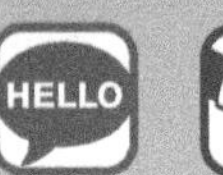

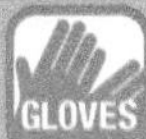

PURPOSE

To administer an intramuscular injection to the newborn effectively

STEPS

1. Prepare medication for injection.
   a. A 1-mL syringe with a 1.5 cm, 25-gauge needle is often used. A small needle reaches the muscle but potentially prevents striking the bone.
2. Put on gloves to protect against contamination with blood.
3. Locate the correct site. The middle third of the vastus lateralis muscle is the preferred site (see illustration).

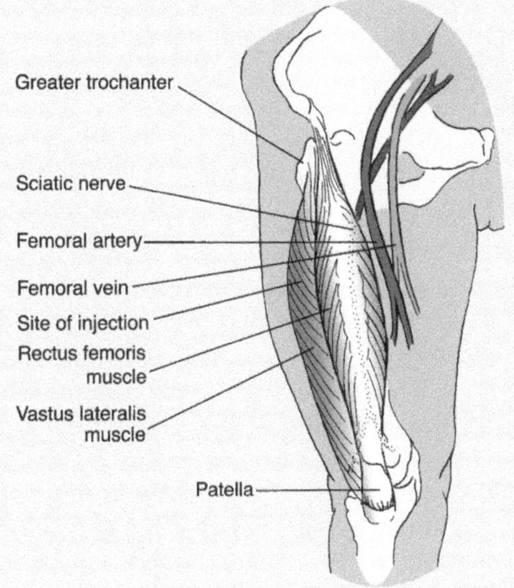

4. Cleanse area with an alcohol wipe.
5. Stabilize leg while holding tissues (upper thigh) between thumb and fingers to prevent sudden movement by the newborn and possible injury. (NOTE: When an injection is administered to the newborn the infant should be held skin-to-skin, breastfed, or given a sucrose solution as pain management strategies.)
6. Insert needle at a 90-degree angle to the thigh.
7. Do not aspirate, and inject rapidly.
8. Remove needle quickly and gently massage site. Massage helps the body absorb medication.
9. Calm and soothe the infant; reposition infant. Remove gloves, perform hand hygiene, and document administration in medical record.

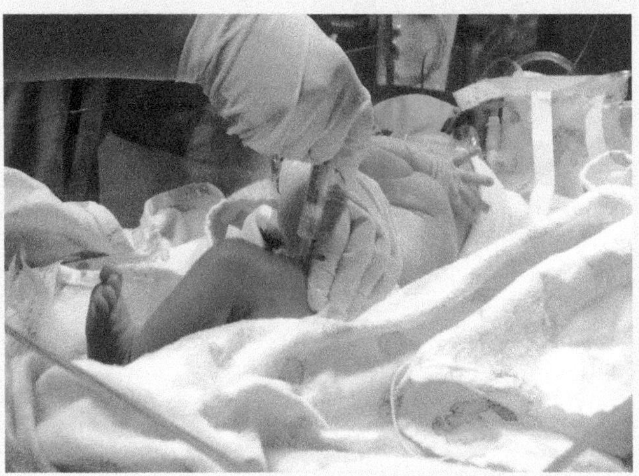

MICROBIOMES AND NURSING CARE DURING LABOUR AND BIRTH

Microbiata are a community of microorganisms, both pathogenic and nonpathogenic, that are in every human body. **Microbiomes** contain the genetic material of a variety of the organisms consisting of bacteria, fungi, and single-cell organisms (archaea) that live in every human body and have an influence on health and disease. The introduction of microbiomes to the newborn infant occurs at birth when the mother transfers these microbiomes to the infant, either by mouth or vaginal contact. The transfer of these microbiomes to the infant plays an important role in the future health of the infant (Dunn, Jordan, Bakar, et al., 2017).

Labour and birth practices can enhance or interfere with this transfer. For example, vaginal birth enhances the transfer of the microbiome, and frequent vaginal examinations or antibiotic administration can interfere with successful transfer of microbiomes. Infants born via Caesarean are not exposed to vaginal microbiota and may be at risk for health problems in later life.

The nurse plays an important role in the care of mothers during labour and birth to promote successful transfer of maternal–newborn microbiomes by supporting vaginal birth and promoting early skin-to-skin contact and breastfeeding in the first hours after birth and beyond (Mutic, Jordan, Edwards, et al., 2017).

Unfolding Case Study

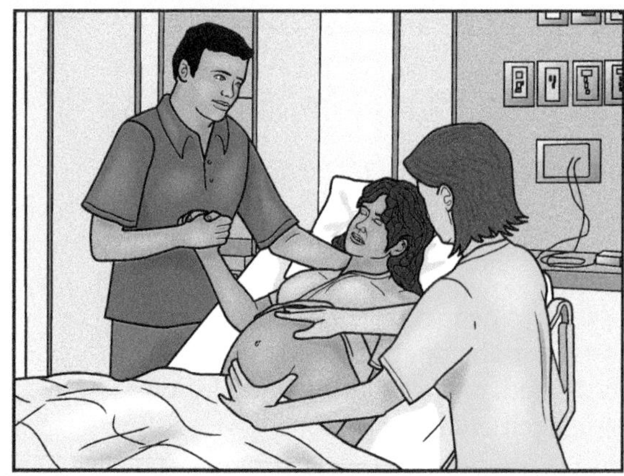

Tess was a patient in the prenatal clinic in Chapter 4 and was followed through Chapter 5 where she came to the clinic with specific concerns. The remainder of her pregnancy was without incident.

Tess is admitted to the obstetrical unit in her fortieth week of pregnancy, stating she has frequent contractions. She states that she felt a sudden gush of fluid from her vagina.

QUESTIONS

1. What is the probable cause of the gush of fluid that she expelled? What is the nursing responsibility when this happens to a woman during pregnancy?
2. What findings would indicate that Tess is close to giving birth to her infant?
3. The nurse performs the Leopold manoeuvre. What information can be obtained through this procedure?
4. The nurse auscultates the fetal heart. What kind of variations of the FHR are normal, and what findings should immediately be reported to the health care provider?
5. If late decelerations of the fetal heart are noted, what nursing action is indicated?
6. Tess's partner, Luis, is standing in the corner of the labour room. How can the nurse offer support to Luis during the labour process?

Get Ready for the Certification Examination!

Key Points

- The five components, or "five *P*s," of the birth process are the **p**owers, the **p**assage, the **p**assenger, maternal **p**osition, and the **p**syche. All interrelate during labour to either facilitate or impede birth.
- True labour and prelabour have several differences; however, the conclusive difference is that true labour results in cervical change (effacement or dilation).
- The woman should go to the hospital if she is having persistent, regular contractions (every 4–5 minutes for nulliparas, and every 5–7 minutes for multiparas); if her membranes rupture; if she has bleeding other than normal bloody show; if fetal movement decreases; or for other concerns not covered by the basic guidelines.
- Three key assessments on admission are fetal condition, maternal condition, and nearness to birth.
- There are four stages of labour, and each stage includes different characteristics. The first stage is dilation, lasting from labour's onset to full (10 cm) cervical dilation. The first stage of labour is subdivided into two phases: latent (early) and active. Second-stage labour, the stage of expulsion, extends from full cervical dilation until birth of the infant. The third stage, the placental stage, is from the birth of the infant until the placenta is delivered. The fourth stage is the immediate postbirth recovery period and includes the first 1 to 2 hours after birth.
- Nursing care during the first and second stages focuses on observing the fetal and maternal conditions and on helping the woman to cope with labour.
- Intermittent auscultation is the recommended method of fetal monitoring for low-risk healthy women. Continuous electronic fetal monitoring is used for women who have increased risk for adverse perinatal outcomes.
- The normal baseline fetal heart rate (FHR) should be between 110 and 160 beats/min.
- An FHR tracing demonstrates the relationship between the baseline FHR and uterine contractions.
- The presence of accelerations and moderate variability in the FHR pattern reassures that the fetus is well oxygenated.
- Abnormal FHR patterns require specific interventions to try to reverse the FHR pattern. If the pattern cannot be changed, the healthcare provider must be notified.
- Labouring women can assume many positions. Upright positions add gravity to the forces promoting fetal descent. Hands-and-knees and leaning-forward positions promote normal internal rotation of the fetus if "back labour" is a problem. Squatting facilitates fetal descent during the second stage. The supine position should be discouraged because it causes the heavy uterus to compress the mother's main blood vessels, which can reduce fetal oxygen supply.
- The main fetal risk during first- and second-stage labour is fetal compromise caused by interruption to the fetal oxygen supply. The main maternal risk during fourth-stage labour is hemorrhage caused by uterine relaxation.
- Nursing care after episiotomy or perineal lacerations includes comfort measures such as cold applications, analgesics, and wound assessment.
- The immediate care of the newborn after birth includes maintaining warmth, maintaining cardiorespiratory function, maintaining skin-to-skin contact, assessing for major anomalies, encouraging parent–infant bonding and breastfeeding, and providing proper identification and documentation.

Additional Learning Resources

evolve Go to your Evolve website (http://evolve.elsevier.com/Canada/Leifer) for the following learning resources:

- Answer Key for Critical Thinking Questions
- Answer Key for Textbook Review Questions
- Audio Glossary
- Fluids & Electrolytes tutorial
- Interactive Review Questions
- Skills Performance Checklists
- Video clips and more!

Online Resources

- Coping with labour: https://www.lamaze.org
- Society of Obstetricians and Gynaecologists of Canada, *Birth plan template:* https://www.pregnancyinfo.ca/your-pregnancy/preparing-for-birth/birth-plan/
- World Health Organization, *Intrapartum Care for a Positive Childbirth Experience:* https://www.youtube.com/watch?v=lPYnPKaqyt4

Review Questions

1. To determine the frequency of uterine contractions, the nurse should note the time from the:
   a. beginning to end of the same contraction.
   b. end of one contraction to the beginning of the next contraction.
   c. beginning of one contraction to the beginning of the next contraction.
   d. contraction's peak until the contraction begins to relax.
2. Excessive anxiety and fear during labour may result in which of the following?
   a. An ineffective labour pattern
   b. An abnormal fetal presentation or position
   c. The release of oxytocin from the pituitary gland
   d. A rapid labour and uncontrolled birth
3. A woman who is pregnant with her first child phones the labour unit and says her "water broke." What should a nurse tell the woman to do?
   a. Wait until she has contractions every 5 minutes for 1 hour.
   b. Take her temperature every 4 hours and come to the hospital if it is over 38°C (100.4°F).
   c. Come to the hospital for assessment.
   d. Call an ambulance to bring her to the hospital.
4. A labouring woman suddenly begins making grunting sounds and bearing down during a strong contraction. What is the nursing prioritiy?
   a. Leave the room to find an experienced nurse to assess the woman.
   b. Look at her perineum for increased bloody show or perineal bulging.
   c. Ask her if she needs pain medication.
   d. Tell her that these are common sensations in late labour.
5. A woman in active labour has contractions every 3 minutes lasting 60 seconds, and her uterus relaxes between contractions. The electronic fetal monitor shows the fetal heart rate to reach 90 beats/min for periods lasting 20 seconds during a uterine contraction. What is the priority nursing action?
   a. continue to monitor closely.
   b. administer oxygen by mask at 10 L/min.
   c. notify the health care provider.
   d. prepare for a Caesarean section.
6. The nurse is caring for a woman in labour. Which of the following observations require immediate nursing intervention? *(Select all that apply).*
   a. Fetal heart rate of 90 beats/min between contractions
   b. Maternal tachysystole with fetal heart rate changes
   c. Contractions lasting 60 seconds with a resting period of 90 seconds
   d. Moderate variability in fetal heart rate

Critical Thinking Question

1. A $G_1T_0P_0A_0L_0$ woman is admitted to the hospital in active labour. She states that she has completed prenatal care and wishes for a natural, unmedicated childbirth. However, she states she now does not feel she can cope with the increasing levels of pain and asks if it is okay if she takes pain medication. What is the best response of the nurse?

REFERENCES

Armson, A., Allan, D., & Casper, R. (2015). SOGC clinical practice guideline: Umbilical cord blood: Counselling, collection and banking. *Journal of Obstetricians & Gynaecologists of Canada, 37*(9), 832–844.

Bohren, M. A., Hofmeyr, G. J., Sakala, C., et al. (2017). Continuous support for women during childbirth. *Cochrane Database of Systematic Reviews,* (7), CD003766. https://doi.org/10.1002/14651858.CD003766.pub6.

Dunn, A., Jordan, S., Bakar, B., et al. (2017). The maternal infant microbiome: Considerations for labor and birth. *MCN: American Journal of Maternal/Child Nursing, 42*(6), 318.

Garofalo, M., & Abenhaim, H. A. (2012). Early versus delayed cord clamping in term and preterm births: A review. *Journal of Obstetrics & Gynaecology Canada, 34*(6), 525–531.

Hutton, E., Cappelletti, A., Reitsma, A., et al. (2015). Outcomes associated with planned place of birth among women with low-risk pregnancies. *Canadian Medical Association Journal, 190*(2), 1–11.

Kotaska, A., Menticoglou, S., Gagnon, R., et al. (2009). Vaginal delivery of breech presentation. *Journal of Obstetrics and Gynaecology Canada, 31*(6), 557–566.

Lee, L., Dy, J., Azzam, H., et al. (2016). SOGC clinical practice guideline: Management of spontaneous labour at term in healthy women. *Journal of Obstetrics and Gynaecology Canada, 38*(9), 843–865.

Liston, R., Sawchuck, D., Young, D., et al. (2018). No. 197b fetal health surveillance: Intrapartum consensus guideline. *Journal of Obstetrics and Gynaecology Canada, 40*(4), e298–e322.

McDonald, S. J., Middleton, P., Dowswell, T., et al. (2013). Effect of timing of umbilical cord clamping of term infants on maternal and neonatal outcomes. *Cochrane Database of Systematic Reviews* (7), CD004074. https://doi.org/10.1002/14651858.CD004074.pub3.

Miller, L., Miller, D., & Tucker, S. M. (2013). *Mosby's pocket guide to fetal monitoring: A multidisciplinary approach* (7th ed.). St. Louis: Mosby.

Moore, D. S., MacDonald, N., & Canadian Paediatric Society (CPS), Infectious Diseases and Immunization Committee. (2015). Preventing ophthalmia neonatorum. *Paediatrics & Child Health, 20*(2), 93–96.

Mutic, A., Jordan, A., Edwards, S., et al. (2017). The postpartum maternal and newborn microbiomes. *MCN American Journal of Maternal/Child Nursing, 42*(6), 326–331.

Neczypor, J. L., & Holley, S. (2017). Providing evidence-based care during the golden hour. *Nursing for Women's Health, 21*(6), 462–472.

Ontario Ministry of Health and Long-Term Care. (2018). *Health Protection and Promotion Act: Regulation 557 Communicable Diseases—General.* Retrieved from: http://www.health.gov.on.ca/en/common/legislation/opth_neo/default.aspx.

Perron, L., Synikas, V., Burnett, M., et al. (2013). SOGC clinical practice guideline: Female genital cutting. *Journal of Obstetrics and Gynaecology Canada, 35*(11), e1–e18.

Public Health Agency of Canada (PHAC). (2018). Care during labour and birth. In *Family-centred maternity and newborn care: National guidelines.* Retrieved from: https://www.canada.ca/en/public-health/services/publications/healthy-living/maternity-newborn-care-guidelines-chapter-4.html.

Rivard, L., & Morin, F. (2017). Fetal health surveillance during labour. In S. Perry, M. Hockenberry, J. Lowdermilk, et al. (Eds.), *Maternal child nursing care in Canada* (2nd ed.). Toronto, ON: Elsevier.

Scamell, M., & Ghumman, A. (2019). The experience of maternity care for migrant women living with female genital mutilation: A qualitative synthesis. *Birth: Issues in Perinatal Care, 46*(1), 15–23.

Selby, C., Valencia, S., Garcia, L., et al. (2012). Activity level during one hour labor check evaluation: Walking vs bed rest. *MCN American Journal of Maternal/Child Nursing, 37*(2), 101–107.

Society of Obstetricians and Gynaecologists of Canada (SOGC). (2009). Policy statement on midwifery. *Journal of Obstetrics and Gynaecology Canada, 31*(7), 662.

Wolfe-Roubatis, E., & Spatz, D. L. (2015). Transgender men and lactation: What nurses need to know. *MCN American Journal of Maternal/Child Nursing, 40*(1), 32–38.

World Health Organization (WHO). (2014). *Fact sheet: Female genital mutilation.* Retrieved from: http://www.who.int/mediacentre/factsheets/fs241/en/.

World Health Organization. (2015). *Postnatal care for mothers and newborns: Highlights from the World Health Organization 2013 guidelines.* Retrieved from: http://www.who.int/maternal_child_adolescent/publications/WHO-MCA-PNC-2014-Briefer_A4.pdf?ua=1.

World Health Organization (WHO). (2017). *Early initiation of breastfeeding to promote exclusive breastfeeding.* Retrieved from: http://www.who.int/elena/titles/early_breastfeeding/en/.

World Health Organization. (2019). *Individualized, supportive care key to positive childbirth experience.* Retrieved from: http://www.who.int/news-room/detail/15-02-2018-individualized-supportive-care-key-to-positive-childbirth-experience-says-who.

Yee, L., Bailit, J., Reddy, U., et al. (2017). Maternal and neonatal outcomes with early compared to delayed pushing among nulliparous women. *OBGYN, 128*(5), 1039–1047.

Pain Management During Labour and Birth

7

Melanie Basso

http://evolve.elsevier.com/Canada/Leifer

Objectives

1. Define each key term listed.
2. List the common types of classes offered to childbearing families.
3. Describe the methods of childbirth preparation.
4. Describe factors that influence a woman's comfort during labour.
5. Discuss the advantages and limitations of nonpharmacological methods of pain management during labour.
6. Explain nonpharmacological methods of pain management for labour, including the nursing role for each.
7. Discuss the advantages and limitations of pharmacological methods of pain management.
8. Explain each type of pharmacological pain management, including the nursing role for each.

Key Terms

Bradley method
cleansing breath
effleurage (ĕf-loo-RĂHZH)
endorphins (ĕn-DŌR-fĭnz)
epidural blood patch (EDP)
focal point
Lamaze method
opioids (Ō-pē-ŏydz)
pain threshold
pain tolerance
postdural puncture headache (PDPH)

Pregnant women are usually interested in how labour will feel and how they can manage the experience. Their preparation for childbirth is important.

CHILDBIRTH EDUCATION

Various classes are offered to women during pregnancy to help them adjust to pregnancy, cope with labour, and prepare for life with an infant (Fig. 7.1). Classes during pregnancy focus on topics that contribute to good outcomes for the mother, family, and infant. The goal of prenatal classes is to help women and their families make informed, safe decisions about pregnancy, birth, and early parenthood. Topics addressed in this chapter include:

- Decision making about and during labour
- Skills for labour
- Pain relief
- Infant and postpartum care
- Breastfeeding
- Parenting skills such as communication

Prenatal education also needs to nurture the appreciation that birth is a normal, healthy event. See the Health Promotion box for other types of classes that may be available.

CHILDBIRTH PREPARATION METHODS

Most childbirth preparation classes are based on one of several methods. The basic method is often modified to meet the specific needs of the women who attend.

Dick-Read Method

Grantly Dick-Read was an English physician who introduced the concept of a fear–tension–pain cycle during labour. He believed that fear of childbirth contributed to

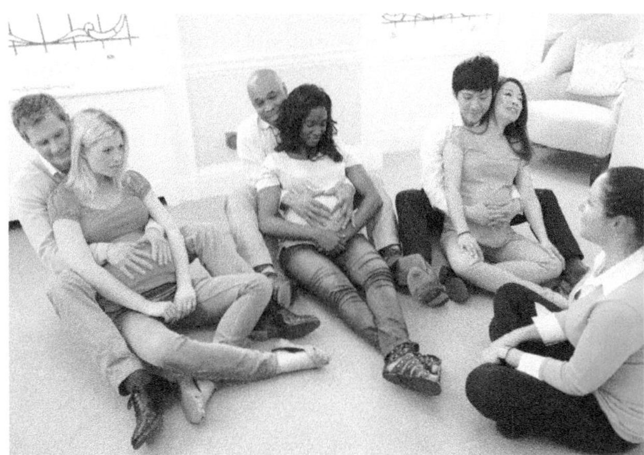

Fig. 7.1 The nurse teaches a group mothers and partners about self-care and comfort measures for labour.

Health Promotion

Types of Childbirth Education and Possible Topics

PRENATAL CLASS
Changes of pregnancy
Fetal development
Prenatal care
Hazardous substances to avoid
Healthy nutrition
Relieving common pregnancy discomforts
Management of labour and birth
Care of the infant, such as feeding methods, choosing a health care provider, and selecting clothing and equipment
Early newborn growth and development

EXERCISE
Enhancing or maintaining pregnancy fitness (see Chapter 4)

SIBLING
Helping children to prepare for their new sibling
Providing tips for parents about helping older children adjust to the new baby after birth

GRANDPARENT
Trends in childbirth and parenting styles
Importance of grandparents to a child's development
Reducing conflict between the generations

BREASTFEEDING
Process of breastfeeding
Feeding techniques
Solving common problems
Some classes with lactation specialists continue after birth

ADOLESCENT PREGNANCY CLASS
Adolescent classes for birth and parenthood preparation

REFRESHER CLASS
Review of information from previous pregnancy
Review of previous birth experience
Sibling preparation

CAESAREAN BIRTH CLASS
Preparation to understand the reason for the procedure and what to expect during the process
Discussion of recovery post–Caesarean birth

VAGINAL BIRTH AFTER CAESAREAN (VBAC)
What to expect during labour when previous childbirth was by Caesarean birth

tension, which resulted in pain. His methods include education and relaxation techniques to interrupt the cycle.

Bradley Method

The **Bradley method** was originally called "husband-coached childbirth" and was the first to include the partner as an integral part of labour. It emphasizes slow abdominal breathing and relaxation techniques.

Lamaze Method

The **Lamaze method** is the basis of many childbirth preparation classes. The goal of Lamaze is to prepare parents by providing evidence-informed information about safe and healthy pregnancy, birth, and early parenting. One aspect of Lamaze education is to use mental techniques that condition the woman to respond to contractions with relaxation rather than tension. Other mental and breathing techniques occupy her mind and limit the brain's ability to interpret labour sensations as painful. The breathing technique should be what works best for the woman, although normally it should be no slower than half of the woman's baseline respiratory rate and no faster than twice the baseline rate.

The Lamaze Healthy Birth Practices are based on research and designed to help keep birth as safe and healthy as possible. The six practices are as follows (Lamaze International, 2018):

- Let labour begin on its own—avoid induction if possible.
- Walk, move around, and change positions throughout labour.
- Bring a loved one, friend, or doula for continuous support.
- Avoid interventions that are not medically necessary.
- Avoid giving birth; follow the body's urges to push.
- Ensure the baby is not separated from the mother; it's best for mother, baby, and breastfeeding.

CHILDBIRTH PREPARATION CLASS CONTENT

Regardless of the specific method taught, most classes are similar in basic content. Many of the techniques covered can also be used to help the unprepared woman during labour. The woman who learns about the changes produced by pregnancy and childbirth is less likely to respond with fear and tension during labour. Information about Caesarean birth is usually included.

Adolescent Childbirth Preparation Classes

A pregnant adolescent's needs are different from those of an adult. Adolescents may be uncomfortable in regular childbirth preparation classes with people who are older than they are. They may be single mothers and have a different perception of birth and child rearing. Some are not old enough to drive or do not have access to a car. They cannot attend classes that target working adults. The content of classes for adolescents is tailored to their special needs and taught in a manner that meets the learning needs of a teenager. Because acceptance by their peer group is important to adolescents, the participants in the class are a significant source of support for one another. Classes may be held in the school setting. Expectant fathers may be included.

Benefits of Exercise

Exercise during pregnancy has been shown to lower the rate of pregnancy complications as well as enhance maternal well-being (Berghella & Saccone, 2017; Mottola,

Davenport, Ruchat, et al., 2019). Conditioning exercises such as the pelvic rock, tailor sitting, and shoulder circling prepare the woman's muscles for the demands of birth. These exercises also relieve the back discomfort that is common during late pregnancy (see Chapter 4).

Pain Control Methods for Labour

The woman and her partner learn a variety of techniques that may be used during labour as needed. These are some examples:

- Skin stimulation, such as massage (Fig. 7.2) or effleurage (Fig. 7.3)
- Diversion and distraction
- Breathing techniques

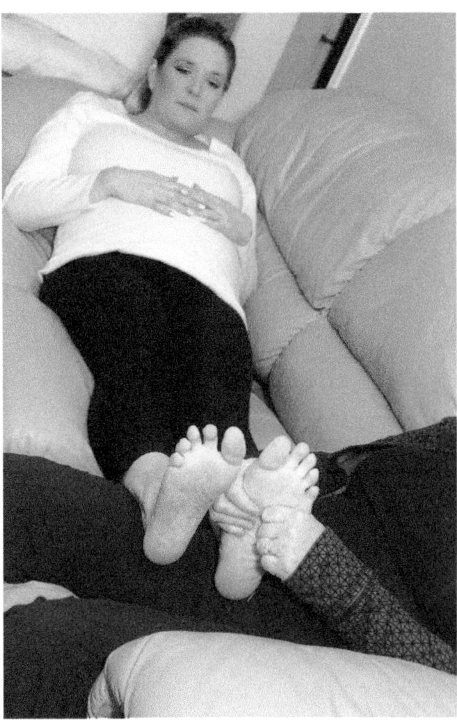

Fig. 7.2 The pregnant woman receiving a foot massage. Massage can be an effective technique for pain relief during labour (Courtesy of Sandy Matos)

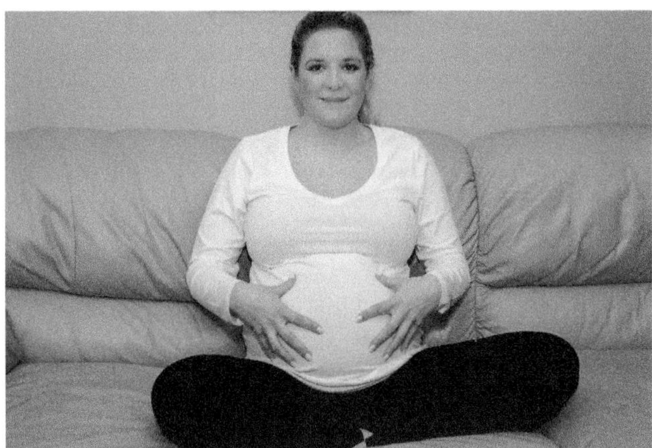

Fig. 7.3 Effleurage. This woman is practicing effleurage, stroking the abdomen with the fingertips in a circular motion. This technique stimulates large-diameter nerve fibres, thus interfering with pain transmission. Fingertip pressure should be firm enough to prevent creating a tickling sensation. (Courtesy of Sandy Matos)

These techniques are most effective if learned before labour begins. Box 7.1 describes selected nonpharmacological pain-relief techniques.

CHILDBIRTH AND PAIN

Pain is an unpleasant and often distressing symptom that is personal and subjective. No one can feel another's pain, but empathic nursing care helps to alleviate pain and helps the woman cope with it.

Several factors distinguish childbirth pain from other types of pain:

- It is part of the normal birth process.
- The woman has several months to prepare for pain management.
- It is self-limiting and rapidly declines after birth.

Pain is usually a symptom of injury or illness, yet pain during labour is an almost universal part of the normal process of birth. Although excessive pain is detrimental to the labour process, pain also can be beneficial. Pain often motivates the woman to assume different body positions, which can facilitate the normal descent of the fetus (see Figs. 6.20 and 6.22). Labour ends with the birth of an infant, followed by a rapid and nearly total cessation of pain.

FACTORS THAT INFLUENCE LABOUR PAIN

Several factors lead to pain during labour and influence the amount of pain a woman experiences. Other factors influence a woman's response to labour pain and her ability to tolerate it.

Pain Threshold and Pain Tolerance

Two terms are often used interchangeably to describe pain, although they have different meanings. **Pain threshold**, also called *pain perception,* is the least amount of sensation that a person perceives as painful. Pain threshold is fairly constant, and it varies little under different conditions. **Pain tolerance** is the amount of pain one is able to endure. Unlike pain threshold, one's pain tolerance can change under different conditions. A primary nursing responsibility is to modify as many factors as possible so that the woman is able to cope with the pain of labour.

Sources of Pain During Labour

The following physical factors contribute to pain during labour:

- Dilation and stretching of the cervix
- Reduced uterine blood supply during contractions (ischemia)
- Pressure of the fetus on pelvic structures
- Stretching of the vagina and perineum

Physical Factors That Modify Pain

Several physical factors influence the amount of pain a woman feels or is able to tolerate during labour.

Box 7.1 Selected Nonpharmacological Pain-Relief Measures

PROGRESSIVE RELAXATION

The woman contracts and then consciously releases different muscle groups.

Technique helps the woman to distinguish tense muscles from relaxed ones.

The woman can assess and then release muscle tension throughout her body.

Technique is most effective if practiced before labour.

NEUROMUSCULAR DISSOCIATION (DIFFERENTIAL RELAXATION)

The woman contracts one group of muscles strongly and consciously relaxes all others.

The partner checks for unrecognized tension in muscle groups other than the one contracted.

This prepares the woman to relax the rest of her body while the uterus is contracting.

Technique is most effective if practiced before labour.

TOUCH RELAXATION

The woman contracts a muscle group and then relaxes it when her partner strokes or massages it.

The woman learns to respond to touch with relaxation.

Technique is most effective if practiced before labour.

RELAXATION AGAINST PAIN

The woman's partner exerts pressure against a tendon or large muscle of the arm or leg, gradually increasing pressure and then gradually decreasing pressure to simulate the gradual increase, the peak, and the decrease in contraction strength.

The woman consciously relaxes despite this deliberate discomfort.

This gives the woman practice in relaxation against pain.

Technique is most effective if practiced before labour.

EFFLEURAGE

The abdomen or other areas are massaged during contractions (see Fig. 7.3).

Massage interferes with transmission of pain impulses, but prolonged continuous use reduces effectiveness. Therefore, the pattern or area massaged should be changed when it becomes less effective.

Massaging in a specific pattern (such as circles or a figure eight) also provides distraction.

OTHER MASSAGE

Massage of the feet, hands, or shoulders often helps relaxation (see Fig. 7.2).

Habituation may occur in any type of massage. Change the area massaged if it occurs.

SACRAL PRESSURE

Technique helps to reduce the pain of back labour.

Obtain the woman's input about the best position. Moving the pressure point a fraction of a centimetre or changing the amount of pressure may significantly improve effectiveness.

Tennis balls in a sock, a warmed plastic container of intravenous solution, or other means may also be used to apply pressure (see Fig. 7.5).

THERMAL STIMULATION

Technique is used to stimulate temperature receptors that interfere with pain transmission.

Either heat or cold applications may be beneficial. Examples are cool cloths to the face and ice or heat packs to the lower back.

POSITIONING

Any position, except the supine position, is acceptable if there is no other indication for a specific position.

Upright positions favour fetal descent and may decrease the length of labour.

Hands-and-knees positions help to reduce the pain of back labour.

Change positions about every 30 to 60 minutes to relieve pressure and muscle fatigue.

DIVERSION AND DISTRACTION

Technique increases mental concentration on something besides the pain. It may take many forms:

Focal point: Concentrating on a specific object or other point

Imagery: Creating an imaginary mental picture of a pleasant environment or visualizing the cervix opening and the infant descending

Music: Serves as a distraction or provides "white noise" to obscure environmental sounds

Scent: Lotions with a particular scent may provide a distraction

HYDOTHERAPY

The heat of the water of a shower, tub, or whirlpool relieves tired muscles and relaxes the woman.

The bouyancy of the water in a tub helps to decrease pain.

Nipple stimulation by shower can increase contraction, because it stimulates the pituitary to release oxytocin.

Gate control theory

The gate control theory explains how pain impulses reach the brain for interpretation. It supports several nonpharmacological methods of pain control. According to this theory, pain is transmitted through small-diameter nerve fibres. However, the stimulation of large-diameter nerve fibres temporarily interferes with the conduction of impulses through small-diameter fibres. Techniques to stimulate large-diameter fibres and "close the gate" to painful impulses include massage, palm and fingertip pressure, change in position, and heat and cold applications.

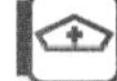

Nursing Tip

Stroking or massage, palm or foot rubbing, pressure, or gripping a cool bed rail stimulate nerve fibres that interfere with the transmission of pain impulses to the brain.

Endorphins

Endorphins are natural body substances similar to morphine. Endorphin levels increase during pregnancy and reach a peak during labour. Endorphins may explain why women in labour often need smaller doses of an analgesic or anaesthetic than might be expected during a similarly painful experience.

Nursing Tip

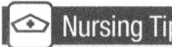

Labouring women often tolerate more pain than usual because they have high levels of endorphins and because they are concerned about the infant's well-being.

Maternal Conditions That Influence Pain

Cervical readiness

The mother's cervix normally undergoes prelabour changes that facilitate effacement and dilation in labour (see Chapter 6). If her cervix does not make these changes (ripening), more contractions are needed to cause effacement and dilation.

Pelvis

The size and shape of the pelvis significantly influence how readily the fetus can descend through it. Pelvic abnormalities can result in a longer labour and greater maternal fatigue. In addition, the fetus may remain in an abnormal presentation or position, which interferes with the mechanisms of labour (see Chapter 6).

Labour intensity

The woman who has a short, intense labour often experiences more pain than the woman whose birth process is more gradual. Contractions are intense and frequent, and their onset may be sudden. The cervix, vagina, and perineum stretch more abruptly than during a gentler labour. Contractions come so fast that the woman cannot recover from one before another begins. In addition, a rapid labour may limit the woman's choices for pharmacological pain control.

Fatigue

Fatigue reduces pain tolerance and a woman's ability to use coping skills. Many women are tired when labour begins, because sleep during late pregnancy is difficult. The active fetus, frequent urination, and shortness of breath when lying down all interrupt sleep.

Fetal presentation and position

The fetal presenting part acts as a wedge to efface and dilate the cervix as each contraction pushes it downward. The fetal head is a smooth, rounded wedge that most effectively causes effacement and dilation of the round cervix. The fetus in an abnormal presentation or position applies uneven pressure to the cervix, resulting in less effective effacement and dilation and thus prolonging the labour and birth process. Various fetal positions and presentations are described in Chapter 6.

The fetus usually turns during early labour so that the occiput is in the front left or right quadrant of the mother's pelvis (occiput anterior positions) (see Figs. 6.9 and 6.10). If the fetal occiput is in a posterior pelvic quadrant, each contraction pushes it against the mother's sacrum, resulting in persistent and poorly relieved back pain (back labour). Labour is often longer with this fetal position (see Chapter 6, Back Labour).

Interventions of caregivers

Although they are intended to promote maternal and fetal safety, several interventions may add to pain during labour. Following are some examples:

- Intravenous (IV) lines
- Continuous electronic fetal monitoring, especially if it hampers mobility
- Amniotomy (artificial rupture of the membranes)
- Vaginal examinations or other interruptions

Psychosocial Factors That Modify Pain

Several psychosocial variables alter the pain a woman experiences during labour. Many of these variables interrelate with one another and with physical factors. For example, poorly relieved pain increases fear and anxiety, thus increasing the secretion of catecholamines and therefore diverting blood flow from the uterus and impairing the normal labour process. Fear in childbirth may lead to tension, which can increase the amount of pain the woman experiences (Fig. 7.4). If this cycle can be broken it can decrease the amount of pain a woman experiences. Decreasing fear by teaching a woman what to expect can help decrease the pain.

Nurses also need to be aware that a woman's cultural background may influence how she feels about pregnancy and birth and how she reacts to pain during childbirth.

NONPHARMACOLOGICAL PAIN MANAGEMENT

Nonpharmacological pain control methods are important to use, even if the woman receives medication or an anaesthetic. Most pharmacological methods cannot be instituted until labour is well established because these methods may slow the progress of labour. Nonpharmacological methods help the woman to cope with labour before it has advanced far enough for her to be given medication. In addition, most medications

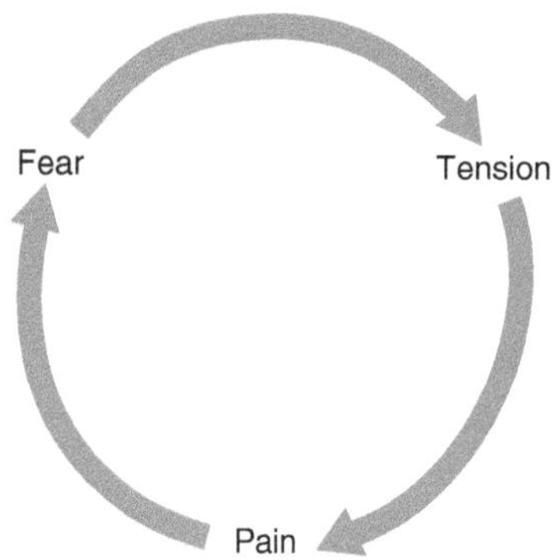

Fig. 7.4 Fear–tension–pain cycle. Breaking this cycle can decrease the amount of pain a woman in labour experiences.

for labour do not eliminate pain, and the woman will need nonpharmacological methods to manage the discomfort that remains. Nonpharmacological methods may be the only option if the woman comes to the hospital in advanced labour or she is giving birth at a hospital with limited pain-relief options (e.g., rural hospitals).

Advantages

There are several advantages to nonpharmacological methods if pain control is adequate. Nonpharmacological methods do not harm the mother or fetus. They do not slow labour if they provide adequate pain control.

Limitations

For best results, nonpharmacological measures should be rehearsed before labour begins. They can be taught to the unprepared woman, preferably during early labour, when she is comfortable enough to learn. The nurse may help the woman use several key techniques of nonpharmacological pain control during labour. If the woman and her partner attended childbirth preparation classes, the nurse can build on their knowledge during labour (see Box 7.1).

Nonpharmacological Techniques

Relaxation techniques

The ability to release tension is a vital part of the expectant woman's "tool kit." Relaxation techniques require concentration, thus occupying the mind while reducing muscle tension. Promoting relaxation is basic to all other methods of pain management and birth preparation, both nonpharmacological and pharmacological. The nurse should adjust the woman's environment and help her with general comfort measures, as discussed in Chapter 6. For example, water in a tub or shower helps to refresh her and promotes relaxation. Validating the woman's discomfort and providing support are essential nursing interventions during all stages of labour.

To reduce anxiety and fear, the woman is oriented to the labour area, any procedures that are done, and what is happening in her body during the normal process of birth. A partnership style of nurse–patient–labour partner is essential in the maternity setting.

Looking for signs of muscle tension and teaching her support person to look for these signs can help the woman who is not aware of becoming tense. She can change position or guide her support person to massage the area where muscle tension is noted. The labouring woman is guided to release the tension specifically, one muscle group at a time, by saying, for example, "Let your arm relax; let the tension out of your neck . . . your shoulders. . . ." Specific instructions are repeated until she relaxes each body part.

The woman should change methods at intervals because constant use of a single technique reduces its effectiveness (habituation).

Massage

Several variations of massage are often used during labour. Most can be taught to the woman and partner who did not attend childbirth preparation classes.

Effleurage. **Effleurage** is a technique that stimulates the large-diameter nerve fibres that inhibit painful stimuli travelling through the small-diameter fibres. The woman or partner strokes her abdomen in a circular movement during contractions (see Fig. 7.3). If fetal monitor belts are on her abdomen, she can massage between them or on her thigh.

Sacral pressure. Firm pressure against the lower back helps relieve some of the pain of back labour. The woman should instruct her partner where to apply the pressure and how much pressure is helpful (Fig. 7.5).

Thermal stimulation

Heat can be applied with a warm blanket or heat pack. Warmth can also be applied in the form of a shower or tub if there is no contraindication to doing so. Most women appreciate a cool cloth on the face. Two or three moistened washcloths are kept at hand and changed as they become warm. Cold can be a more effective pain-relief method than heat. It often lasts longer than heat and is effective for back labour. Ice packs or frozen bottles rolled up the back are useful.

Positioning

Frequent changing of position relieves muscle fatigue and strain. In addition, position changes can promote the normal mechanisms of labour and often speed up the process of labour. It is important to work with the woman to determine what positions are most comfortable. Examples of upright positions include walking, rocking in a chair, the use of a birth ball, squatting, or slow dancing. For helping women with back labour, refer to discussion in Chapter 6 and Fig. 6.20.

Diversion and distraction

Several methods may be used to stimulate the woman's brain, thus limiting her ability to perceive sensations

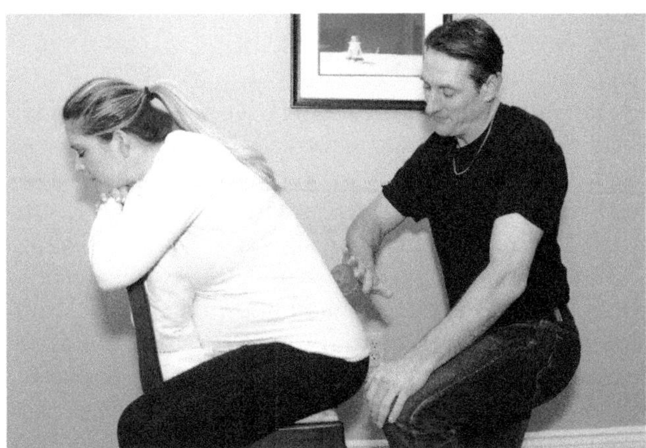

Fig. 7.5 Sacral pressure. The partner applies firm pressure on the lower back of the woman in labour. Using a tennis ball enhances the effect. (Courtesy of Sandy Matos)

as painful. All of these methods direct her mind away from the pain.

Focal point. The woman fixes her eyes on a picture, an object, or simply a particular spot in the room. Some women prefer to close their eyes during contractions and focus on an internal **focal point**.

Imagery. The woman learns to create a tranquil mental environment by imagining that she is in a place of relaxation and peace. Preferred mental scenes often involve warmth and sunlight, although some women imagine themselves in a cool environment. During labour, the woman can imagine her cervix opening and allowing the infant to come out, as a flower opens from bud to full bloom. The nurse can help to create a tranquil mental image, even in the unprepared woman.

Music. Favourite music or relaxation recordings divert the woman's attention from pain. The sounds of rainfall, wind, or the ocean can contribute to relaxation and block disturbing sounds; the woman can also listen to her favourite types of music on a variety of electronic devices.

Intradermal sterile water injections

The use of intradermal water injection has been shown to be an effective method to decrease back pain in labour. A small amount of sterile water (e.g., 0.05 to 0.1 mL) is injected with a fine needle (e.g., 25-gauge) into four locations on the lower back. It probably works according to principles of the gate control theory.

Breathing

Like other techniques, breathing techniques are more effective if practiced before labour. The woman should not use them until she needs them, generally when she can no longer walk or talk through a contraction. She may become tired if she uses them too early or if she moves to a more advanced technique sooner than she must. If the woman has not had childbirth preparation classes, each technique is taught as she needs it.

Each breathing pattern begins and ends with a **cleansing breath**, which is a deep inspiration and expiration, similar to a deep sigh. The cleansing breaths help the woman to relax and focus on relaxing. The breathing discussed here is Lamaze breathing; there are also other types of breathing that may work for a woman in labour. There is no correct way to do the breathing as long as it is working.

First-stage breathing

Slow-paced breathing. The woman begins with a technique of slow-paced breathing. She starts the pattern with a cleansing breath, then breathes deeply and slowly into her belly (Fig. 7.6, *A*). A cleansing breath ends the contraction. An exact rate is not important, but the rate should not be less than half her usual rate to ensure adequate fetal oxygenation and prevent hypoventilation.

Modified-paced breathing. This pattern begins and ends with a cleansing breath. During the contraction, the woman breathes more rapidly and shallowly (Fig. 7.6, *B* and *C*). The rate should be no more than twice her usual rate. She may combine slow-paced with modified-paced breathing. In this variation, she begins with a cleansing breath and breathes slowly until the peak of the contraction, when she begins rapid, shallow breathing. As the contraction abates, she resumes slow, deep breathing and ends with a cleansing breath.

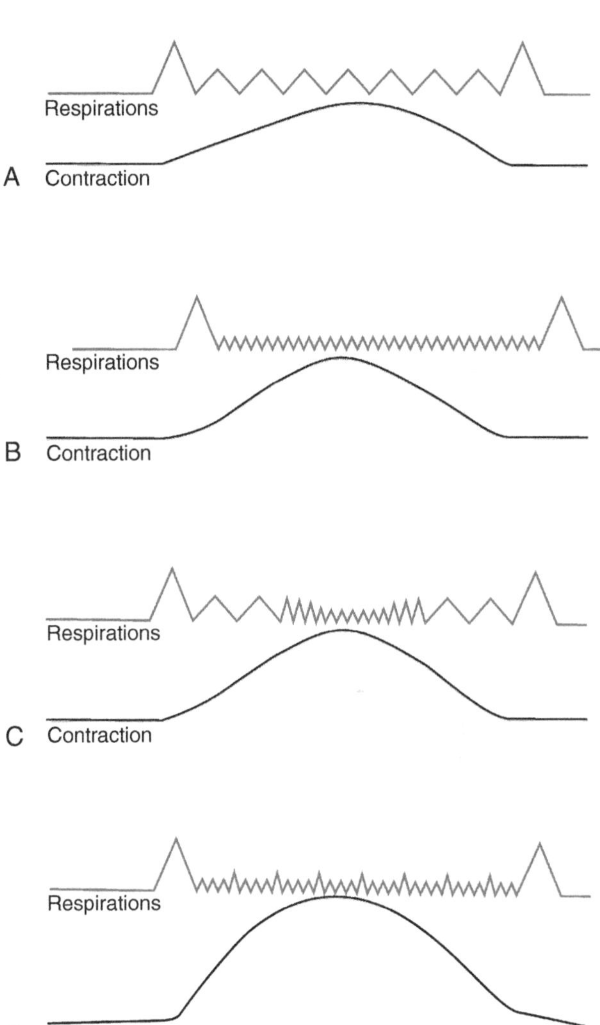

Fig. 7.6 Breathing patterns. **A,** *Slow-paced breathing.* The pattern starts with a cleansing breath as the contraction begins. The woman breathes slowly, not less than half her usual rate, and ends with a second cleansing breath at the end of the contraction. **B,** As labour intensifies, the woman may need to use *modified-paced breathing.* The pattern begins and ends with a cleansing breath. After the opening cleansing breath, the woman breathes rapidly and shallowly during the contraction, no faster than twice her usual respiratory rate, and makes the closing cleansing breath as the contraction subsides. **C,** In this variation of modified-paced breathing, the woman begins with slow-paced breathing at the beginning of the contraction, switching to faster breathing during its peak. A cleansing breath also begins and ends this pattern. **D,** *Patterned-paced breathing* begins and ends with a cleansing breath. During the contraction the woman emphasizes the exhalation of some breaths. She may count and use a specific pattern or may randomly emphasize the blow.

Box 7.2 How to Recognize and Correct Hyperventilation

SIGNS AND SYMPTOMS
Dizziness
Tingling of hands and feet
Cramps and muscle spasms of hands
Numbness around the nose and mouth
Blurring of vision

CORRECTIVE MEASURES
Breathe slowly, especially in exhalation.
Breathe into cupped hands or a paper bag.
Place a moist washcloth over the mouth and nose while breathing.
Hold breath for a few seconds before exhaling.

Hyperventilation is sometimes a problem when the woman is breathing rapidly. She may state that she feels dizziness, tingling, and numbness around her mouth and may have spasms of her fingers and feet. Box 7.2 lists measures to overcome hyperventilation.

Patterned-paced breathing. The technique of patterned-paced breathing is more difficult to teach the unprepared labouring woman because it requires her to focus on the pattern of her breathing. It begins with a cleansing breath, which is followed by rapid breaths as in modified-paced breathing, but the breathing is punctuated with an intermittent longer exhalation (Fig. 7.6, *D*). The woman may maintain a constant number of breaths before the expiration or may vary the number in a specific pattern, as follows:

- *Constant pattern:* 3:1 pattern: IN-OUT/IN-OUT/IN-OUT/IN-BLOW/ and so on.
- *Stairstep pattern:* IN-BLOW, IN-OUT/IN-BLOW, IN-OUT/IN-OUT/IN-BLOW, IN-OUT/IN-OUT/IN-OUT/IN-BLOW, IN-OUT/IN-OUT/IN-OUT/IN-OUT/IN-BLOW

In another variation, her partner calls out random numbers to indicate the number of breaths to take before a blow.

If she feels an urge to push before her cervix is fully dilated, the woman is taught to blow in short breaths to avoid bearing down. Blowing out or panting prevents closure of the glottis and the breath-holding urges that often accompany spontaneous pushing. Pushing before full cervical dilation may cause cervical edema or lacerations, although many women who are allowed to push spontaneously when they feel the urge to push do not have any complications.

Second-stage breathing. When it is time for the woman to push, the woman takes a cleansing breath, then takes another deep breath and pushes down while exhaling to a count of 6. She blows out, takes a deep breath, and pushes again while exhaling (open glottis pushing). Encouraging women to hold their breath during pushing causes a decrease in blood flow to the uterus and also to the fetus, and is not an effective method of breathing for pushing.

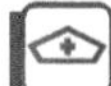 **Nursing Tip**

If a woman is successfully using a nonpharmacological pain-control technique, do not interfere and continue to provide support.

The nurse's role in nonpharmacological techniques

When a woman is admitted to the labour and birth unit, the nurse determines whether she has taken childbirth preparation classes and works with what the woman and her partner learned. The nurse helps them to identify signs of tension so the woman can be guided to release it. Most importantly, the nurse needs to determine the goals of the woman and her partner with respect to the labour and should work to facilitate these goals.

If the woman did not have childbirth preparation classes, the nurse teaches simple breathing and relaxation techniques. If the woman is extremely anxious she may not be able to comprehend verbal instructions. It may be necessary to make close eye contact with her and to breathe with her through each contraction until she can regain her composure.

The nurse needs to minimize environmental irritants as much as possible. The lights should be lowered and the woman kept comfortable by regularly changing the underpads on the bed. The temperature should be adjusted; the nurse can provide a warm blanket if that offers the most comfort. (See Chapter 6 for other general comfort measures to provide during labour.)

All women in labour should receive continuous labour support. *Labour support* describes the caring work or social support provided to a labouring woman. It consists of emotional support (continuous presence, reassurance, and praise), comfort measures (touch, massage, warm baths or showers, encouraging fluid intake and output), advocacy (communicating the woman's wishes), and provision of information (coping methods, update on progress of labour) (Liston, Sawchuck, Young, et al., 2018). Research has shown that support during labour significantly increases a family's satisfaction with the birth experience, reduces the use of medications and interventions, and enhances the positive attitude women need to care for their babies (Public Health Agency of Canada [PHAC], 2018). This support during labour can be provided by the nurse, or a nurse working alongside a doula.

The nurse should be cautious not to overestimate or underestimate the amount of pain a woman is experiencing. The quiet, stoic woman may need analgesia yet be reluctant to ask for it. A tense body posture or facial grimacing may indicate that she needs additional pain-relief measures.

It is most important that labouring women be able to make their own decisions regarding pain-management strategies and not be forced into anything they do not want. Nurses must support the woman to make pain-management choices that support the goals the woman has for her labour. The use of pain scales is not helpful in labour, as the woman may have high levels of pain but may be able to cope with that pain.

PHARMACOLOGICAL PAIN MANAGEMENT

Pharmacological pain-management methods include analgesics, adjunctive medications to improve the effectiveness of analgesics or to counteract their adverse effects, and anaesthetics. *Analgesics* are systemic medications (affecting the entire body) that reduce the sensation of pain without loss of consciousness. *Anaesthetics* cause a loss of sensation, especially of pain. *Regional anaesthetics* block sensation from a localized area by interrupting the nerve impulses to the brain without causing a loss of consciousness. *General anaesthetics* are systemic medications that cause a loss of consciousness and sensation of pain. A specialist in anaesthetic administration may provide other anaesthetics. An *anaesthesiologist* is a physician who specializes in administering anaesthesia. Table 7.1 summarizes intrapartum analgesics and adjunctive medications.

Physiology of Pregnancy and Its Relationship to Analgesia and Anaesthesia

Specific factors in the physiology of pregnancy affect the pregnant woman's response to analgesia and anaesthesia:

- The pregnant woman is at a higher risk for hypoxia caused by the pressure of the enlarging uterus on the diaphragm.
- The sluggish gastrointestinal tract of the pregnant woman can result in increased risk for vomiting and aspiration.
- Aortocaval compression (pressure on the abdominal aorta by the heavy uterus when the woman is in supine position) increases the risk of hypotension and the development of shock.
- The effect on the fetus must be considered. Special consideration must be given to women in preterm labour, as there is an increase in adverse effects on the preterm fetus who is unable to process the effects of medications. Health care providers who are

Table 7.1 Medications for Labour: Intrapartum Analgesics and Related Medications

MEDICATION	USE AND EFFECTS
Opioids	
Morphine sulphate	May be given intramuscularly or intravenously Best used in early labour Fewer adverse effects for the newborn; most infants born within 3 hours of administration will have no adverse effects Administered with dimenhydrinate (Gravol) to counteract effects of nausea and vomiting
Fentanyl (Sublimaze)	Rapid onset and short duration of action **Note:** Sufentanil and alfentanil are *not* the same medication Can cause respiratory depression Often used with epidural analgesia Must be alert for medication interactions, such as with antihistamines, barbiturates, and muscle relaxants Oxygen saturation must be monitored for 30 minutes
Meperidine (Demerol)	May be used for women with allergy to morphine but otherwise **NOT RECOMMENDED** Given to mothers in labour either intravenously, with a 5- to 10-minute peak of action, or intramuscularly, with a 50-minute peak of action
Combination Opioid Agonist-Antagonist	
Nalbuphine (Nubain)	Reduces pain and is thought to cause less respiratory depression than meperidine Should not be used in women who have addictions to substances
Opioid Antagonist	
Naloxone (Narcan)	Opioid antagonist that acts within minutes to decrease adverse effects of opioid given to the mother (e.g., sedation, itching) Duration of action is 1–2 hours, so vital signs of the mother should continue to be observed May cause withdrawal symptoms (e.g., tremors, perspiration, anxiety, irritability, and seizures) if administered to a woman who regularly uses illicit drugs Should NOT be administered to newborns for resuscitation (see discussion in text)
Inhaled Anaesthetic	
Nitrous oxide	Administered via mask controlled by the woman Decreases awareness of pain May cause nausea and dizziness No negative effects on the woman or the developing fetus

Note: Consult drug guide for safe doses of medications.
From Perinatal Services of British Columbia. (2007). *Obstetric guideline 4: Pain management options during labour*. Updated 2010. Retrieved from http://www.perinatalservicesbc.ca/Documents/Guidelines-Standards/Maternal/PainManagementGuideline.pdf; Morin, F., & Rivard, L. (2017). Pain management during labour. In S. Perry, M. Hockenberry, D. Lowdermilk, et al. (Eds.), *Maternal child nursing care in Canada* (2nd ed.). Toronto, ON: Elsevier.

skilled in neonatal resuscitation must be present at the birth of a preterm fetus (Perinatal Services of British Columbia, 2007/2010).

The goal of pain relief is to provide maximum comfort to the labouring woman with minimum effect on the fetus.

Advantages

There are many methods of pharmacological pain management that can provide pain relief and comfort to the labouring woman with minimal adverse effects. For some women, a reduction of pain during birth can help them to be a more active participant in their birth. Decreasing pain sensations can allow the woman to help her focus her energy on working with the pain. It must be acknowledged that pain has a physiological role in childbirth (Bonapace, Gagné, Chaillet, et al., 2018). Parenteral medications do not usually relieve *all* pain and pressure sensations.

In some women, the pain of labour may cause a "stress response" that results in an increase in autonomic activity, a release of catecholamines, and a decrease in perfusion to nonessential organs. This stress response can increase the woman's perception of suffering, which can decrease her labour progress, resulting in the use of obstetrical interventions. Some women experience maternal hyperventilation which can lead to respiratory alkalosis and a feeling of lightheadedness and loss of control. If prolonged, respiratory alkalosis can progress to a compensating metabolic acidosis. Metabolic acidosis in the woman can result in fetal acidosis. Women's perception of pain relief during labour can play an important role in the positive outcome of pregnancy for mother and infant. Women who have decreased stress in labour have a more positive response to their labour experience.

Limitations

Pharmacological methods are effective, but they do have limitations. One important factor to consider is that two persons are medicated—the mother and her fetus. Opioids administered to the mother can affect the fetus, and the effects may be prolonged in the infant after birth. Every effort should be made to administer short-acting opioids to reduce the effects of respiratory depression in the newborn, as this can impact successful breastfeeding initiation because of the need for additional intervention. Some medications may directly affect the fetus, and some may indirectly affect the fetus because of effects on the mother (such as hypotension).

Several pharmacological methods may slow the progress of labour if used early in labour. Some complications during pregnancy limit the pharmacological methods that are safe. For example, a method that requires the infusion of large amounts of IV fluids might overload the woman's circulation if she has heart disease or hypertension. If she takes other medications (legal or illicit), they may interact adversely with the medications used to relieve labour pain.

Analgesics and Adjunctive Medications

Nitrous oxide

Nitrous oxide is a tasteless and odourless gas used as a labour analgesic in some hospitals. It reduces anxiety and increases a feeling of well-being so that pain is easier to cope with. Nitrous oxide is mixed with oxygen and inhaled through a mask. The woman holds the mask herself and decides when she will inhale. It works best when a woman begins inhaling 30 seconds before the start of a contraction.

Adverse effects and risks of nitrous oxide. Nitrous oxide is safe for the mother and the baby. Some women feel dizzy or nauseated while inhaling nitrous oxide, but these sensations go away within a few minutes.

Opioid analgesics

Systemic **opioids** are commonly administered for labour analgesia. Opioids do not provide complete pain relief during labour, but they do help the woman cope with a tolerable level of intermittent labour pains. Medications used are listed in Table 7.1. Special consideration must be given when planning care for a pregnant woman who is a substance user. Nurses must individualize their approach, taking the woman's past history and expressed needs into account. Dosing adjustments should be considered for women who have an increased tolerance level for opioid medications (Ordean, Wong, & Graves, 2017).

Typically, opioids are used in small doses to avoid causing fetal respiratory depression. In general, use of narcotic analgesia is avoided if birth is expected within an hour. An attempt is made to time administration so the medication does not reach its peak effect at the time of birth, or the infant may have respiratory depression that may require interventions such as the ventilation with bag and mask. The nurse must be prepared to support the respiratory efforts of all infants at birth regardless of whether or not the mother received opioids during labour.

> **! Safety Alert!**
>
> When opioids are administered for pain relief, safety protocols must be implemented for maternal safety, such as raising the side rails, close observation, and having naloxone readily available if needed. Naloxone is absorbed not only through intravenous (IV) but also by intramuscular (IM), subcutaneous, endotracheal, sublingual, intralingual, submental, and nasal routes. Via the IV route, onset of action is within 1–2 minutes. The dose is naloxone 0.1 mg IV stat for respiratory rate LESS than 10 and when the patient is sleepy and difficult to rouse.

Resuscitation of a newborn with respiratory depression. The routine use of naloxone to manage respiratory depression in infants born to mothers with opioid exposure in labour is *NOT* recommended (Canadian Paediatric Society [CPS], 2017). The CPS Neonatal Resuscitation Program (NRP) guidelines do not support the administration of naloxone to a newborn with respiratory depression due to maternal opiate exposure, owing to possible complications that include pulmonary edema, cardiac arrest, and seizures (Wyckoff, Aziz, Escobedo, et al., 2015). Epinephrine and volume expanders such as normal saline or O-negative packed red blood cells are used for resuscitation with weight-based dosing (CPS, 2017).

Adjunctive drugs

Adjunctive drugs are not pain relievers but are given to act synergistically with opioid medication to enhance their effectiveness. They also relieve any nausea and vomiting, which are common adverse effects of pain-relief medications. All benzodiazepines can disrupt the variability of the fetal heart rate and delay the newborn infant's ability to regulate temperature (Hawkins & Bucklin, 2017).

Regional Analgesics and Anaesthetics

The membranes around the spinal cord are called the *meninges*. The meninges have three layers:

1. Dura mater
2. Arachnoid mater
3. Pia mater

Epidural and subarachnoid blocks and intrathecal narcotics are given by injecting anaesthetic medications so they bathe the nerves as they emerge from the spinal cord. The spinal cord and nerves are not directly injected. The *epidural space* is located between the dura mater and the inside bony covering of the brain or spinal cord. The *subdural space* is located between the dura mater and the arachnoid mater, and the *subarachnoid space* is located between the arachnoid mater and the pia mater. Regional anaesthesia in obstetrics usually involves placement of an anaesthetic in the epidural or the subarachnoid space (Fig. 7.7).

The role of the RN in caring for a woman with regional analgesia or anaesthesia is to monitor her responses and the status of the fetus. Starting or managing intermittent

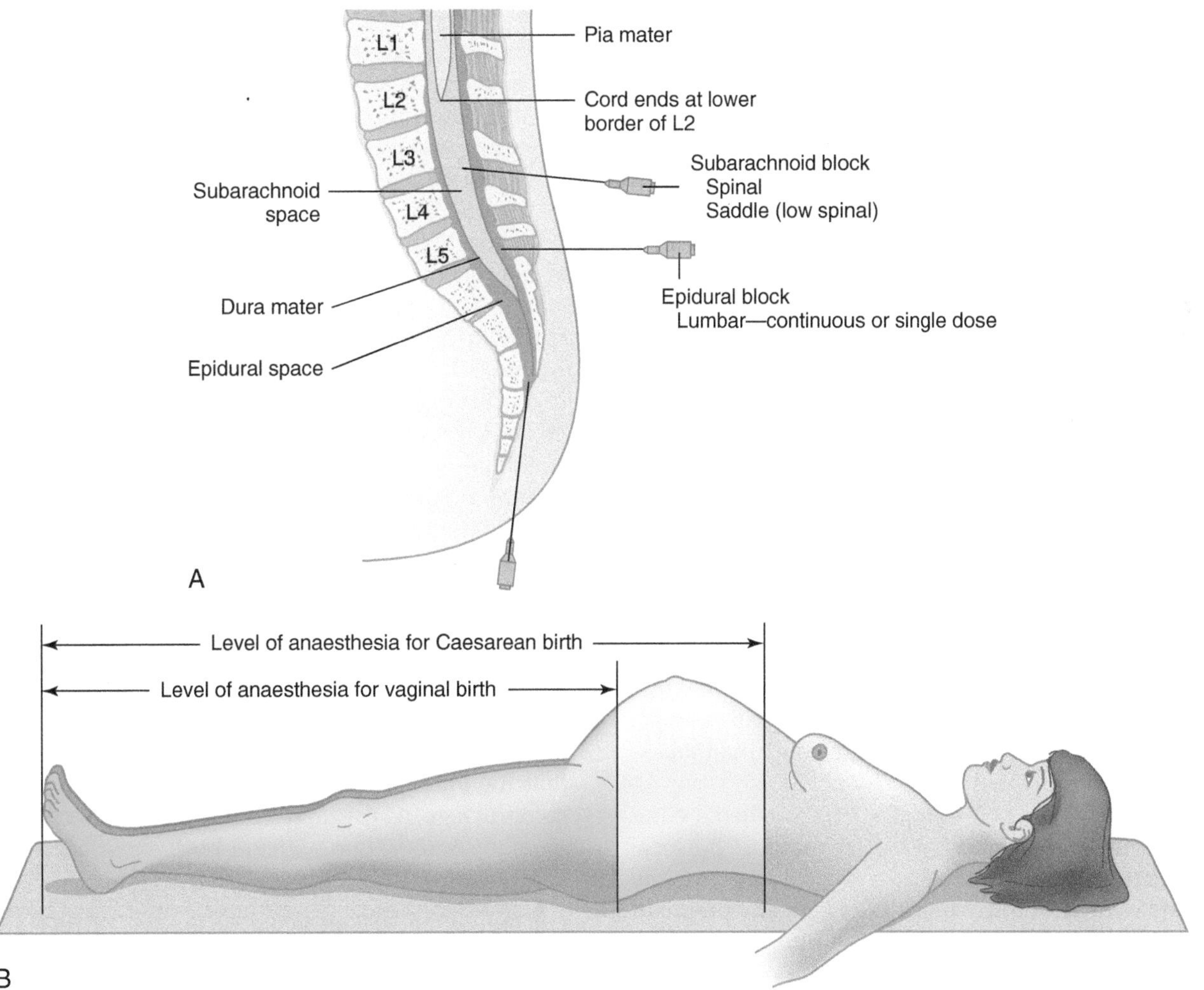

Fig. 7.7 Epidural and spinal anaesthesia. **A,** The insertion sites for the needle in epidural, subarachnoid, and spinal blocks. **B,** Levels of anaesthesia for vaginal birth compared with minimum level required for Caesarean birth. (From Matteson, P. S. [2001]. *Women's health during the childbearing years: A community-based approach*. St. Louis: Mosby.)

dosages of a regional anaesthetic is not within the nursing scope of practice for a practical nurse.

Regional anaesthetics block sensation in varying degrees, depending on the type of regional block used, the quantity of medication, and the medication injected. The woman still feels pressure and may feel some pain. The major advantage of regional anaesthetics is that they provide satisfactory pain relief, yet they allow the woman to be awake and participate in the birthing process.

Epidural block

The epidural space is a small space just outside the dura (outermost membrane covering the brain and spinal cord). The woman is in a sitting or side-lying position for administration of the epidural block. Her back is curved outward, to enhance administration of the epidural catheter.

The anaesthesiologist penetrates the epidural space with a large needle (16- to 18-gauge) called a *Tuohy needle.* A fine catheter is threaded into the epidural space through the bore of the needle (see Fig. 7.7). A test dose (2 to 3 mL) of local anaesthetic agent is injected through the catheter. The woman is not expected to experience effects from the test dose if the catheter is in the right place. Numbness or loss of movement and difficulty taking a deep breath after the small test dose indicate that her dura mater was likely punctured and the medication was injected into the subarachnoid space (as in a subarachnoid block) rather than in the epidural space. The woman will become hypotensive, experience numbness around the mouth, ringing in the ears (tinnitus), and have jitteriness, which are symptoms that suggest injection into a vein.

The test dose is small enough to detect incorrect placement of the needle and thus helps to prevent long-term adverse effects. If the test dose is normal (no effects), a larger amount of anaesthetic agent is injected to begin providing adequate pain relief with the block. A few minutes are needed before the onset of the block. If an epidural block is being used for surgery, such as Caesarean birth, the anaesthesiologist tests for the level of numbness before surgery begins.

Local anaesthetic medications are usually combined with a small dose of an opioid analgesic. The combination of medications allows quicker and longer-lasting pain relief with less anaesthetic agent and minimal loss of movement. An epidural block for labour is more accurately termed *analgesia* (reducing pain) than *anaesthesia* (obliterating all sensation).

The woman can sometimes ambulate when a combination-medication epidural is used, because the local anaesthetic dose is much lower. She can assume any position with this type of block, although any pregnant woman should avoid the supine position. The woman is encouraged to ambulate to the bathroom to empty her bladder rather than have a urinary catheter.

To maintain pain relief during labour, the anaesthetic medication is constantly infused into the catheter via an infusion pump or via programmed intermittent bolus (PIB). Alternatively, intermittently repeated injections of the medication may be given. An epidural block may decrease postpartum depression and reduce the partner's feeling of helplessness, often increasing the partner's participation (Hawkins & Buchlin, 2017).

Dural puncture. The dura lies just below the tiny epidural space. This membrane is sometimes punctured inadvertently with the epidural needle or the catheter that is inserted through it. If a dural puncture occurs, a relatively large amount of spinal fluid can leak from the hole, which may result in a **postdural puncture headache (PDPH)** (see Adverse effects of subarachnoid block, later in the chapter).

Limitations of epidural block. Although it is a popular method of intrapartum pain relief, an epidural block is not used if the woman has any of the following conditions (Perinatal Services of British Columbia, 2007/2010):

- Abnormal blood clotting
- An infection in the area of injection or a systemic infection
- Hypovolemia (inadequate blood volume)
- Low platelet count (below 80×10^9/L)
- Increased intracranial pressure

Adverse effects of epidural block. The most common adverse effects are *maternal hypotension* and *urinary retention*. After initiation of the epidural block, the fetal heart rate and blood pressure should be monitored and documented every 5 minutes for 30 minutes, and then 30 minutes for 1 hour. A bolus (500 mL to 1 000 mL or more) of IV solution, such as normal saline or Ringer's lactate, is no longer recommended unless the woman is dehydrated or has an atypical or abnormal fetal tracing before the block is initiated. When a bolus of IV fluids is given, the nurse should palpate the suprapubic area for a full bladder every 2 hours. The woman should be encouraged to ambulate to the bathroom if she has adequate mobility with her epidural block or she will need to be catheterized if she is unable to void. If the woman requires a catheter, intermittent catheterization is recommended rather than an indwelling catheter.

The woman may feel less of an urge to push in the second stage of labour when she has an epidural block, depending on the density of the local anaesthetic used for her block. Therefore, this stage may be longer if a woman has an epidural block. Maternal and fetal conditions are monitored closely. It is not recommended that the epidural block be turned down or off in the second stage, as this may contribute to a decrease in a woman's satisfaction with her birth experience.

! Safety Alert!

Assess the woman for bladder distention regularly if she has received an epidural or subarachnoid block. A full bladder can delay fetal descent and increase the risks for postpartum hemorrhage.

Subarachnoid (spinal) block

The woman's position for a subarachnoid block is similar to that for the epidural block. The dura is punctured with a thin (25- to 27-gauge) spinal needle called a *pencil point needle.* A few drops of spinal fluid confirm entry into the subarachnoid space (see Fig. 7.7). The local anaesthetic drug is then injected. A much smaller quantity of the drug is needed to achieve anaesthesia using the subarachnoid block than with the epidural block. The effect of anaesthesia occurs quickly and is more profound than that of the epidural block. The woman loses all movement and sensation below the block very quickly. The effect lasts longer than that of the epidural block.

The subarachnoid block is a "one-shot" block, because it does not involve placing a catheter for reinjection of the drug. It is not often used for vaginal births but remains common for Caesarean births. Its limitations are essentially the same as those for an epidural block.

Adverse effects of subarachnoid block. Hypotension and urinary retention are the main adverse effects of subarachnoid block, as with the epidural block. Epidurals and spinal blocks cause low blood pressure due to the effect of the local anaesthetic used. The anaesthetic blocks the nerves that regulate blood pressure, causing blood to pool rather than be pumped around the body. IV fluids are given to reduce the effects of hypotension. Urinary retention occurs owing to a block of the nerves leading to the bladder and feelings of having to void. Frequent bladder assessment is thus important.

A PDPH sometimes occurs, most likely because of spinal fluid loss. The incidence and severity of headache are directly related to the size and design of the needle used. The majority of women who have an inadvertent dural puncture with a Tuohy needle will develop a PDPH severe enough to require an **epidural blood patch (EBP)**; the introduction of small-gauge needles with pencil points has greatly reduced the incidence of headaches after spinal anaesthesia. An epidural blood patch, done by the anaesthesiologist, may provide dramatic relief from PDPH. The woman's blood (10 to 15 mL) is withdrawn from her vein and injected into the epidural space in the area of the subarachnoid puncture (Fig. 7.8). The blood clots and forms a gelatinous seal that stops spinal fluid leakage. The clot later breaks down and is resorbed by the body.

For some women, the PDPH may be self-limiting. Nonetheless, the possibility, however remote, of a serious complication such as a subdural hematoma if the hole in the dura is not sealed has to be kept in mind. The woman may be advised to remain flat for several hours after the block to decrease the chance of PDPH. However, there is no absolute evidence that this precaution is effective. PDPH is worse when the woman is upright, and it often disappears entirely when she lies down. Bed rest, analgesics, and oral and IV fluids help to relieve the headache.

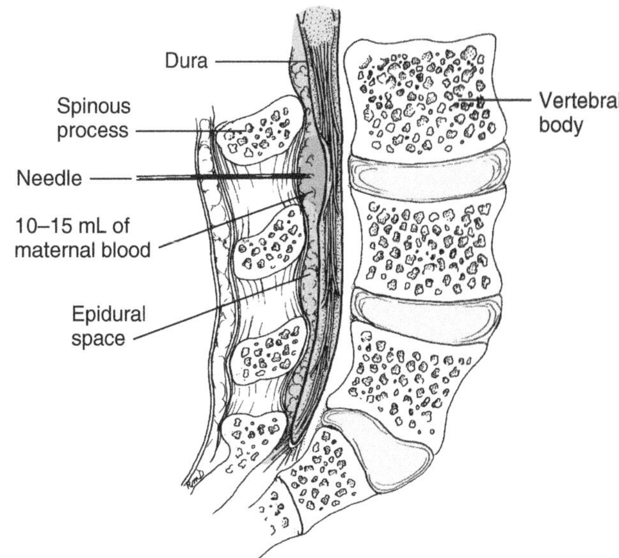

Fig. 7.8 Epidural blood patch. An epidural blood patch may provide dramatic relief from postspinal headache.

Safety Alert!

When spinal anaesthesia is used, assess for numbness of fingers. This can mean the medication has reached the L6–L8 and affects the diaphragm, which will cause respiratory problems.

Combined spinal epidural

The combined spinal-epidural (CSE) is a technique that is similar to epidural block insertion. The difference is that the medication is inserted using an epidural needle and smaller spinal needle to access the subarachnoid space. The spinal needle is withdrawn and the epidural catheter is threaded through, remaining in place for ongoing top-ups. The advantage of the CSE is rapid onset of pain relief with less motor block. Women tend to be more satisfied with the use of CSE for pain relief, as ambulation is possible with this technique (Perinatal Services of British Columbia, 2007/2010).

Local and pudendal blocks

Local and pudendal blocks are administered in the vaginal-perineal area. Local anaesthetic agents for childbirth are similar to those used for dental work. On admission, the nurse should ask each woman if she is allergic to or has had problems with dental anaesthesia. If so, her health care provider should be alerted so she can receive the safest pain-relief measures.

Local block. Injection of the perineal area for an episiotomy may be performed just before birth, when the fetal head is visible. It may also be used after placental expulsion to repair a perineal laceration. There is a short delay between injection of the anaesthetic agent and the loss of pain sensation. The health care provider allows the anaesthetic to become effective before beginning the episiotomy. There are virtually no risks to this procedure if the woman is not allergic to the medication.

Pudendal block. The pudendal block is used for vaginal births, although its use has become less common as the popularity of the epidural block has increased. A pudendal block can be used to provide pain relief during the second stage of labour, as well as for episiotomy and repair, but it does not relieve contraction pain. It is most often used for pain relief for women requiring the use of vacuum or forceps for the birth in the absence of an existing epidural. It provides pain relief in the perineal and lower vagina area. There is a delay of a few minutes between injection of the medication and the onset of numbness (paresthesia).

The health care provider injects the pudendal nerves on each side of the mother's pelvis (Fig. 7.9). The nerves may be reached through the vagina or by injection directly through her perineum. A long needle (13 to 15 cm [5 to 6 inches]) is needed to reach the pudendal nerves, which are near the mother's ischial spines. If the injection is done through the vagina, a needle guide ("trumpet") is used to protect the mother's tissues. The needle is injected only about 1.3 cm (0.5 inch) into the woman's tissues. The perineum is also infiltrated, because the pudendal block alone does not completely anaesthetize the perineum. The advantage to a pudendal nerve block is the lack of effect on maternal cardiovascular system and no effect on fetal heart rate (Morin & Rivard, 2017).

Adverse effects of pudendal block. The pudendal block includes few adverse effects if the woman is not allergic to the medication. A vaginal hematoma (collection of blood within the tissues) sometimes occurs. An abscess may develop, but this is not common.

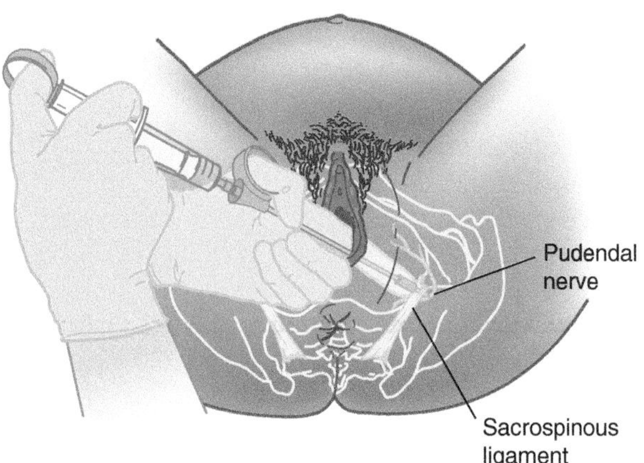

Fig. 7.9 Pudendal block anaesthesia. The two pudendal nerves on each side of the pelvis are injected to numb the vagina and perineum. The illustration shows the technique of inserting the needle beyond the needle guard and passing through the sacrospinous ligament to reach the pudendal nerve. (From Matteson, P. S. [2001]. *Women's health during the childbearing years: A community-based approach.* St. Louis: Mosby.)

General Anaesthesia

General anaesthesia is rarely used for Caesarean births as regional blocks are preferred. However, general anaesthesia may be necessary in the following circumstances:

- Emergency caesarean birth, when there is no time to establish either an epidural or a subarachnoid block
- Caesarean birth in the woman who has a contraindication to epidural or subarachnoid block
- Caesarean birth in the woman who refuses epidural or subarachnoid block

Combinations of general anaesthetic medications (balanced anaesthesia) allow for a quick onset of anaesthesia, minimal fetal effects, and prompt maternal wakening after the medication is stopped.

Adverse effects in the mother

The major risk of general anaesthesia is the same during birth as at any other time: regurgitation with aspiration (breathing in) of the acidic stomach contents. This results in a chemical injury to the lungs, *aspiration pneumonitis,* which can be fatal. Many women begin labour with a full stomach, and their gastric action slows during labour. In addition, the full uterus exerts upward pressure against the stomach. Therefore, every pregnant woman is presumed to have a full stomach for purposes of anaesthesia.

Adverse effects in the newborn

Respiratory depression is the main risk in the newborn, because medications given to the mother may cross the placenta. To reduce this risk, the time from induction of anaesthesia to clamping of the umbilical cord is kept as short as possible. The woman is prepped and draped for surgery, and all personnel are scrubbed, gowned, and gloved before anaesthesia begins. In addition, the anaesthesia is kept as light as possible until the cord is clamped. Personnel trained in neonatal resuscitation are present at the birth in anticipation of the need for resuscitation of the newborn.

Nurse's Role in Pharmacological Techniques

All obstetrical anaesthesia must be supervised by a registered nurse who is prepared to manage unexpected responses in the mother or the newborn. The nurse's responsibility in pharmacological pain management begins at admission (Nursing Care Plan 7.1). Information about the woman's allergies to foods, medications (including dental anaesthetics), and latex must be gathered to identify pain-relief measures that may not be advisable. The woman's preferences for pain-management options for labour and birth should be obtained on admission to the birthing suite. Factors that may have an impact on the choice of pain relief should be noted, such as a history of back surgery, infection in the area where an epidural block would be injected, or blood pressure abnormalities.

Nursing Care Plan 7.1 The Woman Needing Pain Management During Labour

PATIENT DATA

A woman, $G_1T_0P_0A_0L_0$, is in active labour and is 4 cm dilated. She is thrashing in bed and is not responding to coaching from her partner.

Selected Nursing Diagnosis Acute pain as a result of uterine contractions and descent of fetus in pelvis

Goals	Nursing Interventions	Rationales
The woman states that her discomfort is manageable during labour using techniques learned in childbirth preparation classes or taught by the nurse. The woman will have a relaxed facial and body appearance between contractions.	Continuously determine presence and character of pain during labour: • Statement of pain (assess nature of pain, such as location, intensity, whether intermittent or constant, and how well the woman is coping with pain) • Crying, moaning during and/or between contractions • Tense, guarded body posture or thrashing with contractions • "Mask of pain" facial expression	These are common verbal and nonverbal signs of pain; assessment enables the nurse to identify if pain is normal for the woman's labour status and to choose the best interventions for pain relief (nonpharmacological and/or pharmacological measures). Evaluating verbal and nonverbal communication helps the nurse to determine the need for pain relief in women who may not directly communicate their need for pain relief or who do not speak the prevailing language.
	Provide general comfort measures, such as: • Adjust the room temperature and light level for comfort. • Replace wet underpads frequently as needed. • Provide ice chips, Popsicles, or juices to relieve dry mouth. Provide a light diet as tolerated.	These general measures reduce outside distractions that make it harder for the woman to use childbirth preparation techniques and are themselves a source of discomfort. A comfortable environment is conducive to relaxation.
	Encourage the woman to assume positions she finds most comfortable, other than supine.	Position changes promote comfort and help the fetus adapt to the size and shape of woman's pelvis. A supine position can result in supine hypotension, which reduces placental blood flow and fetal oxygenation.
	Observe for a full bladder every 1 to 2 hours, or more often if the woman receives boluses of oral or intravenous (IV) fluids.	A full bladder is a source of discomfort and can prolong labour by inhibiting fetal descent.
	Promote use of techniques learned in childbirth preparation, including labour partner or support person as appropriate: • Do not stand in front of her focal point. • Offer a back rub or firm sacral pressure; ask her about the best location and amount of pressure; use powder to prevent skin irritation. • Encourage the woman to switch to more complex breathing patterns only when simpler ones are no longer effective. • Breathe along with the woman if she has trouble maintaining patterns; make eye contact.	These are examples of how to assist the woman and her partner in using learned methods most effectively. The use of nonpharmacological pain relief prevents problems associated with pharmacological interventions and supplements any medication therapy used. Nonpharmacological pain relief measures also provide the woman and her partner with a sense of control and mastery that enhances the perception of birth as a positive experience.
	If the woman has signs of hyperventilation (dizziness, numbness, or tingling sensations), have her breathe into her cupped hands, a small bag, or a washcloth placed over her mouth and nose.	Hyperventilation often occurs when the woman uses rapid breathing patterns, because she exhales too much carbon dioxide. These measures help her to conserve carbon dioxide and rebreathe it to correct for excess loss.

Continued

Nursing Care Plan 7.1 The Woman Needing Pain Management During Labour—cont'd

Goals	Nursing Interventions	Rationales
	Tell the woman and her partner when labour progresses; for example, if she is pushing and her infant's head becomes visible, let her see or feel it. Use a mirror so she can see the fetal head progress.	Labour does not last forever; her knowing that her efforts are having the desired results gives her courage to continue and helps her tolerate pain.

Selected Nursing Diagnosis Possible unfamiliarity with procedures and expected effects of epidural block

Goals	Nursing Interventions	Rationales
After explanations, the woman will state that she understands what will happen during and after epidural block is administered.	Explain what to expect as the epidural block is administered (reinforcing explanations of the anaesthesiologist) • An IV line will be started, and she will receive fluids to offset the tendency for blood pressure to fall. • The fetus will be monitored by intermittent auscultation, unless there are risk factors for mother or fetus. • The nurse will assist the anaesthesiologist to position the woman; she should remain still and in the desired position for insertion of the epidural catheter. • A small plastic catheter will be taped to her back to allow administration of medication. • Her blood pressure will be checked every 5 minutes when the epidural medication is first inserted.	This list reflects a common sequence of events for starting an epidural block. The anaesthesiologist explains the procedure and expected effects; the nurse reinforces explanations as needed, because the woman in pain may not be able to concentrate. Knowledge reduces anxiety and fear of the unknown. If the woman understands that these procedures are a normal part of an epidural block, she is less likely to interpret them as problems.
	If she needs to remain flat briefly to allow the medication to disperse, put a small pillow under her hip.	Placing a pillow under her hip helps prevent supine hypotension.
	Explain that she will feel less pain but will feel pressure; movement and sensation in her legs and feet will vary.	Explanations help the woman understand that the epidural block is not expected to totally eliminate the pain of labour. Leg movement and sensation are affected to varying degrees. If she understands these possible variations, she is less likely to interpret them as abnormal or as evidence that the block is not working.

Selected Nursing Diagnosis Possible risk for injury due to loss of sensation.

Goals	Nursing Interventions	Rationales
The woman will not have an injury, such as a muscle strain or fall, while her epidural block is in effect.	Check for movement, sensation, and leg strength before the woman starts ambulating; she should ambulate cautiously with an assistant. Assist the woman to change positions regularly.	A fall is more likely if the woman does not have sensation and control over her movements. A change of position prevents muscle strain.
	Observe for signs that birth may be near: increase in bloody show, perineal bulging, or crowning.	Loss of sensation varies among women having an epidural block. Labour may progress more rapidly than expected. These are signs associated with imminent birth that should be evaluated by the experienced nurse, the midwife, or the physician.

CRITICAL THINKING QUESTION

1. A woman, $G_2T_1P_0A_0L_1$, is in active labour. The last vaginal examination determined that her cervix was 7 cm dilated and 1 cm long (75% effaced). She states that her contraction pains are almost unbearable, even with the medication she has received. Because getting up and walking helped her earlier, and she needs to go to the bathroom now, she asks the nurse to help her out of bed to walk to the nearby bathroom. What would be the best response of the nurse?

Safety measures must be put in place for a woman who receives medications for pain relief. Opioids may cause drowsiness or dizziness, so the woman should not be left alone. Regional anaesthetics reduce sensation and movement to varying degrees; therefore, the woman may have less control over her body. Assessment of the woman's mobility is required prior to any attempt at ambulation.

The nurse reinforces the explanations given by the anaesthesiologist regarding procedures and the expected effects of the regional pain-management methods. Women often receive these explanations when they are very uncomfortable and do not remember everything they were told. The woman is assisted to the correct position for the insertion of an epidural, spinal, or combined spinal epidural block. The nurse informs the anaesthesiologist when the woman has a contraction during the insertion process to delay the procedure until after the contraction is completed. The anaesthetic medication is usually injected between contractions.

If an epidural or subarachnoid block is administered, the woman is assessed frequently for the development of hypotension. Hospital protocols vary, but blood pressure is usually measured every 5 minutes after the block begins (and with each reinjection) until her blood pressure is stable. An automatic blood pressure monitor is often used. Some facilities add a pulse oximeter to monitor oxygen saturation. At the same time, the nurse assesses the fetal heart rate for signs associated with fetal compromise (see Chapter 6), because maternal hypotension can reduce placental blood flow. Intermittent auscultation can be used with increased frequency following epidural insertion for a fetus without risk factors.

The epidural block is given during labour and may reduce the mother's sensation of rectal pressure. The nurse coaches her about the right time to start and stop pushing with each contraction if needed. The nurse also observes for signs of imminent birth, such as increased bloody show and perineal bulging, because the woman may not be able to feel the sensations distinctly.

Nursing responsibilities related to general anaesthesia include assessment and documentation of oral intake and administration of medications to reduce gastric acidity. The woman should be told that all preparations for surgery will be performed *before* she is anaesthetized. The nurse should reassure her that she will be asleep before any incision is made. Having a familiar nurse in the operating room full of new people can be reassuring to the woman before surgery.

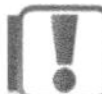

Safety Alert!

The following are important admission assessments related to pharmacological pain management: last oral intake (time and type), adverse reactions to medications (especially dental anaesthetics), other medications taken, and any food allergies or latex allergy.

When a woman receives opioid medications for pain relief in labour, the nurse must closely assess her respiratory rate for depression. Because respiratory depression is more likely to occur in the newborn than in the mother, the newborn is closely observed after birth. Opioid effects in the infant may persist longer than in an adult. The nurse must be prepared to implement the steps of neonatal resuscitation to provide support to a newborn experiencing respiratory depression (Wykoff et al., 2015).

The nurse observes the woman for late-appearing respiratory depression and excessive sedation if she received epidural narcotics after Caesarean birth. This may occur up to 24 hours after administration, depending on the amount and type of medication given. The woman's respiratory rate is monitored hourly, and a pulse oximeter may be applied. Facilities often use a scale to assess for sedation so all caregivers use the same criteria for assessment and documentation. Additional analgesics are given cautiously and strictly as ordered. If mild analgesics do not relieve the pain adequately, the health care provider is contacted for additional orders.

The woman who has received a general anaesthetic is usually awake enough to move from the operating table to her bed after surgery. Her respiratory status is observed every 15 minutes for 1 to 2 hours. A pulse oximeter provides constant information about her blood oxygen level. She is given oxygen by face mask or other means until she is fully awake. Her uterine fundus and vaginal bleeding are observed as for any other postpartum woman. Her urine output from the indwelling catheter should be observed for quantity and colour at least hourly for 4 hours. The nurse needs to assist the woman to ambulate when getting up for the first time to prevent the potential for falling. The woman is monitored closely for bladder distention and hypotension. Frequent ambulation is encouraged once full sensation and full motor control return.

Unfolding Case Study

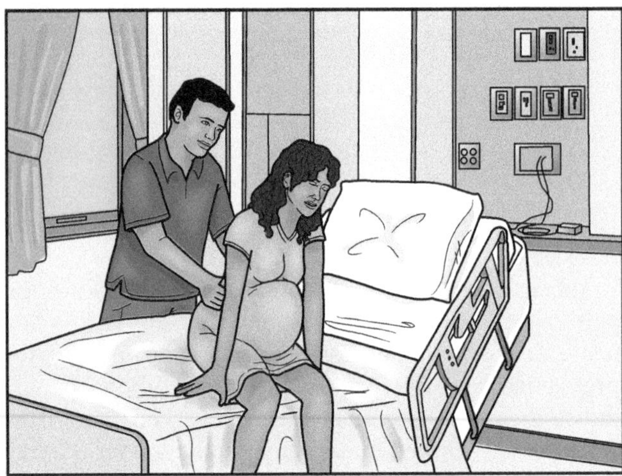

Tess and Luis were introduced to the reader in Chapter 2, and Tess's pregnancy experience has unfolded in each chapter. Refer to earlier chapters for her history and progress.

Tess has been admitted to the labour room in active labour at 40 weeks' gestation. She states that she has very painful contractions. Her partner, Luis, is at her side.

QUESTIONS

1. What causes Tess's labour pain? What factors influence Tess's labour pain?
2. What are some nonpharmacological pain-relief measures that the nurse can suggest to help Tess cope with her pain? With which measures can her partner, Luis, help?
3. What are some pharmacological measures for pain relief during labour? What are the nursing responsibilities involved in each?
4. What is the effect on the newborn of pharmacological pain-relief measures used during the labour process?
5. What are the nursing responsibilities in the care of the newborn that relate to Tess having pharmacological pain relief during labour?

Get Ready for the Certification Examination!

Key Points

- Pain during childbirth is different from other types of pain, because it is part of a normal process that results in the birth of an infant. The woman has time to prepare for it, and the pain is self-limiting.
- A woman's pain threshold is fairly constant. Her pain tolerance varies, and nursing actions aim to support her ability to tolerate pain.
- The pain of labour is caused by cervical dilation and effacement, uterine ischemia, and stretching of the vagina and perineum.
- Poorly relieved pain can decrease maternal satisfaction with the labour process.
- Childbirth preparation classes provide pain-management information and tools for the woman and her partner to use during labour. Some tools, such as breathing techniques and effleurage, can also be taught to the woman at the time of labour.
- The nurse supports the woman to try relaxation during labour because it enhances the effectiveness of all other pain-management methods, both nonpharmacological and pharmacological.
- Any medication taken by the pregnant women may cross the placenta and have an effect on the fetus. Effects may persist much longer after birth in the infant than in an adult.
- Observe the mother and infant for respiratory depression if the mother received opioids, including epidural narcotics, during the intrapartum period.
- Regional anaesthetics are a common choice for pain relief during labour because they allow the mother to remain awake, including for Caesarean birth.
- It is important to determine any medication allergies that the woman has when she is admitted.
- It is important to assess for reactions to dental anaesthetics because medications used for regional anaesthesia are related to those used in dentistry.
- Observe the mother's blood pressure and the fetal heart rate after epidural or spinal block to identify hypotension or fetal compromise. Assess for urinary retention.

Additional Learning Resources

evolve Go to your Evolve website (http://evolve.elsevier.com/Canada/Leifer) for the following learning resources:

- Answer Key for Critical Thinking Questions
- Answer Key for Textbook Review Questions
- Audio Glossary
- Fluids & Electrolytes tutorial
- Interactive Review Questions
- Skills Performance Checklists
- Video clips and more!

Online Resources

- Canadian Association of Perinatal and Women's Health Nurses (CAPWHN): http://www.capwhn.ca
- Lamaze International: https://www.lamazeinternational.org

Review Questions

1. Which of the following is most appropriately used for pain relief during labour when the cervix is dilated less than 4 cm?
   a. Narcan (naloxone) via intramuscular (IM) route
   b. Demerol (meperidine) via IM route
   c. Morphine sulphate (morphine) via IM route
   d. Fentanyl (Sublimaze) via epidural
2. Which technique is likely to be most effective for "back labour"?
   a. Stimulating the abdomen by effleurage
   b. Applying firm pressure in the sacral area
   c. Blowing out in short breaths during each contraction
   d. Rocking from side to side at the peak of each contraction
3. What medication should be immediately available for emergency use in the woman when she receives opioids during labour?
   a. Fentanyl (Sublimaze)
   b. Diphenhydramine (Benadryl)
   c. Lidocaine (Xylocaine)
   d. Naloxone (Narcan)
4. Select the most important nursing assessment immediately after a woman receives an epidural block.
   a. Bladder distention
   b. Condition of intravenous site
   c. Respiratory rate
   d. Blood pressure
5. A woman in labour states she wants to have epidural analgesia. When is the best time for this method of analgesia be given?
   a. Anytime during labour
   b. During prelabour
   c. During the first stage of labour
   d. During the third stage of labour
6. A woman who is in the early first stage of labour asks how she can relieve her discomfort. The nurse knows that nonpharmacological techniques that can relieve discomfort include which of the following? *(Select all that apply.)*
   a. Sacral pressure
   b. Effleurage
   c. Sitz bath
   d. Laxatives
   e. Massage

REFERENCES

Berghella, V., & Saccone, G. (2017). Exercise in pregnancy!. *American Journal of Obstetrics & Gynecology, 216*(4), 335–337.

Bonapace, J., Gagné, G. P., Chaillet, N., et al. (2018). SOGC clinical practice guideline: No. 355—Physiologic basis of pain in labour and delivery: An evidence-based approach to its management. *Journal of Obstetrics & Gynaecology Canada, 40*(2), 227–245. https://doi.org/10.1016/j.jogc.2017.08.003.

Canadian Paediatric Society (CPS). (2017). *2016 Medications for Neonatal Resuscitation Program—Canadian Adaptation.* Retrieved from: https://www.cps.ca/uploads/nrp/Medications_for_NRP_2016_v03.pdf.

Hawkins, J., & Bucklin, D. (2017). Obstetric anesthesia. In S. G. Gabbe, J. R. Niebyl, J. L. Simpson, et al. (Eds.), *Obstetrics: Normal and problem pregnancies* (7th ed.). Philadelphia: Saunders.

Lamaze International. (2018). *Lamaze Healthy Birth Practices.* Retrieved from: https://www.lamazeinternational.org/healthybirthpractices.

Liston, R., Sawchuck, D., Young, D., et al. (2018). No. 197b fetal health surveillance: Intrapartum consensus guideline. *Journal of Obstetrics and Gynaecology Canada, 40*(4), e298–e322.

Morin, F., & Rivard, L. (2017). Pain management during labour. In S. Perry, M. Hockenberry, D. Lowdermilk, et al. (Eds.), *Maternal child nursing care in Canada* (2nd ed.). Toronto, ON: Elsevier.

Mottola, M. F., Davenport, M. H., Ruchat, S., et al. (2019). Canadian guideline for physical activity throughout pregnancy. *British Journal of Sports Medicine, 52*, 1339–1346.

Ordean, A., Wong, S., & Graves, L. (2017). Substance use in pregnancy. *Journal of Obstetrics and Gynaecology Canada, 39*(10), 922–937. https://doi.org/10.1016/j.jogc.2017.04.028. e2.

Perinatal Services of British Columbia. (2007). *Obstetric guideline 4: Pain management options during labour*. Reaffirmed, 2010. Retrieved from: http://www.perinatalservicesbc.ca/Documents/Guidelines-Standards/Maternal/PainManagementGuideline.pdf.

Public Health Agency of Canada (PHAC). (2018). Care during labour and birth. In *family-centred maternity and newborn care: national guidelines*. Ottawa: Author. Retrieved from: https://www.canada.ca/en/public-health/services/publications/healthy-living/maternity-newborn-care-guidelines-chapter-4.html.

Wyckoff, M. H., Aziz, K., Escobedo, M. B., et al. (2015). Part 13: Neonatal resuscitation: 2015 American Heart Association guidelines update for cardiopulmonary resuscitation and emergency cardiovascular care. *Circulation, 132*(Suppl. 2), S543–S560.

8 Nursing Care of Women With Complications During Labour and Birth

http://evolve.elsevier.com/Canada/Leifer

Nancy Watts

Objectives

1. Define each key term listed.
2. Describe each obstetrical procedure discussed in this chapter.
3. Understand the nurse's role in each obstetrical procedure.
4. Describe the nurse's role(s) in a Caesarean birth.
5. Describe factors that contribute to an abnormal labour.
6. Understand the intrapartum complications or emergencies described within this chapter.
7. Discuss the nurse's role in caring for women and families with intrapartum complications.

Key Terms

amniotic fluid embolism
anaphylactoid syndrome
artificial rupture of membranes (AROM)
augmentation of labour
Bishop score
cephalopelvic disproportion (sĕf-ăh-lō-PĔL-vĭc dĭs-prŏ-PŎR-shŭn)
chorioamnionitis (kō-rē-ō-ăm-nē-ō-NĪ-tĭs)
complementary and alternative health modalities (CAHM)
dysfunctional labour
dystocia
external cephalic version (ECV)
fetal fibronectin (fFN) test (fī-brō-NĔK-tĭn tĕst)
hydramnios (hī-DRĂM-nē-ōs)
induction of labour
laminaria (lăm-ĭ-NĂ-rē-ăh)
macrosomia (măk-rō-SŌM-ē-ă)
oligohydramnios (ŏl-ĭ-gō-hī-DRĂM-nē-ōs)
placenta accreta
polyhydramnios
shoulder dystocia (SHŌL-dŭr dĭs-TŌ-sē-ă)
spontaneous rupture of membranes (SROM)
tocolytics (tō-kō-LĬT-ĭks)

Childbirth is a normal, natural event that occurs in the lives of many women and their families. When a woman has a healthy low-risk pregnancy, often she will have a normal labour and birth. However, complications can occur in women with low-risk or high-risk pregnancies and may be unexpected, affecting maternal health, that of their infant, or both.

INDUCTION OR AUGMENTATION OF LABOUR

Induction of labour is the artificial initiation of labour before it begins naturally. The Society of Obstetricians and Gynaecologists of Canada (SOGC) states that the goal of induction is to achieve a successful vaginal birth that is as normal as possible (Leduc, Biringer, Lee, et al., 2013). **Augmentation of labour** is the stimulation of contractions after they have begun naturally.

Labour involves the complex interaction between fetus and mother. Before labour is induced, it is important that fetal maturity be confirmed, as induction is avoided before 39 weeks' and, ideally, after 40 weeks' gestation. Use of a first-trimester ultrasound report can assist with dating this pregnancy to ensure growth and development of the fetus. Amniotic fluid analysis (lecithin/sphingomyelin [L/S] ratio) (see Chapter 5) may be considered if a preterm infant requires induction based on medical indications. The **Bishop score** is used to assess the status of the cervix in determining its response to induction (Table 8.1). The presence of increased fetal fibronectin at the cervix and a Bishop score above 6 determine cervical readiness for labour induction. Continuous assessment of uterine activity and fetal heart rate (FHR) monitoring during labour induction is recommended by the SOGC (Liston, Sawchuck, Young, et al., 2018).

INDICATIONS FOR INDUCTION

Labour is induced if the risk of continuing the pregnancy for the woman or the fetus(es) is greater than the risk associated with the induced labour and birth. The following are some of the indications for labour induction:

- Gestational hypertension (GH) or pre-eclampsia (see Chapter 5)
- Ruptured membranes without spontaneous onset of labour, particularly with group B streptococcus (GBS) colonization
- Infection within the uterus (chorioamnionitis)

Table 8.1 Modified Bishop Scoring System

SCORE	0	1	2	3
Dilation of cervix (cm)	0	1–2	3–4	5–6
Consistency of cervix	Firm	Medium	Soft	—
Length of cervix (cm)	>4	2–4	1–2	1–2
Cervical effacement (%)	0–30	40–50	60–70	80
Position of cervix	Posterior	Midline	Anterior	—
Station of presenting part related to ischial spines	−3	−2	−1 or 0	+1 or +2

NOTE: A high score is predictive of a successful labour induction, because the cervix has ripened, or softened, in preparation for labour. The Society of Obstetricians and Gynaecologists of Canada (SOGC) recommends a score of 6 or above before induction of labour.
Modified from Leduc, D., Biringer, A., Lee, L., et al. (2013). SOGC clinical practice guideline: Induction of labour. *Journal of Obstetrics and Gynaecology Canada, 35*(9), S1–S18. Stables, D., & Rankin, J. (2005). *Physiology in childbearing: With anatomy and related biosciences* (2nd ed.). Edinburgh: Elsevier.

- Medical problems in the woman that worsen during pregnancy, such as diabetes or renal or pulmonary disease
- Fetal concerns, such as intrauterine growth restriction, prolonged pregnancy, or incompatibility between fetal and maternal blood types (see Chapter 5)
- Placental insufficiency
- Intrauterine fetal death

Convenience for the health care provider or the family is not an indication for inducing labour. However, the woman who has a history of rapid labour and lives a long distance from the birth facility may have her labour induced because she has a higher risk of giving birth en route if she awaits spontaneous labour.

CONTRAINDICATIONS TO INDUCTION

Labour is *not* induced in the following conditions:

- Placenta previa (see Chapter 5)
- Umbilical cord prolapse
- Abnormal fetal lie or presentation (e.g., footling breech)
- Active herpes infection externally or in the birth canal, which the infant can acquire during birth
- Pelvic structural deformities
- Suspected fetal macrosomia
- Previous classic (vertical) Caesarean incision or inverted T incision
- Previous uterine rupture

The health care provider may attempt to induce labour in a preterm pregnancy if continuing the pregnancy is more harmful to the woman or the fetus than the hazards of prematurity would be to the infant.

NONPHARMACOLOGICAL METHODS TO STIMULATE CONTRACTIONS

Natural or Complementary Methods of Inducing Labour

Complementary and alternative health modalities (CAHM) offer "natural" methods of stimulating labour that have been practiced for centuries but often lack the rigorous and controlled studies to prove effectiveness. One CAHM therapy that may be suggested by a midwife or doula is nipple stimulation. Stimulating the nipples causes the woman's posterior pituitary gland to secrete oxytocin naturally. This improves the quality of contractions that have slowed or weakened, just as intravenous (IV) administration of synthetic oxytocin does. The woman can stimulate her nipples by doing the following:

- Pulling or rolling them, one at a time
- Gently brushing them with a dry washcloth
- Using water in a whirlpool tub or a shower
- Applying suction with a breast pump

Sexual intercourse may also be used to stimulate labour as orgasm that occurs during sexual intercourse stimulates uterine contractions, and the male ejaculate contains prostaglandins. Acupuncture and acupressure, given by professional practitioners, have been used for centuries to stimulate labour. If contractions become too strong with these techniques, the woman simply stops stimulation.

See Table 4.4 for common herbs contraindicated in pregnancy and lactation.

Position changes

Many women benefit from changing position or ambulation if their labour slows. Walking stimulates contractions, eases the pressure of the fetus on the mother's back, and adds gravity to the downward force of contractions and is a method of augmenting labour. She can sit (in a chair, on the side of the bed, or in the bed), squat, kneel while facing the raised head of the bed for support, or maintain other upright positions. Use of a peanut ball may be helpful in position changes, particularly for those women who have had an epidural for pain management (Fig. 8.1).

Membrane sweeping

Routine sweeping (stripping) of the membranes promotes the onset of labour and involves the insertion of a digit past the internal cervical os with massage or "sweeps" of the membranes. The woman may experience some discomfort and the potential of bleeding postprocedure. In collaboration with the woman, the health care provider could choose to perform this in the clinic or office when the woman is reaching term or postdates before initiating an induction.

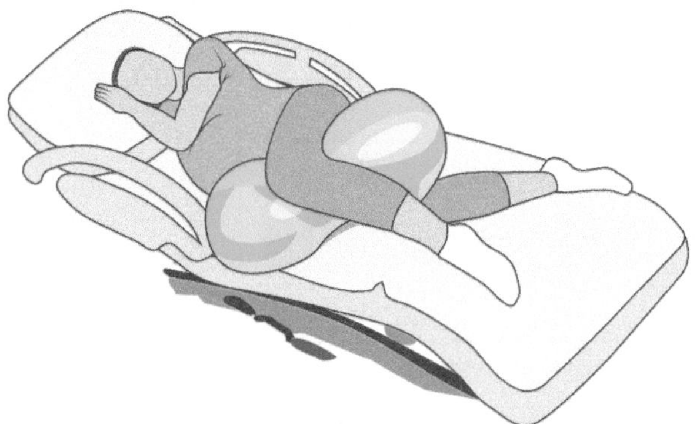

Fig. 8.1 Optimal maternal positioning for fetal descent can be achieved with the use of a peanut ball during labour. In this position the woman has her upper leg as far as possible away from her lower leg (increasing the transverse diameter of the pelvis) and allows the sacrum and coccyx to move back (increasing the anterior-posterior diameter of the pelvis). (Source: © CanStock Photo Inc./bearsky23)

PHARMACOLOGICAL AND MECHANICAL METHODS TO STIMULATE CONTRACTIONS

Cervical ripening is the physical softening of the cervix that leads to effacement and dilation. Induction of labour is more effective if the woman's cervix is "ripe" or prepared for labour (see Table 8.1). These prelabour cervical changes occur naturally in many women toward the end of the third trimester. Methods to hasten the changes, or "ripen" the cervix, ease labour induction because oxytocic drugs may have no effect on the unripe cervix. Oxytocin used to induce labour without a ripe cervix increases the risk of needing a Caesarean birth (Sheibani & Wing, 2017). Cervical ripening can be achieved by pharmacological or mechanical means.

Pharmacological Methods

Prostaglandins act on the cervix by dissolving the collagen structural network of the cervix (ripen the cervix). They are contraindicated in women with a history of uterine myomectomy surgery or previous Caesarean birth because of the risk of uterine rupture (based on the risk of hypertonic contractions). Women with asthma are also at risk with prostaglandin preparations as these medications are bronchodilators and could worsen their condition.

Prostaglandin E_2

Dinoprostone (Cervidil) vaginal insertion is recommended via a sustained-release vaginal insert, as it can be removed if there are adverse effects such as tachysystole. Prostin gel is applied intravaginally or intracervically as alternative methods of cervical preparation with appropriate fetal monitoring before and after the procedure.

Prostaglandin E_1

Misoprostol was designed for treatment of peptic ulcer disease. The use as a preinduction medication both for cervical ripening and labour induction is considered an "off-label" use. It can be administered orally (sublingual or buccal) or intravaginally. Prostaglandin E_1 is more effective at achieving vaginal birth within 24 hours, but it is associated with uterine tachysystole and FHR abnormalities.

Nursing care related to prostaglandin insertion. The procedure should be explained to the woman and her family. An FHR baseline is recorded for 20 minutes. After insertion of the prostaglandin gel or insert, the woman remains in a supine position (with a wedge on one side) for 1 to 2 hours and is monitored for uterine contractions. Vital signs and FHR are also recorded. Oxytocin induction can be started when the insert is removed—usually after 6 to 12 hours. Signs of uterine tachysystole include 10 or more uterine contractions in 20 minutes with or without alteration of FHR or pattern.

The vaginal insert can be removed by pulling on the netted string that protrudes from the vaginal orifice. Some women who receive cervical ripening products begin labour without additional oxytocin stimulation.

Mechanical Methods

Hydroscopic dilators

Laminaria tents and Lamicel are mechanical dilators placed in the lower uterine segment that stimulate the release of prostaglandins from the fetal membranes and maternal decidua. They swell inside the cervix, resulting in mechanical cervical dilation. This is a method most often used for a nonviable fetus or in preparation for a second-trimester termination of pregnancy.

Transcervical balloon dilators

A 16-Fr catheter with a 30-mL balloon is inserted through the cervix and inflated. Mechanical pressure by gentle traction against the cervix dilates the cervix. This can be done as an outpatient procedure with the woman returning in 12 hours to start oxytocin, if needed, or sooner if there are signs of labour or the Foley catheter falls out. FHR monitoring before and after the procedure for 20 to 30 minutes is required. This is often used for women who have had a previous Caesarean birth and having a trial of labour.

Amniotomy

Amniotomy is the **artificial rupture of membranes (AROM)** (amniotic sac) using a sterile, sharp instrument to puncture the amniotic sac and release the amniotic fluid in order to induce or augment labour. It may also be performed to enable internal fetal monitoring (see Chapter 6). A health care provider performs the procedure. The nurse assists the health care provider with the procedure and cares for the woman and fetus afterward. Confirmation of a vertex presentation and the station is essential to prevent umbilical cord prolapse. The amniotomy stimulates prostaglandin secretion, which stimulates labour, but the loss of amniotic fluid may result in umbilical cord compression.

Complications of amniotomy. Three complications associated with amniotomy may also occur if a woman's membranes rupture spontaneously (**spontaneous rupture of**

membranes [SROM]). These complications are prolapse of the umbilical cord, infection, and placental abruption.

Prolapse of the umbilical cord. Prolapse may occur if the cord slips downward with the gush of amniotic fluid. This is considered an obstetrical emergency.

Infection. Infection may occur because the membranes no longer block vaginal organisms from entering the uterus. Once performed, an amniotomy commits the woman to birth within a certain time frame; the health care provider delays amniotomy until reasonably sure that birth will occur before the risk of infection markedly increases.

Placental abruption. Placental abruption (separation of the placenta before birth) is more likely to occur if the uterus is overdistended with amniotic fluid (hydramnios) when the membranes rupture. The uterus becomes smaller with the discharge of amniotic fluid, but the placenta stays the same size and no longer fits its implantation site (see Chapter 5 for more information about placental abruption).

Nursing care after amniotomy. Nursing care after amniotomy is the same as that after spontaneous membrane rupture: assessing the FHR (intermittent auscultation or continuous fetal heart monitoring depending on the woman's risk factors), observing for the colour and amount of fluid, and promoting the woman's comfort.

> **Nursing Tip**
>
> Observe for wet underpads and linens after the membranes rupture. Change them as often as needed to keep the woman relatively dry and to reduce the risk for infection or skin breakdown.

Observing for complications. The FHR is recorded for at least 1 minute after amniotomy. Rates outside the normal range of 110 to 160 beats/min for a term fetus suggest a prolapsed umbilical cord. A large quantity of fluid increases the risk for prolapsed cord, especially if the fetus is high in the pelvis.

The fluid should be clear, possibly with flecks of vernix (newborn skin coating) and lanugo, and should not have a bad odour. Cloudy, yellow, or malodorous fluid suggests infection. Green fluid means that the fetus passed the first stool (meconium) into the fluid before birth. Meconium-stained amniotic fluid is associated with fetal compromise during labour and infant respiratory distress after birth.

The woman's temperature is taken every 2 hours after her membranes rupture, according to facility policy. A maternal temperature of 38°C (100.4°F) or higher suggests infection. An increase in FHR, especially if above 160 beats/min, may precede the woman's temperature increase.

Promoting comfort. When amniotomy is anticipated, several disposable underpads are placed under the woman's hips to absorb the fluid that continues to leak from the woman's vagina during labour. Disposable underpads are changed often enough to keep her reasonably dry and to reduce the moist, warm environment that favours the growth of microorganisms.

Oxytocin Induction or Augmentation of Labour

Initiation or stimulation of contractions with oxytocin (Syntocinon) is the most common method of labour induction and augmentation in women with a favourable or ripe cervix (Sheibani & Wing, 2017). Registered nurses (RNs) who have additional training in the induction of labour and electronic fetal monitoring administer oxytocin. Augmentation of labour with oxytocin follows a similar procedure to other methods of induction.

Oxytocin for induction or augmentation of labour is diluted in an IV solution. The oxytocin solution is a secondary (piggyback) infusion that is inserted into the primary (nonmedicated) IV solution line so it can be stopped quickly while an open IV line is maintained. The infusion of oxytocin solution is regulated with an infusion pump. Administration begins at a very low rate and is titrated upward or downward according to how the fetus responds to labour and to the woman's contractions (as per facility policy or orders). The dose is individualized for every woman. When contractions are well established, it is often possible to reduce the rate of oxytocin. Augmentation of labour usually requires less total oxytocin than induction of labour because the uterus is more sensitive to the medication when labour has already begun.

Continuous electronic monitoring is used to assess and record fetal and maternal responses to oxytocin. Some women may require internal methods of monitoring when oxytocin is used, because it is important to assess for contraction intensity and FHR. Women who are obese or have an increased body mass index (BMI) may require internal monitoring for safe use of oxytocin. Oxytocin checklists have been developed in some institutions to promote safety with the use of oxytocin as a high-alert medication (associated with preventable adverse effects and harm). Vital signs are monitored closely. Oxytocin is also used in the fourth stage of labour to induce contraction of the uterus and to reduce uterine bleeding after the placenta has been delivered.

Complications of oxytocin induction or augmentation of labour

The most common complications related to the use of oxytocin to stimulate contractions are decreased fetal circulation based on too frequent contractions (tachysystole) and uterine rupture. Blood flow to the placenta is reduced if contractions are excessive. Most placental exchange of oxygen, nutrients, and waste products occur between contractions. This exchange is likely to be impaired if the contractions are too long, too frequent, or too intense (more than five in 10 minutes, last longer than 90 seconds, or have less than 60 seconds between contractions).

Water intoxication sometimes occurs, because oxytocin inhibits the excretion of urine and promotes fluid retention. Water intoxication is not likely with the small amounts of oxytocin and fluids given intravenously during labour, but it is more likely to occur if large doses of oxytocin and fluids are given intravenously after birth, for example, with a postpartum hemorrhage.

Oxytocin is discontinued, or its rate reduced, if abnormal or atypical FHRs are noted or excessive uterine contractions occur. FHR outside the normal range of 110 to 160 beats/min, late or repetitive variable decelerations, and decreased variability (see Chapter 6) are the most common signs of fetal compromise.

> **Safety Alert!**
>
> Tachysystole is most often evidenced by greater than five uterine contractions in 10 minutes with or without alteration of fetal heart rate or pattern (Leduc et al., 2013).

The resting tone of the uterus (muscle tension when it is not contracting) is often higher than normal. Internal uterine activity monitoring allows determination of peak uterine pressures and uterine resting tone.

In addition to stopping the infusion or decreasing the oxytocin by half, the RN can choose one or more of the following measures to correct adverse maternal or fetal reactions:

- Increasing the nonmedicated or mainline IV solution
- Changing the woman's position, avoiding the supine position
- Giving oxygen by face mask at 8 to 10 L/min

The health care provider is notified after corrective measures are taken. A tocolytic medication such as nitroglycerine as a one-time spray may be administered by the health care provider if the excessive contractions do not resolve with the above measures (Leduc et al., 2013).

> **Safety Alert!**
>
> Intravenous oxytocin is considered to be a high-alert medication because it has an increased risk of causing significant adverse reactions if used incorrectly.
>
> The nurse must be aware of signs and symptoms of increased uterine activity and must monitor the fetal heart rate (FHR) continuously with documentation every 15 minutes during active labour and every 5 minutes during the pushing phase of the second stage of labour. Safety interventions for oxytocin-induced uterine contractions or FHR abnormalities include the following:
>
> - Notifying the health care provider and the registered nurse
> - Repositioning the woman to left or right lateral position
> - Decreasing the dose of oxytocin to half of the current rate or discontinuing oxytocin (as per hospital policy or orders)
> - Preparing an intravenous bolus of lactated Ringer's or normal saline
> - Administering oxygen at 8 to 10 L/min via a nonrebreather face mask
> - Assessing uterine contractions and FHR every 5 minutes

Nursing care during induction or augmentation

The SOGC recommends that an RN provide one-to-one care for patients undergoing oxytocin-induced labour (Leduc et al., 2013). The FHR must be assessed and recorded every 15 minutes during active labour and every 5 minutes once the woman is pushing in the second stage. Baseline maternal vital signs are assessed, and a fetal monitor tracing is performed to identify contraindications to induction or augmentation before the procedure begins.

If abnormalities are noted in either the mother or fetus, the nurse stops the oxytocin and begins measures to reduce contractions and increase placental blood flow. The woman's blood pressure, pulse rate, and respirations are measured every 30 to 60 minutes. Her temperature is taken every 2 hours if membranes are ruptured. Recording her intake and output hourly helps in identifying potential water intoxication.

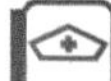

> **Nursing Tip**
>
> Women who have oxytocin stimulation of labour may find that their contractions are more painful more quickly than with the gradual progression of labour. The nurse can help the woman stay focused on breathing and relaxation techniques with each contraction and offer other pain management strategies as requested by the woman, such as an epidural, patient-controlled analgesia (PCA), or hydrotherapy.

OBSTETRICAL PROCEDURES

Nurses assist with several obstetrical procedures during birth; they also care for women after the procedures. Some procedures, such as amnioinfusion, are performed to prevent complications during birth. Other procedures are needed when the woman has a complication that necessitates an intervention to promote a positive outcome for the mother and fetus.

AMNIOFUSION

An *amnioinfusion* is the injection of warmed sterile saline or lactated Ringer's solution into the uterus via an intrauterine pressure catheter during labour after the membranes have ruptured. The goal of this procedure is to increase the amniotic fluid surrounding the baby, decreasing the risk of umbilical cord compression and variable decelerations. Amnioinfusion replaces the "cushion" for the umbilical cord and relieves variable decelerations of the FHR that may occur during contractions when the volume of amniotic fluid is decreased. It can be administered as a onetime bolus for 1 hour or as a continuous infusion. Continuous monitoring of uterine activity and FHR is essential. The nurse providing care changes pads on the bed for patient comfort and assesses colour, amount, and odour of fluid discharged from the vagina following the procedure.

EXTERNAL CEPHALIC VERSION

External cephalic version (ECV) is a method of changing the fetal presentation, usually from breech or oblique to cephalic. There are two methods: external and internal. External version is the more common one. A successful version increases the chances of a woman having a vaginal birth rather than needing a Caesarean birth.

Risks and Contraindications of Version

ECV is not indicated if there is any maternal or fetal reason that vaginal birth should not occur, because that is its goal. The following are examples of maternal or fetal conditions that are contraindications for an external cephalic version:

- Disproportion between the mother's pelvis and fetal size
- Abnormal uterine or pelvic size or shape
- Abnormal placental placement
- Previous Caesarean birth with a vertical uterine incision
- Active herpes virus infection
- Inadequate amniotic fluid
- Placental insufficiency
- Multiple gestation

An ECV may not be attempted in a woman who has a higher risk for uterine rupture, such as several previous Caesarean births or high parity. An ECV is not usually attempted if the fetal presenting part is engaged in the pelvis. The main risk to the fetus is that it will become entangled in the umbilical cord, thus compressing the cord. This is more likely to happen if there is not adequate room to turn the fetus, such as in multifetal gestation (e.g., twins) or when the amount of amniotic fluid is minimal.

Technique

ECV is usually done between 36 and 38 weeks of gestation but before the onset of labour. The procedure begins with a non–stress test (NST) or biophysical profile (BPP; see Table 5.1) to determine whether the fetus is healthy and if there is adequate amniotic fluid to perform the version. The woman may have an IV started in case it is needed for an emergency birth or to receive a muscle relaxant to assist with the external manoeuvres involved in turning the fetus.

Using ultrasound to guide the procedure, the obstetrical health care provider pushes the fetal buttocks upward out of the pelvis while pushing the fetal head downward toward the pelvis in either a clockwise or a counterclockwise turn. The fetus is monitored frequently during the procedure. Rh-negative women receive a dose of $Rh_0(D)$ immune globulin to prevent development of RH-positive antibodies if the fetus is RH positive.

Internal version is an emergency procedure. The health care provider usually performs internal version during a vaginal birth of twins to change the fetal presentation of the second twin.

Nursing Care

Nursing care of the woman having an external version includes assisting with the procedure and observing the mother and fetus afterward for 1 to 2 hours. Baseline maternal vital signs and a fetal monitor strip (NST) are taken before the version. The mother's vital signs and the FHR are observed to ensure return to normal levels after the version is complete.

Vaginal leaking of amniotic fluid suggests that manipulating the fetus caused a tear in the membranes, and this must be reported to the health care provider. Uterine contractions usually decrease or stop shortly after the version. The health care provider is notified if they do not. The nurse needs to review signs of labour with the woman because ECV is performed near term, when spontaneous labour is expected.

EPISIOTOMY AND LACERATIONS

Episiotomy is the surgical enlargement of the vaginal opening. A *laceration* is a tear in the tissues that occurs during birth. Both are discussed in Chapter 6.

FORCEPS AND VACUUM EXTRACTION BIRTHS

A health care provider uses forceps or a vacuum extractor to provide traction and rotation to the fetal head when the mother's pushing efforts are insufficient to accomplish a safe birth. *Forceps* are instruments with curved blades that fit around the fetal head without unduly compressing it (Fig. 8.2). Several different styles are available to assist the birth of the fetal head in a cephalic presentation or the after-coming head in a breech birth. Forceps may also help the health care provider extract the fetal head through the incision during Caesarean birth.

A vacuum extractor uses suction applied to the fetal head so that the health care provider can assist the mother's expulsive efforts (Fig. 8.3). One advantage of the vacuum extractor is that it does not take up room in the mother's pelvis, as forceps do. The rate of assisted vaginal births—births aided by forceps or vacuum—has declined from 17.4% in 1991/92 to 13.2% in 2015/16. Specifically, the rate of vacuum extraction has increased from 6.8 to 9.2%, while the rate of forceps-assisted birth has declined from 11.2 to 3.4% over that same period (Public Health Agency of Canada [PHAC], 2018).

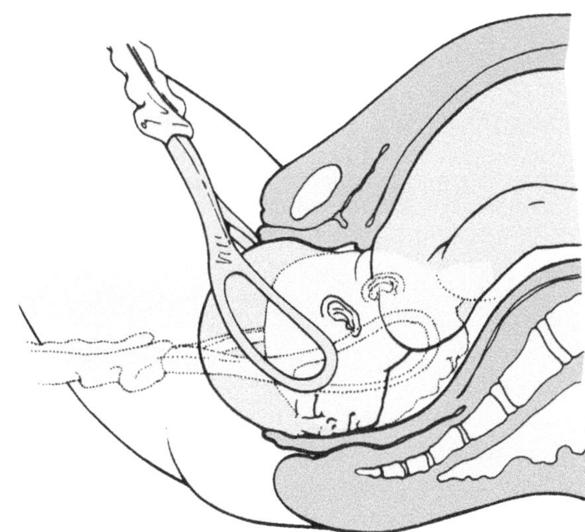

Fig. 8.2 Use of forceps to assist with the birth of the fetal head. After applying the forceps to each side of the fetal head and locking the two blades, the health care provider pulls, following the pelvic curve.

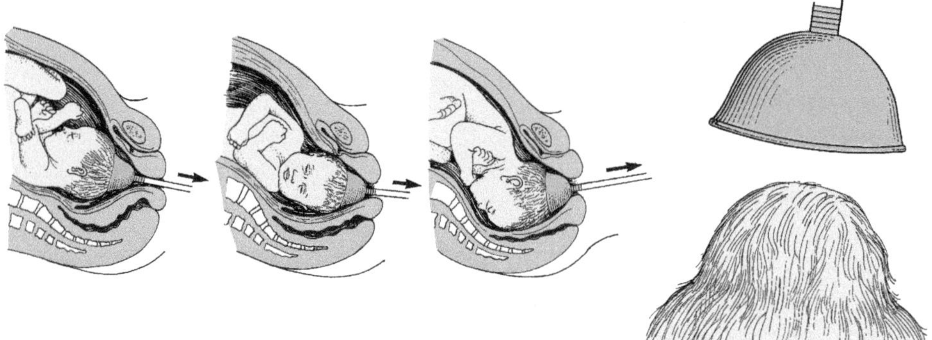

Fig. 8.3 Use of the vacuum extractor to rotate the fetal head and assist with birth. The arrows indicate the direction of traction on the vacuum cup. The vacuum cup is positioned on the midline, near the posterior fontanelle. (From Lowdermilk, D. L., Perry, S. E., & Cashion, K. L. [2013]. *Maternity nursing* [8th ed.]. St. Louis: Mosby.)

Indications

Forceps or vacuum extraction should only be used to end the second stage of labour if it is in the best interest of the mother or fetus. The mother may be exhausted, or she may be unable to push effectively. Women with cardiac or pulmonary disorders may have forceps or vacuum extraction births because prolonged pushing can worsen these conditions. Fetal indications include conditions in which there is evidence of an increased risk to the fetus near the end of labour. The cervix must be fully dilated, the membranes ruptured, the bladder empty, and the fetal head engaged and at +2 station for optimal outcome.

Contraindications

The use of these techniques is not done if they would be more traumatic than Caesarean birth, such as when the fetus is high in the pelvis or too large for a vaginal birth.

Risks

Trauma to maternal or fetal tissues is the main risk when forceps or vacuum extraction is used. The mother may have a laceration or hematoma (collection of blood in the tissues) in her vagina. The infant may have bruising, facial or scalp lacerations or abrasions, cephalohematoma (see Chapter 11), or intracranial hemorrhage. The vacuum extractor causes a harmless area of circular edema on the infant's scalp where it was applied.

> **Nursing Tip**
>
> Many parents are concerned about the marks made by forceps. Reassure them that these marks are temporary and usually resolve without treatment.

Technique

The woman is catheterized to prevent trauma to her bladder and to make more room in her pelvis. After the forceps are applied, the health care provider pulls in line with the pelvic curve. An episiotomy may be required, although usually it is not necessary. After the fetal head is brought under the mother's symphysis pubis, the rest of the birth occurs in the usual way.

Birth assisted with the vacuum extractor follows a similar sequence. The health care provider applies the cup over the posterior fontanelle of the fetal occiput, and suction is created with a machine to hold it there. Traction is applied by pulling on the handle of the extractor cup.

Nursing Care

If the use of forceps or vacuum extraction is anticipated, the nurse places the sterile equipment on the instrument table. After birth, care is similar to that for episiotomy and perineal lacerations. Ice is applied to the perineum to reduce bruising and edema. The health care provider is notified if the woman has signs of vaginal hematoma, which include severe and poorly relieved pelvic or rectal pain.

The infant's head is examined for lacerations, abrasions, or bruising. Mild facial reddening and moulding (alteration in shape) of the head are common and do not require treatment.

Pressure from forceps may injure the infant's facial nerve. This is evidenced by facial asymmetry (different appearance of right and left sides), which is most obvious when the infant cries. Facial nerve injury usually resolves without treatment. The scalp swelling from the vacuum extractor does not require intervention and resolves quickly.

CAESAREAN BIRTH

Caesarean birth is the surgical birth of the fetus through incisions in the mother's abdomen and uterus. Caesarean section is currently the most common major surgical procedure in Canada, with a rate of 28% in 2016–2017 (Canadian Institute for Health Information [CIHI], 2018). Various organizations such as Health Quality Ontario (2018) have produced recommendations around strategies such as the promotion of vaginal birth after Caesarean and normal birth to try to address the rising Caesarean birth rate. Some of these practices include the following:

- Ambulation or position changes in labour
- Epidural analgesia that allows ambulation and birth in various positions (i.e., less motor block)

- Oxytocin augmentation of labour
- Spontaneous open glottis pushing
- Use of operative-assisted birth (e.g., forceps and vacuum), with skills practice for health care providers
- Electronic fetal and uterine monitoring for high-risk pregnancies

Indications

Several conditions may necessitate Caesarean birth:

- Abnormal labour
- Inability of the fetus to pass through the mother's pelvis (**cephalopelvic disproportion**)
- Abnormal fetal presentation (Many breech presentations are born by Caesarean section.)
- Active maternal herpes virus, which may cause serious or fatal infant infection
- Previous surgery on the uterus, including the classic or unknown type of Caesarean incision
- Fetal compromise, including prolapsed umbilical cord and abnormal presentations
- Placenta previa or placental abruption

Contraindications

There are few contraindications to Caesarean birth, but it is not usually performed if the fetus is not viable or too premature to survive or if the mother has abnormal blood clotting. A Caesarean birth should NOT be planned for the convenience of the woman, as there are risks involved.

Risks

Caesarean birth carries risks to both mother and fetus. Maternal risks are similar to those of other types of surgery and include the following:

- Risks related to anaesthesia (see Chapter 7)
- Respiratory complications
- Hemorrhage
- Blood clots
- Injury to the urinary tract
- Delayed intestinal peristalsis (paralytic ileus)
- Infection
- Slower recovery time
- Scarring of the uterus may influence options for future pregnancies.

Risks to the newborn may include the following:

- Inadvertent preterm birth
- Respiratory problems because of delayed absorption of lung fluid
- Injury, such as laceration or bruising

Technique

Caesarean birth may occur under planned, unplanned, or emergency conditions. The preparation is similar for each and includes routine preoperative care such as obtaining informed consent. If the woman wears eyeglasses, they should accompany her to the operating room, because she is usually awake and seeing her infant aids with attachment during the birth process.

Preparations for Caesarean birth

As with other surgeries, several laboratory studies are performed to identify anemia or blood-clotting abnormalities. Complete blood count, coagulation studies, and blood typing and history screening are common, and appropriate consent is obtained. One or more units of blood may be typed and cross-matched if the woman is likely to need a transfusion. The baseline vital signs of the mother and the FHR are recorded. The woman is placed in a supine position with a wedge under the hip to prevent decreased blood flow to the fetus. Medication to reduce gastric acidity and speed gastric emptying is provided and a regional anaesthetic is usually administered. A prophylactic IV antibiotic will be administered before the incision is made. Shaving of the skin or hair removal is not necessary and could increase the risk of infection.

An indwelling Foley catheter is inserted to keep the bladder empty and to prevent trauma to it and should be placed after the anaesthetic is administered. Nursing roles include both circulating and scrubbing and encompass care of the woman and the infant after birth. The circulating nurse or surgeon prepares the abdomen with a scrub solution by using a circular motion that goes outward from the incisional area. The woman's partner may don a hat, mask, and gown and provide support to the mother at the head of the table (Fig. 8.4).

Types of incisions

There are two incisions in Caesarean birth: a skin incision and a uterine incision. The directions of these incisions are not always the same.

Skin incisions. The skin incision is done most often in a transverse direction. In an emergency, the vertical incision can be accomplished more quickly. The transverse, or Pfannenstiel, incision is nearly invisible when healed.

Uterine incisions. The more important of the two incisions is the one that cuts into the uterus. There are three types of uterine incisions (Fig. 8.5): low transverse, low vertical, and classic.

Low transverse incision. A low transverse incision is preferred because it is not likely to rupture during another birth, causes less blood loss, and is easier to repair. It may not be an option if the fetus is large or if there is a placenta previa in the area where the incision would be made. This type of incision makes a trial of labour after Caesarean (TOLOC) possible for subsequent births.

Low vertical incision. A low vertical incision produces minimal blood loss and allows birth of a larger fetus. However, it is more likely to rupture during another birth, although less so than the classic incision.

Classic incision. The classic incision is rarely used, because it involves more blood loss, and of the three types it is the most likely to rupture during another pregnancy. However, it may be the only choice if the fetus is in a transverse lie or if there is scarring or a placenta previa or abnormal placentation such as a percreta in the lower anterior uterus.

Sequence of Events

The SOGC recommends that before initiation of the anaesthesia (usually a spinal is preferred) the surgical team begins the surgical safety checklist as an important part of the obstetrical surgery (Singh, Mehra, & Hopkins, 2018). The nurse is part of the team, introducing him- or herself to the patient and family and identifying key elements of the woman's history to ensure that the rest of the team is aware of allergies and medications. After the woman has received a spinal anaesthetic and has been prepped and draped, the surgeon makes the skin incision. After making the uterine incision, the surgeon ruptures the membranes (unless they are already ruptured) with a sharp instrument. The amniotic fluid is suctioned from the operative area and its amount, colour, and odour are noted.

The surgeon reaches into the uterus to lift out the fetal head or buttocks. Forceps or vacuum extraction may

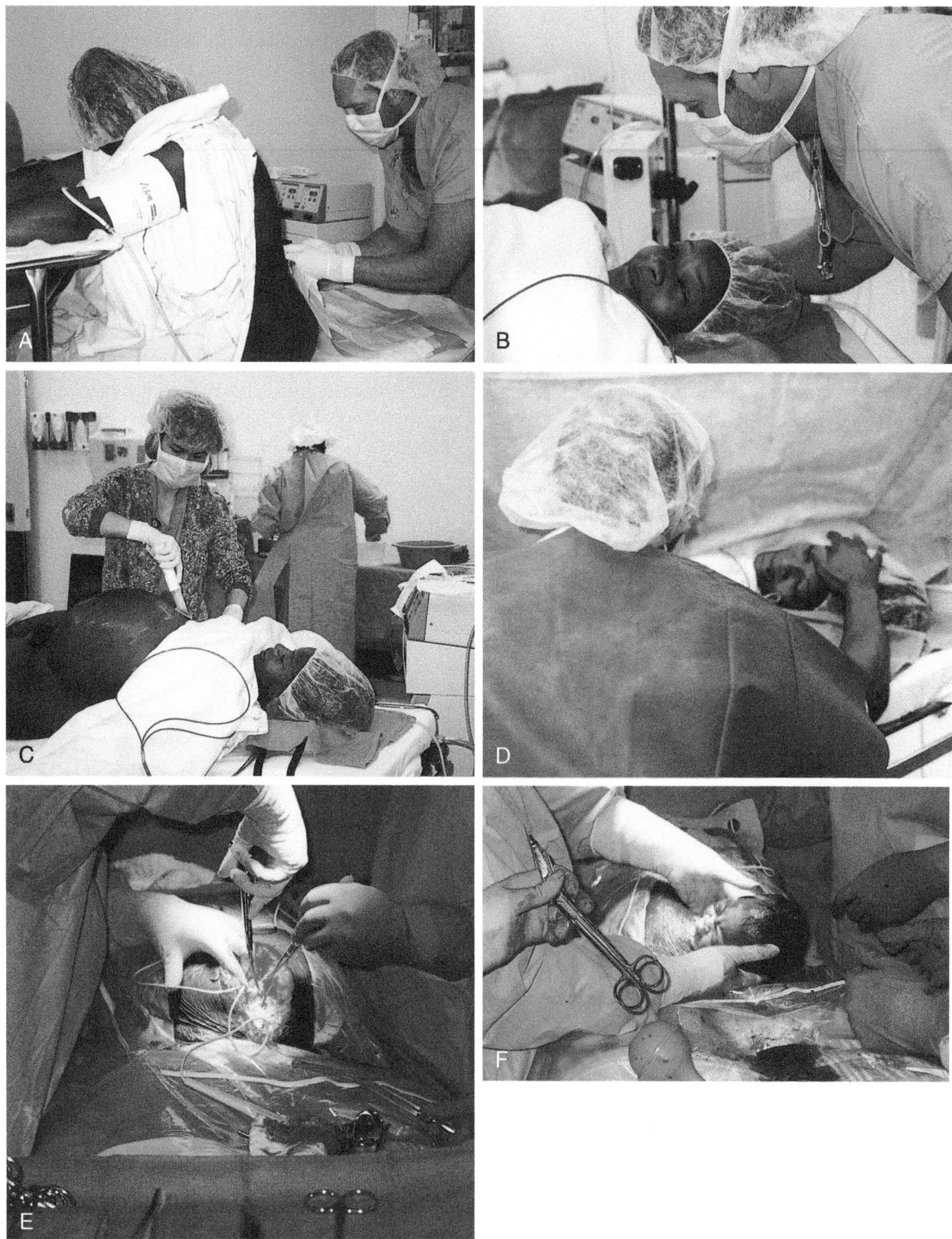

Fig. 8.4 Caesarean birth. **A,** Spinal anaesthetic is given. **B,** The anaesthesiologist provides information throughout the surgery to the woman. **C,** The nurse or health care provider preps the abdomen. **D,** The partner encourages the woman. **E,** A vertical incision is made. **F,** The head of the infant is lifted out of the uterus.

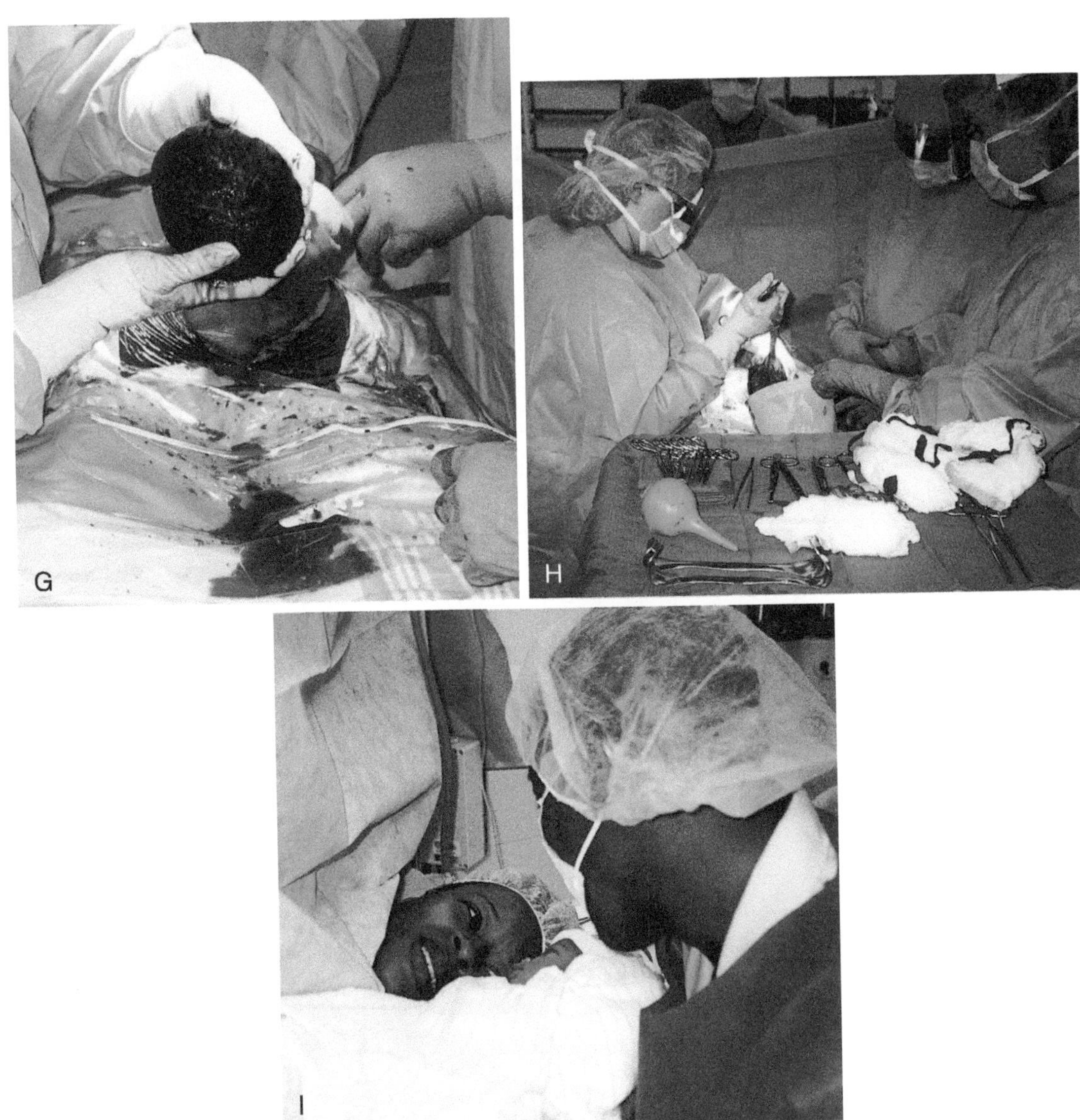

Fig. 8.4, cont'd **G,** The body of the infant is lifted out of the uterus. **H,** The placenta is delivered from the uterus. **I,** The parents and the newborn bond. (Courtesy Pat Spier, RN-C.)

be used to assist with birth of the head. The infant's mouth and nose are wiped, and the cord is clamped. The physician places the infant onto sterile blankets in a radiant warmer. The infant should not be passed to another person, to prevent dropping the newborn. A pediatrician, respiratory technologist, or another nurse should be available for resuscitation or initial baby care.

After the birth of the infant, the surgeon removes the placenta and examines it for intactness. The uterine cavity is sponged to remove blood clots and other debris. The uterine and skin incisions are then closed and secured in layers with sutures or staples.

Nursing Care

The RN assumes most of the preoperative and postoperative care of the woman. This includes obtaining the required laboratory studies, initiating IV access, administering medications, performing preoperative teaching, and preparing the woman for surgery. Women who have unexpected Caesarean births may require greater emotional support than those having vaginal births. They are usually happy and excited about the newborn, but they may also feel grief, guilt, or anger because the expected course of birth did not occur. These feelings may linger and resurface during another pregnancy. Emotional care of the partner and family is essential; they are included in explanations of the surgery as much as the woman wishes. The partner may be frightened when an emergency Caesarean is needed but may not express these feelings because the woman needs so much support. The nurse informs the partner when they may enter the operating room, because 30 minutes or longer may be needed to administer a regional anaesthetic and for surgical preparations if there is no emergency. The partner dons surgical attire or a gown during this time.

The partner may be almost as exhausted as the woman if a Caesarean birth is performed after hours of labour. The thoughtful nurse includes the partner and promotes their emotional and physical well-being.

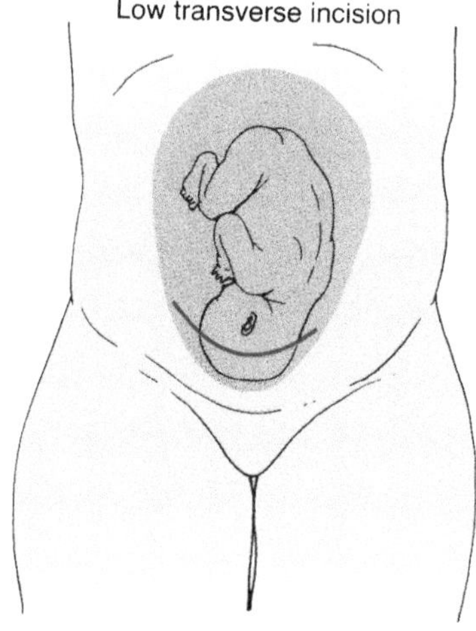

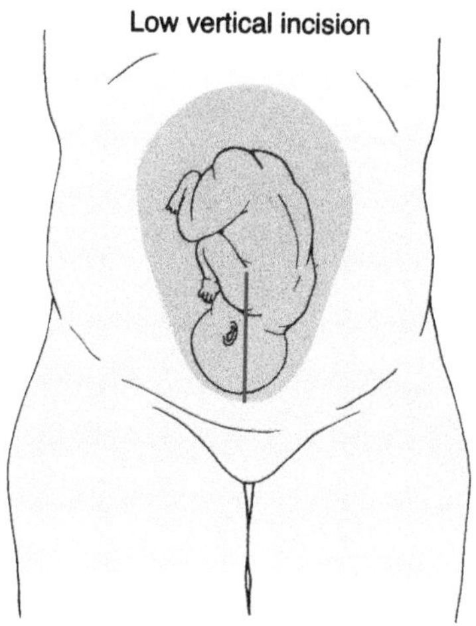

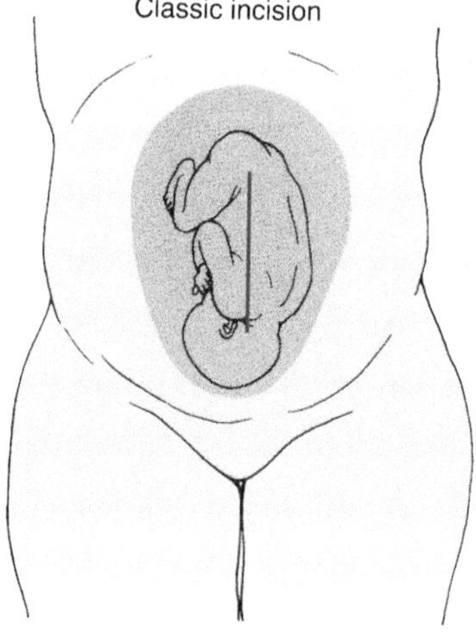

Fig. 8.5 Three types of uterine incisions for Caesarean birth. The low transverse uterine incision is preferred because it is not likely to rupture during a subsequent birth, facilitating a vaginal birth after a Caesarean birth. The low vertical and classic incisions may occasionally be used. The skin incision and uterine incision do not always match.

The mother, newborn, and partner are kept together as much as possible after birth, just as for a vaginal birth. The woman and her partner are encouraged to talk about the Caesarean birth so they can integrate the experience. The nurse answers questions about events surrounding the birth. The focus is on the *birth* rather than on the surgical aspects of the Caesarean.

It is important to balance the requirements for surgical safety with the needs of the infant and the family (PHAC, 2018). What happens in the operating room can influence health and well-being long term in both the parents and the newborn. Keeping the newborn in the operating room skin-to-skin on the upper chest of the mother or, if that is not possible for medical reasons, on the chest of the partner or the chosen support person promotes the same benefits as with a vaginal birth. Separation should occur only if medically indicated by the health of the mother or infant (PHAC, 2018).

Nursing assessments after Caesarean birth are similar to those after vaginal birth, including assessment of the uterine fundus. Assessments are done every 15 minutes for the first 1 or 2 hours and then every 30 minutes for 1 hour according to hospital policy. Recovery room assessments after Caesarean birth include the following:

- Vital signs to identify hemorrhage or shock; a pulse oximeter is used to better identify depressed respiratory function
- IV site and rate of solution flow
- Fundus for firmness, height, and midline position
- Dressing for drainage
- Lochia for quantity, colour, and presence of clots
- Urine output from the indwelling catheter
- Return of sensation to the lower body
- Newborn assessment and initiation of breastfeeding

The fundus is checked as gently as possible. The woman flexes her knees slightly and takes slow, deep breaths to minimize the discomfort of fundal assessments. While supporting the lower uterus with one hand, the fingers of the other hand are gently "walked" from the side of the uterus toward the midline. Massage is not needed if the fundus is already firm.

Safety Alert!

Although assessing the uterus after Caesarean birth causes discomfort, it is important to do so regularly because the woman may have a relaxed uterus that causes excessive blood loss. Explaining the rationale for this assessment as well as asking about pain and offering medication as needed are helpful.

The woman is told to take deep breaths at each assessment and to cough to move secretions from her airways. A small pillow or folded blanket supports her incision when she coughs or moves, which reduces pain. Changing her position every 1 or 2 hours helps expand her lungs and also makes her more comfortable.

Pain relief after Caesarean birth may be administered via a PCA pump or by intermittent injections of opioid analgesics. Epidural narcotics provide long-lasting pain relief but are associated with respiratory depression and itching (see Chapter 7), which vary with the medication injected. The woman is changed to oral analgesics after about the first 24 hours. Nursing Care Plan 8.1 details interventions for selected nursing diagnoses that pertain to the woman with an unplanned Caesarean birth.

Nursing Care Plan 8.1 The Woman With an Unplanned Caesarean Birth

PATIENT DATA

A woman, $G_1T_0P_0A_0L_0$, has been using breathing, relaxation, and imagery techniques during the first stage of labour, and her partner has been helpful and supportive. However, the labour is not progressing, and there is an increasing fetal heart rate baseline with minimal variability noted for the past hour with meconium in the amniotic fluid. The health care provider orders that the patient be prepared for an emergency Caesarean birth.

Selected Nursing Diagnosis Anxiety as a result of development of complications

Goals	Nursing Interventions	Rationales
The woman and her partner will express decreased anxiety after explanations about the planned surgery.	Determine coping level and learning needs.	Provides a database to build on to provide information that will decrease anxiety.
	Reinforce all explanations given by health care provider, expressing them in simpler terms if needed.	Anxiety tends to narrow attention; although the health care provider may have explained the need for surgery, the woman and her partner may not have comprehended everything they were told.
	Encourage the woman to continue using the breathing and relaxation techniques she learned in prepared childbirth classes as long as contractions continue.	Learned pain management techniques increase the woman's sense of control. Control over a situation reduces feelings of helplessness and decreases anxiety.
	Explain to the woman and partner who will be part of the team for the surgery and what the room will look like. Once she moves into the room, explain the purpose of the basic equipment, such as narrow table, monitors for her heart rate and blood pressure, anaesthesia machine, and large overhead lights. Explain that personnel will wear protective equipment such as masks, eye protection, gowns, gloves, hats, and shoe covers.	Commonplace equipment and attire in an operating room can be intimidating for someone who has not seen them before. Unfamiliarity increases anxiety; preparation reduces anxiety and fear of the unknown.
	Describe the usual postoperative care: assessment of vital signs, fundus, vaginal bleeding, dressing, and catheter. Tell her she will be asked to take deep breaths and change position regularly.	If the woman knows what to expect, she is able to understand the need for the care provided, even if assessments are uncomfortable.
	Encourage her partner to be with her during surgery (if this is culturally appropriate), and do not separate family afterward, if possible.	Companionship of familiar persons helps to reduce anxiety; keeping the new family together promotes attachment to the newborn.
	Stay with the woman. Encourage verbalization and support her coping mechanisms.	The presence of a professional person reduces anxiety.

Selected Nursing Diagnosis Pain as a result of increasing stress

Goals	Nursing Interventions	Rationales
The woman will verbalize reduced discomfort or will be able to use effective techniques to decrease perception of pain.	Determine the nature, duration, and location of pain.	Never assume that the pain is related to a contraction. Locating the site of pain helps identify complications that may be occurring (e.g., embolism). Assessing pain and contractions can help identify a prolonged contraction that can cause fetal hypoxia.
	Encourage the woman to continue to use coping mechanisms learned during prenatal classes or with a previous life event that required coping, such as slow breathing or distraction. Use therapeutic touch to increase comfort.	A feeling of loss of control can increase the perception of pain. Reduction of tension can promote comfort.
	Maintain a calm manner and environment.	A calm manner calms the parents and reduces anxieties and tensions that elevate pain perception.

CRITICAL THINKING QUESTION

1. What are the advantages and disadvantages of a transverse abdominal incision compared to the classic midline incision?

ABNORMAL LABOUR

A normal labour shows contractions that result in regular progression in cervical effacement, dilation, and descent of the fetus. The determination of the timing of a normal labour is based on Friedman's work and determination of a labour curve meant for labour assessment. Abnormal labour, called **dysfunctional labour,** does not progress. **Dystocia** is a term used to describe a labour that is progressing slowly.

The "five *Ps*" of labour (see Chapter 6) interact constantly throughout the birth. Abnormalities in the **p**owers, **p**assenger, **p**assageway, maternal **p**osition, or **p**syche may result in a dysfunctional labour. In addition, the length of labour may be unusually short or long. Labour abnormalities may necessitate use of forceps or Caesarean birth, and they are more likely to result in injury to the mother or fetus.

It is essential for nurses to understand the normal birth process so that deviations from normal can be recognized and prompt interventions implemented. Effective support for the woman and her family is part of competent and compassionate care. Risk factors for dysfunctional labour include the following:

- Advanced maternal age (>35 years of age)
- Obesity or high BMI (>40)
- Overdistention of uterus (**polyhydramnios** or multiple gestation)
- Abnormal fetal presentation
- Cephalopelvic disproportion (CPD)
- Overstimulation of the uterus
- Maternal fatigue, dehydration, fear
- Lack of analgesic assistance or extended analgesia/anaesthesia

PROBLEMS WITH THE POWERS OF LABOUR

Increased Uterine Muscle Tone—Hypertonic Labour

Increased uterine muscle tone usually occurs during the latent (early) phase of labour (before 4 cm of cervical dilation) and is characterized by contractions that are frequent, cramp-like, and ineffective. Even between contractions the uterus is tense, which reduces blood flow to the placenta and to the fetus. Hypertonic labour dysfunction is less common than hypotonic dysfunction. Table 8.2 summarizes the differences between hypertonic and hypotonic labour.

Medical treatment

Pharmacological treatment may include mild sedation to allow the woman to rest. Encouraging her to ambulate or to return home may be helpful if all is well with the woman and fetus. Eating and drinking in this stage of labour, taking a shower, and sleeping may facilitate moving into the active phase of labour more easily.

Nursing care

Women with increased uterine muscle tone may be uncomfortable and frustrated. Anxiety about the lack of progress and fatigue can impair their ability to tolerate pain. They may lose confidence in their ability to give birth. The nurse needs to assess what coping strategies the woman and partner have been using up to this point and offer suggestions for comfort measures. Both the woman and partner may be fearful, frustrated, excited, or exhausted from the near-constant discomfort. Warm showers or baths may help to promote relaxation. Individual assessment of the woman's pain and vital signs and fetal assessment can assist with determining the appropriate interventions.

Decreased Uterine Muscle Tone—Hypotonic Labour

A woman who has decreased uterine muscle tone has contractions that are too weak to be effective during active labour. The woman begins labour normally, but contractions diminish during the active phase (after 4 cm of cervical dilation) when the pace of labour is expected to accelerate. This is more likely to occur if the uterus is overdistended, such as with twins, a large fetus, or excess amniotic fluid (polyhydramnios). Uterine overdistention stretches the muscle fibres and thus reduces their ability to contract effectively.

Table 8.2 Differences Between Dysfunctional Labour Caused by Hypertonic and Hypotonic Contractions

HYPERTONIC LABOUR	HYPOTONIC LABOUR
Contractions are frequent and painful.	Contractions are weak and ineffective.
Uterine resting tone between contractions is increased.	Uterine resting tone is not elevated.
It is less common than hypotonic labour dysfunction.	It is more common than hypertonic labour dysfunction.
It is more likely to occur during latent labour, before 4 cm of cervical dilation.	It occurs during the active phase, after 4 cm of cervical dilation. It is more likely if the uterus is overly distended or if the woman has had many other births.
Medical management includes mild sedation.	Medical management includes amniotomy, ambulation, oxytocin augmentation, and adequate hydration.
Nursing interventions include support of labour, assessment of the woman's pain, labour progress, and fetal well-being as well as offering options of comfort measures and pain management.	Nonpharmacological stimulation methods include walking, changing positions, and encouragement.

Medical treatment

The primary health care provider usually performs an amniotomy if the membranes are intact. Augmentation of labour with oxytocin can increase the strength of contractions together with the amniotomy. IV or oral fluids may improve the quality of contractions if the woman is dehydrated.

Nursing care

The woman is reasonably comfortable but frustrated because her labour is not progressing. In addition to providing care related to amniotomy and labour augmentation, the nurse needs to provide emotional support to the woman and her partner. The woman should be encouraged to express her frustrations. The nurse should tell the woman when she is making progress to encourage continuation of her efforts.

Position changes may help to relieve discomfort and enhance progress. Contractions are usually stronger and more effective when the woman assumes an upright position or lies on her side, although they may be less frequent. Walking or nipple stimulation may intensify contractions (Nursing Care Plan 8.2).

Nursing Care Plan 8.2 The Woman With Dysfunctional Labour Caused by Hypotonic Contractions

PATIENT DATA

A woman, $G_2T_0P_0A_0L_0$, is admitted at 1900 because of premature rupture of the membranes. Contractions remain irregular at 0700 the next morning. The woman appears anxious and fearful concerning her lack of progress.

Selected Nursing Diagnosis Risk for infection as a result of ruptured membranes

Goals	Nursing Interventions	Rationales
The woman's temperature will remain under 38°C (100.4°F), and the amniotic fluid will remain clear with no abnormal odour.	Take the woman's temperature every 2 hours, or more often if elevated. At the same time, assess the amniotic fluid drainage for colour, clarity, and odour.	Elevated temperature is a sign of infection; cloudy, yellow, or foul-smelling fluid suggests infection; and meconium (green) staining suggests fetal compromise but is also seen with prolonged pregnancy.
	Observe fetal heart rates (see Chapter 6).	Fetal tachycardia (rate >160 beats/min) may be the first sign of infection. Decreased fetal oxygenation may also occur, especially with abnormal labour.
	Assist the woman in maintaining good perineal hygiene (wiping front to back). Keep underpads clean and dry.	Good hygiene reduces the possibility of introducing bacteria into the birth canal.
	After birth, continue to assess the woman's temperature at least every 4 hours. Assess the lochia (postbirth vaginal drainage) for a foul odour or brown colour.	The woman may not show these signs of infection until after birth.
	Observe the newborn for a temperature below 36.2°C (97°F) or above 38°C (100.4°F). Observe for challenges with feeding, lethargy, irritability, or "not looking right."	The newborn may become infected in utero and display these signs of infection after birth. Neonatal sepsis may occur with prolonged rupture of membranes and is a potentially fatal infection.

Selected Nursing Diagnosis Ineffective coping as a result of frustration with slow labour and delayed birth

Goals	Nursing Interventions	Rationales
The woman will use breathing and relaxation techniques. The woman will verbalize an understanding of what is happening and how she can still participate in the birth process.	If there is no contraindication, encourage the woman to walk or to change positions such as sitting, hands and knees, side-lying, or rocking on a birthing ball.	Upright positions enhance fetal descent. Walking strengthens labour contractions; walking when membranes are ruptured and fetal station is high could lead to umbilical cord prolapse, and vaginal examinations will help to determine safety of ambulation.
	Help the woman to use comfort measures to promote labour, such as a shower or whirlpool if available and not contraindicated.	Water may help the woman relax, which improves labour. All nonpharmacological methods to stimulate labour enhance her sense of control.

Continued

Nursing Care Plan 8.2 The Woman With Hypotonic Dysfunction—cont'd

Goals	Nursing Interventions	Rationales
	Assist the registered nurse with oxytocin augmentation if it is ordered. Observe contractions for excessive frequency (more frequent than every 2 minutes), duration (>90 seconds), or inadequate rest interval (<60 seconds). Observe fetal heart rate for rates outside the normal range of 110 to 160 beats/min.	The primary risks of oxytocin augmentation or induction of labour relate to overstimulating the uterus. Excessive contractions can reduce fetal oxygen supply. These are signs of potential uterine overstimulation.
	Explain to the woman how each method is expected to help her labour advance. Inform her any time she is making progress, either in improved contractions or with increasing cervical dilation.	If the woman understands the reason for any interventions, she will be better able to assist with treatment and feel more in control. Knowing that her efforts are having the desired effect encourages her to continue with her learned coping methods.
	Help the woman relax and use the breathing techniques. Praise and support her when she uses them.	Relaxation promotes normal labour. Praise encourages the woman to continue efforts at managing contractions.
	Reposition frequently. Acknowledge the reality of discomfort.	Feeling supported enhances coping.

CRITICAL THINKING QUESTION

1. A woman, $G_1T_0P_0A_0L_0$, has been admitted with ruptured membranes. Contractions are irregular and ineffective, and progress in dilation and effacement of the cervix is very slow. An oxytocin IV infusion is started after 15 hours. What could happen if the health care provider decides not to augment labour?

Ineffective Maternal Pushing

The woman may not push effectively during the second stage of labour because she does not understand which techniques to use or fears tearing her perineal tissues. Epidural or subarachnoid blocks (see Chapter 7) may also depress or eliminate the natural urge to push. An exhausted woman may be unable to gather her resources to push appropriately.

Nursing care

Nursing care focuses on coaching the woman about the most effective techniques for pushing. If she cannot feel her contractions because of a regional block, the nurse tells her when to push as each contraction reaches its peak.

The exhausted woman may benefit from pushing only when she feels a strong urge. The fearful woman may benefit from explanations of the sensations that accompany fetal descent but that her body is designed to accommodate the fetus. Promoting relaxation, relieving fatigue, changing position, and increasing hydration can help the woman sustain the energy level needed for effective pushing.

PROBLEMS WITH THE PASSENGER

Fetal Size

A large fetus (**macrosomia**) is generally considered to be one that weighs more than 4 000 g (8.8 lb) at birth. The large fetus may not fit through the woman's pelvis. A very large fetus also distends the uterus and can contribute to hypotonic labour dysfunction.

Sometimes a single part of the fetus is too large. For example, the fetus may have hydrocephalus (an abnormal amount of fluid in the brain). In that case, the fetal body size and weight may be normal, but the head is too large to fit through the pelvis. These infants are often in abnormal presentations as well.

Shoulder dystocia may occur, usually when the fetus is large. The fetal head is born, but the shoulders become impacted above the mother's symphysis pubis. A shoulder dystocia is an emergency, because the fetus needs to begin breathing. The head is out, but the chest cannot expand. The cord is compressed between the fetus and the mother's pelvis. The health care provider may request that the nurse apply firm downward pressure just above the symphysis pubis (suprapubic pressure) to push the shoulders toward the pelvic canal. Squatting or sharp flexion of the thighs against the abdomen may also loosen the shoulders. The nurse should document the time of the birth of the head and call for help with positioning the woman to assist with this emergency.

Nursing care

If the woman is able to give birth vaginally to a large infant, both mother and child should be observed for injuries after birth. The woman may have a large episiotomy or laceration. The large infant has an increased risk for a fracture of one or both clavicles (collarbones).

The infant's clavicles are felt for crepitus (crackling sensation) or deformity of the bones, and the arms are observed for equal movement (unilateral Moro reflex). The woman is more at risk for uterine atony and postpartum hemorrhage because after birth, her uterus does not contract well to control bleeding at the placental site. The woman needs assistance in understanding what happened as the bleeding can be frightening (to her partner as well), so providing information afterward is very helpful.

Abnormal Fetal Presentation or Position

Labour is most efficient if the fetus is in a flexed, cephalic presentation and in one of the occiput anterior positions (see Chapter 6). Abnormalities of fetal presentation and position prevent the smallest diameter of the fetal head from passing through the smallest diameter of the pelvis for the effective progress of labour.

The fetus in an abnormal presentation, such as occiput posterior, breech, or face presentation, does not pass easily through the woman's pelvis and interferes with the most efficient mechanisms of labour (see Chapter 6).

After birth, the mother and infant are observed for signs of birth trauma. The mother is more likely to have a hematoma of her vaginal wall if the fetus remained in the occiput posterior position for a long time. The infant may have excessive moulding (alteration in shape) of the head, caput succedaneum (scalp edema; see Chapter 11), and possibly injury from forceps or the vacuum extractor.

In Canada, most fetuses in the breech presentation are born by Caesarean section, although some women do give birth vaginally. The SOGC recommends that a woman with a persistent breech fetus at term should be informed about the options available to her, namely a trial of labour or prelabour Caesarean birth. The respective risks of each option need to be discussed, including the maternal morbidity and mortality associated with birth (Kotaska, Menticoglou, Gagnon, et al., 2009). With careful selection and intrapartum labour management of women with breech fetuses, the risk of a trial of labour to the fetus has been shown to be approximately 2% and perinatal mortality in approximately 1/500 to 1/1 000 trials of labour (PHAC, 2018). During vaginal birth in this presentation, the trunk and extremities are born before the head. After the fetal body is born, the umbilical cord can be compressed between the fetal head and the mother's pelvis. The head, which is the single largest part of the fetus, must be quickly delivered to avoid fetal hypoxia. Fig. 8.6 illustrates the sequence for a vaginal breech birth. The rate of breech presentation is approximately 3 to 4% (PHAC, 2018).

Intrapartum nurses must be prepared to assist with a breech birth, because a woman sometimes arrives at the birth facility in advanced labour with her fetus in a breech presentation. ECV is sometimes used to avoid the need for Caesarean birth in the case of a breech presentation; however, ECV is not always successful, and the fetus sometimes returns to the abnormal presentation.

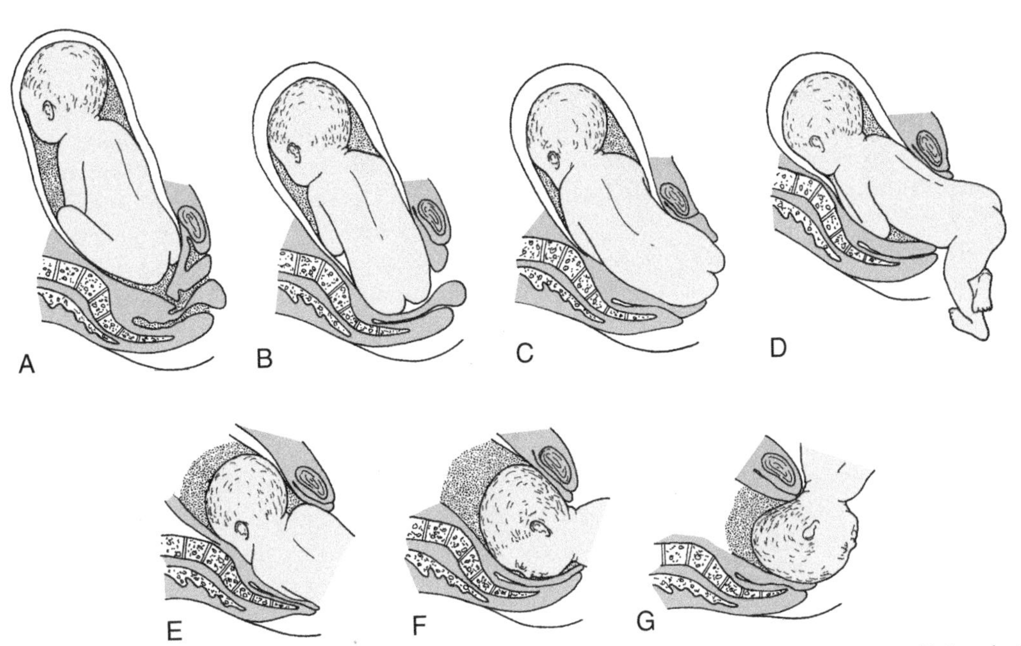

Fig. 8.6 The mechanism of labour in a breech birth. **A,** Breech before onset of labour. **B,** Engagement and internal rotation of buttocks. **C,** Lateral flexion. **D,** External rotation and restitution of buttocks. **E,** Internal rotation of shoulders and head. **F,** Face rotates to sacrum. Note that there is no flexion of the head so that the smallest diameter of the fetal head is not passing through the pelvis. The umbilical cord is compressed between the fetal head and the bony pelvis. **G,** The head is born as the fetal body is elevated. (From Lowdermilk, D. L., Perry, S. E., & Cashion, K. L. [2013]. *Maternity nursing* [8th ed.]. St. Louis: Mosby.)

Multifetal Pregnancy

If the woman has more than one fetus, several factors can make dysfunctional labour likely:

- Uterine overdistention contributes to irregular and inefficient contractions.
- Abnormal presentation or position of one or more fetuses interferes with labour mechanisms.
- Often one fetus is in the cephalic position and the second is breech, unless an internal version is done.

Because of the difficulties inherent in multifetal deliveries, Caesarean birth is not uncommon. Birth is almost always Caesarean if three or more fetuses are involved.

Nursing care

When the woman has a multifetal pregnancy, each fetus is monitored separately during labour. An upright or side-lying position with the woman's head slightly elevated aids breathing and is usually most comfortable. Multiple gestation is considered at increased risk, so continuous fetal monitoring is needed for fetal health as well as assessment of uterine activity.

A team including pediatricians, anaesthesiology, obstetricians, and nurses most often works together to care for the woman and her infants. The partner is kept aware and involved with information and helps with support throughout the process.

PROBLEMS WITH THE PASSAGEWAY

Bony Pelvis

Some women have a small or abnormally shaped pelvis that impedes the normal mechanisms of labour. The gynecoid pelvis is the most favourable for vaginal birth (see Fig. 6.5). Absolute pelvic measurements are rarely helpful to determine whether a woman's pelvis is adequate for birth. A woman with a "small" pelvis may still give birth vaginally if other factors are favourable. She often gives birth vaginally if her fetus is not too large, the head is well flexed, contractions are good, and her soft tissues yield easily to the forces of labour.

The ultimate test of a woman's pelvic size is whether her fetus fits through it at birth. A trial of labour may be indicated, and a Caesarean birth is done if necessary.

Soft Tissue Obstructions

The most common soft tissue obstruction during labour is a full bladder. The woman should be encouraged to urinate every 1 or 2 hours. Catheterization may be needed if she cannot urinate, especially if a regional anaesthetic or large quantities of IV fluids were given, which fill her bladder quickly yet reduce her sensation to void. Often an in-and-out catheter is used initially and a more permanent catheter only placed if needed, based on the length of time of labour, which reduces the potential for a urinary catheter postpartum.

Soft tissue obstructions that are less common include pelvic tumours, such as benign (noncancerous) fibroids. Some women have a cervix that is scarred from previous infections or surgery. The scar tissue may not readily yield to the forces of labour to efface and dilate.

PROBLEMS WITH THE PSYCHE

Labour is stressful, but women who have had prenatal care and have adequate social and professional support usually adapt to this stress and can labour and give birth vaginally. The most common factors that can increase stress and cause dystocia include previous labour that included an emergency or lack of progress, previous experience of intimate partner violence, lack of analgesic control of excessive pain, absence of a support person to assist with nonpharmacological pain-relief measures, immobility and restriction to bed, and lack of ability to carry out cultural traditions.

Increased anxiety releases hormones such as epinephrine, cortisol, and adrenocorticotropic hormone that reduce contractility of the smooth muscle of the uterus. The body responds to stress with a "fight-or-flight" reaction that impedes normal labour by the following mechanisms:

- Using glucose the uterus needs for energy
- Diverting blood from the uterus
- Increasing tension of the pelvic muscles, which impedes fetal descent
- Increasing perception of pain, creating greater anxiety and stress and thus worsening the cycle

Nursing Care

Promoting relaxation and helping the woman conserve her resources for the work of childbirth are the principal nursing goals. The nurse uses every opportunity to spare the woman's energy and promote her comfort. The SOGC notes that one-to-one nursing care with therapeutic presence is critical to encouraging the woman to feel safe and progress in labour and is associated with other benefits such as decreased analgesia and postpartum depression (Liston et al., 2018) (see Chapter 7). Women who have been victims of any type of trauma may not acknowledge the trauma, but treating all women with respect and using a trauma-informed approach may enhance the relationship between the nurse and the woman. It may also help to decrease the risk of retraumatization during the birth experience.

ABNORMAL DURATION OF LABOUR

Prolonged Labour

Any of the previously discussed factors may be associated with a long or difficult labour (dystocia). The average rate of cervical dilation during the active phase of labour is about 1.2 cm/hr for the woman having her first child and about 1.5 cm/hr if she has had a child previously. Descent is expected to occur at a rate of at least 1.0 cm/hr in a first-time mother and 2.0 cm/hr in a woman who has had a child before.

A *Friedman curve* is often used to graph the progress of cervical dilation and fetal descent. The Friedman curve is used as a *guide* to assess and manage the normal progress of labour, rather than as a rigid determination of "normal" length of labour. Nursing interventions such as encouraging a delay in pushing during the second stage of labour until after full cervical dilation has occurred, alternative positioning of the patient during the first and second stages of labour, and electronic fetal monitoring along with the use of epidural anaesthesia all have an impact on either increasing or decreasing the length of the first and second stages of labour. Therefore, the Friedman curve remains a management guide in assessing cervical dilation in relation to the descent of the fetal head along with other factors and assessments. It may be referred to when determining the need for a Caesarean birth.

Prolonged labour can result in several problems, including the following:

- Maternal or newborn infection, especially if the membranes have been ruptured for a long time (usually more than 24 hours)
- Maternal exhaustion
- Postpartum hemorrhage (see Chapter 10)
- Greater anxiety and fear in an ensuing pregnancy

Nursing care

Nursing care focuses on helping the woman conserve her strength and encouraging her as she copes with the long labour. The nurse should observe for signs of infection during and after birth in both the mother (see Chapter 10) and newborn (see Chapter 12).

Precipitate Birth

A precipitate birth is completed in less than 3 hours, and sometimes it may be so quick there is no health care provider present. Labour often begins abruptly and intensifies quickly, rather than having a more subtle onset and gradual progression. Contractions may be frequent and intense, often from the onset. If the woman's tissues do not yield easily to the powerful contractions, she may have cervical lacerations, hematoma, or uterine rupture.

Fetal oxygenation can be compromised by intense contractions because normally the placenta is resupplied with oxygenated blood between contractions. In precipitate labour, this interval may be very short. Birth injury from rapid passage through the birth canal may become evident in the infant after birth. These injuries can include intracranial hemorrhage or nerve damage.

Nursing care

Women who experience precipitate birth may have panic responses about the possibility of not getting to the hospital in time or not having their health care provider present. Although they are relieved after birth, they may require support and reassurance concerning the deviation from their expected experience. After birth, the nurse should observe the mother and the infant for signs of injury. Excessive pain or bruising of the woman's vulva is reported and the woman is carefully assessed for postpartum hemorrhage. Cold applications limit pain, bruising, and edema. Abnormal findings on the newborn's assessment (see Chapter 11) are reported to the health care provider.

OTHER CONSIDERATIONS IN LABOUR

OBESITY

The number of pregnant Canadian women who are obese (BMI >30) is increasing, based on a variety of factors related to lifestyle, financial situation, education, and genetics (Davies, Maxwell, McLeod, et al., 2010). The prevalence of overweight and obesity among Canadian women has increased from 41.3% in 2003 to 46.2% in 2014 (PHAC, 2018). Women who are obese have higher risks for the following (PHAC, 2018):

- Stillbirth or neonatal death
- Prolonged labour or slow progress
- Shoulder dystocia
- Emergency Caesarean birth
- Hemorrhage
- Need for induction

They are also at risk for infection and deep vein thrombosis. Women who are obese should be cared for like all women are—with compassion, respect, and dignity (PHAC, 2018). They also need appropriate resources, such as larger hospital gowns, larger blood pressure cuffs, equipment that will support the weight of the patient, and special dressings to promote healing if Caesarean birth is required. Appropriate consultation with anaesthesiology ahead of time, support in labour with the nursing team, and consideration of intrauterine monitoring to ensure accuracy of contraction assessment are required in the care of these women.

PREMATURE RUPTURE OF MEMBRANES

Premature rupture of membranes (PROM) is spontaneous rupture of the membranes at term (38 or more weeks of gestation) more than 1 hour before labour contractions begin. A related term, *preterm premature rupture of membranes (PPROM)*, is rupture of the membranes before term (before 37 weeks of gestation) with or without uterine contractions. Vaginal or cervical infection may cause prematurely ruptured membranes.

Diagnosis is confirmed by either testing the fluid with nitrazine paper, which turns blue in the presence of amniotic fluid, or placing a sample of vaginal fluid on a slide and sending it to the laboratory or having it viewed by the health care provider; it will show a ferning pattern under the microscope (see Chapter 6). Treatment is based on weighing the risks of early birth of the fetus against the risks of infection in the mother (**chorioamnionitis**, or inflammation of the fetal membranes) and sepsis in the newborn. An ultrasound determines gestational age, and **oligohydramnios** is confirmed if the amniotic fluid index (AFI) is less than 5 cm. Oligohydramnios in a gestation less than 24 weeks can lead to fetal pulmonary and skeletal defects. If ruptured membranes occur at 36 weeks of gestation or later, labour is usually induced within 24 hours. Because the cushion of amniotic fluid is lost, the risk for umbilical cord compression is greater.

Nursing Care

The nurse should observe, document, and report maternal temperature above 38°C (100.4°F), fetal tachycardia, and tenderness over the uterine area. Antibiotic and steroid therapy may be anticipated, cultures may be ordered, and labour may be induced or a Caesarean birth may be indicated. Nursing care for the woman who is not having labour induced immediately primarily involves monitoring and teaching the woman. Teaching combines information about infection and preterm labour and includes the following:

- Report a temperature that is above 38°C (100.4°F).
- Avoid sexual intercourse or insertion of anything in the vagina, which can increase the risk for infection.
- Avoid orgasm, which can stimulate contractions.
- Avoid breast stimulation, which can stimulate contractions because of natural oxytocin release.
- Maintain any activity restrictions prescribed.
- Note any uterine contractions, reduced fetal activity, or other signs of infection (see the section on amniotomy).
- Record fetal kick counts daily and report fewer than six in a 2-hour period.

PRETERM LABOUR

Preterm labour occurs after 20 and before 37 weeks of gestation. The main risks are the problems of immaturity in the newborn. Preterm birth is a major cause of perinatal morbidity and mortality and has a major medical and economic impact. Preterm birth occurs in about 7.9% of all Canadian labours and births (CIHI, 2018). Early prenatal care can assist women and their health care providers in identifying signs and symptoms of preterm labour and identifying women at risk (Box 8.1).

Box 8.1 Some Risk Factors for Preterm Labour

- Underweight or low body mass index (BMI)
- Chronic illness such as pregestational diabetes or hypertension
- Dehydration related to severe nausea or vomiting
- Pre-eclampsia
- Previous preterm labour or birth
- Previous pregnancy losses
- Uterine or cervical abnormalities or surgery
- Uterine distention
- Abdominal surgery during pregnancy
- Infection
- Anemia
- Preterm premature rupture of the membranes
- Inadequate prenatal care
- Inadequate nutrition to meet the needs of pregnancy
- Age less than 18 years or greater than 40 years
- Low education level
- Poverty
- Tobacco use
- Problematic substance use and prescribed opioid use related to chronic pain
- Chronic stress
- Multiple gestation

Signs of Impending Preterm Labour

A transvaginal ultrasound showing a shortened cervix at 20 weeks of gestation may be predictive of impending preterm labour. The ultrasound may be advised for high-risk women such as a woman who has had a previous preterm birth. A cervicovaginal test, the **fetal fibronectin (fFN) test,** is also used to predict preterm labour. Fibronectin is a protein produced by the fetal membranes that can leak into vaginal secretions if uterine activity, infection, or cervical dilation of 2 cm or more occurs. The presence of increased fibronectin in vaginal secretions between 22 and 34 weeks of gestation is predictive of preterm labour. *Diagnosis of preterm labour is based on presence of contractions causing progressive cervical effacement and dilation.*

Maternal symptoms of preterm labour that cause women to seek medical care include the following:

- Contractions that may not feel comfortable
- Menstrual-like cramps
- Constant low backache
- Pelvic pressure or a feeling that the fetus is pushing down
- Presence of increased or a change in vaginal discharge
- Abdominal cramps with or without diarrhea
- Pain or discomfort in the vulva or thighs
- "Just feeling bad" or "coming down with something"

An ultrasound of the fetus to determine maturity, position, and other problems that may exist may be ordered. Treatment of preterm labour is more aggressive at 28 weeks of gestation than at 34 weeks of gestation.

The Alliance for the Prevention of Preterm Birth and Stillbirth is a newly formed partnership in Ontario that is looking at ways to decrease the rates of preventable preterm birth and stillbirth (Katherine & Robson, 2018). They have identified risk factors and developed a proposed model of care that includes the following:

- Risk assessment for all patients at prenatal care intake
- Low-dose aspirin (ASA) recommended for individuals with clinical risk factors
- Cervical length measurement as part of routine mid-pregnancy anatomical ultrasound scan between 16 and 24 weeks
- Natural vaginal progesterone prescribed nightly and until 36 weeks' gestation for anyone with a history of preterm birth or short cervix

- Fetal movement awareness teaching as part of routine pregnancy care
- Use of prompt electronic fetal monitoring when fetal movement is significantly reduced

Further research and details about this initiative will be coming in the future.

Tocolytic Therapy

Tocolysis is the inhibition of myometrial uterine contractions. The goal of **tocolytics** is to stop uterine contractions long enough to enable one or two doses of glucocorticosteroids prior to the infant's birth (24 to 48 hours).

Magnesium sulphate is administered if the woman continues with contractions or signs of labour and birth is imminent. Magnesium sulphate provides fetal neuroprotection, as it has been shown to decrease the risk of developing cerebral palsy (Simhan, Iams, & Romero, 2017). A continuous IV infusion is administered beginning with a bolus, and adverse effects are monitored. The woman should be informed that a warm flush may be perceived during the initiation of therapy. Overdose can affect the cardiorespiratory system, and vital signs are recorded every hour. If the fetus is born during magnesium therapy, drowsiness may be present and resuscitation may be required. The nursery staff should be notified if magnesium sulphate therapy was used within 2 hours before birth. Calcium gluconate should be on hand to treat adverse effects in the woman. When magnesium sulphate is used, the nurse should monitor the patient for respiratory rate and lung sounds and signs of fluid overload, urine output, deep tendon reflexes, and bowel sounds because the intestinal muscles also relax in response to the medication.

Prostaglandin synthesis inhibitors such as indomethacin are a type of medication that can be used to stop or decrease labour contractions. This type of medication causes a reduction in amniotic fluid, which is helpful when polyhydramnios is a problem. However, this medication is not commonly used because it can stimulate the ductus arteriosus to close prematurely, causing fetal death. Close fetal monitoring is essential. Most often it is used for a short time only to enable two doses of corticosteroids to help with lung maturation.

Antimicrobial therapy is usually initiated in women with preterm labour, because studies have shown that subclinical chorioamnionitis is often present and for prevention of GBS infection.

Contraindications

Tocolytics should not be used in women with pre-eclampsia, placenta previa, placental abruption, a fetus of gestational age over 37 weeks, chorioamnionitis, or fetal demise. In these cases, it would not improve the obstetrical outcome to delay birth of the fetus.

Speeding Fetal Lung Maturation

If it appears that preterm birth is inevitable, the health care provider may order the woman to receive steroids (glucocorticoids) to increase fetal lung maturity if the gestation is between 24 and 34 weeks. Glucocorticoids are often used together with tocolytics. Betamethasone may be administered for this purpose in two intramuscular injections 24 hours apart.

Activity Restrictions

Historically, bed rest was often prescribed for women at risk for preterm birth. However, the benefits of bed rest are not clear, and many adverse maternal effects can occur. Therefore, limited activity is usually prescribed for the woman, but no scientific evidence exists about the benefit to the pregnancy.

Nursing Care

Nurses should be aware of the symptoms of preterm labour because they may occur in any pregnant woman, with or without risk factors. Symptoms should be taught and regularly reinforced for women who have increased risk factors. Nursing care of the woman with preterm labour includes positioning the woman on her side when resting for better placental blood flow, assessing vital signs frequently, and notifying the health care provider if contractions or tachycardia occur. Signs of pulmonary edema (chest pains, cough, crackles, or rhonchi) and intake and output should be closely monitored. If the woman is monitored at home, appropriate activities and restrictions are identified, and arrangements for household responsibilities such as childcare should be made with the family or with the help of social services. If birth appears to be imminent, monitoring of the FHR is essential, and preparation for admission to the neonatal intensive care unit is initiated. Full emotional support of the parents needs to be offered because they may be grieving the loss of the normal birth process.

PROLONGED PREGNANCY

A late-term pregnancy lasts between 41 weeks and 41 weeks and 6 days. A post-term pregnancy lasts over 42 weeks. The term *postmature* most accurately describes the infant whose characteristics are consistent with a prolonged gestation (see Chapter 12).

Risks

The greatest risks of prolonged pregnancy are to the fetus. As the placenta ages, it delivers oxygen and nutrients to the fetus less efficiently. The fetus may lose weight, and the skin may begin to peel; these are the typical characteristics of postmaturity. Meconium may be expelled into the amniotic fluid, which can cause severe respiratory problems at birth. Low blood glucose level is also a complication after birth.

The fetus with placental insufficiency does not have the reserves to tolerate labour well. Because the fetus has fewer reserves, the normal interruption in blood flow during contractions may cause more stress on the infant. If the placenta continues to function well, the fetus continues growing. This can lead to a large fetus and the problems accompanying macrosomia.

If placental function remains normal, there is little physical risk to the mother other than labouring with a large fetus. Psychologically, however, she often feels that pregnancy will never end. She may become more anxious about when labour will begin and when her health care provider will "do something."

Medical Treatment

The health care provider will evaluate whether the pregnancy is truly prolonged or if the gestation has been miscalculated. If the woman had early and regular prenatal care, ultrasound examinations have usually clarified her true gestation. Any pregnancy that lasts longer than 41 weeks must be monitored closely with twice-weekly NSTs, AFIs, BPPs, and daily kick counts (see Chapter 5). Oligohydramnios (decreased amniotic fluid) in a post-term pregnancy is an indication for labour induction. If the woman's pregnancy has definitely reached 41 weeks, 6 days, labour is usually induced by oxytocin. Prostaglandin application to ripen the cervix before oxytocin administration increases the probability of successful induction.

Nursing Care

Nursing care involves careful observation of the fetus during labour to identify signs associated with decreased placental blood flow, such as late decelerations (see Chapter 6). After birth, the newborn is observed for respiratory difficulties and hypoglycemia.

EMERGENCIES DURING CHILDBIRTH

Several intrapartum conditions can endanger the life or well-being of the woman or her fetus. They necessitate timely communication between members of the health care team to provide information and initiate appropriate interventions. The obstetrical team of physicians, nurses, and other health care providers work together collaboratively in emergencies for optimal outcomes for the mother and infant.

Women's birth experiences can hold positive or negative influence in their lives for many years. Women may experience giving birth as traumatic despite the lack of harm to themselves or their babies, based on their level of safety; their caregiver's emotional support; clear communication, particularly in an emergency; and their participation in decision making (Lyndon, Malana, Hedli, et al., 2018). As members of the interdisciplinary team nurses need to provide support, including clear communication and development of therapeutic relationships. During emergencies good relationships and communication have been shown to increase the woman's perception of safety during her childbirth experience. Talking with the woman following her experience is also helpful. Nursing staff from the labour and birth area who visit women and their partners postpartum can provide them with support and understanding of their experiences.

Depending on the extent of the emergency, health care providers need support as well. Immediate debriefing to discuss emotional responses and providing further counselling as needed are extremely beneficial for the emotional health of the staff, particularly for nurses who have been with the woman and her family extensively.

PROLAPSED UMBILICAL CORD

The umbilical cord prolapses if it slips downward in the pelvis after the membranes rupture. In this position, it can be compressed between the fetal head and the woman's pelvis, interrupting blood supply to and from the placenta. It may slip down immediately after the membranes rupture, or the prolapse may occur later. A prolapsed cord (Fig. 8.7) can be classified in the following ways:

- *Complete:* The cord is visible at the vaginal opening.
- *Palpated:* The cord cannot be seen but can be felt as a pulsating structure when a vaginal examination is done.
- *Occult:* The prolapse is hidden and cannot be seen or felt; it is suspected on the basis of abnormal fetal heart rates.

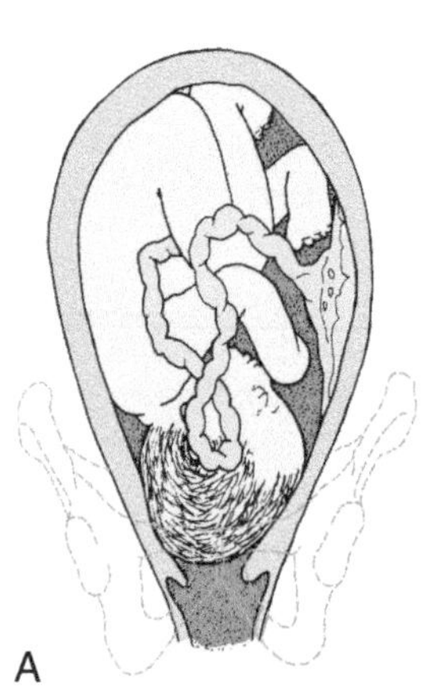

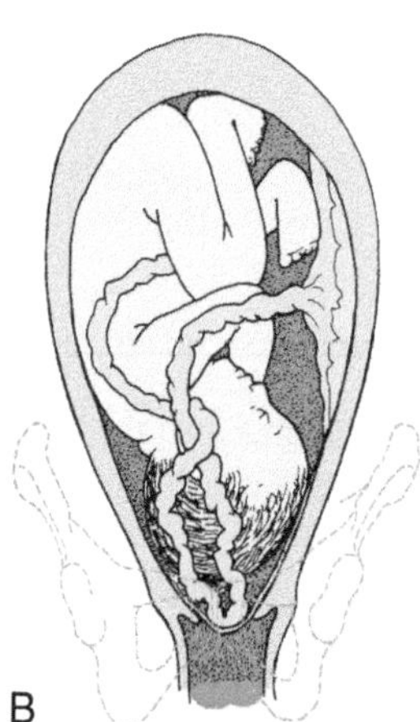

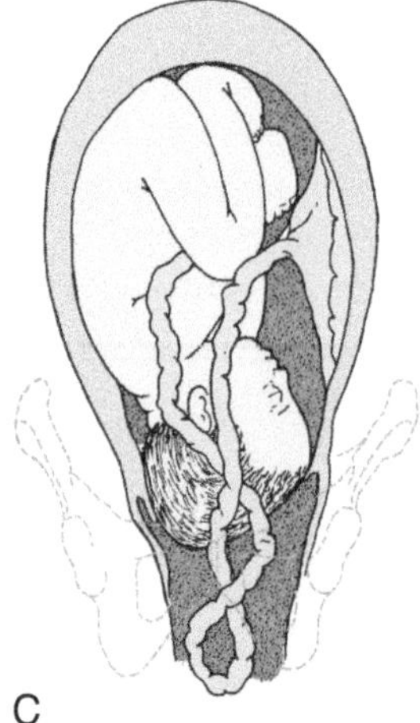

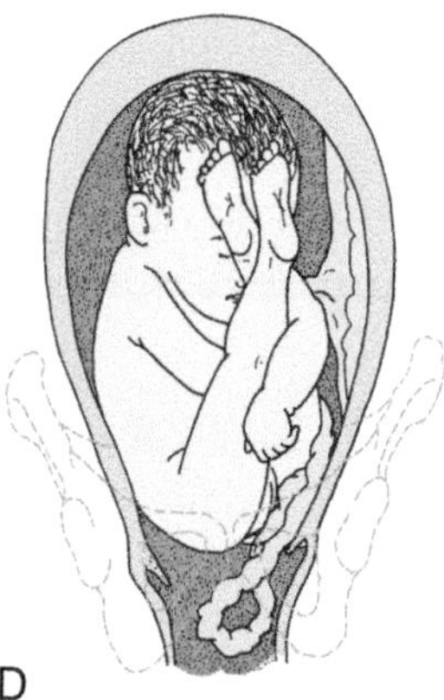

Fig. 8.7 Prolapsed umbilical cord. Note the pressure of the presenting part on the umbilical cord, which will interfere with oxygenation of the fetus. **A,** Occult (hidden) prolapse of cord. The cord will be compressed between the fetal head and the mother's bony pelvis. **B,** Complete prolapsed cord. Note that the membranes are intact. **C,** Cord is presenting in front of the fetal head and may be seen in the vagina. **D,** Frank breech presentation with prolapsed cord. (From Lowdermilk, D.L., Perry, S.E., & Cashion, K. L. [2013]. *Maternity nursing* [8th ed.]. St. Louis: Mosby.)

> **Safety Alert!**
>
> The risk for prolapsed cord is increased if the membranes rupture before the fetal presenting part is completely engaged in the pelvis. Documenting fetal heart rate after the membranes rupture in any labour is an essential nursing responsibility.

Risk Factors

Prolapse of the umbilical cord is more likely if the fetus does not completely fill the space in the pelvis or if fluid pressure is great when the membranes rupture. These conditions are more likely to occur in the following situations:

- Presenting part is not engaged so fetus is high in the pelvis
- Preterm premature rupture of membranes, infant is small
- Abnormal presentations, such as footling breech or transverse lie
- **Hydramnios** or polyhydramnios (excess amniotic fluid) is present.

Treatment and Nursing Care

The primary focus is to ensure birth of the fetus by the quickest means possible, usually via Caesarean birth. The main risk of a prolapsed cord is to the fetus. When a prolapsed cord occurs, the first action is to displace the fetus upward to stop compression against the pelvis. The health care provider who identifies the prolapsed cord with a vaginal examination will keep their hand in place, ensuring the fetal presenting part is not compressing the cord while the woman is being transported to the operating room. Maternal positions such as the knee–chest or Trendelenburg (head down) position can assist with this displacement (Fig. 8.8). Placing the mother in a side-lying position with her hips elevated on pillows also reduces cord pressure.

In addition to prompt corrective actions and assisting with emergency procedures, the nurse should remain calm to avoid increasing the woman's anxiety. Prolapsed cord is a sudden development; anxiety and fear are inevitable reactions in the woman and her partner. Calm, quick actions on the part of nurses can help the woman and her family feel that she is in competent hands. After birth, the nurse can help the woman understand the experience. She may need several explanations of what happened and why.

PLACENTA ACCRETA

Placenta accreta is an abnormal attachment of the placenta to the uterine wall that occurs in 3 of 1 000

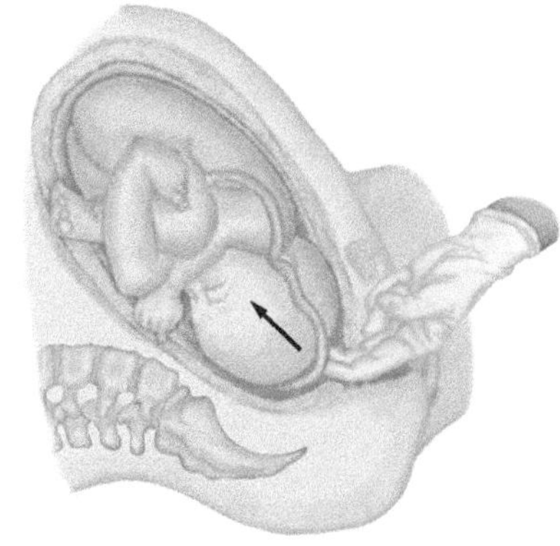

A gloved hand in the vagina pushes the fetus upward and off the cord.

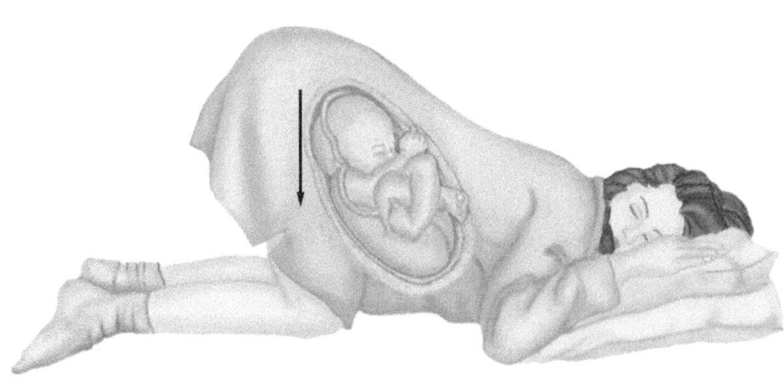

Knee-chest position uses gravity to shift the fetus out of the pelvis. The woman's thighs should be at right angles to the bed and her chest flat on the bed.

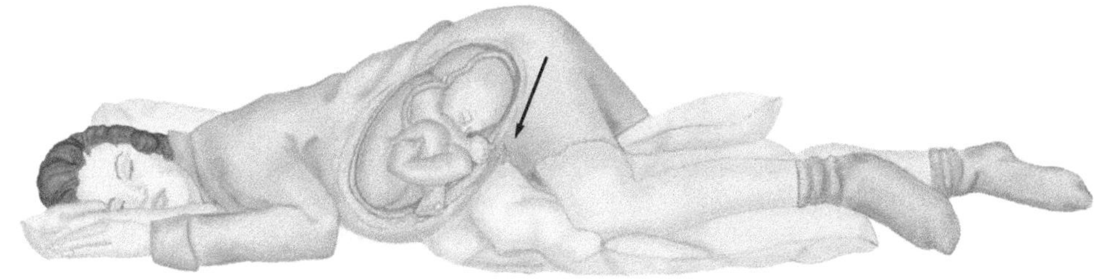

The woman's hips are elevated with two pillows; this is often combined with the Trendelenburg (head down) position.

Fig. 8.8 Positioning of the mother when the umbilical cord prolapses. These positions can be used to relieve pressure on the prolapsed umbilical cord until delivery can take place. (From Murray, S. S., & McKinney, E. S. [2011]. *Foundations of maternal-newborn and women's health nursing* [5th ed.]. St. Louis: Saunders.)

births (Francois & Foley, 2017). It is common with women who have had a previous Caesarean birth, have fibroids, are of advanced maternal age, or have endometrial defects. Symptoms include profuse bleeding during attempts to manually deliver the placenta after the fetus is born and episodes of bleeding during pregnancy. The condition can be diagnosed before birth via ultrasound and interventions used to minimize postpartum blood loss, but often a hysterectomy is required. The nurse should give care and support to the mother, who may not have another opportunity for pregnancy. Nursing responsibilities include monitoring and documenting vital signs, observing for any bleeding vaginally, IV therapy, providing pain relief, and observing the principles of blood transfusion therapy that may accompany similar interventions for other bleeding disorders of pregnancy.

UTERINE RUPTURE

Uterine rupture is defined as the complete separation of the myometrium with or without extrusion of the fetal parts into the maternal peritoneal cavity and it requires emergency Caesarean birth or postpartum laparotomy (Martel, MacKinnon, et al., 2018).

Risk Factors

Uterine rupture is more likely to occur if the woman has had previous surgery on her uterus, such as a previous Caesarean birth. The low transverse uterine incision (goes side to side) (see Fig. 8.5) is least likely to rupture. Because the classic uterine incision (goes up and down) is prone to rupture, a vaginal birth after this type of incision is not recommended. For the woman who has had a previous Caesarean birth and wants to try and give birth vaginally, a trial of labour should be offered after an assessment of her risk factors. But there must be a surgical team available to prevent or treat uterine rupture during labour in case an emergency Caesarean birth is indicated. Surgical intervention must be available within 30 minutes.

Uterine rupture may also occur if tachysystole occurs as a result of labour induction with oxytocin or the woman has sustained blunt abdominal trauma, such as from a motor vehicle collision or from intimate partner violence.

Characteristics

The most common sign or symptom of uterine rupture is atypical or abnormal FHR. Other signs include the following:

- Suddenly unable to feel presenting part on vaginal examination
- Shock caused by bleeding into the abdomen (vaginal bleeding may be minimal)
- Abdominal pain that continues between contractions
- Pain in the chest, between the scapulae (shoulder blades), or with inspiration
- Cessation of contractions
- Abnormal or absent fetal heart tones (may be a prolonged deceleration that does not return to baseline and often the change in FHR is the first sign).
- Palpation of the fetus outside the uterus because the fetus has pushed through the torn area

Medical Treatment

If the fetus is living when the rupture is detected or if blood loss is excessive, the physician performs surgery to deliver the fetus and to stop the bleeding. Hysterectomy (removal of the uterus) is likely to be required for an extensive tear. Smaller tears may be surgically repaired.

Nursing Care

The nurse should be aware of women who are at high risk for uterine rupture, and continuous fetal monitoring during labour is essential for these women, to assess uterine activity as well as the fetus. When uterine rupture occurs, the woman is prepared for immediate Caesarean birth. Measures to alleviate anxiety in the woman and her partner are necessary as emergency measures are being initiated.

Uterine rupture is sometimes not discovered until after birth. In these cases, the woman does not have dramatic symptoms of blood loss. However, she may have continuous bleeding that is brighter red than the normal postbirth bleeding. A rising pulse rate and falling blood pressure reading are signs of hypovolemic shock, which may occur if blood loss is excessive.

AMNIOTIC FLUID EMBOLISM

Amniotic fluid embolism, also known as **anaphylactoid syndrome**, is rare in pregnancy and usually happens in labour or the immediate postpartum. It occurs when there is a massive inflammatory response or maternal immunological response possibly to components of amniotic fluid such as fetal materials (e.g., lanugo, vernix, fetal hair, and sometimes meconium). These particles can enter the maternal circulation through the placental site, and the response is similar to anaphylaxis. Initially, signs and symptoms include agitation, numbness, feeling cold, chest pain, panic, distress, nausea, and vomiting together with a sense of impending doom. Then there is severe and abrupt hypotension, cardiac arrest, respiratory failure, and hemorrhage with changes in the clotting mechanism that can lead to disseminated intravascular coagulation (DIC). Risk factors include induction of labour, advanced maternal age, women with multiple fetuses, operative vaginal birth, Caesarean birth, eclampsia, and placenta previa.

The nurse needs to know the signs and symptoms and to be able to recognize these early in care, notifying the primary health care provider with the patient information. A timely response is key to increasing the patient's chance at recovery rather than her risk of morbidity and mortality. Treatment includes calling for help immediately with the initial signs of respiratory failure and hypotension, with responders such as anaesthesiology providing respiratory support with intubation and mechanical ventilation as necessary, treating shock with electrolytes and volume expanders, and replacing the coagulation factors such as platelets and fibrinogen. Packed red blood cells are sometimes given intravenously. Bringing an interdisciplinary team together to do cardiopulmonary resuscitation, provide transfusions as necessary, and respond to the symptoms is required.

The woman's intake and output are monitored closely. A pulse oximeter monitors oxygen saturation. The woman may be transferred to the critical care unit for closer monitoring and nursing care.

Unfolding Case Study

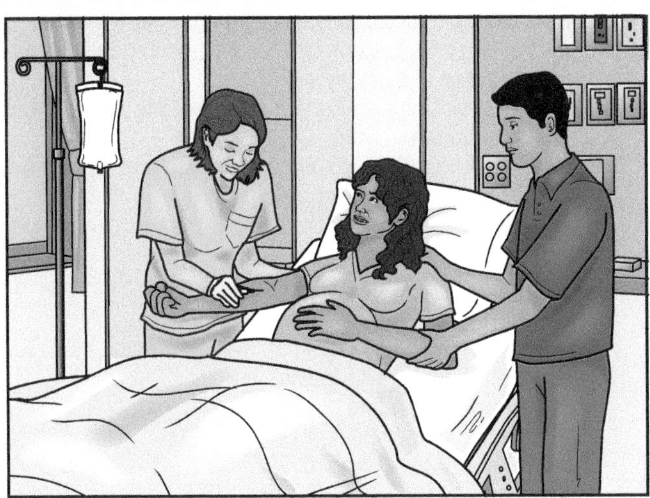

Tess and Luis were introduced to the reader in Chapter 2, and Tess's pregnancy experience has unfolded in each chapter. Refer to earlier chapters for her history and progress.

Tess was admitted to the labour unit and has been in active labour. However, after many hours, her labour contractions stop. The health care provider determines that her labour has stopped progressing (has been at 5 cm for the last 3 hours) and decides to augment her labour.

QUESTIONS

1. What is the difference between induction of labour and augmentation of labour?
2. When is induction or augmentation of labour contraindicated?
3. How can the nurse help Tess stimulate labour contractions using nonpharmacological methods?
4. How can her partner, Luis, help?
5. What nursing responsibilities are involved during the administration of oxytocin during labour?

Get Ready for the Certification Examination!

Key Points

- Induction of labour is the intentional initiation of labour before it occurs naturally.
- Augmentation of labour is the stimulation of contractions after they started naturally.
- A Bishop score above 6 may predict successful labour induction because of a "ripe cervix."
- The nurse observes the character of the amniotic fluid and fetal heart rate (FHR) when the membranes are ruptured. Fluid should be clear, but it may contain bits of lanugo and have a mild odour; the FHR should remain near its baseline level and between 110 and 160 beats/min at term.
- The nurse observes the fetal condition and character of contractions if any methods to stimulate labour are used.
- *Dystocia* is a term used to describe a difficult labour, which can be caused by an abnormality of the *power, passenger, passage, position,* or *psyche* of the woman.
- Nursing measures such as encouraging position changes, aiding relaxation, and reminding the woman to empty her bladder can promote a more normal labour.
- Pharmacological, nonpharmacological, or mechanical methods can be used to stimulate labour.
- After an external cephalic version, the nurse observes for leaking amniotic fluid and for a pattern of contractions that may indicate labour has begun. Before discharge, signs of labour are reviewed with the woman so she will know when to return to the birth centre.
- Nursing care after Caesarean birth is similar to that after vaginal birth, with the addition of assessing the wound, indwelling catheter patency, encouraging ambulation, and intravenous flow. The woman and her partner may need extra emotional support after Caesarean birth.
- Nursing care after births involving instruments (forceps or vacuum extraction) and after abnormal labour and birth include observations for maternal and newborn injuries or infections. Infection is the most common hazard after membranes rupture prematurely, especially if there is a long interval before birth.
- When oxytocin is given to the woman in labour, the nurse must be aware of signs and symptoms of increased uterine activity and monitor the FHR every 15 minutes during active labour and every 5 minutes during the transition phase.
- Induction of labour is more effective if cervical ripening is achieved before oxytocin is administered to stimulate contractions.

- An amnioinfusion is the insertion of fluid directly into the uterus to provide a cushion for the umbilical cord after amniotic membranes have ruptured and fluid decreased.
- Nurses should be aware of the subtle symptoms a woman may experience at the beginning of preterm labour and should encourage her to seek care at the hospital promptly.
- The nurse must be aware of the adverse effects of tocolytic drugs and monitor the mother and fetus closely.
- Anaphylactoid syndrome occurs when amniotic fluid enters the woman's circulation.
- After any type of emergency, the woman and her family need emotional support, explanations of what happened, and patience with their repeated questions.

Additional Learning Resources

evolve Go to your Evolve website (http://evolve.elsevier.com/Canada/Leifer) for the following learning resources:

- Answer Key for Critical Thinking Questions
- Answer Key for Textbook Review Questions
- Audio Glossary
- Fluids & Electrolytes tutorial
- Interactive Review Questions
- Skills Performance Checklists
- Video clips and more!

Online Resource

- Family-Centred Maternity and Newborn Care: National Guidelines: https://www.canada.ca/en/public-health/services/maternity-newborn-care-guidelines.html

Review Questions

1. The nurse notes that a woman's contractions during oxytocin induction of labour are every 2 minutes; the contractions last 95 seconds, and the uterus remains tense between contractions. What action is expected based on these assessments?
   a. No action is expected; the contractions are normal.
   b. The rate of oxytocin administration will be increased slightly.
   c. Pain medication or an epidural block will be offered.
   d. Infusion of oxytocin will be stopped.
2. The nurse can anticipate that which patient may be scheduled for induction of labour?
   a. A woman at 38 weeks' gestation with fetus in transverse lie
   b. A woman at 40 weeks' gestation with fetal macrosomia
   c. A woman at 40 weeks' gestation with gestational hypertension
   d. A woman at 40 weeks' gestation with a fetal prolapsed cord
3. A woman has an emergency Caesarean birth after the umbilical cord was found to be prolapsed. She repeatedly asks similar questions about what happened at birth. The nurse's interpretation of the woman's behaviour is which of the following?
   a. Cannot accept that she did not have the type of birth she planned.
   b. Trying to understand her experience and move on with postpartum adaptation.
   c. Thinks the staff is not telling her the truth about what happened at birth.
   d. Is confused about events because the effects of the general anaesthetic are persisting.
4. Which nursing intervention during labour can increase space in the woman's pelvis?
   a. Promote adequate fluid intake.
   b. Position her on the left side.
   c. Assist her to take a shower.
   d. Encourage regular urination.
5. A woman is being observed in the hospital because her membranes ruptured at 30 weeks of gestation. While providing morning care, the nursing student notices that the draining fluid has a strong odour. What is the priority nursing action?
   a. Caution the woman to remain in bed until her primary health care provider visits.
   b. Ask the woman if she is having any more contractions than usual.
   c. Take the woman's temperature; report it and the fluid odour to the registered nurse.
   d. Help to prepare the woman for an immediate Caesarean birth.
6. Following a vacuum extraction birth, the nurse notices the newborn's head is not symmetrical with swelling over the posterior fontanelle. The appropriate nursing actions would be which of the following? *(Select all that apply.)*
   a. Apply cold compresses to the swollen area.
   b. Notify the charge nurse or healthcare provider.
   c. Document and continue routine observation.
   d. Explain to the parents the swelling will resolve without treatment.

REFERENCES

Canadian Institute for Health Information (CIHI). (2018). *Inpatient hospitalizations, surgeries, newborns and childbirth indicators, 2016–2017*. https://www.cihi.ca/sites/default/files/document/hospch-hosp-2016-2017-snapshot_en.pdf.

Davies, G., Maxwell, C., McLeod, L., et al. (2010). SOGC clinical practice guideline: Obesity in pregnancy. *Journal of Obstetrics and Gynaecology Canada*, *32*(2), 165–173.

Francois, K., & Foley, M. (2017). Antepartum and postpartum hemorrhage. In S. G. Gabbe, J. R. Niebyl, J. L. Simpson, et al. (Eds.), *Obstetrics: Normal and problem pregnancies* (7th ed.). Philadelphia: Elsevier.

Health Quality Ontario. (2018). *Vaginal birth after Caesarean: Care for people who have had a Caesarean birth and are planning their next birth*. https://www.hqontario.ca/portals/0/documents/evidence/quality-standards/qs-vaginal-birth-after-caesarean-clinician-guide-en.pdf.

Katherine, W., & Robson, K. (2018). *The alliance for the prevention of preterm birth and stillbirth in Ontario*. Presented at Best Start Conference. Retrieved from: http://en.beststart.org/sites/en.beststart.org/files/u7/K2B_AlliancePreterm_Feb_7.pdf.

Kotaska, A., Menticoglou, S., Gagnon, R., et al. (2009). SOGC clinical practice guideline: Vaginal delivery of breech presentation. *Journal of Obstetrics & Gynaecology Canada*, *31*(6), 557–566.

Leduc, D., Biringer, A., Lee, L., et al. (2013). SOGC clinical practice guideline: Induction of labour. *Journal of Obstetrics and Gynaecology Canada*, *35*(9), S1–S18.

Liston, R., Sawchuck, D., Young, D., et al. (2018). No. 197b fetal health surveillance: Intrapartum consensus guideline. *Journal of Obstetrics and Gynaecology Canada*, *40*(4), e298–e322.

Lyndon, A., Malana, J., Hedli, L., et al. (2018). Thematic analysis of women's perspectives on the meaning of safety during hospital-based birth. *Journal of Obstetric, Gynecologic and Neonatal Nursing*, *47*, 324–332.

Martel, M., & MacKinnon, C., (2018). SOGC clinical practice guideline: Guidelines for vaginal birth after previous Caesarean birth. *Journal of Obstetrics and Gynaecology Canada*, *40*(3), e195–e207.

Public Health Agency of Canada (PHAC). (2018). *Family centred maternity and newborn care: National guidelines*. Ottawa, ON: Author. https://www.canada.ca/en/public-health/services/maternity-newborn-care-guidelines.html.

Sheibani, L., & Wing, D. (2017). Abnormal labor and induction of labor. In S. G. Gabbe, J. R. Niebyl, J. L. Simpson, et al. (Eds.), *Obstetrics: Normal and problem pregnancies* (7th ed.). Philadelphia: Elsevier.

Simhan, H., Iams, J., & Romero, R. (2017). Preterm labor and birth. In S. G. Gabbe, J. R. Niebyl, J. L. Simpson, et al. (Eds.), *Obstetrics: Normal and problem pregnancies* (7th ed.). Philadelphia: Elsevier.

Singh, S. S., Mehra, N., & Hopkins, L. (2018). SOGC clinical practice guideline: Surgical safety checklist in obstetrics and gynecology. *Journal of Obstetrics and Gynaecology Canada*, *40*(3), e237–e242.

9 Nursing Care of the Woman and Family After Birth

http://evolve.elsevier.com/Canada/Leifer

Jennifer Abbass-Dick and Lisa Keenan-Lindsay

Objectives

1. Define each key term listed.
2. Describe how to individualize postpartum nursing care for different patients and families.
3. Describe how cultural beliefs may impact the postpartum period.
4. Describe postpartum changes that occur in the mother and the nursing care associated with those changes.
5. Modify nursing assessments and interventions for the woman who has a Caesarean birth.
6. Explain the emotional needs of postpartum women and their families.
7. Recognize the needs of a grieving parent.
8. Identify signs and symptoms that may indicate a complication in the postpartum mother.
9. Discuss the elements of informed decision-making related to the choice of breastfeeding or formula-feeding the newborn.
10. Describe nursing interventions to support the breastfeeding and formula-feeding mother.
11. Explain the physiological characteristics of lactation.
12. Compare various maternal and newborn positions used during breastfeeding.
13. Identify principles of breast pumping and milk storage.
14. Discuss the principles of weaning the infant from the breast.
15. Explain the principles of the Baby Friendly Initiative
16. Describe techniques of formula preparation and feeding.
17. Discuss the dietary needs of the lactating mother.
18. Plan appropriate discharge teaching for the postpartum woman.

Key Terms

afterpains
colostrum (kŏ-LŎS-trŭm)
diastasis rectus (dī-ĂS-tă-sĭs RĔK-tus)
episiotomy
foremilk
fundus
galactogogues (gă-LĂK-tō-gŏgz)
hindmilk
involution (ĭn-vō-LŪ-shŭn)
laceration
let-down reflex
lochia (LŌ-kē-ă)
perinatal mood disorders
postpartum blues
puerperium (pū-ŭr-PĔ-rē-ŭm)
rugae
suckling

The postpartum period, or puerperium, is approximately the 6 weeks following childbirth. This period is often referred to as the fourth trimester of pregnancy. This chapter addresses the physiological and psychological changes in the mother and her family.

PROVIDING INDIVIDUALIZED NURSING CARE FOR SPECIFIC GROUPS AND CULTURES

The nurse must adapt care to each individual, whether they are a lone parent or an adolescent, having a multiple birth, are LGBTQ2 or from another culture, or are lacking financial resources.

Adolescents, particularly younger ones, may need help learning parenting skills. Their peer group is very important to them, so the nurse must make every effort during both pregnancy and the postpartum period to help them fit in with their peers and to provide education about parenting. They may also lack family support and financial resources and may require social work support.

A lone parent may lack a strong support system. Often, she must return to work very soon because she is the sole provider for her family.

Families who live with poverty may have difficulty meeting their basic needs before the newborn arrives, and the new family member adds to their strain. The family may need social service referrals to direct them to appropriate resources.

Same-sex couples and transgender parents may have unique experiences in the postpartum period. Being aware of how maternal newborn nursing care has historically taken a heteronormative approach when providing care to these families will help to ensure their unique needs are being addressed.

Families who have twins (or more) face different challenges. The newborns may need intensive care due to a preterm birth, which may delay the parents' close contact and ability to bond and provide daily newborn care. The newborns may require care at a distant hospital if the family does not live close to a centre that can provide the care needed.

Homelessness, defined as a lack of a permanent home, is not limited to women who must live on the street. Some women live in single-room hotels, and others stay with friends or extended family. Homeless women often have difficulty accessing health care, receive care from different health care providers at different sites, and have incomplete medical records. Follow-up is difficult. The nurse can be a key link in facilitating referrals to outreach programs, support services, counselling, shelters, and follow-up medical care. Before discharging a homeless mother with her newborn infant, it is essential to determine that she has a place to go and has a way of accessing help for herself or her newborn.

CULTURAL INFLUENCES ON POSTPARTUM CARE

Canada has a diverse population. Special cultural practices are often most evident at significant life events such as birth and death. The nurse must adapt care to fit the health beliefs, values, and practices of a specific culture to make the birth a meaningful event as well as a physically safe event.

USING TRANSLATORS

The nurse may need an interpreter to understand the woman and her family and provide optimal care to them. If possible, especially when discussing sensitive information, the interpreter should not be a family member, who might interpret selectively. The interpreter should not be of a group that is in social or religious conflict with the patient and her family. Often educational material is available in different languages, and this should be used whenever possible.

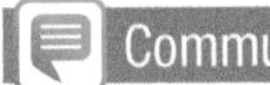 Communication

Cross-Cultural Communication

To verify that a woman (or family) understands what the nurse has told her, the nurse should have the woman repeat the teaching in her own words. An affirmative nod may indicate courtesy, not agreement or understanding, when the primary languages and the cultures of the nurse and family are different.

DIETARY PRACTICES

Some cultures (e.g., Chinese) may adhere to the "hot" and "cold" theory of diet after childbirth. Temperature has nothing to do with the foods that are considered hot and those that are considered cold; it is the believed intrinsic property of the food itself that classifies it. For example, "hot" foods include eggs, chicken, and rice. Women may also prefer their drinking water hot rather than cool or cold. Other hot–cold dietary practices include a balance between *yin* foods (e.g., bean sprouts, broccoli, and carrots) and *yang* foods (e.g., broiled meat, chicken, soup, and eggs).

POSTPARTUM CHANGES IN THE MOTHER

The postpartum woman must make physiological and psychological adaptations to adjust from being pregnant to the postpartum period. The nurse must assess the postpartum woman to ensure that this is a successful transition. Postpartum assessments are done frequently immediately after birth (every 15 minutes × 4, every 1 hour × 1 and then in 4 hours), and once the woman is stable, they are usually done once per shift. The acronym BUBBLLEE will help the nurse to remember parts of the postpartum assessment. See Table 9.1 for a summary of the nursing assessment for a postpartum woman. See Chapter 10 for additional information about postpartum complications.

REPRODUCTIVE SYSTEM

Following the third stage of labour, there is a fall in the blood levels of placental hormones, human placental lactogen, human chorionic gonadotropin, estrogen, and progesterone that help return the body to the prepregnant state. The most dramatic changes after birth occur in the woman's reproductive system. These changes are discussed in the following sections, and the nursing care is discussed for each area as applicable.

Breasts

Both breastfeeding and nonbreastfeeding mothers experience breast changes after birth. Assessments for both types of mothers are similar, but nursing care differs.

Changes in the breasts

During the first 24 hours after birth, the breasts have little or no change in breast tissue and feel soft. Colostrum can be expressed from the breasts. The breasts eventually become fuller and heavier around day 2 to 4 postpartum, with the breasts feeling increasingly firm and fuller as blood flow increases and milk production begins. Breast engorgement can occur in both breastfeeding and nonbreastfeeding mothers. The engorged breast is hard and erect and can be very uncomfortable. The nipple may be so hard that the newborn cannot easily grasp it. Engorgement is temporary and usually lasts for 24 to 48 hours and is caused by increased blood and lymph supply to the breasts as the body produces milk. Engorgement should be treated by expressing enough milk to provide comfort for the mother. Breastfeeding mothers should feed the newborn frequently. Mothers should be educated on how to perform hand expression to ensure they are able to relieve engorgement (Box 9.1).

Table 9.1 Summary of Postpartum Nursing Assessments (BUBBLEE)

ASSESSMENT	VARIATIONS AND DEVIATIONS	NURSING INTERVENTIONS
Breasts May be soft, filling, full, or engorged depending on how many days postpartum Assess for presence of colostrum.	Observe for reddened, tender areas, fissures, and sore nipples. Breast do not become full.	Document and report any alteration; assist with breastfeeding and assess progress; consult lactation nurse, if necessary.
Uterus Observe for firmness, height of fundus, and location.	Check for bladder distention if fundus is not midline; massage a boggy uterus.	Document and report any alterations; teach expectations for descent of fundus; teach mother how to massage fundus; discuss "afterpains."
Bladder Observe for bladder distention and urination.	Observe for burning or pain on urination.	Document and report urine output and abdominal assessment for distended bladder.
Bowels Observe for passage of flatus, bowel sounds, and bowel movement; normal not to have a bowel movement for up to 3 days after birth.	Report lack of bowel sounds or constipation; distended hemorrhoids may be seen.	Encourage fluids, ambulation, and fibre in diet; assist with sitz bath for hemorrhoids; stool softeners may be used for women with a more extensive laceration or episiotomy.
Lochia Observe for amount, colour, odour, and presence of clots.	Observe for large clots and heavy pad saturation; watch for a trickle of bright red blood.	Document firm, midline fundus; report bleeding and large clots; count peripads saturated in 1 hour; teach the lochial changes to expect.
Legs Observe for increased swelling and pain.	Pain in the legs may indicate a VTE; Homans's sign is not routinely assessed because it has limited ability to determine a VTE.	Clinical symptoms and venous ultrasound are diagnostic measures for a VTE.
Episiotomy/Laceration Observe perineum.	Observe for vulvar hematoma, perineal bruising; may see hemorrhoids.	Document wound assessment in relation to REEDA; teach pericare technique; apply cold packs or heat as indicated; teach how to use sitz bath at home.
Emotions or bonding with newborn Evaluate family interaction, support, and physical contact with newborn. Postpartum blues are normal for the first 2 weeks and are evidenced by fluctuating mood.	Observe for postpartum blues; observe for "enface contact" with newborn; teach handling and response to newborn needs; assess cultural practices; assess stage of postpartum adaptation.	Teach parents about newborn behaviour and appearance; teach newborn care; teach self-care and *listen* to patient; provide support, nutrition, and periods of rest to prevent fatigue; encourage skin-to-skin contact.
Vital signs There is a slight increase in heart rate immediately after birth; respirations may be slightly elevated; blood pressure may be slightly elevated but should return to normal shortly after birth.	Abnormalities may be consistent with comorbidities; deviation in vital signs may also indicate the woman is in pain; has pre-eclampsia; assess for shock, infection.	Record and report tachypnea, elevated temperature, and blood pressure abnormalities; assess for pain, and provide medication as indicated; administer analgesics as needed.

REEDA, **R**edness, **e**dema, **e**cchymosis, **d**rainage, **a**pproximation; *VTE,* venous thromboembolism.
Isley, M. M., & Katz, V. L. (2017). Postpartum care and long-term health considerations. In S. G. Gabbe, J. R. Niebyl, J. L. Simpson, et al. (Eds.), *Obstetrics: Normal and problem pregnancies* (7th ed.). Philadelphia: Elsevier.

Nursing care

At each assessment, the nurse checks the woman's breasts for consistency and the presence of colostrum. The nipples are inspected for redness and cracking, a sign of an incorrect latch, which may be painful and damaging to the nipple. Damaged nipples can also provide a port of entry for microorganisms, which can lead to infection. Flat or inverted nipples make it more difficult for the newborn to grasp the nipple and suckle. Breastfeeding mothers should wear a bra to support the heavier breasts. Mothers can be taught to wash the nipple with plain water to avoid the drying effects of soap, which can lead to cracking. The nonbreastfeeding woman can wear a supportive bra, take analgesics, and minimize stimulation when washing her breasts for the first few days after birth. See further discussion of infant feeding later in the chapter.

Uterus

Involution refers to changes that the reproductive organs, particularly the uterus, undergo after birth to return them to their prepregnancy size and condition. The uterus undergoes a rapid reduction in

Box 9.1 Hand Expression

Teach the mother to do the following:
- Perform hand hygiene.
- Get into a comfortable position.
- Gently massage breast and nipple to stimulate let-down reflex.
- Place four fingers supporting lower part of the breast and thumb on top at outer edge of the areola, in the shape of the letter *C*.
- Push thumb and fingers back toward chest and squeeze fingers and thumb together.
- Press and release, moving fingers around the areola in a circle to express from different parts.
- Catch milk in a clean cup, bowl, or jar.
- Switch between breasts every few minutes.

Adapted from Public Health Agency of Canada (PHAC). (2016). Chapter 6—Breastfeeding. In *Family-centred maternity and newborn care: National guidelines*. Retrieved from https://www.canada.ca/en/public-health/services/publications/healthy-living/maternity-newborn-care-guidelines-chapter-6.html.

size and weight after birth. The uterus should return to the prepregnant size by 5 to 6 weeks after birth. The failure of the uterus to return to the prepregnant state after 6 weeks is called *subinvolution* (see Chapter 10).

Descent of the uterine fundus

The uterine **fundus** (the upper portion of the body of the uterus) descends at a predictable rate as the muscle cells contract to control bleeding at the placental insertion site and as the size of each muscle cell decreases. Immediately after the placenta is expelled, the uterine fundus can be felt midline, at or slightly below the level of the umbilicus, as a firm mass (about the size of a grapefruit). A boggy uterus is one that is not firm and increases the risk of postpartum bleeding. The fundus may rise slightly over the umbilicus at 12 hours, but after 24 hours the fundus begins to descend about 1 to 2 cm (one finger's width) each day. By 2 weeks postpartum, the fundus will no longer be palpable. A full bladder interferes with uterine contraction because it pushes the fundus up and causes it to deviate to one side, usually to the right side (Fig. 9.1).

Nursing Tip

If the mother's uterus is boggy, massaging it (while supporting the lower segment) will help the uterus become firm and expel any clots so it will remain contracted. If her bladder is also full, emptying the bladder will assist the uterus in remaining contracted.

Uterine lining

The uterine lining (called the *endometrium* when not pregnant and the *decidua* during pregnancy) is shed when the placenta detaches. A basal layer of the lining remains to generate new endometrium to prepare for future pregnancies. The placental site is fully healed in 6 to 7 weeks.

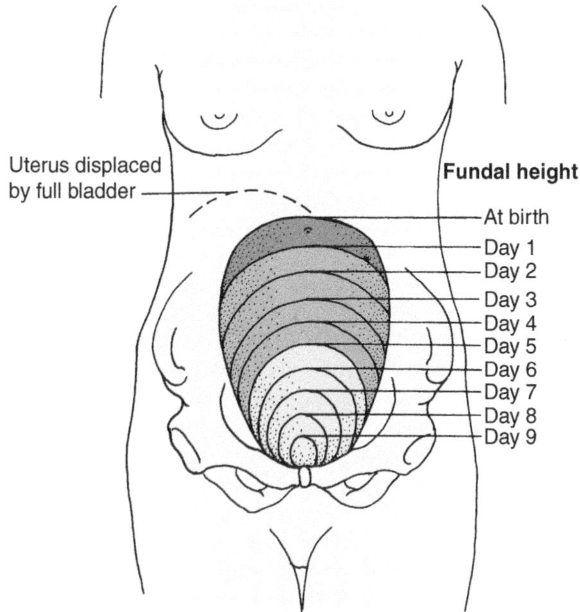

Fig. 9.1 The height of the uterine fundus changes each day as involution progresses.

Afterpains

Intermittent uterine contractions may cause afterpains similar to menstrual cramps. The cramping usually occurs during breastfeeding because **suckling** causes the posterior pituitary to release oxytocin, a hormone that contracts the uterus. The discomfort is self-limiting and decreases rapidly within 48 hours postpartum. **Afterpains** occur more often in multiparas or in women whose uterus was overly distended, for example, for multiple births. Mild analgesics may be prescribed. Aspirin is not used postpartum because it interferes with blood clotting.

Nursing Tip

The nurse should assess the fundus for descent, location, and firmness frequently and should teach the mother about the expected changes.

Lochia

Vaginal discharge after birth, called **lochia**, is composed of endometrial tissue, blood, and lymph. Lochia gradually changes characteristics during the early postpartum period:

- *Lochia rubra* is red because it is composed mostly of blood; it may contain small clots and lasts for about 3 to 4 days after birth.
- *Lochia serosa* is pinkish or brown because it consists of old blood, serum, leukocytes, and tissue debris. It lasts from about the third through the tenth day after birth, although it can last up to 25 days.
- *Lochia alba* is mostly mucus and is yellow or white. It usually starts around the tenth day and can last up to 4 to 6 weeks after birth (Isley & Katz, 2017).

Skill 9.1 Estimating the Volume of Lochia

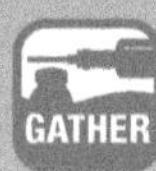

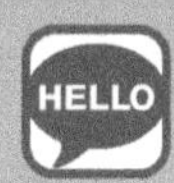

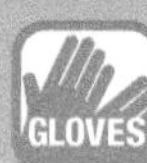

PURPOSE

To determine amount of blood loss during the postpartum period

STEPS

1. Assess lochia for quantity, type, and characteristics. A guideline to estimate and chart the amount of flow on the menstrual pad in 1 hour is as follows (see figure):
   a. *Scant:* Less than a 5-cm (2-inch) stain
   b. *Light:* Less than a 10-cm (4-inch) stain
   c. *Moderate:* Less than a 15-cm (6-inch) stain
   d. *Large or heavy:* Larger than a 15-cm stain or one pad saturated within 2 hours
   e. *Excessive:* Saturation of a perineal pad within 30 minutes
2. Weighing menstrual pads before and after use is a more accurate method of determine blood loss for a woman who is bleeding.

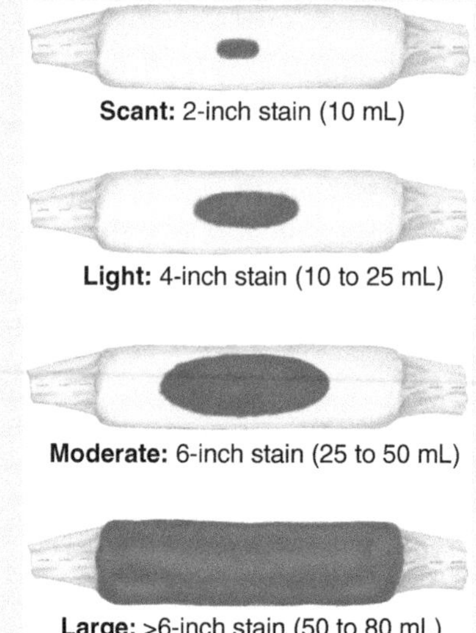

From Murray, S. S., & McKinney, E. S. (2014). *Foundations of maternal-newborn and women's health nursing* (6th ed.). St. Louis: Saunders.

Lochia has a characteristic fleshy or menstrual odour; it should not have a foul odour. The woman's fundus must be assessed for firmness because an uncontracted (boggy) uterus allows blood to flow freely from blood vessels at the placenta insertion site.

Perineal pads must be assessed in order to estimate the amount of blood loss (Skill 9.1). If a mother has excessive discharge of lochia, the fundus should be assessed and a clean pad should be applied and checked within 15 minutes. When bleeding is heavier than normal, the peripads may be counted or weighed to help determine the amount of vaginal discharge. Weighing the pads is a much more accurate method of determining blood loss (see AWHONN online resource in the Additional Learning Resources). One gram of weight equals about 1 mL of blood. The nurse should assess the underpads on the bed to determine if bleeding has overflowed onto the underpad.

The flow of lochia is briefly heavier when the mother ambulates, because lochia pooled in the vagina is discharged when she assumes an upright position. A few small clots may be seen at this time, but large clots should not be present. The quantity of lochia may briefly increase when the mother breastfeeds because suckling causes uterine contraction. The rate of discharge increases with exercise. The absence of lochia is not normal and may be associated with blood clots retained within the uterus or with infection. If lochia rubra persists past the first 4 days, it could indicate retained placenta fragments.

Nursing care

The fundus is assessed at routine intervals for firmness, location, and position in relation to the midline. Women who have a higher risk for postpartum hemorrhage (see Chapter 10) should be assessed more often. While doing initial assessments, the nurse should explain the reason they are done and teach the woman how to assess her own fundus. If her uterus stops descending, this should be reported to her health care provider.

A poorly contracted (boggy) uterus should be massaged until firm to prevent hemorrhage (see Skill 9.2). Lochia flow may increase briefly as the uterus contracts and expels it. It is essential *not* to push down on an uncontracted uterus to prevent inverting it. If a full bladder contributes to poor uterine contraction, the mother should be assisted to void in the bathroom or on a bedpan if she cannot ambulate. Catheterization may be necessary if she cannot void.

The woman should be taught the expected sequence for lochia changes and the amount she should expect. The woman is instructed to report any abnormal conditions, such as:

- Foul-smelling lochia, with or without fever
- Lochia rubra that persists beyond the fourth day
- Unusually heavy flow of lochia
- Lochia that returns to a bright red colour after it has progressed to serosa or alba

Medications that may be given to stimulate uterine contraction include the following (see Chapter 10 for further discussion):

- Oxytocin, usually given routinely after birth via intramuscular injection or intravenous infusion

Skill 9.2 Observing and Massaging the Uterine Fundus

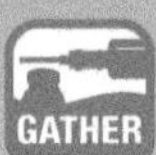

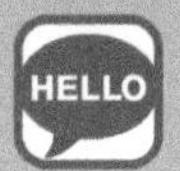

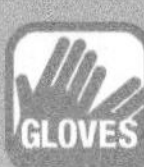

PURPOSE

To prevent excessive postpartum bleeding. This is only to be done when the fundus is not firm.

STEPS

1. Identify the need for fundal massage. The uterus will be boggy and usually higher than the umbilicus. A firm fundus does not need massage.
2. Place the woman in a supine position with the knees slightly flexed. Look at the perineal pad to observe lochia as the fundus is palpated.
3. Place the outer edge of the nondominant hand just above the symphysis pubis, and press downward slightly to anchor the lower uterus.
4. Locate the uterine fundus with the flat portion of the fingers of the dominant hand. If massage is necessary, use side of the hand in a firm, circular motion.
5. When the uterus is not firm, gently push downward on the fundus, toward the vaginal outlet, to expel blood and clots that have accumulated inside the uterus. *Keep the other hand on the lower uterus to avoid inverting it.*
6. If a full bladder contributes to uterine relaxation, have the mother void. Catheterize her (with a health care provider's order) if she cannot void.
7. Document the consistency and location of the fundus before and after massage.
8. Give any prescribed medications, such as oxytocin, to maintain uterine contraction. Have the mother put the newborn to the breast, if she is breastfeeding, to stimulate secretion of natural oxytocin.
9. Report a fundus that does not stay firm.

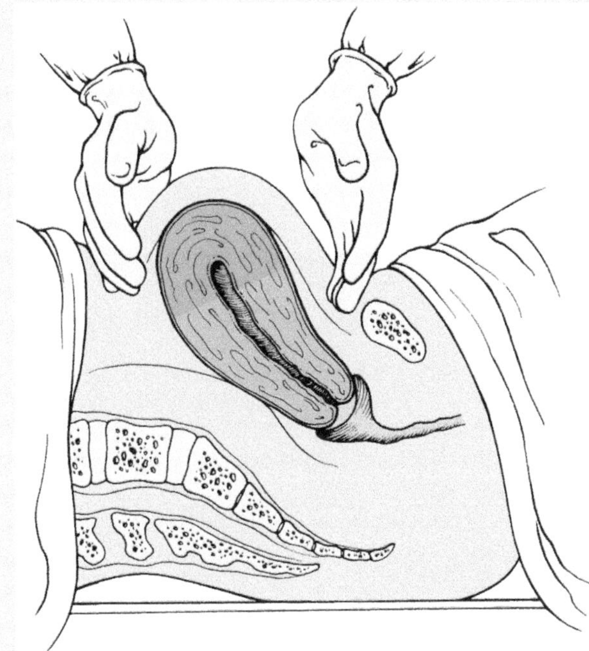

- Methylergonovine (Methergine), given intramuscularly (for postpartum hemorrhage)

A newborn suckling at the breast has a similar effect, because natural oxytocin release stimulates contractions.

Mild analgesics relieve afterpains adequately for most women. The breastfeeding mother should take an analgesic 30 to 60 minutes prior to breastfeeding to maximize the analgesic effect. Afterpains persisting longer than 48 hours after birth should be reported.

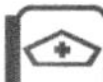 **Nursing Tip**

A firm fundus does not need massage.

Cervix

The cervix regains its muscle tone but never closes as tightly as during the prepregnant state. Some edema persists for a few weeks after birth. A constant trickle of brighter red lochia is not normal and is associated with bleeding from lacerations of the cervix or vagina, particularly if the fundus remains firm.

Vagina

The vagina undergoes a great deal of stretching during childbirth. The **rugae**, or vaginal folds, disappear, and the walls of the vagina become smooth and spacious. The rugae reappear 3 weeks postpartum. Within 6 weeks, the vagina has regained most of its prepregnancy form, but it never returns to the size it was before pregnancy.

Perineum

The perineum is often edematous, tender, and bruised. An **episiotomy** (incision to enlarge the vaginal opening) may have been performed, or a perineal **laceration** may have occurred (see Chapter 6 for further discussion). Women with hemorrhoids often find that these temporarily worsen because of the pressure exerted during the birth process.

Nursing care

The perineum should be assessed for normal healing and signs of complications (Skill 9.3). The REEDA acronym helps the nurse remember the five signs to assess.

Skill 9.3 Assessing the Perineum

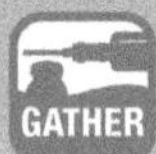

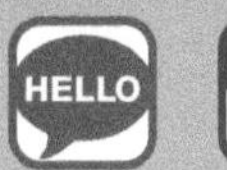

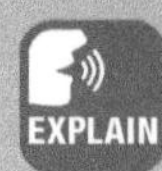

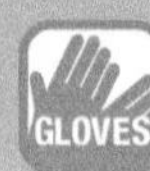

PURPOSE

To observe the perineum, hemorrhoids, and status of healing

STEPS

1. Provide privacy; explain purpose of procedure.
2. Put on gloves (provide protection from contact of bodily fluids).
3. Ask woman to turn on her side and to flex her upper leg, lower perineal pad, and lift up upper buttock; if necessary, use flashlight to inspect perineum.
4. Observe for edema, bruising, and hematoma.
5. Examine laceration or episiotomy for REEDA (redness, edema, ecchymosis, discharge, approximation).
6. Observe hemorrhoids for extent of edema (can interfere with bowel elimination).
7. Apply clean peripads, taking care to only touch edges.
8. Reposition woman into position of comfort.
9. Dispose of soiled contents in appropriate waste container, and perform hand hygiene.
10. Document care provided in medical record.

Memory Jogger

REEDA is **r**edness, **e**dema, **e**cchymosis, **d**ischarge, and **a**pproximation

***R**edness.* Redness without excessive tenderness is probably the normal inflammation associated with healing, but pain with the redness is more likely to indicate infection.

***E**dema.* Mild edema is common, but severe edema interferes with healing.

***E**cchymosis (bruising).* A few small superficial bruises are common. Larger bruises interfere with normal healing.

***D**ischarge.* No discharge from the perineal suture line should be present.

***A**pproximation (intactness of the suture line).* The suture line should not be separated. If intact, it is almost impossible to distinguish the laceration or episiotomy from surrounding skin folds.

Note: The REEDA acronym is also useful when assessing a Caesarean incision for healing.

Comfort and hygienic measures are the focus of nursing care and patient teaching. An ice pack, frozen peripad, or chemical cold pack is applied for the first 24 hours to reduce edema and bruising and to numb the perineal area. The cold pack should be covered with a paper cover or a washcloth to prevent tissue damage. The ice pack should be removed after 20 minutes and left off for 20 minutes before applying another, for maximum effect. In some cultures, women believe that heat has healing properties and may not want to use an ice pack.

After 24 hours, heat in the form of a chemical warm pack or a sitz bath increases circulation and promotes healing (Skill 9.4). The sitz bath circulates either cool or warm water over the perineum to cleanse the area and increase comfort. There is some evidence that sitting in a cool sitz bath and adding ice cubes and remaining in the water for 20 minutes may provide immediate pain relief in the first 24 hours (Isley & Katz, 2017). However, after the first 24 hours heat is more comforting and effective in promoting healing.

The woman is taught to do perineal care after each voiding or bowel movement, to cleanse the area without trauma. A plastic bottle (peri-bottle) is filled with warm water, and the water is squirted over the perineum in a front-to-back direction. The perineum is blotted dry. Perineal pads (peripads) should be applied and removed in the same front-to-back direction to prevent fecal contamination of the perineum and vagina (Skill 9.5).

Topical and systemic medications may be used to relieve perineal pain. Topical application of anaesthetic ointments or spray reduces inflammation or numbs the perineum.

In addition to topical medications, witch hazel pads (Tucks) and sitz baths reduce the discomfort of hemorrhoids.

To reduce pain when sitting, the mother can be taught to squeeze her buttocks together as she lowers herself to a sitting position and then to relax her buttocks.

Nutrition Considerations

Pay special attention to a woman's diet and fluids if she had a third- or fourth-degree laceration. A high-fibre diet and adequate fluids help to prevent constipation that might result in a breakdown of the perineal area where the laceration was sutured.

Return of Menstruation and Contraception

The production of placental estrogen and progesterone stops when the placenta is delivered, causing a rise in the production of follicle-stimulating hormone. Menstrual cycles resume in about 7 to 9 weeks after birth if the woman is not breastfeeding and may not resume for 6 to 12 months if the woman is breastfeeding (Isley & Katz, 2017).

Couples often are hesitant to ask questions concerning resumption of sexual activity after childbirth, and

Skill 9.4 Assisting with a Sitz Bath

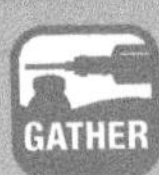

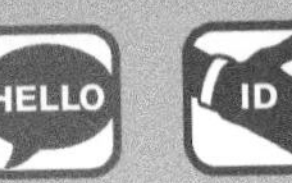

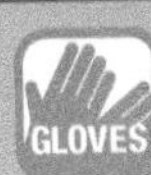

PURPOSE

To aid healing of perineum through application of moist heat or cold

STEPS

1. Perform hand hygiene, explain procedure, and provide privacy.
2. Assess woman's condition; analyze appropriateness of procedure.
3. Place sitz bath on toilet seat; turn flow of water on.
4. Help woman remove pad and sit in flow of water for 20 minutes.
5. When completed, assist woman to pat perineum dry (front to back); apply clean perineal pad.
6. Perform hand hygiene.
7. Record in medical record that sitz bath was taken, condition of woman, and condition of perineum.

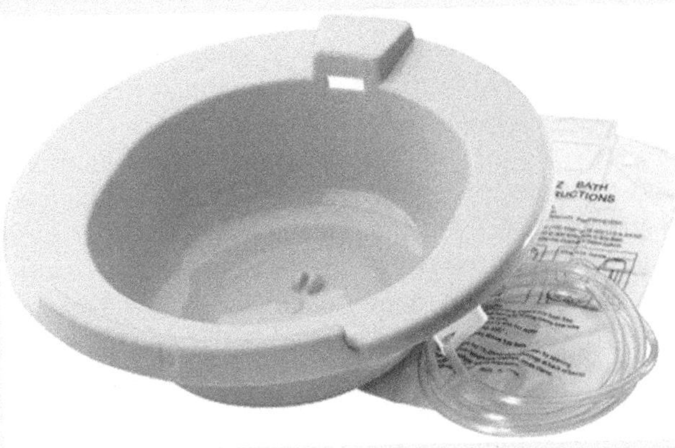

Skill 9.5 Performing Perineal Care

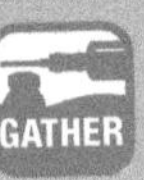

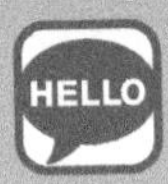

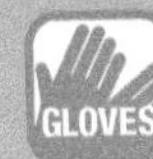

PURPOSE

To teach the woman the proper technique of perineal care to promote healing and prevent infection

STEPS

1. Perform hand hygiene.
2. Explain procedure to the woman.
3. Assist the woman to the bathroom.
4. Instruct woman to perform hand hygiene before and after each perineal care.
5. Remove soiled pad from front to back; discard in appropriate waste container.
6. Teach woman to squeeze peri-bottle or pour warm water or cleansing solution over perineum without opening labia.
7. Pat dry with clean tissue. Use each tissue one time. Pat from front to back, and then discard tissue.
8. Apply medicated ointments or sprays as ordered. Do not apply perineal pad for 1 to 2 minutes (otherwise the medication will be absorbed in the pad).
9. Apply clean perineal pad from front to back, touching only side and outside of pad to lessen risk of infection.
10. Do not flush toilet until woman is standing upright; otherwise, the flushing water can spray the perineum.
11. Always perform perineal care after each voiding, bowel movement, or at least every 4 hours during first 3–4 days.
12. Report clots, increase in lochia flow, or excessive abdominal cramping.

many resume activity before the 6-week checkup. It is important for the nurse to teach the woman that it is considered safe to resume sexual intercourse when bleeding has stopped and the perineum has healed. However, the vagina does not lubricate well in the first 6 weeks after childbirth (or longer in the breastfeeding mother). A water-soluble gel such as K-Y or a contraceptive gel can be used for lubrication to make intercourse more comfortable. Instructing the woman to perform the Kegel exercise correctly can help her strengthen muscles involved in urination, bowel function, and vaginal sensations during intercourse.

Discussion and teaching concerning contraception should be initiated before discharge, because the mother may not return to her health care provider before 6 weeks postpartum. She may resume sexual activity before that appointment, which may result in an unplanned pregnancy, as *ovulation can occur before menstruation is re-established, and pregnancy can result.*

Short intervals between pregnancies may result in poor pregnancy outcomes. The ideal pregnancy spacing should be approximately 2 years apart, as this interval has been associated with decreased risk of preterm birth and low-birth-weight infants, as well as decreased risk for uterine rupture among women attempting a vaginal birth after a Caesarean birth (Gregory, Ramos, & Jauniaux, 2017).

Breastfeeding or the lactational amenorrhea method (LAM) results in 98% contraceptive protection when the woman is exclusively breastfeeding on demand both day and night, her menstrual period has not returned, and the infant is less than 6 months old (Black, Guilbert, et al., 2015; Isley & Katz, 2017). Combined oral or transdermal estrogen-progesterone contraceptives can be taken about 2 to 3 weeks after birth in women who are not breastfeeding, as estrogen suppresses lactation. For breastfeeding women, a low-dose progestin-only contraceptive can be started 4 weeks postpartum if breastfeeding is well established. For a full discussion of contraception see Chapter 2, Contraception and Family Planning.

Pain Management

Following birth, women need to be assessed for pain, and most women require some pain-relief measures. Common causes of pain can be any of the following: perineal laceration or episiotomy, hemorrhoids, breast engorgement, sore nipples, epidural insertion site, or uterine contractions. Pharmacological and nonpharmacological methods of pain relief can be used. Heating pads may help relieve uterine discomfort and ice packs are used for perineal pain during the first 24 hours; after this time heat may be more soothing. Engorgement is best treated with ice packs and frequent feeding or hand expression to comfort. Many women require pharmacological pain management strategies, which include a variety of analgesics, both opioid (narcotic) and nonopioid (e.g., nonsteroidal anti-inflammatory medications [NSAIDs]). Pain management for Caesarean births is discussed later in the chapter.

URINARY SYSTEM

Kidney function returns to normal within a month after birth. A decrease in the tone of the bladder and ureters as a result of pregnancy, combined with intravenous (IV) fluids administered during labour, may cause the woman's bladder to fill quickly but empty incompletely during the postpartum period. This can lead to postpartum hemorrhage (PPH) when the full bladder displaces the uterus, or a possible urinary tract infection because of stasis of the urine in the bladder. It may be normal for a woman not to feel the urge to void for up to 8 hours after birth, especially if epidural anaesthesia was used.

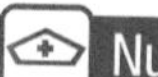 **Nursing Tip**

The woman who voids frequent, small amounts of urine may have increased residual urine, because her bladder does not empty completely. Residual urine in the bladder may promote the growth of microorganisms.

Nursing care

The nurse should regularly assess the woman's bladder for distention. The bladder may not feel full to the woman, yet the uterus is high and deviated to one side. If she can ambulate, the mother should go to the bathroom and urinate. The first two to three voidings after Caesarean birth or after catheter removal are measured. Women who receive IV infusions or have an indwelling catheter continue to have their urine output measured until the infusion or catheter is discontinued. The following measures may help a woman to urinate:

- Provide as much privacy as possible.
- Remain near the woman, but do not rush her by constantly asking her if she has urinated.
- Run water in the sink.
- Have the woman place her hands in warm water.
- Have the woman use the peri-bottle to squirt warm water over her perineal area to relax the urethral sphincter. Be sure to measure the amount of water in the peri-bottle when it is filled so the amount used can be deducted from the amount of urine voided.

Some discomfort with early urination is expected because of the edema and trauma in the area. However, continued burning or urgency of urination suggests bladder infection. High fever and chills may occur with kidney infection.

GASTROINTESTINAL SYSTEM

The gastrointestinal system resumes normal activity shortly after birth when progesterone decreases. The mother is usually hungry after the hard work of birth and usually tolerates a regular diet.

It is normal not to have a bowel movement for 2 to 3 days after birth, as a result of several factors:

- Pain medications may slow peristalsis.
- There is decreased muscle tone in the intestine during labour.
- Abdominal muscles are stretched, making it more difficult for the woman to bear down to expel stool. A Caesarean incision adds to this difficulty.
- Hemorrhoids or soreness and swelling of the perineum may make the woman fear her first bowel movement.
- She may have had slight dehydration and little food intake during labour

Nursing care

The mother is encouraged to drink lots of fluids, add fibre to her diet, and ambulate. Stool softeners may be ordered for women who have a Caesarean birth or a third- or fourth-degree laceration, if required.

CARDIOVASCULER SYSTEM

Cardiac Output and Blood Volume

Because of a 50% increase in blood volume during pregnancy, the woman can usually tolerate the following normal blood loss at birth:

- 300–500 mL in vaginal birth
- 500–1 000 mL in Caesarean birth

Despite the blood loss, there is a temporary increase in blood volume, cardiac output, and stroke volume, because blood that was directed to the uterus and the placenta returns to the main circulation. Added fluid also moves from the tissues into the circulation, further increasing her blood volume. To re-establish normal fluid balance, the body rids itself of excess fluid in the following two ways:

1. Diuresis (increased excretion of urine), which may reach 3 000 mL/day
2. Diaphoresis (profuse perspiration)

Vital signs may change slightly after birth. Pulse may be elevated for the first hour or so after birth and then decreases to normal and blood pressure is altered only slightly. The respiratory rate, which is often elevated during pregnancy, can take up to 6 weeks to return to a normal rate.

After childbirth, resistance to blood flow in the vessels of the pelvis drops. As a result, the woman's blood pressure may fall when she sits or stands, resulting in *orthostatic hypotension*, and she may feel dizzy or lightheaded or may even faint. Guidance and assistance are needed during early ambulation to prevent injury.

Coagulation

Blood clotting factors are higher during pregnancy and for 4 to 6 weeks postpartum, yet the woman's ability to lyse (break down and eliminate) clots is not increased. Therefore, she is prone to venous thromboembolism (VTE), especially if there is stasis of blood in the venous system. This situation is more likely to occur if the woman has had a Caesarean birth or is confined to bed rest after the birth. *Dyspnea* (difficult breathing) and *tachypnea* (rapid breathing) are hallmark signs of a pulmonary embolus and necessitate immediate medical intervention. Most hospitals have standing orders for VTE prophylaxis for women who have increased risk. This may include prophylactic anticoagulant therapy with heparin or pneumatic compression devices on the lower extremities to prevent venous congestion and to promote circulation. Women are encouraged to ambulate early to decrease the risk of VTE (see discussion on preventing thrombophlebitis later in the chapter).

Blood Values

The massive fluid shifts just described affect blood values such as hemoglobin and hematocrit, making them difficult to interpret during the early puerperium. Fluid that shifts into the bloodstream dilutes the blood cells, which lowers the hematocrit. As the fluid balance returns to normal, the values are more accurately interpreted, usually by 8 weeks postpartum.

The white blood cell (leukocyte) count may rise as high as 20 to 25 × 10^9/L, a level that would ordinarily suggest infection. The increase is in response to inflammation, pain, and stress, and it protects the mother from infection as her tissues heal. The white blood cell count returns to normal by 12 days postpartum.

Chills

Many mothers experience tremors that resemble shivering or "chills" immediately after birth. These tremors are thought to be related to a sudden release of pressure on the pelvic nerves and a vasomotor response involving epinephrine (adrenaline) during the birth process. Most women will deny feeling cold. These tremors or "chills" stop spontaneously shortly after birth. The nurse should reassure the woman and cover her with a warm blanket to provide comfort. Chills accompanied by fever after the first 24 hours suggest infection and should be reported.

INTEGUMENTARY SYSTEM

Hyperpigmentation of the skin ("mask of pregnancy," or chloasma, and the linea nigra) fade as hormone levels decrease, but in some women they do not completely disappear. Striae ("stretch marks") do not disappear but fade from reddish purple to silver.

MUSCULOSKELETAL SYSTEM

The abdominal wall has been greatly stretched during pregnancy and many women are dismayed to discover that they still look pregnant after they give birth. They should be reassured that time and exercise can tighten their lax muscles. Also, some women have **diastasis recti**, in which the longitudinal abdominal muscles that extend from the chest to the symphysis pubis are separated. Abdominal wall weakness may remain for 6 to 8 weeks and contribute to constipation. Hypermobility of the joints that normally occurs during pregnancy usually stabilizes within 6 to 8 weeks, but the joints of the feet may remain separated, and the new mother may notice an increase in shoe size. The centre of gravity of the body returns to normal when the enlarged uterus returns to its prepregnant size.

A woman can usually begin light exercises as soon as the first day after vaginal birth. Women who have undergone a Caesarean birth should wait about 4 weeks to do any abdominal exercise. Common postpartum exercises include the following:

- *Abdominal tightening.* In the supine or erect position, the woman inhales slowly and then exhales slowly while contracting her abdominal muscles. After a count of 10, she relaxes the muscles. She should begin with 3 repetitions and increase the number to 5, then 10. This may be done 3 times and then 5 times daily, up to 10 times each day.
- *Head lift.* The woman lies flat on her back on her bed with her knees bent and inhales. While exhaling, she lifts her head, chin to chest, and looks at her thighs. She holds this position to a count of

three, and then relaxes. This is repeated several times. After the third week, the head lift may progress to include the head and shoulders. This may be done 5 to 10 times daily.

- *Pelvic tilt.* While lying supine with her knees bent and feet flat, the woman inhales and exhales, flattening her lower back to the bed or exercise surface and contracting her abdominal muscles. She holds the position to a count of three. She begins with 5 repetitions and works up to 10 repetitions daily.
- *Kegel exercises.* Perineal exercises may be resumed immediately after birth to promote circulation and healing. The mother tightens the muscles of the perineal area, as if to stop the flow of urine, and then relaxes them. She should inhale, tighten for a count of 10, exhale, and relax. Increasing the time spent doing Kegel exercises to 15 minutes twice a day will increase muscle strength. She should not actually stop her urine flow when urinating, however, because this could lead to urine stasis and urinary tract infection.

IMMUNE SYSTEM

Prevention of blood incompatibility and infection are addressed in the postpartum period according to each woman's specific needs.

Rh_0(D) Immune Globulin

The woman's blood type and Rh factor and antibody status are determined during prenatal care. The Rh-negative mother should receive a dose of Rh_0(D) immune globulin within 72 hours after giving birth to an Rh-positive newborn. This prevents sensitization to Rh-positive erythrocytes that may have entered her bloodstream when the newborn was born. *Rh_0(D) immune globulin is given to the mother, not the newborn,* by intramuscular injection.

Rubella (German Measles) Immunization

Rubella titres are done early in pregnancy to determine if a woman is immune to rubella. A titre of 1:8 (or enzyme immunoassay level less than 0.8) indicates nonimmunity to the rubella virus. The mother who is not immune is given the vaccine in the immediate postpartum period. The vaccine prevents infection with the rubella virus during subsequent pregnancies, which could cause birth defects. Informed consent is required before administering the rubella vaccine, and this includes providing information about the teratogenic effect of the vaccine and the importance of using contraception for 1 month after administration. The rubella vaccine is given subcutaneously in the upper arm. The vaccine should not be administered if the woman has a severe life-threatening allergy to eggs or if she or anyone in the home is immunocompromised. Women vaccinated during the postpartum period may breastfeed without adverse effects to the newborn.

ADAPTATION OF NURSING CARE FOLLOWING CAESAREAN BIRTH

The woman who undergoes a Caesarean birth has had surgery as well as given birth. Many of her reactions to the surgical birth depend on whether she expected it. The woman who had an unexpected, emergency Caesarean often has many questions about what happened to her and why, because there may not have been time to answer these questions at the time of birth. In addition, her anxiety may have limited her ability to comprehend any explanations given. Occasionally a woman may feel that she failed if she was unable to give birth after labouring. Terms such as *failed induction* and *failure to progress* imply that the woman herself was not competent in some way, and these words should not be used. Some variations of normal postpartum care are needed for the woman who has experienced a Caesarean birth (Nursing Care Plan 9.1). Assessments after a Caesarean birth are usually done every 15 minutes for 1 to 2 hours until vital signs are stable; this is then done every 4 hours for the first 24 hours and then once per shift.

Uterus

The nurse should check and document the descent and firmness of the fundus as on any new mother; it descends at a similar rate. Checking the fundus when a woman has a skin incision can be very uncomfortable for her. If possible, it is advisable that the woman have pain medication prior to assessment of the fundus. The nurse should gently "walk" the fingers toward the fundus from the side to her abdominal midline. If the fundus is firm and at its expected level, no massage is necessary. Assessing for lochia is an important part of the maternal assessment that can ensure the fundus is well contracted.

Lochia

Lochia is checked at routine assessment intervals, which vary with the time since birth. The quantity of lochia immediately after Caesarean birth is generally less because the uterus is sponged out, removing the contents of the uterus, during the surgery. The changes in the lochia are the same as in a vaginal birth.

Dressing

When a dressing is present, the dressing should be checked for drainage, as with any surgical patient. When the dressing is removed, the incision is assessed for signs of infection. The wound should be clean and dry, and the staples or sutures should be intact. The REEDA acronym previously described is a good way to remember key items to check as related to an incision: **r**edness, **e**dema, **e**cchymosis, **d**rainage, and **a**pproximation. Staples are removed as per primary health care providers' orders. Some practitioners remove staples and apply steri-strips at 48 hours and others wait until 5 days postbirth and up to 7 to 10 days for women with a high body mass index (BMI). This may need to be done in the health care provider's office.

 **Nursing Care Plan 9.1 The Postpartum Woman After a Caesarean Birth**

PATIENT DATA

A 32-year-old woman is admitted to the postpartum unit after giving birth to a healthy 3 800 g boy via Caesarean birth. The woman is lying still in bed and does not want to move because, she states, she fears postoperative pain.

Selected Nursing Diagnosis Pain related to surgical incision and afterpains

Goals	Nursing Interventions	Rationales
The woman will state that pain relief is adequate with pharmacological and nonpharmacological measures.	Use a 0-to-10 scale to evaluate pain level before and after interventions. Encourage the woman to change positions regularly (minimum every 2 hours). Support her body and extremities with pillows as needed. Teach the woman to splint her incision by using a small pillow pressed to her incision when moving or coughing. Provide ordered analgesia: • Patient-controlled anaesthesia pump • Intermittent injections • Oral analgesia	Provides a more objective way for the nurse to evaluate the woman's subjective experience of pain. Evaluates adequacy of pain relief. Reduces discomfort from constant pressure and having her body in one position for too long. Also helps to mobilize respiratory secretions and decrease risk for DVT. Supports the incision, reducing pain. Increases the likelihood that she will cough adequately, which expels respiratory secretions. Reduces the perception of pain, which facilitates moving, coughing, and ambulating. Reduces anxiety and fatigue.

Selected Nursing Diagnosis Risk for infection related to abdominal incision

Goals	Nursing Interventions	Rationales
The woman will have no excessive redness or tenderness and no separation or discharge from incision.	Observe dressing for drainage with each assessment.	Red drainage indicates bleeding, which should not increase. Foul-smelling drainage indicates infection.
	When dressing is removed, assess incision using REEDA criteria. Assess amount of tenderness.	Identifies proper healing of incision. A separating suture line, excessive redness or tenderness, or discharge indicates probable infection.
	Assess temperature every 4 hours.	A temperature higher than 38°C (100.4°F) after 24 hours is associated with infection.
The woman will demonstrate knowledge of self-care measures related to her incision prior to discharge.	Teach woman self-care measures: • Expected progress of healing and how the incision should look Teach her to look at the incision in the mirror when she gets home so she knows if changes have occured. • Avoid lifting anything heavier than the baby for 6 weeks, avoid abdominal exercise for 4 weeks • What to report (signs of bleeding or infection) • When her staples or sutures should be removed if not done before discharge • Follow-up appointment	Women must assume responsibility for their own care because of short hospital stays. These guidelines give the woman a framework for knowing what is and is not normal and how to care for herself to prevent infection. Follow-up appointments allow her health care provider to assess how healing is progressing and to identify complications early.

CRITICAL THINKING QUESTION

1. How will a nurse's discharge teaching for a patient who gave birth by Caesarean section differ from that for a patient who had a vaginal birth?

DVT, Deep vein thrombosis; *REEDA*, **r**edness, **e**dema, **e**cchymosis, **d**rainage, **a**pproximation.

The woman can shower once the dressing is removed (often at 24 hours). Use of a shower chair reduces the risk for fainting.

Urinary Catheter

An indwelling urinary catheter is generally removed within 8 to 12 hours after the surgery. Urine is observed for blood, which may indicate trauma to the bladder during labour or surgery. The blood should quickly clear from the urine as diuresis occurs. Intake and output are measured until both the IV infusion and the catheter are discontinued. The first two to three voidings are measured, and measuring should continue until the woman urinates at least 150 mL. The nurse should observe and teach the woman to observe for the following signs of urinary tract infection, because use of a catheter increases this risk:

- Fever
- Burning pain on urination
- Urgency of urination

Frequency of urination is difficult to assess in any postpartum woman because of normal postpartum diuresis. However, frequent voidings of small quantities of urine, especially if associated with the described signs and symptoms, suggest a urinary tract infection.

Respiratory Care

Lung sounds should be auscultated each shift. Diminished breath sounds, crackles, or wheezes indicate that lung secretions are being retained. When she is confined to bed, the woman should take deep breaths and turn from side to side every 2 hours. She should be encouraged to cough to move secretions out of her lungs. To reduce incisional pain from coughing or other movement, the nurse can have the woman splint the incision by holding a small pillow or folded blanket firmly against her incision. An incentive spirometer may be used to give the woman a "target" for deep breaths. The woman should begin ambulating, usually within no more than 8 hours to mobilize lung secretions.

Preventing Thrombophlebitis

The woman who has undergone a cesarean birth has a greater risk for thrombophlebitis especially if she has other risk factors such as: preterm birth, BMI over 30, stillbirth, smoker, or postpartum hemorrhage (Chan, Rey, Kent, et al., 2014). She may receive prophylactic heparin anticoagulation therapy or pneumatic compression devices may be applied to her lower extremities to decrease venous congestion and promote circulation until ambulation is established. She should do simple leg exercises, such as alternately flexing and extending her feet or moving her legs from a flexed to an extended position when turning. Early and frequent ambulation is the most important intervention to reduce the risk for thrombophlebitis.

Pain Management

Pain control is essential to facilitate movement that can prevent several complications and to enhance recovery. The severity, frequency, character, and location of discomfort are assessed. Use of a 0-to-10 scale helps quantify the subjective experience of pain; zero indicates no pain at all, and 10 is the worst pain ever. The scale helps the nurse choose the most appropriate relief methods and provides a means of evaluating the amount of relief the woman receives from the pain interventions.

Some women receive epidural or spinal narcotics for long-lasting pain relief. These medications can cause respiratory depression many hours after they are administered, sometimes up to 24 hours. Therefore, hourly respiratory monitoring is done for 24 hours. Naloxone (Narcan) should be readily available to reverse the respiratory depression.

If the woman does not have epidural or spinal narcotics for her pain management, she may require further medication as ordered by the health care provider. Some women have a patient-controlled analgesia (PCA) pump to provide them with analgesia. The pump has a syringe with a opioid analgesic inside. It is programmed to deliver a specific dose of the medication when the woman pushes a button. To prevent overdose, there is a lockout interval during which pushing the button has no effect. As with any opioid, the medication inside the PCA pump is counted at shift change, and the facility's protocol for record keeping is followed to account for all medication doses received, remaining, or wasted when the PCA medication is discontinued.

Some women only require oral analgesic after surgery. The woman should be instructed to take medication around the clock rather than waiting until when she becomes uncomfortable. Pain is much harder to relieve if it becomes severe.

The breastfeeding mother should be reassured that the administration of analgesia will not impact the newborn and that taking medication prior to breastfeeding may help to decrease discomfort. Also, adequate pain control helps her to relax so she can breastfeed better and can have the energy to become acquainted with her newborn.

EMOTIONAL CHANGES IN THE MOTHER

The birth of a newborn brings about physical changes in the mother, which can also cause emotional and relationship changes in family members. The transition to motherhood brings many hormonal changes, changes in body image, and psychological acceptance of the self as a mother figure. Rubin (1967) described three phases of postpartum change that have been a framework for nursing care for over 50 years (Table 9.2). More recent studies have shown that women progress through the same three phases, although at a more rapid pace than originally described, probably because of much earlier discharge from the hospital. The nurse can refer to the three phases when providing postpartum care, although it is important to remember that this theory is only a guide and women may vary in length of time in each stage and the stages may overlap. The nurse must use the "teachable moments" when the woman enters the take-hold phase, because the woman will be focused on the newborn's needs and will be most receptive to teaching. Fluctuating hormones in pregnancy and the puerperium have an effect on mood, causing early elation at birth that can be followed by tearfulness, irritability, and fatigue peaking on the third to fifth day postpartum, commonly known as the **postpartum blues**. However, the physiological factors that affect mood can interact with minor anxieties and stresses to result in a **perinatal mood disorder**.

Table 9.2 Rubin's Psychological Adaptation of Postpartum and Related Nursing Interventions

PSYCHOLOGICAL ADAPTATION	NURSING RESPONSES
Taking-in Phase (24 to 48 hours)	
Mother is passive and willing to let others do things for her. Conversation centres on her birth experience. She has interest in newborn but prefers that others care for newborn. She may have little interest in learning. Focus is on need for food, fluids, and restorative sleep.	Provide opportunity for rest and appropriate nutrition. Provide opportunity to discuss birth experience and vent disappointments or share joys.
Taking-Hold Phase (Second or Third Day, Lasts 10 Days to Several Weeks)	
Mother begins to initiate action and becomes interested in caring for newborn. She may be critical about her abilities. She has increased concern about her body functions and assumes self-care needs. She is interested in learning how to care for self and baby.	Provide supportive atmosphere. Identify support system of mother. Use teaching moments. Reinforce self-care and newborn care-taking abilities.
Letting-Go Phase	
Mothers and partners work through giving up their previous lifestyle to incorporate their newborn. Many mothers must give up their ideal of the birth experience and reconcile it with what really occurred. They give up the fantasy child and accept the real child.	Provide a supportive atmosphere. Provide referrals to community agencies as appropriate for assistance needed. Reinforce newborn caregiving abilities.

Source: Rubin, R., (1967). Attainment of the maternal role part 1: Processes. *Nursing Research*, 16, 237–245.

Postpartum Blues

New mothers often experience conflicting feelings of joy and emotional let-down during the first few weeks after birth, often called the *postpartum blues*, or the *baby blues*. Approximately 50 to 80% of women experience the postpartum blues. The woman may feel let down, depression, and fatigue and cry for no reason. The symptoms may last up to approximately 10 to 14 days. When providing discharge teaching, the nurse should prepare the woman and her family that this may occur and reassure them that this is normal and temporary. If the blues last longer than 2 weeks, the family should be instructed to seek help in case it has developed into a perinatal mood disorder.

Perinatal Mood Disorders

Perinatal mood disorders can range from anxiety to depression or psychosis and are discussed further in Chapter 10. When teaching about the postpartum blues, as described earlier, the nurse should explain that persistent depression or anxiety is *not* expected and should be reported to her health care provider. The term *perinatal mood disorder* has replaced *postpartum mood disorders* because the conditions may also occur during pregnancy.

Fatigue

Postpartum assessment typically includes physical assessment and assessment of psychological bonding and must also include evaluation for fatigue. Fatigue is a common postpartum concern for mothers. They may have had a long labour that interfered with sleep prior to birth and then find it difficult to sleep in the hospital because of excitement, noise, or hospital routines. Women need to understand that fatigue is normal and what they can do to help alleviate the symptoms. While they are in the hospital the nurse can offer back rubs and other comfort measures and ensure that pain management is a priority. Nurses need to teach women to sleep when the baby sleeps, try to limit visitors, and to accept help when offered. The home environment and available support persons should be reviewed before discharge.

PARENTHOOD

Becoming a parent requires learning new roles and making adjustments, whether it is a first child or one of several children. Many parents say that parenthood, not marriage, made the greatest change in their lives.

The demands of parenthood can affect communication between the partners, and there is little doubt that children may distract from the relationship at times. It is not unusual for one member to feel left out. The division of responsibility can be a source of conflict, particularly when both parents work. Parents often feel inept, which may cause lower self-esteem, depression, and anger. These feelings can be overwhelming.

Fatigue triggers irritability. Even in the ideal situation, waking up two or three times every night is wearisome for anyone. For the new mother, physiological changes continue to play a part in her emotional lability (instability). Both parents may be concerned with increased economic responsibilities. Loss of freedom and a decrease in socialization may give the couple a sense of loneliness.

Ideally, preparing parents for the lifestyle changes that occur with a new child begins before conception. Parenting courses, group discussions, and support from relatives or friends can be explored. Social service agencies, public health nurses, and other professional resources should be suggested as appropriate.

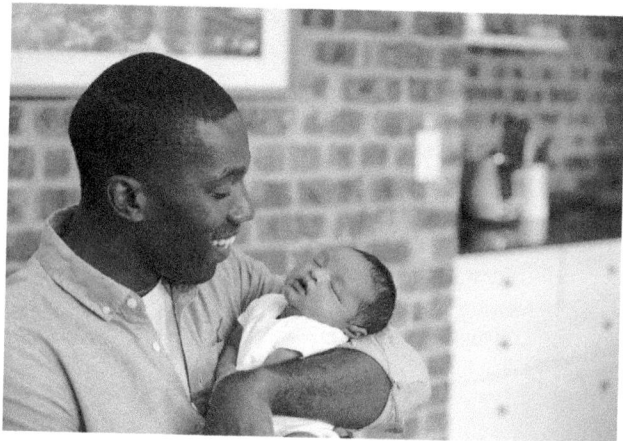

Fig. 9.2 This father shows intense interest in his new newborn *(engrossment)*. The father's reaction to the newborn parallels the mother's. Eye-to-eye contact *(en face position)* helps the bonding process. (istock.com/monkeybusinessimages)

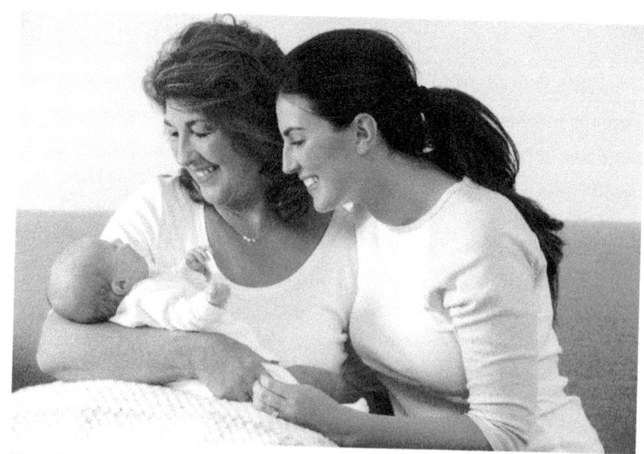

Fig. 9.3 A daughter introducing her mother to her newborn. Grandmothers can reinforce cultural customs, help with newborn care, and assist with household tasks. (istock.com/SolStock)

Encouraging parents to share their concerns and worries with one another and to keep communication lines open is of foremost importance. Re-establishing a relationship in which the newborn fits can be accomplished when the parents identify their own needs, set priorities, maintain their sense of humour, and relax their standards.

These tools can make the transition to parenthood rewarding, regardless of the fact that it is sometimes a difficult experience—one in which the stable family can grow and become stronger. Parents who find themselves at an impasse should seek early intervention with a professional counselor.

PARTNERS

The partner of the woman typically displays intense interest in their new child *(engrossment)* (Fig. 9.2). Their behaviours with their newborn parallel those of the new mother. A partner's relationship with their own parents, previous experiences with children, and relationship to the mother are important influences on how they may relate to the newborn. Goodman (2005) has researched new fathers and found that they often experience four phases of adjustment to fatherhood, characterized by the following:

- Having expectations and personal intentions
- Confronting reality and overcoming frustrations
- Creating one's own personal father role
- Reaping rewards of fatherhood

Adjustment to parenthood is facilitated in the partner by involvement in the newborn's care. Partners should be included when the nurse is sharing instructions about newborn care and handling. The nurse must be supportive of a new parent who is trying to assume their new role.

SIBLINGS

The influence of a new child's birth on siblings depends on the age and developmental level of the older child. Toddlers may respond with regression and anger when the mother's attention turns to the newborn. Preschool children typically look at and discuss the newborn but may hesitate to touch or hold the newborn. Older children often enjoy helping with care of the newborn and are very curious about the newcomer. Parents need to be taught what behaviours are normal in older children so they do not have unreasonable expectations of the children.

GRANDPARENTS

The grandparents' involvement with a new child is often dictated by how near they live to the younger family. Grandparents who live a long distance from the family cannot have the close, regular contact that they may desire. Grandparents also differ in what they expect their role to be, and culture sometimes determines their expected role. Some feel that their child-rearing days are in the past, and they want minimal day-to-day involvement in raising the children. Others expect to have regular involvement in the grandchild's life, second only to the parents (Fig. 9.3). It is important for new parents to have a discussion with grandparents to determine values and beliefs about child-rearing. If parents and grandparents agree on the grandparents' role, little conflict is likely.

THE FAMILY CARE PLAN

The family care plan is similar to the traditional nursing care plan except that the "patient" is the family rather than only the woman in the hospital. It is most appropriate to use a family care plan in perinatal care because the birth of a child will have a profound impact on the family processes. Studying the family as the patient, rather than an individual as the patient, can offer insight into community-based care and can help the nurse integrate knowledge of family structure, culture, and composition into a plan of care.

The data required in a family care plan are listed in Nursing Care Plan 9.2. The new family should be given telephone numbers or online addresses for follow-up questions, a list of community services available, and a list of available breastfeeding classes and "Mommy and Me" programs. Many families will receive follow-up with a public health nurse either by phone call or visit after the birth of the baby, depending on provincial guidelines. Follow-up appointments with the health care provider for both mother and baby should be given to them before they leave the hospital.

LOSS OF AN EXPECTED BIRTH EXPERIENCE

The postpartum period is usually a joyful time, but nurses occasionally care for grieving parents who have experienced a loss. Couples rarely anticipate problems when they begin a pregnancy. Most have specific expectations about how their pregnancy, particularly the birth, will proceed. A high-risk pregnancy may result in the loss of their expected experience. With most of these parents, the nurse should simply listen to them and support them. Therapeutic communication techniques such as open-ended questions or reflection of feelings help the parents express their grief—an early step in resolving it.

It seems strange to talk of grief when a healthy newborn is born, but even a healthy child may be much different in size, sex, or appearance from what parents expected. Most parents eventually come to accept their unique newborn and his or her characteristics. Their feelings about their child are not right or wrong—feelings simply exist. The nurse should accept and encourage their expressions of grief to allow them to move forward and accept the newborn they have.

A woman who has experienced the loss of a newborn may experience guilt, remorse, and sorrow. This can be one of the most difficult kinds of grief. The woman may question what she could have done differently to prevent the loss. Anniversaries of these events may be painful, and feelings often last for many years, if not forever. The birth of a new child may awaken grief that parents thought they had resolved ("We have one child, but we almost had two").

If the condition of a newborn is poor, the parents may wish to have a baptism performed. The minister or priest is notified.

Nursing Care Plan 9.2 The Family Care Plan

PATIENT DATA

A woman is admitted to the postpartum unit after giving birth to a healthy baby girl. The husband, two sons (ages 14 and 10), and the woman's mother are present in the room. The woman tells the nurse she would like to stay in the hospital as long as she can, because she has forgotten everything about baby care.

Selected Nursing Diagnosis Possible change in family coping related to new family member (newborn)

Goals	Nursing Interventions	Rationales
Family members will express satisfaction with adaptation to newborn and be confident in their roles.	Determine relationship of family members to one another.	Can help provide a positive experience to prepare the family for new developmental tasks.
	Provide unlimited visiting privileges for the family and siblings.	Facilitates the attachment and bonding process.
	Provide information about support groups for breastfeeding and child care.	Verbalization of family culture, roles, and perceived responsibilities enables the appropriate person to be included in instruction concerning breastfeeding and child care.
	Provide anticipatory guidance concerning changes to expect and family adaptation options.	Meeting needs concerning housing, equipment, and community resources available for assisting will help the family adapt to changes.
	Discuss sexuality needs and plans for contraception.	Clarification of contraception options acceptable to the cultural group will enhance learning and enable the family to make informed decisions.
	Provide written information and suggested books and websites for siblings concerning the new child. Encourage sibling verbalization.	Including the needs of each family member will promote family coping and adaptation.

CRITICAL THINKING QUESTION

1. How does family care differ from the care of an individual patient?

If the newborn dies, is stillborn, or has a birth defect, the parents' reactions depend on whether the event was expected. If they have known for some time that the fetus was not living, they may have already begun the grief process and may not display all the typical behaviours. If the death was not expected, the nurse may encounter the following reactions typical of any grieving:

- Shock and disbelief
- Anger (may be directed at health care providers; rarely at the newborn)
- Guilt about what the parents could have done differently
- Sadness and depression
- Gradual resolution of the sadness

The nurse may encounter grieving families at any point in their grieving process and in many settings. When the newborn has a birth defect, grieving is often chronic because of the constant reminders of what might have been.

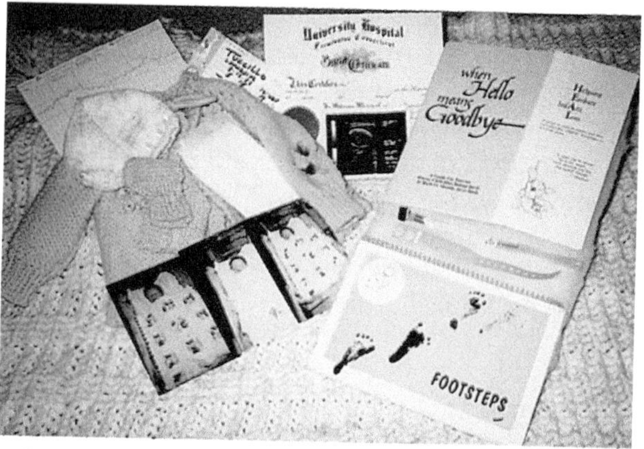

Fig. 9.4 Memory kit. This "memory kit" may include pictures of the newborn, clothing, death certificate, footprints, ID band, fetal monitor printout, and ultrasound picture.

CARING FOR GRIEVING PARENTS

If a newborn dies or is stillborn, nursing units may have a protocol to help parents cope with the loss. Perinatal loss shatters the hopes of human life and severs a unique attachment between mother and fetus. Parents exhibit mourning behaviours associated with the various stages of the grieving process. Health care providers must address these aspects of the grieving process as they work with the parents through interventions, including the following (Hendson, Davies, & Canadian Paediatric Society (CPS), Fetus and Newborn Committee, 2018):

- Allowing parents and family members to remain together in privacy
- Accepting behaviours related to grieving
- Developing a plan of care to provide support to the family
- Offering mementos, such as a footprint, identification (ID) band, and lock of hair (if acceptable to the parents) (Fig. 9.4)
- Providing parents with educational materials and referrals to support groups
- Discussing wishes concerning religious and cultural rituals

The parents should be encouraged to see and hold the newborn if they want to. It should be explained to them that parents may grieve better if they have the opportunity to hold and "parent" their child. The parents should be prepared for the newborn's appearance. For instance, a stillborn newborn may have blue skin, which often is peeling. The nurse should try to keep the newborn warm so he or she feels more natural to the parents. If this is not possible, the parents should be prepared for the coolness of the newborn's skin and the limp body. The newborn should be wrapped in a blanket and the parents should be allowed to unwrap the newborn when and if they want to do so. If an anomaly is present, the newborn should be wrapped so the anomaly is not what the parents see first. They should be encouraged to focus on all the positives of the child first.

The nurse should listen to the parent's responses to determine the level of support needed, to answer questions, and to understand the grief behaviours individual to the family or culture. The support system of the parents (and grandparents) should be assessed, and some information concerning the expected grief process, its influence on behaviour and the ability to perform activities of daily living, coping mechanisms, and resources for follow-up care should be discussed. Referral to social work is often appropriate, and social workers may provide follow-up after discharge.

Many nursing units make a memory packet containing items such as a lock of hair (if acceptable to the parents), footprints, the ID band, photographs, and clothing or blankets (see Fig. 9.4). An organization called *Now I Lay Me Down to Sleep* is a nonprofit group of photographers who offer their services to families who have experienced a loss. Professional-level photographers volunteer their time to capture the only moments parents spend with their babies and provide the pictures to the families free of charge. Parents often find these pictures valuable in the healing process.

Some type of sign, such as a picture of flower or butterfly, is placed on the mother's door to alert personnel from other departments that a grieving family is inside). This reduces the chance that well-intentioned but painful remarks or questions might be made, such as "What did you have, a boy or girl?"

BREASTFEEDING

Nutrition for the newborn is especially important in the first few months of life, because the brain grows rapidly. Energy use is high because of the newborn's rapid growth. More in-depth discussions of the nutritional needs of the newborn are found in Chapters 13 and 14.

Exclusive breastfeeding for the first 6 months of life is the recommended infant feeding method with continuation of breastfeeding to age 2 years and beyond once complementary foods are introduced (Public Health Agency of Canada [PHAC], 2018; Registered Nurses Association of Ontario [RNAO], 2018; World Health Organization WHO], 2018). Regardless of these recommendations, breastfeeding rates in Canada have remained suboptimal; despite the fact that the majority of women initiate breastfeeding, the minority of women practice exclusively to 6 months and continue breastfeeding past 1 year (Gionet, 2015). Of the mothers who initiate breastfeeding, close to 25% stop before their infant is 1 month old. The most common reasons mothers give for stopping breastfeeding before 6 months are "not enough milk" (44%) and "difficulty with breastfeeding technique" (PHAC, 2018). The rate of exclusive breastfeeding to 6 months is 32%, and 19% of women breastfeed past the first year of life. Ninety percent of women initiate breastfeeding (PHAC, 2018). The 10% who do not initiate tend to be single and younger in age and have less formal education, which demonstrates the impact of social determinants of health on breastfeeding practices (RNAO, 2018). Although breastfeeding is natural, it is a learned behaviour that requires support. Supporting women with breastfeeding and providing them with education will assist them in meeting their breastfeeding goals. Nurses, the interprofessional team, family, and peers play integral roles in supporting the initiation, exclusivity, and continuation of breastfeeding (RNAO, 2018).

IMPORTANCE OF BREASTFEEDING

Breastfeeding is important to the health of mothers and of their newborns for some of the following reasons:

- Breastmilk contains all the nutrients that the newborn needs and in the right proportions and is constantly changing to meet the needs of the growing infant.
- Breastmilk is easily digested by the newborn's maturing digestive system.
- Breastfeeding provides natural immunity, because the mother transfers antibodies through the milk. This protects the newborn and assists them in recovering from illness and in developing a strong immune system. Colostrum is particularly high in antibodies and provides important immune protection in the first days of life.
- Breastfed infants have a lower incidence of childhood respiratory and gastrointestinal diseases and otitis media and a reduced risk of diabetes mellitus, childhood leukemia, obesity, and necrotizing enterocolitis.
- Breastfeeding may prevent the development or delay the onset of allergies in the newborn, especially if there is a family history of allergies.
- Breastfeeding may play a significant role in improving brain development of the newborn.
- Breastmilk promotes elimination of meconium, and adequate intake may decrease the risk of jaundice in the early days of life. Breastfed newborns are rarely constipated.
- Suckling at the breast promotes jaw and mouth development.
- Newborn suckling promotes a return of the uterus to its prepregnant state.
- Breastfeeding reduces mothers' risk of developing uterine, breast, and ovarian cancers and osteoporosis.
- Breast milk production uses maternal fat stores, which facilitates maternal weight loss.
- Exclusive breastfeeding for 6 months increases the likelihood of continued LAM to be an effective birth control method.
- Breastfeeding enhances mother–infant bonding.
- Breastfeeding is convenient and economical.
- Breastfeeding eliminates the risks of a contaminated water supply or improper dilution, which are risks of feeding infants breastmilk substitutes (PHAC, 2018; Kim & Froh, 2012; RNAO, 2018).

Infectious Diseases, Medications, and Breastfeeding

Breastfeeding is rarely contraindicated; however, there are a few conditions and situations where this is warranted. Mothers should be advised to talk to their health care providers before breastfeeding if they have a medical condition or are on medication (MacDonald & CPS Infectious Disease and Immunization Committee (2006/2018). Mothers should be supported to maintain lactation during temporary interruption of breastfeeding.

Some contraindications to breastfeeding include the following:

- The mother is infected with the human immunodeficiency virus (HIV) (in resource-rich environments such as Canada with safe, culturally acceptable alternatives, although in developing countries it is often recommended that women breastfeed as this is safer than formula made from unclean water), human T-cell lymphotrophic viruses (HTLV-1 and -2), or Ebola virus (in the mother but with asymptomatic infant) or has untreated brucellosis. For the breastfed infant of an Ebola-infected mother where the infant has developed Ebola or is suspected of having contracted Ebola, the risks of not breastfeeding (considering community infection control and infant nutrition) outweigh any possible benefits of replacement feeding. If the mother is well enough to breastfeed, she should be supported to continue to do so. If the mother is too ill to breastfeed, then replacement feeding is needed (WHO, 2019).
- The mother has herpes lesions on both breasts, active varicella zoster virus (5 days prior to 2 days

after the birth), and untreated infectious tuberculosis (in these cases, the mothers' expressed milk can be provided).
- The mother is using certain substances (e.g., illicit drugs) or is undergoing treatment (chemotherapy, radioactive isotope therapy). Many medications and herbs are safe to take while breastfeeding, thus it is important for mothers to discuss medication options with their health care provider when breastfeeding so safe alternatives can be found.
- Galactosemia in the infant

STAGES OF LACTATION

There are four stages of lactation (Wambach & Riordan, 2014):
- Stage 1 (secretory differentiation)
- Stage 2 (secretory activation)
- Stage 3 (galactopoiesis)
- Stage 4 (involution)

Stage 1: Lactogensis begins in response to the pregnancy hormones and by mid-pregnancy the breast is capable of secreting colostrum, the first milk. Late in pregnancy and for the first few days after birth, colostrum is the milk secreted by the breasts. This yellowish fluid is rich in protective antibodies. It provides protein, vitamins A and E, and essential minerals, but it is lower in calories than milk. It has a laxative effect, which aids in eliminating meconium.

Stage 2: This stage occurs in response to delivery of the placenta, which causes the removal of the inhibitory hormones, including progesterone, and the increased presence of the hormone prolactin. Starting on day 2 or 3 until day 8, the milk will increase in volume and "comes in." This milk-increased synthesis occurs in response to these hormones and occurs regardless of breastfeeding or manual expression of milk.

Stage 3: Approximately 9 days after birth, the milk production alters from the endocrine response described in stages 1 and 2, which occurs in response to changes in hormones occurring in pregnancy and at birth, to autocrine, which is driven by milk removal. The establishment of an adequate milk supply becomes dependent on the continual production and removal of breast milk from the breast. Mothers need to be educated on the process of milk production so that they understand the direct relationship between milk removal and milk production.

Stage 4: Involution occurs, on average, 40 days after the last breastfeed, when breast milk secretion ceases.

MILK PRODUCTION

Hormones

To better support the breastfeeding mother, the nurse must understand how breast milk production occurs and how the milk changes with time. The hormones prolactin and oxytocin have a major role in the production and expulsion of breast milk:

- *Prolactin* from the anterior pituitary gland is necessary for the secretion of breastmilk in the cells of the alveoli (Fig. 9.5). During pregnancy, the glandular tissue of the breasts grows under the influence of several hormones. The woman also secretes high levels of prolactin, which is the hormone that is needed for milk production. However, other hormones from the placenta inhibit the breasts' response to prolactin. The influence of prolactin is unopposed after birth and after the expulsion of the placenta. Prolactin is released in response to suckling and stimulates the production of milk by the alveoli. Prolactin concentration in the plasma is highest at night, which aids milk production, therefore nighttime breastfeeding can aid the establishment of an adequate milk supply. While breastfeeding is being established, increased prolactin increases the production of milk. Over time, prolactin levels do not reach the same levels in response to suckling later on in lactation, and although it still plays a role in the production, the amount of prolactin does not correlate to the amount of breast milk.
- *Oxytocin* from the posterior pituitary gland causes the milk to be delivered, as it causes the contraction of the muscles around the alveoli sacs (milk-producing

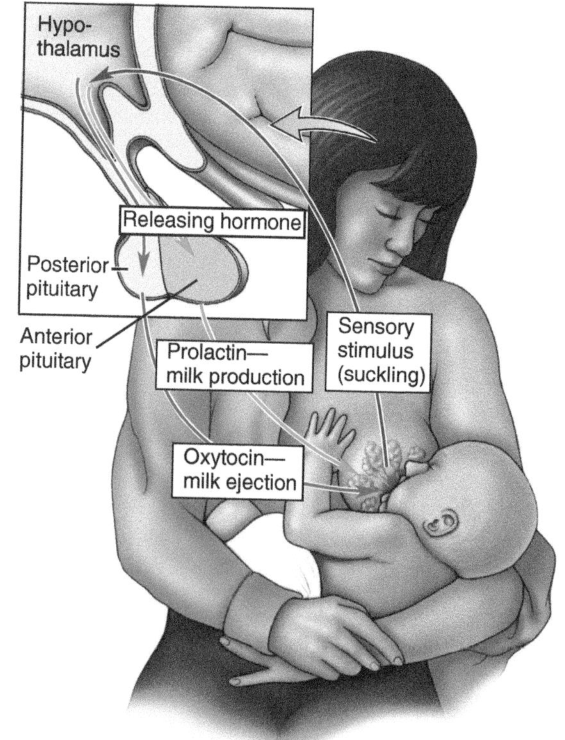

Fig. 9.5 Lactation reflex arc. The newborn suckling on the breast stimulates nerve fibres in the areola of the nipple that travel to the hypothalamus. The hypothalamus stimulates the anterior pituitary to secrete prolactin; this stimulates milk production and stimulates the posterior pituitary to release oxytocin, which causes a "let-down" reflex, contracting the lobules in the breast and squeezing milk out into the nipple and to the newborn. (From Herlihy, B. [2018]. *The human body in health and illness* [6th ed.]. St. Louis: Saunders.)

sacs), which sends the milk through the duct system to the nipple (*milk ejection*, or **let-down reflex**). The mother usually feels a tingling in her breasts and sometimes abdominal cramping as her uterus contracts, as oxytocin also causes the uterus to contract (see Fig. 9.5). Multiple milk ejections occur during a breastfeeding session.

Supply and Demand

Milk is produced on a supply-and-demand basis, with the more milk being removed, the more milk the breast will make. The *feedback inhibitor of lactation* (FIL) plays a role in this. This FIL is a whey protein found in breastmilk. As the alveoli become distended with milk, when it is not removed, the accumulation to this inhibits further milk secretion. Conversely, when the milk is being removed and not concentrated in the alveoli, milk continues to be secreted. This chemical feedback loop assists with regulating the volume of milk to meet the newborn's needs. Therefore, feedings that are infrequent or too short can reduce the amount of milk produced. Additionally, supplementing feedings with liquids other than the mother's milk can impact this supply-and-demand system and the body's ability to determine the amount of milk needed for the baby. Given this supply-and-demand process, a mother can produce enough milk for twins or multiples, as the more milk removed, the more milk the breast will make. Very little milk is stored in the breast between feedings; most is manufactured as the newborn breastfeeds.

Changes in Fat Content in Breastmilk Throughout the Feed

The composition of milk changes in fat content from the beginning of a feeding until the end of that feeding, as follows:

- The milk in the breast at the beginning of the feeding is lower in fat and has been referred to as **foremilk**. It is watery and quenches the newborn's thirst. The fat concentration is lowest when the breast is at its fullest.
- As the breast continues to make and deliver milk during a feed, the milk becomes higher in fat content. When the baby drains the breast well and the volume of milk decreases in the breast, the fat content of this milk is higher; this high-fat breastmilk has been referred to as **hindmilk**. This high-fat milk helps satisfy the newborn's hunger. Feedings that are too short may not drain the breast enough to result in this high-fat breastmilk. Watching the newborn and allowing the infant to feed off the same breast until they show signs of satiation or come off will help the baby regulate the amount of fat they get from the breastmilk. Cue-based feeding and offering the second breast only once the baby is finished on the first will assist with ensuring that the baby receives the high-fat milk and calories they need for growth and development.

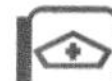 **Nursing Tip**

Anticipatory guidance concerning possible problems associated with breastfeeding helps the mother to see these challenges as common occurrences and not as complications.

NURSING CARE FOR THE BREASTFEEDING MOTHER

Newborns are more likely to be breastfed and to breastfeed longer if they had skin-to-skin contact and initiated breastfeeding in the birthing room (RNAO, 2018) (Fig. 9.6). Skin-to-skin contact and early breastfeeding initiation:

- Promotes mother–newborn bonding
- Maintains newborn temperature

Newborn suckling stimulates oxytocin release to contract the mother's uterus and control bleeding.

The newborn should be put to the breast within the first hour when in the alert state, as this allows for suckling and bonding. Breastfeeding should ideally be initiated within the first hour, but if the mother is too tired or uncomfortable to nurse at this time, or if the newborn seems disinterested, she should be reassured that she can still breastfeed successfully. If the newborn and the mother are separated, hand expression can begin in the first hours postpartum. The nurse can reviews techniques of hand expression with the new mother (see Box 9.1).

The focus of the nurse in the early hours of breastfeeding should be to help the mother get the colostrum flowing and to position the newborn correctly and to help the newborn obtain an open, gaping mouth in preparation for suckling (Table 9.3). Prior to discharge from the hospital or other childbirth settings, a full breastfeeding session must be observed and assessed to determine the quality of the positioning and latch, including the mother's level of comfort (RNAO, 2018). Frequent reassurance and praise of the mother's efforts are essential.

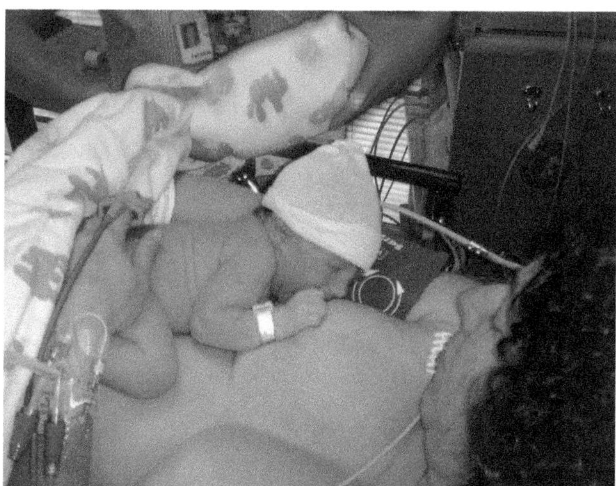

Fig. 9.6 Placing the naked newborn on the bare chest of the mother, covered by a blanket, encourages both breastfeeding and bonding.

Cultural Considerations

Galactogogues

Mothers from many cultures use **galactogogues** (breast-milk stimulators), and nurses should be aware of these practices. Beer, brewer's yeast, rice, gruel, fenugreek tea, and sesame tea are commonly used postpartum. Garlic eaten by the mother to prevent newborn illness will flavour her breast milk but will not harm the newborn. Cultural practices should be respected and education provided to enable women to make informed choices. Although beer was thought to increase milk supply, this has been disproven. Because alcohol in beer is ingested in the breastmilk, this practice is no longer recommended. Additionally, some herbs can have effects on the newborn. The mother should discuss with her health care provider any medications or herbs she is taking to increase her milk supply.

Assisting Mothers With Breastfeeding Positions

Assisting mothers in getting into a comfortable position, lying skin-to-skin, reclined, supporting the newborn's bottom, back, and neck, and allowing the baby to crawl and to "root" (a newborn instinct in which they move up and down, pecking or bobbing, looking for the nipple) may assist the newborn in self-attaching to the breast. This has been referred to as *baby-led nursing* or *laid-back breastfeeding* (Fig. 9.7, *A*). This allows the newborn to use instinctive behaviours to find the breast and begin to breastfeed. For some mothers, this works very well.

Mothers can breastfeed in a variety of positions that may work well for them and their infant. Some general principles to keep in mind are as follows (Box 9.2):

1. The mother should perform hand hygiene before each breastfeeding session.
2. The newborn's body should be in "chest-to-chest" position with the mother, with the head and neck in alignment facing the mother; if the head and neck are not aligned, the newborn will have to turn their head to the side to grasp the breast nipple. This position makes swallowing difficult for the newborn.
3. The newborn should be brought to the normal resting level of the breast nipple to allow for comfort and easy flow of milk. The mother should bring the newborn to the breast and not bring the breast to her newborn. The mother should feel comfortable supporting the newborn's weight in her arms; pillows can be used to help support the mother's arm and bring the baby to the level of the breast, if needed.

Table 9.3 Teaching the New Mother How to Breastfeed

INSTRUCTION	RATIONALE
Perform hand hygiene before feeding; teach mother to wash nipples with warm water and no soap when bathing.	Prevents infection of the newborn and breast; use of plain water prevents nipple cracking and irritation.
Sit comfortably in a chair or raised bed with back and arm support; hold newborn with cradle hold, football hold, or laid-back position, supported by pillows.	Pillow support of mother's back and arm and the newborn's body in any position reduces fatigue; newborn is more likely to remain in a good position for breastfeeding.
If in side-lying position, use a pillow beneath the head, arm above head; support newborn in side-lying position.	Side-lying position reduces fatigue and pressure on abdominal incision.
Turn body of the newborn to face the mother's breast.	Prevents pulling on nipple or poor position of mouth on nipple.
Stroke newborn's top lip with the nipple.	Elicits rooting reflex to cause newborn to open mouth wide.
Newborn should take in a big mouthful of breast, which includes the areola.	Compresses ducts and stimulates milk production and delivery, lessens tension on nipples.
Avoid strict time limits for breastfeeding; continue to offer the breast until newborn stops sucking vigorously and shows signs of satiation.	Let-down reflex may take 5 minutes; a too-short feeding will yield newborn foremilk only, not the hunger-satisfying hindmilk. Strict time limits do not prevent sore nipples.
Use a bracelet or safety pin on the bra as a reminder about which breast to start with at the next feeding.	Alternating breasts increases milk production and helps ensure that both breasts have an adequate milk supply.
Lift newborn or breast slightly if breast tissue blocks nose or pull the newborn's hip in and the chin will go deeper into the breast and the nose will be not touching the breast. This is an asymmetrical latch (Fig. 9.8, *D*).	Provides a small breathing space and allow the baby to bring more areola into the mouth to suckle on, which will increase hormone release in the brain and milk production and delivery.
Break suction by placing finger in the corner of newborn's mouth or by indenting breast tissue.	Removing newborn in this way prevents nipple trauma.
Breastfeed the newborn in the first hour after birth and at least eight times in 24 hours.	Early, regular, and frequent nursing establishes milk supply and reduces breast engorgement. Early suckling stimulates oxytocin from the mother's pituitary to contract her uterus and control bleeding. Frequent stimulation and breast emptying establishes an efficient milk supply.
Trying burping newborn halfway through feeding and following feeding.	Rids stomach of air bubbles and reduces regurgitation.

4. Lining the newborn up so that their nose aligns with the nipple will enable the newborn to take in a big mouthful of breast tissue below the nipple and aim the nipple to the back of the newborn's mouth. When the newborn's mouth is wide open before latch-on, a more effective latch-on will occur as the mother moves her arm to bring the newborn's chin in close to the breast (see Fig. 9.8).
5. In preparing for the breastfeed, if the mother has flat or inverted nipples, manually stimulating the nipple may draw it out and make it easier for the infant to latch on. As well, expressing a few drops of colostrum may increase the newborn's interest in feeding.
6. Alternating the breast that the feeding begins on will ensure both breasts are stimulated equally when the newborn is most hungry. This will assist in having a similar milk supply in each breast.
7. If the mother is going to support her breast, she should support her breast in a "C position," with the thumb above the nipple and the fingers below it. The thumb and fingers should be well back, away from the nipple, and the nipple should not tip upward. This will enable the newborn to take a big mouthful of breast tissue, without the hand getting in the way. The hand should be holding the breast gently and not putting pressure on the breast tissue as this could block the flow of milk and lead to a blocked duct. Mothers with larger breasts may need to provide support to the breast.
8. The mother should watch the newborn's hunger cues and begin the feeds with early cues and not wait until the newborn is crying and frantic, as this is a late cue (Box 9.3). Mothers should be advised to watch the baby, not the clock (Wambach & Riordan, 2014).
9. The principles described above should apply to all breastfeeding positions, which include the cradle hold, football (clutch) hold, cross-cradle, and side-lying position (Fig. 9.7, *B–E*). The cross-cradle provides good head control and allows the mother to have more control and easily bring the newborn to the breast. The football hold, also called the clutch hold, can be used for smaller babies and mothers who have had a Caesarean birth, as there is good head control and less pressure on the mother's incision. The side-lying hold can help the mother rest while feeding, and the classic hold can seem like a familiar hold to support the infant in. These last two positions do not allow the mother to control the head and latch as well and may be used more comfortably once the newborn is older and able to latch on effectively and comfortably.

The latch

As stated earlier, to elicit latch-on, the mother aligns the newborn's nose to her nipple and holds her breast so the nipple brushes against the newborn's upper lip. A hungry newborn usually opens the mouth wide with this stimulation. This is called the *rooting reflex*. As

Box 9.2 Essential Techniques in Breastfeeding

- Proper body alignment of newborn—the newborn is chest-to-chest with the mother
- Newborn's mouth is wide open to grasp a large mouthful of breast tissue
- Proper hand position of mother on the breast
- Newborn's mouth moves in a rhythmic motion to compress areola
- Audible swallow is heard
- Mother is in a relaxed, supported position
- Room is warm and private
- Newborn ends feeding relaxed and appears satiated
- Mother has soft breasts at end of the feeding

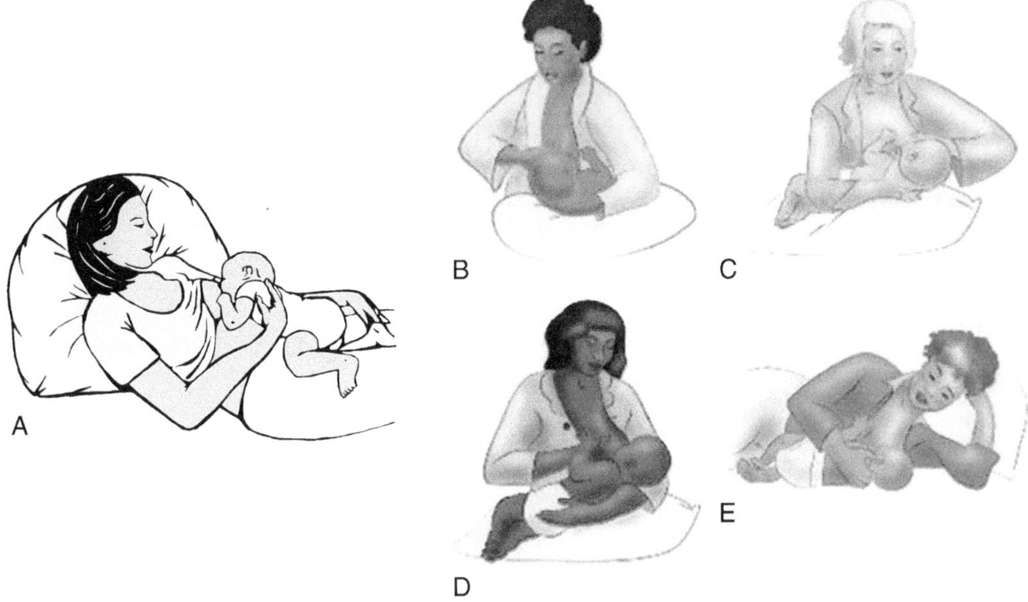

Fig. 9.7 Positions for breastfeeding. **A**, Laid-back breastfeeding. **B,** Football hold (clutch). **C,** Cross-cradle. **D**, Cradling. **E**, Side-lying position. (Reprinted with permission by the Best Start Resource Centre.)

soon as the newborn's mouth opens wide, the mother should bring the newborn close to her breast and aim the nipple to the back of the newborn's mouth so that the newborn has a big mouthful of breast tissue. The latch is often asymmetrical, with the baby having more of the breast tissue below the nipple in their mouth than above. The nose may be touching the breast. The newborn should have a deep latch and suckle on the areola and breast tissue below the nipple to stimulate the release of hormones in the brain that make and deliver the milk. The newborn's lips should flare outward (Fig. 9.8).

Suckling patterns

Suckling is the term that specifically relates to giving or taking nourishment at the breast. Newborns have different suckling patterns when they breastfeed. There are times of non-nutritive sucking, when the newborn is getting less breastmilk and is stimulating milk production, and times of nutritive suckling, which occurs after the milk ejection reflex. There are a number of milk ejections per breastfeed. Mothers should be made aware of the different sucking patterns and signs of nutritive sucking, or drinking. These include hearing a soft "ka" or "ah" sound, which indicates that the newborn is swallowing colostrum or milk; seeing the infant's jaw drop and pausing before swallowing, indicating a full mouth; or seeing the baby swallow. Noisy sucking or smacking sounds or dimpling of the cheeks usually indicates improper mouth position. "Fluttering" sucking motions indicate non-nutritive suckling.

Removing the newborn from the breast

The newborn will often come off the breast when finished feeding; however, if the mother should need to remove the newborn from the breast due to discomfort or for another reason, she should break the suction and remove the newborn quickly. This will prevent the nipple from becoming damaged. She can break the suction by inserting a finger in the corner of the newborn's mouth or by indenting her breast near the mouth (Fig. 9.9).

Evaluating intake of the newborn

Often the mother must be reassured that she is providing adequate milk for her newborn, because she cannot see the milk consumed as she can with bottle feeding. Signs that breastfeeding is successful and that the newborn is receiving adequate milk intake include the following:

- The breast feels firm before feedings and softer afterward.
- "Let-down" reflex occurs—a tingling sensation and possibly milk dripping from the breast that is not being fed on.
- The newborn stays awake feeding at the breast until satiated, a minimum of eight times a day.
- A frequent audible swallow is heard as the newborn sucks.
- The newborn cues to feed, stays awake during feeds, and shows signs of satiation after feeds, which may include being relaxed and calm.
- The newborn has six to eight wet diapers per day by age 6 days. The frequency and quantity of the urine should increase by one wet diaper each day after birth until day 6, then it will remain consistent. Diapers should be heavy and the urine clear, not concentrated (Fig. 9.10).
- The newborn passes stool several times a day. The stool changes appearance over the first days, from meconium at birth, to transitions stool, which is greenish in colour, to breastmilk stool, which is yellow, seedy, and soft.
- Newborns may lose 5 to 10% of their birth weight in the first days, as they have excess fluid at birth. If the infant loses more than 7%, it may indicate the mother needs more breastfeeding assistance. By day 4 babies should be gaining a minimum of 20 g/day and should regain their birth weight by 14 days postpartum (Wambach & Riordan, 2014).

Box 9.3 Recognizing Hunger Cues in Newborns

- Hand-to-mouth movements
- Mouth and tongue movements
- Sucking motions
- Rooting movements
- Clenched fists
- Kicking of legs
- Crying (a late sign of hunger; may result in shut-down and poor feeding if needs are not met)

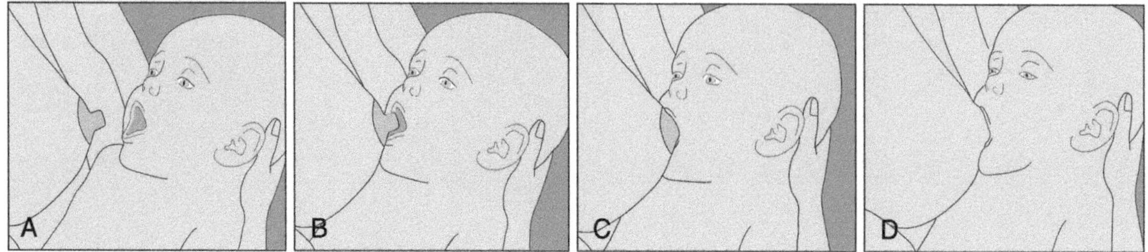

Fig. 9.8 **A,** The newborn responds to touch on the lips and opens the mouth wide. **B,** After the mouth is open, the newborn is quickly pulled close to enable latch-on. **C,** The baby should have as much areola in their mouth as possible, not just the nipple. **D,** Correct attachment (latch-on) at breast. (Monica Schroeder/Science Source.)

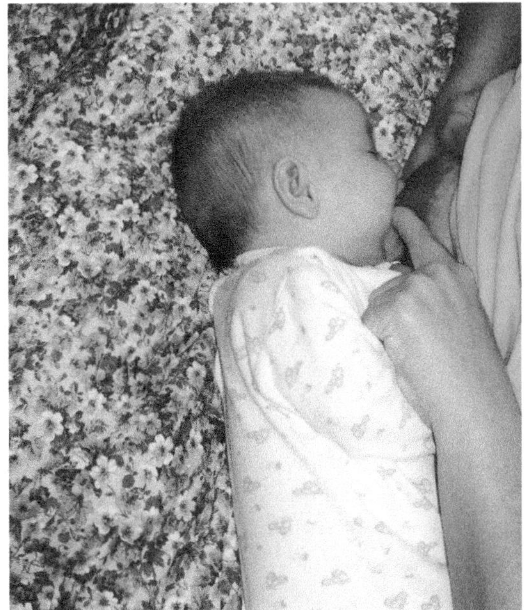

Fig. 9.9 Breaking suction. The mother should always first break the suction before removing the newborn from the breast. She can break the suction by inserting a finger in the corner of the newborn's mouth.

Frequency and duration of feedings

Breastfed newborns breastfeed at least 8 to 12 times a day; usually they will get hungry and cue to feed every 1.5 to 3 hours during the early weeks, because their stomach capacity is small and breastmilk is easily digested. Some newborns cluster several feedings at frequent intervals and then wait a longer time before breastfeeding again. It is best to feed in response to hunger cues during the early weeks. Responsive cue-based breastfeeding (also known as "baby-led breastfeeding") is a type of breastfeeding pattern in which the frequency and length of feeds are unrestricted and based on the infant's cues and sleep duration and is the best way to feed babies (RNAO, 2018). However, if the newborn is not showing adequate signs of hydration or waking on their own to nurse, the mother should gently waken the newborn and try to breastfeed after about 3 hours. A newborn who has medications in their system from labour or is not getting enough milk may be sleepy and not have enough energy to wake up and cue to feed. Mothers need to watch their newborn's behaviour to determine if they are not waking on their own.

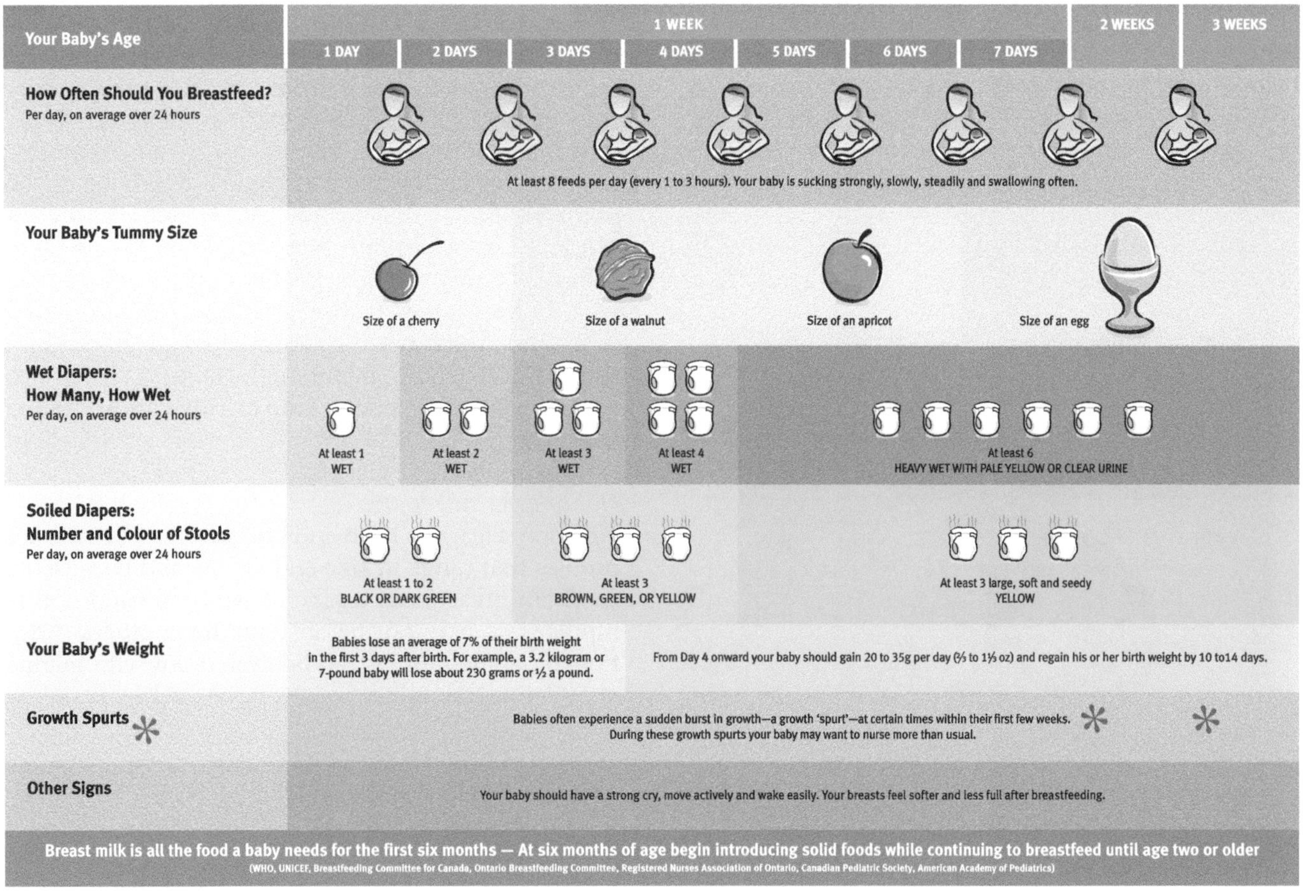

Your Baby's Age	1 WEEK							2 WEEKS	3 WEEKS
	1 DAY	2 DAYS	3 DAYS	4 DAYS	5 DAYS	6 DAYS	7 DAYS		
How Often Should You Breastfeed? Per day, on average over 24 hours	At least 8 feeds per day (every 1 to 3 hours). Your baby is sucking strongly, slowly, steadily and swallowing often.								
Your Baby's Tummy Size	Size of a cherry		Size of a walnut		Size of an apricot		Size of an egg		
Wet Diapers: How Many, How Wet Per day, on average over 24 hours	At least 1 WET	At least 2 WET	At least 3 WET	At least 4 WET	At least 6 HEAVY WET WITH PALE YELLOW OR CLEAR URINE				
Soiled Diapers: Number and Colour of Stools Per day, on average over 24 hours	At least 1 to 2 BLACK OR DARK GREEN		At least 3 BROWN, GREEN, OR YELLOW		At least 3 large, soft and seedy YELLOW				
Your Baby's Weight	Babies lose an average of 7% of their birth weight in the first 3 days after birth. For example, a 3.2 kilogram or 7-pound baby will lose about 230 grams or ½ a pound.			From Day 4 onward your baby should gain 20 to 35g per day (⅔ to 1⅕ oz) and regain his or her birth weight by 10 to14 days.					
Growth Spurts *	Babies often experience a sudden burst in growth—a growth 'spurt'—at certain times within their first few weeks. During these growth spurts your baby may want to nurse more than usual.							*	*
Other Signs	Your baby should have a strong cry, move actively and wake easily. Your breasts feel softer and less full after breastfeeding.								

Breast milk is all the food a baby needs for the first six months — At six months of age begin introducing solid foods while continuing to breastfeed until age two or older
(WHO, UNICEF, Breastfeeding Committee for Canada, Ontario Breastfeeding Committee, Registered Nurses Association of Ontario, Canadian Pediatric Society, American Academy of Pediatrics)

Fig. 9.10 Guidelines for nursing mothers regarding how often to feed and how to know the baby is getting enough to eat. (Courtesy Best Start, retrieved from https://www.beststart.org/resources/breastfeeding/pdf/magneng.pdf. Reprinted with permission by the Best Start Resource Centre.)

In this case, it will be necessary to wake them for feedings.

Burping

Newborns who breastfeed usually do not swallow very much air. Some newborns will need to burp throughout the feed, while others may not have the need. It is a good idea to provide the newborn with an opportunity to burp. Some babies show signs of discomfort and fuss when they need to burp, and this may be in the middle or at the end of the feeding. The mother can hold the newborn, supporting the head in a sitting position on her lap, and pat or rub the back to assist with getting the air up (Fig. 9.11). Alternately, the newborn can be placed against the mother's shoulder for burping. A soft cloth protects the adult's clothing from any spit-ups.

Overcoming Challenges

Teaching can help new mothers prevent many difficulties with breastfeeding. Nipple pain and perception of an insufficient milk supply are the two most common breastfeeding issues. If the mother can avoid difficulties in breastfeeding, she is less likely to become discouraged and stop breastfeeding early. Lactation consultants are available in many birth settings to help with breastfeeding concerns. Mother-to-mother breastfeeding support groups and local chapters of La Leche League may be available to the mother for ongoing support after discharge. "Warm lines," public health nurses, and community and hospital-based breastfeeding clinics are also excellent resources to help with breastfeeding and the common issues that occur after birth. Breastfeeding initiation and continuation can be influenced by the support and attitudes of partners, family members, and peers, so it is important for women to seek out good support (RNAO, 2018).

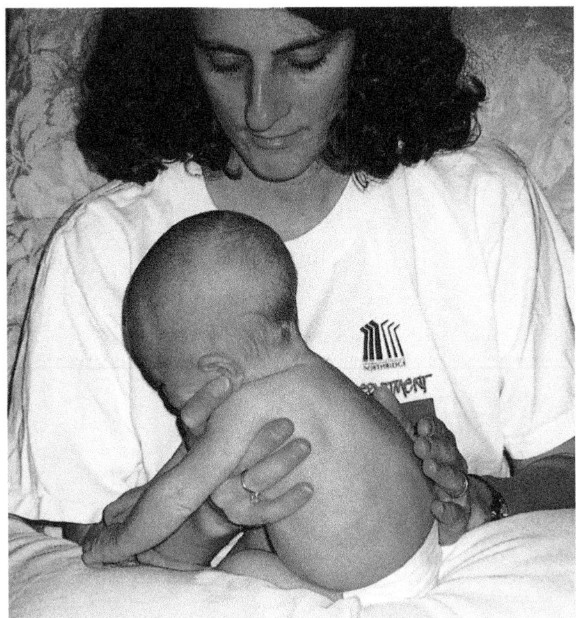

Fig. 9.11 The mother can burp the newborn by holding the newborn in a sitting position on her lap, supporting the chin and chest, and gently patting or rubbing the back.

The sleepy newborn

If the newborn is sleepy and is not waking up on their own to breastfeed at least eight times in 24 hours, the mother can be encouraged to wake the baby to feed until the infant is waking on their own and gaining weight. The longest stretch of sleep for the newborn should be no more than 4 hours. Mothers should be advised to watch for feeding cues and to bring the baby to the breast when they cue and show early signs of hunger (see Box 9.3). To bring the newborn to an alert state in preparation for feeding, the newborn can be unwrapped, the diaper can be changed, the mother can hold the newborn skin-to-skin and talk softly to the child, or she may provide a gentle massage. Hand expressing milk at the beginning of the feed may assist in getting the newborn interested in feeding by getting a taste of the milk, and using breast compressions (gently squeezing the breast with a hand to increase the flow of milk when milk flow is slow) may help the newborn stay awake at the breast.

The fussy newborn

Newborns cry for a variety of reasons. Crying is a late hunger cue, so parents should be encouraged to stay close to their newborns to observe for early hunger cues (see Box 9.3). If a newborn is fussy and crying, they may need to be calmed before breastfeeding. Holding the newborn skin-to-skin and talking calmly to the infant will often calm them. Gentle rocking and swaying can also calm the baby. When the newborn calms, feeding can begin. Breast compressions may be used to keep the newborn calm and more interested in feeding. If the newborn cries during feeds and has difficulties latching, the mother can see a health provider or lactation consultant to rule out additional concerns.

Flat or inverted nipples

Newborns learn to latch and breastfeed on breasts and nipples that range in size and shape, and because the newborn breastfeeds on the breast tissue and not the nipple, this may not be an issue for mothers. Additionally, some nipples can be drawn out with manual stimulation, pumping, and the newborn breastfeeding. If mothers have flat or inverted nipples that create difficulties with latching, they should consult a lactation consultant for support.

Supplemental feedings

Supplemental feedings of formula or water should not be offered to the healthy newborn who is breastfeeding unless medically necessary and the mother's expressed or banked breastmilk is not available. Successful breastfeeding is based on supply and demand. The hungry newborn will breastfeed and stimulate maternal milk production to meet their physiological needs. If the newborn has been fed supplemental feeds, they will not be hungry to breastfeed, which is required to stimulate milk production. Additionally, formula feeding carries risks that should be communicated to the mother so she can make an informed decision regarding supplementation.

Concerns with transitioning between bottles and breast
Newborns feed differently at the breast than with a bottle. The bottle nipple is smaller, the flow is faster, and feeding is effortless. Some newborns have difficulty transitioning to the breast where they need to have a wide open mouth with a large mouthful of breast. Additionally, the flow is not consistent, and they must actively breastfeed to stimulate the breast to make and deliver the milk. These differences can lead to the newborn being less effective breastfeeding, and if they have a smaller mouth at the breast, this can result in nipple pain and trauma. There is no way to know which newborns will have difficulty with this transition and which will be able to make it effortlessly. Pacifiers can have a similar impact on the latch and decrease stimulation at the breast. When pacifiers are used to space out feedings, this can have a negative impact on the milk supply. Although some parents choose to use pacifiers, they should be informed of the risks their use (Ponti & CPS Community Pediatrics Committee, 2003/2018).

Breast engorgement
Engorgement occurs due to an increased blood and lymph supply to the breasts as the body produces milk. When the milk comes in on day 2 or 3, the supply of breastmilk exceeds the newborn's needs, or the mother misses a feeding, engorgement can occur. If this occurs in the early days, it usually lasts only a few days, while the breasts regulate the volume to the newborn's needs. Mothers should be encouraged to breastfeed often, eight or more times in 24 hours, ensure the newborn has a good latch and is drinking, and offer both breasts at each feed. If the breast is still full and uncomfortable after the feed, or if the newborn only nurses from one breast, the mother can be encouraged to hand express or pump the breast to comfort. If the breast and areola are very tense and distended, the mother can hand express or pump her breasts to get the milk flow started and soften the areola. This will assist the newborn in getting a good latch. Cold applications between feedings reduce discomfort and engorgement. It is important to remove the milk, as the pressure in the breast from engorgement can cause problems such as blocked ducts, mastitis, and abscesses.

Sore nipples
Nipple pain should not occur during breastfeeding. Although some mothers may feel stretching or a little discomfort in the first days, pain is a sign of a problem. The most common cause is the latch and placement of the nipple in the newborn's mouth causing it to be rubbed and damaged. A deep latch may prevent the pain and damage, as the nipple will be at the back of the mouth where it is free from harm. If the nipple is not placed correctly in the mouth, cracks, blisters, redness, and bleeding may occur. Positioning of the newborn correctly will prevent further damage. Additional tips to aid healing include rubbing a small amount of breast milk onto the nipples, exposing the nipples to air, and keeping the nipples dry. Sometimes there are additional causes of nipple pain, and if the pain is not improving, the mother should consult a lactation consultant, who can help the mother adjust feeding techniques and ensure no additional causes are present.

Special Breastfeeding Situations

Multiple births
The mother's body adjusts the milk supply to the greater demand of multiple newborns. Twins can be fed one at a time or simultaneously. Feeding one at a time gives the mother time to bond with each baby, whereas feeding them together can save time. The mother should be encouraged to accept help from family and friends in the early days as she may feel that breastfeeding is taking up a great deal of time. The mother may want to use the double clutch hold when nursing simultaneously (Fig. 9.12). She will need help to position two newborns at the breasts in a double cradle hold in each arm. She positions the first newborn in a cradle hold, then her helper positions the second newborn at the other breast in the crook of her arm. Their bodies cross over each other. An alternative position is the cradle clutch where both newborns' bodies are facing in the same direction (Fig. 9.12). Pillows can be used to support the

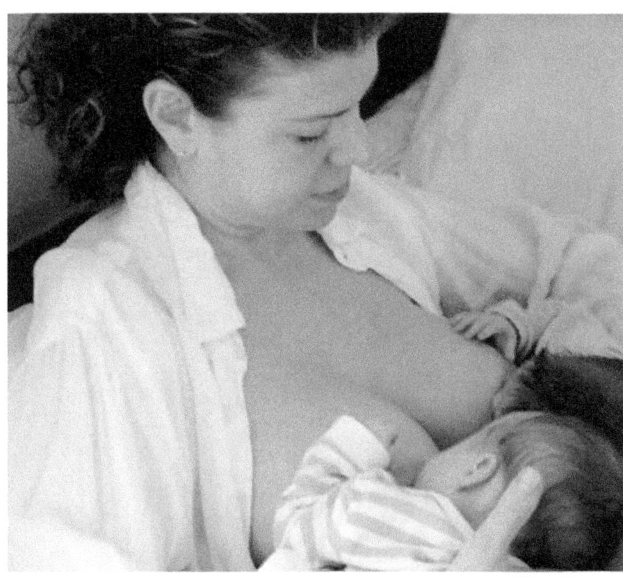

Fig. 9.12 Breastfeeding twins (© Beth Dixson/Alamy Stock Photo.)

newborns and the mother. The nurse should assess each newborn breastfeeding separately.

Premature birth

Breastfeeding is especially important to the health and development of a preterm newborn because of its immunological advantages (see Chapter 12 for more information on the preterm newborn). If the newborn cannot breastfeed, the mother can pump her breasts and freeze the milk for gavage (tube) feedings. When breastfeeding the preterm or small newborn, the mother may prefer the cross-cradle hold, football or clutch hold. In these positions, the mother can support the newborn's head with her hand and use her other hand to support the weight of the breast.

Breast surgery

Previous breast surgery for breast augmentation or reduction may influence successful breastfeeding and milk production. The extent to which the surgery can impact the milk supply depends on the type of surgery, location of the incision, and damage to ducts or nerves. The degree of impairment to the lactation system cannot be predetermined. The mother should try to breastfeed and build her milk supply while working closely with a health care provider and lactation consultant. The newborn will need to be monitored closely with frequent weight checks to determine the success the mother is having with building her milk supply and meeting the nutritional needs of her newborn.

Delayed feedings and using a breast pump

When breastfeeding must be temporarily delayed, a mother will be away from her baby, an alternative method of milk removal is required because the infant is not being able to suckle, or additional milk removal is required to simulate increased milk production, the mother should be taught how to pump her milk to continue full breastfeeding (Fig. 9.13). Portable breast pumps enable the mother to return to work and continue pumping and storing the breast milk to be available later for the infant. The mother should be taught how to assemble, disassemble, and clean the breast pump. The double pumping system increases milk production (Newton, 2017). Pumping should last approximately 10 to 15 minutes on each breast eight or more times in 24 hours. The nurse should teach the mother how to centre the flanges of the pump over the breast with the nipple in the centre of the flange opening, making an air-tight seal. Proper positioning will help prevent nipple trauma. The pump should be started on high speed and low suction. When milk flow starts ("let down"), the pump is adjusted to medium speed and comfort level. The breasts should be drained and feel soft after pumping. Daily milk production after breastfeeding is established should be approximately 750 to 1 050 mL (25–35 ounces) in a 24-hour period. Weaning from the pump should be gradual. The mother should not suddenly stop pumping, or discomfort and engorgement may occur (Newton, 2017).

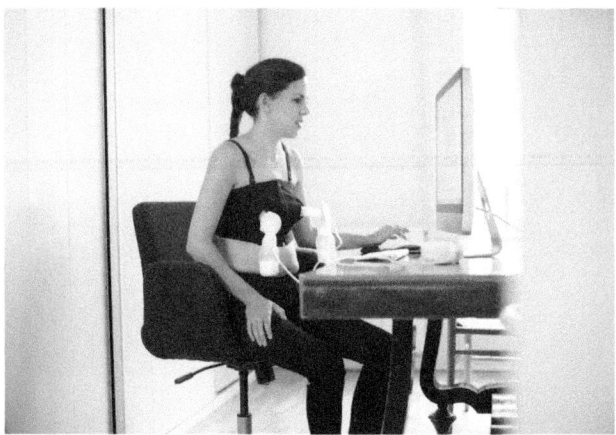

Fig. 9.13 Electric breast pump. One or both breasts can be pumped, and suction pressure is adjustable. Most hospitals and breastfeeding clinics help new mothers establish breastfeeding and breast pumping schedules to fit their individual needs. (iStock.com/Orbon Alija)

Storing and Freezing Breast Milk

While fresh breastmilk is best, milk can be stored for use later if needed. Various commercial containers are available for the storage of breastmilk, each with advantages and disadvantages. The container size should hold about as much milk as the infant will consume at one feeding. Milk may be safely stored in glass or hard plastic containers that are bisphenol A (BPA)–free. Plastic bags made for breast-milk storage can be used; however, bottle liners are not designed for storage

Milk can be thawed in the refrigerator for 24 hours (best to preserve immunoglobulins) or by holding the container under running lukewarm water or placing it in a container of lukewarm water, rotating (not shaking) the bottle often. Microwaving is not advised, because it destroys some immune factors and lysozyme contained in the milk. It can also cause hot spots to develop from uneven heating, and these hot spots can cause mouth burns in the infant. Milk can be stored at room temperature optimally for 4 hours, although 6 to 8 hours is acceptable in very clean conditions; in the back of the refrigerator (4°C [39°F]) for up to 96 hours (4 days); or in a freezer (−4°C [−18°F]) for 6 to 12 months (Best Start, 2018). Please refer to the Best Start resource (Additional Learning Resources) for more details on storing breast milk. Freezing can destroy some antimicrobial factors in the breast milk. Thawed milk should not be stored in the refrigerator longer than 24 hours, and if warmed for a feeding, it should be discarded in 1 to 2 hours. Containers should be labelled with the date and should not be refrozen after thawing.

Maternal Nutrition

Mothers should eat a well-balanced diet to promote postpartum healing and establish an adequate milk supply. They should choose foods according to Canada's *Food Guide* (see Appendix C)

To maintain her own nutrient stores while providing for the infant, the mother needs a little more food each day, usually one extra snack is enough (Government of Canada, 2019). An indicator of adequate caloric intake is a stable maternal weight and a gradually increasing infant weight. The maternal protein intake should be the same as during pregnancy so the growing infant has adequate protein. Some breastfeeding mothers will continue to take their prenatal vitamins. Mothers who do not eat meat, fish, eggs, or milk may require a vitamin B_{12} supplement (HealthLinkBC, 2019). Fluid intake should be sufficient to relieve thirst.

Some foods eaten by the mother may change the taste of the milk or cause the infant to have gas. Foods that often cause problems are chocolate, cabbage, beans, and broccoli. If the mother suspects that a particular food is causing fussiness or gas in the infant, she can eliminate it from her diet for a few days to determine whether the infant has less distress. These problems do not indicate an allergy to breastmilk but only an irritation with some food by-product contained in the milk. Excessive caffeine intake should be avoided, as well as alcohol intake, which may impair the milk ejection reflex. Lactating mothers should be instructed that many types of medications or herbs can be secreted in varying amounts in the breastmilk. Medications should be taken only with the health care provider's advice. Mothers should inform their health care providers of any vitamins or herbal supplements she is taking.

Weaning

Gradual weaning is preferred to abrupt weaning, which can cause engorgement, lead to mastitis, and be upsetting to the newborn. There is no particular "best" time to wean; this is a personal decision and should be when both the mother and baby are ready.

The nurse can teach mothers the following tips when they want to wean their newborns:

- Eliminate one feeding at a time. Wait several days and before eliminating another one. Depending on the age of the baby, the feed will need to be replaced. If younger than 6 months, this may be stored breast milk or formula from a bottle; the older baby may be weaned from the breast to a cup and may eat additional solids.
- Omit daytime feedings first, starting with the one in which the baby is least interested.
- Eliminate the baby's favourite feeding last. This will often be the early morning or bedtime feeding.
- Expect the baby to need "comfort nursing" if the child is tired, ill, or uncomfortable.
- If the mother must wean abruptly for some reason, the following tips may help: wearing a supportive bra, using cold packs and analgesics, or hand expressing or pumping to relieve breast fullness. Mothers should monitor for plugged ducts and breast infection while weaning abruptly. Mothers may need to express or pump to comfort for several days. Some mothers report that applying cool, raw cabbage leaves to the breasts may relieve engorgement and discomfort (Grueger & CPS Community Paediatrics Committee, 2013/2018; Wambach & Riordan, 2014).

THE BABY-FRIENDLY HOSPITAL INITIATIVE

The Baby-Friendly Hospital Initiative (BFI) was launched in 1991 by UNICEF and the World Health Association (WHO) with a goal of supporting, protecting, and promoting breastfeeding. A *baby-friendly hospital* is defined as a facility that meets specific criteria and has been recognized to have met the recently revised 10 steps to successful breastfeeding (Box 9.4) (Tran, 2017). The Breastfeeding Committee for Canada (BCC) works with organizations in Canada to become BFI designated and adhere to the International Code for Marketing Breast-milk Substitutes. The BFI has demonstrated a

Box 9.4 Baby-Friendly Initiative (BFI) 10 Steps for Hospitals and Community Health Services

1. Have a written infant feeding policy that is routinely communicated to all staff, health care providers, and volunteers.
2. Ensure that all staff, health care providers, and volunteers have the knowledge and skills necessary to implement the infant feeding policy.

KEY CLINICAL PRACTICES

3. Inform pregnant women and their families about the importance and process of breastfeeding.
4. Place babies in uninterrupted skin-to-skin contact with their mothers immediately following birth for at least an hour or until completion of the first feeding or as long as the mother wishes. Encourage mothers to recognize when their babies are ready to feed, offering help as needed.
5. Assist mothers to breastfeed and maintain lactation should they face challenges, including separation from their infants.
6. Support mothers to exclusively breastfeed for the first 6 months unless supplements are medically indicated.
7. Facilitate 24-hour rooming-in for all mother–infant dyads: mothers and infants remain together.
8. Encourage responsive, cue-based breastfeeding. Encourage sustained breastfeeding beyond 6 months with the appropriate introduction of complementary foods.
9. Support mothers to feed and care for their breastfeeding babies without the use of artificial teats or pacifiers (dummies or soothers).
10. Provide a seamless transition between the services provided by the hospital, community health services, and peer support programs. Apply principles of primary health care and population health to support the continuum of care and implement strategies that affect the broad determinants that will improve breastfeeding outcomes.

Source: Breastfeeding Committee for Canada (2017). *The BFI 10 Steps and WHO code for outcome indicators for hospitals and community health services.* Retrieved from http://breastfeedingcanada.ca/documents/Indicators%20-%20complete%20June%202017.pdf

positive impact on breastfeeding initiation and exclusivity in developed and developing countries (RNAO, 2018). The RNAO (2018) states all of the BFI principles must be integrated into perinatal health care settings, both within hospitals and the community, to better ensure support for mothers beyond hospital discharge.

Human Rights Protections for Breastfeeding Mothers

Breastfeeding is protected by the Canadian Human Rights Commission; it is illegal to discriminate because a women is breastfeeding. Women returning to employment should be accommodated in a variety of ways to support their breastfeeding, including (1) providing a clean, suitable place to breastfeed or express and store milk, (2) longer or extra breaks for breastfeeding or expressing breastmilk, and (3) allowing for alternative work arrangements (Canadian Human Rights Commission, 2010). These accommodations should be provided in other settings as well. Breastfeeding mothers have the right to breastfeed in public spaces and cannot be asked to move or cover up. These places include parks, stores, restaurants, schools, and public transit (Ontario Human Rights Commission, 2018).

FORMULA FEEDING

Women choose to formula feed for many reasons. Some feel uncomfortable breastfeeding or may have little social support. Others find it difficult when they cannot see the amount of milk the newborn takes at each feeding. Women who have many other commitments and cannot maintain the flexibility needed when lactation is established may find that formula feeding is the only realistic choice. A few women must take medications or may have other illnesses that make breastfeeding unwise. When a woman who has been fully informed about the advantages of breastfeeding for both the mother and the infant chooses to formula feed, regardless of the reason for choosing to formula feed, the nurse should fully support the mother and reassure her that her infant can receive adequate nutrition and emotional closeness.

TYPES OF INFANT FORMULAS

Most formulas are modifications of cow's milk. Infants who do not tolerate cow's milk formulas or who come from a family with many allergies may be prescribed a specialty formula. Many formulas are available to meet special needs, such as those of the preterm infant or the infant with phenylketonuria (PKU). Common formulas are available in three forms:

1. Ready-to-feed, either in cans or in glass bottles
2. Concentrated liquid
3. Powdered

Powdered infant formula is not sterile and is therefore not recommended for infants at greatest risk (e.g., preterm, low birth weight, or immunocompromised). Commercially produced liquid infant formulas (either concentrated or ready-to-use) are recommended for these infants as these products are sterile (Government of Canada, 2010). If a child must be fed powdered formula, strictly following the recommendations for boiling water is warranted.

PREPARATION

The parent should perform hand hygiene before preparing formula and feeding the infant. Bottles, nipples, and spoons should be sterilized by boiling in an open pan of water for 2 minutes. They are then allowed to air dry and cool. Water to make the formula needs to be boiled for 2 minutes and the water cooled to 70°C, prior to adding the powder (Government of Canada, 2012). Bottles of formula can be prepared one at a time, or a 24-hour supply can be prepared. Formula should be refrigerated promptly and kept refrigerated at 4°C for a maximum of 24 hours (Government of Canada, 2012). See Table 14.1 for further information on formula preparation.

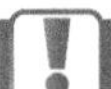
Safety Alert!

Overdilution or underdilution of concentrated liquid or powdered formulas can result in serious illness.

Bottled cow's milk and evaporated milk are nutritionally inadequate for use as infant formula and stress the kidneys of the newborn and young infant and should not be used.

FEEDING THE INFANT

Formula is digested more slowly than breastmilk, so formula-fed infants may initially feed less frequently than a breastfed newborn. Like the breastfeeding mother, the formula-feeding mother should be encouraged to avoid rigid scheduling and should feed on demand based on infant hunger cues (Skill 9.6).

Many mothers prefer to warm the formula somewhat, but this is not necessary. Placing the bottle in a container of hot water takes the chill off the milk. Microwave heating of infant formula is *not* recommended because heating is uneven and may result in hot spots that can cause mouth burns in the infant. The temperature of the formula should be checked on the inside of the wrist before feeding the baby to ensure it is not too hot.

The nurse should caution parents not to prop the bottle, even when the infant is older. Propping the bottle may cause the infant to aspirate formula and is associated with dental caries (cavities) and ear infections.

Partners are encouraged to assist with feedings. When teaching new parents about infant care, the partner or other support person should be involved to add their involvement and attachment to the infant as well as to enhance support for the mother. Tips concerning safe bottle feeding of the infant can be found in Chapter 14.

DISCHARGE PLANNING

Discharge planning begins on admission or even earlier, when parents attend childbirth classes. Because mothers and infants are discharged quickly after birth, usually within 24 hours, self-care and infant care teaching must often begin before the mother is psychologically ready to learn. Some birth facilities use *clinical pathways* (also called *care maps, care paths,* or *multidisciplinary action plans [MAPs]*) to ensure that important care and teaching are not overlooked (Couplet Care Plan 9.1). These plans guide the nurse in identifying areas of special need that require referral and offer a way for the parents to keep up with the many facets of routine care needed after birth. The nurse must take every opportunity to provide relevant teaching during the short stay in the birth facility. Ample written materials and online sources regarding both the new mother and infant care should be provided to refresh the memory of parents who may be tired and uncomfortable when teaching occurs. Nurses need to learn to use "teachable moments" to enhance learning. Parents often do not retain information well if all the information is provided in one session; it needs to be spread out over the hospital stay and provided when the parents show interest in certain topics.

POSTPARTUM SELF-CARE

The nurse must teach the new mother how best to care for herself to reduce her risk for complications.

Skill 9.6 Bottle Feeding the Newborn

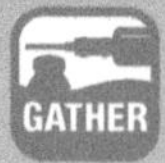

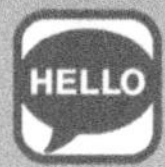

PURPOSE

To provide nutrients for growth and development in the formula-feeding newborn

STEPS

1. Perform hand hygiene.
2. Identify newborn.
3. Verify formula prescribed and expiration date on the bottle.
4. Select an appropriate nipple. Cross-cut nipple offers rapid feedings and should only be used in special situations; single-hole nipple offers regular milk flow; preemie nipple offers softer nipple that requires less sucking effort from the newborn.
5. Open bottle (you should hear a "pop" to indicate bottle was previously unopened); place selected nipple on the bottle and tighten securely. Use room-temperature formula.
6. Hold newborn in "cradle position" with newborn's head slightly elevated above the body (see figure).
7. Touch the newborn's lip with nipple and gently insert nipple along newborn's tongue. Hold bottle so nipple always has formula in it.
8. Feed the newborn slowly. Stop to burp newborn after feeding 30 to 45 mL and at end of feeding.
9. If formula runs out of the side of the mouth during feeding, the nipple holes may be too large. The nipple should be discarded and replaced with a different one.
10. To burp the newborn, sit the newborn on your lap with their body leaning slightly forward. Support the head and gently pat the middle or upper back (see Fig. 9.13).
11. Place the newborn in the crib on their back after feeding.
12. Leftover formula should be discarded because microorganisms from the newborn's mouth grow rapidly in warm formulas.
13. Document the amount taken; type of formula; any regurgitation; sucking strength; and parent teaching that was provided.

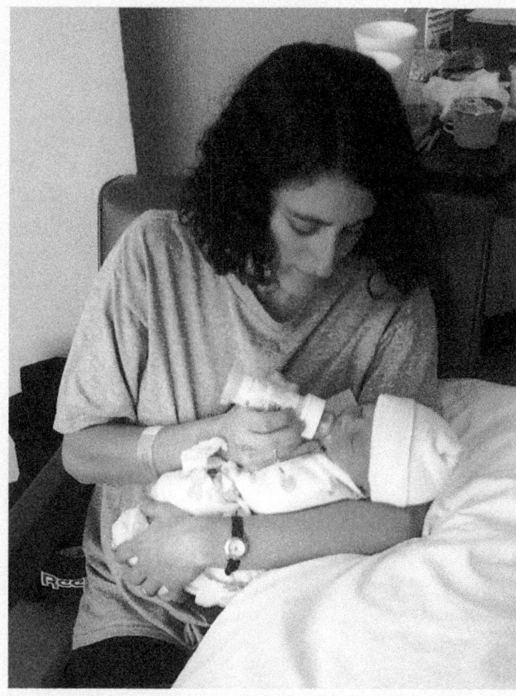

Hygiene

A shower is refreshing and cleanses the skin of perspiration that may be more profuse in the first days after birth. Perineal care should be continued until the flow of lochia stops. Douches and tampons should not be used for sanitary protection until after lochia stops.

Diet and Exercise

A well-balanced diet and moderate exercise promote healing and recovery from birth. Because constipation may be a concern, the mother is taught about high-fibre foods (e.g., whole-grain breads, and fruits and vegetables with the skins). Moderate exercise can aid in returning the uterus to its prepregnancy state and promoting a feeling of well-being. Most health care providers recommend that new mothers continue any prescribed prenatal vitamins until at least the 6-week checkup.

Follow-up Appointments

Most health care providers want to see the postpartum woman for a specific check-up 6 weeks after giving birth, although this may be earlier if there are specific concerns, and most women will have a breastfeeding assessment appointment prior to 6 weeks. The nurse should emphasize the importance of attending these

Couplet Care Plan 9.1

A 28-year-old woman who is $G_1T_0P_0A_0L_0$ has given birth by Caesarean section. Cervical dilation ceased at 5 cm and the woman was given an oxytocin infusion to augment labour. No progress occurred in labour and a Caesarean birth was done. The skin was closed with staples. Estimated blood loss was 700 mL. She gave birth to a 3 400 gm female infant, 52 cm in length, APGAR 8 at 1 minute, 9 at 5 minutes. Mother and infant are on the postpartum unit.

Nursing Diagnosis Acute pain related to tissue trauma from Caesarean birth

Healthcare Provider and Nursing Orders	Intervention	Rationale	Expected Outcome
Tylenol 650 mg po, q4–6 hrs prn for mild pain	Using pain scale of 0 to 10, assess patient's pain along with vital signs.	To ensure appropriate interventions are implemented.	Mother will rate pain level less than 3 or state it is at an acceptable level; no obvious signs of discomfort, e.g., frequent repositioning, grimacing or moaning
Naproxen 250 mg 1–2 tabs po q6 hr for moderate pain	Assess location of pain	Assists in determining nursing interventions to minimize pain.	Medication administered around the clock to maintain pain at a low level.
	Administer analgesics based on assessment.	To ensure adequate pain relief is experienced by the mother.	
	Assess pain level 30 minutes after analgesics are given.	To determine if adequate relief was experienced or if further interventions are needed.	The mother has received adequate pain relief.
	Reinforce splinting of incision site whenever moving or coughing.	Minimizes level of pain mother would experience.	Mother states she is able to move more easily using splinting.

Nursing Diagnosis Need for education related to postpartum, infant care, safety, and follow-up

Healthcare Provider and Nursing Orders	Intervention	Rationale	Expected Outcome
Review hand expression techniques with mother	Educate about hand expression of milk and use of compresses in the event of engorgement.	Compresses help promote comfort; hand expression of milk helps relieve engorgement.	Breasts will be soft and nontender after each feeding; she understands when she should apply compresses and self-express milk to minimize breast discomfort.
	Provide and review infant care pamphlet.	Enhances learning and encourages questions.	Mother will be able to demonstrate or verbalize proper breast and infant care.
Provide breastfeeding support	Observe mother breastfeeding the infant.	To assess the latch, assess for signs of swallowing and intake and mother's comfort.	Mother is able to latch infant to the breast comfortably and identify when the infant is drinking (nutritive suckling).

Continued

Couplet Care Plan 9.1

Healthcare Provider and Nursing Orders	Intervention	Rationale	Expected Outcome
Infant: exclusive breastfeeding	Review how milk is made and feeding frequency, e.g., breastfeed on demand and reading infant cues.	Breastfed infants require frequent feedings and will cue when hungry. Responding to these cues with frequent feeds are needed to produce adequate amounts of milk for the infant.	Mother reads infant's cues and infant feeds eight or more times in a 24-hour period after day 1 postpartum. The infant feeds with signs of satiety after feeds.
Use teachable moments during contact with mother and infant	Educate regarding umbilical care, e.g., fold diaper below umbilical cord, appearance of cord as it dries and then falls off.	To minimize risk of infection or trauma to umbilical site.	Mother demonstrates correct use of the techniques taught; she appreciates teaching provided.
Discuss safety issues related to infant care	Reinforce importance of "back to sleep" for infant.	Minimizes risk of sudden infant death syndrome (SIDS).	
	Review importance of car seats and their proper use and proper method of carrying infant.	To ensure safe transport of infant while in an auto or baby carrier and to increase awareness of the need for safety in the care of the newborn.	Parents demonstrates correct use of safety techniques during the day of care.
Teach parents normal infant behaviours	Reaffirm throughout the day as infant sleeps, wakes, feeds and, voids/stools.		Parents demonstrates ability to be alert for infant cues and meet infant needs throughout the day.
Provide follow-up appointments for mother and infant	Ensure that family can travel to appointments. Discuss signs and symptoms in infant that warrant calling or returning for health care.	Ensure follow-up care of mother and infant	Parents have the appointments for mother and infant on their smartphone calendars.

follow-up appointments, where the health care provider will verify that involution is proceeding normally and identify any complications as soon as possible. Signs of problems the woman should report have been discussed in previous sections, and danger signs are discussed below.

At the 6-week appointment, the mother's general health and recovery from birth are assessed. The healing of the mother's perineum or Caesarean incision is assessed. Birth control options should be reviewed again at this time. Occasionally a complete blood count is done, and vitamins or iron supplements, or both, are ordered if anemia is present.

The woman has the opportunity to discuss any physical or psychological issues she may be having. The health care provider and the nurse usually inquire about how she is adapting to motherhood. Is she getting enough rest? How is breastfeeding progressing? Does she have help at home? How is the partner adapting to this new role? Women should be assessed for a perinatal mood disorder and the 6-week appointment is often a good time to do this. The Edinburgh Postnatal Depression Scale is a screening tool that can be used to assess for depression. If the woman screens positive, further assessment and referral may be necessary (see Chapter 10 for further discussion).

Danger Signs

By teaching the mother about changes to expect as she returns to the prepregnant state, the nurse gives her a framework for recognizing when something is not progressing normally. Hemorrhage, infection, and thrombosis are the most common complications (see Chapter 10 for further discussion). The mother should report the following:

- Fever higher than 38°C (100.4°F)
- Persistent lochia rubra or lochia that has a foul odour
- Bright red bleeding, particularly if the lochia has changed to serosa or alba
- Prolonged afterpains, pelvic or abdominal pain, or a constant backache
- Signs of a urinary tract infection
- Pain, redness, or tenderness of the calf
- Localized breast tenderness or redness
- Discharge, pain, redness, or separation of any suture line (Caesarean, perineal laceration, or episiotomy)
- Sudden onset of headaches
- Prolonged and pervasive feelings of depression or being let down; generally, not enjoying life

Unfolding Case Study

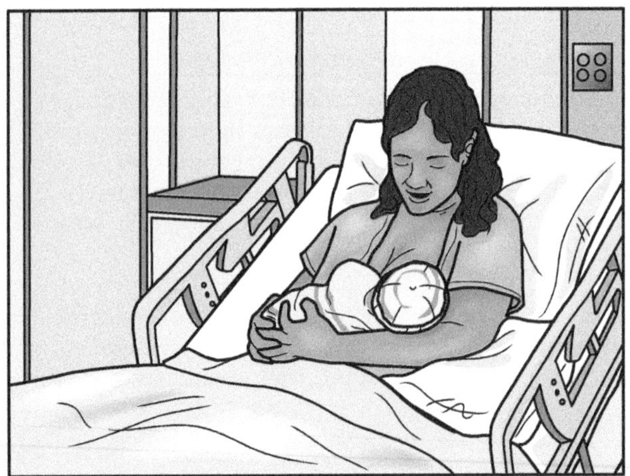

Tess and Luis were introduced to the reader in Chapter 2, and Tess's pregnancy experience has unfolded in each chapter. Refer to earlier chapters for her history.

Tess has given birth to twins! Baby A, a girl named Sofia, has been admitted to the neonatal intensive care unit (NICU) and will be discussed in Chapter 12. Partner Luis follows Sofia to the NICU with his cell phone, taking pictures of the unexpected event. Baby B, a boy named Marco, is admitted to the maternal child unit with his mother Tess. Tess is tired but very talkative about her birth experience, which included a laceration. She states that she is having afterpains that seem to be worse during breastfeeding. She is also worried that she is having vaginal bleeding; she thought her menstrual period would not return so quickly.

QUESTIONS

1. Explain (according to Rubin's theory of psychological changes during the puerperium) why Tess is so talkative after the birth and state how these stages influence when parent teaching would be most effective.
2. What are afterpains and why do they often worsen during breastfeeding?
3. Explain how the nurse can evaluate Tess's vaginal bleeding after childbirth and state what the nurse will teach Tess about what she can expect in the next few days and weeks concerning her vaginal discharge.
4. How will the nurse assess the perineum after Tess's laceration and what nursing care can be implemented?

Get Ready for the Certification Examination!

Key Points

- It is essential to consider all patients individually to better incorporate their culture and special needs into the plan of care.
- From its level at the umbilicus, the uterus should descend about one finger's width per day after birth. It should no longer be palpable at approximately 14 days postpartum.
- A slight increase in maternal heart rate is common in the first hour after birth. A maternal pulse rate that continues to be high may indicate hemorrhage or infection in the postpartum patient.
- A full bladder interferes with uterine contraction, which can lead to hemorrhage.
- Measures to promote bowel movements should be emphasized at each assessment: fluid intake, a high-fibre diet, and activity.
- $Rh_o(D)$ immune globulin is given within 72 hours to the Rh-negative mother who gives birth to an Rh-positive newborn.
- The postpartum check should include the status of fundus, lochia, breasts, perineum, bowel and bladder elimination, vital signs, pain, and evidence of parent–newborn attachment.
- The ideal interval between pregnancies is 24 months to prevent adverse outcomes in subsequent pregnancies.
- Bonding and attachment require contact between parents and newborn. The nurse should promote this contact whenever possible.
- Skin-to-skin contact should be initiated immediately after birth at least until the first breastfeeding occurs.
- More breast milk removed means more milk is produced. Early, regular, and frequent nursing promotes milk production and lessens engorgement.
- Newborns should be fed on demand, using infant cues to determine when they need to be fed.
- The breastfeeding mother needs an extra snack each day plus enough fluid to replace liquid lost via breastfeeding; mothers should drink to thirst.
- Weaning from the breast should be gradual, starting with the feeding the infant is least interested in and ending with the one in which he or she has the most interest.
- Commercially prepared formulas are available in ready-to-feed, concentrated liquid or in powdered form. Dilution, if required, must be followed exactly according to instructions.
- Discharge planning should take place with every instance of mother or newborn nursing care as the nurse teaches the mother normal findings, significance, and what to report. Written materials should be provided to augment all teaching.

Additional Learning Resources

evolve Go to your Evolve website (http://evolve.elsevier.com/Canada/Leifer) for the following learning resources:

- Answer Key for Critical Thinking Questions
- Answer Key for Textbook Review Questions
- Audio Glossary
- Fluids & Electrolytes tutorial
- Interactive Review Questions
- Skills Performance Checklists
- Video clips and more!

Online Resources

- AWHONN, *Quantification of Blood Loss*: https://www.youtube.com/watch?v=F_ac-aCbEn0&list=UUPrOhL3Od7ZeFDq27ycS00g
- Best Start, *Expressing and Storing Breast Milk:* https://www.beststart.org/resources/breastfeeding/Expressing_Fact%20Sheets_Eng_rev2.pdf
- Best Start, *Resources and Research:* http://en.beststart.org/resources-and-research
- International Lactation Consultant Association: https://www.ilca.org
- La Leche League International: https://www.llli.org
- Stanford Medicine, *Successful Breastfeeding Begins Right at Birth:* http://med.stanford.edu/newborns/professional-education/breastfeeding/breastfeeding-in-the-first-hour.html
- Toronto Public Health, *Breastfeeding Protocols for Health Care Providers:* http://breastfeedingresourcesontario.ca/resource/breastfeeding-protocols-health-care-providers
- World Health Organization, *International Code of Marketing of Breast-milk Substitutes:* https://www.who.int/nutrition/publications/code_english.pdf

Review Questions

1. Which maternal assessment is expected to be seen at 24 hours after birth?
   a. Scant amount of lochia alba on the perineal pad.
   b. Fundus firm and in the midline of the abdomen.
   c. Breasts distended and hard with flat nipples.
   d. Bradycardia.
2. Breastfeeding the newborn promotes uterine involution because it does which of the following?
   a. It uses maternal fat stores accumulated during pregnancy.
   b. It stimulates additional secretion of colostrum.
   c. It causes the pituitary to secrete oxytocin to contract the uterus.
   d. It promotes maternal formation of antibodies
3. Eight hours postpartum a woman states she prefers that the nurse takes care of her newborn. The woman talks in detail about her birthing experience on the phone and to anyone who enters her room. She states she is hungry, thirsty, and sleepy and is unable to focus on the newborn care teaching offered to her. The nurse would interpret this behaviour as which of the following?
   a. Inability to bond with the newborn.
   b. Development of postpartum psychosis.
   c. Inability to assume the parenting role.
   d. The normal taking-in phase of the postpartum period.
4. Which of the following is a nursing intervention that does not require the written order of the primary health care provider? *(Select all that apply.)*
   a. Administer an analgesic for pain.
   b. Teach the patient how to perform perineal care.
   c. Apply topical anaesthetic for perineal suture pain.
   d. Turn the patient every 2 hours.

REFERENCES

Best, Start (2018). *Expressing and storing breast milk.* Toronto, ON: Author. Retrieved from https://www.beststart.org/resources/breastfeeding/Expressing_Fact%20Sheets_Eng_rev2.pdf.

Black, A., Guilbert, E., et al. (2015). SOGC clinical practice guideline: Canadian contraception consensus (Part 2 of 4). *Journal of Obstetrics and Gynaecology Canada, 37*(11), S1–S39.

Canadian Human Rights Commission. (2010). *Pregnancy & human rights in the workplace—Policy and best practices.* Ottawa: Author. Retrieved from https://www.chrc-ccdp.gc.ca/eng/content/policy-and-best-practices-page-2.

Chan, W., Rey, E., Kent, N. E., et al. (2014). SOGC clinical practice guideline: Venous thromboembolism and antithrombotic therapy in pregnancy. *Journal of Obstetrics & Gynaecology Canada, 36*(6), 527–553.

Gionet, L. (2015). *Breastfeeding trends in Canada.* Health at a Glance. Statistics Canada Catalogue no, 82–624-X.

Goodman, J. H. (2005). Becoming an involved father of an infant. *Journal of Obstetric, Gynecologic, & Neonatal Nursing, 34,* 190–200.

Government of Canada. (2010). *Recommendations for the preparation and handling of powdered infant formula (PIF).* Retrieved from https://www.canada.ca/en/health-canada/services/food-nutrition/healthy-eating/infant-feeding/recommendations-preparation-handling-powdered-infant-formula-infant-feeding.html.

Government of Canada. (2012). *Infant formula.* Retrieved from https://www.canada.ca/en/health-canada/services/infant-care/infant-formula.html.

Government of Canada. (2019). *Healthy eating and pregnancy.* Retrieved from https://www.canada.ca/en/public-health/services/pregnancy/healthy-eating-pregnancy.html.

Gregory, K., Ramos, D., & Jauniaux, E. (2017). Preconceptual and prenatal care. In S. G. Gabbe, J. R. Niebyl, J. L. Simpson, et al. (Eds.), *Obstetrics: Normal and problem pregnancies* (7th ed.). Philadelphia: Elsevier.

Grueger, B., & Canadian Paediatric Society (CPS), Community Paediatrics Committee. (2013). Position statement: Weaning from the breast. *Paediatrics & Child Health, 18*(4), 210 Reaffirmed 2018.

HealthlinkBC. (2019). *Nutrition while breastfeeding.* Retrieved from https://www.healthlinkbc.ca/health-topics/hw130509.

Hendson, L., Davies, D., & Canadian Paediatric Society (CPS), Fetus & Newborn Committee. (2018). *Practice point: Supporting and communicating with families experiencing a perinatal loss.* Retrieved from https://www.cps.ca/en/documents/position/perinatal-loss.

Isley, M. M., & Katz, V. L. (2017). Postpartum care and long-term health considerations. In S. G. Gabbe, J. R. Niebyl, J. L. Simpson, et al. (Eds.), *Obstetrics: Normal and problem pregnancies* (7th ed.). Philadelphia: Elsevier.

Kim, J. H., & Froh, E. B. (2012). What nurses need to know regarding nutritional and immunobiological properties of human milk. *Journal of Obstetric, Gynecologic, & Neonatal Nursing, 41*(1), 122–137.

MacDonald, N., & Canadian Pediatric Society (CPS), Infectious Diseases and Immunization Committee. (2006). Practice point: Maternal infectious diseases, antimicrobial therapy or immunizations: Very few contraindications to breastfeeding. *Paediatrics & Child Health, 11*(8), 489–491. Reaffirmed 2018.

Newton, E. (2017). Lactation and breastfeeding. In S. G. Gabbe, J. R. Niebyl, J. L. Simpson, et al. (Eds.), *Obstetrics: Normal and problem pregnancies* (7th ed.). Philadelphia: Elsevier.

Ontario Human Rights Commission. (2018). *Pregnancy and breastfeeding*. Toronto, ON: Author. Retrieved from http://www.ohrc.on.ca/sites/default/files/Pregnancy%20and%20breastfeeding_English_accessible.pdf.

Ponti, M., & Canadian Pediatric society (CPS), community pediatrics committee. (2003). Position statement: Recommendations for the use of pacifiers *Paediatrics & Child Health, 8*(8), 515–519. Reaffirmed 2018. Retrieved from https://www.cps.ca/en/documents/position/pacifiers.

Public Health Agency of Canada [PHAC]. (2018). Chapter 6—Breastfeeding. In *Family-centred maternity and newborn care: National guidelines*. Ottawa, ON: Author. Retrieved from https://www.canada.ca/en/public-health/services/publications/healthy-living/maternity-newborn-care-guidelines-chapter-6.html.

Registered Nurses' Association of Ontario (RNAO). (2018). *Promoting and supporting the initiation, exclusivity, and continuation of breastfeeding for newborns, infants, and young children* (3rd ed.). Toronto (ON): Author.

Rubin, R. (1967). Attainment of the maternal role. Part 1: Process. *Nursing Research, 16*, 237–245.

Tran, A. (2017). Becoming a baby friendly hospital. *Maternal Child Nursing Journal MCN, 42*(1), 36–42.

Wambach, K., & Riordan, J. (2014). *Breastfeeding and human lactation* (5th ed.). Sudbury, MA: Jones & Bartlett Publishers.

World Health Organization (WHO). (2018). *Protecting, promoting and supporting breastfeeding in facilities providing maternity and newborn services: The revised Baby-Friendly Initiative.* Geneva: Author. Retrieved from http://www.who.int/nutrition/publications/infantfeeding/bfhi-implementation-2018.pdf?ua=1.

World Health Organization (WHO). (2019). *Nutritional care of children and adults with Ebola virus disease in treatment centres.* Geneva: Author. Retrieved from http://www.who.int/elena/titles/nutrition_ebola/en/.

Nursing Care of Women With Complications After Birth

10

Katie Lindsay

http://evolve.elsevier.com/Canada/Leifer

Objectives

1. Define each key term listed.
2. Describe signs and symptoms for each postpartum complication.
3. Identify factors that increase a woman's risk for developing each complication.
4. Explain nursing measures that reduce a woman's risk for developing specific postpartum complications.
5. Describe the medical and nursing management of postpartum complications.
6. Explain general and specific nursing care for each complication.
7. Compare and contrast mood disorders in the postpartum period.

Key Terms

atony (ĂT-ŏ-nē)
curettage (KYŪ-rĕ-tăhzh)
endometritis (ĕn-dō-mē-TRĪ-tĭs)
hematoma (hē-mă-TŌ-mă)
hypovolemic shock (hī-pō-vō-LĒ-mĭk shŏk)
involution (ĭn-vō-LŪ-shŭn)
mastitis (măs-TĪ-tĭs)
psychosis (sī-KŌ-sĭs)
puerperal sepsis (pū-ĔR-pŭr-ăl SĔP-sĭs)
subinvolution (sŭb-ĭn-vō-LŪ-shŭn)

Most women who give birth recover from pregnancy and childbirth without any problems. However, occasionally complications can arise after birth that slow their recovery and may interfere with their ability to assume their new role as mother. The most common complications related to childbirth fall into one of four categories:

1. Postpartum hemorrhage
2. Thromboembolic disorders
3. Puerperal infections
4. Mood disorders

POSTPARTUM HEMORRHAGE

Postpartum hemorrhage (PPH) has been traditionally defined as blood loss greater than 500 mL after vaginal birth or 1 000 mL after Caesarean birth, resulting in signs or symptoms of hypovolemia. More recently, PPH has been defined as any amount of blood loss with the potential to produce hemodynamic instability (Society of Obstetricians and Gynaecologists of Canada [SOGC], 2014). Because the average-size woman has 1 to 2 litres of added blood volume from pregnancy, she can tolerate up to these amounts of blood loss better than would otherwise be expected.

Early PPH is more common and occurs within 24 hours of birth. *Late PPH* occurs after 24 hours and up to 12 weeks after birth (American College of Obstetricians & Gynecologist [ACOG], 2017). The four *T's* mnemonic can be used to identify and address the four most common causes of PPH: **t**one (uterine atony; **t**rauma (laceration, hematoma, inversion, rupture); **t**issue (retained tissue or invasive placenta); and **t**hrombin (coagulopathy) (Evensen, Anderson, & Fontaine, 2017). Uterine atony (tone), or when the uterus fails to contract after birth, accounts for 70 to 80% of cases and should usually be considered first (ACOG, 2017). The major risk of hemorrhage is hypovolemic (low-volume) shock, which interrupts blood flow to body cells. This prevents normal oxygenation, nutrient delivery, and waste removal at the cellular level. Although a less dramatic problem, anemia is likely to occur after hemorrhage. PPH is a leading cause of postpartum death around the world.

EARLY POSTPARTUM HEMORRHAGE

Early PPH usually results from one of the following three causes:

1. Tone
   - Uterine atony (the most common cause)
2. Trauma
   - Hematomas in the reproductive tract
   - Lacerations (tears) of the reproductive tract
3. Thrombin
   - Coagulopathies (discussed later in section)

Table 10.1 summarizes the common types of early PPH.

Table 10.1 Causes of Early Postpartum Hemorrhage

UTERINE ATONY	LACERATIONS	HEMATOMA
Characteristics		
Soft, high uterine fundus that is difficult to feel through a woman's abdominal wall Heavy lochia, often with large clots or sometimes a persistent moderate flow Bladder distention that causes uterus to be high and usually displaces it to one side Possible signs of hypovolemic shock	Continuous trickle of blood that is brighter than normal lochia Fundus that is usually firm Onset of hypovolemic shock that may be gradual and easily overlooked	If visible, appears as blue or purplish mass on vulva Severe and poorly relieved pain and/or pressure in vulva, pelvis, or rectum Large amount of blood lost into tissues, which causes signs and symptoms of hypovolemic shock Lochia that is normal in amount and colour
Contributing Factors		
Bladder distention Abnormal or prolonged labour Overdistended uterus Multiparity (five or more births) Use of oxytocin during labour Medications that relax uterus Operative birth Low placental implantation	Rapid labour Use of instruments such as forceps or vacuum during birth	Prolonged or rapid labour Large infant Use of forceps or vacuum

LATE POSTPARTUM HEMORRHAGE

Late PPH (bleeding that occurs 24 hours to 12 weeks after childbirth) usually occurs after discharge from the hospital and usually results from the following:

1. Tone
   - Subinvolution of the uterus
2. Tissue
   - Retention of placental fragments

HYPOVOLEMIC SHOCK

Hypovolemic shock occurs when the volume of blood is depleted and cannot fill the circulatory system. The woman can die if blood loss does not stop and if the blood volume is not corrected.

Body's Response to Hypovolemia

The body initially responds to a reduction in blood volume with increased heart and respiratory rates. These reactions increase the oxygen content of each erythrocyte (red blood cell) and faster circulation of the remaining blood. *Tachycardia (rapid heart rate) is usually the first sign of inadequate blood volume (hypovolemia).* The first blood pressure change is a narrow pulse pressure (a falling systolic pressure and a rising diastolic pressure). The blood pressure continues falling and eventually cannot be detected.

Blood flow to nonessential organs gradually stops to make more blood available for vital organs, specifically the heart and brain. This change causes the woman's skin and mucous membranes to become pale, cold, and clammy (moist). As blood loss continues, flow to the brain decreases, resulting in anxiety, confusion, restlessness, and lethargy. As blood flow to the kidneys decreases, they respond by conserving fluid. Urine output decreases and eventually stops.

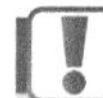

Safety Alert!

Because postpartum women often have a slow pulse rate, the caregiver should investigate for the possibility of hypovolemic shock or infection if the pulse rate is greater than 100 beats/min.

Medical Management and Nursing Care

Management of hypovolemic shock resulting from hemorrhage may include any of the following actions:

- Stopping the blood loss by:
  - Uterine massage
  - Administration of medications such as oxytocin to contract the uterus
- Notifying primary health care provider
- Giving intravenous (IV) fluids to maintain the circulating volume and to replace fluids
- Giving blood transfusions to replace lost erythrocytes
- Giving oxygen to increase the saturation of remaining blood cells; a pulse oximeter is used to assess oxygen saturation of the blood
- Placing an indwelling (Foley) catheter to assess urine output, which reflects kidney function

Routine postpartum nursing care involves assessing vital signs every 15 minutes until stable so that the signs of PPH are identified as early as possible. The woman should be observed closely for early signs of shock, such as tachycardia, pallor, cold and clammy hands, and decreased urine output. Decreased blood pressure may be a late sign of hypovolemic shock. Routine frequent assessment of lochia in the fourth stage of labour helps identify early PPH. When the amount and character of lochia are normal and the uterus is firm but signs of hypovolemia are still evident, the cause may be a large hematoma. Excessive bright red bleeding despite a firm fundus may indicate a cervical or vaginal laceration. The occurrence of petechiae, bleeding from venipuncture sites, or oliguria may indicate a blood clotting problem. In the woman who is bleeding heavily, the perineal pad should be weighed to determine a more accurate output amount, with 1 g equaling 1 mL (see Skill 9.1). Intake and output should be recorded and IV therapy monitored.

Safety Alert!

Saturation of a peripad within 15 minutes to 1 hour after birth must be promptly reported.

Careful explanations to the mother and family are essential, and providing emotional support and maintaining the integrity of the woman's support system are key nursing roles. Intensive care may be required to allow invasive hemodynamic monitoring of the woman's circulatory status. Even if the mother is separated from her infant, information concerning the infant's condition should be readily accessible. Rooming-in should be established as soon as the woman's condition permits. Nursing Care Plan 10.1 specifies interventions for the woman at high risk for altered tissue perfusion related to hemorrhage.

NORMAL POSTPARTUM CHANGES

The postpartum uterus is a large, hollow organ with three layers of muscle. The middle layer includes interlacing "figure-eight" fibres. The uterine blood supply passes through this network of muscle fibres to supply the placenta. After the placenta detaches, the uterus normally contracts and the muscle fibres compress bleeding vessels.

After a full-term birth, the uterus should easily be felt through the abdominal wall as a firm mass about the size of a grapefruit. After the placenta is expelled, the fundus of the uterus is at the umbilicus level and then begins descending at a rate of about one finger's width (1 cm) each day.

Lochia should be rubra. The amount of lochia during the first few hours should be no more than one saturated perineal pad per hour. A few small clots may appear in the drainage, but large clots are not normal.

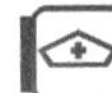

Nursing Tip

Perineal pads containing cold packs absorb less than regular perineal pads.

Nursing Tip

To determine blood loss most accurately, weigh perineal pads before and after applying them: 1 g in weight equals about 1 mL in volume of blood lost.

Nursing Care Plan 10.1 The Woman With Postpartum Hemorrhage

PATIENT DATA

A woman is admitted to the postpartum unit. She appears anxious and frightened, and her lochia has saturated three perineal pads in the past hour.

Selected Nursing Diagnosis Risk for hypovolemic shock as a result of excessive blood loss

Goals	Nursing Interventions	Rationales
The woman's blood pressure and pulse rate will be within 10% of her values when she was admitted.	Identify whether woman has added risk factors for postpartum hemorrhage.	Women who have risk factors should be assessed more often than those who do not.
	Observe the following: • Fundus for height, firmness, and position • Distended bladder • Lochia for colour, quantity, and clots; count pads and degree of saturation (weigh pads for greater accuracy); check blood pressure, pulse rate, and respiratory rate per hospital protocol	The fundus must be firm to compress bleeding vessels at the placenta site. Bladder distention interferes with uterine contraction and causes the fundus to be high and displaced to one side. Observing lochia provides an estimate of actual blood loss. A rising pulse rate is often the first sign of inadequate blood volume. Blood pressure may also decrease. Most blood lost after birth is visible rather than concealed.
	Observe for less obvious signs of bleeding: • Constant trickle of brighter red blood with a firm fundus • Severe, poorly relieved pain, especially if accompanied by changes in vital signs or shock signs and symptoms	Most postpartum hemorrhage is caused by uterine atony, which often produces dramatic blood loss. However, blood loss from a laceration or hematoma can be significant, even though it is less obvious.

Continued

Nursing Care Plan 10.1 The Woman With Postpartum Hemorrhage

The woman will not have signs or symptoms of hypovolemic shock.	Observe for other signs and symptoms of hypovolemic shock.	Excessive blood loss can result in hypovolemic shock.
	If signs of hemorrhage are noted, take appropriate actions according to the probable cause for hemorrhage: • *Uterine atony:* Massage uterus until firm—do not overmassage; expel blood from uterine cavity when uterus is firm; have woman breastfeed infant; notify health care provider for orders and medication if uterus does not become firm and stay firm. • *Lacerations:* Notify health care provider to examine woman. • *Hematomas on the vulva:* Place cold pack on the area.	Hemorrhage can cause death of a mother if not promptly corrected. Most minor episodes of uterine atony are easily corrected with fundal massage and infant suckling. If the uterus does not remain firm, the health care provider examines the woman to identify and correct the cause of bleeding. Oxytocin infusions are often ordered to contract the uterus. Other medications, such as methylergonovine (Methergine) or prostaglandin, may be needed. Excessive massage of the uterus can tire it, possibly resulting in inability to contract. Trauma such as laceration or hematoma may necessitate repair by the health care provider. Small hematomas on the vulva can be limited by cold applications, because these applications reduce blood flow to the area; cold also numbs the area and makes the woman more comfortable.

Selected Nursing Diagnosis Fear, as a result of an unexpected complication

Goals	Nursing Interventions	Rationales
Woman will be able to cope with the unexpected complication. Anxiety will be decreased.	Identify woman's reaction to unexpected complication and correct misconceptions and provide information.	Supplying factual information reduces fear. Identifying the reaction establishes basis for intervention.
	Be calm and reassuring when in contact with the woman.	Anxiety can be transferred by voice or body language.
	Encourage woman to verbalize her fears and perceptions.	This helps establish a basis for patient teaching and identification of fears.
	Stay with the woman and her partner.	Having a knowledgeable person present promotes a feeling of security.

CRITICAL THINKING QUESTION

1. A woman is admitted to the postpartum unit after the birth of an infant weighing 4 600 g. She voids 600 mL. The fundus is difficult to locate, and lochia is heavy. What are the priority nursing actions?

Subinvolution of the Uterus

Involution is the return of the uterus to its nonpregnant condition after birth. Normally the uterus descends at the rate of 1 cm (one finger's width) per day and is no longer palpable by 2 weeks postpartum. The placental site heals by approximately 6 weeks postpartum. **Subinvolution** is a slower-than-expected return of the uterus to its nonpregnant condition and a common cause of late PPH. Infection and retained fragments of the placenta are the most common causes. Typical signs of subinvolution include the following:

- Fundal height greater than expected for the amount of time since birth
- Persistence of lochia rubra or a slowed progression through the three phases
- Pelvic pain, heaviness, fatigue

Treatment

Medical treatment is selected to correct the cause of the subinvolution. It may include the following:

- Methylergonovine to maintain firm uterine contraction
- Antibiotics for infection
- Dilation of the cervix and curettage to remove fragments of the placenta from the uterine wall

Nursing care

The mother will almost always have been discharged when subinvolution of the uterus occurs. All new mothers should be taught about the normal changes to expect so they can recognize a departure from the normal pattern. Women should report fever, persistent pain, persistent red lochia (or return of bleeding after it

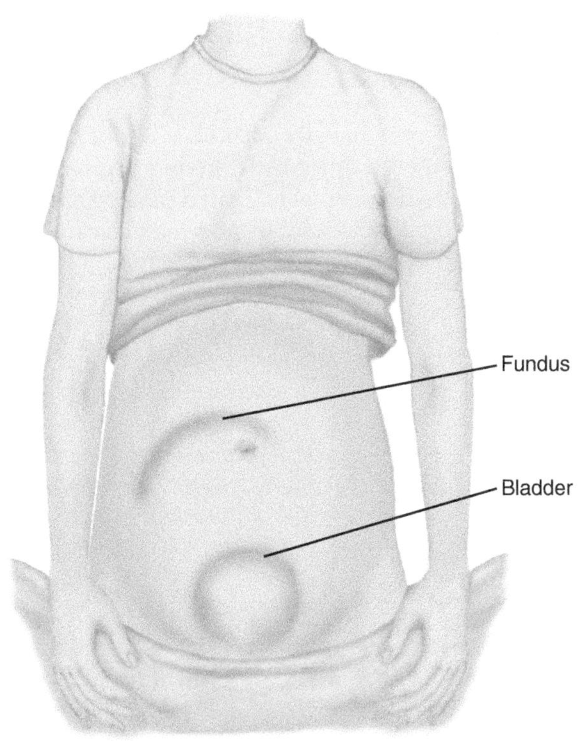

Fig. 10.1 A distended bladder pushes the uterus upward and usually to one side of the abdomen. The fundus may be boggy or firm. If not emptied, a distended bladder can result in uterine atony and hemorrhage, because it interferes with normal contraction of the uterus. (From McKinney, E. S., James, S. R., Murray, S. S., et al. [2013]. *Maternal-child nursing* [4th ed.]. St. Louis: Saunders.)

has changed), or foul-smelling vaginal discharge. The woman should be taught how to palpate the fundus.

The woman with subinvolution may be admitted to the hospital. Nursing care involves assisting with medical therapy and providing analgesics and other comfort measures. Specific nursing care depends on whether the subinvolution results from infection or another cause.

TONE

Uterine **atony** describes a lack of normal muscle tone. If the uterus is atonic, the muscle fibres are flaccid and do not compress the blood vessels causing the placenta site to bleed freely and massively. Uterine overdistention (due to large-for-gestational-age fetus, multiple birth, or polyhydramnios), prolonged labour, or the use of medications during labour that relax the uterus may cause atony.

When uterine atony occurs, the woman's uterus is difficult to feel and, when found, it feels boggy (soft). The fundal height is high, often above the umbilicus. If the bladder is full, the uterus is higher and pushed to one side (usually the right side) rather than located in the midline of the abdomen (Fig. 10.1). A full bladder interferes with the ability of the uterus to contract and, if not corrected, eventually leads to uterine atony.

Lochia is increased and may contain large clots. The bleeding may be dramatic but may also simply be slightly above normal for a long time. Some lochia will be retained in the relaxed uterus, because the cavity is enlarged. Thus, the true amount of blood loss may not be immediately apparent. Collection of blood within the uterus further interferes with contraction and worsens uterine atony and PPH. A woman who has risk factors for PPH (see Table 10.1) should have more frequent postpartum assessments of the uterus, lochia, and vital signs.

Medical Management and Nursing Care

Care of the woman with uterine atony combines nursing and medical measures. When the uterus is boggy, it should be massaged until firm (see Skill 9.2), but it should not be overly massaged. Because the uterus is a muscle, excessive stimulation to contract it will tire it and can actually worsen uterine atony. If the uterus is firmly contracted, it should be left alone. Pressing toward the vagina should expel any clots or blood pooled in the vagina *after the uterus is firm.*

Bladder distention is an easily corrected cause of uterine atony. The nurse should catheterize the woman if she is unable to urinate on the toilet or in a bedpan. Most health care providers include an order for catheterization to prevent delaying this corrective measure. First, the uterus is massaged to firmness, and then the bladder is emptied to keep the uterus firm.

The infant suckling at the breast stimulates the woman's posterior pituitary gland to secrete oxytocin, which causes uterine contraction. A dilute oxytocin IV infusion is the most common medication ordered to control uterine atony. Other medications to increase uterine tone include methylergonovine (Methergine) or prostaglandins such as carboprost (Hemabate) or misoprostol (Cytotec). Methylergonovine increases blood pressure and should not be given to a woman with hypertension. Tranexamic acid (Cyklokapron) may also be given, in addition to other uterotonic medications, to prevent PPH following vaginal and Caesarean birth (Novikova, Hofmeyr, & Cluver, 2015). Tranexamic acid inhibits the break-up of clots that form and therefore supports the developing blood clot that is necessary to control hemorrhage if administered within 3 hours of birth (WOMAN Trial Collaborators, 2017).

Excessive bleeding may also be managed by providing a uterine tamponade (packing), using an intrauterine balloon, selective arterial embolization, or surgical ligation of the artery. IV calcium gluconate may be used to counteract a tocolytic medication that may have been administered to relax the uterus during labour.

The health care provider may examine the woman in the birthing or operating room to determine the source of her bleeding and to correct it. Rarely, a hysterectomy is needed to remove the bleeding uterus that does not respond to any other measures. The woman should have nothing by mouth (NPO) until her bleeding is controlled.

Safety Alert!

The woman who develops a hemorrhagic complication should be kept NPO until the health care provider evaluates her condition, because she may need general anaesthesia for correction of the problem.

TRAUMA

Lacerations of the Reproductive Tract

Lacerations of the perineum, vagina, cervix, or area around the urethra (periurethral lacerations) can cause postpartum bleeding. The vascular beds are engorged during pregnancy, and bleeding can be profuse. Trauma is more likely to occur if the woman has a rapid labour or if forceps or a vacuum extractor is used. Blood lost in lacerations is usually a brighter red than lochia and flows in a continuous trickle. Typically, the uterus is firm.

Treatment

The health care provider should be notified if the woman has signs of a laceration, for example, bleeding with a firmly contracted uterus. The injury is usually sutured in the birthing or operating room.

Nursing care

Signs and symptoms of a bleeding laceration should be reported. A continuous trickle of blood can result in as much or more blood loss than the dramatic bleeding associated with uterine atony. The woman should be kept NPO until further orders are received, because she may need a general anaesthetic for repair of the laceration. Genital trauma can cause long-term effects such as cystocele, prolapsed uterus, or urinary incontinence.

Hematomas of the Reproductive Tract

A **hematoma** is a collection of blood within the tissues. Hematomas resulting from birth trauma are usually on the vulva or inside the vagina. They may be easily seen as a bulging bluish or purplish mass. Hematomas deep within the vagina are not visible from the outside.

Discomfort after childbirth is normally minimal and easily relieved with mild analgesics. The woman with a hematoma usually has severe, unrelenting pain that analgesics do not relieve. Depending on the amount of blood in the tissues, she also may describe pressure in the vulva, pelvis, or rectum. She may be unable to urinate because of the pressure.

The woman does not have unusual amounts of lochia, but she may develop signs of concealed blood loss if the hematoma is large. Her pulse and respiratory rates rise, and her blood pressure falls. She may develop other signs of hypovolemic shock if blood loss into the tissues is substantial. See Table 10.1 for risk factors for the development of a hematoma.

Treatment

Small hematomas usually resolve without treatment. Larger ones may require incision and drainage of the clots. The bleeding vessel is ligated or the area packed with a hemostatic material to stop the bleeding.

Nursing care

An ice pack to the perineum is sufficient for most small perineal hematomas. The nurse should observe and report for the classic symptom: excessive, poorly relieved pain. Signs of concealed blood loss accompanied by maternal symptoms of severe pain, perineal or vaginal pressure, or the inability to void should be reported. The woman is kept NPO until the health care provider examines her and prescribes treatment.

TISSUE

Placental fragments are more likely to be retained if the placenta does not separate cleanly from its implantation site after birth or if there is disruption of the placental scab. Clots form around these retained fragments and slough several days later, sometimes carrying the retained fragments with them. Retention of placental fragments is more likely to occur if the placenta is manually removed (removed by hand rather than being pushed away from the uterine wall spontaneously as the uterus contracts). These placental fragments are also more likely to exist if the placenta grows more deeply into the uterine muscle than is normal. Retained placenta is a common cause of subinvolution (see discussion later in the chapter).

Treatment

Treatment consists of the administration of medications such as oxytocin, methylergonovine, or prostaglandins such as carboprost to contract the uterus. Firm uterine contraction often expels the retained fragments and no other treatment is needed. Ultrasound may be used to identify remaining fragments. If bleeding continues, **curettage** (scraping or vacuuming the inner surface of the uterus) is performed to remove small blood clots and placental fragments. This procedure is known as dilation and curettage (D&C) or dilation and evacuation (D&E). Antibiotics are prescribed if infection is suspected.

Nursing Care

The nurse should teach each postpartum woman what to expect about changes in the lochia (see Chapter 9). The woman should be instructed to report the following signs of PPH to her health care provider:

- Persistent bright red bleeding
- Return of red bleeding after it has changed to pinkish or white
- Soaking a pad in 1 hour or less

THROMBIN (COAGULAPATHIES)

Coagulopathy is another cause of PPH. Causes of coagulopathies may be pre-existing or pregnancy related, such as idiopathic or immune thrombocytopenia (ITP), thrombocytopenia with pre-eclampsia, von Willebrand disease, and disseminated intravascular coagulation (DIC). Coagulopathies may also develop as a result of fetal demise, severe infection, or amniotic fluid embolus (SOGC, 2014).

Treatment

Primary medical management in all cases of DIC involves correction of the underlying cause (e.g., removal of the dead fetus, treatment of existing infection or of pre-eclampsia or eclampsia, or removal of a placental abruption). Treatment includes volume replacement, blood component replacement, ensuring optimum oxygenation and perfusion status, and continued reassessment of laboratory results. Resolution of DIC often begins with the birth of the newborn (SOGC, 2014). Tranexamic acid is given to women with von Willebrand disease half an hour before the birth (or when fully dilated). Consequently, fibrinolysis is inhibited and excessive bleeding is reduced. Tranexamic acid is an antifibrinolytic agent that has been shown to reduce excessive bleeding.

Nursing Care

Nursing care includes assessing for signs of bleeding, administering fluid or blood replacement as ordered, observing for signs of complications from the administration of blood and blood products, and protecting the woman from injury. Because renal failure is one consequence of DIC, urinary output is monitored, usually by insertion of an indwelling urinary catheter. Urinary output must be maintained at more than 30 mL/hr (Andrews, 2017).

THROMBOEMBOLIC DISORDERS

The levels of fibrinogen and other clotting factors normally increase during pregnancy, whereas levels of clot-dissolving factors (such as plasminogen activator and antithrombin III) are normally decreased, resulting in a state of hypercoagulability. Therefore, there is an increased susceptibility to develop blood clots. If the woman has varicose veins or obesity or is on bed rest, her state of hypercoagulability places her at increased risk for thrombus formation. Complete bed rest is no longer recommended for any pregnant woman because of this increased risk. Blood vessel injury during Caesarean birth can also cause a thrombus.

Venous thromboembolism (VTE) is a disease that includes deep vein thrombosis (DVT) and pulmonary embolism (PE). VTE remains an important cause of maternal morbidity and mortality in Canada, with an overall incidence of DVT and PE of 12.1 per 10 000 and 5.4 per 10 000 pregnancies, respectively (Chan, Rey, Kent, et al., 2014).

Box 10.1 Risk Factors for Venous Thromboembolism

MATERNAL PREPREGNANCY RISK FACTORS
Body mass index (BMI) >30 kg/m^2 at first antenatal visit
Smoking more than 10 cigarettes per day
Maternal cardiac disease
System lupus erythematosus (SLE)
Sickle cell disease
Inflammatory bowel disease
Varicose veins

RISK FACTORS RELATED TO PRESENT PREGNANCY
Pre-eclampsia
Preterm birth
Intrauterine growth restriction (IUGR)
Gestational diabetes
Placenta previa
Stillbirth

RISK FACTORS RELATED TO BIRTH AND POSTPARTUM PERIOD
Emergency Caesarean birth
Any Caesarean birth
>1 L postpartum hemorrhage or transfusion postpartum

COMBINED RISK FACTORS
Pre-eclampsia + IUGR

Source: Chan, W., Rey, E., Kent, N. E., et al. (2014). SOGC clinical practice guideline: Venous thromboembolism and antithrombotic therapy in pregnancy. *Journal of Obstetrics & Gynaecology Canada*, *36*(6), 527–553.

Clinical traits of DVT and PE are as follows:

1. DVT can involve veins from the feet to the femoral area and is characterized by pain, calf tenderness, leg edema, colour changes, and pain when walking. An increase in leg circumference greater than 2 cm accompanied by redness, tenderness, and edema should be promptly reported. Diagnosis is confirmed via ultrasound with or without a Doppler (Chan et al., 2015).
2. PE occurs when the pulmonary artery is obstructed by a blood clot that breaks off (embolizes) and lodges in the lungs. It may have dramatic signs and symptoms, such as sudden chest pain, cough, dyspnea (difficulty breathing), decreased level of consciousness, and signs of heart failure. A small PE may have nonspecific signs and symptoms, such as shortness of breath, palpitations, hemoptysis (bloody sputum), faintness, and low-grade fever. *A PE is a medical emergency.*

Preventive measures include use of pneumatic compression devices on the lower extremities and prophylactic heparin. Risk factors for postpartum VTE are listed in Box 10.1. The level of preventative measures should be considered on an individual basis to determine whether pharmacological intervention is required (Chan et al., 2014).

Treatment

DVT is treated with administration of analgesics, local application of heat, and elevation of the legs to promote venous drainage, and the addition of subcutaneous or IV anticoagulation medications such as heparin or warfarin (Coumadin). Warfarin can only be used in the postpartum period due to the transmission across the placenta to the fetus during pregnancy. Low-molecular-weight heparin (LMWH) may be used because it is long-acting and requires less frequent doses and laboratory testing. LMWH anticoagulants are contraindicated with regional anaesthesia.

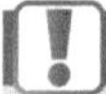
Medication Safety Alert!

The antidote for a warfarin overdose is vitamin K.

Nursing Care

The woman should be observed before and after birth for signs and symptoms that suggest venous thrombosis. Dyspnea, coughing, and chest pain suggest PE and must be reported immediately.

Prevention of thrombi is most important. Pregnant women should be encouraged not to cross their legs because this impedes venous blood flow. When the legs are elevated, there should not be a sharp flexion at the groin or pressure in the popliteal space behind the knee, which would restrict venous flow. Measures to promote venous flow should be continued during and after birth because levels of clotting factors remain high for several weeks.

Early ambulation is valuable in preventing thrombus formation in the postpartum woman. Antiembolic stockings may be used if varicose veins are present. The nurse should teach the woman how to put on the stockings properly because rolling or kinking of the stocking can further impede blood flow. If stirrups are used during birth or episiotomy repair, they should be padded to prevent pressure at the popliteal angle.

The woman who will be undergoing anticoagulant therapy at home should be taught how to give herself the medication and about signs of excess anticoagulation (prolonged bleeding from minor injuries, bleeding gums, nosebleeds, unexplained bruising). She should use a soft toothbrush and avoid minor trauma that can cause prolonged bleeding or a large hematoma.

INFECTION

PUERPERAL SEPSIS

Puerperal sepsis is an infection or septicemia after childbirth and is the sixth leading cause of maternal mortality in Canada (Public Health Agency of Canada [PHAC], 2013). Tissue trauma during labour, the open wound of the placental insertion site, prolonged ruptured membranes, surgical incisions, cracks in the nipples of the breasts, and increased pH of the vagina after birth are all risk factors for the postpartum woman. Inflammation of the inner lining of the uterus is called **endometritis**. The danger of postpartum infection is that a localized infection of the perineum, vagina, or cervix can ascend the reproductive tract and spread to the uterus, fallopian tubes, and peritoneum, causing peritonitis, which is a life-threatening condition. Table 10.2 lists characteristics, medical treatment, and nursing care for these infections. Regardless of their location or the causative organism, postpartum infections have several common features.

Manifestations

Puerperal (postpartum) fever is defined as a temperature of 38°C (100.4°F) or higher after the first 24 hours and for at least 2 days during the first 10 days after birth. Slight temperature elevations with no other signs of infection often occur during the first 24 hours because of dehydration. The nurse should look for other signs of infection if the woman's temperature is elevated, regardless of the time since birth. A pulse rate that is higher than expected and an elevated temperature often occur when the woman has an infection. Other signs and symptoms of infection may be localized (in a small area of the body) or systemic (throughout the body). The assessment of any Caesarean section wound, episiotomy wound, using the REEDA mnemonic R (redness), E (**e**dema), E (**e**cchymosis), D (**d**ischarge), A (**a**pproximation), or hardening of the operative area should be promptly reported and documented. Fever, pain, foul odour, or abnormal findings on routine postpartum assessment must be reported to the health care provider.

White blood cells (leukocytes) are normally elevated during the early postpartum period to about 20 to 25 × 10^9/L, which limits the usefulness of the blood count to identify infection. Blood culture samples are a more accurate form of identifying infection. Leukocyte counts in the upper limits are more likely to be associated with infection than lower counts.

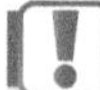
Safety Alert!

Proper hand hygiene is the primary method to prevent the spread of infectious organisms. Gloves should be worn when in contact with any blood or body fluid or any other potentially infectious materials.

Treatment

The goals of medical treatment are to limit the spread of infection, to prevent it from reaching the blood and other organs, and to eliminate the infection. A culture and sensitivity sample from the suspected site of infection is taken to determine the antibiotics that will be most effective. IV antibiotics will be ordered and the woman may be placed on bed rest.

Nursing Care

Nursing care objectives focus on preventing infection. If an infection occurs the focus is on facilitating medical treatment. To achieve these goals, the nurse should do the following:

- Use and teach hygienic measures to reduce the number of organisms that can cause infection (e.g., hand hygiene, perineal care), including teaching hand hygiene to the patient and visitors.

Table 10.2 Postpartum Infections

WOUND INFECTIONS	ENDOMETRITIS (UTERUS)	URINARY TRACT INFECTIONS	MASTITIS (BREAST)
Characteristics			
Signs of inflammation (redness, edema, heat, pain) Separation of suture line Purulent drainage	Tender, enlarged uterus Prolonged, severe cramping Foul-smelling lochia Fever and other systemic signs of infection Signs of uterine subinvolution	Cystitis (bladder) Low-grade fever Burning, urgency, and frequency of urination Pyelonephritis (kidneys) High fever with pattern of spikes Chills Pain in costovertebral angle or flank Nausea and vomiting	Reddened, tender, hot area of breast Edema and feeling of heaviness in breast Purulent drainage (may occur if an abscess forms)
Medical Management			
Culture and sensitivity of wound exudate Antibiotics	Culture and sensitivity test of cervix Antibiotics by intravenous (IV) route initially	Clean-catch or catheterized urine specimen for culture and sensitivity testing Antibiotics (initially by IV route for pyelonephritis)	Antibiotics (usually oral, although may be IV initially if woman has abscess) Incision and drainage of abscess
Nursing Care			
Use aseptic or sterile technique for all wound care as indicated. Teach proper perineal hygiene to reduce fecal contamination.	Teach woman the usual progression of lochia, because infection often occurs after discharge. Use Fowler's position to facilitate drainage of infected lochia. Administer analgesics. Observe for absent bowel sounds, abdominal distention, and nausea or vomiting, which suggest spread of infection.	Teach perineal hygiene. Encourage fluid intake of 3 L/day. Teach which foods increase acidity of urine, such as apricots, cranberry juice, plums, and prunes.	Teach effective breastfeeding techniques. Encourage moist heat applications. Use warm shower before nursing to start milk flow. Massage affected area to reduce congestion and start milk flow. Encourage regular and frequent nursing or pumping to keep breasts empty.

- Promote adequate nutrition for healing.
- Observe for signs of infection.
- Teach signs of infection that the woman should report after discharge.
- Teach the woman to take all of the antibiotics prescribed rather than stopping them after her symptoms are eliminated.
- Teach the woman how to apply perineal pads (front to back).

Women should be taught to perform hand hygiene before and after performing self-care that may involve contact with secretions. The nurse should explore ways to help the woman get enough rest.

Ultimately, a woman's own body must overcome infection and heal any wound. Nutrition is an essential component of her body defenses. The nurse, should teach her about foods that are high in protein (meats, cheese, milk, legumes) and vitamin C (citrus fruits and juices, strawberries, cantaloupe) because these nutrients are especially important for healing. Foods high in iron to correct anemia include meats, enriched cereals and breads, and dark green, leafy vegetables.

MASTITIS AND BREASTFEEDING

Mastitis is an infection of the breast. It usually occurs about 2 or 3 weeks after giving birth (Fig. 10.2). Mastitis occurs when organisms from the skin or the infant's mouth enter small cracks in the nipples or areolae. These cracks may be microscopic. Mastitis usually involves only one breast.

Signs and symptoms of mastitis include the following:

- Redness and warmth in the breast
- Tenderness
- Edema and a heaviness in the breast
- Purulent drainage (may or may not be present)

The woman usually has fever, chills, and other systemic signs and symptoms. If not treated, the infected area becomes encapsulated (walled off) and an abscess forms. The infection is usually outside the ducts of the breast, and the milk is not contaminated.

Treatment

Antibiotics and the continued removal of milk from the breast are the primary treatments for mastitis. Mild

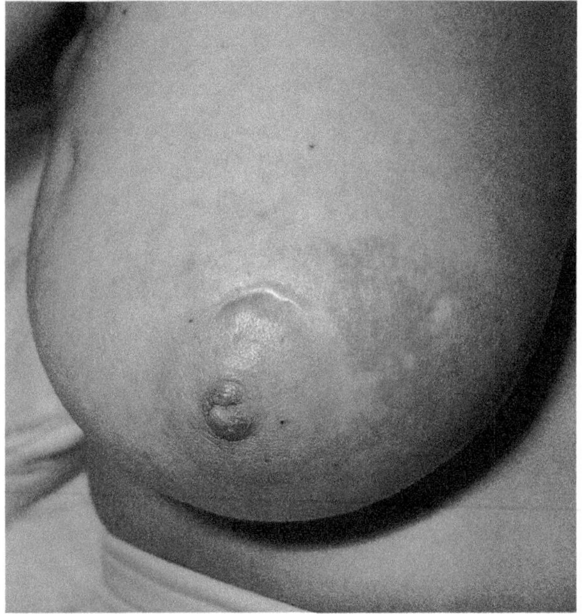

Fig. 10.2 Mastitis typically occurs several weeks after birth in the woman who is breastfeeding. Bacteria usually enter the breast through small cracks in the nipples. Breast engorgement and milk stasis increase the risk for mastitis. (From Swartz, M. H. [2009]. *Textbook of physical diagnosis: History and examination* [6th ed.]. Philadelphia: Saunders.)

analgesics make the woman more comfortable. The woman may need an incision and drainage of the infected area and IV antibiotics if an abscess forms. The mother is encouraged to continue to breastfeed. If she should stop nursing for any reason, she should pump her breasts. She should not wean her infant when she has mastitis because weaning leads to engorgement and stasis of milk, which will increase her discomfort.

Nursing Care

The breastfeeding mother should be taught proper breastfeeding techniques to reduce the risk for mastitis (see Chapter 9). Nursing care for mastitis centres on relieving pain and on maintaining lactation. Heat promotes blood flow to the area and enhances comfort. Moist heat can be applied with chemical packs. Placing a warm, wet cloth in a plastic bag and applying it to the breasts can create an inexpensive warm pack. A warm shower provides warmth and cleanliness and stimulates the flow of milk if taken just before breastfeeding.

Patient Teaching

Mastitis

- Perform thorough hand hygiene before breastfeeding.
- Wash breasts with water only (no soap) to avoid drying.
- Keep nipples dry and expose to air when possible.
- Ensure correct newborn latch-on and removal from breast.
- Frequently breastfeed to encourage milk flow.
- If an area of the breast is distended or tender, breastfeed from the uninfected side *first* at each feeding (to initiate let-down reflex in the affected breast).
- Massage distended area as the newborn nurses.
- Report redness and fever to the health care provider.
- Apply ice packs or moist heat to relieve discomfort.

If the affected breast is too painful for the mother to breastfeed, she can use a breast pump to empty it (see Chapter 9). She can massage the area of inflammation to improve milk flow. Breastfeeding first on the unaffected side starts the milk flow in both breasts and can improve emptying with less pain. Other nursing measures include the following:

- Encouraging fluid intake
- Advising the woman to wear a good supportive bra to support the breasts and limit movement of the painful breast
- Supporting the woman emotionally and reassuring her that she can continue to breastfeed

PERINATAL MOOD DISORDERS

Perinatal mood disorders (PMD) were previously known as *postpartum depression* or *postpartum mood disorders*. It has been found that many women develop these symptoms during pregnancy so the term *perinatal* rather than *postpartum* identifies this as more than just a postpartum concern. A PMD can be evidenced by depression, anxiety, or psychosis so the term *mood disorder* is more inclusive. Postpartum blues or "baby blues" are not part of PMD, as this is normal to occur after birth (see Chapter 9 for further discussion). The woman has periods when she feels let down, but overall, she finds pleasure in life and in her new role as mother. *Postpartum blues* occurs in about 50 to 80% of women, appearing shortly after birth and usually disappearing by day 14 (Registered Nurses' Association of Ontario [RNAO], 2018). Her roller-coaster emotions are usually self-limiting as she adapts to the changes in her life. The changes in emotions may be due to the rapid decrease in estrogen and progesterone levels following childbirth (RNAO, 2018).

Perinatal anxiety, depression, and psychosis are disorders that are not normal and are more serious than postpartum blues. Many women feel especially guilty about having depressive feelings at a time when they believe they should be happy. They may be reluctant to discuss their symptoms or their negative feelings toward the infant (Andrews, 2017). There is also stigma surrounding mental illness, which causes women to keep their feelings to themselves. Women with current depression or anxiety, a history of PMD, or risk factors for PMD warrant particularly close monitoring, evaluation, and assessment (ACOG, 2015).

PERINATAL ANXIETY

Anxiety and insomnia are common forms of PMD. Anxiety disorders include generalized anxiety disorder, obsessive-compulsive disorder, panic disorder and panic attacks, specific phobias, social anxiety disorder, and post-traumatic stress disorder. Common characteristics of these disorders are irrational fear, worry, and tension; physical symptoms such as trembling, nausea and vomiting, dizziness, dyspnea, and insomnia are often seen (Andrews, 2017). Asking a

Box 10.2 Risk Factors for Perinatal Depression

STRONG RISK FACTORS
- Previous history of mental health concerns
- Prenatal symptoms of anxiety or depression

MODERATE RISK FACTORS
- Stressful life events
- Newly moved to Canada
- Low social support
- History of physical or sexual abuse
- Victim of intimate partner violence
- Grief from miscarriage, stillbirth, or infant loss
- Substance use, including tobacco

WEAK RISK FACTORS
- Low socioeconomic status
- Lone parent
- Unplanned or unwanted pregnancy
- Breastfeeding challenges; lack of social support or health care provider's support

Adapted from Registered Nurses Association of Ontario. (2018). *Assessment and interventions for perinatal depression* (2nd ed.). Toronto, ON: Author. Retrieved from https://rnao.ca/sites/rnao-ca/files/bpg/Perinatal_Depression_FINAL_web_0.pdf.

woman whether she is having intrusive or frightening thoughts or is unable to sleep even when her infant is sleeping can be helpful in diagnosing these disorders.

PERINATAL DEPRESSION

Perinatal depression is a depressive illness that usually manifests within 2 to 4 weeks after birth, although it can occur during pregnancy. The onset of depression during this time may interfere with the mother's ability to respond to her infant's cues and interferes with the developing maternal–infant bonding. ACOG (2015) recommends that women be screened at least once during the perinatal period for depression and anxiety symptoms. Also, routine prenatal visits during the perinatal period are important opportunities to identify any woman at risk. Although formal postpartum screening for depression is not standard practice in Canada, the RNAO (2018) states that all women should be routinely screened with a valid tool such as the Edinburgh Postnatal Depression Scale (EPDS) (see RNAO link for EPDS in Online Resources). If the woman screens positive for depression, she should be referred to the appropriate resource for counselling and treatment.

Risk factors for perinatal depression are listed in Box 10.2. Those having close contact with the woman often notice the depression first. Signs and symptoms may include the following:
- Lack of enjoyment in life
- Disinterest in others; loss of normal give-and-take in relationships
- Intense feelings of inadequacy, unworthiness, guilt, inability to cope
- Loss of mental concentration; inability to make decisions
- Disturbed sleep or appetite
- Constant fatigue and feelings of ill health
- Crying—difficulty managing activities of daily living

Perinatal depression strains the coping mechanisms of the entire family at a time when all are adapting to the birth of a child. As a result of the strained relationships, communication is often impaired, and the depressed woman may withdraw further, which distances her even further from her support system. The nurse should observe for signs and symptoms during clinic visits and in the postpartum period and screen if required.

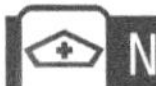 **Nursing Tip**

If a postpartum woman seems depressed, the nurse should not assume that she has the common "baby blues" or that she will "snap out of it." She should be assessed with a valid perinatal depression screening tool.

Treatment

A combination of psychotherapy and antidepressants is often the course of therapy on an outpatient basis. For the breastfeeding mother there are medications that are safe to take while breastfeeding; this requires consultation with her health care provider. The nurse should provide support, observe the woman's behaviour, and be alert to the possibility of self-harm by the woman. The woman should be informed about self-care strategies that may be effective methods to decrease PPD. These methods include time for self, exercise, relaxation, and ensuring adequate sleep (RNAO, 2018). Herbs, dietary supplements, massage, aromatherapy, and acupuncture are complementary and alternative health modalities (CAHM) that may help in the management of perinatal depression, although research on effectiveness is lacking for some of these strategies. Persons with PPD symptoms need and benefit from social support from partners, family members, and social networks (e.g., friends, community partners, or work colleagues) where appropriate. This type of support has been shown to improve a person's ability to cope with their depression symptoms (RNAO, 2018). Peer support can be in person, via telephone, or online. Through interaction with peers who share similar experiences of PPD women can gain knowledge and lessen feelings of hopefulness regarding overcoming the depression symptoms (RNAO, 2018). Referral for follow-up to available community mental health support services and facilities is a nursing responsibility to ensure ongoing care and support. Counselling should include the woman's partner and family.

PERINATAL PSYCHOSIS

Women experiencing a perinatal **psychosis** have an impaired sense of reality. Psychosis is quite rare, occurring in 0.1 to 0.5% of postpartum women (RNAO, 2018). The onset of psychosis is usually rapid, with symptoms presenting as early as the first 48 to 72 hours postpartum, and the majority of episodes develop within the first 2 weeks postpartum. The symptoms are typically depressed or elated mood (which can fluctuate rapidly), disorganized behaviour, mood lability, delusions, and hallucinations (RNAO, 2018). Postpartum psychosis is most commonly associated with the diagnosis of bipolar (or manic-depressive) disorder (Andrews, 2017).

Perinatal psychosis can be fatal for both the mother and infant, especially if she is having delusions or suicidal thoughts. Postpartum psychosis carries a relatively good prognosis with early detection and aggressive treatment. Women with acute postpartum psychosis need to be treated as a medical emergency and are cared for in an inpatient psychiatric treatment centre until symptoms have stabilized.

NURSING CARE

Nursing care for PMDs involves educating all women and their partners and families about the symptoms of PMDs, when they should seek help, and appropriate resources. If women and families have the correct knowledge they may feel more empowered to seek help when needed. It is important that women and their partners know the symptoms of PMDs, as they often occur when the woman has been discharged and may not understand what is happening. Seeking treatment is important for the health of the mother, baby, and family. Families need to be aware of this, as it can encourage follow-up care and reduce stigma in the family.

Women who develop a PMD along with their families, need reassurance that it is not their fault and that there are resources and supports to help them. The key to providing appropriate nursing care is screening women for PMD, as they may not openly admit the feelings they are having. Women who are at higher risk for developing a PMD should be referred for follow-up care when they are discharged from the hospital.

Unfolding Case Study

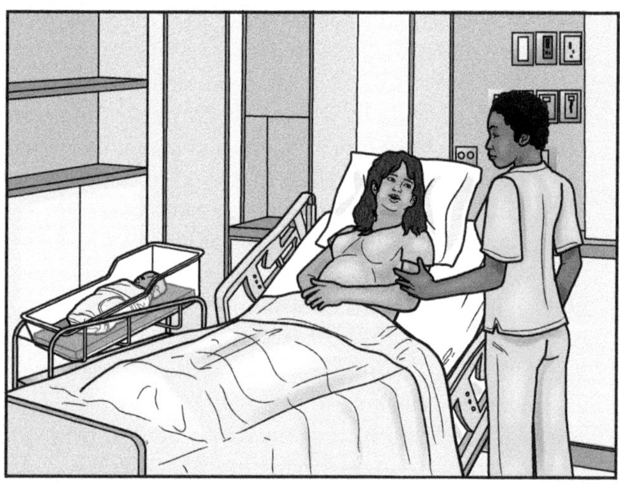

Tess and Luis were introduced to the reader in Chapter 2, and Tess's pregnancy experience has unfolded in each chapter. Tess has given birth to twins and has been transferred to the postpartum unit with one twin infant, while her partner, Luis, stays with the other twin infant in the NICU.

Tess has been resting in the postpartum unit for 4 hours with the infant at her bedside. She states that she is worried that her lochia is heavy and still red, and she believes she may be bleeding too heavily. She has not ambulated at all, because she says she is too tired.

QUESTIONS

1. What factors during birth may contribute to postpartum hemorrhage for Tess?
2. What assessments would the nurse make to determine if her lochia is excessive?
3. Since Tess has not yet ambulated to the bathroom, what safety precautions need to be initiated for Tess?
4. What safety precautions need to be initiated for the baby?
5. What teaching would the nurse offer?

Get Ready for the Certification Examination!

Key Points

- The nurse must be aware of women who are at higher risk for postpartum hemorrhage and assess them more often.
- The risk factors for postpartum hemorrhage include the four T's: tone, trauma, tissue, and thrombin.
- A constant small trickle of blood can result in significant blood loss, as can a larger one-time hemorrhage.
- Pain that is persistent and more severe than expected is characteristic of a hematoma in the reproductive tract.
- It is essential to identify and limit a local infection before it spreads to the blood or other organs.
- The nurse should teach new mothers about normal postpartum changes and indications of problems that should be reported.
- Early ambulation can prevent thrombosis formation.

- Careful assessment and listening can help the nurse identify a new mother who has a perinatal mood disorder (PMD).
- Women and their families require education about PMDs, including the symptoms and when it is important to seek help.
- Perinatal psychosis is a serious disorder that is potentially life-threatening to the woman and others, including her infant.

Additional Learning Resources

evolve Go to your Evolve website (http://evolve.elsevier.com/Canada/Leifer) for the following learning resources:

- Answer Key for Critical Thinking Questions
- Answer Key for Textbook Review Questions
- Audio Glossary
- Fluids & Electrolytes tutorial
- Interactive Review Questions
- Skills Performance Checklists
- Video clips and more!

Online Resource

- Registered Nurses' Association of Ontario, *Assessment and Interventions for Perinatal Depression* (2nd ed.): https://rnao.ca/sites/rnao-ca/files/bpg/Perinatal_Depression_REVISED_web_final.pdf

Review Questions

1. Which early sign of postpartum hypovolemic shock would a nurse assess first?
   a. Low blood pressure.
   b. Rapid pulse rate.
   c. Pale skin colour.
   d. Soft uterus.

2. Which of the following signs would most likely indicate a bleeding laceration?
   a. A soft uterus that is difficult to locate.
   b. Low pulse rate and blood pressure.
   c. Bright red bleeding and a firm uterus.
   d. Profuse dark red bleeding and large clots.

3. A nurse assessing the white blood cell (leukocyte) count during the postpartum period should find which of the following?
   a. Higher than normal.
   b. Lower than normal.
   c. Unchanged.
   d. Unimportant.

4. A postpartum mother who is breastfeeding has developed mastitis. She states that she does not think it is good for her infant to drink milk from her infected breast. Which one of the following topics should a nurse providing teaching to the mother include?
   a. Breastfeed the infant from only the unaffected breast until the infection clears up.
   b. Discontinue breastfeeding and start the infant on formula.
   c. Continue breastfeeding the infant.
   d. Apply a tight breast binder to the infected breast until the infection subsides.

5. A woman has given birth to a newborn several hours previously, and her uterus is boggy. Which medications should a nurse anticipate that the health care provider may prescribe to increase uterine tone and firm the uterus? *(Select all that apply.)*
   a. Methylergonovine
   b. Hemabate
   c. Magnesium sulphate
   d. Oxytocin

6. A nurse should be alert to subinvolution of the uterus as a cause of late postpartum bleeding. The nurse would report and document which of the following signs? *(Select all that apply).*
   a. Fundal height higher than expected for date
   b. Persistence of lochia rubra
   c. Low blood pressure
   d. Persistence of lochia alba

REFERENCES

American College of Obstetricians and Gynecologists (ACOG). (2015). Screening for perinatal depression. Committee Opinion No. 630. American College of Obstetricians and Gynecologists. *Obstetrics & Gynecology, 125*, 1268–1271.

American College of Obstetricians and Gynecologists (ACOG). (2017). *ACOG expands recommendations to treat postpartum hemorrhage*. Retrieved from: https://www.acog.org/About-ACOG/News-Room/News-Releases/2017/ACOG-Expands-Recommendations-to-Treat-Postpartum-Hemorrhage.

Andrews, J. (2017). Postpartum complications. In S. Perry, M. Hockenberry, D. Lowdermilk, et al. (Eds.), *Maternal child nursing care in Canada* (2nd ed.). Toronto, ON: Elsevier.

Chan, W., Rey, E., Kent, N. E., et al. (2014). SOGC clinical practice guideline: Venous thromboembolism and antithrombotic therapy in pregnancy. *Journal of Obstetrics & Gynaecology Canada, 36*(6), 527–553.

Evensen, A., Anderson, J. M., & Fontaine, P. (2017). Postpartum hemorrhage: Prevention and treatment. *American Family Physician, 95*(7), 442–449.

Novikova, N., Hofmeyr, G. J., & Cluver, C. (2015). Tranexamic acid for preventing postpartum haemorrhage. *Cochrane Database of Systematic Reviews*, (6), CD007872. https://doi.org/10.1002/14651858.CD007872.pub3.

Public Health Agency of Canada (PHAC). (2013). *Maternal mortality in Canada*. Ottawa: Author. Cat.: HP32-7/2011E-PDF.

Registered Nurses' Association of Ontario (RNAO). (2018). *Assessment and interventions for perinatal depression* (2nd ed.). Toronto, ON: Author. Retrieved from: https://rnao.ca/sites/rnao-ca/files/bpg/Perinatal_Depression_REVISED_web_final.pdf.

Society of Obstetricians and Gynaecologists of Canada. (2014). *Advances in labour and risk management (ALARM) course syllabus* (21st ed.). Ottawa, ON: Author.

WOMAN Trial Collaborators. (2017). Effect of early tranexamic acid administration on mortality, hysterectomy, and other morbidities in women with post-partum haemorrhage (WOMAN): An international, randomised, double-blind, placebo-controlled trial. *The Lancet, 389*(10084), 2105–2116. https://doi.org/10.1016/S0140-6736(17)30638-4.

The Term Newborn

11

Lisa Keenan-Lindsay

http://evolve.elsevier.com/Canada/Leifer

Objectives

1. Define each key term listed.
2. Describe the initial assessment of the normal newborn.
3. Describe three normal reflexes of the newborn, including the approximate age of their disappearance.
4. State methods of newborn pain management.
5. Demonstrate the details of physical assessment of the newborn.
6. Describe the nursing care that would be provided to a newborn.
7. State four methods of maintaining the body temperature of a newborn.
8. Define the following skin manifestations in the newborn: lanugo, vernix caseosa, Mongolian spots, milia, acrocyanosis, and desquamation.
9. State the cause and describe the appearance of physiological jaundice in the newborn.
10. State the methods of preventing infection in newborns.
11. State the ways to prevent occurrence of sudden infant death syndrome (SIDS).
12. Review appropriate discharge teaching regarding newborn care.

Key Terms

acrocyanosis (ăk-rō-sī-ă-NŌ-sĭs)
attachment
bonding
caput succedaneum (KĂP-ŭt sŭk-sĕ-DĀ-nē-ŭm)
cephalohematoma (sĕf-ă-lō-hē-mă-TŌ-mă)
circumcision (sŭr-kŭm-SĬZH-ŭn)
cold stress
Epstein pearls
fontanelles (fŏn-tă-NĔLZ)
head lag
lanugo (lă-NŪ-gō)
meconium (mĕ-KŌ-nē-ŭm)
milia (MĬL-ē-ă)
Mongolian spots
Moro reflex
moulding
physiological jaundice
rooting reflex
scarf sign
sutures
tissue turgor
tonic neck reflex
vernix caseosa (VŪR-nĭks kā-sē-Ō-să)
walking reflex

ADJUSTMENT TO EXTRAUTERINE LIFE

Initial care of the newborn is discussed in Chapter 6. This chapter focuses on care of the newborn beyond the period immediately after birth. The arrival of the newborn begins a transition period during which many psychological and physiological adjustments to life outside the uterus must be made. The *transition period* is the first 6 to 8 hours following birth in which the child is making the adaptation to extrauterine life. The stages of the transition period are as follows:

First period of reactivity. The first 30 to 60 minutes of life is the best time to initiate breastfeeding and bonding between parents and the newborn. Often seen during this period are the following:

- Tachycardia, gradually lowering to a normal rate within 30 to 60 minutes
- Irregular respirations
- Crackles may be present on auscultation
- Newborn is alert; frequent Moro (startle reaction) reflex, tremors, crying, increased motor activity (often due to response to light)
- Hypoactive bowel sounds
- Sucking reflex is present

Period of decreased responsiveness (1 to 3 hours after birth). The infant either sleeps or becomes less active, and the following may occur:

- Decreased motor activity
- Respirations up to 60 breaths/min
- Normal heart rate for term newborn
- Audible bowel sounds

Second period of reactivity. After a deep sleep, the infant again becomes responsive and alert between 3 and 8 hours after birth, along with the following:

- Abrupt, brief changes in colour and muscle tone
- Increased respiratory (tachypnea) and heart rate (tachycardia) are normal

- Presence of oral mucus (can cause gagging)
- Responsiveness to external stimuli
- Often passage of meconium

The infant's genetic background, the health of the mother during pregnancy, and what happens during the birth contribute to this adjustment to extrauterine life. When a child is born, an orderly, continuous adaptation from fetal life to extrauterine life takes place. All the body systems undergo some change. Respirations are stimulated by exposure to a cold environment and by chemical changes within the blood. Sensory and physical stimuli also appear to play a role in respiratory function. The first breath opens the alveoli. The infant then breathes air independently rather than depending on the placenta for oxygen. This process also initiates cardiopulmonary interdependence. The newborn's ability to metabolize food is hampered by the immaturity of the digestive system, particularly because of deficiencies in enzymes from the pancreas and liver. The kidneys are structurally developed, but their ability to concentrate urine and maintain fluid balance is limited because of a decreased rate of glomerular flow and limited renal tubular reabsorption. Most neurological functions are primitive (see discussion of the individual body systems in this chapter).

ADMISSION ASSESSMENT

If the newborn is stable, the infant usually remains undisturbed while they and the parents become acquainted. The nurse can usually assess temperature, heart rate, and respirations while the parents hold their newborn skin-to-skin. The nurse will complete a physical and gestational age assessment of the newborn within the first few hours but if the newborn is healthy skin-to-skin contact is more important in the initial period of life. The nurse can play a vital role in educating new parents about normal growth and development, health care and the developmental needs of their newborn while performing assessments and providing care.

Observing for Injuries or Anomalies

The nurse notes signs of injury or anomalies while performing an assessment. The newborn's movements and facial expression during crying are observed for symmetry and equality of movement. The head and face should be assessed for trauma, especially if forceps were used. A small puncture wound may be apparent on the scalp if an internal spiral electrode was used for fetal monitoring (see Chapter 6). If the newborn was born vaginally in a breech presentation, the buttocks may be bruised.

Many anomalies, such as spina bifida (open spine) or a cleft lip, are immediately obvious. The fingers and toes should be counted to identify abnormal numbers or webbing. The feet should be observed for straightness or to determine if deviated feet can be returned to the straight position. The length of arms and legs should also be checked for equality. Urination or meconium passage, which confirms patency, must also be noted.

SUPPORTING THERMOREGULATION

The normal temperature of the term newborn is between 36.5° and 37.5°C (97.7° and 99.5°F) (axillary). Maintenance of body temperature is very important to the newborn, who has an unstable heat-regulating system and is aided by the metabolism of brown adipose tissue (brown fat); this process is called *nonshivering thermogenesis*. Hypothermia (low body temperature) can lead to **cold stress** in the newborn, which is evident by the following:

- Hypoglycemia (low blood sugar), because the newborn uses glucose to generate heat
- Respiratory distress, because the higher metabolic rate consumes more oxygen, sometimes beyond the newborn's ability to supply it

Hypoglycemia can be both the cause and the result of hypothermia; therefore, the nurse must evaluate both factors. Respiratory distress can also require more glucose for the increased work of breathing, causing hypoglycemia.

Heat is lost by any of the following four means:

- *Evaporation* of liquids from the skin
- *Conduction* caused by direct skin contact with a cold surface
- *Convection* of heat away from the body by drafts
- *Radiation* caused by being near a cold surface, although not in direct contact with it

Conduction, convection, and radiation can also be used to add heat to the body. Newborns lose heat quickly after birth, because amniotic fluid evaporates from their body, drafts move heat away, and they may contact cold surfaces (Table 11.1).

The newborn should be dried after birth and placed skin-to-skin with the mother. If the mother is unable to receive the infant, the partner can also put the baby skin-to-skin. The first bath is delayed for at least 8 to 12 hours, although the World Health Organization (WHO) recommends waiting at least 24 hours, when the body temperature is stabilized at 36.5° to 37°C (97.7° to 99.5°F) (WHO, 2015).

The newborn's hands and feet are not used as guides to determine warmth because the infant's extremities are cooler than the rest of the body. *Acrocyanosis* (*acro*, "extremity," and *cyanosis*, "blue colour") is also evident because of sluggish peripheral circulation and this is normal for the first few weeks of life. The newborn cannot adapt well to changes in temperature.

Because the sweat glands do not function effectively during the neonatal period, the newborn infant is at risk for developing an elevated temperature if overdressed or if placed in an overheated environment. A red skin rash may develop in response to overheating. A quivering or shivering-like tremor of the chin may be noticed in the newborn, which is evidence of

Table 11.1 Nursing Interventions to Prevent Heat Loss in Newborns

MECHANISM OF HEAT LOSS	SOURCES OF HEAT LOSS	INTERVENTIONS
Evaporation (conversion from liquid to vapour)	Wet skin from amniotic fluid at birth evaporates from skin	Dry newborn quickly. Dry and cover head of newborn.
Conduction (transfer of heat to a cooler surface)	Cool surface of bed, scale, stethoscope	Prewarm radiant warmer and stethoscope before use. Place scale paper on scale, and place warm blanket on other surfaces.
Convection (loss of heat to surrounding cooler air)	Drafts from window, air conditioning, oxygen vents	Place crib away from windows and vents.
Radiation (loss of heat to surrounding cold environment)	Cold environment of walls, windows	Place crib away from cold walls. Keep room temperature warm.

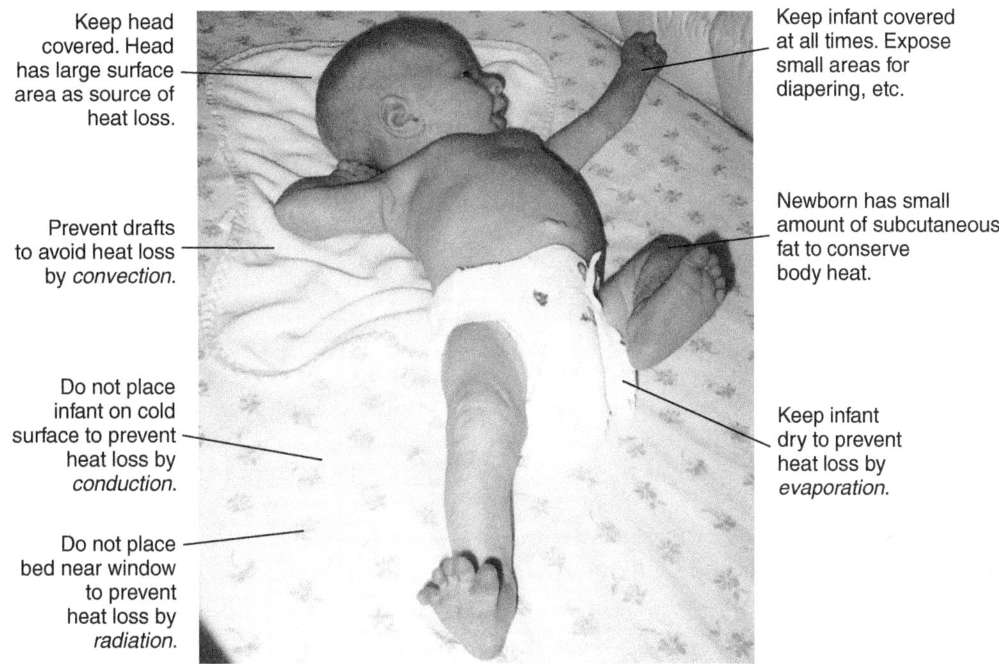
Keep head covered. Head has large surface area as source of heat loss.
Prevent drafts to avoid heat loss by *convection*.
Do not place infant on cold surface to prevent heat loss by *conduction*.
Do not place bed near window to prevent heat loss by *radiation*.
Keep infant covered at all times. Expose small areas for diapering, etc.
Newborn has small amount of subcutaneous fat to conserve body heat.
Keep infant dry to prevent heat loss by *evaporation*.

Fig. 11.1 Maintaining body temperature of the newborn. Chilling causes "cold stress"—an increased metabolism and oxygen consumption in the newborn—because the infant cannot shiver, as the adult can, to raise body temperature.

an immature neurological system, not an indication of response to a cold environment. Measures to take to maintain body temperature in the newborn are shown in Fig. 11.1.

EVALUATING GESTATIONAL AGE

A thorough gestational age assessment is done using a scale such as the Ballard form (see Chapter 12, Fig. 12.2). The nurse can do a quick assessment to evaluate whether the newborn seems to be of the appropriate gestational age. Characteristics to assess include the following:

- *Skin.* Is the skin thin and somewhat transparent (preterm) or peeling (post-term or possible intrauterine growth restriction [IUGR])?
- *Vernix.* Is this cheesy substance covering most of the skin surface (preterm), is it present only in skin creases (term), or is it absent (post-term)? Greenish vernix indicates that meconium was passed before birth, which may indicate that the newborn is post-term or had poor placental support.
- *Hair.* Is the skin heavily covered with fine lanugo hair (preterm), or is hair only in a few places (term)? Dark-skinned newborns often have more lanugo than light-skinned ones.
- *Ears.* When folded toward the lobe, do the ears spring back slowly (preterm) or quickly (term or post-term)?
- *Breast tissue.* Is there no or minimal breast tissue under the nipple (preterm), or is there a palpable mass of tissue 5 mm or more (term)? (A millimetre is about the thickness of a dime.)
- *Genitalia.* For males, is the scrotum smooth and small (preterm) or pendulous and covered with rugae or ridges (term)? For females, are the labia majora and labia minora of nearly equal size (preterm), or do the labia majora cover the labia minora (term)?

- *Sole creases.* Are the sole creases on the anterior third of the foot only (preterm), over the anterior two-thirds (term), or over the full foot (term or post-term)? Peeling skin may be obvious on the feet in post-term or IUGR newborns.

OBTAINING VITAL SIGNS

Observation of vital signs begins while parents and newborn are bonding and can be done while the newborn is skin-to-skin with a parent. They are measured at 15- to 30-minute intervals at first, then hourly, and every 4 to 8 hours after the newborn is stable.

With some minor alterations in vital signs the first intervention is often to put the newborn skin-to-skin with a parent. Vital signs may improve; if not, then further intervention may be necessary at that time. If significant distress or cyanosis is noted, the newborn requires more thorough interventions and skin-to-skin contact would not be appropriate.

Respiratory Rate

The normal respiratory rate for newborn infants is 30 to 60 breaths per minute. For best accuracy, the respiratory and heart rates are assessed before disturbing the newborn. The respirations are counted for 1 full minute. Newborn respirations are difficult to count because they are shallow and irregular. The rate can be auscultated by listening with a stethoscope. Placing a hand lightly over the abdomen or watching the abdomen rise and fall also helps to identify each breath. If the newborn is crying, a gloved finger to suck may quiet the infant so the respiratory rate can be counted accurately.

Further assessment is required in the following situations:

- Respirations greater than 60 breaths/min or less than 30 breaths/min
- Noisy (grunting) respirations
- Nasal flaring or chest retractions

A slight increase in respirations is normal during the transition of the newborn period. If no other signs of distress are evident, routine assessment is all that is necessary.

Nursing Tip

In the past, newborns were placed in a prone position to facilitate drainage of mucus. Because the prone position has been associated with sudden infant death syndrome (SIDS), it is recommended that newborns be placed on their back to sleep. It is important to teach all parents this information.

Heart Rate

The newborn's apical pulse rate is counted before the temperature is taken because the infant is apt to cry when disturbed. Fig. 11.2 illustrates the apical pulse rate being obtained from a newborn infant. The newborn's pulse is irregular and rapid and varies from 110 to 160 beats/min. A pediatric stethoscope is used, if possible, to limit extraneous noise. The nurse should count the heartbeat for 1 minute. If the child is in a deep sleep, the heart rate may be as low as 90 to 100 beats/min and if crying, the heart rate may be greater than 160 beats/min. These results should be reassessed within 30 minutes of initial assessment if all other vital signs are normal. A consistently low or high heart rate can indicate a pathological condition.

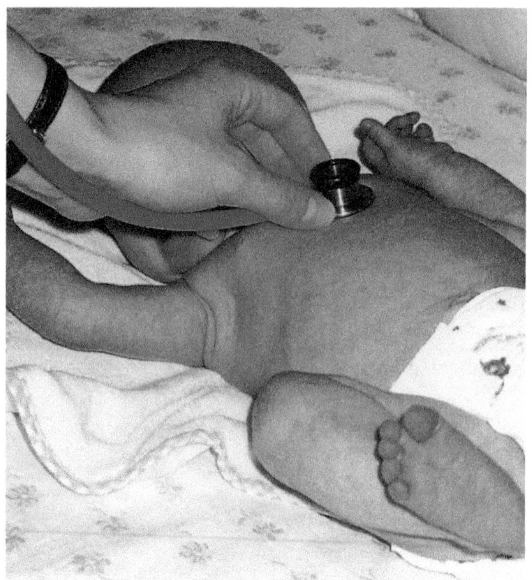

Fig. 11.2 Assessing an apical pulse. The most accurate method of assessing the heart rate in the newborn is by determining the apical pulse rate.

Temperature

An axillary temperature is commonly used for newborns, although a temporal artery thermometer has been used with success in some hospital settings. Normal temperature ranges from 36.5° to 37.5°C (97.7° to 99.5°F). The rectal temperature technique is no longer recommended because of the risk of injury (see Chapter 20 for temperature monitoring techniques). To obtain the axillary temperature, the thermometer is held firmly in the centre of the newborn's axilla. During this time, the arm is held against the infant's side. If the temperature is below 36.5 or greater than 37.5°C the newborn should be placed skin-to-skin and reassessed within 30 minutes. A persistently low temperature in a newborn can indicate infection.

Blood Pressure

A healthy newborn's blood pressure is not normally assessed, but if required it is measured with an electronic instrument. If cardiovascular symptoms are present (tachycardia, central cyanosis, or murmur) a four-extremity blood pressure and preductal and postductal oxygen saturation levels may be taken (see Chapter 12). The normal range of blood pressure is between 65 and 95 mm Hg systolic over 30 to 60 mm Hg diastolic in term newborns (see Chapter 20 for blood pressure measurement techniques).

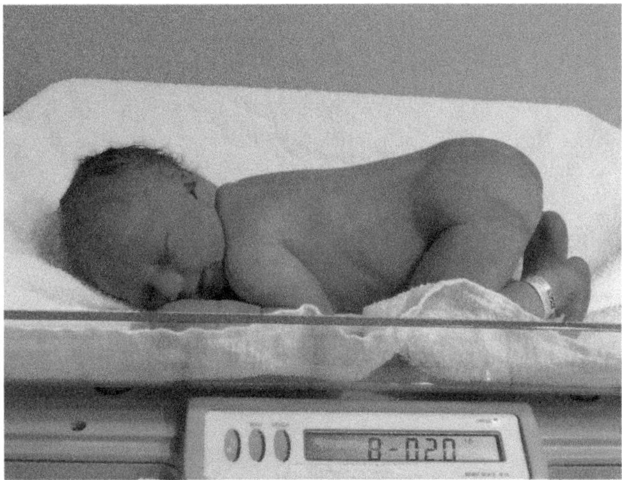

Fig. 11.3 Weighing the infant. The infant is placed prone on the scale, which is covered with a blanket. (Courtesy Lisa Keena-Lindsay).

Nursing Tip

When measuring blood pressure in the lower extremity, remember that the artery runs on the posterior aspect of the leg, so the cuff must be placed appropriately.

OBTAINING WEIGHT AND OTHER MEASUREMENTS

Weight

The newborn is usually weighed in the birthing room (Fig. 11.3). Disposable paper is put on the scale, and the scale is balanced to zero according to its model. The unclothed newborn is then placed on the scale. The nurse's hand should not touch the newborn but should be kept just above the infant to prevent falls.

The weight varies from 2 500 to 4 000 g. In general, girls weigh a little less than boys. In the first 3 to 4 days after birth, the infant may lose up to 7 to 10% of the birth weight. This may result from withdrawal from maternal hormones, fluid shifts, and the loss of feces and urine. Mothers should be prepared for this and reassured that this is normal and that the infant should regain birth weight by 14 days of age. Newborns are often only weighed prior to discharge. The following demonstrates how to determine percentage weight loss:

$$\frac{\text{Birth weight - current weight}}{\text{Birth weight}} \times 100 = \%\text{ weight loss}$$

If weight loss is more than 10%, the newborn feeding needs to be assessed more thoroughly (see Chapter 9).

Measurements

Length and head circumference are normally assessed. A disposable tape measure is used. To avoid giving a paper cut, the tape should not be pulled out from under the newborn. Measurements are noted in centimetres.

Length

There are several ways to measure the length of the newborn. Some facilities have a tape measure applied to the clear wall of a bassinet. The nurse places the newborn's head at one end, extends the leg, and notes where the heel ends. Another method is to lay the newborn down and to make a mark at the top of the head; the body and leg are extended, and a mark is made where the foot is located. Length is measured between the marks. Still another method involves placing the zero end of the tape at the newborn's head, extending the body and leg, and stretching the tape to the heel (see Chapter 13, Skill 13.1). The length of the average newborn is 45 to 55 cm.

Head circumference

The fullest part of the newborn's head is measured just above the eyebrows. Moulding of the head may affect the accuracy of the initial measurement. The average head circumference is 33 to 35 cm, although normal variations range from 32 to 36.8 cm (Skill 11.1).

ONGOING ASSESSMENT AND CARE OF THE NEWBORN

In this section, the ongoing assessments by body system and care of the healthy newborn are addressed. Newborns stay in the mother's room most of the time unless either mother or newborn has a problem that necessitates separation. Routine assessments and care provide an opportunity for the nurse to teach the parents normal newborn characteristics, signs of problems that should be reported, and how to provide care for the newborn. Involving the parents in care of their newborn helps them to learn most successfully. The nurse should praise the parent's efforts while providing education during provision of care.

If the newborn is breastfed, the nurse should discuss with the mother how well the newborn is nursing, the frequency and duration of the nursing sessions, and any difficulty she is having. If the newborn is fed formula, the mother should be asked how many millilitres the newborn has taken since the previous assessment. Newborn feeding is discussed more in depth in Chapter 9.

When observing the newborn, the nurse identifies expected normal findings as well as *variations* of normal and *deviations from* normal, which must be reported to the health care provider.

NERVOUS SYSTEM

Reflexes

The nervous system directs most of the body's activity. Newborns can move their arms and legs vigorously but cannot control them and at rest are normally well flexed. When the infant is lifted from the bed, the head will fall back, because the newborn cannot maintain neutral position of the head. This is called

Skill 11.1 Taking Head and Chest Measurements

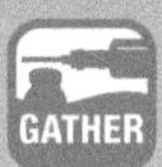
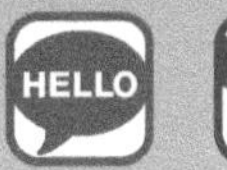

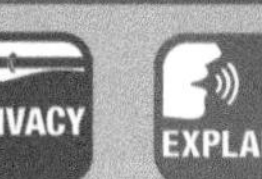

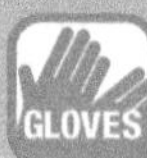

PURPOSE

To determine baseline measurements of the head and the chest

STEPS

1. The circumference of the head is measured from the top of the eyebrow to the widest part of the occiput.

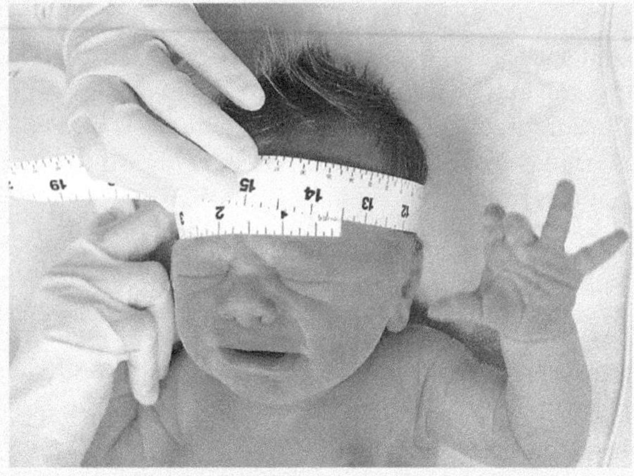

From Hockenberry, M. J., & Wilson, D. (2009). *Wong's essentials of pediatric nursing* (8th ed.). St. Louis: Mosby.

2. To obtain the size of the fontanelle, measure the widest point of the width and widest point of the length, add the measurements together, and divide by 2.

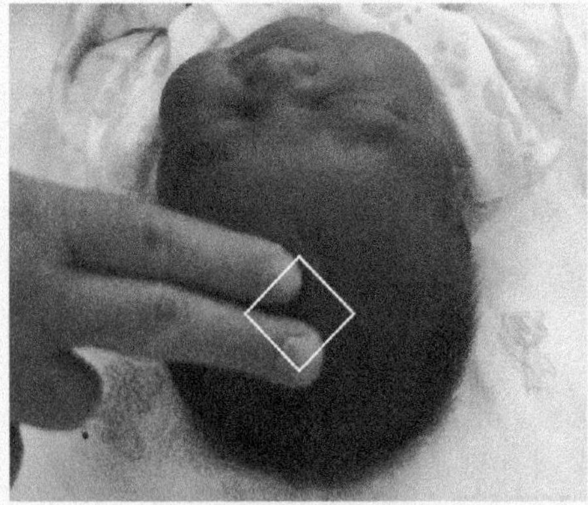

From Hockenberry, M. J., & Wilson, D. (2009). *Wong's essentials of pediatric nursing* (8th ed.). St. Louis: Mosby.

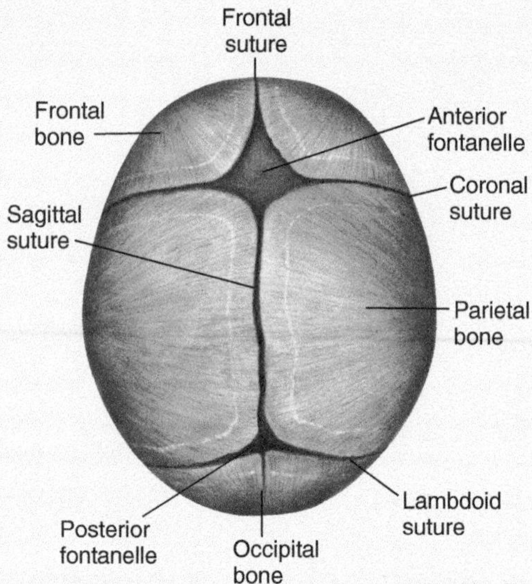

From Hockenberry, M. J., & Wilson, D. (2009). *Wong's essentials of pediatric nursing* (8th ed.). St. Louis: Mosby.

3. The normal anterior fontanelle in a newborn is approximately 3.6 to 6 cm. The fontanelles should appear flat with the contour of the skull. A bulging fontanelle may indicate increased intracranial pressure. A depressed fontanelle may indicate dehydration and should be reported to the health care provider.
4. When measuring the chest circumference, the measuring tape is placed at the nipple line.

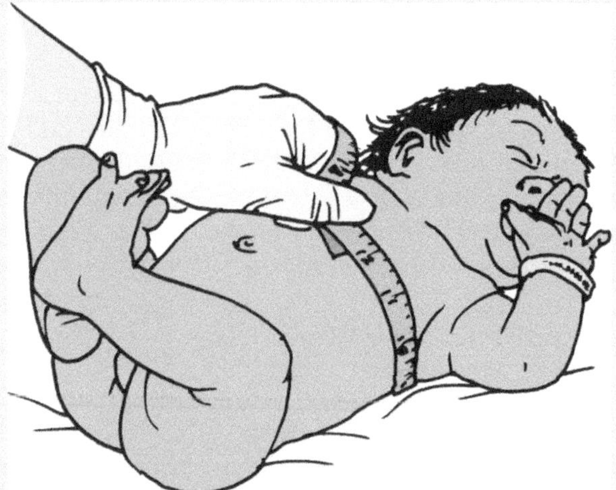

From Leifer, G. (2011). *Maternity nursing: an introductory text* (11th ed), Philadelphia: Elsevier/Saunders.

5. Lift the infant to remove the paper tape in order to prevent paper cuts to the infant's skin.
6. Document findings and report any abnormal measurements.

Note: The head circumference should be equal to and no more than 2 cm greater than the chest circumference until age 2. See normal growth charts to compare findings and to determine need for follow-up referral.

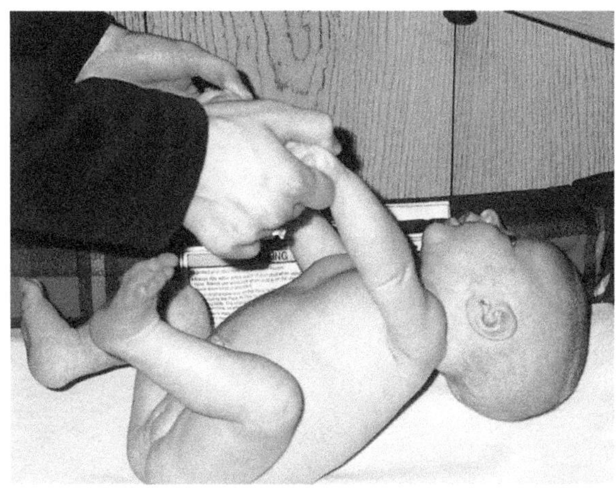

Fig. 11.4 Head lag. The newborn has some ability to control the head in some positions. When placed on the abdomen, the newborn may be able to raise the chin from the bed briefly. However, head lag and hyperextension normally occur when the newborn is raised from the bed in a supine position. Significant head lag after age 6 months indicates a need for follow-up care.

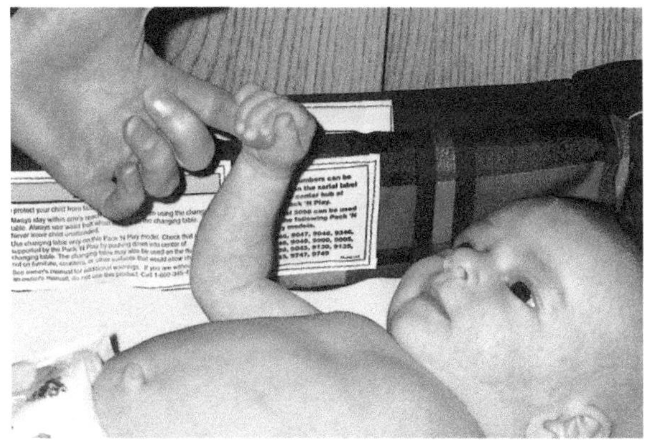

Fig. 11.5 Grasp reflex. Touching the hands near the base of the fingers causes a reflex flexion of the hands. This grasp reflex is replaced after age 3 months by a voluntary grasp.

head lag (Fig. 11.4). The reflexes that full-term infants are born with, such as blinking, sneezing, gagging, sucking, and grasping (Fig. 11.5), help to keep them alive. They can cry, swallow, and lift their heads slightly when lying on their abdomen.

If the newborn is startled by a loud noise or movement, they will draw their legs up and the arms fan out and then come toward midline in an embrace position. This is a normal response, called the Moro reflex (Fig. 11.6). Its absence may indicate abnormalities of the nervous system. The rooting reflex causes the infant's head to turn in the direction of anything that touches the cheek. The nurse uses this when helping a mother to breastfeed her infant. A breast touching the cheek causes the infant to turn toward it to find the nipple (see Chapter 9).

The tonic neck reflex is a postural reflex in which the head is turned to one side, the arm and leg are extended on the same side, and the opposite arm and leg are flexed in a "fencing" position. This reflex disappears by 3 to 4 months of life (Fig. 11.7). Stepping movements of the legs, seen when an infant is held upright on the examining table, are termed the *stepping* or walking

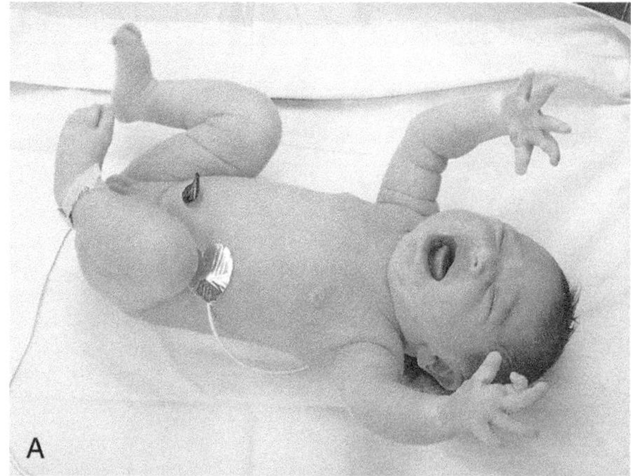

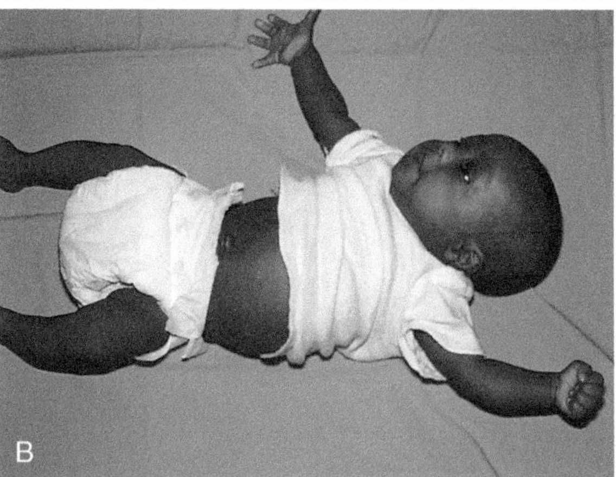

Fig. 11.6 **A,** Moro reflex. Sudden jarring causes extension and abduction (an embracing motion) of the extremities and spreading of the fingers, with the index finger and the thumb forming a *C* shape. A unilateral (one-sided) Moro reflex may indicate a fractured clavicle. Absence of the Moro reflex may indicate a pathological condition of the central nervous system. **B,** Abnormal Moro reflex. Note the clenched fist of one hand that does not follow a symmetrical embracing motion. This infant requires follow-up care. (**A,** from Murray, S. S., McKinney, E. S., & Gorrie, T. M. (2002). *Foundations of maternal-newborn nursing* (3rd ed.). Philadelphia: Saunders. **B,** from Zitelli, B. J., & Davis, H. W. (2012). *Zitelli and Davis' atlas of pediatric physical diagnosis* (6th ed.). St. Louis: Saunders.)

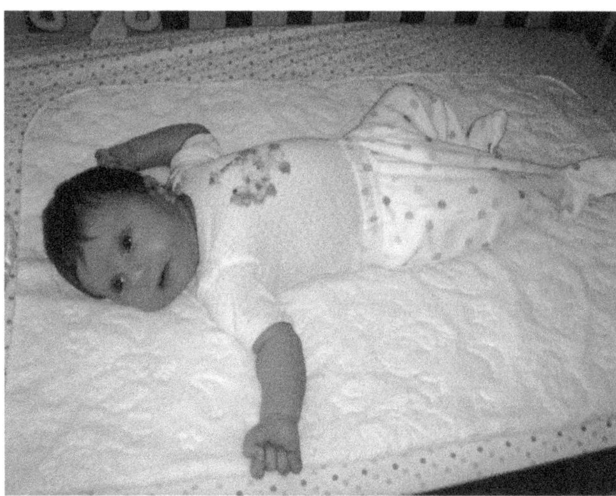

Fig. 11.7 Spontaneous tonic neck reflex. The infant turns the head to one side, and the arm and leg are extended on that side. The opposite arm and leg flex. Often called the "fencing" reflex.

Table 11.2 Ages of Appearance and Disappearance of Neurological Signs Unique to Infancy

RESPONSE	HOW TO ELICIT	AGE AT TIME OF APPEARANCE	AGE AT TIME OF DISAPPEARANCE
Reflexes of Position and Movement			
Moro reflex	A loud noise, bumping the surface of crib, or suddenly lowering the head while holding will cause the infant to symmetrically extend and abduct the arms and then adduct in an embracelike motion (see Fig. 11.6).	Birth	3–6 months
Tonic neck reflex	Turn infant's head to one side, and the arm and leg will extend on that side with flexion of the opposite arm and leg (see Fig. 11.7). (This is a postural reflex that is assumed by sleeping infants.)	Birth	Complete response disappears by 3–4 months
Palmar grasp reflex	Place object in hand of the newborn and newborn will grasp it tightly (plantar reflex involves curling of the toes when pressure is applied to the sole of the foot).	Birth	3–4 months for palmar grasp Plantar grasp lessens by 8 months
Babinski reflex	Stroke side of the foot: the big toe will dorsiflex, and the toes will flare out.	Birth	Variable, but before the infant begins walking†
Responses to Sound			
Blinking response	The infant will blink on hearing a loud noise.	Birth	NA
Turning response	The infant will turn their head toward the source of the noise.	Birth	NA
Reflexes of Vision			
Eye opening	Holding the newborn infant upright, under the arms, and tipping the infant forward will induce eye opening.	Birth	3 months
Blinking to threat	Bringing an object close to the eye at a fast pace will induce blinking.	6–7 months	NA
Horizontal following	Moving an object side to side within the infant's visual field will elicit this response.	4–6 weeks	NA
Vertical following	Moving a colourful object up and down within the visual field of the infant will induce this response.	2–3 months	NA
Eating Reflexes			
Rooting response	Infant's head turns in the direction of anything that touches the cheek in anticipation of food.	Birth	3–4 months
Sucking response	Infant will suck on a finger or nipple placed in the mouth.	Birth	7–12 months
Other Signs			
Stepping or "walking" reflex	Hold infant upright above a table: the infant will lift the foot up on contact with firm surface of the table.	Birth	2–3 weeks

NA, Not applicable. **Note:** Absence of these reflexes or prolonged appearance may indicate a neurological problem and requires further follow-up.
†Usually of no diagnostic significance until after age 2 years.

reflex. Table 11.2 lists the ages at which the neurological signs of infancy appear and disappear.

Head

The brain grows rapidly before birth, thus the newborn's head is large in comparison with the rest of the body. The head may be out of shape from moulding (the conforming of the fetal head to the size and shape of the birth canal) (Fig. 11.8, *A*). There may also be swelling of the soft tissues of the scalp, which is termed caput succedaneum. This swelling crosses the suture lines and gradually subsides without treatment within a few days. Occasionally, a cephalohematoma (*cephal,* "head," *hemato,* "blood," and *toma,* "tumour") protrudes from beneath the scalp (see Fig. 11.8, *B* and *C*). This condition is caused by a collection of blood beneath the periosteum of the cranial bone. It may be seen on one or both sides of the head but does not cross the suture line. This condition usually recedes within 3 to 6 weeks without treatment and is considered a normal finding.

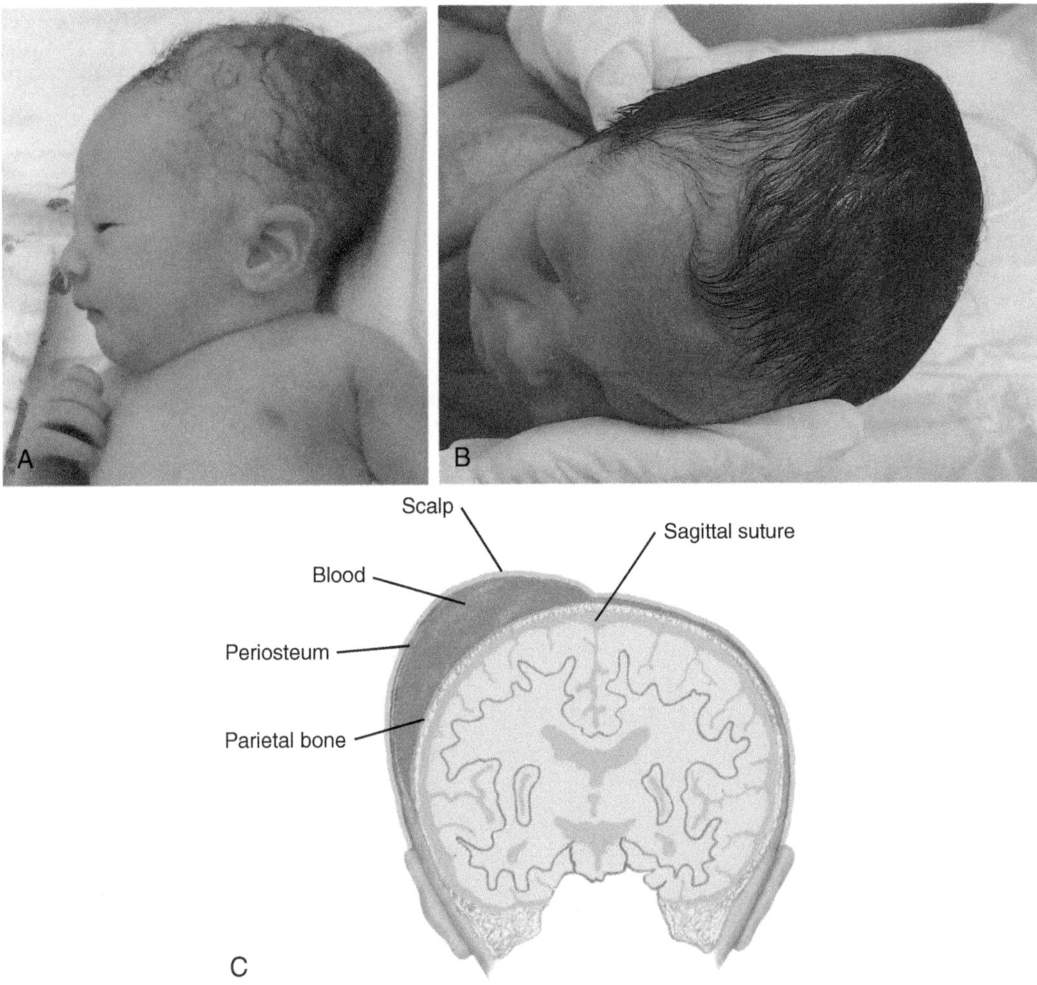

Fig. 11.8 **A,** Moulding of the head occurs as a result of the parietal bones overriding one another as the head passes through the birth canal. Often a collection of fluid under the scalp caused by edema of the presenting part (caput succedaneum) causes the head to appear longer than normal and soft to the touch. This condition disappears without treatment within a few weeks. **B,** Cephalohematoma appears as a lump on one side of the head. **C,** With a cephalohematoma, the blood collects between the surface of the cranial bone and the periosteal membrane. The swelling does not cross the suture lines and may take several weeks to disappear. (**A,** from Beischer, N. A., Mackey, E. V., & Colditz, P. B. (1997). *Obstetrics and the newborn* (3rd ed.). Philadelphia: Saunders. **B,** from McKinney, E. S., James, S. R., Murray, S. S., & Ashwill, J. W. (2013). *Maternal-child nursing* (4th ed.). Philadelphia: Saunders.)

The newborn's head is composed of several bones separated by strong connective tissue, called **sutures** (see Fig. 6.7). A wider area, called a *fontanelle,* is formed where the sutures meet. The **fontanelles** are unossified spaces or soft spots on the cranium of a young infant. They protect the head during birth by permitting the process of moulding and allow for further brain growth during the next 1½ years. The *anterior fontanelle* is diamond shaped and is located at the junction of the two parietal and two frontal bones. It usually closes by age 12 to 18 months. The *posterior fontanelle* is triangular and is located between the occipital and parietal bones. It is smaller than the anterior fontanelle and is usually ossified between the second and third months. A tough membrane covers these areas, and there is little chance of their being injured during ordinary care. The sutures lines should also be assessed. They may be found to be overriding in the newborn as the skull moulded its way through the birth canal; this is a normal finding. If there is a large space between the sutures, the primary health care provider should be notified, as this could be a sign of hydrocephalus. The features of the newborn's face are small. The mouth and lips are well developed because they are necessary to obtain food. The newborn can both taste and smell. In fact, the newborn can recognize the scent of the mother's milk.

Eyes

The healthy newborn can see and can fixate on points of contrast; although they see up to 50 cm, the best visual acuity is 17 to 20 cm. The newborn shows a preference for observing a human face and follows moving objects. *Visual stimulation* is thus an important aspect of newborn care. Contrasting colours, such as black and white, attract the newborn.

Many newborns appear cross-eyed because their eye muscle coordination is not fully developed. This may last until about 9 months, at which point the infant will need to be assessed for strabismus by a pediatric care provider if it continues. At first, the eyes may appear to be blue or grey; the permanent colouring becomes fixed usually between ages 6 and 12 months. Tears do not appear until approximately age 1 to 3 months because of the immaturity of the lacrimal gland ducts.

A small conjunctival hemorrhage may be seen in the eye, or mild conjunctivitis may be seen as a result of a response to eye medication instilled at birth, but these conditions are considered variations rather than deviations from normal, usually require no specific follow-up, and will resolve spontaneously.

Ears

The ears are well developed but small at birth. The ears are assessed for placement because low-set ears may indicate a congenital abnormality in another part of the body. An imaginary line drawn from the outer canthus of the eye should be even with the upper tip of the pinna of the ear (Fig. 11.9). An "ear tag" is a small skin tag or pit on the outside of the ear that is sometimes seen as a variation in newborns. Although its presence should be documented on the physical assessment record, it is rarely of medical significance. The hearing ability of the newborn is well developed at birth, but the sick or premature newborn may not respond to sounds that are heard. The presence of amniotic fluid in the ear canal can diminish hearing, but normal drainage and sneezing that occur shortly after birth help clear the ear canal.

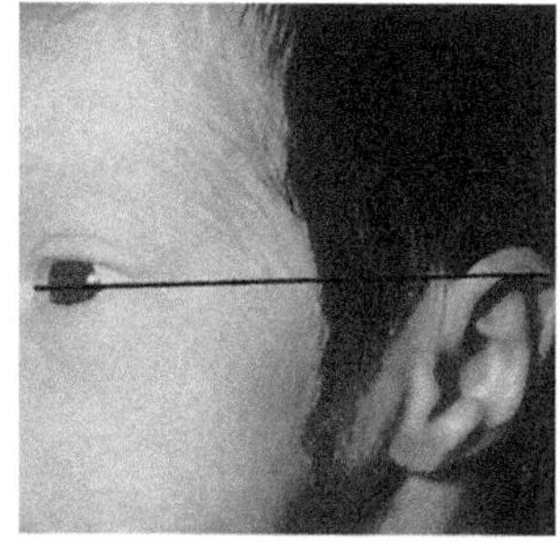
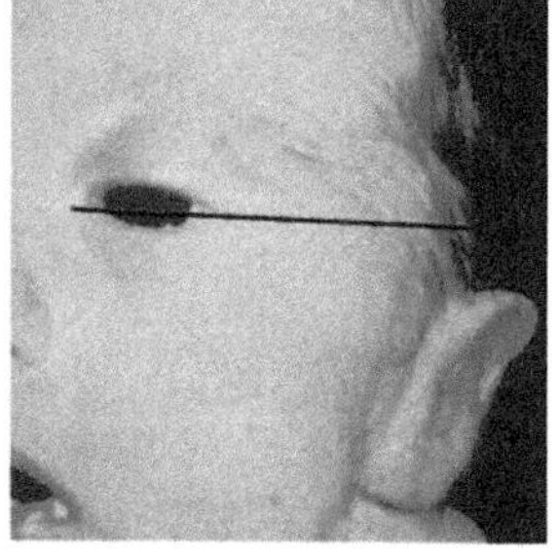

Fig. 11.9 Ear position. The ears are assessed for placement because low-set ears may indicate a congenital abnormality. (From Thureen, P. J., Deacon, J., O'Neill, P., & Hernandez, J. A. [2005]. *Assessment and care of the well newborn* [2nd ed.]. Philadelphia: Saunders.)

The newborn will react to a sudden sound with an increase in pulse rate and respirations or a display of the startle reflex. Infants will show increased responses to vocal stimulation, particularly higher-pitched female voices. The ability to discriminate between the voice of a parent and the voices of others may occur as early as age 3 days. Hearing is important to the development of normal speech.

Permanent hearing loss occurs in about 2 of 1 000 live births. The Canadian Paediatric Society (CPS) recommends routine hearing screening for all newborns prior to discharge, although it is not mandatory in all provinces (CPS, 2016). Hearing screening done early ensures that the child has access to earlier diagnosis and intervention. The initial screening is usually done with the evoked otoacoustic emissions (EOAE) test that measures sounds from the cochlea in response to sound stimulation (Fig. 11.10). If the initial test is abnormal, the auditory brainstem response (ABR) test is done, in which brain wave responses to sound are assessed. A computer is used to compare the response to normal responses, and a pass/fail score is recorded. If these tests are abnormal, further testing is required.

The ears and nose need no special attention except for cleansing with a soft cloth during the bath. Occasionally they may be externally cleansed with a cotton ball moistened slightly with water. The bony canal of the external ear is not well developed, and the tympanic membrane is vulnerable to injury. The nurse should *not* insert applicators and should teach the parents this as well. Insertion of applicators may cause serious injury to the tympanic membrane if they are inserted too far into the ear canal or if the infant moves suddenly.

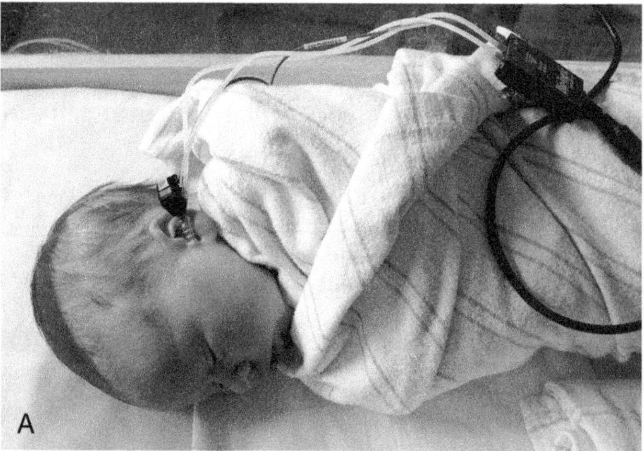

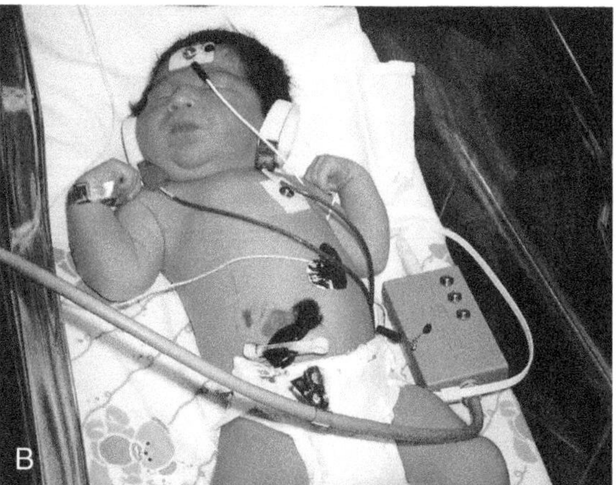

Fig. 11.10 The evoked optoacoustic emissions (EOAE) test. During newborn hearing screening the screener sends a series of soft clicking sounds to a device placed in the newborn's outer ear. The healthy ear will "echo" the sound back to an ear piece. Newborns with an abnormal result will have an auditory brainstem response (ABR) test performed and, depending on the results, may be referred for follow-up evaluation. (A, Courtesy Julie and Darren Nelson. B, Courtesy Dee Lowdermilk.)

Sensory Overload

Sensory overload can occur if there is too much stimulation. This detrimental overload can occur in the hospital environment, where lights are bright and voices carry. The nurse can help to modify this situation by turning lights down when possible, responding quickly to call bells and alarms, and speaking quietly when working near the infant.

Sleep–Wake Cycles

Newborns sleep approximately 15 to 20 hours a day. There is a gradual change in the quantity and quality of sleep as the newborn matures. The environment plays a large role in the infant's sleep behaviour. The nurse can convey to parents that normal conversational tones can quiet a newborn, whereas high noise levels may cause increased crying.

In the early newborn period, infants tend to alternate periods of sleep and wakefulness that resemble their fetal inactivity and activity patterns. Variations in the state of consciousness of infants are called sleep–wake states (O'Flaherty, 2017).

- *Deep sleep:* The infant sleeps and does not move.
- *Light sleep (rapid eye movement [REM] sleep):* Respirations are more irregular during REM sleep. Eye movements are evident beneath the eyelid, and limb and mouth movement may be seen.
- *Drowsy:* The infant may be quiet and relaxed but not very responsive to the environment.
- *Quiet alert:* The infant is awake, relaxed, and quiet. In this state, the infant is most responsive to stimulation and responds to people talking to them.
- *Active alert:* The infant displays diffuse motor activity.
- *Crying:* The infant's cry is accompanied by vigorous motor activity of extremities.

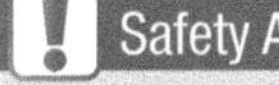
Safety Alert!

Even the youngest of infants can roll off a changing table or bed when left unattended.

Pain

In the past, it was believed that newborns did not experience pain, because of immaturity of the nerve pathways to the brain. It is now thought that fibres that conduct pain stimuli to the spinal cord are in place early in fetal life. These are called *nociceptors* (*noci,* "pain," and *ceptus,* "to receive"). The newborn also produces catecholamines and cortisol in response to stress. Heart rate and respiratory rates change. Blood pressure increases, and blood glucose levels rise. Newborns should be medicated for pain when discomfort is anticipated.

The nurse is responsible for understanding the physiological and behavioural responses to pain and providing appropriate pain-relief measures. Untreated pain in early infancy can have long-term effects, because the pain pathways and structures required for long-term memory are well developed by 24 weeks of gestation. Unrelieved pain can also cause exhaustion and irritability and can slow the healing process. Some infants may be too weak to demonstrate a visible response to pain and so behavioural responses and physiological changes must both be monitored. There are several pain assessment tools available for assessing pain in preterm and term infants, although it is important to note that many pain scales for infants are subjective. Pain assessment tools appropriate for the older child are discussed in Chapter 19. Examples of pain assessment tools for infants include the following:

- *CRIES:* This 10-point scale (with each component scored from 0 to 2) includes facial expression, cry, movement of the arms and legs, consolability, and oxygen saturation in its scoring. Letters of the acronym are defined as follows: **C** = **c**ry, **R** = **r**equires oxygen, **I** = **i**ncreased vital signs, **E** = **e**xpression on face, **S** = **s**leeplessness.
- *FLACC:* This pain tool measures the pain of infants. The parameters include **f**ace, **l**egs, **a**ctivity, **c**ry, and **c**onsolability. Each parameter is scored from 0 to 2, with a higher cumulative score indicating increased distress.
- *PIPP:* The **P**remature **I**nfant **P**ain **P**rofile is based on scales similar to the CRIES scale. This rates eye squeeze, nasal labial furrow, heart rate, oxygen saturation, and the brow furrow on a 0-to-3 scale, with 21 indicating the worst level of pain.
- *NIPS:* The **N**eonatal **I**nfant **P**ain **S**cale is based on scales similar to the CRIES scale. This scale rates facial expression, arm movement, cry, leg movement, respiration, and arousal on a 0-to-2 scale, with a score of 7 indicating the worst level of pain.
- *NPASS:* The **N**eonatal **P**ain, **A**gitation, and **S**edation **S**cale considers the previous criteria, in addition to behaviour, and is considered to be a very reliable and valid assessment tool, even for premature infants on ventilators. Scores are given for crying or irritability, behavioural state, facial expression, tone of extremities, vital signs, and oxygen saturation. Scores in each category range from −2 for sedated infants to +2 for agitated infants. A normal response indicating no pain or sedation is scored as 0 (zero).

The pain assessment findings should be documented and appropriate nursing interventions implemented.

Adequate pain relief in newborns who undergo painful procedures (e.g., blood work or circumcision) is very important. Evaluation of pain in the newborn can be based on changes in vital signs and behaviour of the infant as well as decreased oxygen saturation rates (Fig. 11.11). Nonpharmacological pain-relief methods should be used when required. Oral sucrose, nonnutritive sucking, skin-to-skin contact, and breastfeeding are effective pain-relief methods for newborns (Cignacco, Sellam, Stoffel, et al., 2012; Stevens, Yamada, Ohlsson, et al., 2016). Combining some of these

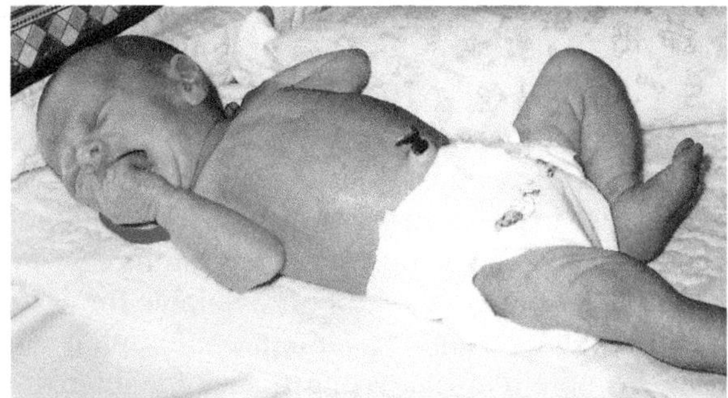

Fig. 11.11 Pain in the newborn. Note furrowed brow, clenched fist, irritability or cry, chin quiver, increased muscle tone and activity, tightly closed eyes, facial grimace, raised cheeks, deepened nasolabial fold, and open mouth. Diaphoresis; rapid, shallow respirations; and increased heart rate and blood pressure also can be observed in the newborn experiencing pain. Pain relief for the newborn during any medical procedure is very important to carry out.

strategies is more effective in reducing pain. Other strategies can include touch, massage, rocking, holding, and low noise and light. Medications include non-opioids (e.g., acetaminophen) and topical anaesthetics for mild to moderate pain, and morphine or fentanyl can be used safely for severe pain. The nurse must be aware of safe dosage ranges and must observe infants receiving these medications closely for adverse effects.

Conditioned Responses

A conditioned response or reflex is one that is learned over time. It is an unconscious response to an external stimulus. An example is the hungry infant who stops crying merely at the sound of the caregiver's footsteps, even though food is not yet available. Emotions are particularly subject to this type of conditioning. As an infant matures, the mere sight of an object that once caused pain can precipitate fear.

RESPIRATORY SYSTEM

The unborn fetus is completely dependent on the mother for all vital functions. The fetus needs oxygen and nourishment to grow. These nutrients are supplied through the bloodstream of the pregnant woman by way of the placenta and the umbilical cord. The fetus is relieved of the waste products of metabolism by the same route. The lungs are not inflated and are almost completely inactive. The circulatory system is adapted only to life within the uterus. Little blood flows through the pulmonary artery because of natural openings within the heart and vessels that close at birth or shortly thereafter (see Chapter 3, Fetal Circulation).

When the umbilical cord is clamped and cut, the lungs take on the function of breathing oxygen and removing carbon dioxide. The first breath helps to expand the collapsed lungs, although full expansion does not occur for several days. The newborn should be placed on the mother's chest if stable, and the nurse can assess the newborn in this position. Using a towel to rub the newborn can help to stimulate breathing, if needed. Any mucus that is seen draining from the nose or mouth can be wiped away.

The nurse must complete a thorough assessment of the newborn approximately every 4 to 8 hours once the infant is stable. Respiratory distress may be evidenced by the rate and character of respirations, colour (cyanosis), sternal retractions, grunting, nasal flaring, and a change in behaviour (see Chapter 12).

CIRCULATORY SYSTEM

The mother's blood carried essential oxygen to the placenta, which sent it to each cell of the fetus while in the uterus. This supply is cut off when the umbilical cord is cut. Thereafter the newborn depends on their own systemic circulation and pulmonary circulation (see Fig. 3.7).

The newborn has approximately 300 mL of circulatory blood volume. The circulation of blood in the fetus differs from that in the newborn in that most fetal blood bypasses the lungs (see Chapter 3, Fetal Circulation). Some of the blood goes from the right atrium to the left atrium of the heart through an opening (the foramen ovale) in the septum. Some passes from the pulmonary artery to the thoracic aorta by way of the ductus arteriosus. These normal openings close soon after birth. If they fail to close, the infant may be cyanotic because part of the blood continues to bypass the lungs and does not pick up oxygen.

Murmurs are sounds heard when auscultating the heart and are caused by blood leaking through openings that have not yet closed. Murmurs may be functional (innocent) or organic (caused by improper heart formation). Functional murmurs result from blood passing through normal valves. Organic murmurs are caused by blood passing through abnormal openings. The majority of heart murmurs are not serious, but they should be checked periodically to rule out other pathological conditions.

Acrocyanosis, or peripheral blueness of the hands and feet, is normal for the first few weeks and results from poor peripheral circulation. Central body areas are not cyanotic in normal newborns. Pallor is not normal and should be reported because it may indicate neonatal anemia or another more serious condition.

MUSCULOSKELETAL SYSTEM

The bones of the newborn are soft because they are composed mostly of cartilage, in which there is only a small amount of calcium. The skeleton is flexible, and the joints are elastic to accommodate the passage through the birth canal. Because the bones of the infant are easily moulded by pressure, the infant's position must be changed frequently. If the infant spends much of the day lying on their back, the bones of the head can become flattened. This condition is called *plagiocephaly* (flattening of the head) and requires treatment as the child gets older (see further discussion in Chapter 14).

The movements of the newborn are random and uncoordinated. The newborn lacks the muscular control to hold the head steady. The development of muscular control proceeds from head to foot and from the centre of the body to the periphery (see the discussion of cephalocaudal and proximodistal control in Chapter 13). Therefore, the infant holds the head up before sitting erect. In fact, the head and neck muscles are the first ones to come under control. The newborn's legs are small and short and may appear bowed. There should be no limitation of movement. Fingers clenched in a fist should be separated and observed.

An examination of the newborn for gestational maturity includes checking for the scarf sign (see Fig. 12.3, *D*). This refers to the full-term infant's resistance to attempts to bring one elbow farther than the midline of the chest. No resistance is observed in the preterm infant. The infant stretches, sucks, and makes faces and vigorously moves the entire body when crying. Tremors of the lips and extremities during crying are normal. Constant tremors during sleep may be pathological. These are often accompanied by eye movements, are not related to particular stimuli, and should be reported to the health care provider. When handled, the infant should not feel limp.

GENITOURINARY SYSTEM

The kidneys function at birth but are not fully developed. The glomeruli are small. Renal blood flow is only about one-third that of the adult. The ability to handle a water load is reduced, as is the excretion of drugs. The renal tubules are short and have a limited capacity for reabsorbing important substances such as glucose, amino acids, phosphate, and bicarbonate. There is a decrease in the ability to concentrate urine and to cope with fluid imbalances. It is important to note the first voiding of the newborn. This may occur right after birth or may not occur for several hours. If a newborn urinates in the birthing or operating room, the voiding should be documented on the birth record. If voiding does not occur within the first 24 hours, the health care provider is notified. The colour of urine may look cloudy after the initial voiding; this is due to mucus in the urine and is not a concern. The newborn should have one wet diaper on the first day of life. This amount will increase by one diaper per day until 5 days of age, when six to eight wet diapers per day are expected (see Fig. 9.11).

Male Genitalia

The genitalia of the male are developed at birth, although their maturation varies. The testes of the male descend into the scrotum before birth. Occasionally, they remain in the abdomen or the inguinal canal. Nurses must assess the newborn for the presence of the testes. This condition is called *cryptorchidism*, or undescended testes, and is described in Chapter 29. With proper surgical treatment, the prognosis is good. The location of the urethral opening should be at the tip of the penis in newborn boys. Any deviations from this should be noted (see Chapter 29 for discussion of hypospadias and epispadias). A white cheesy substance called *smegma* is found under the foreskin and is thought to be bacteriostatic. The foreskin should not be retracted until it is done easily, often not until the age of 2 to 3. Full retraction may not be possible before puberty.

Circumcision

Circumcision is the surgical removal of the foreskin on the penis. The benefits of circumcision include possible prevention of penile cancer, fewer urinary tract infections in males less than 1 year of age, and fewer occurrences of sexually transmitted infections, particularly human immunodeficiency virus (HIV) later in life (Carlo, 2016; Sorokan, Finlay, Jefferies, et al., 2015). The risks of circumcision include pain, bleeding, and infection. Circumcision is usually performed in the first 2 weeks of life and often on an outpatient basis, although some hospitals perform them during the first few days of life. Infants with congenital anomalies of the penis, such as *hypospadias* (the opening of the urethra is on the undersurface of the penis), should not be circumcised because the skin may be needed for surgery.

The infant should be physiologically stabilized before a circumcision. The newborn is restrained on a circumcision board (Fig. 11.12, *A*). The *Gomco clamp* and the *Plastibell clamp* are two devices commonly used for performing circumcisions. If the Gomco clamp is used, a thin layer of petroleum jelly or petroleum jelly–impregnated gauze may be applied to the end of the penis to protect it from moisture and from sticking to the diaper. The area is observed for bleeding, infection, and irritation. The first voiding is noted.

When a Plastibell clamp is used, the foreskin is tied over a fitted plastic ring and the excess prepuce cut away. The rim usually drops off 5 to 8 days after circumcision. Parents are instructed not to remove it prematurely. No special dressing is required, and the infant must be sponge bathed until the circumcision heals. A dark brown or black ring encircling the plastic rim is natural. This disappears when the rim drops off. Parents are instructed to consult their pediatric health care provider if there are any questions, if there is increased swelling, or if the ring has not fallen off within 8 days; parents should contact their health care provider immediately if the ring has slipped onto the shaft of the penis.

The Jewish religious custom of circumcision is performed on the eighth day after birth if the newborn's condition permits (see Fig. 11.12, *B*). Families of the Muslim faith also believe in circumcision, and it is considered a rite of passage for many African tribes. Rates of circumcision have decreased over the past few decades, with the current rate of circumcision in Canada at around 32% (Public Health Agency of Canada [PHAC], 2009).

The nurse's role in circumcision includes assessing parental knowledge, checking to see that the surgical consent has been signed, and preparing the newborn. The infant is usually not fed for 2 to 3 hours before the procedure to prevent possible vomiting and aspiration.

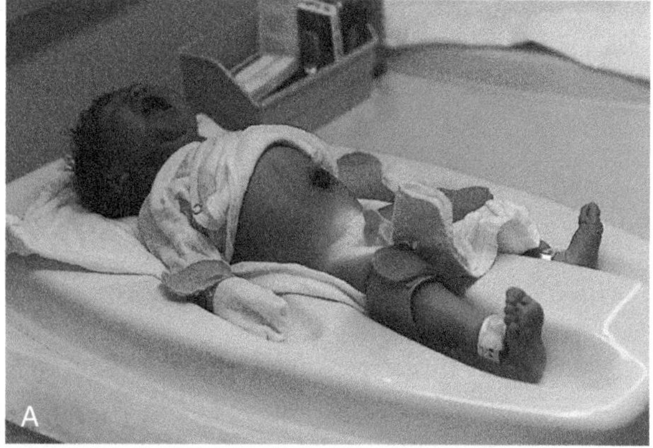

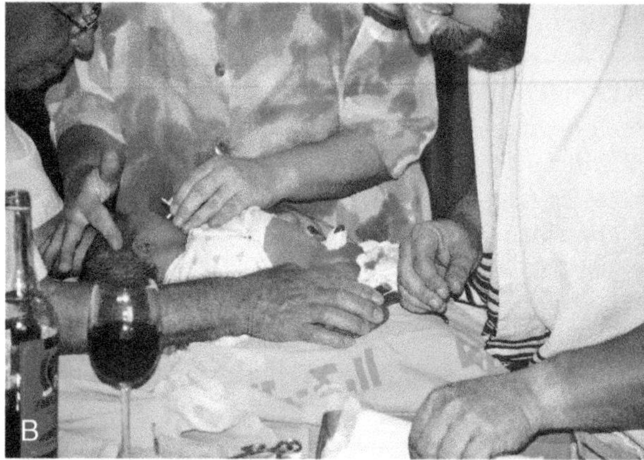

Fig. 11.12 Circumcision. **A,** A circumcision board is used to restrain the newborn during circumcision. A eutectic mixture of local anaesthetics (EMLA) is a local skin anaesthetic that may be used before the procedure. A sucrose-sweetened pacifier is a helpful pain-relief measure during this procedure. **B,** A ritual circumcision. In the Jewish faith, a circumcision is called a *bris milah* and is performed at home on the eighth day of life. It is performed by a specially trained individual called a *mohel* (seen in this picture wearing a *tollis*, or religious scarf). The person who restrains the newborn during the procedure is known as the *sandek* (pictured on the left); this honour is often bestowed on an elder in the family. A few drops of the wine in the foreground are fed to the newborn by a nipple for pain relief during the procedure. Understanding and respecting the rituals and traditions of others is an integral part of cultural competence. (**A,** from Hockenberry, M. J., Wilson, D., Winkelstein, M., & Klein, M. E. (2003). *Wong's nursing care of infants and children* (7th ed.). St. Louis: Mosby.)

A bulb syringe is kept handy in case suctioning is required. A light blanket is placed under the infant on the circumcision board, and the diaper is removed. Three types of anaesthesia and analgesia are used in newborns undergoing circumcision: ring block, dorsal penile nerve block (DPNB), and topical anaesthetic such as eutectic mixture of lidocaine and prilocaine (EMLA) (prilocaine-lidocaine), although DPNB is the most effective for pain management. Nonpharmacological methods such as concentrated oral sucrose, non-nutritive sucking, containment, and swaddling may be used to enhance pain management (Gladding, 2017).

If bleeding occurs, gentle pressure is applied to the site with a sterile gauze pad and the health care provider is notified. The amount and characteristics of the urinary stream are recorded, because edema could cause an obstruction. Parents should be provided with written instructions concerning the care of the circumcised penis.

A discussion of the pros and cons of circumcision is included as part of prenatal and postpartum education. In 2015, the CPS position on circumcision stated that although there are some medical benefits of circumcision for some boys in high-risk populations, the data are not sufficient to recommend routine circumcision (Sorokan et al., 2015). The CPS believes circumcision is a parental decision. Parents, and later all males, at an appropriate age, should be taught daily hygiene of the genitalia. This includes special attention to skin folds, retraction and replacement of the foreskin, cleansing of the penis, and examination for lumps or swelling of the penis or the scrotum (see Patient Teaching box).

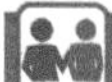 Patient Teaching

Home Care of the Penis

CARE OF THE CIRCUMSCRIBED PENIS

Keep area clean; change diaper frequently.
Wash area with warm water; avoid alcohol-containing wipes.
Do not remove yellow crust from penis.
Apply diaper loosely to prevent pressure.
Report redness and bleeding or drainage.
Observe for voiding appropriate amount per day.

CARE OF THE UNCIRCUMSCRIBED PENIS

Do not retract the foreskin over the glans.
Wash penis with water. White lumps (smegma) are normal.
At toddler age, gently retract the foreskin, if done easily, after bathing to prevent moisture collection; be sure to replace foreskin after retraction.
At school age, the child can be taught to gently retract foreskin for cleansing during bathing.
Retraction of the foreskin should never be forced.

Female Genitalia

The female genitalia may be slightly swollen. A thin, white or blood-tinged mucus (*pseudomenstruation*) may be discharged from the vagina. This discharge is caused by hormonal withdrawal from the mother at birth. The nurse cleanses the vulva from the urethra to the anus, using a clean cotton ball or different sections of a washcloth for each stroke to prevent fecal matter from infecting the urinary tract. Parents need to be taught the importance of this method of cleansing.

INTEGUMENTARY SYSTEM

Skin

Tissue turgor refers to the hydration or dehydration of the skin. To test tissue turgor (elasticity), the nurse gently grasps and releases the skin (Fig. 11.13). It should spring back into place immediately in the well-hydrated infant. When the skin remains distorted ("tented"), tissue turgor is considered poor.

The body is usually covered with fine hair called lanugo, which tends to disappear during the first week of life. This is more evident in premature infants. Vernix

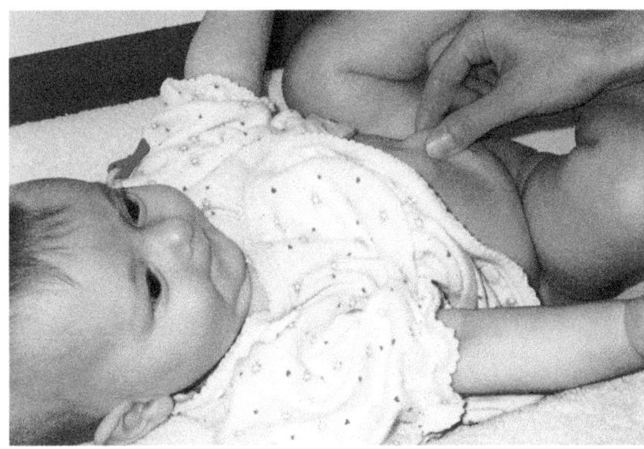

Fig. 11.13 Testing tissue turgor. The term *turgor* refers to the elasticity of the skin, which is affected by the extent of hydration. The nurse tests skin turgor by gently grasping the skin. When the skin is released, it should instantly spring back into place; if it does not, tissue turgor is considered poor.

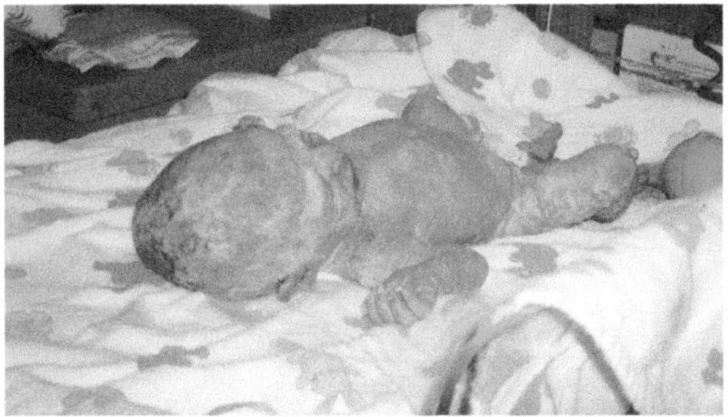

Fig. 11.14 Vernix is the thick, white, cheesy substance covering the skin of the newborn. Preterm newborns are heavily covered in vernix, whereas post-term newborns have little vernix protection on their skin. Note the heavy covering of vernix on this newborn.

caseosa, a cheeselike substance that covers the skin of the newborn, is made of cells and glandular secretions; it is thought to protect the skin from irritation and the effects of a watery environment in utero (Fig. 11.14). To preserve skin integrity, vigorous removal of all remnants of vernix is not advised. There will be less vernix present on the skin of the term newborn.

White pinpoint "pimples" caused by the obstruction of sebaceous glands may be seen on the nose and chin. These are called milia and disappear within a few weeks. Lesions on the midline of the hard palate of the milia type are called Epstein pearls and are caused by a collection of epithelial cells. *Telangiectatic nevi* (stork bites) are flat, red areas seen on the nape of the neck and on the eyelids. They result from the dilation of small vessels. See Table 11.3 for other skin manifestations seen in the newborn and the appropriate nursing care.

Mongolian spots, which are bluish discolorations of the skin, are common in non-white infants. They are usually found over the sacral and gluteal areas (see Table 11.3). They disappear spontaneously during the early years of life. Mongolian spots can be differentiated from a hematoma resulting from abuse, because the hematoma will change colour each day, but the Mongolian spot remains the same colour and hue and may last for one year up to many years. *Desquamation*, or peeling of the skin, occurs during the early weeks of life.

Initial skin care after the newborn's condition is stable involves wiping off the blood and amniotic fluid that may be present on the newborn's skin. Until the newborn's first bath and shampoo, the nurse must wear gloves while handling the newborn. The buttocks need special attention. A wet diaper should be changed immediately to prevent chafing. The buttocks are washed and dried well. Care of the skin of the newborn is discussed later in the chapter.

Jaundice

The newborn's skin should be observed for jaundice at each assessment. Physiological jaundice, also called *hyperbilirubinemia*, is characterized by a yellow tinge of the skin. It is caused by the rapid destruction of excess red blood cells, which the infant does not need now because the infant is in an atmosphere that contains more oxygen than was available during prenatal life. The breakdown of red blood cells releases bilirubin into the bloodstream. High levels of bilirubin cause yellow skin colour, starting at the head and progressing downward on the body. Extremely high levels of bilirubin can cause kernicterus (see Chapter 12).

Plasma levels of bilirubin increase to an average of 85–100 mcmol/L between the second and fourth days (Table 11.4). Physiological jaundice becomes evident between the second and the third days of life and lasts for about 1 week. This is a normal process in 60% of term infants and 80% of preterm infants and is not harmful to the infant. However, ethnic factors (higher risk in Indigenous and Asian infants), method of feeding, and gestational age may affect its severity. Evidence of jaundice should be reported and charted, and the newborn evaluated frequently to ensure safety (Skill 11.3).

Jaundice can be assessed using the following:

1. *Transcutaneous bilirubin measurement (TcB):* Transcutaneous measurement of jaundice is noninvasive. TcB is an adequate screening device with a more accurate blood test or follow-up required when the newborn screens high.
2. The CPS recommends that all healthy newborns over 35 weeks' gestation have blood work drawn using hour-specific serum bilirubin levels prior to discharge from the hospital. The result of this test will determine the risk of developing hyperbilirubinemia and whether further follow-up is indicated (Barrington, Sankaran, & CPS, 2007/2016).

Pathological jaundice and treatment are discussed further in Chapter 12.

 **Safety Alert!**

Jaundice that appears in the first day of life is not normal and should be recorded and reported.

Table 11.3 Common Skin Manifestations of the Newborn

	APPEARANCE	INTERVENTION
Acrocyanosis		
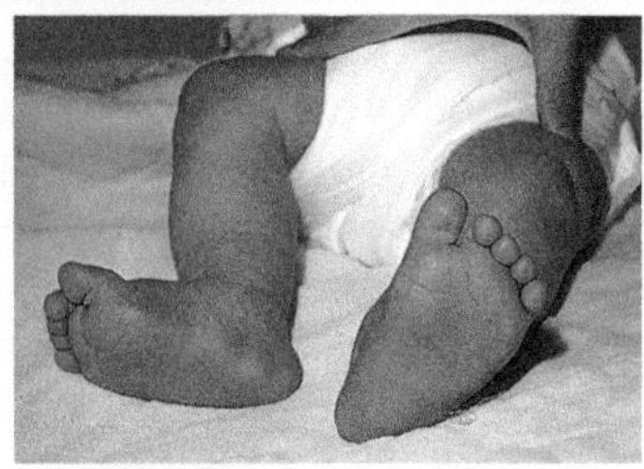	Cyanosis of the hands and feet in the first week of life is caused by a combination of a vasomotor instability and capillary stasis. Often occurs when infant is cold	Parent education concerning this normal phenomenon is helpful.
Cutis Marmorata		
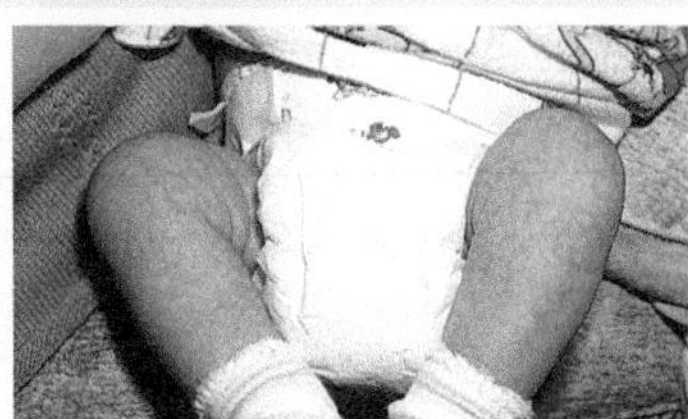	Lacelike red or blue pattern on the skin surface of a newborn's body	Normal vasomotor response to low environmental temperature. Warm infant by putting skin-to-skin with parent. Intense or persistent appearance should be reported.
Desquamation		
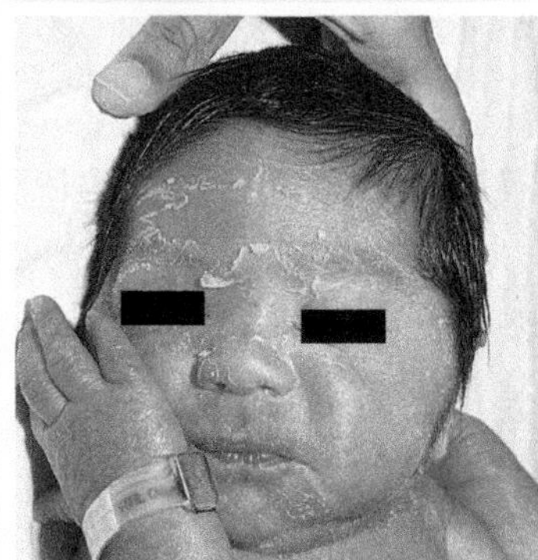	Peeling of the skin at birth may indicate postmaturity. Early removal of vernix can be followed by desquamation in term newborns.	Instruct parents to avoid harsh soaps. It is recommended that vernix not be removed from skin of newborns but allowed to absorb into the skin.
Epstein Pearls		
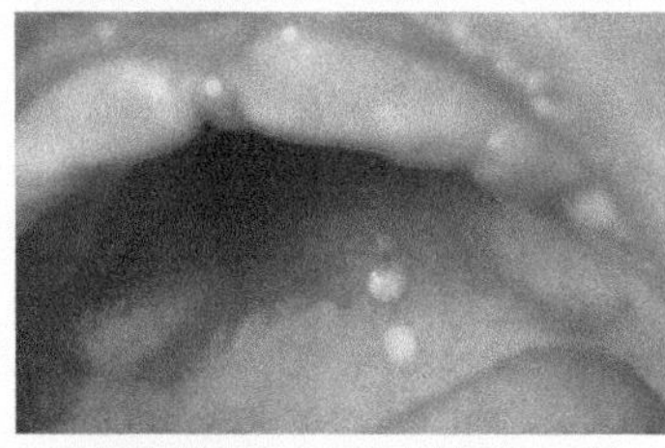	Pearly white pinpoint papules in midline of upper palate	Distinguish from a thrush lesion (see Chapter 28).
Erythema Toxicum (Newborn Rash)		
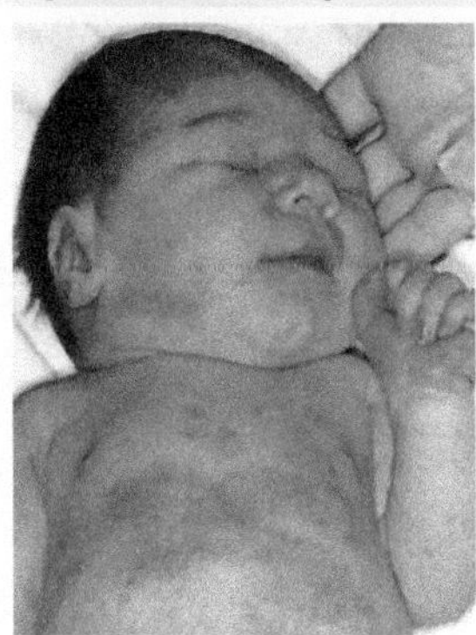	Splotchy erythema with firm yellow-white papules that have a red base	Can occur at age 2 days; no intervention is required because erythema will spontaneously clear.

Table 11.3 Common Skin Manifestations of the Newborn—cont'd

	APPEARANCE	INTERVENTION
Forceps Marks		
	Bruised area on skin in the shape of forceps	Bruising and swelling fade within a few days and do not necessitate intervention other than parental support and teaching.
Harlequin Colour Change		
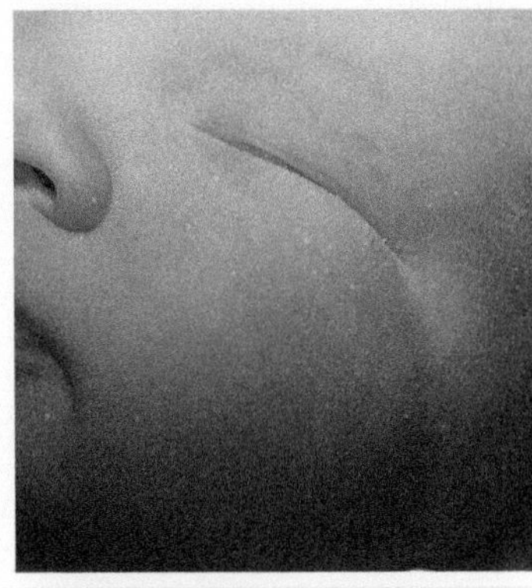	Imbalance of autonomic vascular regulatory mechanism; deep red colour over half of body; pallor on longitudinal half of body; usually occurs with preterm infants who are placed on their side	Phenomenon disappears with muscular activity. Changing position of infant is helpful. Condition is temporary and does not usually indicate a problem.
Milia		
	Pearly white pinpoint papules on face and nose of newborn	No treatment is needed; it will spontaneously disappear. Educate parents not to attempt to "squeeze out" the white material because infection can occur.
Mongolian Spots		
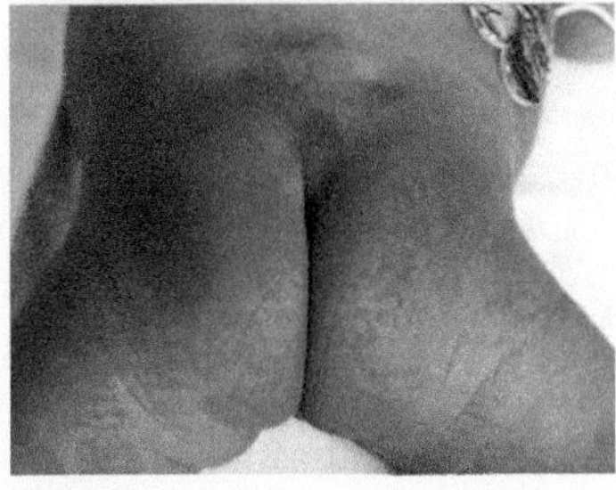	Dark blue or slate grey discolorations most commonly found in lumbosacral area; intensity and hue of colour remain until fading occurs	Caused by melanin deposits in dark-skinned persons and will gradually disappear in a few years.
Nevi		
	Known as *stork bites;* pink, easily blanched patches that can appear on eyelids, nose, lips, and nape of neck (see Chapter 30)	Marks gradually fade and are of no clinical significance.
Port-Wine Stain		
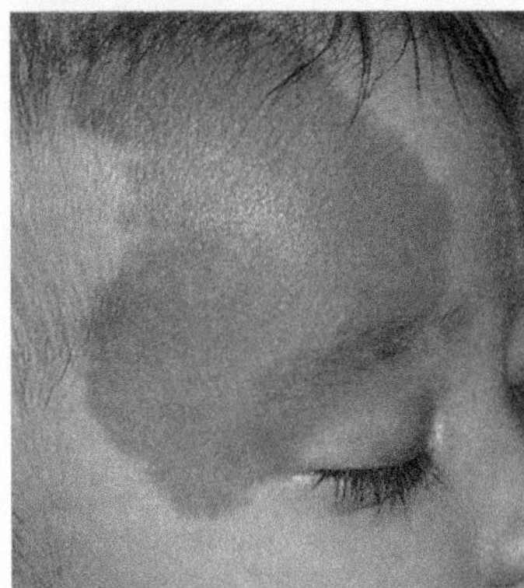	Known as *nevus flammeus;* a collection of capillaries in the skin. It is a flat, red-purple lesion that does not blanch on pressure.	This is a permanent skin marking that darkens with age and can become elevated and vulnerable to injury. If a large area of face or neck is involved, laser surgery may be indicated to preserve the child's self-image. It can be associated with genetic disorders.

Unnumbered Figures 1, 2, 3, 6: From Eichenfield, L. F., Friden, I. J., & Esterly, N. B. (2001). *Textbook of neonatal dermatology*. Philadelphia: Saunders; unnumbered Figures 4 and 7: From Zitelli, B. J., et al. (2012). *Atlas of pediatric physical diagnosis* (6th ed.). St. Louis: Mosby; unnumbered Figure 5: From Swartz, M. H. (2006). *Textbook of physical diagnosis* (5th ed.). Philadelphia: Saunders; unnumbered Figure 8: From Murray, S. S., & McKinney, E. S. (2014). *Foundations of maternal-newborn and women's health nursing* (6th ed.). St. Louis: Saunders; unnumbered Figure 9: From Swartz, M. H. (2014). *Textbook of physical diagnosis* (7th ed.). Philadelphia: Saunders.)

Table 11.4 Changing Laboratory Values

	NEWBORN	1–2 MONTHS	2–6 MONTHS
Hemoglobin (Hgb) (g/L)	140–240	120–200	100–170
Hematocrit (Hct) Volume fraction (%)	0.37–0.48	0.34–0.43	0.30–0.39
White blood cell count (WBC) × 10^9/L	9–30		
Bilirubin (mcmol/L)	<100		

Pagana, K. D., Pagana, T. J., & Pike-MacDonald, S. A. (2013). *Mosby's Canadian manual of diagnostic and laboratory tests* (1st Canadian ed.). Toronto, ON: Elsevier.

GASTROINTESTINAL SYSTEM

Stools

The intestinal tract functions as an outlet for amniotic fluid as early as the fifth month of fetal life. The normal functions of the gastrointestinal tract begin after birth. Food is digested and absorbed into the blood, and waste products are eliminated. **Meconium**, the first stool, is a mixture of amniotic fluid and secretions of the intestinal glands. It is dark greenish black, thick, and sticky (tarry) and should be passed by 8 to 24 hours after birth. By the third day the stools gradually change and become loose and are greenish yellow with mucus. These are called *transitional stools* (Fig. 11.15). By the fourth day after birth the stools of a breastfed infant are bright yellow, soft, and pasty. There may be three to six stools a day. The number of stools decreases with age. The bowel movements of a formula-fed infant are more solid than those of the breastfed infant. They vary from yellow to brown and are generally fewer in number. There may be one to four a day at first, but this gradually decreases to one or two a day. The stools are darker when an infant is receiving oral iron supplements, and they are green when an infant is under the phototherapy lamp for jaundice. Small, puttylike stools or diarrhea and bloody stools are abnormal and a health care provider needs to be notified about these.

The nurse needs to explain to parents that straining in the newborn period results from undeveloped abdominal musculature. This is normal, and no treatment is required. In the first month of life, a breastfed infant will pass at least four stools a day. After the second month of life, the infant will increase stool volume and decrease stool frequency. Older infants differ in regularity. Some pass a soft stool every other day. This is not constipation. Even if 5 to 6 days pass without a stool, it is not considered constipation if the stool passed is soft or pasty in character. *Constipation* refers to the passage of hard dry stools. Constipation is sometimes seen as the infant matures and if a formula change is made. If the older infant is eating solid foods, an increased intake of fruits, vegetables, and whole-grain cereals is usually sufficient to help the situation. The nurse should encourage mothers to contact their health care provider's office when questions arise and to ask to speak to the nurse. This is particularly emphasized for new mothers, who may be afraid of appearing "ignorant." Very often a simple solution can relieve hours of anxiety.

Digestion

Breastfeeding and formula feeding are discussed in Chapters 9 and 14. Breastfed infants should be put to the breast in the first hour after birth for psychological benefits and to help stimulate milk production. Formula feedings are begun when the newborn shows evidence of hunger cues such as crying, restlessness, fist sucking, and a rooting reflex. The capacity of the newborn's stomach on day 1 is less than 30 mL and peristalsis is rapid. Emptying time can depend on the temperature of the food as well as the volume of the feeding. The *gastrocolic reflex* is often stimulated with feeding, which results in the infant passing a stool.

The immature cardiac sphincter of the stomach may cause regurgitation to occur. Deficiency of pancreatic enzymes such as lipase limits fat absorption. Breastmilk contains some lipase enzyme that aids infant digestion.

Skill 11.2 Assessing for Jaundice

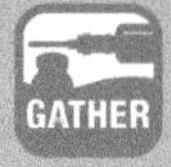

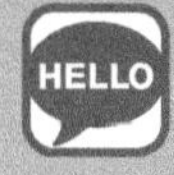

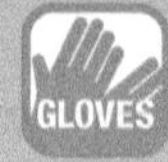

PURPOSE

To determine if a blood test for bilirubin level is indicated

STEPS

1. Observe skin in a well-lit room.
2. Press skin over the nose or sternum with the thumb until the skin blanches (lightens).
3. Observe the level of jaundice. Note: There is a cephalocaudal progression of jaundice in term infants. As the bilirubin level increases, the jaundice progresses from the head toward the feet (Ambalavanan & Carlo, 2016).
4. Jaundice seen below the sternum or present in the arms, lower abdomen, or feet may indicate that a serum bilirubin test is required (Ambalavanan & Carlo, 2016).

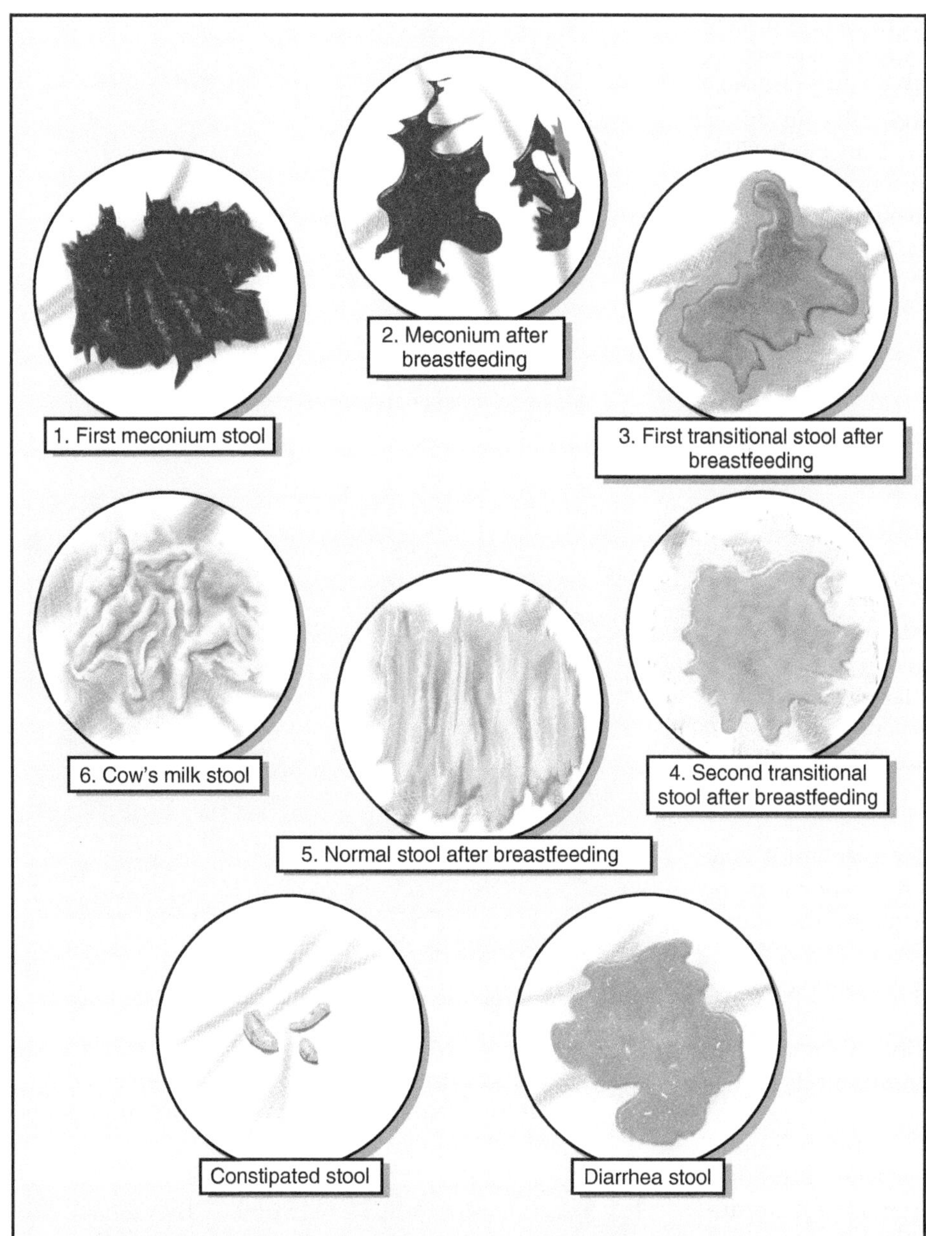

Fig. 11.15 The normal infant stool cycle. The first meconium is dark, black, and tarry. It gradually changes to a greenish yellow transitional stool. The breastfed infant's "milk" stool is golden yellow, whereas the formula-fed infant has a pale yellow stool. A green, watery stool is indicative of diarrhea and should be reported to the health care provider. (Redrawn from Clinical Education Aid #3. Courtesy Ross Laboratories, Columbus, Ohio, 1978.)

Whole cow's milk does not contain this enzyme and thus should not be fed to newborns or young infants.

The salivary glands do not secrete saliva until the infant is age 2 to 3 months. Drooling in the newborn is considered a sign of pathological disturbance and should be reported. The liver is immature, especially in its ability to conjugate bilirubin, regulate blood glucose, and coagulate blood.

Vitamins

Breastmilk contains all the vitamins newborns need except for vitamin D. All breastfed, healthy term infants in Canada should receive a daily vitamin D supplement of 10 mcg (400 IU) and this dosage should continue until the infant receives adequate vitamin D from the diet (Health Canada, CPS, & Dietitians of Canada and Breastfeeding Committee for Canada, 2015). Vitamin D is added to formula so supplementation is not required by the formula-fed newborn.Hiccoughs

Hiccoughs appear frequently in newborns and are normal. Most disappear spontaneously and there is nothing that can be done to help alleviate them.

Hypoglycemia

The brain is totally dependent on a steady supply of glucose for its metabolism. Until newborns begin regular feedings, they must use the glucose stored in their bodies. In healthy newborns, blood glucose levels fall after birth and may be as low as 2.0 mmol/L at birth. By 2 hours after birth the glucose level should be 2.6 mmol/L. The first intervention for a hypoglycemia is usually to put the newborn skin-to-skin with the mother and encourage breastfeeding. If the blood sugar does not increase, further intervention may be necessary. Infants with low blood glucose for 3 to 4 days should be evaluated for endocrine disorders. Newborns with the following conditions may be at risk for low blood glucose after birth: preterm, post-term, small for gestational age (SGA), large for gestational age (LGA), newborns of diabetic mothers, and any newborn who is stressed because of hypoxia.

These at-risk newborns should have close observation and monitoring of blood glucose after an initial feeding and at 2 hours of age (Aziz, Dancey, & CPS, 2004/2014). There is no need to monitor glucose levels of healthy term infants. Frequent feedings early and often help to maintain glucose levels.

Signs of hypoglycemia in the newborn include the following:

- Jitteriness
- Poor muscle tone
- Sweating
- Respiratory difficulty
- Low temperature (which can also cause hypoglycemia)
- Poor suck
- High-pitched cry
- Lethargy
- Seizures

If these signs are present, further testing may be required. A heel stick is performed when obtaining capillary blood for the glucose-screening test. The heel stick should avoid the centre of the heel where bone, nerves, and blood vessels are near the surface (Fig. 11.16).

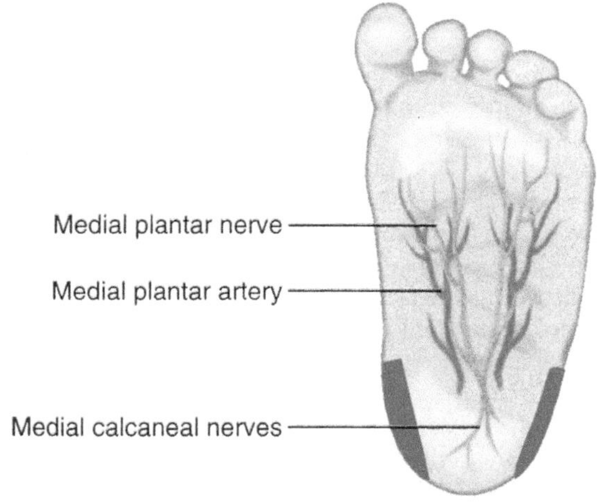

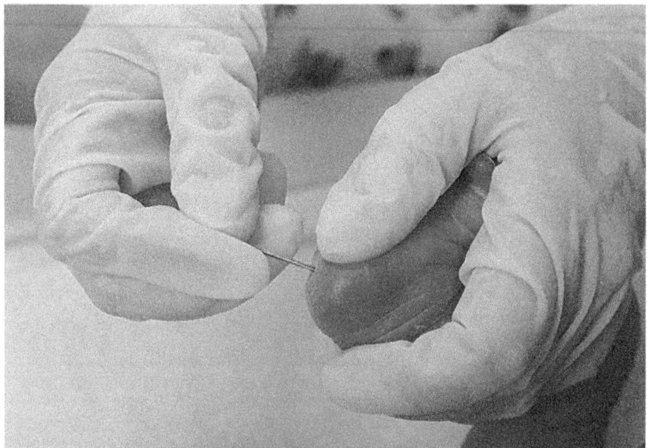

Fig. 11.16 Heel stick. The shaded areas at the sides of the heel are used for heel sticks in newborns to avoid nerves, blood vessels, and bony areas. Warming the heel before puncture will promote better blood flow.

PREVENTING INFECTION

Infections that are relatively harmless to an adult may be fatal to the newborn. The newborn's response to inflammation and infection is slow because of the immaturity of the immune system, as follows:

- Immunoglobulin G (IgG) is an immunoglobulin that crosses the placenta and provides the newborn with passive immunity to infections to which the mother was immune. This type of immunity rarely lasts longer than 3 months.
- Immunoglobulin M (IgM) is an immunoglobulin produced by the newborn and reaches the adult level by 2 years of age. It is important for immunity against bloodborne infections; an elevated level suggests serious infection.
- Immunoglobulin A (IgA) is an immunoglobulin present in breastmilk that provides some resistance to respiratory and gastrointestinal infections.

Measures to prevent infections in the infant include using routine precautions, hand hygiene, cleansing and replacement of equipment, and proper disposal of soiled diapers and linens. Newborns who need to go to a neonatal intensive care unit (NICU) require extra care. Provisions governing space, control of temperature and humidity, lighting, and safety from fire and other hazards are considered in the NICU. Each newborn has an individual crib, bath equipment, and linen supply.

Hand hygiene is the most reliable precaution available. The nurse caring for the newborn must perform hand hygiene between handling different babies. The nurse should stress to parents the need for proper hand hygiene in the home.

The nurse who has signs of a cold, earache, skin infection, or intestinal upset should not work with infants or ill children. Visitors should be instructed not to come to the hospital or be around hospital patients if they are not feeling well.

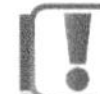 **Safety Alert!**

The nurse must adhere to routine precautions while working in all maternal–child departments. These guidelines are of particular importance during the initial care of the newborn when exposure to secretions, blood, and amniotic fluid is high.

NEWBORN SCREENING

Newborn screening is done for up to 40 conditions, although this number varies across provinces. Many of these conditions, if detected early, can be treated to prevent significant health problems. An example is testing for phenylketonuria (PKU), which is mandatory in all provinces. If the newborn has this disorder, a special formula begun early in life can reduce disability and prevent severe cognitive deficiencies in most cases. Newborn screening is usually done between 24 and 48 hours of life. Other tests may include those for hypothyroidism, galactosemia, sickle cell disease, thalassemia, maple syrup urine disease, critical congenital heart disease, and congenital hearing loss. Hearing screening is discussed earlier in the chapter, in the section on ears.

PROVIDING FOR SECURITY

Identifying the Newborn

Wristbands with preprinted numbers are placed on the mother, the newborn, and often the partner or another support person in the birthing room as the primary means of identifying the newborn. The nurse should check to be sure that all numbers in the set are identical (Fig. 11.17). Other identifying information such as the mother's name, birth attendant's name, date and time of birth, sex of the newborn, and usually the mother's hospital identification number should be completed. The bands are applied relatively snugly on the newborn with only a finger's width of slack because newborns lose weight after birth.

If the newborn is separated from the mother at any point, the nurse must check the preprinted band numbers to see that they match. The nurse should either look at the numbers to see that they are identical or have the mother read her own band number while the nurse reads the newborn's band. The identification bands must be checked every time a newborn assessment is completed.

The possibility of abduction must be addressed in any facility that cares for newborns and children. In the maternal–newborn setting, newborns are often given an extra security band that alerts the staff if the child is near the doors of the unit, either by beeping or by locking the doors. These security bands are removed just prior to discharge.

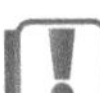

Safety Alert!

Do not check bands by asking, "Is your band number...?" The mother who is sleepy, sedated, or simply distracted may answer affirmatively and receive the wrong newborn.

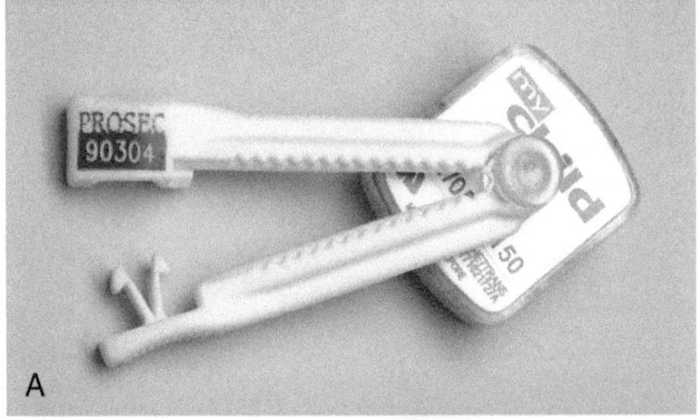

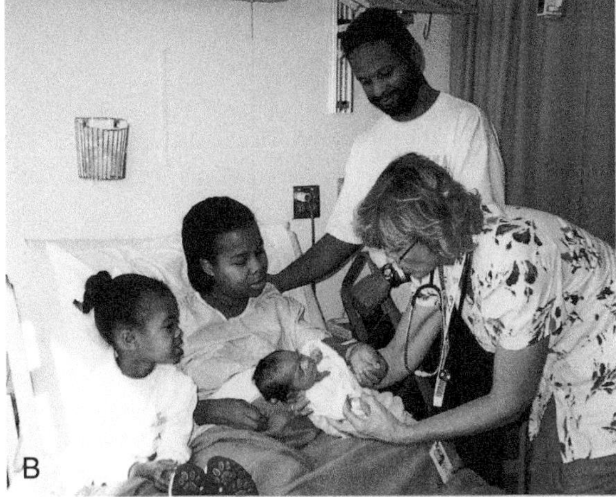

Fig. 11.17 Identification. **A,** This umbilical clamp can be used as identification (with an identical numbered wristband for the mother) and also as protection from abduction because it has a lightweight transponder attached to the clamp. When the transponder is moved out of the unit, an alarm sounds unless the transponder is neutralized. **B,** The nurse compares the identification bracelet of the newborn with the bracelet on the mother's wrist as the father and sibling look on. (Courtesy Pat Spier, RN-C.)

Recognition of Employees

Parents should be able to recognize employees who are authorized to work in the maternal–child unit. Employees wear photo identification badges, and maternal–newborn staff may have an additional badge. They may wear distinctive uniforms. The family is taught how to recognize an employee who is allowed to take the newborn and to refuse to release their newborn to any other person. Security measures should be reinforced when providing care.

Other Security Measures

The mother should not leave her newborn alone in the room for any reason. If she is alone in her room, she should leave the bathroom door ajar while she toilets or take the newborn to the nurse's station if she showers. These measures also reduce the risk that the high-risk newborn would aspirate mucus because no one was present for suctioning.

PROMOTING BONDING AND ATTACHMENT

Bonding and *attachment* are terms often used interchangeably, although they differ slightly. **Bonding** refers to a strong emotional tie that forms soon after birth between the parents and the newborn. **Attachment** is an affectionate tie that occurs through time as newborn and caregivers interact. It is important for nurses to promote these processes to help parents claim the newborn as their own. Bonding actually begins during pregnancy as the fetus moves, and parents are able to see individual characteristics on the ultrasound.

The parents should view, hold, and—most important—*touch* the newborn as soon as possible after birth. They must do this to reconcile the fantasy child of pregnancy with the real child they now have. Many parents are not surprised regarding the sex of their newborn at birth if the ultrasound showed it earlier. However, some do not want to know the newborn's sex before birth, and some are surprised when the predicted sex differs from the actual one.

To prevent newborn hypothermia, the unclothed newborn is put on the mother or partner's skin, and both are covered with a warm blanket (skin-to-skin contact) (see Fig. 9.6). Parents soon identify individual characteristics, such as a nose that looks like Grandpa's, long fingers like the father's, or a cry just like that of an older sibling. All of these parental behaviours help to identify the newborn as a separate individual.

For some, parental feelings take time to develop. Difficulty in bonding, rejection, or indifference in one or both parents should be recorded, and a referral to social services should be considered.

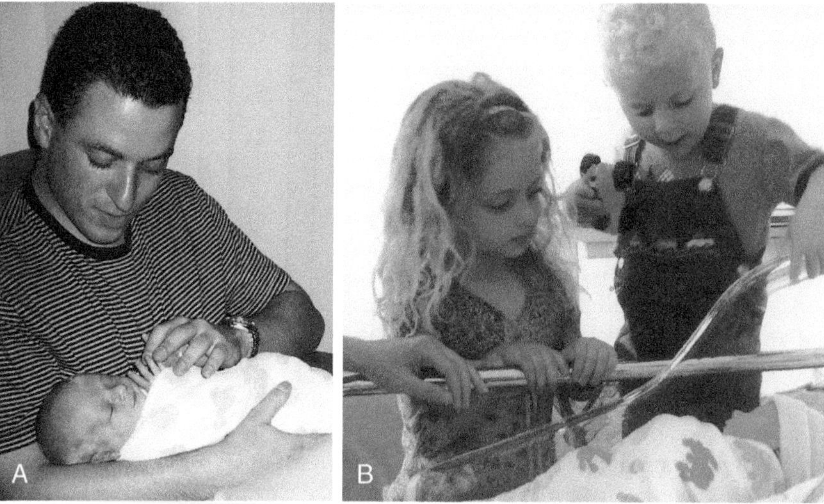

Fig. 11.18 **A,** An uncle bonds with the newborn as he examines features and fingers. **B,** Siblings get their first introduction to their newborn brother.

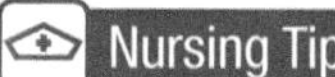

Nursing Tip

Observe the interaction between parents and newborn to assess the attachment process.

Nursing Care to Promote Bonding and Attachment

The nurse needs to observe parenting behaviours, such as the amount of affection and interest shown to the newborn. The amount of physical contact, stimulation, eye-to-eye contact (*en face position;* see Fig. 9.2), and time spent interacting with the newborn are significant. Adults tend to talk with newborns in high-pitched voices. The extent to which the parents encourage involvement of siblings and grandparents with the newborn should be noted. This information provides a basis for nursing interventions that may encourage bonding and foster positive family relationships (Fig. 11.18).

Parents must learn what their newborn's communication cues mean. Soon after birth, most parents begin to recognize when a newborn is signalling discomfort from hunger as opposed to discomfort from other causes, such as a wet diaper or boredom. In addition, the parents usually are able to distinguish their newborn's cry from the cries of other newborns.

The nurse should observe for parent–newborn interactions that dictate a need for additional interventions. Some of these include indifference to the newborn's signals of hunger or discomfort, failure to identify their newborn's communication, avoidance of eye contact with the newborn, or discussing the newborn in negative terms.

Nursing interventions to facilitate parent–newborn attachment vary. Calling the newborn by name, holding the newborn en face, encouraging skin-to-skin contact, and talking in gentle, high-pitched tones help the nurse to model behaviour for the parent. Role modelling is especially important for adolescent mothers who may feel self-conscious when interacting with their child. Expected newborn behaviours should be discussed and unique characteristics pointed out to enhance the bonding process. This is especially important if the parents' "fantasy" child differs from the real child in sex, physical attributes, or health.

DISCHARGE PLANNING AND PARENT TEACHING

Discharge teaching ideally begins with the admission of the woman to the hospital or birthing centre. Because of short stays after birth, the nurse should teach the family newborn care at every opportunity. Discharge teaching will then be more of a summary than an attempt to crowd all teaching into a short time.

Many hospitals have flow sheets that are helpful in ensuring that all topics have been addressed and that patients understand what has been explained to them. Areas of teaching include the following:

- Basic care of the infant, including bathing, cord care, circumcision care, temperature assessment, feeding, and elimination
- Safety measures, including position for sleep and prevention of sudden infant death syndrome (SIDS)
- Immunization schedules
- Breastfeeding resources, such as the local health department or La Leche League
- Return appointments for well-baby care
- Proper use of car safety seats
- Signs and symptoms of problems and who to contact
- How to suction mucus with a bulb syringe (Skill 11.2) in case of respiratory infection

The nurse should guide the parents in assessing, bathing, and feeding the newborn so that questions can be answered early and parents can demonstrate understanding of skills and behaviours. New parents should be given written instructions because they are often overwhelmed at the volume of information provided in such a short time. They should be given resources—for example, the public health department phone number they can call, and online resources—if they need to refresh their memory when they forget what they were told to do.

Skill 11.3 Bulb Suctioning

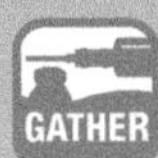

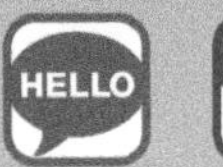

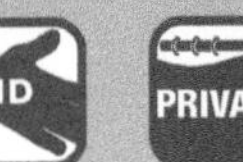

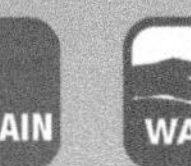

WASH
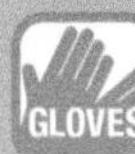

PURPOSE

To clear the airway of mucus

STEPS TO TEACH THE PARENTS

1. Compress the ball of the bulb syringe.
2. Insert the narrow portion of the bulb syringe into the side of the infant's mouth to avoid stimulating the gag reflex. Suction the mouth first to prevent inhalation and aspiration of mucus during a gasp reflex, which is stimulated by nasal suctioning.
3. Release the pressure on the ball of the bulb syringe and listen for the sound of mucus being suctioned.
4. Remove the bulb syringe and empty the contents into a receptacle by compressing the bulb.
5. Compress the bulb syringe and insert into one nostril; then release pressure on the bulb to suction the mucus out.
6. Remove the bulb syringe and empty it into a receptacle. Repeat for the other nostril.
7. The nurse should demonstrate to parents the technique of suctioning with a bulb syringe and review cleaning and storage of the bulb syringe.

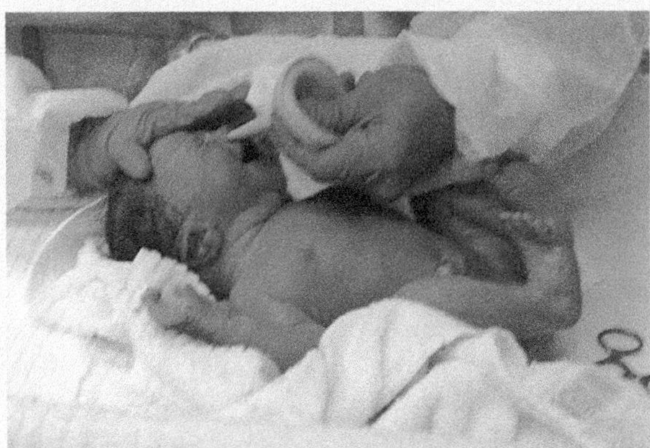

For families that require extra support, the social worker may be helpful in accessing resources. The community health nurse is a key member of the interdisciplinary health care team who can help with after-discharge needs of the family.

FOLLOW-UP CARE

Most newborns are checked by a pediatric health care provider at birth and before discharge. The newborn is assessed at this early check for jaundice, feeding adequacy, urine and stool output, and behaviour. Most healthy newborns are discharged between 24 and 48 hours of age and should then be seen by a health care provider within 2 days of discharge to assess the newborn for feeding, elimination, and jaundice because the bilirubin level usually peaks between 3 and 5 days of age. The frequency of visits to a health care provider will be individualized after this point, as it depends on the needs and concerns of the infant and parents.

Newborns are usually seen again at 2 months after birth to begin well-baby care. When providing discharge teaching, the nurse should emphasize the value of these visits. It should be explained that immunizations are administered to prevent many illnesses. The health care provider assesses the newborn for growth and development, nutrition, and any problems the parents or newborn are having. Teaching parents about the newborn's upcoming needs (anticipatory guidance) helps them to plan ahead to prevent injuries and to promote healthy growth and development.

Parents need to be instructed to call the pediatric health care provider if any of the following symptoms occur, for further follow-up: temperature greater than 38°C (100.4°F) by axilla, refusal of two feedings in a row, two green watery stools, frequent or forceful vomiting, lack of voiding or stooling, and a change in usual behaviour.

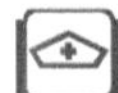
Nursing Tip

Advise parents, if possible, to try to avoid the newborn's exposure to crowds during the early weeks of life because newborns have difficulty forming antibodies against infection until about 2 months of age. Parents should be taught to ask visitors to wash their hands before touching the newborn.

HEALTH TEACHING

The Newborn Bath

Once the infant is able to maintain a normal body temperature, initial skin care is done, which involves washing blood and amniotic fluid from the skin. This bath should not be given until at least 8 to 12 hours after birth, although the WHO recommends waiting until 24 hours after birth, if possible (WHO, 2015). There is some evidence that delaying the bath until at least 12 hours enhances breastfeeding rates in the hospital (Preer, Pisegna, Cook, et al., 2013). Some hospitals are not doing baths at all while the newborn is in the hospital, so before the parents go home they need to be given appropriate resources to access, so they have the information they need for bathing their infant. Until the infant's first bath and shampoo, the nurse needs to wear gloves when handling the newborn, to protect the nurse from exposure to blood and body substances (Skill 11.4).

Skill 11.4 Bathing the Newborn

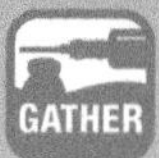

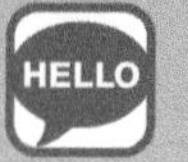

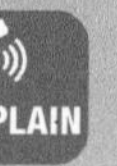

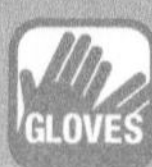

PURPOSE

To cleanse the skin and interact with the newborn

A tub bath is recommended for all newborns unless there is a healing circumcision site. Newborns cry less and stay warmer with tub baths than in sponge baths.

- Give bath between feedings at most convenient time for baby and family.
- Complete baths are not necessary more than two or three times a week because specific areas are washed after diaper changes and when milk is spit up.
- After the bath, the baby may sleep.
- A bath should not be given immediately after feeding, because excessive handling may cause regurgitation.
- Carefully wash and dry each area to prevent heat loss.
- Keep the baby warm by exposing only the area you are washing.

STEPS

Tub Bath

1. Use a plastic tub or a clean sink for the bath.
2. Place a small blanket or pad at the bottom of the tub for comfort and to prevent slipping.
3. Fill the tub to cover as much of the newborn's body as possible and is at a comfortable level for caregiver. The water temperature should be approximately 37°C. A bath thermometer can be used; many have preset temperature alerts. If not available then check the temperature with the elbow. The water should feel comfortably warm.
4. Using a clean, dampened washcloth, wash eyes and face with plain water. Use a separate clean area of the washcloth (or use cotton ball) to wipe each eyelid. Use a clean area to wash outer ear (do not put anything inside ear or nose).
5. Place the baby in the tub. The baby may seem frightened and cry when first put in the water. Holding the baby securely and talking with a soft voice will often help baby adjust to the bath, which is a new experience. Covering the baby with a warm wet cloth will often make the newborn feel more secure.
6. Wash the baby from clean to dirty.
   a. Wash behind ears, where milk that is spit up may accumulate.
   b. Put hand under the baby's shoulders and lift slightly. This allows the creases of the neck to be washed.
   c. Wash the vulva of a female newborn by wiping from front to back to prevent contamination of the vagina or urethra by rectal content. In the male newborn, do not retract the foreskin of the uncircumcised penis. Clean the penis and scrotal area gently. It is important to clean under the scrotum and the folds of the scrotum.
7. Be sure all soap is rinsed off the baby before removing them from the tub.
8. Remove newborn from the tub and immediately wrap in a dry towel.
9. With the baby wrapped in a towel and held in a football hold, gently shampoo the hair; rinse thoroughly with warm water and dry with a clean towel. Hair can also be washed at the beginning or at the end of the bath but ensure that head is well dried after.

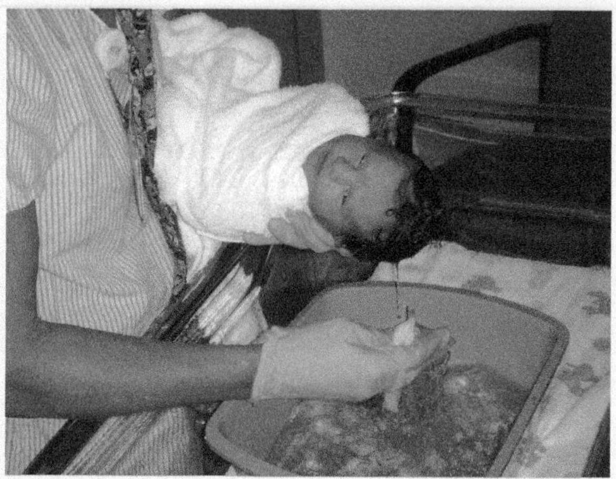

Sponge Bath

1. Test bath water. (It should be approximately 37.2° to 38°C.)
2. Proceed from the cleanest to the most soiled area of the body: from eyes and face to the trunk and extremities and finally to the diaper area. Shampooing the hair could be done first (and well dried) or last to prevent excessive heat loss from the head.
   a. Wash the baby's face with clear water. Use a separate clean area of the washcloth (or use cotton ball) to wipe each eyelid. Use a clean area to wash outer ear (do not put anything inside ear or nose).
   b. Wash behind ears, where milk that is spit up may accumulate.
   c. Put hand under the baby's shoulders and lift slightly. This allows the creases of the neck to be washed.
   d. Wash the vulva of a female newborn by wiping from front to back to prevent contamination of the vagina or urethra by rectal content. In the male newborn, do not retract the foreskin of the uncircumcised penis. Clean the penis and scrotal area gently. It is important to clean under the scrotum and the folds of the scrotum.
3. Dry each part of the body before moving to the next to keep newborn warm.

The bath provides an opportunity for teaching as well as assessment of the infant and infant–parent interaction. The bath is an excellent time for parent–infant social interaction; parents should be taught some of the normal behaviours of the newborn to enhance this experience. The nurse should emphasize certain basic principles of care, such as hand hygiene, cleansing the tub, organizing supplies to be within easy reach, safe water temperature, and techniques for holding the wet infant securely. Teaching such principles can foster good bathing technique at home. Principles of eye and ear care are also reviewed—for example, cotton swabs should not be inserted into the ear or the nose.

The infant needs to be bathed only two or three times a week. Use of alkaline soaps, oils, and lotions is not advised, as they can alter the normal pH of the newborn's skin, making it vulnerable to bacterial infection. Use of powders should be avoided because of the high risk of aspiration of small particles. Some parents prefer to give sponge baths until the umbilical cord falls off and heals (about 1 to 2 weeks), but tub baths are the recommended method of bathing a newborn as they result in less heat loss and less crying (Association of Women's Health, Obstetric and Neonatal Nurses [AWHONN], 2013). Male newborns who are circumcised should have sponge baths until the circumcision heals.

The temperature of the bath water should be approximately 37°C (98.6°F) in a warm room environment at 24° to 27°C. Parents should be taught to test the water with their elbow; the water should feel just comfortably warm. The temperature should not be tested with the hands, as they are not as sensitive to temperature. Special care should be taken to keep the infant covered as much as possible to prevent chilling. Parents should be taught to start bathing the face and then proceed in a cephalocaudal (head-to-toe) direction. The bath should also be done from clean to dirty: Eyes are washed first and genitals last. The nurse can teach the parents to observe the cues and responses of the infant to the warmth of the water and the touch of the washcloth, drying, and dressing. Learning these cues will promote parent–infant bonding.

The nurse may wrap the infant in a towel and use a football hold to shampoo the hair. The shampooing can be done first or last, but the head needs to be well dried because the large surface area of the head predisposes the infant to heat loss.

Nursing Tip

The infant bath provides not only cleaning but also an opportunity to assess the infant and for parents to bond with the infant.

Diaper Care

Disposable diapers are most commonly used in hospitals and homes. They have an outer waterproof layer. Cotton diapers are available in contoured shapes or prefolded styles. Diaper liners are specially treated tissues placed within the cloth diaper. When diapers are soiled, the liner and stool are rinsed into the toilet. The diapers are soaked in cold water, washed with a mild laundry soap, rinsed thoroughly, and dried in a clothes dryer or outdoors in the sun.

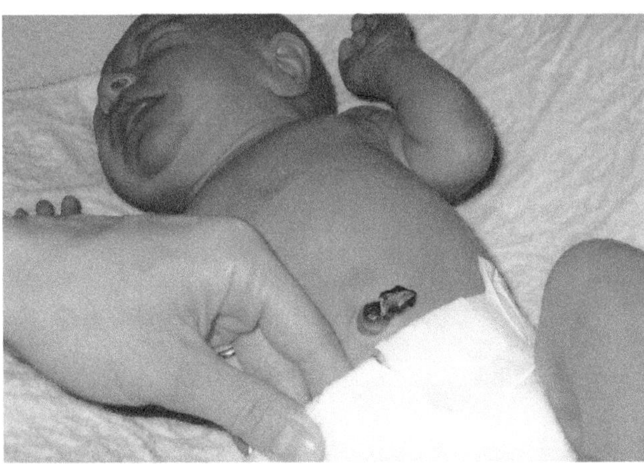

Fig. 11.19 Note that the diaper is folded so that it does not touch the umbilical cord stump. The umbilical cord stump is kept dry and it usually falls off between 1 and 2 weeks after birth.

Diapers that have been improperly washed and rinsed may aggravate rashes. If a rash is present, the buttocks need to be kept exposed to the air as often as possible. Also, diapers should be changed as soon as they are wet. If a rash becomes increasingly worse, the health care provider should be consulted.

Umbilical Cord Care

Umbilical cord care is aimed at preventing infection. Keeping the cord clean and dry shortens the time to cord separation. The use of triple dye or alcohol to promote drying of the cord is no longer recommended. The diaper should be fastened low to allow air circulation to the cord. Fig. 11.19 shows how the diaper is folded so that the edge is below the umbilical cord stump to keep the cord clean and dry. The cord should become dry and brownish black as it dries. The clamp may be removed prior to discharge, although many hospitals send the newborn home with the umbilical clamp in place. It falls off when the umbilical stump falls off. The parents should be taught to report redness of the area or a moist, foul-smelling umbilical cord.

While it is safe to get the umbilical cord wet in the bath, the cord must be dried thoroughly after the bath (Skill 11.5).

Prevention of Sudden Infant Death Syndrome (SIDS)

SIDS is defined as the sudden death of an infant less than 1 year of age that remains unexplained after a thorough case investigation (PHAC et al., 2012). The incidence of SIDS is higher among infants who are male, premature, or of low birth weight, as well as for infants from socioeconomically disadvantaged or Indigenous families.

The following guidelines are recommended to enhance safe sleep and decrease the risk of SIDS:

- Infants must be placed on their back to sleep (for all sleep)
- Infants should not be exposed to tobacco smoke, before and after birth

Skill 11.5 Umbilical Cord Care and Observation

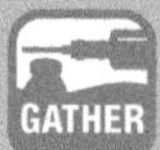

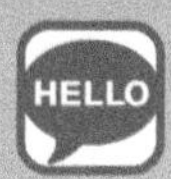

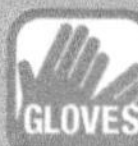

PURPOSE

To assist the cord in drying and falling off

STEPS

1. Check umbilical clamp placement for tight closure. There should be no bleeding or discharge from the cord.
2. Keep cord dry and exposed to the air.
3. Assess the cord for presence of vessels. There should be two arteries and one vein.
4. If the cord becomes soiled, a cotton tip swab and warm water gently washes away the soil, start from the base of the cord and gently wipe upward and outward. Lift the cord away from the newborn's abdomen to facilitate observation or cleansing of all areas, if needed.
5. Observe cord and abdominal area for redness, discharge, or foul odour.
6. Diaper newborn, and be sure the upper end of diaper is folded down *below* the cord so it does not rub against the cord.
7. Document observations, condition of the cord, teaching of the parents, and the parents' response.

- Infants should sleep in a crib, cradle, or bassinet that meets current Canadian Safety Association (CSA) standards.
- Pillows, stuffed animals, bumper pads, and blankets should not be placed in the crib of the newborn.
- Infants should not be overdressed, or overheated by blankets, as this increases the risk for SIDS.
- Infants should share a room (but not bed) with a parent or caregiver for 6 months.
- Breastfeeding provides some protection for newborns from the risk of SIDS.
- Pacifiers appear to provide a protective effect for SIDS. Their use does not seem to impair breastfeeding; however, delaying the introduction of a pacifier is best left until breastfeeding is well established.
- *Bed sharing* is when a newborn sleeps on the same sleeping surface, such as an adult bed, sofa, or armchair, as that of an adult or another child. Sharing a sleeping surface increases the risk of SIDS. The risk is particularly high for infants less than 4 months of age. Thus bed sharing is not recommended.

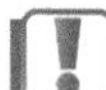
Safety Alert!

Instruct parents about the danger of suffocation if the infant sleeps in the same bed with the parents.

Clothing

Newborns need the same amount of clothing that an adult needs and not any extra layers. A cap is used because the newborn's head is the largest body surface area and can be a source of significant heat loss. Clothing should be soft, washable, and easy to put on and take off. Parents should be instructed to launder new clothing and sheets before using them, to prevent skin irritation. Use of nightgowns with drawstring necks is to be avoided because this may lead to strangulation. Fig. 11.20 illustrates the simplest way to dress the newborn.

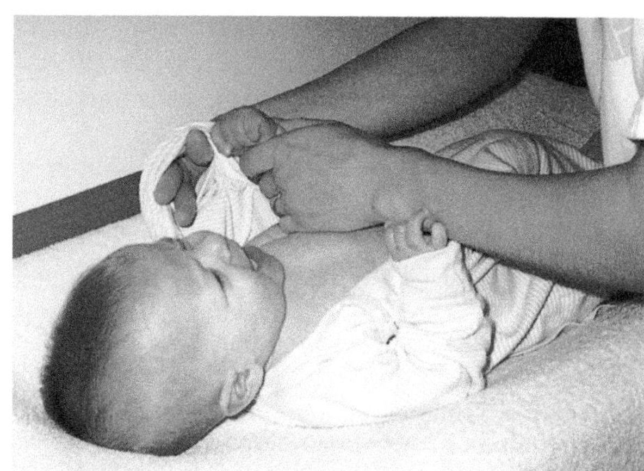

Fig. 11.20 Dressing the newborn. The simplest technique of dressing the newborn is to place the hand through the sleeve, grasp the infant's hand, and gently pull it through the sleeve.

Swaddling has been used to keep infants warm but can be associated with various risks to the infant. For instance, wrapping babies tightly in blankets can cause overheating, which can put them at greater risk of SIDS. A blanket can also become unravelled and cover the baby's face, increasing the risk for suffocation. A blanket that is too tight can cause hip dysplasia and limit chest expansion (Di Constanzo, 2014). The CPS (2018) has developed safe swaddling guidelines that include the following:

- Don't overdress the baby. Use light blankets so the baby doesn't overheat.
- Stop swaddling when the baby shows signs of rolling over.
- Make sure the baby's nose and mouth are not covered.
- Make sure the baby can still move their legs, to avoid hip dysplasia (abnormality of the hip joint where the socket does not fully cover the ball portion, which can increase the risk for dislocation).

Siblings

Mothers who have other children at home often worry about how they will introduce the new baby to the other children and how they will cope with another child. Parents can try having the new baby give the older children a present when they first visit; this is often an effective strategy for helping older children to accept the new baby. Younger children often exhibit regression in toilet independence behaviour or wanting to sleep in a crib. Parents need to understand that this is normal and not to punish the child for the behaviour but rather to ignore it and reward positive behaviour. Mothers need to spend more time with a newborn, so it is a good time for partners and other family members to spend more time with the older children.

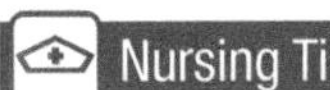

Nursing Tip

If siblings are waiting when mother and baby return from the hospital, it is helpful if the partner arrives carrying the newborn. This leaves the mother's arms free for hugs before turning attention to the new child.

Car Seat Safety

The nurse should teach parents the importance of using newborn car safety seats and how to use them correctly (Fig. 11.21). The newborn must be placed in a car seat in a semi-reclining position in the car's back seat (never in the front), facing the rear until the child is 10 kg and able to walk unassisted (Government of Canada, 2018). The seat's harness is snugly fastened, and the seat is secured to the automobile seat with the seat belt. Parents should consult their car's instruction manual for specific instructions on securing safety seats. See Additional Learning Resources at the end of this chapter for more information from the Government of Canada on car seat safety.

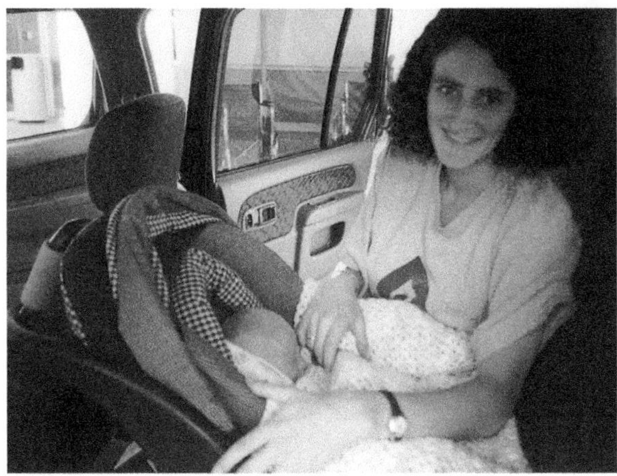

Fig. 11.21 A new mother prepares to leave the birth facility. The newborn is placed in a car seat that will be rear-facing and secured by the car's seat belt for the ride home.

The nurse must emphasize to parents that even in a low-impact accident, the newborn can be thrown from the car safety seat if the newborn is improperly restrained and will become a "missile" within the car or will even be ejected from it. While air bags can prevent serious injuries to older children and adults in motor vehicle accidents, the air bag thrusts a newborn toward the rear, causing a whiplike motion that can seriously injure the infant's neck or head.

Unfolding Case Study

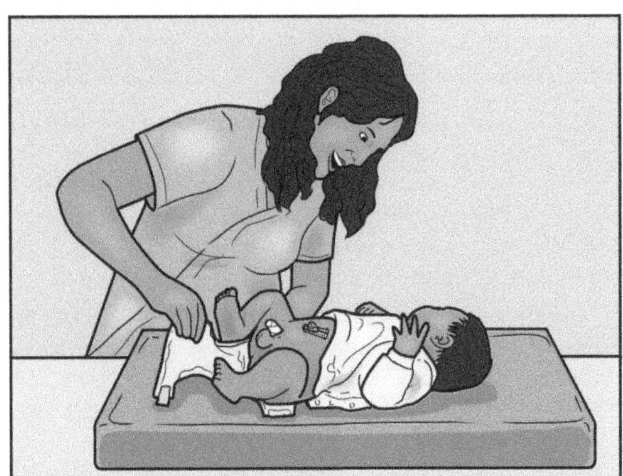

Tess and her partner, Luis, were introduced to the reader in Chapter 2, and each chapter has followed Tess through her labour and birth. She has given birth to twins. Their daughter, Sofia, was admitted to the NICU, accompanied by Luis. (Sofia will be discussed in Chapter 12.) After 1 hour in the labour and birth room, their son Marco was admitted to the postpartum unit with Tess.

Baby Marco's weight is 3.19 kg and he has had one black-green tarry stool and one void since birth. The cord clamp is in place and the umbilical cord stump is clean and dry. Tess is planning on breastfeeding the twins.

QUESTIONS

1. What can the nurse tell Tess about the normal changes in the appearance of her infant's stool that she will see in the next week when she is at home?
2. What will the nurse tell Tess about the care of the umbilical cord when she is at home? How should Tess modify the diapering technique while the umbilical cord stump is still in place?
3. Tess is worried that she will not have enough breastmilk for the twins. How can she tell if the infants are receiving enough breastmilk when they are discharged and at home?
4. Tess states that Marco must be cold because she sees his chin quiver and his hands are a bit blue, so she wants to delay bathing the baby. What can the nurse teach Tess about her baby's quivering chin, his blue hands, and how often baths should be given to newborn infants?
5. Tess asks about the risks and benefits of circumcision. What does the nurse teach Tess?
6. What does the nurse teach Tess and Luis about the prevention of SIDS?

Get Ready for the Certification Examination!

Key Points

- Assessment of the newborn includes gestational age, weight and length measurements, reflexes, system assessment, and bonding with parents.
- Transition of the newborn occurs during the first 6 to 8 hours of life, when the newborn makes the transition to extrauterine life.
- The newborn has an unstable heat-regulating system and must be kept warm.
- Heat loss occurs in the newborn via conduction, convection, evaporation, and radiation.
- The newborn is born with certain reflexes. Three of these are the Moro reflex, the rooting reflex, and the tonic neck reflex.
- Physiological jaundice becomes evident after the second and third days of life and lasts for about 1 week.
- Although the kidneys function at birth, they are not fully developed. Likewise, the immune system is not fully activated.
- Vernix caseosa is a cheeselike substance that covers the skin of the newborn at birth.
- Meconium, the first stool of the newborn, is a mixture of amniotic fluid and secretions of the intestinal glands. These stools change in colour from tarry greenish black, to greenish yellow (transitional stools), to yellow gold (milk stools).
- Proper hand hygiene is essential for preventing infection in newborn infants.
- The hydration status of newborns can be evaluated by determining the number and consistency of stools, frequency of voiding, appearance of sunken fontanelles, and status of tissue turgor.
- The normal newborn infant will lose about 10% of the birth weight in the first few days of life but will return to the birth weight by the age of 2 weeks.
- The fontanelles are spaces between the skull bones of the newborn that allow for moulding and provide space for the brain to grow. They are known as "soft spots" on the infant's head.
- Caput succedaneum is edema of the infant's scalp that occurs during the birth process.
- Cephalohematoma is a collection of blood under the periosteum of a cranial bone. The swelling does not cross the suture lines of the skull bones.
- Newborn screening tests such as the phenylketonuria (PKU) test are used to identify disorders that can be treated to reduce or prevent disability.
- The nurse must always keep the possibility of newborn abductions in mind when providing care.
- Discharge teaching begins before birth and continues to discharge date. It includes infant care, follow-up visits, community resources, and safety.
- The infant bath time is used to cleanse the skin, assess the newborn, and teach about newborn behaviours to the parents.
- Umbilical cord care involves observing the cord for infection and bleeding and keeping the cord dry until it falls off naturally.
- Newborns should sleep on their back in order to decrease the risk of sudden infant death syndrome (SIDS).
- When swaddling the infant, the hips and knees should remain in a flex, abducted position.

Additional Learning Resources

evolve Go to your Evolve website (http://evolve.elsevier.com/Canada/Leifer) for the following learning resources:

- Answer Key for Critical Thinking Questions
- Answer Key for Textbook Review Questions
- Audio Glossary
- Interactive Review Questions
- Skills Performance Checklists
- Video clips and more!

Online Resources

- Health Canada, *Child Car Seat Safety:* https://www.tc.gc.ca/en/services/road/child-car-seat-safety.html
- Public Health Agency of Canada, Health Canada, Canadian Paediatric Society, Canadian Foundation for the Study of Infant Deaths & Canadian Institute of Child Health, *Joint Statement on Safe Sleep: Preventing Sudden Infant Deaths in Canada:* https://www.canada.ca/en/public-health/services/health-promotion/childhood-adolescence/stages-childhood/infancy-birth-two-years/safe-sleep/joint-statement-on-safe-sleep.html

Review Questions

1. Which would be the best way for a nurse to maintain a newborn's temperature immediately after birth?
   - **a.** Dry the newborn thoroughly, including the head.
   - **b.** Give the newborn a bath using warm water.
   - **c.** Place the newborn under a radiant warmer.
   - **d.** Feed 30 to 60 mL of warmed formula
2. A mother of a newly born infant reports to a nurse that her infant has had a black tarry stool. The nurse would tell the mother which of the following?
   - **a.** This is most likely caused by blood the infant may have swallowed during the birth process.
   - **b.** The health care provider will be promptly notified.
   - **c.** The infant will be given nothing by mouth (remain NPO) until a stool culture is taken.
   - **d.** This is a normal stool in newborn infants.
3. Which assessment finding of a newborn infant should be promptly reported to the health care provider? *(Select all that apply.)*
   - **a.** Grunting respirations
   - **b.** Temperature of 36.9°C
   - **c.** Pulse rate of 80 beats/min.
   - **d.** Nasal flaring

e. Acrocyanosis

4. Infections in the newborn require prompt intervention because of which of the following?
   a. They spread more quickly.
   b. Infections that are relatively harmless to an adult can be fatal to the newborn.
   c. The portals of entry and exit are more numerous.
   d. The newborn has few defenses against infection.
5. The mother states that her newborn has white pinpoint "pimples" on his nose and chin and she plans to squeeze them to make them disappear. What would be the best response by a nurse?
   a. "Be sure to wipe the area with an alcohol sponge to avoid infection."
   b. "Ask your health care provider to prescribe an antibiotic ointment for the pimples."
   c. "These pimples are called *Epstein pearls* and are a normal occurrence."
   d. "These pimples are called *milia* and will disappear on their own in a week or two."
6. Which observation of the newborn should be reported to the health care provider?
   a. A swelling beneath the scalp on one side of the head
   b. A respiratory rate of 60 breaths/min
   c. Flaccid muscle tone
   d. Cyanosis of the hands and feet
7. A nurse documents the following observations on a newly born infant. Which of the following should be immediately reported to the health care provider? *(Select all that apply).*
   a. Unilateral Moro reflex
   b. Small blood tinged mucous discharge from the vagina
   c. Drooling
   d. Acrocyanosis

Critical Thinking Question

1. A new mother brings her 5-day-old infant to the clinic and states she wants to stop breastfeeding and start formula because her infant weighs less now than he did at birth. She states that her breasts are small anyway, so she probably is not providing enough milk to help him gain weight. What is the best response of the nurse?

REFERENCES

Ambalavanan, N., & Carlo, W. A. (2016). Jaundice and hyperbilirubinemia in the newborn. In R. Kliegman, B. Stanton, J. St. Geme, & et al. (Eds.), *Nelson textbook of pediatrics* (20th ed.). Philadelphia: Saunders.

Association of Women's Health, Obstetric and Neonatal Nurses (AWHONN). (2013). *Neonatal skin care: Evidence-based clinical practice guideline* (3rd ed.). Washington, DC: Author.

Aziz, K., Dancey, P., & Canadian Paediatric Society (CPS). (2004). Screening guidelines for newborns at risk for low blood glucose. *Paediatrics & Child Health, 9*(10), 723–729. Reaffirmed February 1, 2014.

Barrington, K. J., Sankaran, K., & Canadian Paediatric Society (CPS). (2007). Guidelines for detection, management and prevention of hyperbilirubinemia in term and late term newborn infants [35 or more weeks gestation]. *Paediatrics & Child Health, 12*(Suppl. B), 1B–12B. Reaffirmed 2016.

Canadian Paediatric Society (CPS). (2016). *Newborn hearing screening*. Retrieved from: https://www.cps.ca/en/status-report/newborn-hearing-screening.

Canadian Paediatric Society (CPS). (2018). *Swaddling*. Retrieved from: https://www.caringforkids.cps.ca/handouts/swaddling.

Carlo, W. (2016). The newborn infant. In R. Kliegman, B. Stanton, J. St. Geme et al (Eds.), *Nelson textbook of pediatrics* (20th ed.). Philadelphia: Saunders.

Cignacco, E. L., Sellam, G., Stoffel, L., et al. (2012). Oral sucrose with facilitated tucking is effective pain control for preterm infants: A randomized control trial. *Pediatrics, 129*(2), 299–308.

Di Constanzo, M. (2014). A safer sleep. *Registered Nurse Journal, 26*(3), 10–14. Retrieved from: http://www.who.int/maternal_child_adolescent/publications/WHO-MCA-PNC-2014-Briefer_A4.pdf?ua=1.

Gladding, I. (2017). Nursing care of the newborn and family. In S. Perry, M. Hockenberry, D. Lowdermilk, et al. (Eds.), *Maternal child nursing care in Canada* (2nd ed.). Toronto, ON: Elsevier.

Government of Canada. (2018). *Installing and using a child car seat, booster seat, or seat belt.* Retrieved from: https://www.tc.gc.ca/en/services/road/child-car-seat-safety/installing-using-child-car-seat-booster-seat-seat-belt.html.

Health Canada, Canadian Paediatric Society, & Dietitians of Canada and Breastfeeding Committee for Canada. (2015). *Nutrition for healthy term infants: Birth to six months.* Ottawa: Health Canada. Retrieved from: http://www.hc-sc.gc.ca/fn-an/nutrition/infant-nourisson/recom/index-eng.php.

O'Flaherty, P. (2017). Physiological adaptations of the newborn. In S. Perry, M. Hockenberry, D. Lowdermilk, et al. (Eds.), *Maternal child nursing care in Canada* (2nd ed.). Toronto, ON: Elsevier.

Preer, G., Pisegna, J., Cook, J., et al. (2013). Delaying the bath and in-hospital breastfeeding rates. *Breastfeeding Medicine, 8*(6), 485–490. https://doi.org/10.1089/bfm.2012.0158.

Public Health Agency of Canada (PHAC). (2009). *What mothers say: The Canadian maternity experiences survey*. Ottawa: Author. Retrieved from: http://www.phac-aspc.gc.ca/rhs-ssg/pdf/survey-eng.pdf.

Public Health Agency of Canada (PHAC), Canadian Paediatric Society, Canadian Foundation for Study of Infant Deaths, Canadian Institute for Child Health, & Health Canada. (2012). *Joint statement on safe sleep: Preventing sudden infant deaths in Canada*. Ottawa: Author. Retrieved from: http://www.phac-aspc.gc.ca/hp-ps/dca-dea/stages-etapes/childhood-enfance_0-2/sids/pdf/jsss-ecss2011-eng.pdf.

Sorokan, S. T., Finlay, J. C., Jefferies, A. L., et al. (2015). Newborn male circumcision. *Paediatric & Child Health, 20*(6), 311–315.

Stevens, B., Yamada, J., Ohlsson, A., et al. (2016). Sucrose for analgesia (pain relief) in newborn infants undergoing painful procedures. *Cochrane Database of Systematic Reviews*, (7), CD001069. https://doi.org/10.1002/14651858.CD001069.pub5.

World Health Organization (WHO). (2015). *Postnatal care for mothers and newborns: Highlights from the World Health Organization 2013 guidelines.* Retrieved from: http://www.who.int/maternal_child_adolescent/publications/WHO-MCA-PNC-2014-Briefer_A4.pdf?ua=1.

12 High-Risk Newborns

http://evolve.elsevier.com/Canada/Leifer

Jola Berkman

Objectives

1. Define each key term listed.
2. Differentiate between the preterm and the low–birth weight newborn.
3. List three causes of preterm birth.
4. Describe selected problems and needs of preterm newborns and the nursing goals associated with each problem.
5. Describe the symptoms of cold stress and methods of maintaining thermoregulation.
6. Contrast the techniques for feeding preterm and full-term newborns.
7. Discuss two ways to help facilitate maternal–infant bonding for a preterm newborn.
8. Describe possible family reactions to preterm infants and nursing interventions.
9. List three characteristics of the post-term infant.
10. Outline the causes and treatment of hemolytic disease of the newborn (erythroblastosis fetalis).
11. Devise a plan of care for a newborn receiving phototherapy.
12. Describe home phototherapy.
13. Discuss the care related to neonatal opioid withdrawal syndrome.
14. Discuss the assessment and nursing care of a newborn with macrosomia.
15. Discuss the care of the newborn with Down syndrome.
16. Discuss the dietary needs of a newborn with phenylketonuria.

Key Terms

apnea (ĂP-nē-ă)
Ballard scoring system
birth defects
bradycardia (brăd-ĕ-KĂHR-dē-ă)
bronchopulmonary dysplasia (brŏn-kō-PŬL-mŏ-năr-ē dĭs-PLĀ-zhă)
classic phenylketonuria
cold stress
early term infant
full-term infant
galactosemia
gestational age
hemolytic disease of the newborn (HDN)
hyperbilirubinemia (hī-pŭr-bĭl-ē-rū-bĭ-NĒ-mē-ă)
hypocalcemia (hī-pō-kăl-SĒ-mē-ă)
hypoglycemia (hī-pō-glī-SĒ-mē-ă)
hypoxia
icterus (ĬK-tŭr-ŭs)
intracranial hemorrhage
kangaroo care
kernicterus
lanugo (lă-NŪ-gō)
late-term infant
macrosomia (măk-rō-SŌ-mē-ă)
meconium aspiration syndrome (MAS)
necrotizing enterocolitis (NEC) (NĔK-rō-tīz-ĭng ĕn-tĕr-ō-kō-LĪ-tĭs)
neonatal opioid withdrawal syndrome (NOWS)
neutral thermal environment
phototherapy
post-term infant
preterm infant
previability
pulse oximetry
respiratory distress syndrome (RDS)
retinopathy of prematurity (ROP)
sepsis (SĔP-sĭs)
surfactant (sŭr-FĂK-tănt)
tachypnea
thermoregulation
transient tachypnea of the newborn (TTN)

At birth, all infants need to transition from intrauterine life to extrauterine life. This transition involves changes in their respiratory, cardiovascular, metabolic, and neurological systems. Some infants may experience delayed transition due to prematurity, postmaturity, growth restriction, or various other factors. Any infant that experiences a delay in transition may require additional observation and care.

In the past, a newborn was classified solely by birth weight. The emphasis is now on gestational age and level of maturation. Fig. 12.1 shows two different term infants of the same gestational age. One newborn would be classified as small for gestational age (SGA), which may be the result of intrauterine growth restriction (IUGR), because of its weight and size. Term infants over 4 000 g (8 lb 13 oz) may be classified as large for gestational age (LGA). Current data also indicate

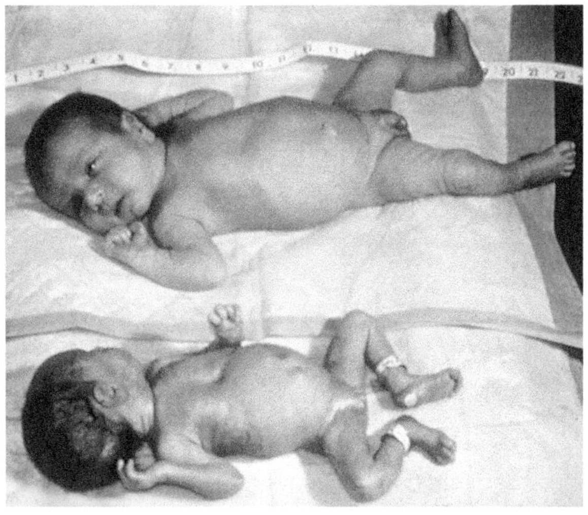

Fig. 12.1 Two different term infants of the same gestational age. These infants are discordant twins. The variation in size and weight resulted from a malformation of the placenta. (From Zitelli, B. L., & Davis, H. W. [2012]. *Zitelli and Davis' atlas of pediatric physical diagnosis* [6th ed.]. St. Louis: Saunders.))

that intrauterine growth rates are not the same for all infants and that individual factors must be considered. **Gestational age** refers to the actual time, from conception to birth, that the fetus remains in the uterus. For the **preterm infant** this is less than 37 weeks. Infants born between 34 and 37 weeks are called *late preterm infants*. These infants may have difficulties with transition that requires admission to a neonatal intensive care unit (NICU). Infants born prior to 33 weeks' gestation have even greater difficulty with transition and may require admission to a tertiary-level NICU. An **early term infant** is born between 37 weeks and 38 weeks, 6 days of gestation. The **full-term infant** is born between 39 and 40 weeks, 6 days, and the **late-term infant** is born between 41 weeks and 41 weeks, 6 days. The **post-term infant** is born beyond 42 weeks. The American College of Obstetricians and Gynecologists Committee on Obstetric Practice and Society for Maternal-Fetal Medicine (2013/2017) redefined "term pregnancy" and "term infant" to emphasize that every week in utero up to 39 weeks is important for optimal fetal development. A low–birth weight infant weighs 2 500 g (5 lb 8 oz) or less. Low birth weight can be caused by IUGR or just be a trait of an SGA newborn, and both are treated as high-risk newborns.

One standardized method used to estimate gestational age within the first 1 to 2 weeks of age is the **Ballard scoring system**, which is based on the infant's external characteristics and neurological development (Figs. 12.2 and 12.3). The Ballard score, the estimated gestational age based on the mother's last normal menstrual period, and ultrasound evaluations all are methods used to evaluate the gestational age of the newborn infant.

Level of maturation refers to how well developed the infant is at birth and the ability of the organs to function outside the uterus. The health care provider can determine much about the maturity of the newborn through careful physical examination, observation of behaviour, and family history. An infant who is born at 34 weeks of gestation, weighs 1 590 g (3 lb 8 oz) at birth, does not have multifactorial birth defects, and has had a good placenta may be healthier than a full-term, "small-for-date" infant whose placenta was insufficient for any number of reasons. Such an infant is also probably in better condition than the heavy but immature infant of a diabetic mother. Each infant has different and distinct needs.

THE PRETERM NEWBORN

The preterm newborn is the most common admission to the intensive care nursery. With increased specialization and sophisticated monitoring techniques, many infants who in the past would have died are now surviving. The nurse's role continues to be increasingly complex, with greater emphasis placed on subtle clinical observations and on technology. In acquainting the student with the preterm infant, one goal of this chapter is to encourage an appreciation of the preterm infant's struggle for survival and the intense responsibility placed on those entrusted with their care. In this discussion the words *preterm* and *premature* are used synonymously. Any newborn whose life or quality of existence is threatened is considered high risk and requires close supervision by professionals in a special NICU. Preterm newborns constitute a majority of these patients. Preterm birth is responsible for more deaths during the first year of life than any other single factor. Preterm infants also have a higher percentage of birth defects. Prematurity and low birth weight are often concomitant, and both factors are associated with increased newborn morbidity and mortality. The less an infant weighs at birth, the greater the risks to life during birth and immediately thereafter.

CAUSES OF PRETERM BIRTH

The predisposing causes of preterm birth are numerous; in many instances, the cause is unknown. Prematurity may be caused by multiple births; illness of the mother (e.g., malnutrition, heart disease, diabetes mellitus, or infectious conditions); or complications of pregnancy itself, such as gestational hypertension, placental abnormalities that may result in premature rupture of the membranes, placenta previa (in which the placenta lies over the cervix instead of higher in the uterus), and premature separation of the placenta (placental abruption). If the mother had a previous preterm infant she is also at higher risk of giving birth to another preterm infant. Studies indicate relationships between prematurity and poverty, smoking, alcohol consumption, and the use of licit and illicit substances during pregnancy. Adequate prenatal care to prevent preterm birth is extremely important.

MATURATIONAL ASSESSMENT OF GESTATIONAL AGE (New Ballard Score)

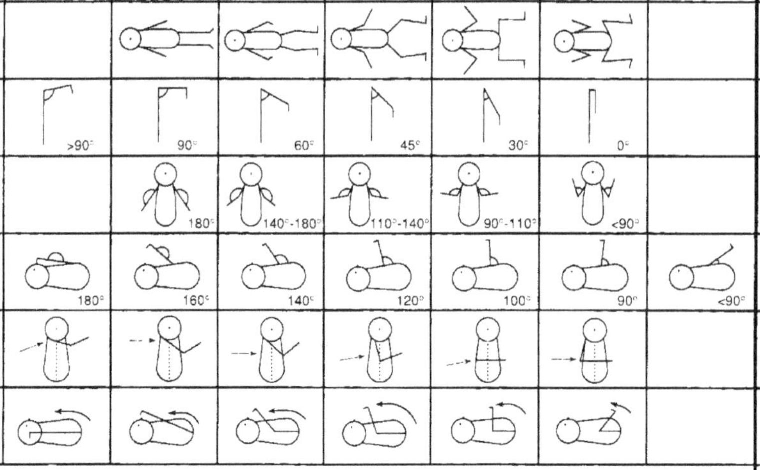

NEUROMUSCULAR MATURITY

NEUROMUSCULAR MATURITY SIGN	SCORE -1	0	1	2	3	4	5	RECORD SCORE HERE
POSTURE								
SQUARE WINDOW (Wrist)	>90°	90°	60°	45°	30°	0°		
ARM RECOIL		180°	140°-180°	110°-140°	90°-110°	<90°		
POPLITEAL ANGLE	180°	160°	140°	120°	100°	90°	<90°	
SCARF SIGN								
HEEL TO EAR								
							TOTAL NEUROMUSCULAR MATURITY SCORE	

A

PHYSICAL MATURITY

PHYSICAL MATURITY SIGN	SCORE -1	0	1	2	3	4	5	RECORD SCORE HERE
SKIN	sticky friable transparent	gelatinous red translucent	smooth pink visible veins	superficial peeling &/or rash, few veins	cracking pale areas rare veins	parchment deep cracking no vessels	leathery cracked wrinkled	
LANUGO	none	sparse	abundant	thinning	bald areas	mostly bald		
PLANTAR SURFACE	heel-toe 40-50 mm:-1 <40 mm:-2	>50 mm no crease	faint red marks	anterior transverse crease only	creases ant. 2/3	creases over entire sole		
BREAST	imperceptible	barely perceptible	flat areola no bud	stippled areola 1-2 mm bud	raised areola 3-4 mm bud	full areola 5-10 mm bud		
EYE/EAR	lids fused loosely: -1 tightly: -2	lids open pinna flat stays folded	slightly curved pinna; soft; slow recoil	well-curved pinna; soft but ready recoil	formed & firm instant recoil	thick cartilage ear stiff		
GENITALS (Male)	scrotum flat, smooth	scrotum empty faint rugae	testes in upper canal rare rugae	testes descending few rugae	testes down good rugae	testes pendulous deep rugae		
GENITALS (Female)	clitoris prominent & labia flat	prominent clitoris & small labia minora	prominent clitoris & enlarging minora	majora & minora equally prominent	majora large minora small	majora cover clitoris & minora		
							TOTAL PHYSICAL MATURITY SCORE	

B

SCORE

Neuromuscular ________

Physical ________

Total ________

MATURITY RATING

score	weeks
-10	20
-5	22
0	24
5	26
10	28
15	30
20	32
25	34
30	36
35	38
40	40
45	42
50	44

GESTATIONAL AGE (weeks)

By dates ________

By ultrasound ________

By exam ________

C

Fig. 12.2 The new Ballard scale estimates gestational age based on the newborn's neuromuscular maturity **(A)** and physical maturity **(B)**. A newborn will score 45 for a 42-week gestation, or only 20 for a 32-week gestation **(C)**. An accurate assessment of the newborn's maturity can aid in the development of an individualized plan of care for that newborn infant. (From Ballard, J. L., Khoury, J., Wedig, K., et al. [1991]. New Ballard score expanded to include extremely premature infants, *Journal of Pediatrics, 119*, 417–423.)

After birth, early parental interaction with the infant is recognized as essential to the bonding (attachment) process. The presence of parents in special care nurseries is commonplace. Multidisciplinary care that is family centred is vital, particularly because current studies indicate a correlation between high-risk births and child abuse and neglect.

CARE AT BIRTH

The pediatric health care provider appraises the physical status of the preterm newborn at birth. The immediate needs are to clear the infant's airway and to provide warmth. If the infant requires any resuscitation, the Neonatal Resuscitation Program Algorithm will be

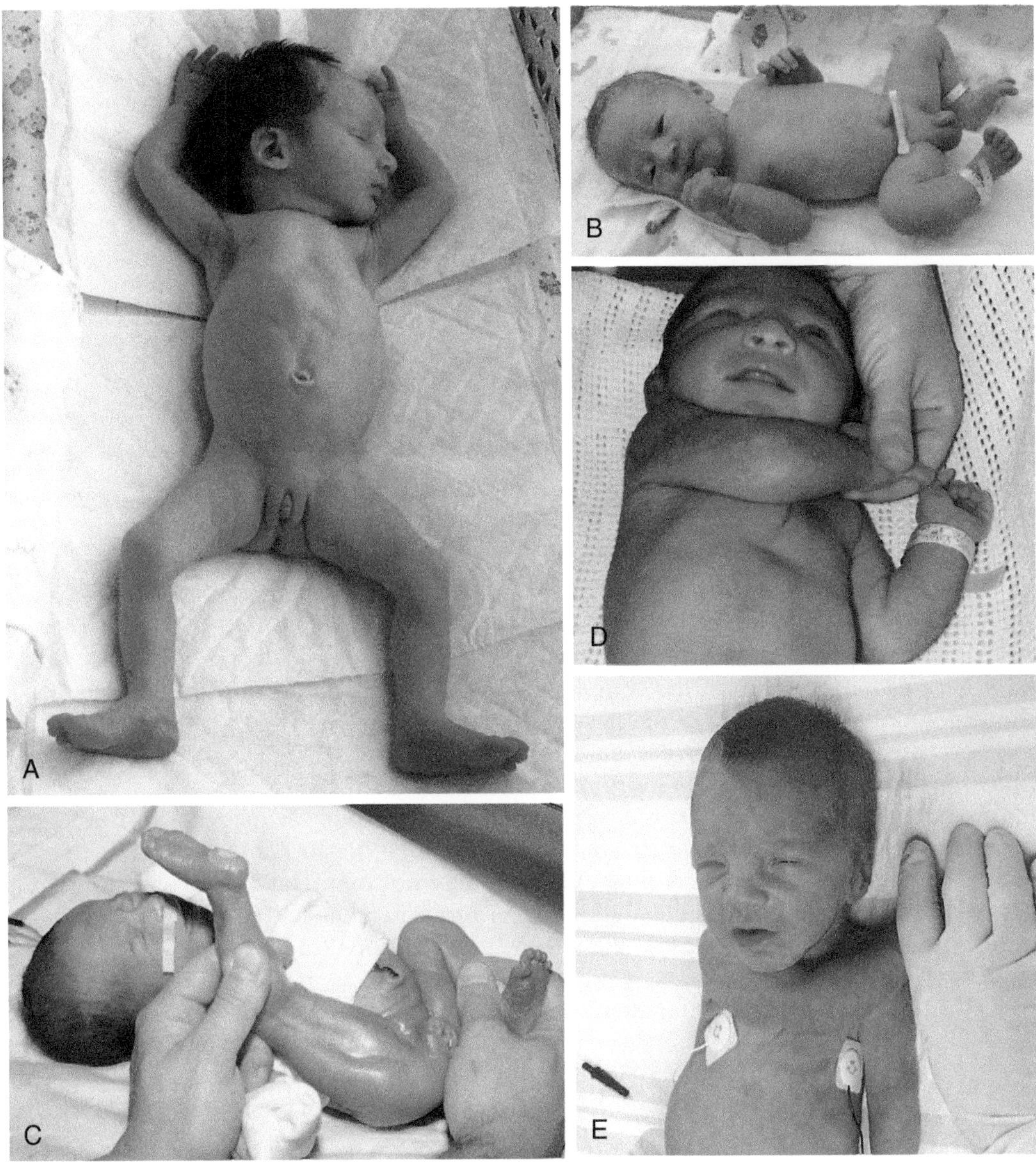

Fig. 12.3 **A,** The preterm newborn. This infant evidences the extended posture of the arms and legs characteristic of the preterm infant. The skin is thin and transparent, and the labia are open and gaping. (See Ballard scale, Fig. 12.2.) **B,** The full-term newborn. The completely flexed arms and legs evidence good muscle tone. The flexed position of the newborn limits the loss of body heat, as less skin surface is exposed to the air. **C,** Popliteal angle. This heel-to-ear manoeuvre demonstrates the easy extension of the leg consistent with a 30-week gestation infant. A full-term infant would show muscle resistance to this manoeuvre. (See Ballard scale, Fig. 12.2.) **D,** When the arm of the full-term infant is pulled across the chest, the elbow goes only as far as the chin in the midline. This is called the *scarf sign.* **E,** When the arm is pulled across the chest of the preterm infant, it can be pulled into a straight line, with the elbow passing the chin at the midline (abnormal scarf sign). (**C** and **D,** from Zitelli, B. L., & Davis, H. W. [2012]. *Zitelli and Davis' atlas of pediatric physical diagnosis* [6th ed.]. St. Louis: Saunders. **E,** from Murray, S. S., & McKinney, E. S. [2014]. *Foundations of maternal-newborn and women's health nursing* [6th ed.]. St. Louis: Saunders.)

followed. Infants born prior to 32 weeks' gestation may be wrapped in a special plastic wrap to prevent insensible water loss and hypothermia (American Academy of Pediatrics & American Heart Association, 2016). For all preterm infants, care must be taken to dry the head thoroughly and put a warm cap on it. The appropriate dose of vitamin K is also administered, with babies weighing 1 500 g or less receiving 0.5 mg intramuscularly (IM), and babies weighing more than 1 500 g receiving 1.0 mg IM (McMillan & Canadian Paediatric Society [CPS] Fetus and Newborn Committee, 1997/2018). Depending on provincial health legislation eye prophylaxis may be administered. After this the baby is identified and then transferred in a special transport isolette to the nursery. The nurse in charge receives a report on the general condition of the newborn, the type of birth, and any complications that have occurred. Box 12.1 lists some nursing goals for care of the preterm newborn.

Box 12.1 Nursing Goals for the Preterm Newborn

The nursing goals in caring for the preterm newborn include the following:
- Improve respiration.
- Maintain body heat (keep the "preemie" warm).
- Conserve energy.
- Prevent infection.
- Provide proper nutrition and hydration.
- Give good skin care.
- Observe the infant carefully and record observations.
- Support and encourage the parents.

Many hospitals transfer their preterm infants to special medical centres geared toward caring for them. The transport team is briefed by the neonatologist and is dispatched to the referring hospital. A life-support infant-transport isolette that can be carried by ambulance (and sometimes helicopter) is used (Fig. 12.4).

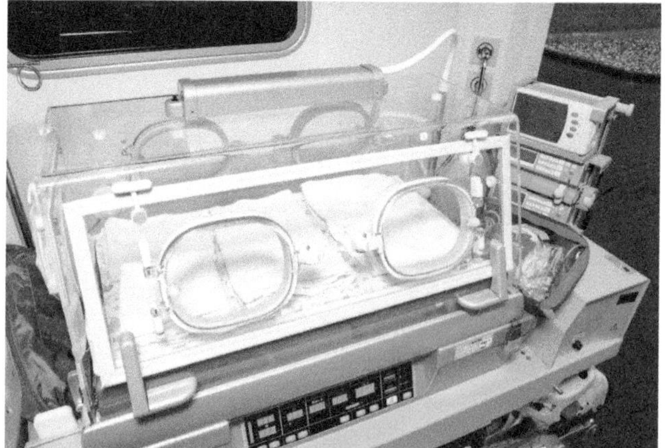

Fig. 12.4 Transport isolette. (iStock.com/ollo)

PHYSICAL CHARACTERISTICS

Preterm birth deprives the newborn of the complete benefits of intrauterine life. The infant in the isolette may resemble a fetus of 7 months of gestation. The skin is transparent and loose. Superficial veins may be seen beneath the abdomen and scalp. There is a lack of subcutaneous fat, and fine hair (*lanugo*) covers the forehead, shoulders, and arms. At birth the cheeselike vernix caseosa is abundant. The extremities appear short. The soles of the feet have few creases, and the abdomen protrudes. The nails are short. The genitalia are small. In girls, the labia majora may be open (see Fig. 12.3, *A*).

RELATED PROBLEMS

Inadequate Respiratory Function

Important structural changes occur in the fetal lungs during the second half of the pregnancy. The alveoli, or air sacs, enlarge, which brings them closer to the capillaries in the lungs. The failure of this phenomenon to occur leads to many deaths attributed to previability. In addition, the muscles that move the chest are not fully developed; the abdomen is distended, creating pressure on the diaphragm; the stimulation of the respiratory centre in the brain is immature; and the gag and cough reflexes are weak because of immature nerve supply. Oxygen may be required and can be administered via endonasal catheter or isolette. The oxygen must be warmed and humidified to prevent drying of the mucous membranes. Mechanical ventilation may be required. Oxygen saturation levels should be monitored. The infant requires close observation and is admitted to the NICU.

Respiratory distress syndrome

Respiratory distress syndrome (RDS) is a result of anatomical and biochemical lung immaturity, which leads to decreased gas exchange. In this disease, there is a deficient synthesis or release of surfactant, a chemical in the lungs. For adequate gas exchange the alveoli need to remain open. Surfactant reduces the surface tension in the alveoli, allowing them to remain open for adequate gas exchange (Davis, Barrington, & CPS Fetus and Newborn Committee, 2005/2015).

Manifestations. In general, the symptoms of respiratory distress are apparent after birth, but they may not manifest for several hours (Fig. 12.5). Respirations increase to 60 breaths/min or more. Rapid respirations (**tachypnea**) are accompanied by gruntlike sounds, nasal flaring, cyanosis, and intercostal and sternal retractions. Edema, lassitude, and apnea occur as the condition becomes more severe. Mechanical ventilation may be necessary. The treatment of these infants should be carried out in the NICU.

Treatment. Surfactant begins to appear in the fetal alveoli at approximately 24 weeks of gestation and is at a level to enable the infant to breathe adequately at birth by 34 weeks of gestation. If a woman presents with possible preterm labour, it is possible to increase the production of surfactant by giving the mother injections of corticosteroids such as betamethasone. Administration of this medication 1 or 2 days before birth may reduce the chances of RDS.

The infant may require pressure support to keep the alveoli open by using a continuous positive airway pressure (CPAP) machine. If the infant is unable to breath adequately they will be placed on a ventilator. In preterm newborns, surfactant can be administered via endotracheal (ET) tube at birth or when symptoms of RDS occur, with improvement of lung function seen over 72 hours. Surfactant production is altered during episodes of cold stress, hypoglycemia, or hypoxia and when there is poor tissue perfusion; such conditions are often present in the preterm infant in the first days of life.

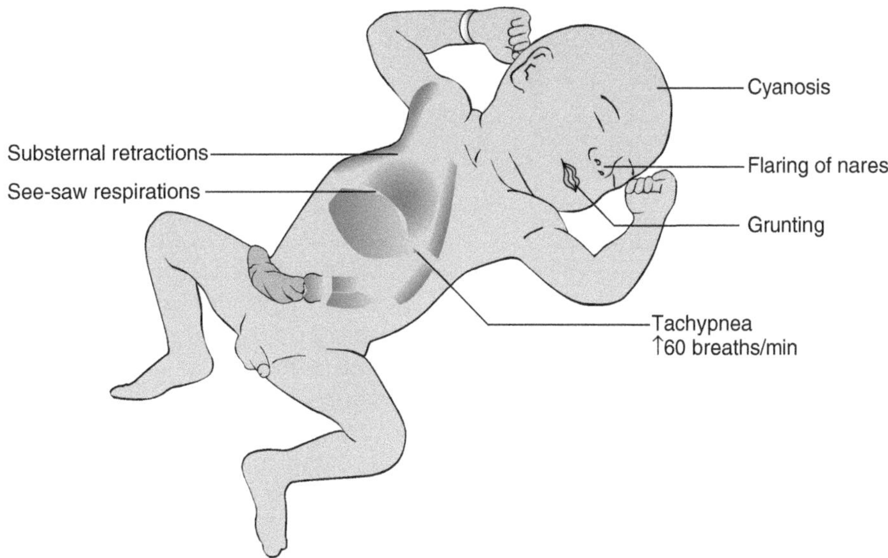

Fig. 12.5 Signs of respiratory distress in a preterm infant.

Vital signs are monitored closely, arterial blood gases are analyzed, and the infant is placed in a warm isolette with gentle and minimal handling so that the infant can conserve energy. The concept of *cluster care* involves combining and coordinating the handling required for assessment and treatments to provide adequate blocks of time for uninterrupted rest. Intravenous (IV) fluids are prescribed, and the nurse observes for signs of overhydration or dehydration. Oxygen therapy may be given via isolette, CPAP machine, or ventilator in concentrations necessary to maintain adequate tissue perfusion. Oxygen toxicity is a high risk for infants receiving prolonged treatment with high concentrations of oxygen. **Bronchopulmonary dysplasia** is the toxic response of the lungs to oxygen therapy. A high concentration of oxygen can lead to atelectasis, edema, and thickening of the lung membranes, which in turn leads to ineffective ventilation of the lung. This situation often results in prolonged dependence on supplemental oxygen and ventilators and has long-term complications.

Apnea

Apnea is defined as the cessation of breathing for 20 seconds or longer. It is not uncommon in the preterm newborn and is believed to be related to immature chemoreceptors in the brain. An apneic episode may be accompanied by **bradycardia** (heart rate of fewer than 100 beats/min) and cyanosis. Apnea monitors can alert nurses to this complication. Gentle rubbing of the infant's feet, ankles, and back may stimulate breathing after this occurrence. When these measures fail, moderate stimulation and, if indicated, suctioning of the nose and mouth as well as raising of the infant's head to a semi-Fowler's position usually facilitates breathing. If breathing does not begin, positive pressure ventilation with a t-piece or self-inflating bag is indicated. A daily dose of caffeine may be prescribed to prevent apnea of prematurity and thus decrease the need for mechanical ventilation (Abdel-Hady, Nasef, Shabaan, et al., 2015).

Neonatal hypoxia

Neonatal **hypoxia** is inadequate oxygenation at the cellular level in a newborn infant. A deficiency of oxygen in the arterial blood is known as *hypoxemia*. The degree of hypoxemia present can be detected by means of a noninvasive pulse oximetry reading. **Pulse oximetry** is defined as the measure of oxygen on the hemoglobin in the circulating blood divided by the oxygen capacity of the hemoglobin. A pulse oximeter saturation level of 90 to 93 % is normal for a preterm infant (Skill 12.1). Although rare, anemia and abnormal fetal hemoglobin may result in normal saturation values in the presence of hypoxia. If the infant is receiving oxygen, the oxygen saturation should not be allowed to go above 95%, to prevent potential effects of oxygen toxicity (Askie, Darlow, Davis, et al., 2017). It is important to set alarm limits to respond to low levels of oxygen saturations (hypoxemia), and to high levels of oxygen saturation if the infant is receiving oxygen.

Sepsis

Sepsis is a generalized infection of the bloodstream. Preterm newborns are at risk for developing this complication because of the immaturity of many body systems. The liver of the preterm infant is immature and forms antibodies poorly. There is little or no immunity received from the mother, and stores of nutrients, vitamins, and iron are insufficient. There may be no local signs of infection, which also hinders diagnosis. Some signs of sepsis include temperature instability (increased or decreased), lethargy or irritability, poor feeding, apnea, and respiratory distress. Maternal infection and complications during labour can also predispose the preterm infant to sepsis.

Good hand hygiene before and after caring for the preterm infant; maintaining strict routine precautions;

Skill 12.1 Applying a Pulse Oximeter

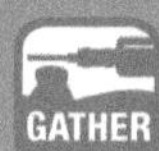

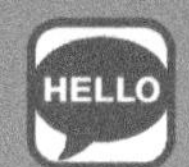

PRIVACY
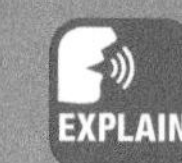

PURPOSE

To determine oxygen saturation of the blood

STEPS

1. Prepare the infant and explain procedure to the family.
2. Turn on oximeter.
3. Set alarm switch to minimum acceptable oxygen saturation (Sao_2) of approximately 92–95%.
4. Apply the oximeter sensor to the toe or the side of the foot (see illustration).

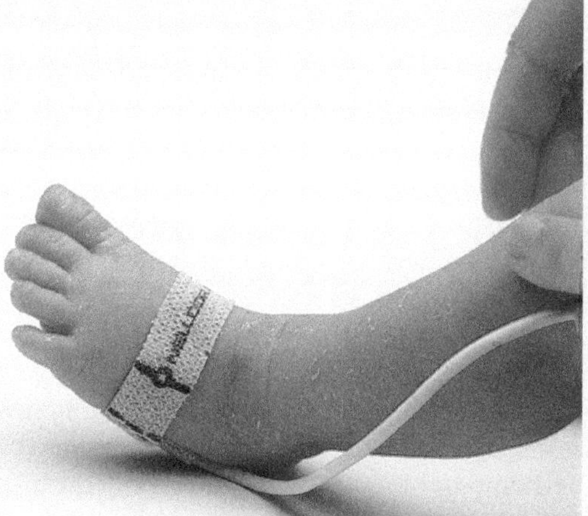

Step 4 (Copyright © 2014 Covidien. All rights reserved. Used with permission of Covidien.)

5. The probe must be flush with the skin and be secured firmly with the wing tapes.
6. The sensors, a light-emitting diode and photo detector, must be lined up opposite each other to obtain an accurate reading. Use the circles on the external surface of the lead to align the sensors. A red light passes from one sensor on the toe or foot through the vascular bed and registers on the sensor on the opposite side.
7. Check the monitor reading for level of oxygen saturation.
8. Compare the heart rate reading on the monitor with the infant's heart rate. Matching heart rates indicate that the saturation level reading is accurate. If heart rates do not match, reapply or adjust sensors.
9. Document time that oximetry is initiated, heart rate and oxygen saturation readings, and location of sensor on the infant's body. Any oxygen administered and method of administration should also be recorded.

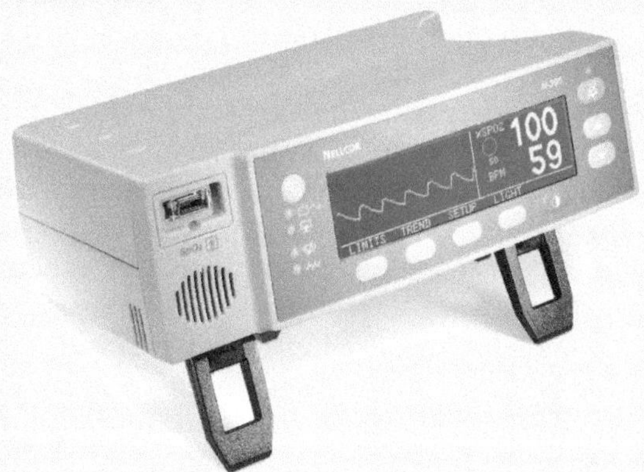

(Figures copyright © 2014 Covidien. All rights reserved. Used with permission of Covidien.)

and monitoring staff, volunteers, and family members for communicable infections are important prevention strategies. Cellular phones have been identified as a source of microbial contamination, and standard cleaning procedures should be considered for all cell phones that will come into the NICU (Kirkby & Biggs, 2016). Close monitoring of vital signs and any other subtle changes in the infant's condition can alert the NICU nurse to the possibility of infection. A septic workup that may include blood work, urinalysis, examination of cerebrospinal fluid, and X-rays will assist in making the diagnosis.

Treatment involves administration of IV antibiotics, maintenance of warmth and nutrition, and close monitoring of vital signs, including blood pressure. Keeping nursing care as organized as possible will help the infant conserve energy. An isolette separates the infant from other infants in the unit and facilitates close observation.

Poor Control of Body Temperature

Keeping the preterm infant warm is a nursing challenge. Heat loss in the preterm infant causing hypothermia (*hypo*, "less than" and *thermia*, "temperature") results from the following factors:

- The preterm infant has a lack of brown fat, which is the body's insulation.
- There is excessive heat loss by radiation from a surface area that is large in proportion to body weight. The large surface area of the head predisposes the infant to heat loss.
- The heat-regulating centre of the brain is immature.
- The sweat glands are not functioning to capacity.
- The preterm infant is inactive, has muscles that are weak and are less resistant to cold, and cannot shiver.
- The posture of the preterm infant's extremities is one of arm and leg extension. This increases the surface area exposed to the environment and increases heat loss.

- Metabolism is high, and the preterm infant is prone to low blood glucose levels (hypoglycemia).

These and other factors make the preterm newborn vulnerable to **cold stress**, which increases the child's need for oxygen and glucose. Early detection can prevent complications.

> **Nursing Tip**
>
> Signs and symptoms of cold stress include the following:
> - Decreased skin temperature
> - Increased respiratory rate with periods of apnea
> - Bradycardia
> - Mottling of skin
> - Lethargy

Nursing care

Maintaining a **neutral thermal environment** is essential to prevent hypothermia or cold stress and to promote optimal growth. This can be done by careful monitoring and documentation of the ambient and infant temperature (**thermoregulation**), appropriate use of clothing and hats and blankets, skin-to-skin care, and, if indicated, placing the infant in an isolette or under a radiant heater. The World Health Organization (WHO) recommends skin-to-skin care routinely for newborns weighing 2 000 g or less at birth and that it should be initiated in health care facilities as soon as newborns are clinically stable (WHO, 2017). The infant's skin temperature will decrease before the core temperature falls. Core temperature is monitored by placing the thermometer in the axilla. A skin probe can be used to measure the infant's skin temperature when utilizing servo control while this infant is in an isolette or placed under a radiant warmer. The skin temperature probe can be placed on the abdomen, flank, or axilla (Schafer et al., 2014). A reflective protector should be used over the skin probe when the infant is in a radiant warmer so that the probe does not measure the temperature within the warmer unit. To protect the infant from potential skin damage, only protectors with a hydrogel base should be used.

The temperature of the isolette or radiant warmer is adjusted so that the infant's body temperature is at an optimal level, between 36.5 and 37.5°C (97.7 and 99.5°F) (WHO, 1997).

Nurses must understand how to use the isolettes available in the nurseries to which they are assigned (Fig. 12.6). The temperature of the isolette is adjusted to a level that will maintain an optimal body temperature in the infant. Smaller infants may require higher isolette temperatures. The nurse records the temperature of the infant and the isolette every 2 to 3 hours depending on unit policy. Overheating should also be avoided because it increases the infant's oxygen and caloric requirements.

Radiant warmers that supply overhead heat have the advantage of providing easier access to the infant while maintaining a neutral thermal environment. The use of a plexiglass shield with the radiant warmer and swaddling the infant are not recommended as they may block infrared heat.

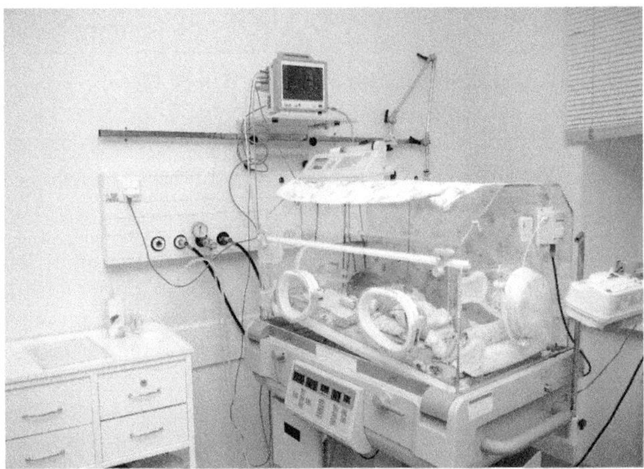

Fig. 12.6 The isolette. The infant is dressed only in a diaper. Portholes facilitate routine infant care without disturbing the atmospheric conditions in the isolette. The infant can be assessed through Plexiglas windows. Levers under the mattress can place the bed in Fowler's position. Openings at the head and foot of the isolette can be used to remove soiled linen. The door of the isolette can be lowered to form a platform that makes the infant accessible for special treatments or tests. To promote circadian rhythms, a blanket may be placed over the top of the isolette to shield the infant from environmental lights. (Fanfo/Shutterstock.com)

Nursing Care Plan 12.1 lists nursing interventions for selected nursing diagnoses pertinent to care of the preterm newborn.

Kangaroo care

Kangaroo care is a method of care for preterm infants that uses skin-to-skin contact (Skill 12.2). The infant, wearing only a diaper and a small cap, rests on the mother or father's naked chest. The skin provides warmth and calms the child, and the contact promotes bonding. Kangaroo care has been shown to be superior to holding a blanket-wrapped infant in enhancing the stabilization of infants and promoting later development (Jefferies & CPS Fetus and Newborn Committee, 2012/2017; Neu, Robinson, & Schmiege, 2013). Skin-to-skin contact is an important practice in hospitals that are designated "baby friendly" (see Chapter 9 for further discussion of baby-friendly initiative).

Hypoglycemia and Hypocalcemia

Hypoglycemia (*hypo*, "less than," and *glycemia*, "sugar in the blood") is common among preterm infants. They have not remained in the uterus long enough to acquire sufficient stores of glycogen and fat. This condition is aggravated by the need for increased glycogen in the brain, the heart, and other tissues due to asphyxia, sepsis, RDS, unstable body temperature, or similar conditions. Any condition that increases energy requirements places more stress on these already deficient stores. In an infant, plasma glucose levels lower than 2.6 mmol/L after 2 hours of age indicate hypoglycemia (Aziz, Dancey, & CPS Fetus and Newborn Committee, 2004/2018).

Nursing Care Plan 12.1 The Preterm Newborn

Patient Data A newborn infant born at 34 weeks + 6 days' gestation or earlier is admitted to the neonatal intensive care unit (NICU). Some infants born between 35 and 37 weeks may also require admission to the NICU. The infant is placed in a prewarmed isolette, and cardiorespiratory sensors are applied.

Selected Nursing Diagnosis Hypothermia as a result of decreased subcutaneous tissue and immature thermoregulation

Goals	Nursing Interventions	Rationales
Infant's temperature will remain at 36.5° to 37°C.	Monitor temperature with skin probe or by axillary method.	These methods provide the best indication of the infant's core temperature and are less invasive.
	Adjust isolette or radiant warmer to maintain skin temperature.	A neutral thermal environment allows the infant to maintain a normal core temperature with minimum oxygen consumption and caloric expenditure.
	Observe for signs of cold stress, such as decreased temperature, pallor, and lethargy.	Preterm infants have little or no muscular activity; they remain in an extended posture because of lack of muscle tone; they cannot shiver.
	Use discretion in bathing.	The temperature of a wet infant drops quickly as a result of evaporation.
	Avoid cold surfaces.	Conductive heat loss occurs when an infant is weighed on a cold scale; prewarm surfaces or use a blanket for protection.

Selected Nursing Diagnosis Potential for skin breakdown as a result of immature skin, inadequate nutrition, and immobility

Goals	Nursing Interventions	Rationales
Skin will remain intact.	Change position regularly.	This prevents skin breakdown and aids respiration and circulation.
	Remove dressings, tape, and electrodes only if indicated. Be gentle when removing anything from the preterm infant's skin.	The preterm infant's skin is fragile and bruises easily; use as little tape as possible.
	Cleanse skin with clear water or approved cleansers.	Avoid using hexachlorophene cleaners because of their toxic effect; all products must be carefully assessed before use, because permeability of the preterm infant's skin fosters absorption of ingredients.
	Observe skin for signs of infection while recognizing that there may be no local inflammatory response but only vague signs and symptoms.	Heel pricks and other invasive procedures are often necessary; the preterm infant's immune system is immature, and healing becomes difficult.

CRITICAL THINKING QUESTION

1. A mother comes to visit her preterm son in the NICU. She states that she wants to see her infant, but she is afraid to touch anything and fears she will hurt her fragile newborn. What is the nurse's best response?

The brain needs a steady supply of glucose, thus hypoglycemia must be anticipated and treated promptly. Any condition that increases metabolism increases glucose needs. Preterm infants may be too weak to effectively feed and often require gavage or parenteral feedings to supply adequate caloric needs. Nursing responsibilities include frequent glucose monitoring, and administering of oral, gavage, or parenteral feedings. Maintaining a neutral thermal environment and preventing hypoxia or infection will also prevent hypoglycemia.

Nursing care

Hypoglycemia in the newborn can cause many other problems, such as hypothermia and worsening RDS, and can lead to potential brain damage. It is important to identify the infant at risk for hypoglycemia, encourage early and adequate feeding, and regularly check their blood sugar levels. A blood sugar less than 2.6 mmol/L must be reported to the registered nurse immediately.

Infants at risk for hypoglycemia are as follows:

- Preterm infants and SGA infants, owing to insufficient levels of glycogen and fat stores
- Infants of diabetic mothers, because of the abrupt loss of maternal glucose and hypertrophy of the pancreatic islet cells, which result in a temporary overproduction of insulin
- LGA infants, as mothers of these infants may have undiagnosed diabetes.
- Any sick infant, owing to increased energy needs

Skill 12.2 Kangaroo Care

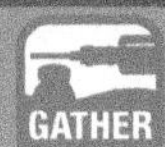
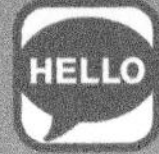

PURPOSE

To maintain skin-to-skin contact to promote warmth and bonding

STEPS

1. Explain the rationale and principles of care to the parents.
2. Provide a comfortable chair and privacy.
3. Have parent wear a top that opens in the front, leaving the chest bare.

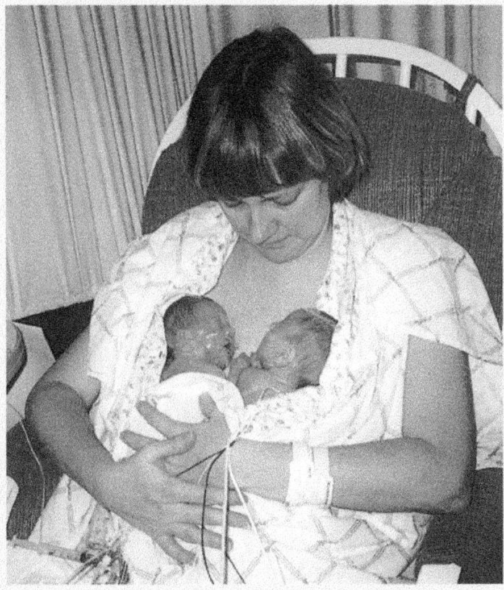

The mother provides kangaroo care for her preterm infants. Skin-to-skin contact is provided, with warmth maintained by the outer covering.

4. Remove newborn's clothes except for diaper.
5. Place newborn in a vertical position between the breasts of the bare chest of the parent.
6. Place a blanket over the newborn.
7. Monitor the temperature of the newborn throughout this form of care.
8. Document the procedure, the infant's vital signs, and responses.

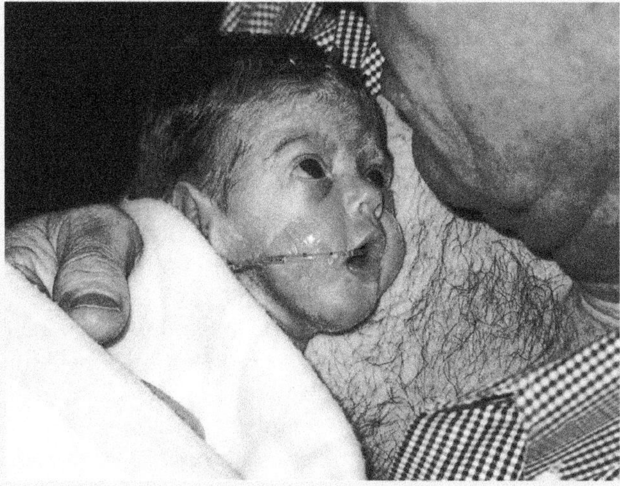

The father can also provide effective kangaroo care. The infant shows a positive response to this contact. (Courtesy Loma Linda University Medical Center, Loma Linda, CA.)

Nursing Tip

Signs of hypoglycemia in the preterm infant include the following:

- Tremors or jitteriness
- Plasma glucose level lower than 2.6 mmol/L after 2 hours of age
- Weak cry
- Lethargy
- Convulsions

Hypocalcemia (*hypo,* "below," and *calcemia,* "calcium in the blood") is also seen in preterm infants born before 32 weeks and in sick newborns. Calcium is transported across the placenta throughout pregnancy, but in greater amounts during the third trimester. Early birth can result in infants with lower serum calcium levels.

In early hypocalcemia, the parathyroid fails to respond to the preterm infant's low calcium levels. Infants stressed by hypoxia or birth trauma are at high risk for this problem. Infants born to mothers who are diabetic or who have had low vitamin D intake are also at risk for developing early hypocalcemia.

IV calcium is the treatment for early hypocalcemia. During IV therapy, the nurse should monitor the infant for bradycardia. The nurse should also frequently check the IV site for extravasation, to avoid subcutaneous tissue necrosis.

Late hypocalcemia is rare and usually occurs about age 1 week in newborns and can be caused by certain vitamin deficiencies, hypoparathyroidism, and cow's milk–based formula feeding. Treatment of late-onset hypocalcemia will vary depending on the cause and may be a lifelong condition.

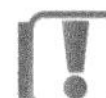

Safety Alert!

When an infant is given intravenous calcium gluconate, the registered nurse should monitor the heart rate closely and report bradycardia if it occurs. The infant should be in the NICU for increased surveillance.

Increased Tendency to Bleed

Preterm infants are more prone to bleeding than full-term infants because their blood is deficient in prothrombin, a factor of the clotting mechanism. Fragile capillaries of the head are particularly susceptible to injury during birth, causing intracranial hemorrhage. Preterm infants are especially susceptible to intraventricular hemorrhages caused by episodes of hypoxia, fast delivery of IV boluses, unstable blood pressure, and Trendelenburg position. Ultrasound is used to diagnose intracranial hemorrhages. The nurse should monitor the neurological status of the infant and report bulging fontanelles, lethargy, poor feeding, and seizures. The preterm infant bed should be in a slight Fowler's position, and unnecessary stimulation that can cause increased intracerebral pressure should be avoided. Depending on the grade and location of the intracranial hemorrhage the infant may have long-lasting deficits.

Retinopathy of Prematurity

Retinopathy of prematurity (ROP) is a disorder of the developing retina in premature infants that can lead to blindness. It is the leading cause of blindness in newborns weighing less than 1 500 g (3 lb 5 oz). The condition can be caused by many factors, but premature infants are more commonly at risk, because their immature retinas are incompletely vascularized at birth.

After birth, the retina completes an abnormal vascularization process that causes fibrous tissue to form behind the lens of each eye, resulting in blindness and retinal detachment. Full-term infants who have fully developed vascular systems in the retina at birth are usually not affected, but infants with an unstable course should be monitored for ROP. The Canadian Paediatric Society (CPS) recommends routine retinal examination by a certified ophthalmologist in the NICU for infants with birth weight less than 1 250 g or gestational age less than 30 weeks. The first screening for ROP should occur at 31 weeks postnatal age for infants born before 27 weeks' gestation and a week or two later for infants between 28 and 30 weeks' gestation (Jefferies & CPS Fetus and Newborn Committee, 2016). Frequency and timing of follow-up examination are decided by the examining ophthalmologist. The objective of ROP screening is the early detection and prompt treatment of abnormal vascularization of the retina. Retinal ablative therapy using laser photocoagulation of the fibrous tissue, or intravitreal injection of bevacizumab, has been used with success in preventing blindness (American Academy of Pediatrics, 2013; Jefferies & CPS Fetus and Newborn Committee, 2016). Follow-up for other eye problems such as strabismus, refractive errors, or cataracts should be provided within 4 to 6 months after discharge from the NICU. The nurse must teach the parents concerning the importance of follow-up care.

Prevention of preterm births and the problems that beset preterm infants are key to preventing ROP. Careful monitoring of oxygen saturation in high-risk infants with a pulse oximeter continues to be a priority in the nursery (see Skill 12.1). It is the level of oxygen in the blood, rather than the amount of oxygen received, that is of importance in oxygen therapy. There is no "safe" level of oxygen. Oxygen saturation levels should not exceed 95% while the infant is receiving oxygen therapy. Optimal nutrition, promoting a breast milk–only diet, and maintaining a sufficient level of vitamin E may also reduce the risk for ROP (Fang, Sorita, Carey, et al., 2016).

Nursing Tip

During oxygen administration the oxygen saturation levels of the preterm infant must not exceed 95%, to prevent the development of ROP. Every NICU should have an evidence-based ROP screening guideline to ensure that all infants born before 30 weeks or with a birth weight less than 1 250 g are screened by a skilled ophthalmologist.

Nutrition Concerns

The stomach capacity of the preterm infant is small. The sphincter muscles at both ends of the stomach are immature, which contributes to regurgitation and vomiting, particularly after overfeeding. Sucking and swallowing reflexes are immature. The infant's ability to absorb fats is poor (this includes fat-soluble vitamins). The inadequate store of nutrients in the preterm infant and the need for glucose and nutrients to promote growth and prevent brain damage contribute to the nutritional problems of the preterm infant. Parenteral or orogavage feedings (via a tube placed through the nose or mouth into the stomach) are usually required until the infant is strong enough to tolerate oral feedings without compromising cardiorespiratory status.

Human milk is the ideal food for the premature infant because the fat and other nutrients are absorbed readily. Breast milk may be manually expressed by the mother. If the mother is unable to supply breast milk, donor breast milk may be ordered, or a special preterm breast milk substitute can be used. Often these infants are fed while still in the isolette. Early initiation of feedings reduces the risk of hypoglycemia, hyperbilirubinemia, and dehydration.

If the infant is gavage fed, the nurse must check that the tube is in the stomach by aspirating and checking the pH of the aspirate. The gastric tube is correctly placed in the stomach if the gastric aspirate has a pH 5.5 or less. Milk can be delivered by gravity or by using a feeding pump if a longer duration of delivering the milk is required. Since there is an increased risk of accidental tube dislodgement and aspiration, the nurse should remain at the patient's bedside during the feed. The tube and tube position also needs to be changed regularly. IV fluids may be provided to meet fluid, calorie, and electrolyte needs in small, weak preterm infants.

Signs that indicate readiness for oral feeding include a strong gag reflex and sucking and rooting reflexes.

Nipple feedings are started slowly, and some initial weight loss may be noted due to the energy expenditure of oral feedings. Breastfeeding is the best way to feed the premature baby and should be attempted whenever the infant displays feeding readiness cues. If feeding by bottle, the infant is placed in a side-lying position to allow easier control of fluid volume by the infant. The suck–swallow–breathing rhythm is not usually present in the preterm infant until 33 to 34 weeks' gestation, so the nurse must ensure that the infant takes a breath after a sucking burst to avoid choking. Since infants will feed reflexively, it is important not to force feed these babies, as this can lead to oral aversion later on. As soon as the infant shows any signs of tiring, the oral feed must be discontinued and completed by gavage. Placing the infant on the right side or abdomen after feeding promotes gastric emptying and decreases aspiration if vomiting occurs.

Necrotizing Enterocolitis

Necrotizing enterocolitis (NEC) is an acute inflammation of the bowel that leads to bowel necrosis. Preterm newborns are particularly susceptible to NEC. Factors implicated include a diminished blood supply to the lining of the bowel wall because of hypoxia or sepsis that causes a decrease in protective mucus and results in bacterial invasion of the delicate tissues. A source for bacterial growth can occur when the infant is fed a breast milk substitute. Oral immune therapy (OIT), where a drop of the mother's colostrum is delivered between the cheek and the gum of the infant, will also protect the preterm infant from NEC and other infections (Gephart & Weller, 2014).

Signs of NEC include abdominal distention, decrease or absent abdominal sounds, bloody stools, diarrhea, and bilious vomitus. Specific nursing responsibilities include observing vital signs, careful assessment of the abdomen including listening for bowel sounds, and maintaining infection-control techniques. Treatment includes antimicrobials and the use of parenteral nutrition to rest the bowels. Surgical removal of the necrosed bowel may be indicated.

Immature Kidneys

Improper elimination of body wastes contributes to electrolyte imbalance and disturbed acid–base relationships. Dehydration occurs easily. Tolerance to salt is limited, and susceptibility to edema is increased.

The nurse should document the intake and output for all preterm infants. The nurse should weigh the dry diaper and subtract its weight from the infant's wet diaper to determine the urine output. The urine output should be between 1 and 3 mL/kg/hr. The infant should be observed closely for signs of dehydration or overhydration. The nurse should document the status of the fontanelles, tissue turgor, weight, and urine output.

Jaundice

The liver of the newborn is immature, which contributes to a condition called **icterus** or jaundice. Jaundice causes the skin and the whites of the eyes to assume a yellow-orange cast. The liver is unable to clear the blood of bile pigments that result from the normal postnatal destruction of red blood cells. The higher the blood bilirubin level is, the deeper the jaundice, and the greater the risk for neurological damage. Visible jaundice and rapidly rising total serum bilirubin (TSB) of more than 86 mcmol/L per day is considered pathological jaundice and requires additional investigation and surveillance (Yaworski, Van Meer, & Wong, 2018). Physiological jaundice is normal and responds well to an increase in fluid intake and phototherapy, if indicated. Pathological jaundice is more serious, occurs within 24 hours of birth, and is secondary to an abnormal condition such as ABO-Rh incompatibility (see discussion later in this chapter) or glucose-6-phosphate dehydrogenase (G6PD) deficiency. In preterm infants, the normal rise in bilirubin levels (icterus neonatorum) is slower than in full-term infants and lasts longer, which predisposes the infant to **hyperbilirubinemia** (*hyper,* "excessive," *bilirubin,* "bile," and *emia,* "blood"), or excessive bilirubin levels in the blood.

There is more evidence of jaundice in infants who are breastfed. Breastmilk jaundice begins to be seen about the fourth day, when the mother's milk supply develops. The newborn usually does well but is carefully monitored to rule out problems. Breastfeeding should *not* be discontinued as it can lead to early discontinuation of exclusive breastfeeding. In early-onset jaundice of the breastfed infant, inadequate infant suckling at the breast causes jaundice and necessitates an increase in breastfeeding. Glucose water feeding is contraindicated and should *not* be offered to the infant, because this practice may decrease milk intake and can serve to further increase bilirubin levels. In late-onset jaundice of the breastfed infant, the breast milk itself may inhibit conjugation of bilirubin, but interruption of breastfeeding is not recommended. Continued breastfeeding while receiving phototherapy is not associated with any adverse outcomes (Barrington, Sankaran, & CPS, 2007/2018). The TSB level typically peaks 3 to 5 days after birth.

The early discharge of a newborn necessitates universal screening for risk to develop hyperbilirubinemia and follow-up visits within 2 days to check TSB and to prevent the development of kernicterus (Barrington, et al., 2007/2018).

Visual assessment of jaundice is an unreliable method to diagnose jaundice; a timed TSB measurement and consideration of the gestational age of the infant is the best method to predict severe hyperbilirubinemia.

Nursing care for hyperbilirubinemia consists of observing the infant's skin, sclera, and mucous membranes for jaundice (blanching the skin over bony prominences enhances the evaluation for jaundice) and following universal screening for hyperbilirubinemia guidelines.

The goals of treatment for hyperbilirubinemia are to avoid the continued increase of bilirubin levels in the blood and prevent kernicterus (a serious neurological complication that can cause brain damage, which is also known as *bilirubin encephalopathy*). Treatment includes increase in fluids and phototherapy. Intravenous immunoglobulin (IVIG) transfusion and exchange transfusion are considered for treatment of severe hyperbilirubinemia (TSB 375–425 mcmol/L). A test for G6PD deficiency should be considered in all infants with severe hyperbilirubinemia (Barrington et al., 2007/2018).

Phototherapy is the use of a strong light source to change the bilirubin in the blood to a water-soluble form that can be excreted. The light source needs to emit more than 30 mcW/cm^2/nm to be effective. Either a standard phototherapy light source or a fibre-optic blanket can be used to deliver effective (also called intensive) phototherapy. Depending on the TSB, double intensive phototherapy may be ordered. Double intensive phototherapy is administered by delivering intensive light to the anterior (phototherapy light) and posterior (fibre-optic blanket) surface of the infant's body.

The nurse needs to monitor and report bilirubin laboratory values and document the response of the infant to phototherapy. Greater fluid intake may be necessary by increasing the frequency of breastfeeding or increasing the volume of measured feeds or IV therapy. The infant will need special eye protectors as the phototherapy lights may cause retinal damage. It is important to remove the eye protectors during feeding. Eyes must be checked regularly for any discharge. The infant's diapers need to be changed often and the buttocks monitored for any skin breakdown due to an increase in stooling related to phototherapy. See Chapter 11 and Skill 11.2 for assessing jaundice.

Positioning and Nursing Care

In the NICU environment with close observation, the preterm newborn can be positioned on the side or prone, with the head of the mattress slightly elevated unless contraindicated. In this position, the abdominal contents do not press against the diaphragm and impede breathing.

Positioning the preterm infant should be compatible with the drainage of secretions and the prevention of aspiration. Propping the infant on the side or placing the infant prone can decrease the work of breathing, improve oxygenation, promote a more organized sleep pattern, and lessen physical activity that burns up energy needed for growth and development. An enclosed space, or *nesting,* can provide a calming, supportive environment that promotes body flexion for the preterm infant (Fig. 12.7). Infants should be gradually weaned from the prone position when the physical condition becomes stable, and they should be placed in the supine position well before discharge from the NICU. In addition, it is important to teach the parents about the importance of the "back-to-sleep" concept to prevent sudden infant death syndrome (SIDS).

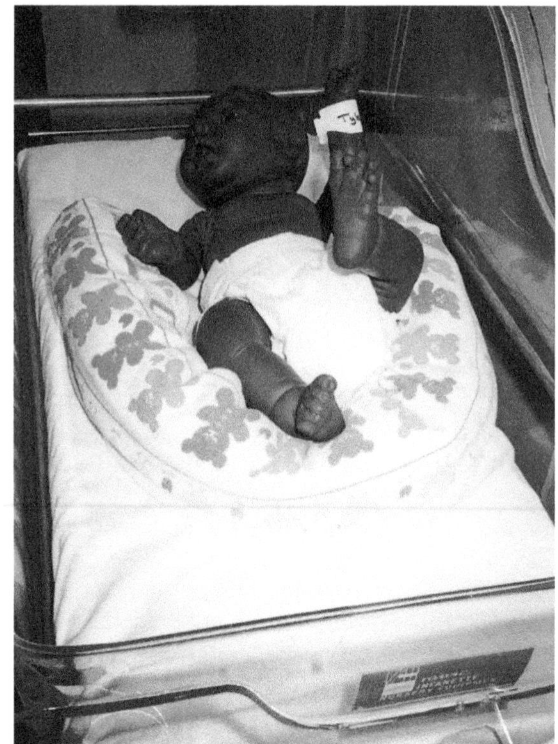

Fig. 12.7 Infant nesting. An enclosed space bounded by small blanket rolls encircling the preterm infant provides a calming, supportive environment.

The nurse should change the position of the preterm infant to prevent breakdown from pressure on the infant's delicate skin. If such a breakdown should occur, the area is exposed to the air, and a suitable ointment is applied as prescribed by the health care provider. Alkaline-based soap, alcohol, and medicated wipes should not be used on the preterm infant's thin and sensitive skin. Hydrocolloid adhesives or using gauze or cotton under adhesive tape is advisable. General skin and other care may include, if indicated, cleansing of the eyes with normal saline, mouth care using sterile water or expressed breast milk especially if the infant is NPO, and cleaning of the diaper area with every diaper change. Approved barrier creams are applied in order to manage diaper rash. Baths two or three times per week are also part of good skin care. Sponge baths with water only are for the very preterm infant, and tub baths using unit-approved cleansers are for the more mature infant (see Chapter 11 for a more extended discussion of the skin of the newborn).

The health care provider will examine the preterm newborn and write specific orders for treatment and nursing care. The nurse is then responsible for reporting any significant changes in the infant's condition. Table 12.1 lists the *general* observations to guide care of the preterm newborn. Sudden changes should be reported immediately.

Table 12.1 **Nursing Observations in Care of the Preterm Infant**

OBSERVATION	SIGNS TO REPORT
General activity	Increase or decrease in movements, lethargy, twitching, frequency and quality of cry, hyperactivity
Fontanelles	Sunken, flat, or bulging
Eyes	Discharge
Respirations	Regularity, apnea, sternal retractions, laboured breathing
Pulse	Rate and regularity
Abdomen	Distention
Cord	Discharge; odour
Feeding	Sucking ability, vomiting or regurgitation, degree of satisfaction
Voiding	Initial, frequency
Stools	Frequency, colour, consistency
Mucous membranes	Dryness of lips and mouth, signs of thrush
Colour	Paleness, cyanosis, jaundice
Skin	Rashes, irritations, pustules, edema

Every effort should be made to maintain a quiet environment and organize nursing care so that overstimulation of the preterm infant is avoided. Blankets can be placed over the top of the isolette to reduce external stimulation and to establish a normal *circadian rhythm* (night–day sleep pattern), and dimmer switches on lights can encourage the infant to open their eyes and become responsive to the environment. Eye patches can be placed over the infant's eyes to protect against the bright procedure lights. Observing physical and behavioural responses of the preterm infant enables a developmentally appropriate care plan to be developed. The preterm infant should be awakened slowly and gently for procedures or nursing care and should be moved gently, maintaining flexion of the arms close to the midline of the infant's body. Non-nutritive sucking is beneficial to the infant.

Some studies have shown that cobedding of twins (placing them together in one isolette) may improve their growth and development, but further research is needed to determine the risks related to SIDS.

Use of Complementary and Alternative Health Modalities in the NICU

Aromatherapy is often used in the NICU, by placing an article of clothing with the mother's natural body odour next to the newborn in the isolette (Kassity-Kritch & Jones, 2014). Music therapy may also be effective in calming the infant and enhancing language development, especially if the parent sings softly to the infant. Gentle therapeutic touch and gentle massage are beneficial to the preterm infant, by reducing motor activity and energy expenditure as well as promoting bonding with the parents (Badr, Abdallah, & Kahale, 2015).

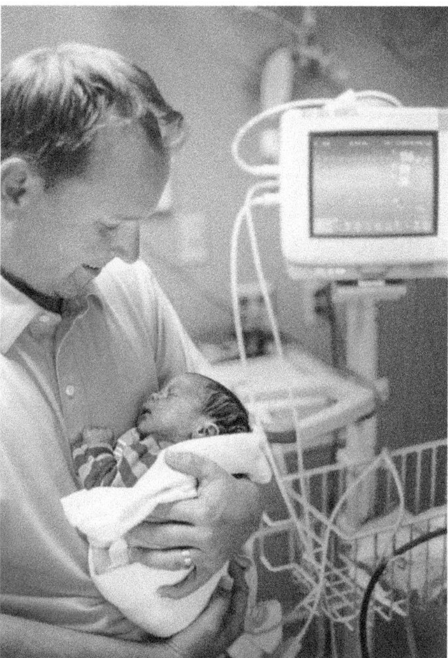

Fig. 12.8 This father holds his preterm infant in a moment of bonding. (istock.com/Yobro10)

PROGNOSIS

In the absence of severe birth defects and complications, the growth rate of the preterm newborn nears that of the term infant by about the second year. Very low–birth weight infants may not catch up, especially if there has been chronic illness, insufficient nutritional intake, or inadequate care taking (Carlo, 2016). Additional studies are needed to determine the effects of these factors at various age levels. Parents must be prepared for comments on the infant's small size and slower development. In general, growth and development of the preterm infant are based on current age minus the number of weeks before term that the infant was born—for example, if born at 36 weeks of gestation, a 1-month-old infant would be at a newborn's achievement level. This calculation ensures that no one has unrealistic expectations of the infant.

FAMILY REACTION

The nurse should assist the parents in coping with their responses to having a small, preterm infant. Parents need guidance throughout the infant's hospitalization to help prepare them for this new experience. They may be disheartened by the appearance of the preterm newborn. They may believe that they are to blame for the infant's condition. They may fear that the infant will die but may be unable to express their feelings. They need time to look at and touch the infant and begin to see the child as uniquely their own (Fig. 12.8). This touching and the immediate human contact are vital for the infant as well. The mother is usually concerned about her ability to care for such a small and helpless individual. When she feels ready, she can be encouraged to assist the nurse in diapering, bathing, feeding, and other activities. Other aspects of infant care are also stressed during this time.

Nursing care of the preterm infant includes measures to provide short periods of stimulation during the alert phase of activity. The parents can be taught to provide stimulation by using a black-and-white mobile; stroking the child gently; talking to the infant; rocking the infant; or providing range-of-motion activity, massage, or kangaroo care. A pacifier may be used during gavage feeding to provide non-nutritive sucking. Care should be taken not to overly stimulate or tire the infant. There should be minimal stimulation during feeding to enable the infant to concentrate energy on the sucking and swallowing process. Mild stimulation and interaction with parents should be provided between feedings.

The nurse should collaborate with pediatricians, nurse practitioners, social workers, nutritionists, psychologists, and staff from other disciplines to plan and coordinate follow-up care of the preterm infant after discharge. Often a mother is discharged without her infant. This is difficult for the entire family and makes attachment and bonding more complicated. The nurse should encourage the family to keep in touch by telephone and visits. Parents can help siblings to accept the infant by addressing the child by name, sharing news of progress, taking pictures of the infant, and encouraging communication by means of drawings and cards. Listening to what siblings are saying provides information for discussion.

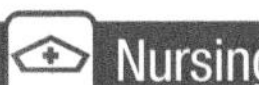

Nursing Tip

Encourage parents to talk about their feelings and fears concerning the preterm infant. Answer questions about home care.

DISCHARGE OF THE HIGH-RISK PRETERM NEWBORN

Discharge planning for the high-risk newborn begins at birth. The preterm infant is ready for discharge when medically stable, able to maintain oxygen saturations greater than 90% in room air, is apnea free for 72 hours, is able to maintain normal body temperature clothed and in a cot, is feeding successfully (breast or bottle), and has sustained weight gain (Jefferies & CPS Fetus and Newborn Committee, 2014). Prior to discharge the nurse ensures that all the necessary screening has been done, including ROP screening, cranial ultrasounds if indicated, assessment for respiratory syncytial virus (RSV) prophylaxis and administration, if indicated, and hearing screening. Referral needs to be made for follow-up with the public health nurse to monitor feeding and weight gain after discharge.

The parents will need to demonstrate and practice routine and, if indicated, specialized care. Continued medical supervision is important. The nurse needs to stress the importance of well-baby examinations, immunizations, and prevention of infection. Good prenatal care for subsequent pregnancies should also be emphasized (especially after a preterm birth, because the mother is at high risk for future preterm births).

Parents are often anxious about taking their high-risk newborn home. The nurse must familiarize the parent with the newborn's care. The newborn's behavioural patterns are discussed, and realistic expectations concerning the preterm infant's catch-up development are reviewed. Communication regarding newborn care can be maintained with "warm-lines" and "hot-lines" provided to parents, and the social services department may be of help in ensuring that the home environment is satisfactory and that the infant's special needs can be met. Support-group referrals are given to parents, and newborn cardiopulmonary resuscitation (CPR) techniques are reviewed. Parents are often given a room attached to the NICU where they can provide care to the infant for a few days before discharge to enhance their confidence and have extra support when needed from nursing staff.

THE POST-TERM NEWBORN

The newborn is considered *post-term* if the pregnancy goes beyond 42 weeks. *Postmaturity* refers to the infant showing characteristics of the postmature syndrome. Identification of infants who are not tolerating the extra time in the uterus is the major goal of treatment. Death of the post-term infant is uncommon today because of early detection and intervention and many women have their pregnancy induced between 41 and 42 weeks so it is unusual to have a fetus go beyond 42 weeks gestation. The cause of postmaturity is not yet clear; however, it is known that the placenta does not function adequately as it ages, which could result in fetal distress. The mortality rate of late infants is higher than that of newborns who are born at term. Morbidity rates are also higher. After the infant survives birth, the risks are fewer.

The late birth can be a psychological strain on the mother, the partner, and other members of the family, who are eagerly awaiting the arrival of the child. The nurse can encourage parents to verbalize their feelings and concerns about the delay. Very large newborns, such as those of diabetic mothers, are not necessarily postmature but are larger than normal because of rapid, abnormal growth before birth.

The following problems are associated with postmaturity:

- Asphyxia caused by chronic hypoxia while in the uterus because of a deteriorated placenta
- Meconium aspiration: hypoxia and distress may cause relaxation of the anal sphincter, and meconium can be aspirated into the fetal lungs
- Poor nutritional status; depleted glycogen reserves cause hypoglycemia

- Increase in red blood cell production (polycythemia) because of intrauterine hypoxia
- Difficult birth because of larger size of the infant
- Seizures as a result of the hypoxic state

PHYSICAL CHARACTERISTICS

The post-term infant is long and thin and looks as though weight has been lost. The skin is loose, especially about the thighs and buttocks. There is little lanugo (downy hair) or vernix caseosa. The loss of the cheeselike vernix caseosa leaves the skin dry; it cracks, peels, and is almost like parchment in texture. The nails are long and may be stained with meconium. The infant may have a thick head of hair and look alert.

NURSING CARE

Labour induction or Caesarean births are commonly performed if testing determines that the pregnancy is past 42 weeks or if there are signs of fetal distress or maternal risk. Many post-term infants suffer few adverse effects from the delay, but they still require careful observation. Nursing care involves observing for respiratory distress (usually because of aspiration of meconium-stained amniotic fluid), hypoglycemia (caused by depleted glycogen stores), and hyperbilirubinemia (as a result of polycythemia). The infant may be placed in an isolette, because fat stores have been used in utero for nourishment and the infant is vulnerable to cold stress.

TRANSPORTING THE HIGH-RISK NEWBORN

Transportation of the high-risk newborn to a regional neonatal centre requires the organization and expertise of a special team. A nurse and sometimes a pediatric health care provider accompany the infant unless specialists in emergency medical transport are part of the transport team. Stabilization of the infant before transport is important; this may include intubation and placement of IV lines. Baseline data, such as vital signs and blood work (blood gases and glucose levels), are obtained. The infant is weighed if this is not contraindicated. Copies of all records are made, including the infant's record, the mother's prenatal history and birth record, and pertinent admission data. A transport isolette is provided for warmth, and its batteries are kept fully charged (see Fig. 12.4).

The nurse is responsible for placing an identification band on the infant before transport and verifying the identification name and number with the mother's identification band. The mother should be reassured that the identification will stay with the infant. If possible, one of the parents should accompany the infant to the referring hospital. If not, the parents should be given the name and location of the receiving hospital and a name and telephone number to contact for follow-up information and visits.

Box 12.2 Terms Helpful in Understanding Rh Sensitization

Antigen (*anti*, "against," and *gen*, "to produce"): A substance that induces the formation of antibodies; the antigen–antibody reaction is the basis of immunity

Coombs' test: Indirectly measures Rh-positive antibodies in the mother's blood; directly measures antibody-coated Rh-positive red blood cells in the infant's blood

Hemolytic disease of the newborn (HDN): The severe form of this disease produces anemia in the fetus as a result of incompatibility between the red blood cells of the mother and those of the fetus

Rh_0(D) immune globulin: Immunoglobulin given to an Rh-negative mother after the birth of an Rh-positive fetus to prevent the maternal Rh immune response

Sensitization (isoimmunization): The phenomenon in which an Rh-negative mother develops antibodies against an Rh-positive fetus

Parents are shown the newborn before departure. If the mother is unable to hold the infant because of the baby's condition, the isolette is wheeled to her bedside for her observation. A picture can be taken and given to the parents. On occasion, a mother is unable to see her infant because of her own unstable condition. Such situations require special empathy from nursing personnel. After the infant has safely reached its destination, the parents are contacted by telephone. It is also thoughtful for the receiving hospital personnel to provide feedback to the transport team so that they may enjoy hearing the results of their efforts.

PERINATAL CONDITIONS

HEMOLYTIC DISEASE OF THE NEWBORN

Pathophysiology

Hemolytic disease of the newborn (HDN) is one of many congenital hemolytic diseases found in the newborn. It is caused when an Rh-negative mother and an Rh-positive father produce an Rh-positive fetus. Although fetal and maternal blood does not mix during pregnancy, small leaks may allow fetal blood to enter the maternal circulation and sensitize the mother. The mother's body responds by producing antibodies that cross the placenta and destroy the blood cells of the fetus, causing anemia and possible heart failure. If large numbers of antibodies are present, the infant may be severely anemic. In the gravest form, the progressive hemolysis causes anemia, fetal hypoxia, anasarca (generalized edema) and heart failure (hydrops fetalis) (see Chapter 5). This condition is rare today because of early prophylaxis and detection methods, which involve isoimmunization and sensitization (Box 12.2). The incidence of HDN has greatly decreased as a result of the protective administration of an Rh immune globulin to women at risk (see following discussion of prevention). Incompatibility of ABO factors are now more common and generally less severe than Rh incompatibility (Box 12.3).

The process of maternal sensitization is depicted in Fig. 12.9. The mother accumulates antibodies with each pregnancy. Therefore, the chance that complications may occur increases with each gestation.

Diagnosis and Prevention

An extensive maternal health history is obtained. Of particular interest are previous Rh sensitizations, an ectopic pregnancy, abortion, blood transfusions, or children who developed jaundice or anemia during the newborn period. The mother's blood titre is carefully monitored. An *indirect Coombs'* test on the mother's blood will indicate previous exposure to Rh-positive antigens.

Diagnosis of the disease in the prenatal period is confirmed by amniocentesis and monitoring of bilirubin levels in the amniotic fluid if the fetus is at risk. Information gained from these tests helps to determine the necessity of early interventions such as induction of labour or intrauterine fetal transfusions that allow the fetus to remain in utero until the lungs mature. Repeated transfusions may be required (Maheshwari & Carlo, 2016). Fetal Rh_0(D) status can be determined noninvasively via free DNA in maternal plasma, also known as noninvasive prenatal testing (NIPT). This technique can be used in other areas of genetic testing as well.

Prevention of HDN by the use of Rh_0(D) immune globulin is now routine. An IM injection is given to the mother within 72 hours of birth of a Rh-positive infant. Rh_0(D) immune globulin is also given to the pregnant woman at 28 weeks of gestation. When appropriate, it is also administered after a spontaneous or therapeutic abortion, after amniocentesis, and to women who have bleeding during pregnancy, because fetal blood may leak into the mother's circulation at these times.

Nursing Tip

Rh_0(D) immune globulin is administered to Rh-negative mothers by the intramuscular route after a birth, after an ectopic pregnancy, or after an abortion to prevent the development of Rh-positive antibodies. Rh_0(D) immune globulin has no effect on existing Rh-positive antibodies.

Box 12.3 ABO Incompatibility

Hemolytic disease with symptoms similar to those of hemolytic disease of the newborn (HDN) can occur with ABO incompatibility. A mother who has an O blood type and who gives birth to an infant with an A or B blood group constitutes the most commonly seen ABO incompatibility. Treatment and nursing care are the same as for HDN.

Manifestations

At the time of birth, a sample of the infant's cord blood is sent to the laboratory, although this may only be done if the mother is Rh negative. The *direct Coombs' test* detects damaging antibodies. The symptoms of HDN vary with the intensity of the disease. Anemia and jaundice may be present. The anemia is caused by hemolysis of large numbers of erythrocytes. This *pathological jaundice* differs from *physiological jaundice*

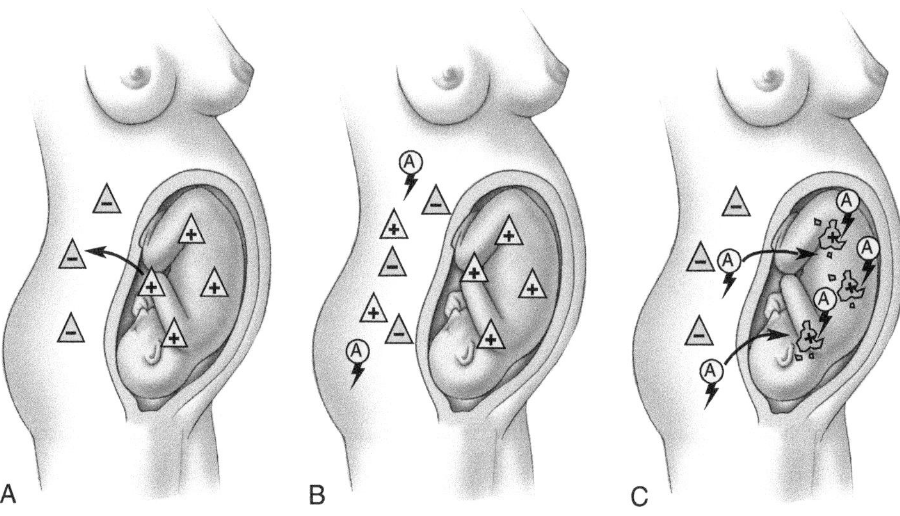

Fig. 12.9 Maternal sensitization producing hemolytic disease in the newborn. **A,** During the first pregnancy, the mother is sensitized to the Rh-positive antigen from the fetus. **B,** The mother produces Rh antibodies to the Rh antigen to which she was exposed. **C,** During a second pregnancy, these Rh antibodies cross the placenta to the fetus and destroy the fetal Rh-positive blood cells. (From Herlihy, B., & Maebius, N. K. [2011]. *The human body in health and illness* [4th ed.]. Philadelphia: Saunders.)

in that it becomes evident within 24 hours after birth. The liver is unable to handle the massive hemolysis, and bilirubin levels rise rapidly, causing hyperbilirubinemia. Early jaundice is immediately reported to the primary health care provider. Techniques of assessing for jaundice are discussed earlier in this chapter, in the Preterm Infant section.

Enlargement of the liver and spleen and extensive edema may develop. The circulating blood usually contains an excess of immature nucleated red blood cells (erythroblasts) caused by the infant's attempts to compensate for the destruction of cells. The oxygen-carrying power of the blood is diminished, as is the blood volume, and thus shock or heart failure may result. Jaundice (with symptoms such as irritability, lethargy, poor feeding, and high-pitched shrill cry), muscle weakness progressing to opisthotonos positioning (arched back), and seizures are indications of bilirubin toxicity that could lead to kernicterus. **Kernicterus** or acute bilirubin encephalopathy (accumulation of bilirubin in the brain tissues) may cause serious brain damage and permanent disability.

Safety Alert!

Jaundice that occurs on the first day of life is always pathological and necessitates prompt intervention.

Treatment and Nursing Care

Treatment of the infant is in the NICU and includes prompt identification, laboratory tests, medication therapy after birth, phototherapy, and exchange transfusion, if indicated. In the developing fetus, when the ultrasound of the middle cerebral artery and the percutaneous umbilical artery blood sampling indicates a high risk of anemia and fetal cardiac failure (*hydrops fetalis*), an in utero intravascular (umbilical vein) transfusion of packed red blood cells is given. For the infant after birth, the hemoglobin level and degree of hyperbilirubinemia determine if exchange transfusion is necessary via umbilical vein. IV administration of IVIG at birth may reduce red blood cell destruction in the newborn, thereby reducing hyperbilirubinemia and the need for exchange transfusion (Maheshwari & Carlo 2016).

Phototherapy (see discussion earlier in chapter) may be used to reduce serum bilirubin levels. It may be used alone or in conjunction with an exchange transfusion (Fig. 12.10). The nursing care of the infant receiving phototherapy is presented in Nursing Care Plan 12.2. If phototherapy and IVIG administration fail to keep the TSB at acceptable levels to prevent kernicterus, an exchange transfusion may be indicated.

During an exchange transfusion, a plastic catheter is inserted into the umbilical vein of the newborn, small amounts of blood (10 to 20 mL) are withdrawn, and equal amounts of Rh-negative blood are injected. The amount of donor blood used is about twice the infant blood volume, to a limit of 500 mL. In this way, healthy cells are added to the infant's blood and antibodies are removed. Additional small transfusions may be necessary later. After a second exchange transfusion, approximately 85% of the infant's blood will have been replaced. Antibiotics may be given to prevent infection.

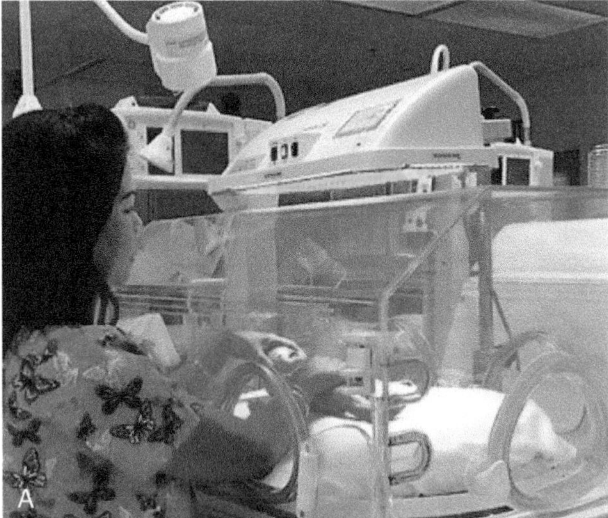

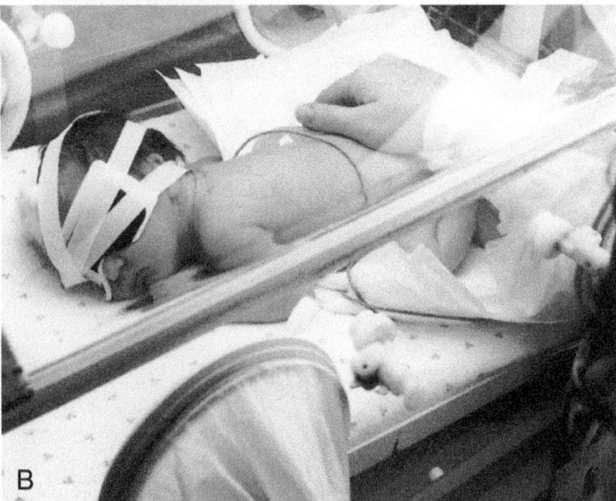

Fig. 12.10 Phototherapy. **A,** The bililight provides a high-intensity, narrow band of blue light that helps break down excess bilirubin. A second light is available to change from conventional to intense phototherapy treatment. **B,** When an infant receives phototherapy in an isolette, the eyes are protected from the lights and the infant may only be dressed in a diaper. The infant is turned frequently so that all skin surfaces are exposed to the lights.

The NICU nurse is usually responsible for the following: observing the newborn's colour and reporting any evidence of jaundice during the first and second days; stressing to mothers the importance of good prenatal care for subsequent pregnancies; helping to interpret the treatment to parents by giving reassurance as needed; and observing and assisting the health care provider with the exchange transfusion.

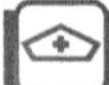

Nursing Tip

All newborns who are visibly jaundiced in the first 24 hours of life should have their serum bilirubin level determined.

Nursing Care Plan 12.2 The Infant Receiving Phototherapy

Patient Data A newborn, 36 hours of age, is diagnosed with hyperbilirubinemia and is placed in an isolette for phototherapy.

Selected Nursing Diagnosis Potential for injury to eyes as a result of phototherapy

Goals	Nursing Interventions	Rationales
Infant does not have eye drainage or irritation.	Apply eye patches over infant's closed eyes before placing infant under lights.	Closing eyes prevents corneal abrasion and protects the retina from damage by high-intensity light.
	Inspect eyes at least once per shift to assess eyes for conjunctivitis.	Facilitates early detection of inflammation
	Remove patches to allow eye contact during feeding.	Provides for visual stimulation and bonding.

Selected Nursing Diagnosis Impaired skin integrity as a result of immature structure and function, immobility

Goals	Nursing Interventions	Rationales
Skin will remain intact as evidenced by absence of skin rash, excoriation, or redness.	Observe for maculopapular rash.	Rashes and burns have been known to occur as a result of phototherapy.
	Check diaper regularly and clean peri-anal area when needed.	Frequent stools may cause breakdown of skin; loose stools are a result of increased bilirubin excretion.
	Observe for jaundice or bronzing. (NOTE: Serum bilirubin level may be high, even though infant may not appear jaundiced under lights.)	Jaundice may be an initial sign of hyperbilirubinemia.
	Observe for pressure areas.	Early intervention prevents skin breakdown.

Selected Nursing Diagnosis Potential for reduced fluid volume as a result of increased water loss through skin and loose stools

Goals	Nursing Interventions	Rationales
Infant will not become dehydrated, as evidenced by good skin turgor, normal fontanelles, and moist tongue and mucous membranes.	Assessment per shift of skin turgor, fontanelles, and mucous membranes. Monitor oral and intravenous fluid intake as well as urine output and bowel movements.	Increase in oral and/or intravenous (IV) fluids is sometimes used to manage or prevent dehydration, as dehydration can increase the serum bilirubin.
Weight maintenance and urine output will be satisfactory.	Encourage frequent feeding.	Adequate hydration facilitates elimination and excretion of bilirubin.
	Measure weights daily.	Assesses progress; helps to determine extent of dehydration.

Selected Nursing Diagnosis Potential risk for hyperthermia or hypothermia

Goals	Nursing Interventions	Rationales
Infant will not become overheated or chilled; temperature will be maintained between 36.5° and 37.4°C.	Monitor infant's temperature at minimum of every 4 hours and adjust isolette temperature accordingly.	Hyperthermia and hypothermia are common complications of phototherapy.

Selected Nursing Diagnosis Potential for injury (neurological) as a result of hyperbilirubinemia

Goals	Nursing Interventions	Rationales
Infant will show no signs of neurological involvement (e.g., lethargy, twitching).	Anticipate measurement of daily bilirubin blood levels.	Phototherapy success is determined by frequently measuring serum bilirubin levels.
	Turn off phototherapy lights when blood is being drawn, to prevent false readings.	Promotes accuracy of blood test.

Continued

Nursing Care Plan 12.2 The Infant Receiving Phototherapy—cont'd

Goals	Nursing Interventions	Rationales
	Observe parameters for neurological deficit (e.g., twitching, lethargy).	Kernicterus (brain damage) is rare but is evidenced by neurological sequelae such as hypotonia, diminished reflexes, twitching, and lethargy.

Selected Nursing Diagnosis Possible imbalanced nutrition due to poor feeding behaviour

Goals	Nursing Interventions	Rationales
Infant will receive adequate nutrients as evidenced by stabilization of weight and laboratory reports.	Provide feedings as ordered.	Early feedings within the first hour after birth tend to decrease high bilirubin levels and provide nourishment.

Selected Nursing Diagnosis Parental anxiety resulting from inadequate knowledge regarding having an infant with jaundice

Goals	Nursing Interventions	Rationales
Parents express fears concerning infant's welfare.	Explain procedures and treatment. Provide reassurance. Provide follow-up care.	Information decreases parental stress. Parents are in need of support persons. Follow-up care is reassuring to parents and medical personnel that family is progressing well without complications.

Home phototherapy

Where available, home phototherapy programs are being used for newborns with mild to moderate physiological (normal) jaundice. These programs are advocated because bilirubin levels generally begin to increase on the third day after birth, when the mother and newborn are discharged. An increase in bilirubin levels may necessitate the newborn's return to the hospital and the possible separation of mother and infant.

A phototherapy blanket in a bassinet (Fig. 12.11) or a fibre-optic pad (Fig. 12.12) can be used. These allow for holding the infant and decrease the risk of eye damage. Written instructions are given to the parents. Parents keep a daily record of their infant's temperature, weight, intake and output, stools, and feedings (see Nursing Care Plan 14.2). Daily monitoring of bilirubin levels is important, to make sure that the bilirubin level is coming down. Phototherapy tips are listed in Box 12.4.

INTRACRANIAL HEMORRHAGE

Pathophysiology

Intracranial hemorrhage, the most common type of birth injury, may result from trauma or anoxia. It occurs more often in the preterm infant, whose blood vessels are fragile. Blood vessels within the skull are broken, and bleeding into the brain occurs. When the diagnosis is made, the specific location of the hemorrhage may be noted (i.e., subdural, subarachnoid, or intraventricular). This injury may also occur during precipitate (rapid) birth or prolonged labour or when the newborn's head is large in comparison with the mother's pelvis.

Manifestations

The signs of intracranial hemorrhage may occur suddenly or gradually. Some signs or all signs may be present, depending on the severity of the hemorrhage, and can include poor muscle tone, lethargy, poor sucking reflex, respiratory distress, cyanosis, twitching, forceful vomiting, a high-pitched shrill cry, and convulsions. Opisthotonos posturing may be observed (see Fig. 23.13). The fontanelle may be tense and under pressure rather than soft and compressible. The pupil of one eye is likely to be small (constricted) and the other large (dilated).

If the symptoms are mild, most patients have a good chance of complete recovery. Death results if there is a massive hemorrhage. The infant who survives an extensive hemorrhage may suffer residual effects such as developmental delays or cerebral palsy. The diagnosis is established by the history of the birth, computed tomography (CT) scan, magnetic resonance imaging (MRI), evidence of an increase in intracranial pressure (ICP), and the symptoms and course of the disease.

Treatment and Nursing Care

The newborn is placed in an isolette, which allows proper temperature control, ease in administering oxygen, and continuous observation. The infant is handled gently and as little as possible. The head is elevated. The health care provider may prescribe vitamin K to control bleeding and phenobarbital if twitching or convulsions are apparent. Prophylactic antibiotics and vitamins may be used. The infant is fed carefully because the sucking reflex may be affected. The infant

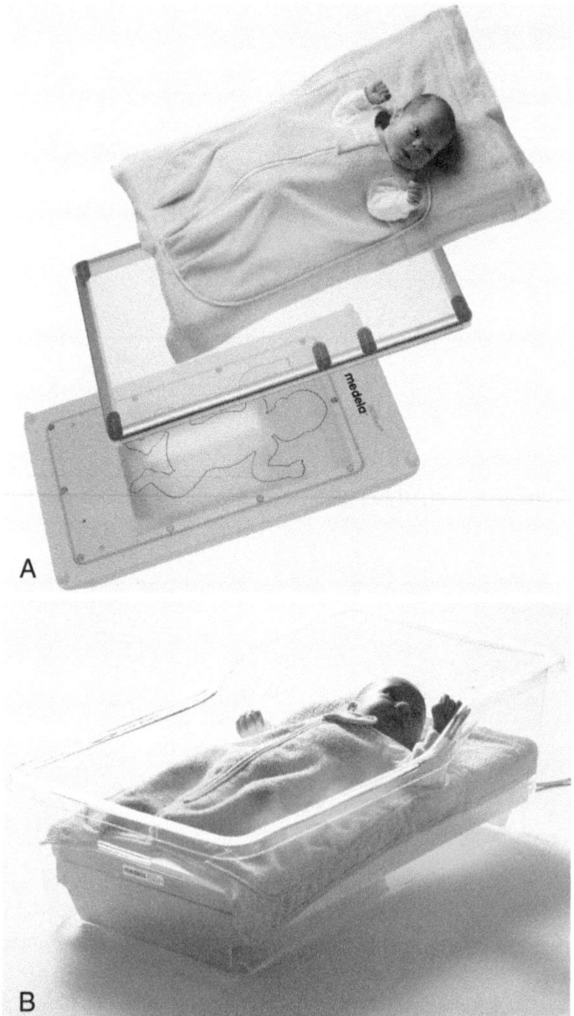

Fig. 12.11 Phototherapy Bilibed. **A,** The infant is diapered and placed in the therapy blanket, which fits on a light-permeable infant support. This plastic support is placed over the irradiation unit, which fits into the standard bassinet instead of the mattress. **B,** The infant in the Bilibed can be with the mother and requires no eye-patch protection. The therapeutic light focuses directly on the infant's skin through the underside of the phototherapy blanket. (Photos courtesy Medela.)

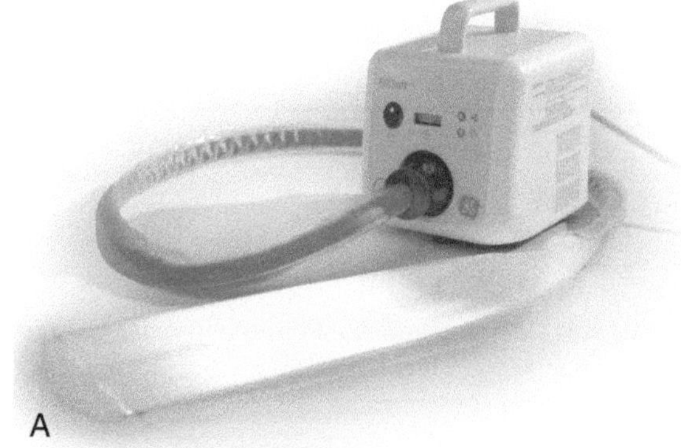

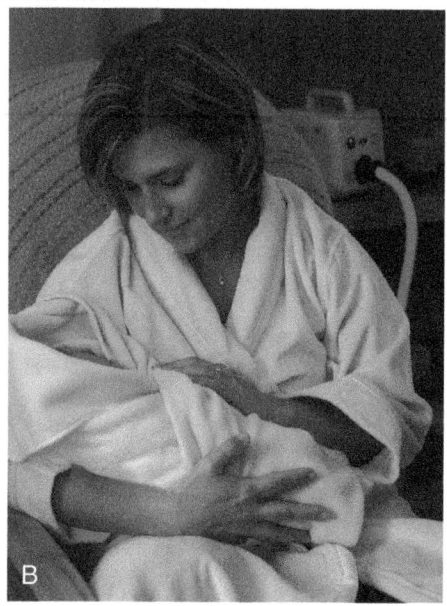

Fig. 12.12 Biliblanket plus high-output phototherapy system. **A,** A pad of woven fibres is used to transport light from a light source to the infant. This fibre-optic pad is wrapped directly on the infant's skin to bathe the skin in light. **B,** The infant can then be diapered, clothed, held, and nursed during treatment at home. (Photos courtesy Medela.)

vomits easily. The nurse needs to observe the infant for signs of increased ICP (see Chapter 23) and convulsions and assists the primary health care provider with procedures such as lumbar punctures and aspiration of subdural hemorrhage. Performing neurological assessments, monitoring vital signs and head circumference, and palpating fontanelles are essential.

Convulsion or seizures may occur. Newborn seizures are very subtle and can be difficult to diagnose. They include eye blinking or fluttering; sucking, lip smacking, chewing, and protruding tongue; bicycling movements of the legs; apnea; and thrashing movements. Clonic movement involves rhythmic movements of part of the face, tongue, arms, or legs. During tonic movement the infant turns their head or eyes to one side and stretches the arms or legs.

If a convulsion occurs, observation of its character can aid the health care provider in diagnosing the possible location of the bleeding. The following are of particular importance: Were the arms, legs, or face involved? Was the right or left side of the body involved? Was the convulsion mild or severe? How long did it last? What was the condition of the infant before and after the seizure? The nurse records observations and notifies the team leader or health care provider.

TRNASIENT TACHYPNEA OF THE NEWBORN

Transient tachypnea of the newborn (TTN) usually occurs after a Caesarean birth or a rapid vaginal birth of a term or near-term infant. It is characterized by tachypnea (rapid respirations) and may also include chest retractions, grunting, and mild cyanosis. The condition is often referred to as "wet lung." The distinctive feature of this condition is that it typically resolves after 3 days. TTN is thought to be caused by slow absorption of the fluid in the lungs after birth. Treatment is supportive, providing warmth, energy conservation, and, if indicated, respiratory pressure support with a CPAP machine and supplemental oxygen.

Box 12.4 Phototherapy Tips

IF THE INFANT IS IN AN ISOLETTE
- Measure the irradiance level of the lights once per shift to ensure that the lights emit the correct dose.
- Cover the infant's eyes while under lights.
- Place a small diaper over the gonad area.
- The infant does not need to be dressed or wrapped because the isolette environment will prevent chilling.
- Distinguish loose, greenish stools caused by photo degradation products from true diarrhea.

IF THE INFANT IS WRAPPED IN A BILIBLANKET
- Put the light source on a flat, nonabsorbent surface and not on a carpet or crib mattress.
- Use a three-pronged plug for safety, and set the intensity knob on the light box to the highest setting.
- Measure the irradiance level at the beginning of the treatment to ensure that the blanket emits the correct dose.
- Do not put anything on top of the light source box or the fibre-optic cable.
- Expose as much of the infant's skin as possible to the biliblanket while keeping a diaper in place.
- Be sure there is a clean, disposable cover between the light-emitting side of the pad and the infant's skin.

MECONIUM ASPIRATION SYNDROME

Meconium aspiration syndrome (MAS) is a group of symptoms that occur when the fetus or newborn aspirates meconium-stained amniotic fluid into the lungs.

In utero, the fetus often expels some meconium into the amniotic fluid during a prolonged labour process, especially if there is cord compression or another condition that temporarily interrupts fetal circulation. If asphyxia and acidosis occur in utero, the fetus may make gasping movements that draw meconium-stained amniotic fluid into the lungs. Meconium aspiration can be prevented by promoting identification of fetal distress and rapid birth when the fetal heart tracings show an abnormal tracing.

Amnioinfusion during labour (see Chapter 8) and suctioning the newborn after birth are not reliably effective. Respiratory distress is the primary symptom of MAS, including nasal flaring, retractions, cyanosis, grunting, rales, and rhonchi (See Fig. 12.5). The tachypnea may persist for several weeks. Treatment includes supportive care with warmth, supplemental oxygen, and energy-conserving plans of care. Intubation and mechanical ventilation may be necessary, and the infant is transferred to the NICU.

NEONATAL OPIOID WITHDRAWAL SYNDROME

Neonatal opioid withdrawal syndrome (NOWS), previously called *neonatal abstinence syndrome (NAS)*, occurs when the fetus has prenatal exposure to opiates while in utero. Because opioids cross the placenta, the infant exposed to opioids in utero is physiologically dependent on the drugs and suffers withdrawal symptoms after birth. Body tremors and hyperirritability are the principal signs of this condition in the newborn. Wakefulness, diarrhea, poor feeding, sneezing, and yawning may also be present. Unless medically indicated, the mother and baby should be kept together.

The nurse needs to educate the mother in nonpharmacological strategies as a first line of treatment. Nonpharmacological strategies include skin-to-skin care with the mother; swaddling and holding the infant in a C position; vertical rocking; and decreasing environmental stimulation. Breastfeeding should be encouraged unless contraindicated because of HIV infection or polydrug use. Breastfeeding has shown to delay the onset and decrease the severity of the symptoms of withdrawal. Often these babies will show impaired feeding behaviours that may require more frequent and smaller feeds, supplementation with concentrate to increase the caloric intake, and gavage feeding (Lacaze, O'Flaherty, & CPS Fetus and Newborn Committee, 2018). Treatment with medication may be indicated if withdrawal symptoms are not controlled.

Fetal alcohol spectrum disorder (FASD) and parent teaching are discussed in Chapter 5.

INFANT OF A DIABETIC MOTHER

Diabetes in the mother presents various problems for the newborn. These are determined by the severity and duration of the disease in the mother, the degree of control of her condition, and the gestational age of the infant. Diabetes in pregnancy is discussed in Chapter 5. When diabetes of the mother is under good control from conception and throughout the pregnancy, the adverse effects on the newborn infant are minimal.

Some newborn infants of diabetic mothers have serious complications. When the mother is hyperglycemic, large amounts of glucose are transferred to the fetus. This makes the fetus hyperglycemic. In response, the fetal pancreas (islet cells) produces large amounts of fetal insulin. Hyperinsulinism, along with excess production of protein and fatty acids, often results in a newborn infant who weighs more than 4 000 g (9 lb). Such an infant is designated LGA, and this condition is termed macrosomia (*macro*, "large," and *soma*, "body"). This infant is prone to injuries at birth because of their size (Fig. 12.13).

After birth, the infant often has low blood glucose levels because of the abrupt loss of maternal glucose and hypertrophy of the pancreatic islet cells, which results in a temporary overproduction of insulin. The infant has a characteristic cushingoid appearance because of increased subcutaneous fat. The face is round and appears puffy, and the infant appears lethargic.

The size of these newborn infants makes them appear healthy, but this is deceptive because they often have developmental deficits and may suffer complications of RDS or congenital anomalies. In contrast, some infants born to a mother with severe diabetes may be SGA because of poor placental perfusion. These infants often have hypoglycemia, hypocalcemia, and hyperbilirubinemia.

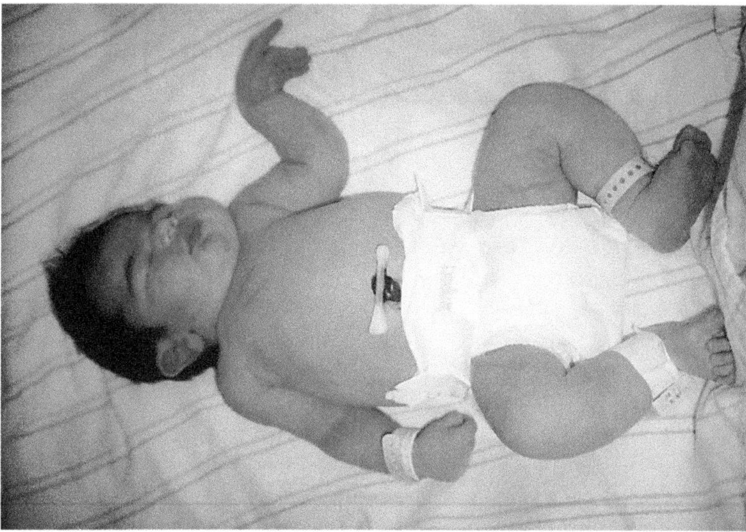

Fig. 12.13 Macrosomia. A newborn with macrosomia caused by maternal diabetes mellitus during pregnancy. This infant weighed 5.5 kg (11 lb) at birth. Macrosomic infants often have respiratory disorders and other problems. (Courtesy Pat Spier, RN-C.)

The nursing care of the infant of a diabetic mother includes close monitoring of vital signs, early feeding, and frequent assessment of blood glucose levels for the first 2 days of life. Hypoglycemia in the first days of life is defined as a blood glucose level that falls below 2.6 mmol/L. It can result in rapid and permanent brain damage. The infant should be closely watched for signs of irritability, tremors, and respiratory distress.

BIRTH DEFECTS

Birth defects, or abnormalities that are apparent at birth, occur in 3 to 4% of all live births. The rate is even higher if the defects that become evident later in life are counted. An abnormality of structure, function, or metabolism may result in a physical or mental disability, may shorten life, or may be fatal. Box 12.5 shows the system of classification of birth defects. Most of these conditions are discussed in detail in the pediatric section of this textbook. FASD and environmental influences on fetal growth are discussed in Chapter 5. Congenital heart disease is discussed in Chapter 26.

Defects present at birth often involve the skeletal system; limbs may be missing, malformed, or duplicated. Some abnormalities (e.g., developmental dysplasia of the hip) are more subtle, and the nurse must be alert to detect them. *Inborn errors of metabolism* include a number of inherited diseases that affect body chemistry. There may be an absence or a deficiency of a substance necessary for cell metabolism. The deficient substance is usually an enzyme. Almost any organ of the body may be damaged. Examples of inborn errors of metabolism include cystic fibrosis and phenylketonuria (PKU). In *disorders of the blood,* there is a reduced or missing blood component or an inability of a component to function adequately. Sickle cell disease, thalassemia, and hemophilia fall in this category. *Chromosomal abnormalities* number in the thousands. Most involve some type of cognitive disability, and others are incompatible with life. The newborn with Turner syndrome or Klinefelter syndrome may have impaired physical growth and sexual development. *Perinatal injuries* have many causes and are seen in various forms, the most common of which is premature birth.

The majority of birth defects are thought to result from an interplay between environment and heredity, depending on inherited susceptibility, stage of pregnancy, and degree of environmental hazard. Newborns with

Box 12.5 Classification of Birth Defects

MALFORMATIONS PRESENT AT BIRTH

Structural Defects

Hydrocephalus, spina bifida, congenital heart malformations, cleft lip and palate, clubfoot, developmental dysplasia of the hip, tracheoesophageal fistula, hypospadias, and others

Metabolic Defects (Body Chemistry)

Cystic fibrosis, phenylketonuria, Tay-Sachs disease, family hypercholesterolemia (high cholesterol that often causes early heart attack), and others

Blood Disorders

Sickle cell disease, hemophilia, thalassemia, defects of white blood cells and immune defense, and others (see Chapter 27)

Chromosomal Abnormalities

Down syndrome, Klinefelter syndrome, Turner syndrome, trisomies 13 and 18, and many others; most involve some combination of cognitive disability and physical malformations that range from mild to fatal

Perinatal Conditions

Infections, drugs, maternal disorders, abnormalities unique to pregnancy (e.g., Rh disease, difficult labour or birth, premature birth)

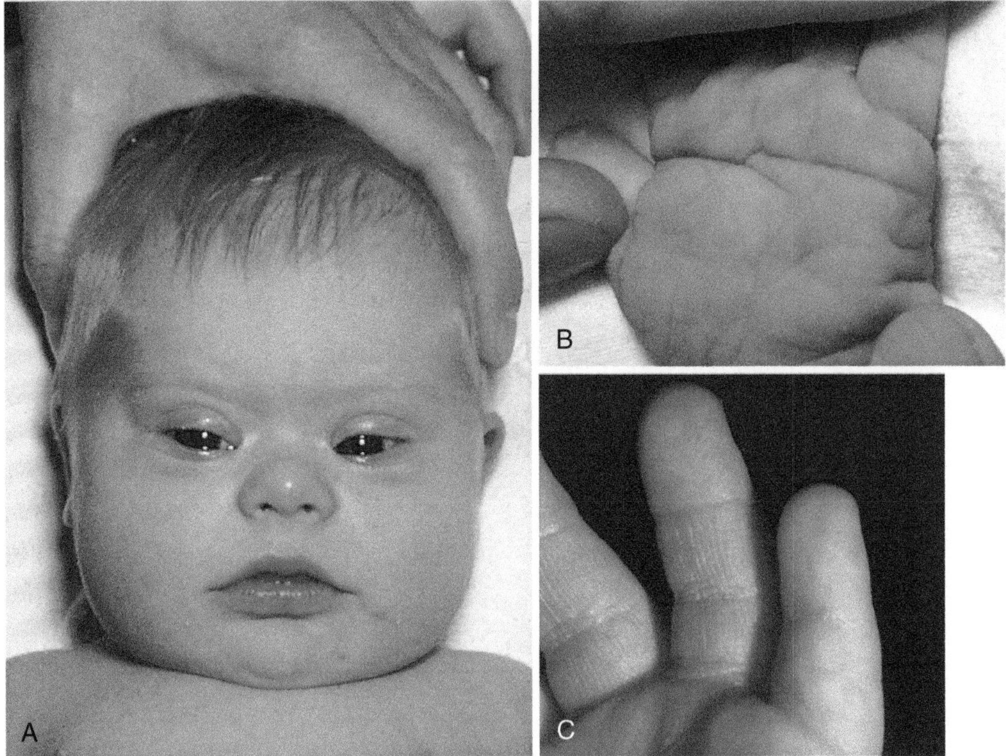

Fig. 12.14 Down syndrome. **A,** The typical facial appearance of an infant with Down syndrome shows the upward slant of the canthal folds of the eyes, protruding tongue, and short, thick neck. **B,** The straight simian crease in the palm of the hand is a typical finding in children with Down syndrome. **C,** The short fifth finger is a typical finding in children with Down syndrome. The tip of the fifth finger does not extend to the distal joint of the adjoining finger. (From Zitelli, B. L., & Davis, H. W. [2012]. *Zitelli and Davis' atlas of pediatric physical diagnosis* [6th ed.]. St. Louis: Saunders.)

birth defects may need to remain in the NICU for an extended period of time for intensive care and treatment.

CHROMOSOMAL ABNORMALITIES

Down Syndrome

Pathophysiology

Down syndrome is one of the most common chromosomal abnormalities. In Canada its incidence is approximately 1 in 750 live births (Public Health Agency of Canada [PHAC], 2017). It is the most common cause of genetic intellectual disability, and children born with this birth defect may also have some physical abnormalities.

There are three phenotypes (genetic makeups) of Down syndrome: trisomy 21, mosaicism, and translocation of a chromosome. The most common type, trisomy 21 syndrome, accounts for 95% of patients. In this instance, there are three number 21 chromosomes rather than the normal two. This is a result of *nondisjunction,* the failure of a chromosome to follow the normal separation process into daughter cells. The earlier in the embryo's development this occurs, the greater the number of cells affected. When nondisjunction occurs late in development, both normal and abnormal cells are present in the newborn. This condition is *mosaicism,* and individuals tend to be less severely affected in physical appearance and intelligence. The third condition is *translocation.* In translocation, a piece of chromosome in pair 21 breaks away and attaches itself to another chromosome. Translocation has the highest rate of reoccurrence in a future pregnancy (Bacino, & Lee, 2016).

Screening for Down syndrome is offered between 11 and 14 weeks of pregnancy and includes an ultrasound assessment of the thickness of the fetal nuchal fold (called *nuchal translucency*) along with blood work. This early screening allows parents to discuss options of terminating or continuing the pregnancy with preparation for the outcome. A positive screening test may indicate the need for amniocentesis to confirm the diagnosis (see Chapter 4).

Manifestations

Down syndrome can be diagnosed by the clinical manifestations, but a chromosomal analysis will confirm the specific type. The signs of Down syndrome, which are apparent at birth, are close-set and upward-slanting eyes, small head, round face, flat nose, protruding tongue that interferes with sucking, and mouth breathing (Fig. 12.14, *A*). There is often a deep, straight line across the palm, which is called a *simian crease* (see Fig. 12.14, *B*). The hands of the infant are short and thick, and the little finger is curved (see Fig. 12.14, *C*). There is also a wide space between the first and the second toes. The undeveloped muscles and loose joints enable the child to assume unusual positions. Physical growth and development may be slower than normal. The child is limited intellectually. Some children have been found to have intelligence quotients (IQs) in the borderline to low-average range. Congenital heart deformities are also associated with this condition.

Children with Down syndrome are very lovable. Their resistance to infection is poor, and they are prone to respiratory and ear infections as well as speech and hearing problems. The lifespan of children with Down syndrome has increased with the widespread use of antibiotics. The incidence of acute leukemia is higher in these children than in the normal population, and Alzheimer disease is common to those who reach middle adult life (Jackson, Vessey, & Schapiro, 2009).

The limp, flaccid posture of the infant is caused by hypotonicity of the muscles; it makes positioning and holding more difficult and contributes to heat loss from the exposed surface areas. The infant should be warmly wrapped to prevent chilling. The hypotonicity of muscles also causes respiratory problems and excess mucus accumulation. Bulb suctioning may be necessary before feedings. In addition, the hypotonicity of muscles contributes to the development of constipation, which can be controlled by dietary intervention.

Nursing care

Counselling parents. The counselling of families of Down syndrome children is ongoing. Nurses must be aware of their own feelings before they can effectively support parents. They, too, may feel saddened at the birth of an imperfect child. They may identify with the parents. It is appropriate to express one's feelings of initial helplessness, and it may encourage the parents to verbalize their concerns. The nurse must listen and provide honest, tactful, and compassionate support.

Empathy from the nurse is particularly important. Involving family in the care and planning for the infant from the start facilitates bonding. The need for the staff's warm concern cannot be overestimated.

Counselling siblings. Siblings of the patient must be informed and included in discussions about the newborn. Even very young children are aware of parental distress, and the situations the children imagine can be more frightening than the reality. Early and open communications will prevent isolation and misconceptions and promote an easier transition period. The effects on siblings have been identified, and not all effects are negative. Some siblings state a deeper understanding of others who are different and are more appreciative of what they themselves have (Hyunkyung & VanRiper, 2013). Social support from friends and parent–child relationships, which may be influenced by family demands, should be recognized and resources in the community identified (Hyunkyung & VanRiper, 2013). The nurse should connect the family with a Down syndrome support group in their area if there is one. Other parents with a Down syndrome child are an important resource. The Canadian Down Syndrome Society is one organization that provides education and support to families.

METABOLIC DEFECTS

The infant with an inborn error of metabolism has a genetic defect that may not be apparent before birth. As the infant adjusts to the birth process and begins to ingest nourishment, symptoms can rapidly emerge that quickly become life-threatening. Symptoms such as lethargy, poor feeding, hypotonia, a unique odour to the body or urine, tachypnea, and vomiting must be reported by the nurse to prevent long-term or life-threatening sequelae. The nurse must also be prepared to offer psychological support and to help parents deal with the impact of having an infant with a genetic problem.

Phenylketonuria

Pathophysiology

Classic phenylketonuria (PKU) is a genetic disorder caused by the faulty metabolism of phenylalanine, an amino acid that is essential to life and is found in all protein foods. This inborn error of metabolism, which is transmitted by an autosomal recessive gene, is associated with abnormally high blood phenylalanine levels. The hepatic enzyme phenylalanine hydrolase, which is normally needed to convert phenylalanine into tyrosine, is missing. When the infant is fed breastmilk or formula, phenylalanine begins to accumulate in the blood. It can increase to as high as 20 times the normal amount. Its byproduct, phenylpyruvic acid, appears in the urine within the first weeks of life.

Classic PKU can result in severe cognitive disability that is evidenced in infancy if not detected and treated early. By the time the urine test is positive, brain damage has already occurred. The infant appears normal at birth but begins to show delayed development at about 4 to 6 months of age. The child may show evidence of failure to thrive, have eczema or other skin conditions, have a peculiar musty odour, or have personality disorders. About one third of the children have seizures. PKU occurs mainly in blonde and blue-eyed children; these features result from a lack of tyrosine, a necessary component of the pigment melanin. Less severe forms of the disorder are now recognized. They are designated as "atypical PKU" and "mild hyperphenylalaninemia."

Diagnosis

The *Guthrie blood test* is widely used and is currently considered the most reliable test for PKU. All babies in Canada are screened for PKU unless screening is declined by the parents. If parents are unsure and are considering declining, it is important to explain to them that the risk associated with the collection of the blood sample is minimal and the screening test is in the best interest of the child. Blood is obtained from a simple heel stick. A few drops of capillary blood are placed on filter paper and mailed to the laboratory for screening. It is recommended that the blood be obtained between 24 and 48 hours of life. If the infant is discharged before

24 hours, the test should be done prior to discharge and repeated by 2 weeks of life. Since blood transfusion can affect the test, it is best to collect a blood sample for screening before the transfusion (Perinatal Service BC, 2018). Confirmation of the diagnosis requires quantitative elevations of phenylalanine compound in the blood (Rizvani & Ficicioglu, 2016). Screening programs for pregnant women have also been advocated, to detect elevated phenylalanine levels that could have an effect on the newborn.

Treatment and nursing care

Treatment of PKU consists of close dietary management and frequent evaluation of blood phenylalanine levels. Because phenylalanine is found in all natural protein foods, a food that provides enough protein for growth and tissue repair, but little phenylalanine, must be substituted. The goals of the diet are to provide enough essential proteins to support growth and development while maintaining phenylalanine blood levels between 120 and 360 mmol/L.

There is a low phenylalanine content in milk, and infants can be partially breastfed and supplemented with Lofenalac while phenylalanine blood levels are monitored. Solid foods that are low in phenylalanine are added at the same age that solid foods are added for infants without PKU. A dietitian may be consulted concerning parental guidance and support in maintaining the dietary regimen, especially for the school-age child and adolescent. Eventually the child learns to assume full management of the diet. While a single can of diet cola containing NutraSweet or Equal (aspartame) will not significantly raise blood levels of phenylalanine, the intake of most meat, dairy products, and diet drinks must be restricted. An exchange list for food selection can aid the child in participating in and monitoring their progress. Flavouring the milk substitute with a fruit-flavoured powder or chocolate flavouring can increase the palatability for the child. Sapropterin dihydrochloride (Kuvan) is the first medication on the market to treat this inherited disorder and is designed to break down excess phenylalaline in the blood and convert it to tyrosine. The tablets or powder is dissolved in juice and administered by mouth.

Genetic counselling is important for the affected child for future family planning. Women of childbearing age who have PKU must follow a low-phenylalanine diet before conception to prevent brain damage of the fetus during development. Phenylalanine levels greater than 360 mmol/L in pregnant women can affect development of the embryo.

> **! Safety Alert!**
>
> Children with PKU must avoid the sweetener aspartame (NutraSweet or Equal) because it is converted to phenylalanine in the body.

Maple Syrup Urine Disease

Pathophysiology

Maple syrup urine disease is caused by a defect in the metabolism of branched-chain amino acids, leading to marked serum elevations of leucine, isoleucine, and valine. This results in acidosis, cerebral degeneration, and death within 2 weeks if left untreated.

Manifestations

The infant with maple syrup urine disease appears healthy at birth but soon develops feeding difficulties, loss of the Moro reflex, hypotonia, irregular respirations, and convulsions. The infant's urine, sweat, and cerumen (earwax) have a characteristic sweet or maple syrup odour. This is caused by ketoacidosis, a process similar to that which may occur in diabetic children, and causes a fruity odour of the breath. However, the condition does not resolve with the correction of blood glucose levels. Because the urine contains high levels of leucine, isoleucine, and valine diagnosis is confirmed by blood and urine tests.

Treatment and nursing care

Early detection by universal screening 24 to 48 hours after birth in the newborn period is extremely important. The nurse should report any newborn whose urine has a sweet aroma. Initial treatment consists of removing these amino acids and their metabolites from the tissues of the body through hydration and peritoneal dialysis to decrease serum levels. The patient is placed on a lifelong diet that is low in the amino acids leucine, isoleucine, and valine. Several formulas specifically for this disease are available. Exacerbations are most often related to the degree to which the leucine level is abnormal. These exacerbations are frequently related to infection and can be life-threatening. The nurse must frequently assess the patient and instruct parents about the need to prevent infections.

Galactosemia

Pathophysiology

In galactosemia the body is unable to use the carbohydrates galactose and lactose. In the healthy person, the liver converts galactose to glucose. In the patient with galactosemia, an enzyme is defective or missing and there is a disturbance in a normally occurring chemical reaction. The result is an increase in the amount of galactose in the blood (*galactosemia*) and in the urine (*galactosuria*). This condition can cause cirrhosis of the liver, cataracts, and developmental delays if left untreated. Because galactose is present in milk sugar, early diagnosis is necessary so that a milk substitute can be used.

Manifestations

The symptoms of galactosemia begin abruptly and worsen gradually. Early signs consist of lethargy, vomiting, hypotonia, diarrhea, and failure to thrive. These commence as the newborn begins breastfeeding or ingesting formula. Jaundice may be present. Diagnosis is made by observing galactosuria, galactosemia, and evidence of decreased enzyme activity in the red blood cells. Screening tests are available.

Treatment and nursing care

Milk and lactose-containing products are eliminated from the diet of the patient with galactosemia. The nursing mother must discontinue breastfeeding. Lactose-free formulas and those with a soy-protein base are often substituted. The nurse needs to realize the frustration and anxiety that this diagnosis can create. Parents can experience periods of feeling overwhelmed and inadequate. They can also become totally absorbed in the dietary program. Managing a rare disease can create feelings of isolation and uncertainty. Because surveillance is ongoing, some of the emotional characteristics of the family with a child who has a chronic disease are pertinent.

Unfolding Case Study

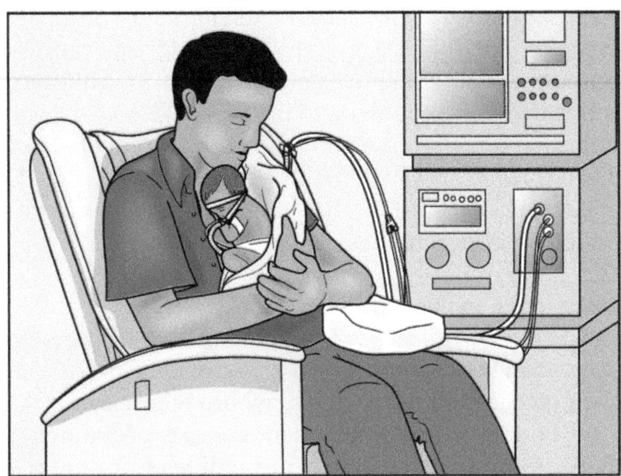

Tess and her husband Luis were introduced to the reader in Chapter 2, and each chapter has followed Tess through her labour and birth. She has delivered twins. Baby Marco is in the postpartum unit with Tess. Baby Sofia showed signs of respiratory distress and was transported to the NICU, accompanied by Tess's partner Luis.

Sofia was admitted to the NICU and has been diagnosed with respiratory distress and inadequate thermoregulation. She has been placed in an isolette.

QUESTIONS

1. What are the signs of respiratory distress in the newborn?
2. What are the nursing responsibilities involved in applying a pulse oximeter and monitoring Sofia's oxygen saturation?
3. The health care provider has suggested kangaroo care for baby Sofia. What is kangaroo care? Can Sofia's father give kangaroo care to Sofia? What guidance and teaching will the nurse offer Sofia's father?
4. While in the NICU, Sofia's vital signs will be monitored. What are the normal vital signs of a newborn infant?
5. Sofia's respiratory distress has resolved but increasing jaundice is now noted and the bilirubin level is reported to be 280 mcmol/L. She has been diagnosed with hyperbilirubinemia. Sofia is diapered and placed in an isolette under phototherapy lights. What factors led to hyperbilirubinemia in Sofia?
6. What are the signs of bilirubin toxicity that leads to kernicterus that the nurse should watch for and document?
7. What are the safety measures involved in the nursing care of Sofia while she is in the isolette?
8. What are the priorities of nursing care for Sofia? Can she be fed breast milk?
9. Based on Sofia's diagnosis, what treatment should Sofia's mother have prior to discharge?

Get Ready for the Certification Examination!

Key Points

- Every week in utero up to 39 weeks' gestation is important for optimal fetal development.
- Early identification of the high-risk fetus facilitates treatment and nursing care.
- Studies indicate that there is a relationship between prematurity and poverty, smoking, alcohol consumption, opioid use, and lack of prenatal care.
- Preterm infants have poor muscle tone and less subcutaneous fat but more vernix and lanugo than full-term infants.
- The preterm infant is observed for jaundice, low oxygen saturation levels, and unstable vital signs. The intake and output of all preterm infants is monitored.
- The care of preterm infants is organized and "clustered" to minimize handling and stimulation.
- Blanket rolls are used to provide an enclosed space for preterm infants.
- Nurses must support parents and encourage participation in care when the parents are ready.
- Respiratory distress syndrome has a high mortality rate, and it may precipitate long-term effects.
- Hypoxia is lack of oxygen on the cellular level, and hypoxemia is decreased oxygen in the circulating blood.
- Problems associated with prematurity include asphyxia, meconium aspiration, hypoglycemia, hypocalcemia, hemorrhage from fragile vessels, poor resistance to infection, and inadequate nutrition.
- Hypoglycemia is defined as glucose level lower than 2.6 mmol/L.

- Thermoregulation is essential for the preterm newborn's survival. Cold stress is to be avoided.
- Nursing goals in caring for the preterm newborn are improving respirations, maintaining body heat, conserving the infant's energy, preventing infection, providing nutrition and hydration, providing good skin care, and supporting and encouraging the parents to provide care.
- Kangaroo care promotes stabilization of the infant and can enhance their later development.
- Retinopathy of prematurity is a disorder of the developing retina that can lead to blindness in the preterm infant.
- The post-term newborn is born after 42 weeks of gestation and shows certain characteristics that place the infant at risk, such as hypoxia, poor nutritional stores, and polycythemia.
- The post-term newborn has little lanugo and vernix, and the skin is dry and peeling.
- Rh immune globulin is given to an Rh-negative mother after giving birth to an Rh-positive fetus to prevent maternal Rh sensitization.
- Hyperbilirubinemia results from rapid destruction of red blood cells.
- Jaundice that occurs in the first 24 hours of life is considered pathological.
- Distinguishing pathological jaundice from physiological jaundice can facilitate early intervention and prevent serious complications.
- Macrosomia is a condition in which the infant is large for gestational age and usually occurs in infants of diabetic mothers.
- Newborn infants are routinely screened for phenylketonuria and other metabolic condtions.

Additional Learning Resources

evolve Go to your Evolve website (http://evolve.elsevier.com/Canada/Leifer) for the following learning resources:

- Answer Key for Critical Thinking Questions
- Answer Key for Textbook Review Questions
- Audio Glossary
- Fluids & Electrolytes tutorial
- Interactive Review Questions
- Skills Performance Checklists
- Video clips and more!

Online Resources

- Canadian PKU & Allied Disorders: http://canpku.org/
- Canadian Paediatric Society: https://www.cps.ca/

Review Questions

1. Some preterm infants are fed by gavage because of which of the following reasons?
   a. Confinement to the isolette
   b. Overdeveloped gag and cough reflexes
   c. Refusal of formula
   d. Weak sucking and swallowing reflexes
2. A characteristic sign of necrotizing enterocolitis (NEC) in the newborn is which of the following?
   a. Bloody diarrhea
   b. Necrosis of the abdomen
   c. Projectile vomiting
   d. High fever
3. Which of the following observations of a preterm newborn would indicate presence of respiratory distress? *(Select all that apply.)*
   a. Substernal retractions
   b. Respiratory rate of 70/min
   c. Grunting
   d. Lethargy
4. An infant is born at 43 weeks' gestation. A nurse should monitor the infant for which of the following common problems? *(Select all that apply.)*
   a. Respiratory distress caused by possible meconium aspiration
   b. Increased weight gain resulting from increased glucose availability
   c. Hypoglycemia resulting from decreased glucose reserves
   d. Presence of increased amounts of lanugo
5. A nurse observes that a preterm infant has a pulse rate of 96 and a pulse oximetry reading of 89%. The *first* action of the nurse should be to do which of the following?
   a. Call the health care provider.
   b. Gently rub the infant's back.
   c. Call a Code.
   d. Continue observation and documentation, as this is normal.
6. Which complementary therapies may be used in the NICU? *(Select all that apply.)*
   a. Place a sweet-smelling room deodorizer in the room that has a calming effect.
   b. Use baby oil on the infant's skin.
   c. Place an article of the mother's clothing in the infant's crib.
   d. Use gentle touch to calm the infant.
7. When caring for an infant with Down syndrome, which of the following characteristic symptoms would the nurse would assess for? *(Select all that apply.)*
   a. Seizures
   b. Curved pinky finger
   c. Straight simian crease
   d. Cognitive delay

REFERENCES

Abdel-Hady, H., Nasef, N. N., Shabaan, A. E., et al. (2015). Caffeine therapy in preterm infants. *World Journal of Clinical Pediatrics*, *4*(4), 81–93.

American Academy of Pediatrics. (2013). Screening premature infants for ROP. *Pediatrics*, *131*(1), 189–195.

American Academy of Pediatrics and American Heart Association. (2016). *Textbook of neonatal resuscitation* (7th ed.). Elk Grove Village, IL: American Academy of Pediatrics.

American College of Obstetricians and Gynecologists Committee on Obstetric Practice & Society for Maternal-Fetal Medicine. (2013). *Committee opinion: Definition of term pregnancy*. Reaffirmed 2017. Retrieved from https://www.acog.org/Clinical-Guidance-and-Publications/Committee-Opinions/Committee-on-Obstetric-Practice/Definition-of-Term-Pregnancy.

Askie, L. M., Darlow, B. A., Davis, P. G., et al. (2017). Effects of targeting lower versus higher arterial oxygen saturations on death or disability in preterm infants. *Cochrane Database of Systematic Reviews*, (Issue 4), CD011190. https://doi.org/10.1002/14651858.CD011190.pub2.

Aziz, K., Dancey, P., & Canadian Paediatric Society (CPS), Fetus and Newborn Committee (2004). Screening guidelines for newborns at risk for low blood glucose. *Paediatrics & Child Health*, *9*(10), 723–729. Reaffirmed 2018.

Bacino, C. A., & Lee, B. (2016). Cytogenetics. In R. M. Kliegman, B. F. Stanton, J. St. Geme, et al. (Eds.), *Nelson textbook of pediatrics* (20th ed.). Philadelphia: Saunders.

Badr, L., Abdallah, B., & Kahale, L. (2015). Meta-analysis of preterm infant massage: An ancient practice with a contemporary application. *Maternal Child Nursing MCN*, *40*(6), 344–357.

Barrington, K. J., Sankaran, K., & Canadian Paediatric Society (CPS) (2007). Guidelines for detection, management and prevention of hyperbilirubinemia in term and late term newborn infants [35 or more weeks gestation]. *Paediatrics & Child Health*, *12*(Suppl. B), 1B–12B Reaffirmed 2018.

Carlo, W. A. (2016). The high risk infant. In R. M. Kliegman, B. F. Stanton, J. St. Geme, et al. (Eds.), *Nelson textbook of pediatrics* (20th ed.). Philadelphia: Saunders.

Davis, D. J., Barrington, K. J., & Canadian Paediatric Society (CPS), Fetus and Newborn Committee (2005). CPS position statement: Recommendations for neonatal surfactant therapy. *Paediatrics & Child Health*, *10*(2), 109–116 Reaffirmed 2015.

Fang, J. L., Sorita, A., Carey, W. A., et al. (2016). Interventions to prevent retinopathy of prematurity: A meta-analysis. *Pediatrics*, *137*(4), 1–15.

Gephart, S. M., & Weller, M. (2014). Colostrum as oral immune therapy to promote neonatal health. *Advances in Neonatal Care*, *14*(1), 44–51.

Hyunkyung, C., & VanRiper, M. (2013). Siblings of children with Down syndrome: An integrative review. *Maternal Child Nursing: MCN*, *38*(2), 72–78.

Jackson, P., Vessey, J., & Schapiro, N. (2009). *Primary care of the child with a chronic condition* (5th ed.). St. Louis: Mosby.

Jefferies, A. L., & Canadian Paediatric Society (CPS), Fetus and Newborn Committee (2012). Kangaroo care for the preterm infant and family. *Paediatrics & Child Health*, *17*(3), 141–143. Reaffirmed 2017. Retrieved from https://www.cps.ca/en/documents/position/kangaroo-care-for-preterm-infant.

Jefferies, A. L., & Canadian Paediatric Society (CPS), Fetus and Newborn Committee (2014). Going home: Facilitating discharge of the preterm infant. *Paediatrics & Child Health*, *19*(1), 31–36.

Jefferies, A. L., & Canadian Paediatric Society (CPS), Fetus and Newborn Committee (2016). Retinopathy of prematurity: An update on screening and management. *Paediatrics & Child Health*, *21*(2), 101–104.

Kassity-Kritch, N., & Jones, J. (2014). Complementary and integrative therapies. In C. Kenner, & J. Lott (Eds.), *Comprehensive neonatal nursing care* (6th ed.). New York: Springer.

Kirkby, S., & Biggs, C. (2016). Cell phones in the neonatal intensive care unit: How to eliminate unwanted germs. *Advances in Neonatal Care*, *16*(6), 404–409.

Lacaze-Masmonteil, T., O'Flaherty, P., & Canadian Paediatric Society (CPS), Fetus and Newborn Committee (2018). *Management of infants born to mothers who have used opioids during pregnancy*. Retrieved from https://www.cps.ca/en/documents/position/opioids-during-pregnancy.

Maheshwari, A., & Carlo, W. (2016). Blood disorders. In R. M. Kliegman, B. F. Stanton, J. St. Geme, et al. (Eds.), *Nelson textbook of pediatrics* (20th ed.). Philadelphia: Saunders.

McMillan, D., & Canadian Paediatric Society (CPS), Fetus and Newborn Committee (1997). CPS position statement: Routine administration of vitamin K to newborns. *Paediatrics & Child Health*, *2*(6), 429–431. Reaffirmed 2018.

Neu, M., Robinson, J., & Schmiege, S. (2013). Influence of holding practice on preterm infant development. *Maternal Child Nursing MCN*, *38*(3), 136–138.

Perinatal Services, B. C. (2018). *Neonatal guideline: Newborn metabolic screening*. Retrieved from http://www.perinatalservicesbc.ca/Documents/Guidelines-Standards/Newborn/NewbornScreeningGuideline.pdf.

Public Health Agency of Canada (PHAC). (2017). *Down syndrome surveillance in Canada, 2005–2013*. Retrieved from https://www.canada.ca/en/public-health/services/publications/healthy-living/down-syndrome-surveillance-2005-2013.html.

Rizvani, I., & Ficicioglu, C. H. (2016). Phenylalanine. In R. M. Kliegman, B. F. Stanton, J. St. Geme, et al. (Eds.), *Nelson textbook of pediatrics* (20th ed.). Philadelphia: Saunders.

Schafer, D., Boogart, S., Johnson, L., et al. (2014). Comparison of neonatal skin sensor temperatures with axillary temperature: Does skin sensor placement really matter? *Advances in Neonatal Care*, *14*(1), 52–60.

World Health Organization (WHO). (1997). *Thermal protection of the newborn: A practical guide*. Geneva: Author.

World Health Organization (WHO). (2017). *WHO recommendations on newborn health: Guidelines approved by the WHO Guidelines Review Committee*. Geneva: Author. Retrieved from https://apps.who.int/iris/bitstream/handle/10665/259269/WHO-MCA-17.07-eng.pdf;jsessionid=EE9EAEEE627170A856A2481781AA5E4A?sequence=1.

Yaworski, A., Van Meer, A., & Wong, E. (2018). *Neonatal hyperbilirubinemia. MacMaster Pathophysiology Review*. Retrieved from http://www.pathophys.org/neonatal-hyperbilirubinemia/.

An Overview of Growth, Development, and Nutrition

13

Lisa Keenan-Lindsay

http://evolve.elsevier.com/Canada/Leifer

Objectives

1. Define each key term listed.
2. Discuss the nursing implications of growth and development.
3. Explain the differences between growth, development, and maturation.
4. Recognize and read a growth chart for children.
5. List five factors that influence children's growth and development.
6. Discuss the importance of family-centred care in pediatrics.
7. Recognize the influence of the family and cultural practices on growth, development, nutrition, and health care.
8. Describe three developmental theories and their impact on planning the nursing care of children.
9. Discuss the nutritional needs of growing children.
10. Differentiate between permanent and deciduous teeth, and list the times of their eruption.
11. Describe the characteristics of play at various age levels.
12. Describe the relationship of play to physical, cognitive, and emotional development.
13. Understand the importance of limiting screen time.
14. Define therapeutic play.
15. Understand the use of play as an assessment tool.

Key Terms

adolescent
cephalocaudal (sĕf-ă-lō-KĂW-dăl)
cognition (kŏg-NĬ-shŭn)
community
competitive play
cooperative play
deciduous (dĕ-SĬD-ū-ŭs)
Erikson's stages
extended family
fetus
fluorosis (flū-RŌ-sĭs)
growth
height
infant
Kohlberg
length
Maslow
maturation
metabolic rate
newborn
nuclear family
nursing caries
parallel play
personality
Piaget (pē-ă-ZHĀ)
preschool
proximodistal (prŏk-sĭ-mō-DĬS-tăl)
school-age
therapeutic play
toddler

GROWTH AND DEVELOPMENT

When caring for a child, it is important to acknowledge that the child is in a continuous process of growth and development. While not steadily paced, this process is orderly and proceeds from simple to more complex behaviours (Box 13.1). Plateaus often follow growth spurts—the most noticeable growth spurts occur during infancy and at the time of puberty. The rate of growth varies with the individual child, and siblings within a family vary in growth rate. Growth is measurable and can be observed and studied by comparing height, weight, increase in vocabulary, physical skills, and other parameters. There are variations in growth within the body systems and the subsystems; not all parts mature at the same time. Skeletal growth approximates whole-body growth, whereas the brain, lymph, and reproductive tissues follow distinct and individual sequences.

THE IMPACT OF GROWTH AND DEVELOPMENT ON NURSING CARE

The pediatric nurse is required to have special skills in many areas. While adult acute care units in a hospital

Box 13.1 Emerging Patterns of Behaviour from Age 1 to 5 Years

12 MONTHS
Motor: Walks with one hand held; rises independently; takes several steps
Adaptive: Picks up pellet with pincer action of thumb and forefinger; releases object to another person on request
Language: Says "mama," "dada," and a few similar words
Social: Plays simple ball game; makes postural adjustment to dressing

15 MONTHS
Motor: Walks alone; crawls up stairs
Adaptive: Makes tower of three cubes; makes a line with crayons; inserts pellet in bottle
Language: Jargon; follows simple commands; may name a familiar object (ball)
Social: Indicates some desires or needs by pointing; hugs caregivers

18 MONTHS
Motor: Runs stiffly; sits on small chair; walks upstairs with one hand held; explores drawers and wastebaskets
Adaptive: Makes tower of four cubes; imitates vertical stroke; imitates scribbling; dumps pellet from bottle
Language: 10 words (average); names pictures; identifies one or more parts of body
Social: Feeds self; seeks help when in trouble; may be unhappy when wet or soiled; kisses caregivers with pucker

2 YEARS
Motor: Runs well; walks up and down stairs, one step at a time; opens doors; climbs on furniture; jumps
Adaptive: Tower of seven cubes (six at 21 months); circular scribbling; imitates horizontal stroke; folds paper once imitatively
Language: Puts three words together (subject, verb, object)
Social: Handles spoon well; often tells immediate experiences; helps to undress; listens to stories with pictures; plays in parallel with other children

2½ YEARS
Motor: Goes up stairs alternating feet
Adaptive: Tower of nine cubes; makes vertical and horizontal strokes but generally will not join them to make a cross; imitates circular stroke, forming a closed figure
Language: Refers to self by pronoun "I"; knows full name
Social: Helps put things away; pretends in play

3 YEARS
Motor: Rides tricycle; stands momentarily on one foot
Adaptive: Tower of 10 cubes; imitates construction of "bridge" of three cubes; copies a circle; imitates a cross
Language: Knows age and sex; counts three objects correctly; repeats three numbers or a sentence of six syllables
Social: Plays simple games (cooperative play is highly imaginative); helps in dressing (unbuttons clothing and puts on shoes); washes hands

4 YEARS
Motor: Hops on one foot; throws ball overhand; uses scissors to cut out pictures; climbs well
Adaptive: Copies bridge from model; imitates construction of "gate" of five cubes; copies cross and square; draws a man with two to four parts besides head; identifies longer of two lines
Language: Counts four coins accurately; tells a story
Social: Plays with several children with the beginning of social interaction and role playing; goes to toilet alone

5 YEARS
Motor: Skips
Adaptive: Draws triangle from copy; identifies heavier of two weights
Language: Names four colours; repeats sentence of 10 syllables; counts 10 coins correctly
Social: Dresses and undresses; asks questions about meaning of words; domestic role playing

may contain a separate neurology unit, cardiac unit, medical unit, and surgical unit, on the pediatric acute care unit in the general hospital all medical-surgical specialties are usually housed on this unit—for patients ranging from newborn to adolescent. The nurse must consider the developmental needs of the child and how this will impact the child's response to illness and incorporate this knowledge into developing a plan of care. Choosing the right words to explain to a child what will happen is essential. For example, if the nurse states that the child will be "put to sleep" before the operation, will the child relate that to a pet at home being "put to sleep" and never heard from again? The fractured jaw of an 8-month-old may affect their developmental process more seriously than the same injury in a 4-year-old, because the 8-month-old is in the oral phase of development.

Because the child differs from the adult both anatomically and physiologically, differences in response to therapy as well as in manifestations of illness can be anticipated. The nurse must understand normal growth and development to recognize deviations within any age group and to plan care that takes these developmental differences into consideration (Box 13.2).

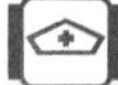 **Nursing Tip**

The developmental level of the child and family values should assist the nurse when planning care.

An understanding of growth and development, including its predictable nature and individual variation, has value in the nursing process. Such knowledge is the basis of the nurse's anticipatory guidance for parents. For example, the nurse who knows when the infant is likely to crawl can, at the appropriate age, expand teaching on safety precautions. The nurse also incorporates these precautions into nursing care plans in the hospital. Age-appropriate care cannot be administered without a good understanding of growth and development.

Box 13.2 Nursing Process Applied to Growth and Development

DATA COLLECTION

Obtain height and weight and plot a standard growth chart.
Record developmental milestones achieved as they relate to age.
Observe infant; interview parents.

ANALYSIS AND NURSING DIAGNOSIS

Determine appropriate nursing diagnoses related to parenting, coping skills, and unmet developmental needs.

PLANNING

Offer guidance and teaching to family, school personnel, and child to meet child's developmental needs. For example, the toddler and preschooler may have specific needs related to safety or the use of age-appropriate toys.

IMPLEMENTATION

Interventions that foster growth and development in the hospital setting can include encouraging age-appropriate self-care. In the home, the school-age child with diabetes may be taught to participate in performing blood glucose tests and administering insulin.

Anticipatory guidance may be given to parents so they understand changes in behaviour, eating habits, and play of the growing child.

EVALUATION

Ongoing evaluation of growth and development of the child and follow-up of teaching and guidance offered at previous clinic/home visits are essential.

While explaining various aspects of child care to families, the nurse needs to stress the importance of individual differences. Parents sometimes compare their children's development and behaviour with those of other children and with information found in books or on the Internet. This may relieve their anxiety, or it may cause them to impose impossible expectations and standards.

The nurse who understands that each child is born with an individual temperament and "style of behaviour" can help teach parents about their child's individual behaviour.

The nurse provides teaching in order to prevent disease and accidents. For example, the nurse may assess a child's immunization status, review poison prevention strategies with parents of a toddler, or teach the effects of alcohol and other substances on an unborn fetus. Knowing that specific diseases are prevalent in certain age groups, the nurse can be alert to these conditions when assessing patients. This approach, based on developmental knowledge, experience, effective communication, and incorporation of the family, helps to ensure a family-centred care approach. Finally, the nurse must understand how to provide nursing care to children of various ages to enhance their physical, mental, emotional, and spiritual development according to their specific needs and comprehension.

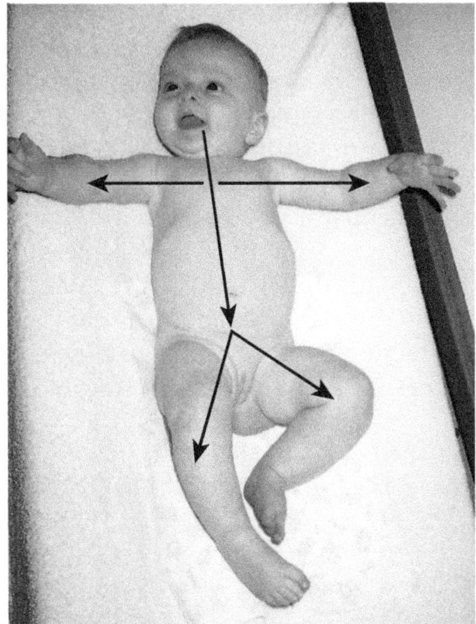

Fig. 13.1 The development of muscular control proceeds from head to foot (cephalocaudally) and from the centre of the body to its periphery (proximodistally).

TERMINOLOGY

The following stages of growth and development are referred to throughout this text:

- **Fetus**: Ninth gestational week to birth
- **Newborn**: Birth to 4 weeks
- **Infant**: 4 weeks to 1 year
- **Toddler**: 1 to 3 years
- **Preschool**: 3 to 5 years
- **School-age**: 5 to 12 years
- **Adolescent**: 12 to 18 years

Growth refers to an increase in physical size and is measured in centimetres and kilograms. *Development* refers to a progressive increase in the function of the body (e.g., the infant's increasing ability to digest solids). **Maturation** (*maturus*, "ripe") refers to the total way in which a person grows and develops, as dictated by genetics. The timing of maturation may be affected by the physical and psychological environment.

DIRECTIONAL PATTERNS

Directional patterns are fundamental to all humans. **Cephalocaudal** development proceeds from head to toe. The infant is able to raise the head before being able to sit, and they gain control of the trunk before walking. The second pattern is **proximodistal**, or from midline to the periphery. Development proceeds from the centre of the body to the periphery (Fig. 13.1). These patterns occur bilaterally, and development proceeds from the general to the specific. For example, the infant grasps with the hands before pinching with the fingers.

DEVELOPMENTAL CONSIDERATIONS

Height

Height refers to standing measurement, whereas **length** refers to measurement while the infant is in a recumbent position. At birth, the newborn has an average length of about 45 to 55 cm. Linear growth is caused mainly by skeletal growth. Growth fluctuates until maturity is reached. Infancy and puberty are both rapid growth periods. Height is generally a family trait, although there are exceptions. Good nutrition and general good health are instrumental in promoting linear growth. Height is measured during each well-child visit (Skill 13.1). The length of the infant usually increases about 2.5 cm (1 inch) per month for the first 6 months. By age 1 year, the birth length increases by about 50% (mostly in the trunk area).

Weight

Weight is another good index of health. However, the weight of a newborn infant does not always imply gestational maturity (see Chapter 12 and Fig. 12.1). The average full-term newborn weighs 2.5 to 4.0 kg (5.5 to 8.8 lb). Approximately 7 to 10% of the birth weight is lost by age 3 or 4 days as the result of the passage of stools, urine, and fluid overload that accumulated during labour. The infant should regain their birth weight by age 2 weeks. *Birth weight usually doubles by age 6 months and triples by age 1 year.* After the first year, weight gain levels off to approximately 1.82 to 2.73 kg (4 to 6 lb) per year, until the pubertal growth spurt begins.

Skill 13.1 Assessing the Length and Height of Infants and Children

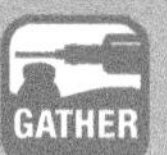

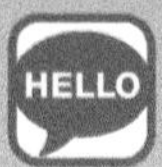

PURPOSE

To determine height in order to calculate body surface area (BSA) measurement and to determine status on growth chart

STEPS

Infants From Birth Until 2 Years

1. Measure infants from birth until age 2 years in the recumbent position.
2. Exert *mild* pressure on the knee to straighten the leg for crown–heel measurement. Use a tape measure or measuring mat (the leg should *not* be "pulled" to straighten by exerting pressure on the ankle.)
3. Plot the measurement on an established growth chart.
4. Document findings and report any abnormalities.

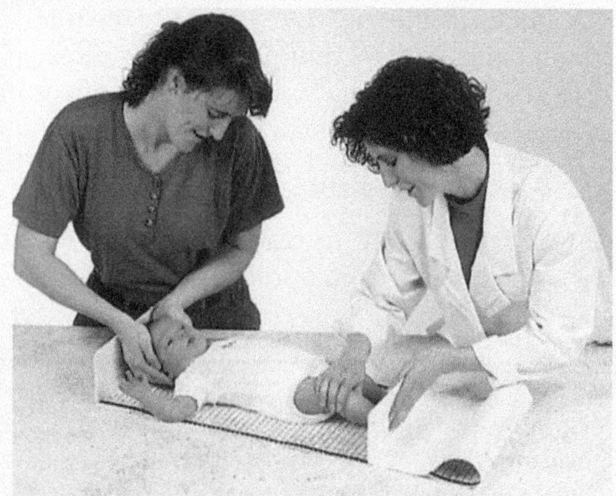

Infants from birth to age 2 years are measured in the recumbent position.

Children From 2 to 18 Years

1. Measure children ages 2 to 18 years in the standing position. The body should be in alignment, with the head erect and the child looking straight ahead, and shoulders, buttocks, and heels touching the wall. The child should not be wearing shoes and should stand on a paper barrier.
2. Plot the measurement on an established growth chart.
3. Document findings and report any abnormalities.

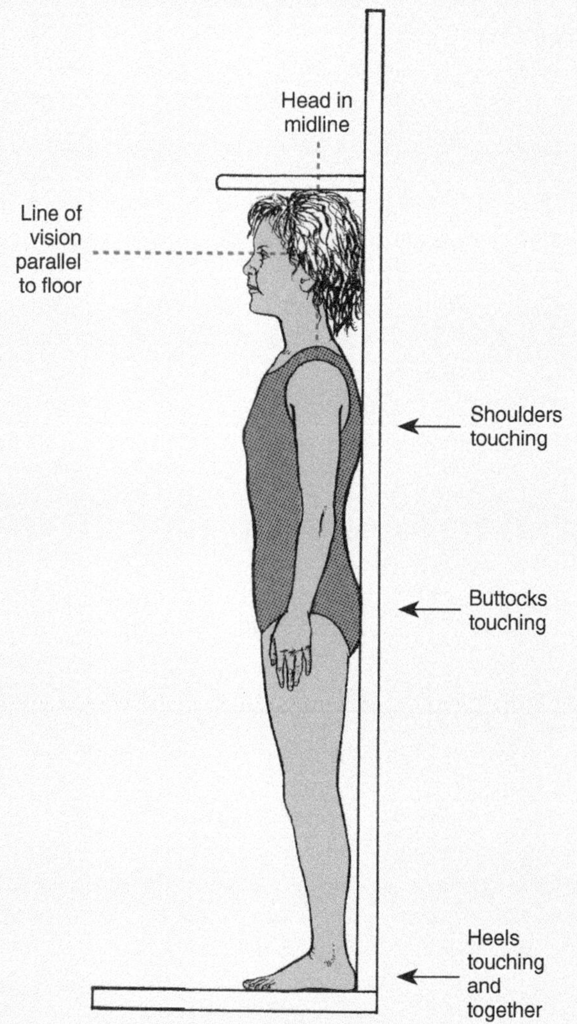

Children from 2 to 18 years are measured in the standing position.

Weight is measured at each office visit. A marked increase or decrease necessitates further investigation. The body weight of a newborn is composed of a higher percentage of water than in the adult. This extracellular fluid falls from 40% in the newborn to 20% in the adult. The high proportion of extracellular fluid in the infant can cause a more rapid loss of total body fluid; therefore, every infant must be closely monitored for dehydration. (See technique of weighing infants in Chapter 11 and Fig. 11.3.)

Body Proportions

Body proportions of the child differ greatly from those of the adult (Fig. 13.2). The head is the fastest growing portion of the body during fetal life. During infancy the trunk grows rapidly, whereas during childhood, growth of the legs becomes the predominant feature. At adolescence, characteristic male and female proportions develop as childhood fat disappears. Alterations in proportions in the size of head, trunk, and extremities are characteristic of certain disturbances.

Metabolic Rate

The metabolic rate (energy use and oxygen consumption) is higher in children than in adults. Infants require more calories, minerals, vitamins, and fluid in proportion to weight and height than adults. Higher metabolic rates are accompanied by an increased production of heat and waste products. The body surface area (BSA) of young children is far greater in relation to body weight than that of adults. The young child loses relatively more fluid from the pulmonary and integumentary systems.

Respirations

The respirations of infants are irregular and abdominal. Small airways can become easily blocked with mucus. The short, straight eustachian tube connects with the ear and predisposes the infant to middle ear infections. The chest wall is thin, and the muscles are immature, thus pressure on the chest can interfere with respiratory efforts.

Cardiovascular System

In newborns, the muscle mass of the right and left ventricles of the heart is almost equal. An increased need for cardiac output is often met by an increase in heart rate. Newborns have high oxygen consumption and require a high cardiac output in the first few months of life. The presence of fetal (immature) hemoglobin in the first months of life also contributes to the need for a high cardiac output. The disappearance of fetal hemoglobin along with the loss of maternal iron stores contributes to the development of physiological anemia in infants after 6 months of age.

Immunity

For the first 3 months of life, the newborn is protected from illnesses to which the mother was exposed. The infant gradually produces his or her own immunoglobulin; 40% of the adult level of immunoglobulin G (IgG) is reached by 1 year of age and adult levels of IgM are reached by 9 months of age (O'Flaherty, 2017). Therefore, care must be taken to prevent health care–acquired infections (HAIs) and exposure to pathogens. Immunizations against common childhood communicable diseases are discussed in Chapter 32.

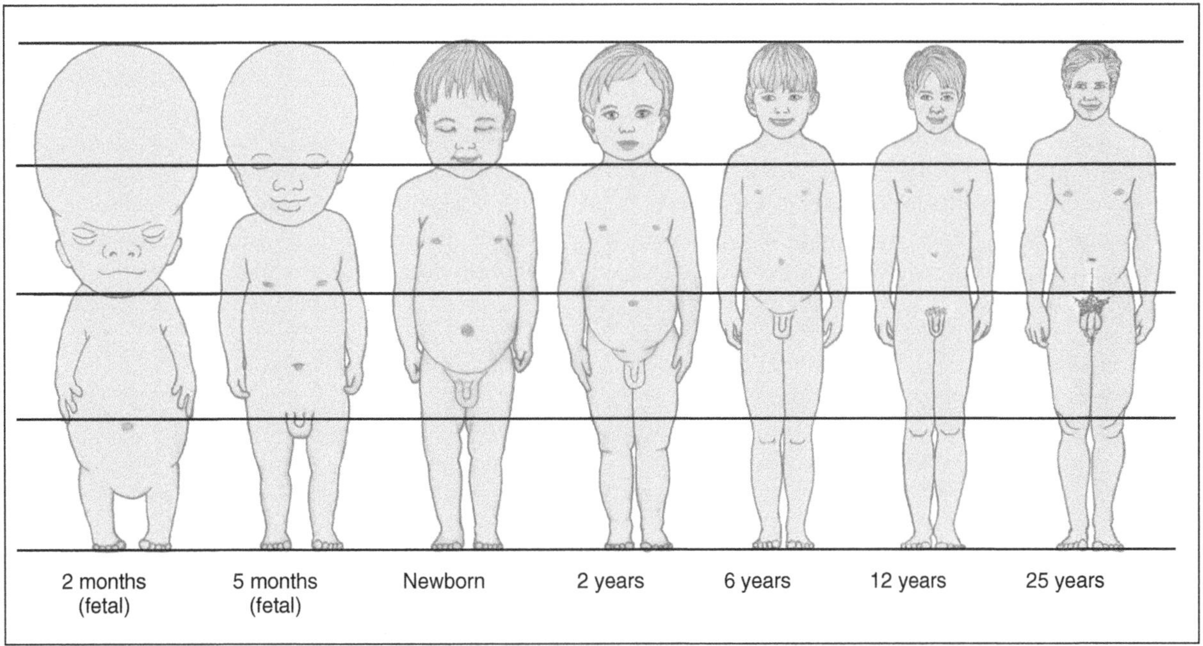

Fig. 13.2 Changes in body proportions. Approximate changes in body proportions from fetal life through adulthood are shown. (From McKinney, E. S., Ashwill, J. W., Murray, S. S., James, S. R., Gorrie, T. M., & Droske, S. C. [2013]. *Maternal-child nursing* [4th ed.]. Philadelphia: Saunders.)

Kidney Function

Kidney function is not mature until the end of the second year of life. Therefore, medications that are eliminated via the kidney can accumulate in the body to dangerous levels before age 2 years. Immature kidney function also predisposes the infant to dehydration. Nursing responsibilities for children less than 2 years of age include monitoring for dehydration and observing closely for toxic effects of medication therapy.

Nervous System

Maturation of the brain is evidenced by increased coordination, skills, and behaviours in the first years of life. Purposeful controlled movement such as voluntarily grasping an object within view replaces primitive reflexes such as the involuntary grasp reflex. Head circumference increases 1.5 cm per month to an approximate total of 43 cm at age 6 months. During the second 6 months of life, head circumference increases 0.5 cm per month to an approximate total of 46 cm at 1 year of age. The choice of age-appropriate toys is correlated with nervous system maturation. When selecting play activities, the nurse should consider the diagnosis and the child's developmental level and abilities, to be sure the toy is safe.

Sleep Patterns

Sleep patterns vary with age. The newborn may sleep as much as 18 hours a day, for 2 to 3 hours at a time. Toddlers may sleep between 11 and 14 hours per day and this may include one daytime nap (Canadian Paediatric Society [CPS], 2017a). The 7-year-old usually requires 11 to 13 hours of sleep and rarely has a daytime nap. These patterns may be altered by cultural practices. For example, Israeli *kibbutzim* often have family members nap after work or school, before dinner.

Bone Growth

Bone growth provides one of the best indicators of biological age. Bone age can be determined by X-ray studies. In the fetus, bones begin as connective tissue, which later is converted to cartilage. Cartilage is converted to bone through ossification. The rate of bone growth and the age of maturity vary among individuals, but the progression remains the same. Growth of the long bones continues until epiphyseal fusion occurs. Bone is constantly synthesized and resorbed. In children, bone synthesis is greater than bone destruction. Calcium reserves are stored in the ends of the long bones. Vitamin A, vitamin D, and fluorine as well as various growth hormones are necessary for the growth and development of skeletal bone.

CRITICAL PERIODS

There appear to be certain periods when environmental events or stimuli have their maximum impact on the child's overall development. The embryo, for example, can be adversely affected during times of rapid cell division. Certain viruses, medications, and other agents are known to cause congenital anomalies during the first 3 months after conception. It is also believed that issues such as developing a sense of trust, particularly during the first year of life, and learning readiness occur at critical periods, and experiences during these periods will influence the future growth and development of the child.

Integration of Skills

As the infant grows and learns new skills, they are combined with those previously mastered. The toddler who is learning to walk may sit, pull the body up to a table by grasping it, balance, and take a cautious step. Tomorrow the toddler may take three steps! Children connect and perfect each skill in preparation for learning a more complex one.

GROWTH STANDARDS

Growth is measured in dimensions such as height, weight, body mass index (BMI), and head circumference. Measurement alone, without any standard of comparison, limits the interpretation of the data. When the data are compared to a standard, developmental progress can be assessed. The Canadian Paediatric Society (CPS), Dietitians of Canada, College of Family Physicians of Canada, Community Health Nurses of Canada, and Canadian Pediatric Endocrine Group (2014) have developed pediatric growth charts that are based on the 2007 World Health Organization (WHO) reference growth charts and are used as tools to assess the child's overall growth and development (see Appendix D).

Some pointers in reading and interpreting growth charts are as follows:

- Children who are in good health tend to follow a consistent pattern of growth.
- At any age, there are wide individual differences in measured values.
- A solid black line designates the median (middle) or fiftieth percentile. Percentile levels show the extent to which a child's measurements deviate from the fiftieth percentile or middle measurement.
- A child whose weight is at the seventy-fifth percentile line is *one percentile above* the median. A child whose height is at the twenty-fifth percentile is *one percentile below* the median.

DEVELOPMENTAL SCREENING

Developmental screening is a vital component of child health assessment. One tool that is used is the Nipissing District Developmental Screen (NDDS). This tool assesses the developmental status of children during the first 6 years of life at 13 different stages. The NDDS assesses skills in the following areas: vision; hearing; speech and language; communication; gross motor and fine motor; cognitive; social/emotional; and self-help. Its purpose is to identify children who are unable to perform at a level comparable to their age-mates. A low score merely indicates a need for further evaluation. Parents, caregivers, nurses, or other health care providers can use this test. Proper administration and interpretation will aid in developing an individualized plan of care for the child. See Online Resources at the end of the chapter for more information on the NDDS. There are other developmental screening tools that are available, and it is often health care provider's preference that determines which tool is used.

> **Nursing Tip**
>
> *Catch-up growth* refers to the process by which a child who has been sick or malnourished and whose growth has slowed or stopped experiences a period of more rapid growth after recovery as the body attempts to compensate.

FACTORS THAT INFLUENCE GROWTH AND DEVELOPMENT

Growth and development are influenced by many factors, such as heredity, culture, ordinal position in the family, gender, environment, and other social determinants of health. These factors are closely related and dependent on one another in their effect on growth and development. They make each person unique. If a child is ill, physically or emotionally, the developmental processes may be delayed.

Socioeconomic Status

It is well known that people who have lower income and social status have poorer health (Government of Canada, 2013). According to Statistics Canada (2017a), nearly 1.2 million Canadian children younger than 18 (17.0%) lived in a low-income household in 2015. One in every two Indigenous child also lives in poverty. The impact of poverty on the health of a child is significant. Families who live in poverty have issues with food insecurity, housing, and poorer health (Canada Without Poverty, 2019). Strategies need to be developed to lower the childhood poverty rate. Some provinces pay for prescription medications for children, particularly in families who have lower income. This should have a significant impact on the health of children.

The Homeless Family

The homeless family with children is a modern-day concern that has an impact on the growth, development, and health of the child. Every night in Canada approximately 35 000 people are homeless, and family homelessness (and, therefore, homelessness among dependent children and youth) is a significant, yet hidden, part of the crisis. Numerous studies have shown that many families are forced to live in overcrowded, substandard housing and regularly make the choice between paying the rent and feeding their children (Gulliver-Garcia, 2016). Support systems and financial resources are often lacking. The community nurse or emergency department nurse may be the first to identify the status of this family. Community referrals to provide shelter, food, education, and financial aid are primary needs that must be met before health teaching can be effective. Especially for these families, it is imperative that nurses work with the strengths of the family while attending to its weaknesses.

Environment

The physical environment is an important determinant of health that can influence the health of children. At certain levels of exposure, contaminants in air, water, food, and soil can cause a variety of adverse health effects, including cancer, birth defects, respiratory illness, and gastrointestinal ailments. Indigenous children in particular may not have access to clean water, and the food they eat may have toxins in it. These factors contribute to the lower level of health among Indigenous children.

The prenatal environment also influences the physical condition of the newborn. The health of the mother at the time of conception and the amount and quality of her diet during pregnancy play large roles in proper fetal development. Infections or diseases may lead to malformations of the fetus.

The home environment can influence the child's physical and emotional growth and development. When an added member financially strains a family's resources or the parents are unable to provide nourishing food and suitable housing, the child's growth and development are directly affected. For example, a parent may be unaware of how to cook foods properly to preserve their nutritional value. Immunizations and other medical attention may not be priorities. An infant may sense tension within the family and develop less trust as a result.

Social Environment

The community, region, province or territory, and country provide resource sharing and social networks that create safety nets and improve overall health for community members (Government of Canada, 2018). Families are greatly influenced by the communities in which they reside. Nurses must understand the culture of the **community** in which they work or to which the patient will return. Assessment of the community is particularly important in creating discharge plans for families. Their lives may be broadened or restricted depending on the facilities within the community. A few factors to consider are housing, access to public transportation, city services, safety, and health care delivery systems. The nurse has immediate access to the patient and therefore becomes an important liaison between various agencies that address specific needs.

Culture

Ethnic differences extend into many areas of a child's life, including growth, speech, food preferences, family structure, religious orientation, health beliefs, and code of conduct. An important factor related to culture is that a person's beliefs may influence their health choices. The nurse should ascertain cultural beliefs and practices when collecting data for nursing assessment. Culturally competent care includes not making assumptions about someone of a certain culture, because not everyone practices the same beliefs and values within cultures.

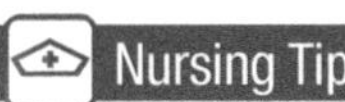
Nursing Tip

Acceptance of the child's value system and cultural beliefs will assist in positive nurse–child interactions.

Hereditary Traits

Characteristics derived from our ancestors are determined at the time of conception by countless genes within each chromosome. Each gene is made of a chemical substance called *deoxyribonucleic acid (DNA)*, which plays an important part in determining inherited characteristics. Examples of inherited traits are eye colour, hair colour, and physical resemblances within families. Certain diseases are also passed down through generations.

Gender

The male infant often weighs more and is slightly longer than the female. He grows and develops at a slightly different rate. Parents and relatives may treat boys differently from girls by providing "gender-appropriate" toys and play and by having different expectations of them. Current trends promote unisex activities in play and career development. Many health issues are a function of gender-based social status or roles (Government of Canada, 2013).

The Family

The *family* has been defined in many different ways and fulfills many different purposes. There is not a universal definition of family; a family is what an individual considers it to be (Keenan-Lindsay, 2017). Families do not have to be related by blood, but the members of the family share mutual responsibility for care of the members of the group. It is important to remember that a change (or illness) in one family member will affect the entire family in some way. Traditionally, the **nuclear family**, or biological family, has been the basic unit of structure in North American society (mother, father, siblings). This type of family unit is steadily decreasing in today's society, as many families do not share the same household because of lone parenthood, divorce, and remarriage. The **extended family** refers to three generations: grandparents, parents, and children. Because of an increasing lifespan, however, there are a greater number of living grandparents and great-grandparents, and the proportion of them living in the family home may increase. In Canada, same-sex marriage has been legal since 2005, and many of these couples also have children, either through adoption or one of the partners having offspring. Transgender couples may also have children through the use of fertility medication, adoption, or the transman discontinuing hormones and becoming pregnant. Table 13.1 lists the various types of families and gives a description of each.

Table 13.1 Variations in Types of Families

TYPE OF FAMILY	DESCRIPTION
Nuclear	Male and female partner with children (natural or adopted)
Extended or multigenerational	Grandparents, parents, children, relatives, living in same house
Lone parent	Women or men establish separate households through individual preference, divorce, or death of other parent
Foster parent	Parents who care for children requiring parenting because of having no family or individual or family problems
Blended	Remarriage of persons with children
Same-sex parent families	Two persons of the same sex adopt children, undergo insemination, or have children from a previous marriage
Common-law families	Heterosexual or LGBTQ2 couples live together but remain unmarried
Alternative	Communal family

The *interactions* of family unit members are by far the most influential aspect of family life in the growth and development of the child. The nurse must understand the interaction of the family unit to be able to develop strategies and work alongside the family. Some families have solid support systems and use available community resources to maintain health. Other families may lack support systems and require closer follow-up care and encouragement by the health team. Parenting is a learned behaviour, often modelled by past experience and modified by the acceptance of specific roles and responsibilities. Some families may not know how to provide for the optimum physical, psychological, and emotional health of the child. A nurse can work with these families to teach them how to be successful in their efforts and interactions.

It is common in today's society that both parents work outside the home. The parents may be absent for most of the day because of long commutes or the demands of the working environment. Both parents may share child care and domestic chores.

Divorce, separation, personal decision, and death of a parent have led to an increasing number of lone-parent families. The percentage of children aged 0 to 14 years living in lone-parent families in 2016 was 19.2%

(Statistics Canada, 2017b). Of those families 15.6% were headed by a female and 3.6% were headed by a male parent (Statistics Canada, 2017b). Most single-wage families have an economic disadvantage, but families with women as the sole wage earner often have considerably lower incomes than those in which men are sole wage earners. The problem of providing good, affordable child care is a serious one for both dual-career families and lone parents. Relatives and the noncustodial parent may assist in raising the child. Many lone parents remarry, creating the *blended* family. The addition may be merely a stepfather or stepmother, or two families may unite. These family units must make many adjustments. To succeed, parents and children have to learn problem-solving techniques, communication skills, and flexibility.

A *family APGAR,* first described by Smilkstein, Ashworth, and Montano (1984), is a tool that can be used as a guide to assess family functioning. This assessment is valuable in determining the approach to home care needs:

- *Adaptation:* How the family helps and shares resources
- *Partnership:* Lines of communication and partnership in the family
- *Growth:* How responsibilities for growth and development of children are shared
- *Affection:* Overt and covert emotional interactions among family members
- *Resolve:* How time, money, and space are allocated to prevent and solve problems

Questions concerning each of these areas should be posed and the answers assessed. The goal in family assessment is to enable the nurse and family to develop strategies that aid the family in achieving a healthier adaptation to their child's health needs or problems.

Nursing Tip

An infant who is hypersensitive to noise or touch needs the parent to understand the importance of quiet surroundings. A chronically depressed parent may interpret fussiness or lack of smiling as rejection. Therefore, an assessment of parent–child interaction is essential in the home, clinic, or hospital setting.

Ordinal position in the family

Whether the child is the youngest, middle, or oldest child in the family has some bearing on growth and development. The youngest and middle children learn from their older siblings. However, motor development of the youngest may be delayed if the others in the family pamper the child. The child without siblings or the oldest child in the family may excel in language development because their conversations are mainly with adults. These children are often the objects of greater parental expectations.

Health Inequities

Health care is an important factor in children's achieving normal growth and development, from birth through adolescence, especially for children at special risk. Children living in remote communities may have limited access to health care, clean water, and electricity. Immigrants, refugees fleeing from war-torn countries, or families who do not speak the dominant language may not be able to identify and use community resources that would help their children, and children affected by violence, war, or natural disasters may lack health care assessment of or treatment for special needs that affect their growth and development. Nurses need to work to increase accessibility to health care education, participate in community care services, and empower communities to strive for adequate health care that promotes children's normal growth and development. Nurses should use available teaching opportunities at every patient contact and maintain awareness of how nurses can contribute to improved global health of families.

Indigenous children

Indigenous children and youth are one of the most vulnerable populations in Canada. They lag behind their non-Indigenous peers on almost every measure of health, including infant mortality, early childhood development, acute health care needs, chronic medical conditions, and mental health (Starkes, Baydela, & CPS First Nations, Inuit and Metis Health Committee, 2014/2017). Increased rates of substance use (i.e., tobacco, prescription drugs, and alcohol) and suicide reflect the more pressing disparities facing Indigenous adolescents in this important transitional phase of life (Starkes et al., 2014/2017). Many of these health inequities are due to lack of access to social determinants of health that promote good health. For Indigenous young people, additional determinants include kinship and support networks, racism, and the loss of traditional language, land, and social identity (Starkes et al., 2014/2017). These unique factors must be considered when looking at the health of Indigenous children.

LGBTQ2 adolescents

Adolescence is a time when children are figuring out their sexuality. It is important that nurses and other health care providers assess a teen's sexual orientation in order to help the teen achieve optimal growth and development. Children who identify as LGBTQ2 may have increased mental health concerns as they deal with stigma and how to tell their family about their sexuality. These issues can have an impact on self-esteem and identity formation. Physical health concerns are similar for all adolescents, although LGBTQ2 teens may have an increased risk of sexually transmitted infections (STIs), and they are more likely to start using tobacco, alcohol, and other substances at an earlier age (Kaufman & CPS Adolescent Health Committee, 2008/2016).

PERSONALITY DEVELOPMENT

Personality is a unique organization of characteristics that determine the individual's typical or recurrent pattern of behaviour. No two persons are exactly alike. An individual's personality is the result of interaction between biological and environmental heritages.

Although no one group of theories can explain all human behaviour, each can make a useful contribution in understanding it. Many experts have devoted their lives to understanding why children and families behave as they do. Some experts, called *systems theorists,* believe that everyone in the family or system is affected by each of its members. This theory focuses on the interrelatedness of the various persons, instead of an analysis of an individual in the group. Nurses using systems theory focus on caring for the child by caring for the whole family. They see the family as protector, educator, resource, and health provider for the child. In turn, they see the child's health as having an impact on each member of the family as a whole.

Many experts see human development through a composite lens of various theories. The hierarchy of needs developed by Abraham Maslow is depicted in Fig. 13.3, and the developmental theories of Erik Erikson, Sigmund Freud, Lawrence Kohlberg, Harry Stack Sullivan, and Jean Piaget are presented in Table 13.2. Other theorists are briefly contrasted within appropriate chapters devoted to specific age groups. Theories provide a framework for the practitioner; however, humans are not a gathering of isolated parts to be disassembled and reassembled according to some theoretical set of instructions, and nurses need to bear this in mind.

COGNITIVE DEVELOPMENT

Cognition (*cognoscere,* "to know") refers to intellectual ability. Children are born with inherited potential, but the potential must be developed. Opportunities for successful exploration enhance the child's cognitive development. The development of logical thinking and conceptual understanding is a complex process. One outstanding authority on cognitive development was Piaget, a Swiss psychologist. He proposed that intellectual maturity is attained through four orderly and distinct stages of development, all of which are interrelated: sensorimotor (birth to 2 years), preoperational (2 to 7 years), concrete operations (7 to 11 years), and formal operations (11 to 15 years). The ages for each stage are approximate, and each stage builds on the preceding one.

Piaget believed that intelligence must be developed through interactions and learning to cope with the environment. Infants begin their interaction by reflex response. As they grow older, their use of symbolism (particularly language) increases. Gradually they acquire a here-and-now orientation (concrete operations)

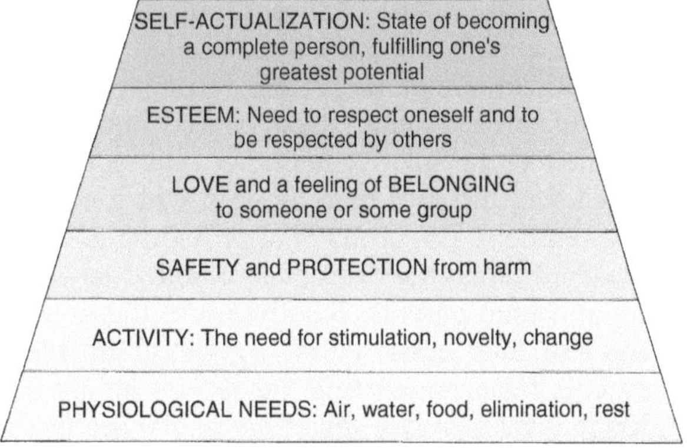

Fig. 13.3 Maslow's hierarchy of basic needs. The needs at the bottom of the pyramid must be met before one can fulfill needs at the next higher level.

and finally a fully abstract comprehension of the world (formal operations). Table 13.3 relates Piaget's theory to feeding and nutrition. It is a good example of how knowledge of development can help in understanding the behaviour of a child at a particular time.

MORAL DEVELOPMENT

Lawrence Kohlberg, a childhood theorist, suggests that moral development in children is sequential. His theories on moral development are based on Piaget's cognitive development investigations. He describes three levels: *preconventional, conventional,* and *postconventional.* In the preconventional stage (4 to 7 years), children try to be obedient to their parents because of fear of punishment. During the conventional phase (7 to 11 years), children show conformity and loyalty, and they focus on obeying rules. In the postconventional level (12 years and older), *moral values* are developed to solve complex problems. There is an emphasis on the conscience of the individual within the society. Although rules are still important, changing them to meet the needs of a culture is considered.

THE GROWTH AND DEVELOPMENT OF A PARENT

Table 13.4 shows the tasks of the parent as they relate to the child's developmental tasks in Erikson's system of stages, as well as some suggestions for nursing interventions that can aid the growth and development of a parent and a child.

Erikson's stages of child development demonstrate the various tasks that must be mastered at each age to achieve optimum maturity. Each stage builds on the successful completion of the previous stage. Achievement of the tasks of childhood does not occur in isolation. Parents must *interact* appropriately to help the child to achieve tasks successfully at the child's developmental level (Fig. 13.4). For example, if the parent constructs a school project for a child, the child will not achieve a sense of industry.

Table 13.2 **Comparison of the Developmental Theories of Erikson, Freud, Kohlberg, Sullivan, and Piaget**

DEVELOPMENTAL PERIOD	ERIKSON	FREUD	KOHLBERG	SULLIVAN	PIAGET
Infancy	*Trust versus mistrust* Getting needs met Tolerating frustration in small doses Recognizing caregiver as distinct from others and self	*Orality*—understanding the world by exploring with the mouth	*Preconventional/Premoral*—cannot distinguish right from wrong	Security Patterns of emotional response Organization of sensation	*Sensorimotor stage* (birth to 2 years)—at birth, responses are limited to reflexes; begins to relate to outside events; concerned with sensations and actions that affect self directly
Toddler	*Autonomy versus shame and doubt* Trying out own powers of speech Beginning acceptance of reality versus pleasure principle	*Anality*—learning to give and take	*Punishment/Obedience*—performance based on fear of punishment	Mastery of space and objects	*Preoperational* (2 to 7 years)—child is still egocentric; thinks everyone sees world as self does
Preschooler	*Initiative versus guilt* Questioning Exploring own body and environment Differentiation of sexes	*Phallic/Oedipal phase*—becoming aware of self as sexual being	*Morality*—rules are absolute; breaking rules results in punishment; behaviour is based on rewards	Speech and conscious need for playmates, interpersonal communication	*Perceptual* (4 to 7 years)—capable of some reasoning but can concentrate on only one aspect of a situation at a time
School-age	*Industry versus inferiority* Learning to win recognition by producing things Exploring, collecting Learning to relate to own sex	*Latency*—focusing on peer relations; learning to live in groups and to achieve knowledge	*Conventional morality*—rules are created for the benefit of all; adhering to rules is the right thing to do (7 to 11 years)	Friendship, one-to-one relationship, self-esteem, compassion	*Concrete operations* (7 to 11 years)—reasoning is logical but limited to own experience; understands cause and effect
Adolescence	*Identity versus role diffusion* Moving toward own identity; sexual identity emerges Selecting vocation Beginning separation from family Integrating personality (e.g., altruism)	*Genitality*	*Principled morality* (autonomous stage) (12 years and older)—acceptance of right or wrong based on own perceptions of world and personal conscience	Capacity to love, empathy, partnership (sexuality)	*Formal operations* (11 to 16 years)—acquires ability to develop abstract concepts for self; oriented to problem solving

Parents should be guided not to attempt to prevent frustration in the lives of their children. Experiences in handling challenges and disappointments prepare the child to function independently in adulthood. Parents should encourage a child to manage successes and failures, should provide socially acceptable outlets, and should intervene only if the frustrations become overwhelming. The parent's task is to provide the child with the skills and tools appropriate at each age level that are needed to deal with life's events.

NUTRITION

FAMILY NUTRITION

Good nutrition begins before conception. Nutritional needs during pregnancy are discussed in Chapter 4. The quality of the child's food intake is dependent for many years on the food choices made by adults, whose eating habits may be influenced by income level, beliefs, folklore, fads, misinformation, or religious, cultural, and ethnic preferences. Table 13.5 describes some

Table 13.3 Piaget's Theory of Cognitive Development in Relation to Feeding and Nutrition

DEVELOPMENTAL PERIOD	COGNITIVE CHARACTERISTICS	RELATIONSHIP TO FEEDING AND NUTRITION
Sensorimotor (birth to 2 years)	Progression is from newborn with automatic reflexes to intentional interaction with the environment and the beginning use of symbols.	Progression is made from sucking and rooting reflexes to the acquisition of self-feeding skills. Food is used primarily to satisfy hunger, as a medium to explore the environment, and to practice fine motor skills.
Preoperational (2 to 7 years)	Thought processes become internalized; they are unsystematic and intuitive. Use of symbols increases. Reasoning is based on appearances and happenstance. Approach to classification is functional and unsystematic. Child's world is viewed egocentrically.	Eating becomes less the centre of attention than social, language, and cognitive growth. Food is described by colour, shape, and quantity, but there is limited ability to classify food into "groups." Foods tend to be classed as "like" and "don't like." Child can identify food as "good for you," but reasons are unknown or mistaken.
Concrete operations (7 to 11 years)	Child can focus on several aspects of a situation simultaneously. Cause–effect reasoning becomes more rational and systematic. Ability to classify, reclassify, and generalize emerges. Decrease in egocentrism permits child to take another's view.	Child begins to realize that nutritious food has a positive effect on growth and health but has limited understanding of how or why this occurs. Mealtimes take on a social significance. Expanding environment increases opportunities for, and influences on, food selection (peer influence rises).
Formal operations (11 to 16 years)	Hypothetical and abstract thought expands. Understanding of scientific and theoretic processes deepens.	The concept of nutrients from food functioning at physiological and biochemical levels can be understood. Conflicts in making food choices may be realized (knowledge of nutritious food versus preferences and non-nutritive influences).

From Mahan, L. K., & Raymond, J. (2017). *Krause's food, and the nutrition care process* (14th ed.). Philadelphia: Elsevier.

common food patterns of various cultures found in Canada. Some families cannot afford nutritious foods, others have inadequate facilities to prepare foods, and some rely on convenience foods to save time. For some families access to healthy and affordable food can be a concern, especially if they live in a remote community.

Some families do not consider providing healthy food a priority. However, optimum nutrition is essential for the child to reach their growth potential; a lack of adequate nutrition can lead to intellectual disabilities. Unhealthy eating leading to childhood obesity may leave these children subject to decreased motor skills and to peer rejection, both of which can contribute to low self-esteem.

The nurse is in a position to identify children at risk for poor nutrition and to help families modify eating habits to ensure proper nutrition. An important resource for the nurse is the dietitian in the community or on staff at the health facility where the nurse is employed.

HEALTHY NUTRITION

Good nutrition is vital to good health and essential for normal growth and development. In 2019, Health Canada developed a new *Canada's Food Guide* (see Appendix C), which translates the science of nutrition and health into a healthy eating pattern for children older than 2 years of age. A healthy, balanced, nutrient-dense diet, combined with adequate physical activity, is at the core of *Canada's Food Guide*. The emphasis is on choosing a variety of foods, including more plant-based proteins, avoiding processed foods, and reading labels to avoid added sodium, sugars, or saturated fat. The *Food Guide* also encourages eating at home, eating together as a family, and including children in food preparation.

These dietary guidelines are intended to help people make informed decisions about what they eat. Families who use the *Food Guide* to determine meal plans are educating their children by good example. Appendix C shows suggested content of a healthy food plate, with fruits and vegetables taking up half the plate.

For families who are vegetarian, the nurse can use teaching tools that respect these families' dietary limitations while also encouraging them to select appropriate foods. A well-balanced vegetarian diet can provide for the needs of children and adolescents. Supplementation may be required in cases of strict vegetarian diets with no intake of any animal products (Amit & CPS Community Paediatrics Committee, 2010/2016). Children who eat vegetarian diets often consume large amounts of high-fibre foods. High-fibre foods cause increased losses of calcium, zinc, magnesium, and iron in the stool and may necessitate the intake of supplements. A diet containing meat, poultry, or fortified foods lessens this nutrient deficiency (see Nutrition Considerations box). Vegetarian diets are discussed in Chapter 20.

Table 13.4 **Growth and Development of a Parent**

CHILD'S TASKS (ERIKSON'S STAGES)	PARENTS' TASKS	NURSING INTERVENTION
First Prenatal Trimester		
Growth	Develop attitude toward newborn: • Happy about child? • Parent of one disabled child? • Lone parent? These factors and others will affect the developing attitude of the parent.	Assist in developing positive attitude in parents concerning expected birth of child. Use referrals and agencies as needed.
Second Prenatal Trimester		
Growth	Mother focuses on infant because of fetal movements felt. Parents picture what infant will look like, what future the child will have, and other ideas.	Parents' focus is on child care and needs and providing physical environment for expected infant's arrival. Therefore, information concerning care of the newborn should be provided at this time.
Third Prenatal Trimester		
Growth	Mother focuses attention on what labour is going to be like.	Detailed information should be presented at this time concerning the birth processes, preparation for birth, breastfeeding, and care of sibling(s) at home.
Birth		
Adjust to external environment	Elicit positive responses from child and respond by meeting child's need for food and closeness. If parents receive only negative responses (e.g., sleepy infant, crying infant, difficult feeder, congenital anomaly), development of the parent will be inhibited.	Encourage early touch, feeding, and other practices. Explain behaviour and appearance of newborn to allay fears. Help parents to identify positive responses. (Use infant's reflexes, such as grasp reflex, to elicit a positive response by placing parents finger into infant's hand.)
Infant		
Develop trust	Learn "cues" presented by infant to determine individual needs of infant.	Help parents assess and interpret needs of infant (prevent feelings of helplessness or incompetence). Help parents cope with problems such as colic.
Toddler		
Autonomy	Try to accept the pattern of growth and development. Accept some loss of control but maintain some limits for safety.	Help parents cope with transient independence of child (e.g., allow child to go on tricycle but do not yell "Don't fall" or anxiety will be radiated).
Preschool-Age		
Initiative	Learn to separate from child.	Help parents show standards but "let go" so child can develop some independence. A preschool experience may be helpful.
School-Age		
Industry	Accept importance of child's peers. Parents must learn to accept some rejection from child at times. Patience is needed to allow children to do for themselves, even if it takes longer. Do not *do* the school project *for* the child. Provide chores for child appropriate to their age level.	Help parents understand that child is developing their own limits and self-discipline. Parents should be there to guide child but not constantly intrude, and help child get results from their efforts at performance.
Adolescent		
Establishing identity Accepting pubertal changes Developing abstract reasoning Deciding on career Investigating lifestyles Controlling feeling	Parents must learn to let child live their own life and not expect total control over the child. Expect, at times, to be discredited by teenager. Expect differences in opinion and respect them. Guide but do not push.	Help parents adjust to changing role and relationship with adolescent (e.g., as child develops their own identify). Parents can expose child to varied career fields and life experiences. Parents should help child to understand emerging emotions and feelings brought about by puberty.

Nutrition Considerations

Fibre Needs of the Child

The Canadian Paediatric Society recommends intake of 0.5 g of fibre/kg/day to avoid dilution of calories and interference with absorption of minerals and essential nutrients (Amit & CPS Community Paediatrics Committee, 2010/2016). High-fibre foods can fill the small stomach capacity and they provide few of the nutrients and calories needed by the active, growing child.

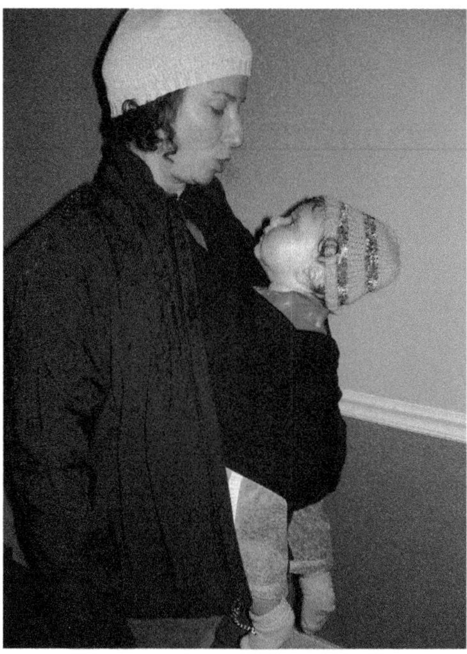

Fig. 13.4 Infant carriers enable face-to-face interaction between the young infant and parent. An older infant can be turned in the carrier to face outward and interact with the environment.

Different types of fibre are contained in foods (Table 13.6). The water-soluble fibre found in oats, apples, and citrus fruits delays intestinal transit and decreases serum cholesterol levels. The water-insoluble fibre found in whole-grain breads, wheat bran, and some cereals accelerates intestinal transit and slows starch digestion.

A well-balanced diet supplies all essential nutrients in the necessary amounts. Food provides heat and energy, builds and repairs tissues, and regulates body processes. A given food is a mixture of elements such as minerals (e.g., calcium, phosphorus, sodium, iron), compounds (carbohydrates, fats, proteins, some vitamins),

Table 13.6 High-Fibre Foods for Relief of Mild Constipation in Children Older Than 12 Months

TYPE OF FOOD	SERVING SIZE	EXAMPLE
Cereals	30 mL (1 oz)	Raisin Bran, Grape-Nuts, Shredded Wheat, Bran Chex*
Bread	1 slice 1 medium 2.5cm (1-inch) piece	Whole-grain bread Bran muffin Corn bread square
Fruits	120 mL (½ cup)	Cooked prunes
Vegetables	120 mL (½ cup)	Spinach
	1 medium	Corn on the cob
Meat substitute	120 mL (½ cup)	Beans (baked, black, garbanzo, kidney, lima, pinto, lentil)

*All products indicated are registered trademarks of their respective companies.
From Mahan, L. K., & Raymond, J. (2017). *Krause's food and the nutrition care process* (14th ed.). Philadelphia: Elsevier.

Table 13.5 Culturally and Religious Diverse Food Patterns of Some Canadians

CULTURE	HISTORICAL DIETARY PATTERN
Black Canadians	All meats, fish, and chicken. Vegetables may be cooked in salt pork for long periods; grits and cornbread muffins. There is some lactose intolerance. Popular vegetables include collard greens, beet greens, and sweet potatoes.
Chinese	Rich in vegetables (bean sprouts, broccoli, bamboo shoots, and mushrooms). Vegetables are cooked until crisp; meat is consumed in small portions with other food. Soy sauce, tofu, peanut butter; limited milk and cheese; fish is baked with native spices; soups with egg, meat, and vegetables. Rice is staple of diet.
Jewish	Diet varies according to whether family is Orthodox, Conservative, or Reform. For an Orthodox family, food must be kosher (must conform to dietary laws); meat is soaked in salt water to remove blood; only meat eaten is that of divided-hoofed animals that chew a cud; fish without scales (shellfish) and pork are prohibited; milk and meat cannot be combined.
Italian	All meats, fish, and chicken, including cold cuts (salami, mortadella) and Italian pork sausage; pasta (staple of diet), breads, olive oil, wine, cheese, and all varieties of fruits and vegetables.
Japanese	Fish and seafood (fresh, smoked, and raw) and beef. Many vegetables are eaten, such as seaweed, bamboo shoots, onions, beans, and dried mushrooms (shitake); enjoy pickled vegetables. Rice is national staple. Little cheese, milk, butter, or cream is consumed. Chief cooking fat is soybean oil or rice oil.
Indigenous people	Meats and fish include caribou, deer, moose, bear, seal, goose, duck, wild turkey, pheasant, and many kinds of fish; other foods include blackberries, blueberries, corn, squash, potatoes, barley, bannock, oatmeal, and wild rice.

Data from Unlockfood.ca. (2018). Traditional food for aboriginal people. Retrieved from http://www.unlockfood.ca/en/Articles/Aboriginal-Health/Traditional-Food-for-Aboriginal-People.aspx; Mahan, L. K., & Raymond, J. (2017). *Krause's food and the nutrition care process* (14th ed.). Philadelphia: Elsevier.

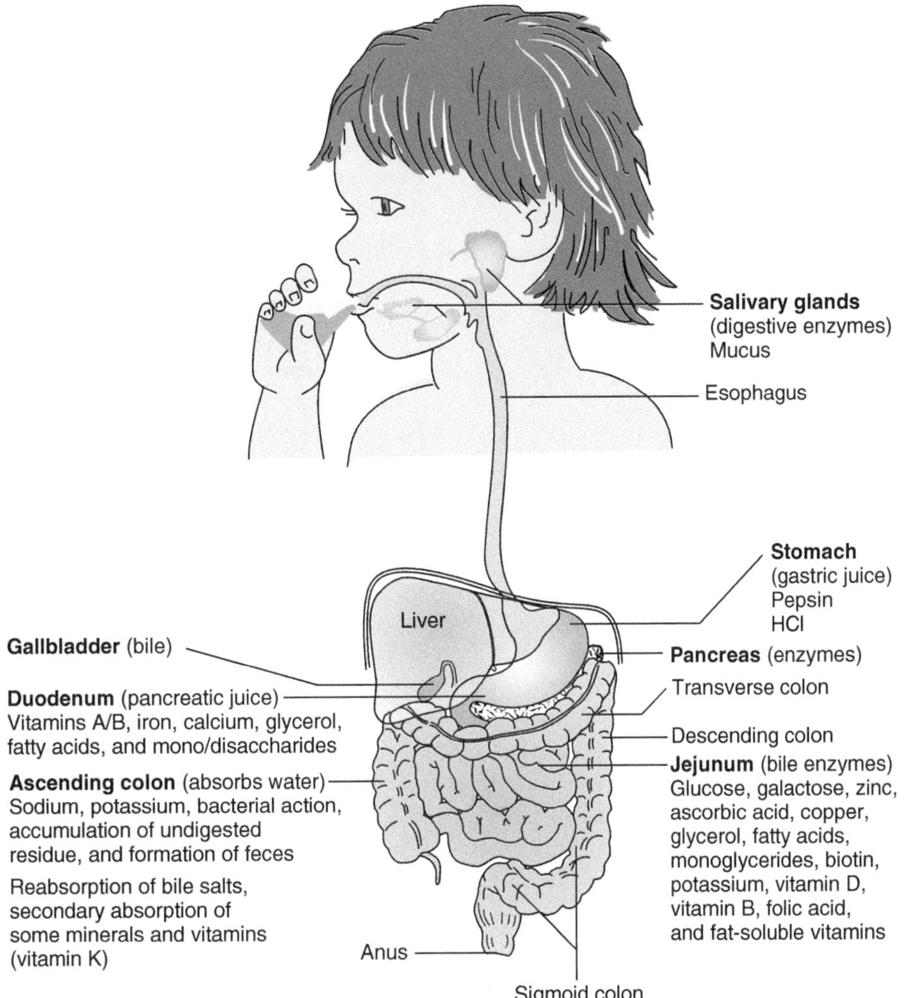

Fig. 13.5 Nutrient digestion. The sites of absorption of major nutrients are shown in this illustration. Most nutrient absorption occurs in the duodenum and jejunum of the small intestine. Most water absorption occurs in the large intestine. Absorption of nutrients depends on adequate secretion of digestive enzymes, normal motility, and normal villi on the mucosal surface of the intestines. Portal circulation, lymphatic circulation, and hormones also play a role in the digestion and absorption of nutrients.

and water. The body needs approximately 50 nutrients, which it absorbs at various sites (Fig. 13.5).

Nutrition Considerations

Enhancing Absorption of Minerals Foods

Foods containing essential minerals such as iron, zinc, and calcium should be combined with citrus, fish, or poultry to enhance absorption of the minerals. Vitamin D and lactose sugars also enhance mineral absorption in the body.

Children are susceptible to nutritional deficiencies because they are growing and developing. Infants require more calories, protein, minerals, and vitamins in proportion to their weight than do adults. Fluid requirements are also higher for infants. Water is the recommended fluid to drink with meals and juices should be avoided. Eating a variety of foods ensures good health for children. Children should be offered small meals and snacks at regular times throughout the day, and they should be allowed to decide how much food they want to eat (Government of Canada, 2019a). Children often eat more at certain meals or at times when activity levels are higher or during growth spurts; parents need to be taught that this is normal. There are no known advantages to consuming excessive amounts of any nutrients, and there are risks for overdoses.

Gluten-Free Diet

A gluten-free diet requires a major lifestyle change because traditional grains cannot be used, and the flours made from corn, rice, soy bean, tapioca, and other foods have a different texture and flavour that may require adjustment. Gluten is a primary ingredient of many foods during processing, such as "hydrolyzed vegetable protein," which contains wheat and corn. Careful scrutiny of food labels is also required. In order for a food to be labelled "gluten free," it must contain less than 20 ppm (parts per million) of gluten (Government of Canada, 2017). Supplementation with vitamin B_{12}, fat-soluble vitamins, and folic acid may be needed (Mahan & Raymond, 2017). Gluten-free diets are becoming more popular and many food companies and restaurants have expanded offers of gluten-free foods. Parents should watch for traces of food with gluten appearing

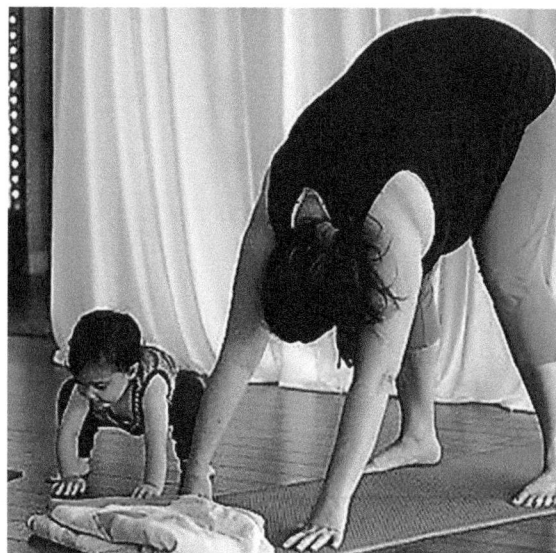

Fig. 13.6 Toddlers enjoy joining exercise activities with parents.

in common toasters, condiment jars, bulk bins, buffet tables, and deep-fried foods in restaurants. A dietitian may be necessary to provide education for the family.

NUTRITION AND DEVELOPMENT

The digestive system of the newborn is immature and functions minimally during the first 3 months. Saliva is minimal; hydrochloric acid and renin in the stomach and trypsin in the intestines aid in the digestion of milk. Amylase (a pancreatic enzyme) and lipase are not present in adequate quantity to digest non-milk foods before age 5 months, thus complex carbohydrates and fats cannot be digested effectively. Excess fibre intake in the young infant results in loose, bulky stools. The ability of the liver to function is limited in the first year of life. The teeth are not present for chewing before 6 to 8 months of age.

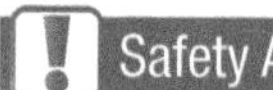

Safety Alert!

Raw fruits that contain seeds or some raw vegetables and nuts may not be appropriate foods for infants and young children because of the risk of choking.

The physiology of digestion is the basis for food introduction in the first year of life. Exclusive breastfeeding is the feeding method of choice for the first 6 months, and it is recommended that breastfeeding be continued for up to 2 years of life. If breastmilk is not provided to the infant, iron-fortified formula is the other option. Breastfeeding and formula feeding are discussed in Chapters 9 and 14. Introducing food before age 6 months does not serve any nutritional purpose and, in fact, a link between overnutrition and obesity has been found in adults. Children should be offered water when thirsty (CPS, 2019). High sodium intake in children is a risk factor for developing high blood pressure as an adult. The effects of childhood nutrition on adult health and illness patterns, such as heart disease, have been established. Home preparation of food for infants is discussed in Chapter 14.

NUTRITION AND HEALTH PROMOTION

Starting healthy dietary patterns in childhood can help prevent conditions such as atherosclerosis in later life. Some foods should be avoided as they can promote dental caries, while others should be encouraged as they contain protective fibres that can prevent some diseases. However, restrictive diets are not advised for infants and young children. Fat and cholesterol are needed for calories and development of the central nervous system. Infants should not receive added sodium in their food; the average diet contains adequate sodium. Some food additives, such as aspartame (an artificial sweetener), may be harmful to children with phenylketonuria. Food additives that prolong the shelf life of foods and food dyes that make food look more attractive should be minimized in the child's diet.

The role of grandparents in providing a diet that may lead to obesity may need to be addressed, because the principles of good nutrition that they were raised with may no longer be valid.

Parents and children need to know how to read food labels to be better informed of the food's ingredients. For instance, fast-food restaurants, often preferred by adolescents, make available to the consumer the nutrient content of the foods they serve. The caloric content of the menu often depends on the foods selected and the toppings added. Therefore, a "salad bar" is not necessarily synonymous with a low-calorie meal.

The child's height and weight should be plotted on a growth chart regularly to enable early identification of health problems related to dietary intake.

There is increasing concern regarding the level of cholesterol in children. Methods to reduce cholesterol in families are listed in the Health Promotion box and are discussed further in Chapter 26.

Health Promotion

Methods to Reduce Cholesterol in School-Age Children

- Exercise more with your children (Fig. 13.6).
- Provide fresh fruits and vegetables rather than empty calories such as those found in doughnuts and store-bought pastries.
- Minimize trips to fast-food restaurants.
- Switch to low-fat foods; use vegetable oil cooking sprays instead of butter; bake or broil foods instead of frying them.
- Seek the advice of a dietitian.
- If there is a family history of cardiovascular risk factors such as a positive family history of dyslipidemia or cardiovascular disease, obesity, smoking, hypertension, or type 2 diabetes, the child's cholesterol level should be tested.

Special Diets

Therapeutic diets, such as the diabetic diet, are well established in medical care. Dietary supplements, breastmilk fortifier, formulas, and nutritional support techniques for preterm infants, children with cancer, and those with long-term disorders (e.g., cystic fibrosis) have become sophisticated and are used successfully. Total parenteral nutrition allows the health care provider to choose preparations ranging from amino acids and intravenous fats to complete multivitamins. Total parenteral nutrition and enteral feedings allow children who need nutritional support to be cared for at home, thus greatly enhancing their quality of life.

An oral rehydration solution (ORS) is recommended for treating acute diarrhea in children. It is composed mainly of electrolytes, glucose, and water and enhances the absorption of water and sodium. One example of an ORS commercial preparation available in Canada is Pedialyte. See Chapter 28 for a detailed discussion of oral rehydrating solutions.

FEEDING THE HEALTHY CHILD

Table 13.7 specifies the nursing interventions that help to meet the nutritional needs of children from infancy to adolescence. For more detail on nutrition for each age group see the specific chapter for each age group.

The Infant

Infants require more calories, protein, minerals, and vitamins in proportion to their weight than do adults. Their fluid requirements are also high. Breastmilk is an excellent food for meeting all of these needs, thus a nursing mother should be encouraged to continue breastfeeding even when her infant is hospitalized. Breastmilk can be manually expressed and refrigerated at the hospital and then given in the mother's absence.

Soy-based infant formula is indicated only for those infants who have galactosemia or who cannot consume dairy-based products for cultural or religious reasons. Other infant formulas for special medical purposes should only be used when the infant has or is suspected to have the indicated condition (Health Canada, CPS, Dietitians of Canada, & Breastfeeding Committee for Canada, 2015). Most products come in dry and liquid forms; parents must be made aware of the concentrations that the health care provider recommends. Solid food is introduced at age 6 months. This first food should be high in iron (Fig. 13.7).

The nurse must be aware of the problems of underfeeding and overfeeding infants. Restlessness, crying, and failure to gain weight suggest underfeeding. Overfeeding is manifested by symptoms such as regurgitation, mild diarrhea, and too rapid weight gain. Diets high in fat delay gastric emptying and cause abdominal distention. Diets too high in carbohydrates may cause distention, flatus, and excessive weight gain. Constipation may be the result of too much fat or protein or a deficiency in bulk. Increased amounts of age-appropriate whole grains, fruits, vegetables, and fluids can often correct this problem.

If the parents plan to prepare their own baby food at home, the nurse should discuss the choice of foods, their preparation, and safe storage. Blenders, strainers, and mashers are equipment often used, and ice cube trays may be used to freeze portions for storage. Most fresh and frozen unsalted foods are appropriate. Water or juice used in cooking can also be used to thin blended food, but overblending should be avoided because it can cause overoxidation of nutrients and make the food too mushy. Prepared foods can be stored in the refrigerator for 48 hours or frozen for several months. Home-prepared foods are less expensive, contain less salt and sugar, and help the infant become familiar with the cultural tastes of the family.

Most infants naturally adapt to a schedule of three meals a day by the first birthday. At this time, the appetite fluctuates as the growth rate slows somewhat. The child may not be interested in eating. Spills are frequent as the 1-year-old child may not be able to manipulate a spoon well.

In the hospital, children in highchairs are secured with safety belts. The nurse remains in constant attendance. Developmental advancements that change eating patterns should be explained to parents to prevent feeding difficulties.

Nursing Tip

Whole cow's milk should not be introduced before 9 to 12 months of age. Low-fat milk should not be introduced before 2 years of age, as fats are needed to complete neurological development.

The Toddler

Toddlers can feed themselves by the end of the second year although some children do this earlier (Fig. 13.8). This is important in developing a sense of independence. The toddler may be rebellious at times, and food may be pushed away or completely refused. Toddlers benefit from the caregivers' presence at mealtime. It is important that toddlers are given small portions so they are not overwhelmed. Feeding difficulties may result from the anxieties of parents and a lack of time planned for meals. Mealtimes should be a pleasurable experience and not used as a time for discipline.

The Preschool Child

Preschoolers and toddlers enjoy finger foods. Dawdling and regression are common in this age group. They may have foods they prefer for several weeks in a row and parents should be instructed to continue feeding this to the child as long as it is nutritious (Dietitians of Canada, 2014).

The School-Age Child

School-age children need a variety of different types of food but in increased quantities to meet energy requirements. The best strategy to ensure healthy eating is for families to eat together for meals as much as possible.

Table 13.7 Nursing Interventions for Meeting the Nutritional Needs of Children

CHARACTERISTICS	NURSING INTERVENTIONS
Newborns and Infants	
High-energy maintenance because of immature systems (e.g., heat loss)	• Assist mother with breastfeeding. • Assist family with bottle feeding. • Teach formula preparation if required.
Immature digestive system	• Burp infant frequently.
Nutrient requirements related to body size	• Observe infant for tolerance to formula. • Teach about vitamin D supplementation for breastfed infants. • Anticipate iron deficiencies after 6 months of age in breastfed infants.
Need for additional nutrients, satiety	• Introduce solids at 6 months, starting with food that is iron-rich. • Teach parents not to add salt or sugar to baby foods to prevent high sodium and calorie intake.
Danger of choking decreases as swallowing matures	• As teething progresses, junior or chopped foods can be provided. • Explain selection and makeup of soy-based formulas if prescribed.
Prevention of dental decay	• Encourage use of fluorides (after age 6 months) only if fluoride content of community water supply is less than 0.3 ppm (parts per million) and child is considered at risk for dental caries. • Encourage use of cup to prevent bottle-mouth caries. • Rinse infant's mouth after feedings.
Continued requirements for basic nutrition education	• Assess the educational and financial needs of the family.
Toddlers and Preschoolers	
Slower rate of growth; although body needs are still high, energy requirements decrease	• Emphasize that from a nutrition viewpoint, child can regulate intake if appropriate foods are offered.
Picky eater	• Provide nutritional snacks. • Respect need for independence; do not force child to eat. • Use coloured straws; if milk is refused, offer cheese, yogurt; add milk to potatoes. • Offer meat in bite-sized portions. • Add fruit to cereal. • Reduce sweets. • Invite playmate to lunch. • Relax at meals. • Promote harmony.
School-Age Children	
Growth rate that continues to be slow but steady until puberty, some spurts and plateaus	• Maintain education in nutrition. • Introduce new foods when eating out. • Assist child in preparing nutritious lunches. • Provide fruits and raw vegetables for snacks. • Encourage parents to include children's participation in meal planning and preparation and food shopping.
Adolescent Girls	
Girls' caloric requirements are less than those of boys Concern with body image may lead to anorexia or bulimia	• Emphasize that skipping meals can lead to decrease in essential nutrients. • Encourage physical exercise to maintain body weight. • Educate regarding proper nutrients to maintain body weight (e.g., skim milk, fruits). • Avoid high-calorie fast foods. • Consider emotional components related to foods (e.g., difficulty with peers, need for love and approval).
Athletic activities	• See interventions for adolescent boys.
Adolescent pregnancy	• Educate concerning increased nutritional needs to complete growth and nourish fetus, and increased requirement for folic acid (see Chapter 4).
Adolescent Boys	
Concern with body image, bodybuilding	• Instruct regarding proper nutrition for sports. • Promote proper conditioning, well-balanced diet (increased calories), proper hydration without supplements.

Table 13.7 Nursing Interventions for Meeting the Nutritional Needs of Children—cont'd

CHARACTERISTICS	NURSING INTERVENTIONS

Overnutrition	• Explain that this can lead to adult obesity.
	• Teach that to lose weight, the following are advised:
	  • Eat a variety of foods low in calories and high in nutrients.
	  • Eat less fat and fewer fatty foods.
	  • Eat less sugar and fewer sweets.
	  • Drink less alcohol.
	  • Eat more fruits, vegetables, whole grains.
	  • Increase physical activity.

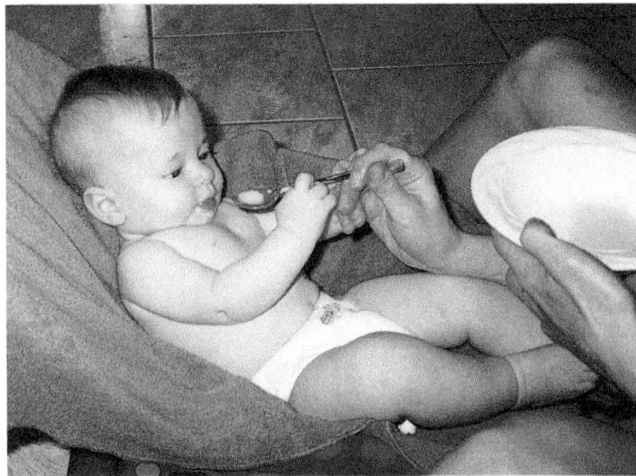

Fig. 13.7 Spoon feeding. Solid foods should be introduced at age 6 months and can be fed by spoon to the infant. Cereal should not be mixed into the formula bottle when feeding the healthy infant.

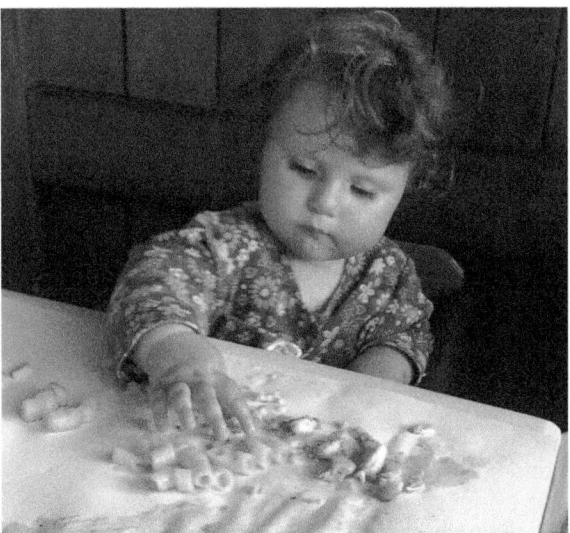

Fig. 13.8 The self-feeding toddler.

The intake of sweets decreases the appetite and provides empty calories so they are not recommended. Children should not be offered more than 250 to 375 mL of juice per day, and water should be encouraged as the drink when thirsty.

The Health Promotion box on nutrition resources in the community lists nutrition services that are available to children of various ages.

The Adolescent

Nutrition is particularly important during the adolescent years. Teenagers grow rapidly and expend large amounts of energy; therefore, their food needs are great. The nurse needs to involve the hospitalized teenager in selecting foods that are nutritious and appetizing by reviewing choices made on the daily menu. Sometimes it helps to stress how important good nutrition is to physical appearance and fitness given the heightened need for peer approval during adolescence. Food fads and skipped meals may result in malnutrition. Fatigue is a common concern at this age. If it is accompanied by a lack of appetite and irritability, anemia should be suspected. If the teen is concerned about their weight they should be encouraged to speak to a health care provider before trying to lose weight. Weight loss is not always recommended during a period of growth, and an unhealthy approach to weight loss can be harmful to mental and physical health (Dietitians of Canada, 2018). Some adolescents consult computer chat rooms for weight loss information, which can lead to anorexic behaviour.

OBESITY

Obesity rates among children have tripled in the past 30 years. Between 1978/79 and 2004, the combined prevalence of overweight and obesity among those aged 2 to 17 years increased from 15 to 26%. Increases were highest among youth aged 12 to 17 years, with overweight and obesity more than doubling for this age group, from 14 to 29% (Public Health Agency of Canada [PHAC], 2012). There are numerous health problems for obese children, including the following (Government of Canada, 2019b):

Physical health problems:
- High blood pressure or heart disease
- Type 2 diabetes
- Sleep apnea and other breathing problems
- Abnormal or missed menstrual cycles
- Bone and joint problems
- Reduced balance

Emotional health problems:
- Low self-esteem and negative body image
- Depression
- Feeling judged
- Being teased or bullied

Health Promotion

Nutrition Resources Within the Community

PROGRAM	ELIGIBILITY	PROGRAM CONTENT
Canadian Prenatal Nutrition Program	Pregnant women, new mothers, and babies facing challenging life circumstances.	Provides nutrition counselling, prenatal vitamins, food and food coupons, counselling in prenatal health and lifestyle, breastfeeding education and support, food preparation training, education and support on infant care and child development, and referrals to other agencies and services.
Aboriginal Head Start Urban and Northern Initiative	Provides comprehensive experiences for Indigenous children up to 6 years of age and their families, with primary emphasis on preschoolers, 3 to 5 years of age. The program has six components, and nutrition is one of these.	Provides children with the essential nutrients they require to grow, develop, and be active; feeds children appropriately for the period of time each day that they are at the Project; provides children and parents with opportunities to learn about and further develop nutritious and healthy eating habits.
Aboriginal Head Start on Reserve (AHSOR)	Promotes child wellness by supporting services that supplement those of the home and community. Provides a daily program for children on reserve.	Head Start's child nutritional services assist families in meeting each child's nutrition needs and in establishing healthy eating habits that nurture healthy development and promote health throughout the child's life.
Canadian Child and Youth Nutrition Program Network	Support for children through grants for childhood nutrition programs and provides support for families with a child with a disability.	Supports children with disabilities by providing financial grants for essential specialized equipment and essential therapists. Provides school-based breakfast, lunch, and snack programs across Canada.
Canadian Feed the Children	Works in partnership with Indigenous communities to support community-led food security programs. These are designed to reduce childhood hunger by increasing access to good food and traditional food practices, and by encouraging healthy eating.	School nutrition program; provides nutrition education; school gardens; Fresh for Less produce boxes.

Excessive weight in childhood is related to obesity in adulthood. Rates of obesity are higher among Indigenous children and the influence of socioeconomic status is clear. For example, young people in households where no members had more than a high school diploma were more likely to be overweight or obese than were those in households where the highest level of education was postsecondary graduation. The prevalence of poor health or poor health behaviours is less common at every step up the socioeconomic scale. This is a critically important fact to acknowledge and address, as programs that fail to address these factors can inadvertently increase disparities in health status or behaviours (PHAC, 2012).

The instrument to determine obesity is the body mass index (BMI) percentile (Skill 13.2). To determine the level of obesity, the child's BMI needs to be graphed on a BMI chart. A BMI between the eighty-fifth and ninety-seventh percentile in children over age 5 is considered overweight. Above the 97th percentile to 99.9th percentile is obese, and greater than 99.9th percentile is severely obese (Dietitians of Canada, 2019). The cause of obesity is most often related to diet and inactivity, although some causes can include illness syndromes. Monitoring, counselling, and follow-up are essential. One factor that may be related to obesity is the use of sports drinks and caffeinated energy drinks. The CPS has stated that these drinks pose potential risks for the health of children and adolescents and that children need to be counselled that water is the best option to drink (Pound, Blair, & CPS Nutrition and Gastroenterology Committee, 2017).

In order to prevent childhood obesity the following are recommended:

- Eat five fruits and vegetables per day.
- Limit screen time to 2 hours per day.
- Get 1 hour of physical activity per day.
- Take in no sugary drinks (Fig. 13.9).

FEEDING THE ILL CHILD

Children in the hospital continue in the process of growing. Well-nourished children can be characterized as follows:

- Nearly always show steady gains in weight and height
- Are alert
- Have shiny hair
- Have no fatigue circles beneath the eyes
- Have a skin colour within normal limits
- Have an erect posture

Skill 13.2 Calculating Body Mass Index (BMI)

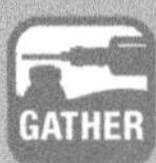
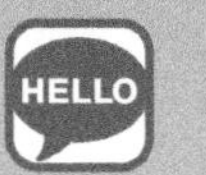
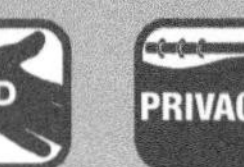
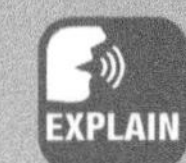

PURPOSE

To estimate a healthy body weight for an individual based on height and to indirectly measure body fat percentage to determine obesity or underweight status

OBTAINING A BMI

A child greater than 2 years of age should be weighed and measured at every health checkup to determine growth and nutritional status. Any deviation from the trend that is plotted on the growth chart may indicate a developing health problem. The following formulas can be used to obtain a BMI:

$$\text{BMI} = \frac{\text{Weight in Kilograms}}{(\text{Height in metres})^2} \text{ OR}$$

$$\text{BMI} = \frac{\text{Weight in pounds}}{(\text{Height in inches})^2} \times 703$$

NOTE: Once the BMI is determined, the nurse must plot the result on an appropriate BMI chart (see https://www.dietitians.ca/your-health/assess-yourself/assess-your-bmi/bmi-children.aspx).

- Have well-developed muscles
- Have mouth and gum mucous membranes that are firm and pink, not swollen or bleeding
- Have no mouth or tongue lesions
- Have teeth that are erupting on schedule
- Have a generally good appetite and eliminate regularly
- Usually sleep well at night, have energy and vitality, and are not irritable

This picture changes somewhat during illness, but the child who is basically well nourished can easily be distinguished from one who is malnourished.

Many hospitalized children have poor appetites. This may be because of age, the nature of the illness, the type of diet, sudden exposure to strange foods and a strange environment, a reaction to hospitalization, or the degree of satisfaction obtained during mealtimes. The child may also refuse to eat in an attempt to manipulate the parents, particularly if lack of appetite was a concern in the past.

The nurse needs to observe the patient's tray to determine if the food is the right consistency. Does the child have any teeth? Do lesions in the mouth prevent chewing? Can the child use a knife and fork? Children with bandaged limbs or those receiving intravenous fluids require assistance. The size of servings is important as large servings may overwhelm the child.

The nurse should avoid showing personal dislikes because negative attitudes are easily transmitted. The nurse should proceed slowly with unfamiliar children to determine their level of mastery. Food is served warm and sufficient time must be allotted. Sweet drinks and snacks should not be served just before meals. Treatments such as chest physiotherapy should not be scheduled immediately after a meal. Infants who are placed NPO (nothing by mouth) should be provided with a pacifier to meet their sucking needs if this is approved by the parents. Some children prefer to use their thumb for non-nutritive sucking (Fig. 13.10).

Medication Interactions

Whenever a child is ill and treated with prescription medications, the nurse is responsible for monitoring medication interactions, medication–food interactions, and medication–environment interactions. Monitoring medication interactions involves knowledge of the adverse effects of each medication prescribed. Medication–environment interactions involve the effects of a medication on the response of the patient to their environment. For example, certain antibiotics have photosensitivity as an adverse effect. The nurse needs to advise the patient or parent to avoid prolonged exposure to sunlight. Medication–food interactions are often overlooked but can have an impact on treatment and the growth and development of the child. For example, cranberry, pomegranate, and blueberry juices contain flavonoids that can interfere with absorption of medications such as ibuprofen, phenytoin, and fluvastatin. Grapefruit juice interacts with the metabolism of atorvastatin and simvastatin; orange juice and apple juice may also interact with the absorption of specific medications (Shirasaka, Schichiri, Mori, et al., 2013). The malabsorption of carbohydrates and the amount of fructose and sorbitol in juice can be the cause of flatulence and diarrhea in young children. Prune juice and apple juice contain sorbitol and can be useful in preventing constipation in children. In general, the nurse should remain alert to any medication interactions while caring for the sick child.

THE TEETH

DECIDUOUS TEETH

The development of the 20 **deciduous**, or baby, teeth begins at about the fifth month of intrauterine life. The health and diet of the expectant mother can affect the development of the teeth. Primary teeth erupt during the first 2.5 years of life. It is a normal process and is generally accompanied by little or no discomfort. Wide

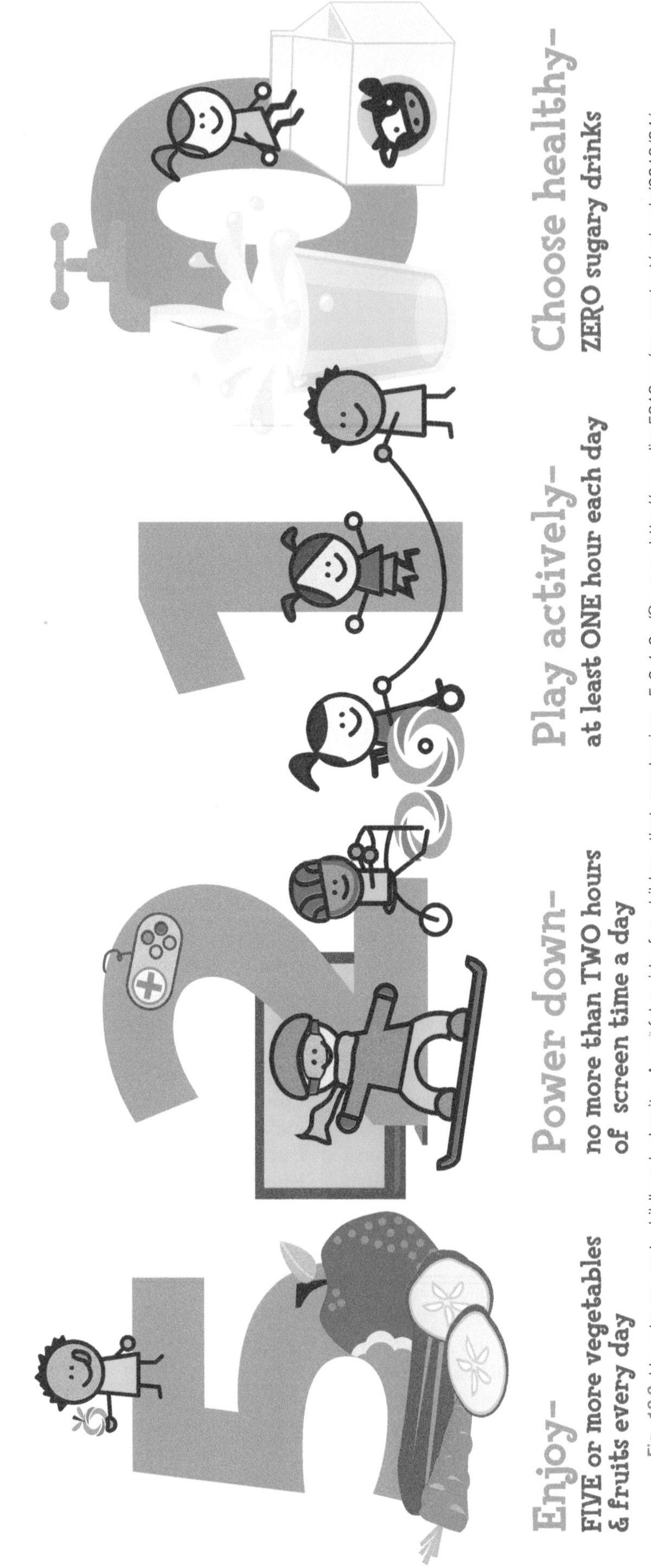

Enjoy-
FIVE or more vegetables & fruits every day
Power down-
no more than TWO hours of screen time a day
Play actively-
at least ONE hour each day
Choose healthy-
ZERO sugary drinks

Fig. 13.9 How to prevent childhood obesity. A useful guide for children that emphasizes 5-2-1-0. (Source: http://www.live5210.ca/wp-content/uploads/2010/04/5210-kids-text.png.)

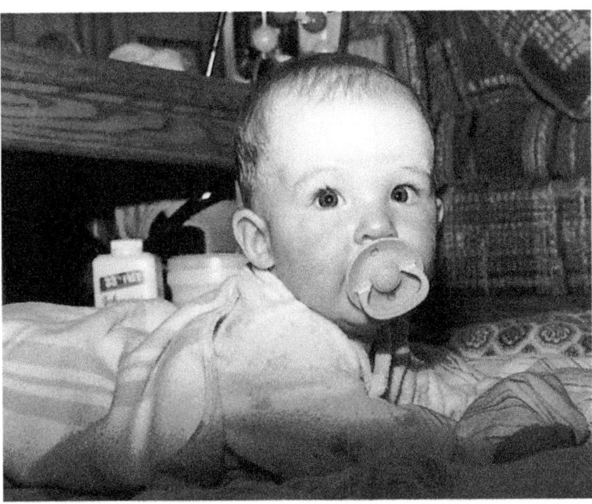

Fig. 13.10 Non-nutritive sucking. Non-nutritive sucking involving the finger or a pacifier is common in infants less than 1 year of age and fulfills the needs of the oral phase of development. In general, malocclusion from non-nutritive sucking will not be a problem if the habit is discontinued by 5 years of age.

individual differences in tooth eruption occur in normal, healthy infants. Occasionally an infant is born with teeth; newborn teeth are removed to prevent the possibility of choking should they fall out. A delay in teething is significant if other forms of immaturity or illness are present. The health care provider evaluates the process of teething during the infant's regular health checkups. Tetracycline antibiotics stain developing teeth a yellowish brown and are to be avoided during pregnancy and in the first 8 years of life.

The first tooth generally appears at about the sixth or seventh month. The 1-year-old has about six teeth, four above and two below. The order in which the teeth appear is almost always the same (Fig. 13.11). They are shed in about the same order in which they appear (i.e., lower central incisors first, and so forth). The Canadian Dental Association (CDA) recommends that the first dental visit occur 6 months after the eruption of the first tooth or by 1 year (CDA, 2019b).

The deciduous teeth serve not only in the digestive process but also in the development of the jaw. When the deciduous teeth are lost early because of neglect, the permanent teeth may become poorly aligned.

PERMANENT TEETH

The 32 permanent teeth develop just before birth and during the first year of life. They do not begin to erupt through the gums, however, until the sixth year. Nutrition and general health during the first year of life affect the formation of permanent teeth. This process is not completed until the wisdom teeth appear, at about 17 to 21 years of age. The first permanent teeth do not replace any of the deciduous teeth but appear behind the deciduous molars. Cavities in them are often neglected because they are mistaken for baby teeth. The most common site of decay in children is the fissures of the molar teeth. These areas can be protected by the professional application of plastic sealants.

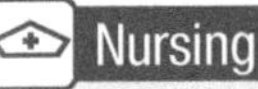 **Nursing Tip**

To assess the number of teeth a child under age 2 years is expected to have, use the following formula:

Age in months – 6.

(Example: 20 months – 6 = 14 teeth.)

ORAL CARE IN HEATH AND ILLNESS

Good dental care begins with a proper diet that supplies adequate nutrients while the teeth are developing in the jaws, especially during the prenatal period and the first year. The many essential elements found in milk include calcium, phosphorus, vitamins A and B complex, and protein. Vitamin D (the "sunshine vitamin") and vitamin C (found in citrus fruits) are also valuable. Dietary practices influence the development of cavities, and parents are encouraged to limit their child's frequency of fermentable carbohydrate intake.

In the past, total carbohydrate consumption was thought to be the most important dietary consideration for dental health. Today, more attention is given to the frequency with which sweets are eaten and how long they stick to the teeth. Sticky foods have more potential to cause caries (cavities) than do sugared drinks that are quickly cleared from the mouth. Oral care after eating sticky foods is recommended. Recommended snack foods include cheese, peanuts, milk, sugarless gum, and raw vegetables. Items to be avoided include sugared gum, dried fruits, sugared soft drinks, cakes, and candy. If a child does eat a sugary food or drink, teeth should be cleaned afterward.

Parents should start cleaning the infant's mouth even before teeth are present (see Health Promotion box). They should take a clean, damp facecloth or soft brush and rub all of the gums and teeth (if present). Toothpaste should not be used until teeth are present (CDA, 2019a). Parental supervision of tooth brushing should occur until 6 years of age. It is important that all children brush their teeth before bedtime.

Of most importance in preventing caries is the use of fluoride. Ideally, fluorides are present naturally in the water supply or are added to it. Too much fluoride may cause the teeth to become permanently "mottled" (**fluorosis**). Supplemental fluoride should be administered only from the age of 6 months, and only if the following conditions prevail (Godel & CPS Nutrition and Gastroenterology Committee, 2002/2019):

- The concentration of fluoride in drinking water is less than 0.3 ppm;
- The child does not brush their teeth (or have them brushed by a parent or guardian) at least twice a day; and
- If, in the judgement of a dentist or other health provider, the child is susceptible to high caries activity (family history, caries trends and patterns in communities or geographic areas).

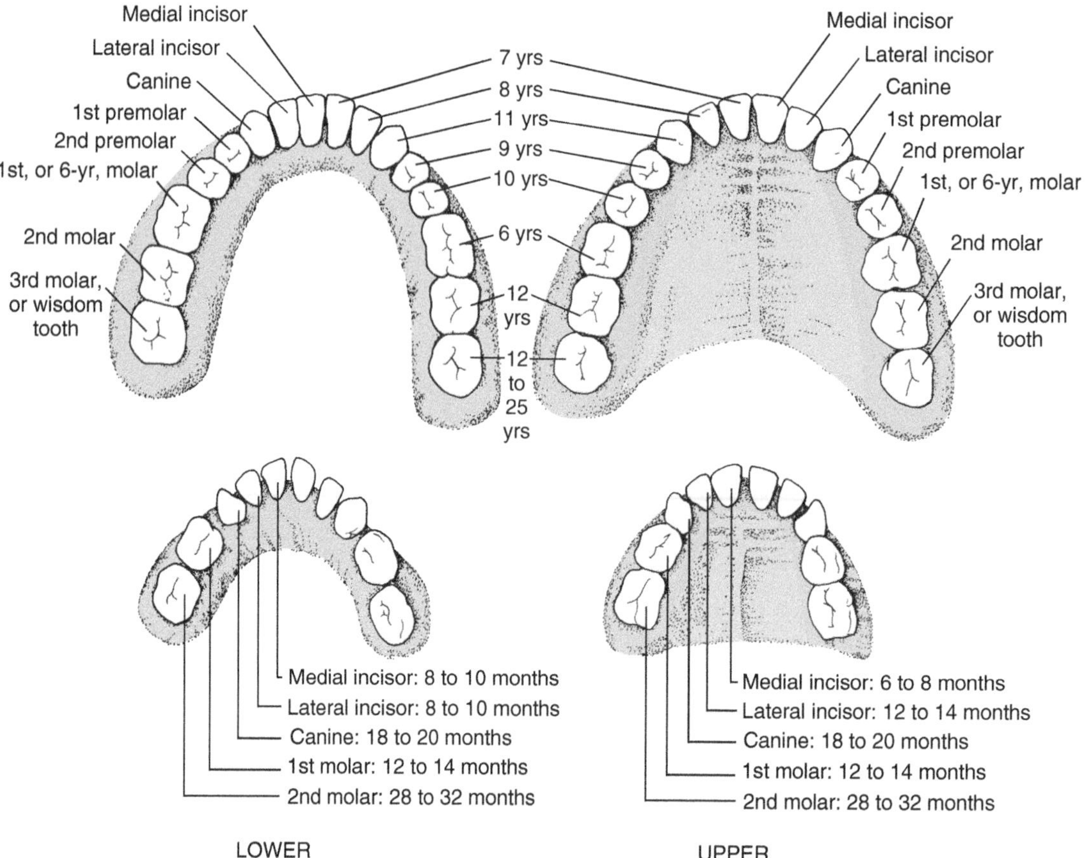

Fig. 13.11 Permanent and deciduous teeth and age of eruption.

Children who are between 6 months and 3 years of age should use a fluoridated toothpaste if they are assessed to be at risk for tooth decay. Children 3 to 6 years of age should only use a pea-sized amount of fluoridated toothpaste.

Another aspect of tooth care is the prevention of *nursing bottle syndrome* or **nursing caries** (Fig. 13.12). This condition occurs when the infant is put to bed with a bottle of milk or juice. Sugar pools within the oral cavity, causing severe decay. It is seen most often in children between 18 months and 3 years of age. Eliminating the bedtime bottle or substituting water in the bottle is recommended. The use of an open cup early (from 6 months) may help avoid prolonged bottle feeding. Severe childhood caries is defined as smooth-surface caries in a child younger than 3 years old. Signs of early decay include chalky white spots on tooth enamel near the gum line of maxillary incisors. Brown discoloration signals more advanced decay. Tooth decay can cause dental abscesses, which can result in serious complications.

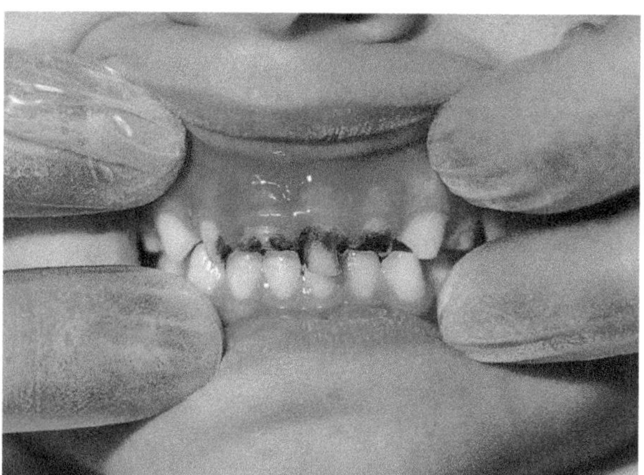

Fig. 13.12 Nursing caries. During sleep, saliva production decreases and the teeth become more vulnerable to decay. When the infant is put to sleep with a bottle containing milk or sweetened juice, the sugar combines with the bacterial flora in the mouth to cause tooth decay. This is known as "milk caries." Parents should be taught to use water as the only liquid in a bottle at bedtime. (From Swartz, M. H. [2014]. *Textbook of physical diagnosis: history and examination* [7th ed.]. Philadelphia: Saunders.)

The maintenance of good oral health is an integral part of comprehensive care for a sick pediatric patient. Education, prevention, and referral in the home, school, or hospital setting must be part of the child's plan of care. Untreated dental caries or malposition of the erupting teeth can cause periodontal disease in later years if not treated promptly. Delayed or early eruption of teeth can be indicative of certain endocrine disorders or other pathological conditions and should be recorded and reported. Parents and caregivers should avoid "tasting" baby food fed to infants

 Health Promotion

Developmental Dental Hygiene

FIRST YEARS OF LIFE
- The infant's gums are wiped daily from shortly after birth with a moist cloth or soft brush.
- Gentle brushing is performed each night with a soft, small toothbrush.
- Use of fluoride toothpaste (amount equivalent to a grain of rice) is begun at 6 months *only if there is high risk for dental caries and if water is not fluoridated.*
- The child is not put to bed with a bottle of milk or juice. If the infant must have a bottle, water is used.

1 TO 3 YEARS
- Parents introduce toothpaste in addition to the soft toothbrush. Fluoridated toothpaste should not be used unless there is a high risk for caries.

3 TO 6 YEARS
- Deciduous teeth erupt, and baby teeth start to loosen and fall out toward the end of this period.
- Parents assist children and remind them to brush and floss until at least age 6 years. A small, soft toothbrush is used. Toothpaste with fluoride is introduced at age 3 using only a pea-sized amount of toothpaste to minimize fluoride ingestion.
- Bedtime routine of brushing is established, because salivary flow rates slow during sleep, reducing natural protective mechanisms.
- Parents are advised to assist the child in brushing the child's teeth at least once a day and to clean teeth that are in contact with each other with dental floss.
- Sweets are limited to daytime meals, when saliva content is high.

6 TO 12 YEARS
- First permanent molars appear. The pits and fissures of molars make them the primary site for caries. Sealants (plastic coating) professionally applied to molars provide a mechanical barrier against bacteria.
- Children should continue with brushing and flossing and reduce *frequency* of exposure to fermentable carbohydrates. Adolescent gingivitis (*gingiv,* "gum," and *itis,* "inflammation of"), characterized by redness, swelling, and bleeding, is common in children and adolescents and may be aggravated by hormonal changes at puberty.
- Orthodontic treatments place children at high risk for gingivitis and caries around appliances or braces.
- Mouth protectors should be used to prevent dental injuries from contact sports.

and young children because the transmission of acid-producing bacteria from their mouths can be passed on to the food or feeding utensils and can contribute to tooth decay in the infant. Children should brush before bedtime because the protective bacteriocidal effects of saliva decrease during sleep, and bacterial growth can cause tooth decay. Fever (body temperature exceeding 38.1°C) is not usually associated with teething and should be evaluated for other causes.

Parents and children should be educated concerning the care of the toothbrush to provide maximum effectiveness of the tooth brushing activity:
- Replace toothbrush every 3 to 4 months.
- Replace toothbrush after a viral illness.
- Avoid rinsing bristles in hot water.
- Do not use a closed container for toothbrush storage.
- Avoid sharing toothbrushes among children.

A properly sized toothbrush will aid in developing good tooth brushing technique. A soft brush with a small amount of toothpaste is appropriate. Dental flossing should be done with an up-and-down motion. A back-and-forth "sawing" motion can cause injury to gingival tissues. Children need assistance and supervision with flossing until at least age 6 years.

Trauma to the teeth often occurs in school-age children. Appropriate protective devices can prevent injury during sports activities. If a primary tooth is knocked out (avulsed) because of trauma, the child should be referred to a dentist for a "spacer" that will maintain tooth alignment until the permanent tooth erupts. If a permanent tooth is avulsed because of trauma, the tooth should be immersed in cold milk or placed in saliva (under the parent's or child's tongue) and brought with the child to the dentist for immediate care. Open wounds to oral tissues may require tetanus prophylaxis or antibiotics. All tooth fractures should be referred to a dentist for evaluation and treatment.

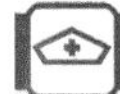 Nursing Tip

When a tooth is "knocked out" or avulsed traumatically, the tooth should be gently cleansed of obvious dirt and placed in cold milk or saliva until dental care is obtained.

Dental problems that often occur with adolescents include puberty gingivitis, medication-related gingivitis, and hyperplastic gingivitis associated with orthodontic therapy. Temporomandibular joint (TMJ) problems and malocclusion caused by missing teeth necessitate a dental referral. Orthodontic appliances such as fixed braces can trap plaque and food and can increase tooth decay. Meticulous oral hygiene, brushing, and flossing are part of comprehensive orthodontic care.

A team approach to dental care for the child receiving chemotherapy or radiation therapy includes the dentist, the health care provider, the nurse, the parent, and the patient. Brushing and flossing when the platelet count is more than 20×10^9 and using moist gauze when the platelet count is less than 20×10^9 are advised to prevent infection and bleeding. The use of chlorhexidine may be prescribed to reduce oral lesions.

Table 13.8 Medical Problems and Dental Health

MEDICAL PROBLEM	EFFECT ON TEETH
Asthma	Sucrose content of medication can cause decay
Hemophilia Cancer	Can cause oral bleeding, impaired healing
Seizure disorders	Causes decreased saliva; gingival overgrowth (use of phenytoin)
Medications that depress the central nervous system	Decrease salivary flow, increasing susceptibility to dental caries
Juvenile rheumatoid arthritis	Sucrose-containing medications increase risk of caries
Bulimia	Erosion of teeth caused by acid contact during vomiting episodes
Chemotherapy	Oral ulcerations
Fluoride ingestion	Excess fluoride can cause fluorosis (mottling of teeth)

Table 13.8 reviews medical problems that have an effect on dental health.

Children who have a disability can master independent tooth brushing by modifying the toothbrush. Using padded tongue depressors to visualize the oral cavity and an aspirating catheter attached to the toothbrush and connected to a suction machine can assist in providing dental care for a child who has a more severe disability. Battery-operated toothbrushes can help to achieve optimum brushing technique.

PLAY

Play is the business of children. Observing the child at play can aid in assessing growth and development and understanding the child's relationship with family members. Any plan of care for a hospitalized child of any age should include a play activity that either encourages growth and development or encourages the expression of thoughts and feelings. Playrooms in the hospital pediatric unit can be used for children who have conditions that are not communicable. Medications and treatments should not be administered in the playroom setting. Play can also be therapeutic and aid in the recovery process. An example of **therapeutic play** is the game of having the child "blow out" the light of a flashlight as if it were a candle, to promote deep breathing. Table 13.9 reviews age-appropriate play behaviours.

Art is an appropriate play activity at almost any age and provides an avenue for experimentation as well as for creative expression and a feeling of accomplishment in the child. Computer programs are popular with all age groups, providing problem-solving games, manipulative skills, and opportunities for new learning. Both of these activities must be balanced with active play experiences.

Nursing interventions should focus on encouraging optimal play activities and experiences that are age appropriate. Parents may need guidance concerning the value of play and that play may not always be a neat and clean activity. Helping parents to select appropriate toys that are safe as well as appropriate to the age and illness is essential. For example, a stuffed animal may not be the toy of choice for an asthmatic child. In the health care setting, a blood pressure cuff can give the child a "hug." Children can play with the equipment they see in their environment to provide stress relief.

Children are spending more time in front of computer or television screens, and this can affect the amount of time they actually have to play and interact with others. This sedentary behaviour also limits the amount of physical activity that a child gets. The CPS (2017b) along with the World Health Organization (2019) have made the following recommendations regarding young children's screen time:

- Screen time for children younger than 2 years is not recommended.
- For children 2 to 5 years, limit routine or regular screen time to less than 1 hour per day.
- Ensure that sedentary screen time is not a routine part of child care for children younger than 5 years.
- Maintain daily "screen-free" times, especially for family meals and book sharing.
- Avoid looking at screens at least 1 hour before bedtime, given the potential for melatonin-suppressing effects.

TRAVELLING WITH CHILDREN

Travelling and exploring the outdoors are popular activities. Parents are encouraged to bring their children when out hiking or vacationing. Safety equipment for small children is available for most outdoor activities (Fig. 13.13). Air travel has also become a part of some families' lifestyle. Air travel often upsets a child's set of routines, such as eating and sleeping, with new surroundings, strange cribs, unfamiliar faces, and restricted movement. Jet lag may not be an issue for an infant or child's travel. Sedation with antihistamines should not be used during air travel as it can increase restlessness and result in excessive crying. Overfeeding should be avoided during flight as air in the stomach expands by 20% due to lower cabin pressure, causing abdominal discomfort and an increase in crying. Air conditioning in the cabin of the plane can result in the child appearing to have dry skin and lips, but dehydration is not an issue during routine flights. Parents should try to provide a warm, comfortable resting place with familiar small toys, appropriate

Table 13.9 **Development of Play**

AGE GROUP	TYPE OF PLAY	SUGGESTED PLAY ACTIVITY
Infants	Explore, imitate	Provide visual stimuli for newborns, touch stimuli for infants, and toys involving manipulation for 1-year-olds.
1 to 2 years	**Parallel play**	Children play next to each other but not with each other. Provide each child with toys that reflect activities of daily living.
3 to 5 years	**Cooperative play** Creative play	Children play with each other, each taking a specific role: "You be the mommy and I'll be the daddy." A simple box can become a train to a 3-year-old.
5 to 7 years	Symbolic group play; secret clubs	Secret codes, "knock-knock" jokes, and rhymes are popular at this age.
7 to 10 years	**Competitive play**	Children at this age start to accept competition with structured rules and highly interactive physical activity.
10 to 13 years	Group sports and explorative Internet activities, electronic or computer games	Monitored Internet contact.
13 to 18 years	Fantasy play; cliques	Leadership activities such as babysitting or tutoring are popular. Daydreaming occurs. Board games are popular. Interactive social activities in "cliques" occur at and after school.

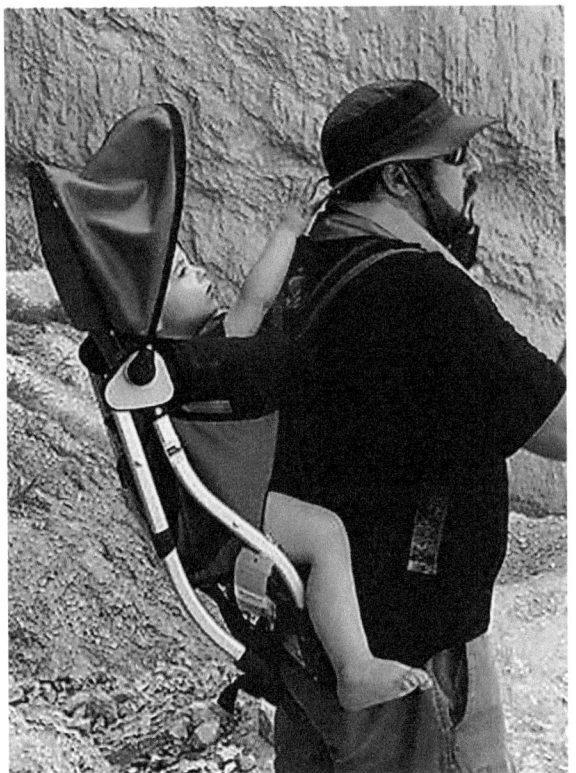

Fig. 13.13 Hiking and exploring the outdoors is a healthy family pursuit.

treats, handheld electronics, and a pacifier. A parent can walk with the child in the aisles when appropriate and sing and play quiet games when seated. To prevent ear pain during ascent or descent, the parent can encourage the child's swallowing starting 30 minutes before descent begins, using breastfeeding, sucking on a bottle or pacifier for young children, or chewing gum for older children. Older children can also be taught the Valsalva manoeuvre (blowing the nose firmly while pinching the nostrils shut and keeping the mouth closed while swallowing). Children under 2 years of age can sit unrestrained on a parent's lap, but an approved child restraint system is recommended by Transport Canada.

ONGOING HEALTH SUPERVISION

Children of all ages should receive ongoing health checkups every 1 to 2 years until 18 years of age. Specific health care recommendations for each age group are discussed in Chapters 14 through 18.

Get Ready for the Certification Examination!

Key Points

- Growth and development are orderly and sequential, although there are spurts and plateaus.
- Cephalocaudal development proceeds from head to toe.
- Motor development follows a predictable sequence.
- Children are susceptible to nutritional deficiencies because they are in the process of growth and development.
- Social determinants of health influence the growth and development of children.
- Maslow depicted human development based on a hierarchy of needs.
- A family is two or more persons that interact together and share mutual responsibility for care of the members of the group.
- A nurse is an advocate, educator, and collaborator in a family-centred care environment.
- Developmental theories can serve as guides to nursing intervention; however, each child grows and develops at an individual pace.
- Freud's theories portrayed personality development as phases of psychosexual development.
- Piaget described phases of cognitive development.
- Erikson described eight stages of psychosocial development from birth to adulthood.
- Parent–child interactions affect positive growth and development.
- Optimal nutrition is essential to physical and neurological growth and development.
- Nutritional practices of early childhood tend to persist through adulthood.
- The nurse should provide counselling focusing on positive nutritional practices that work within the family's culture, religion, and lifestyle.
- Obesity is a serious concern among Canadian children. Nurses have a role in decreasing obesity rates.
- Deciduous teeth are baby teeth. The proper care of the teeth depends on supervision by the caregiver according to the child's physical level of development and mastery.
- The availability of age-appropriate toys enhances physical, emotional, and mental development in infants, children, and adolescents.
- Computer games can foster problem solving, cognitive development, and motor coordination but should be balanced with active play activities.
- Many hospitals have playrooms, which must be kept safe from painful or invasive experiences.

Additional Learning Resources

evolve Go to your Evolve website (http://evolve.elsevier.com/Canada/Leifer) for the following learning resources:

- Answer Key for Critical Thinking Questions
- Answer Key for Textbook Review Questions
- Audio Glossary
- Interactive Review Questions
- Skills Performance Checklists
- Video clips and more!

Online Resources

- Canadian Paediatric Society, *Vegetarian diets for children and teens:* https://www.caringforkids.cps.ca/handouts/vegetarian_diets_for_children_and_teens
- Nipissing District Developmental Screen (NDDS): https://lookseechecklist.com/

Review Questions

1. How many erupted teeth would the nurse expect a healthy 8-month-old infant to have?
   a. 2
   b. 4
   c. 6
   d. 8
2. During the first week of life, the newborn's weight may do which of the following?
   a. Increase by about 7 to 10%
   b. Decrease by about 7 to 10%
   c. Stabilize
   d. Fluctuate widely
3. The nurse should encourage the parent to introduce tooth brushing to the child by which age?
   a. 6 months
   b. 1 year
   c. 3 years
   d. 2 months
4. To meet the needs (as described by Erikson) of a school-age child diagnosed with diabetes, the nurse should do which of the following?
   a. Explain carefully to the mother the need to adhere rigidly to dietary modifications.
   b. Allow the child to eat whatever they want and administer insulin to maintain optimum glucose levels.
   c. Allow the child to perform their own Accuchecks and administer their own insulin.
   d. Perform Accuchecks four times a day and at bedtime.
5. It is most appropriate to first introduce competitive games at which age?
   a. 3 to 5 years
   b. 5 to 6 years
   c. 7 to 9 years
   d. 12 to 15 years
6. Which of the following foods contains sorbitol, which can prevent constipation in young children? *(Select all that apply.)*
   a. Prunes
   b. Apple juice
   c. Tea
   d. Watermelon

REFERENCES

Amit, M., & Canadian Paediatric Society (CPS), Community Paediatrics Committee. (2010). Vegetarian diets in children and adolescents. *Paediatrics & Child Health, 15*(5), 303–314. Reaffirmed in 2016.

Canada without Poverty. (2019). *Just the facts*. Retrieved from: http://www.cwp-csp.ca/poverty/just-the-facts/.

Canadian Dental Association (CDA). (2019a). *Cleaning teeth*. Retrieved from: https://www.cda-adc.ca/en/oral_health/cfyt/dental_care_children/cleaning.asp.

Canadian Dental Association (CDA). (2019b). *Your child's first visit*. Retrieved from: http://www.cda-adc.ca/en/oral_health/cfyt/dental_care_children/first_visit.asp.

Canadian Paediatric Society (CPS). (2017a). *Healthy sleep for your baby and child*. Retrieved from: https://www.caringforkids.cps.ca/handouts/healthy_sleep_for_your_baby_and_child.

Canadian Pediatric Society (CPS). (2017b). Screen time and young children: Promoting health and development in a digital world. *Paediatrics & Child Health, 22*(8), 461–468.

Canadian Paediatric Society (CPS). (2019). *Healthy eating for children*. Retrieved from: https://www.caringforkids.cps.ca/handouts/healthy_eating_for_children.

Canadian Paediatric Society (CPS), Dietitians of Canada, College of Family Physicians of Canada, Community Health Nurses of Canada, & Canadian Pediatric Endocrine Group. (2014). *WHO growth charts adapted for Canada. Summary of changes—March 2014*. Retrieved from: http://www.dietitians.ca/Downloads/Public/WHO-Growth-Charts-Summary-of-Change-March-2014.aspx.

Dietitians of Canada. (2014). *Tips on feeding your picky toddler or preschooler*. Retrieved from: https://www.dietitians.ca/Downloads/Factsheets/Tips-Feeding-Picky-Toddler.aspx.

Dietitians of Canada. (2018). *Healthy weights for teens*. Retrieved from: https://www.dietitians.ca/Your-Health/Nutrition-A-Z/Teens/5-Steps-to-Healthy-Eating-for-Youth-12-18.aspx.

Dietitians of Canada. (2019). *BMI for children/teens*. Retrieved from: https://www.dietitians.ca/your-health/assess-yourself/assess-your-bmi/bmi-children.aspx.

Godel, J., & Canadian Paediatric Society (CPS), Nutrition and Gastroenterology Committee. (2002). The use of fluoride in infants and children. *Paediatrics & Child Health, 7*(8), 569–572. Reaffirmed 2019. Retrieved from: https://www.cps.ca/en/documents/position/fluoride-use.

Government of Canada. (2013). *What makes Canadians healthy or unhealthy?* Retrieved from: https://www.canada.ca/en/public-health/services/health-promotion/population-health/what-determines-health/what-makes-canadians-healthy-unhealthy.html#income.

Government of Canada. (2017). *Canadian food inspection agency (CFIA) compliance and enforcement of gluten-free claims*. Retrieved from: http://www.inspection.gc.ca/food/labelling/food-labelling-for-industry/allergens-and-gluten/gluten-free-claims/eng/1340194596012/1340194681961.

Government of Canada. (2018). *Social determinants of health and health inequalities*. Retrieved from: https://www.canada.ca/en/public-health/services/health-promotion/population-health/what-determines-health.html.

Government of Canada. (2019a). *Canada's food guide*. Retrieved from: https://food-guide.canada.ca/en/.

Government of Canada. (2019b). *Childhood obesity*. Retrieved from: https://www.canada.ca/en/public-health/services/childhood-obesity/childhood-obesity.html.

Gulliver-Garcia, T. (2016). *Putting an end to child & family homelessness in Canada*. Toronto: Raising the Roof. Retrieved from: https://www.raisingtheroof.org/wp-content/uploads/2015/10/CF-Report-Final.pdf.

Health Canada, & Canadian Paediatric Society (CPS), Dietitians of Canada, and Breastfeeding Committee for Canada. (2015). *Nutrition for healthy term infants: Recommendations from six to 24 months*. Retrieved from: https://www.canada.ca/en/health-canada/services/food-nutrition/healthy-eating/infant-feeding/nutrition-healthy-term-infants-recommendations-birth-six-months/6-24-months.html.

Kaufman, M., & Canadian Paediatric Society (CPS), Adolescent Health Committee. (2008). Adolescent sexual orientation. *Paediatrics & Child Health, 13*(7), 619–623. Reaffirmed 2016.

Keenan-Lindsay, L. (2017). The family and culture. In S. Perry, M. Hockenberry, D. Lowdermilk, et al. (Eds.), *Maternal child nursing care in Canada* (2nd ed.). Toronto, ON: Elsevier.

Mahan, L. K., & Raymond, J. (2017). *Krause's food and the nutrition care process* (14th ed.). St. Louis: Elsevier.

O'Flaherty, P. (2017). Physiological adaptations of the newborn. In S. Perry, M. Hockenberry, D. Lowdermilk, et al. (Eds.), *Maternal child nursing care in Canada* (2nd ed.). Toronto, ON: Elsevier.

Pound, C. M., Blair, B., & Canadian Paediatric Society (CPS), Nutrition and Gastroenterology Committee. (2017). Energy and sports drinks in children and adolescents. *Paediatrics & Child Health, 22*(7), 406–410. https://www.cps.ca/en/documents/position/energy-and-sports-drinks.

Public Health Agency of Canada (PHAC). (2012). *Curbing childhood obesity; a federal, provincial and territorial framework for action to promote healthy weights*. Retrieved from: http://www.phac-aspc.gc.ca/hp-ps/hl-mvs/framework-cadre/pdf/ccofw-eng.pdf.

Shirasaka, Y., Schichiri, M., Mori, T., et al. (2013). Major active components in grapefruit, orange and apple juice responsible for OATP2BI-mediated drug interactions. *Journal of Pharmaceutical Science, 102*(9), 3418–3426.

Smilkstein, G., Ashworth, C., & Montano, D. (1984). The validity and reliability of the family APGAR as a test of family function. *Journal of Family Practice, 15*, 303.

Starkes, J. M., Baydala, L. T., & Canadian Paediatric Society (CPS), First Nations, Inuit and Métis Health Committee. (2014). Health research involving First Nations, Inuit and Métis children and their communities. *Paediatrics & Child Health, 19*(2), 99–102. Reaffirmed 2017. Retrieved from: https://www.cps.ca/en/documents/position/health-research-first-nations-inuit-metis-children.

Statistics Canada. (2017a). *Children living in low income households*. Ottawa: Government of Canada. Retrieved from: http://www12.statcan.gc.ca/census-recensement/2016/as-sa/98-200-x/2016012/98-200-x2016012-eng.cfm.

Statistics Canada. (2017b). *Portrait of children's family life in Canada in 2016*. Ottawa: Government of Canada. Retrieved from: http://www12.statcan.gc.ca/census-recensement/2016/as-sa/98-200-x/2016006/98-200-x2016006-eng.cfm.

World Health Organization. (2019). *To grow up healthy, children need to sit less and play more*. Geneva: Author. Retrieved from: https://www.who.int/news-room/detail/24-04-2019-to-grow-up-healthy-children-need-to-sit-less-and-play-more.

14 The Infant

http://evolve.elsevier.com/Canada/Leifer

Lisa Keenan-Lindsay

Objectives

1. Define each key term listed.
2. Discuss the major aspects of cognitive development in the first year of life.
3. Describe normal vital signs for a 1-year-old infant.
4. Describe the physical and psychosocial development of infants from age 1 to 12 months, listing age-specific events and guidance when appropriate.
5. Identify the approximate age for each of the following: posterior fontanelle has closed; central incisors appear; birth weight has tripled; child can sit steadily alone; child shows fear of strangers.
6. Relate the nursing responsibilities in health promotion and illness prevention of infants during the first year of life.
7. Discuss the approach to and the specifics of care of an infant with colic.
8. Discuss the development of favourable sleep patterns.
9. Discuss the nutritional needs of growing infants.
10. Describe nutritional counselling for the infant's family.
11. List four common concerns of parents about the feeding of infants.
12. Discuss the health teaching related to breastfeeding and formula feeding.
13. Describe how to select and prepare solid foods for the infant.
14. Discuss the development of feeding skills in the infant.
15. Discuss safety issues in the care of infants.
16. Identify age-appropriate toys and their developmental or therapeutic value.

Key Terms

colic
extrusion reflex (ěks-TRŪ-zhŭn RĒ-flěks)
grasp reflex
milestones
norms
object permanence
oral stage
parachute reflex
pincer grasp
prehension
satiety (să-TĪ-ĕ-tē)
weaning

Physical, emotional, and cognitive growth and the development of motor abilities occur rapidly during the first year of life. **Milestones** of growth and development describe general patterns of achievements at various stages of infancy. These milestones, or patterns, are referred to as **norms**. While norms can vary greatly for the individual child, the nurse must understand the normal range for milestone achievement to assess the progress of growth and development of the infant and initiate early referral for follow-up care.

Myelinization of the cortex of the brain begins at 7 to 8 months' gestation and continues through adolescence and is the basis of maturation of the sensory, motor, and associative pathways (Feigelman, 2016). The establishment of sleep–wake cycles, feeding preferences, and social interactions form during infancy and affect cognitive and emotional development throughout life. Inadequate dietary intake, caregiver interaction, or lack of environmental stimuli during infancy can result in permanent deficits.

During the newborn phase of development, the chief tasks mastered are the establishment of effective feeding patterns and a somewhat predictable sleep–wake cycle. Infants who have unmet hunger needs can become irritable, may not perceive feeding as pleasurable, and may fail to develop trust in the caregiver. Parental bonding and social interaction begin in the newborn phase but heighten when the infant begins to respond with a social smile.

By the time the infant is age 4 to 6 months, the positive parental interaction with the infant should be noticeable during clinic visits. If the parent does not appear to enjoy the developmental changes in the infant at this age or does not appear relaxed during interactions with the infant, further follow-up of possible family dysfunction or social or mental stresses should be initiated.

By age 9 months, control of feeding may become an issue of conflict between parent and infant. The parent needs to "let go" and introduce the infant to finger foods and initiate drinking from a cup. Offering limited

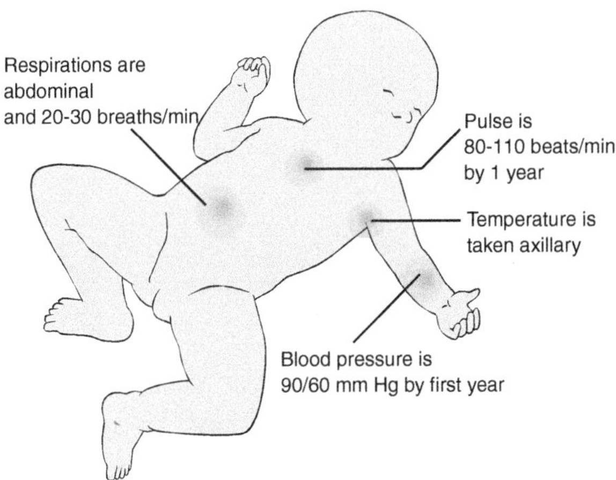
Respirations are abdominal and 20-30 breaths/min
Pulse is 80-110 beats/min by 1 year
Temperature is taken axillary
Blood pressure is 90/60 mm Hg by first year

Fig. 14.1 Average vital signs of the infant.

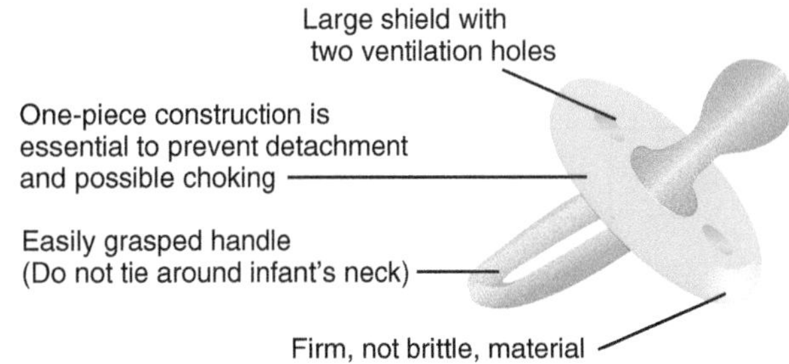
Large shield with two ventilation holes
One-piece construction is essential to prevent detachment and possible choking
Easily grasped handle (Do not tie around infant's neck)
Firm, not brittle, material

Fig. 14.2 Pacifiers provide non-nutritive sucking to meet the needs of the oral phase of infancy. A safe pacifier is illustrated. Note the one-piece construction.

choices can reduce conflict as the infant reaches toward autonomy. If the nurse notices an overly neat and orderly approach during feeding, parental guidance may be necessary. Separation anxiety (see Chapter 15) can be expected by the ninth-month clinic visit, and the nurse should expect to spend some time playing with the infant and getting to know the infant to establish the rapport necessary for a successful physical assessment.

Children at this age who are hospitalized are in the process of growing. To provide total patient care, the nurse must be able to recognize a patient's needs at various stages of growth and development and be aware of normal vital signs for an infant (Fig. 14.1; see Appendix A). The nurse must try to meet individual needs effectively and administer the specialized nursing care required for the particular patient. A cause for concern about a child is a sudden slowing of any aspect of development.

GENERAL CHARACTERISTICS

ORAL STAGE

Sucking is a normal reflex in the newborn. The **oral stage** of personality development is important for the infant's physical and psychological development. The nurse, knowing the importance of sucking to the infant, should hold the infant during feedings and allow sufficient time to suck. The nurse should also teach parents the importance of holding the infant during feeding. The infant who is fed intravenous fluids or gastric feedings should be given added attention and a pacifier, if approved by the parents, to provide the opportunity for non-nutritive sucking (Fig. 14.2). When the teeth appear, the infant learns to bite and enjoys objects that can be chewed. Gradually, the infant begins to put their fingers into their mouth. When infants can use their hands more skillfully, they will not suck their fingers as often and will be able to derive pleasure from other sources. The need for close supervision to maintain safety increases as the child learns to use their hands purposefully to grasp objects and put them into their mouth. Teaching parents about household safety should begin early.

MOTOR DEVELOPMENT

The **grasp reflex** (see Fig. 11.5) is seen when one touches the palms of the infant's hands and flexion occurs. This reflex disappears at about 3 months. **Prehension**, the ability to grasp objects between the fingers and the opposing thumb, occurs later (at 8 months) and follows an orderly sequence of development (Fig. 14.3).

The **parachute reflex** appears by age 8 months. This is a protective arm extension that occurs when an infant is suddenly thrust downward when prone. By age 1 year the **pincer grasp** coordination of index finger and thumb is well established.

EMOTIONAL DEVELOPMENT

Love and security are vital needs of infants. Babies require the continuous affection of their caregivers. If trust is to develop, consistency must be established. Parents need to be assured that they need not be afraid of spoiling their infants by attending promptly to their needs. Infants who are consistently picked up in response to crying show fewer crying episodes when they are toddlers and less aggressive behaviour at 2 years of age. Loving adults affirm that the world is a good place in which to live, and the infant learns to imitate and trust caregivers. A sense of trust is vital to the development of a healthy personality (see Table 13.2). Many consider it to be the foundation of emotional growth. The child who does not develop a sense of trust has a difficult time learning to develop trusting relationships, which could have a permanently negative effect on personality development.

Parents should be encouraged to talk, sing, and touch their infant while providing care. Infants will easily accomplish various activities if they are not forced before they reach readiness. When an infant shows readiness to learn a task or skill, parents should provide encouragement.

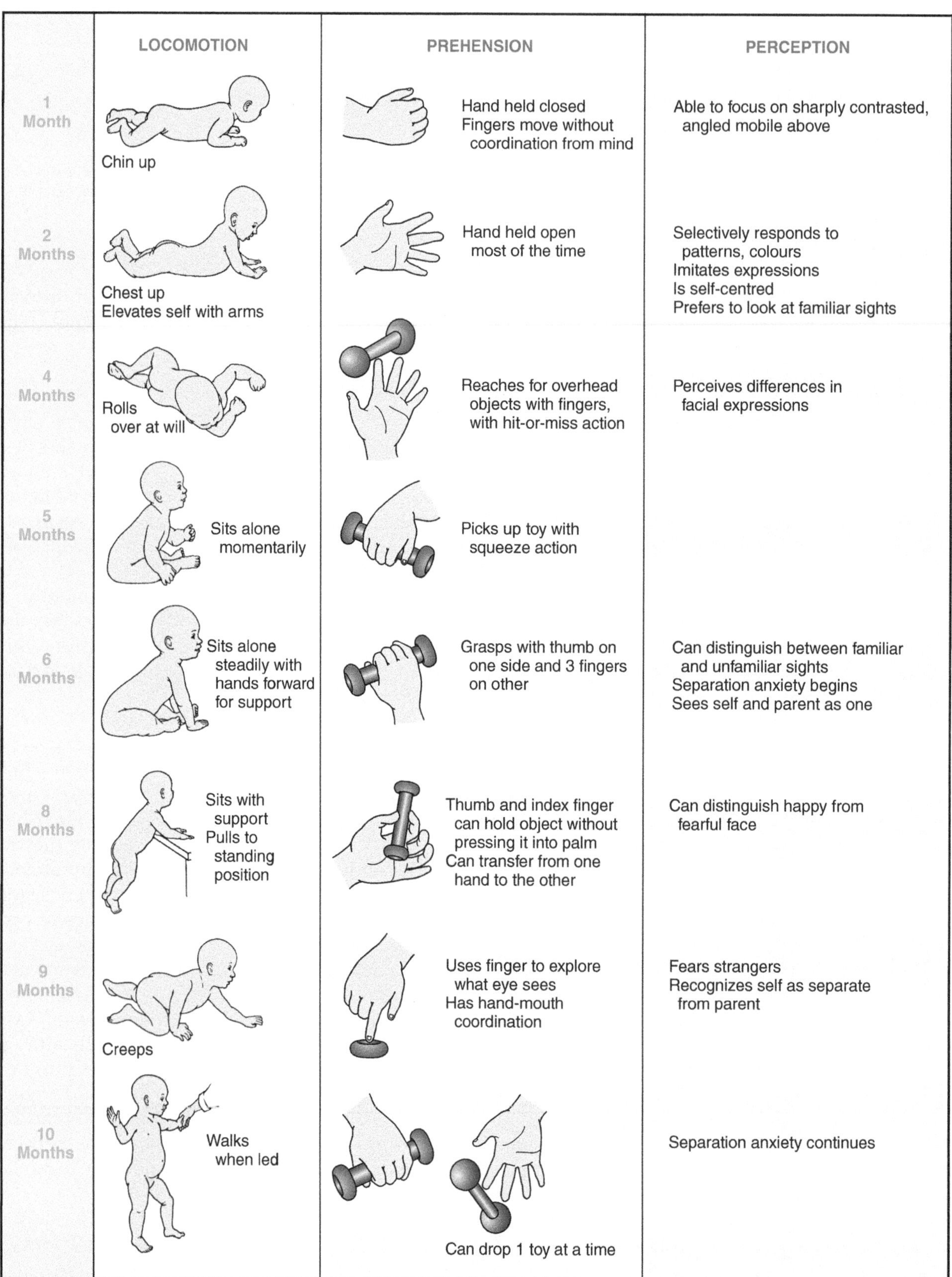

	LOCOMOTION	PREHENSION	PERCEPTION
1 Month	Chin up	Hand held closed Fingers move without coordination from mind	Able to focus on sharply contrasted, angled mobile above
2 Months	Chest up Elevates self with arms	Hand held open most of the time	Selectively responds to patterns, colours Imitates expressions Is self-centred Prefers to look at familiar sights
4 Months	Rolls over at will	Reaches for overhead objects with fingers, with hit-or-miss action	Perceives differences in facial expressions
5 Months	Sits alone momentarily	Picks up toy with squeeze action	
6 Months	Sits alone steadily with hands forward for support	Grasps with thumb on one side and 3 fingers on other	Can distinguish between familiar and unfamiliar sights Separation anxiety begins Sees self and parent as one
8 Months	Sits with support Pulls to standing position	Thumb and index finger can hold object without pressing it into palm Can transfer from one hand to the other	Can distinguish happy from fearful face
9 Months	Creeps	Uses finger to explore what eye sees Has hand-mouth coordination	Fears strangers Recognizes self as separate from parent
10 Months	Walks when led	Can drop 1 toy at a time	Separation anxiety continues

Fig. 14.3 The development of locomotion, prehension, and perception.

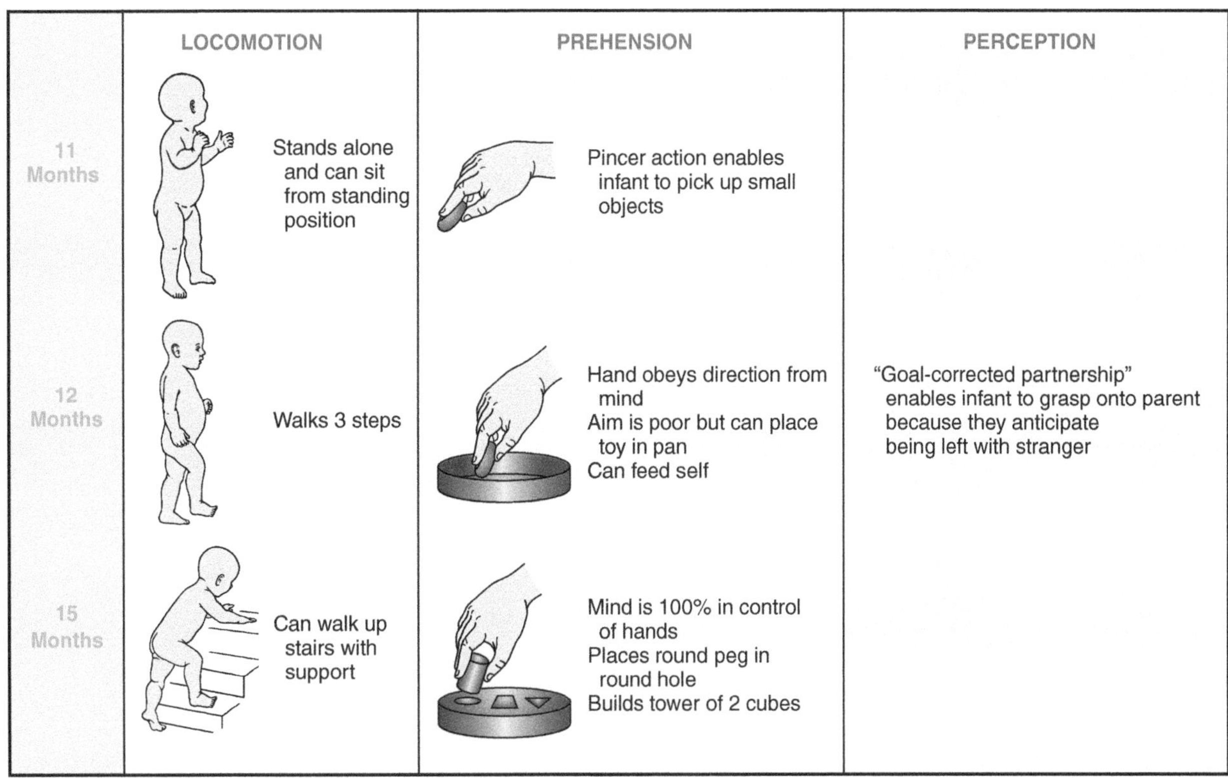

LOCOMOTION
PREHENSION
PERCEPTION
11 Months
Stands alone and can sit from standing position
Pincer action enables infant to pick up small objects
12 Months
Walks 3 steps
Hand obeys direction from mind
Aim is poor but can place toy in pan
Can feed self
"Goal-corrected partnership" enables infant to grasp onto parent because they anticipate being left with stranger
15 Months
Can walk up stairs with support
Mind is 100% in control of hands
Places round peg in round hole
Builds tower of 2 cubes

Fig. 14.3, cont'd

> **Nursing Tip**
>
> Parental approval is important to the infant, and setting limits early is essential. Principles of discipline at this age include the following:
> - Lowering the voice to say no firmly
> - Removing the child from the situation
> - Distraction
> - Consistency

NEED FOR CONSTANT CARE AND GUIDANCE

The full-time caregiver needs and deserves the understanding of and kind support from family at home and from the nurse in the hospital. Pediatrics involves caring for the family as well; a nurse can provide a short break from pressures, which may provide renewed energy for the parent to enjoy the infant and provide sensory stimulation. Such stimulation is essential for the development of the infant's thought processes and perceptual abilities. The infant who is constantly left in a crib or playpen and is not introduced to a variety of learning experiences may become shy and withdrawn.

If a parent is unable to room in with the hospitalized infant, personnel should try to imitate the parent's care by promptly fulfilling the infant's physical and emotional needs. The nurse should feed the infant who appears hungry, rather than delaying feeding to adhere to a specific routine. Wet diapers are changed as soon as possible. The crying child is soothed. The exactness of time or method of bathing or feeding the infant is less important than the care with which it is done. The infant easily recognizes warmth and affection or the lack thereof.

DEVELOPMENT AND CARE

Box 14.1 is a guide to infant care from the first month to the first birthday. Some aspects of care (e.g., safety measures) are important throughout the entire year. The nurse needs to explain to parents that physical patterns cannot be separated from social patterns and that abrupt changes do not take place with each new month. Human development cannot be separated into specific areas any more than the body's structure can be separated from its function.

No two infants are exactly alike at a certain age; Box 14.1 should be viewed as just a guide. However, individual variations fall within a range about central norms that serve as guidelines in the evaluation of an infant's or child's progress. See Table 13.4 for an outline of the parental tasks involved in guiding the infant through the stages of growth and development.

HEALTH PROMOTION

Infant health care encompasses periodic health appraisal, immunizations, assessment of parent–child interaction, teaching about the developmental processes, identification of families at risk (e.g., for child abuse), health education and anticipatory guidance, referrals to various agencies, and follow-up services.

Text Continues on p. 360

Box 14.1 Physical Development, Social Behaviour, and Care and Guidance of Infants

1 MONTH

Physical Development

Has regained weight lost after birth by 2 weeks and then gains approximately 140 to 200 g weekly for first 6 months. Gains about 2.5 cm in length per month for the first 6 months. Lifts head slightly when placed on stomach. Pushes with toes. Turns head to side when prone. Head wobbles. Head lags when infant is pulled from lying to sitting position. Clenches fists. Stares at surroundings.

Vaginal discharge in girls and breast enlargement in boys and girls from maternal hormones received in utero are not unusual and disappear without treatment.

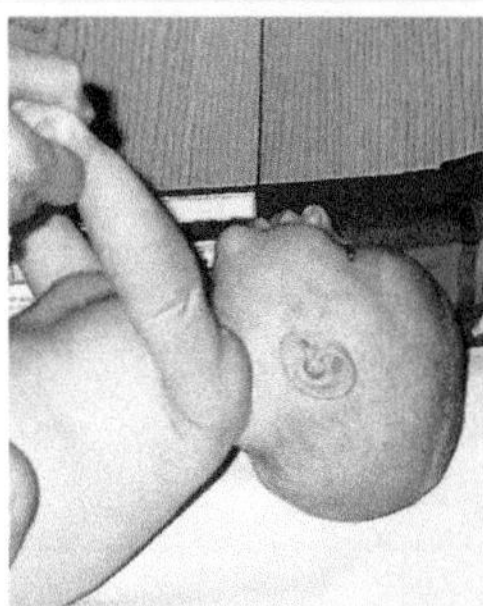

Note head lag of 1-month-old.

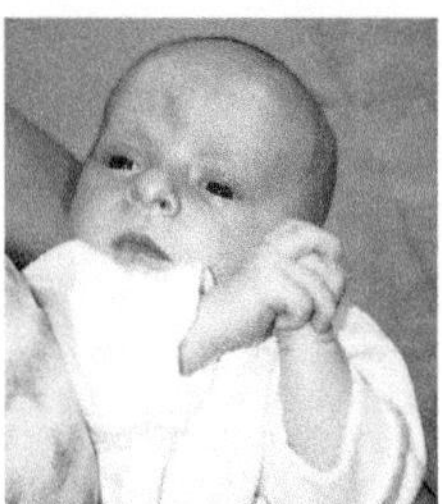

Infant keeps hands at midline.

Social Behaviour

Makes small throaty noises. Cries when hungry or uncomfortable. Sleeps approximately 20 of 24 hours. Wakes several times at night for feedings.

Care and Guidance

Sleep: On back; in a crib that meets Canadian Safety Association standards, with a firm, tight-fitting mattress in a crib with bars properly spaced. Do not use a pillow or bumper pads or place anything else in the crib with the infant (e.g., stuffed animals or bumper pads).

Diet: Breastmilk on demand or iron-fortified formula on demand. Vitamin D (400 international units [IU]/day) in breastfed infants, or infants who are not drinking 1 L/day of formula with vitamin D. May need more than 400 IU if live north of the 55th parallel. Burp infant well.

Exercise: Provide fresh air and sunshine whenever possible. Children under 6 months should be kept out of the sun. Sunscreen is not recommended for children under 6 months. Support head and shoulders when holding infant. Attend promptly to physical needs. Provide colourful hanging toys out of infant's reach for sensory stimulation.

2 MONTHS

Physical Development

Posterior fontanelle closes between second and third month. Tears appear. Can hold head erect in midposition for brief period. Follows moving light with eyes. Holds a rattle briefly. Legs are active.

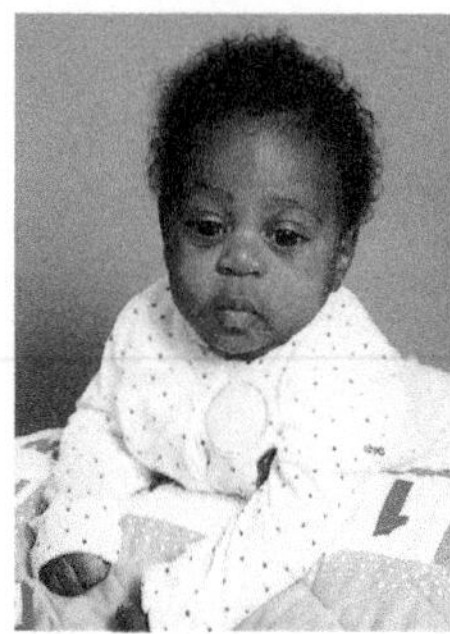

The 2-month-old can hold the head erect in midline for brief periods.

Care and Guidance

Sleep: Develops own pattern; may sleep from feeding to feeding.

Diet: Breastmilk or formula on demand.

Exercise: Provide a safe, flat place to kick and be active. Do not leave infant alone, particularly on any raised surface. Should have a visit with primary health care provider.

Immunization: First diphtheria, tetanus, and whooping cough (DTaP), injectable polio vaccine (IPV), *Haemophilus influenzae* type b (Hib), and second hepatitis B virus (HBV) vaccine (if given as newborn) (see Chapter 32).

Hiccoughs: Are normal and subside without treatment.

Colic: Consists of paroxysmal abdominal pain, irritable crying. Usually disappears after 3 months. Place infant prone over arms (see Fig. 14.4). Massage back. Relieve caregiver periodically (see Nursing Care Plan 14.1).

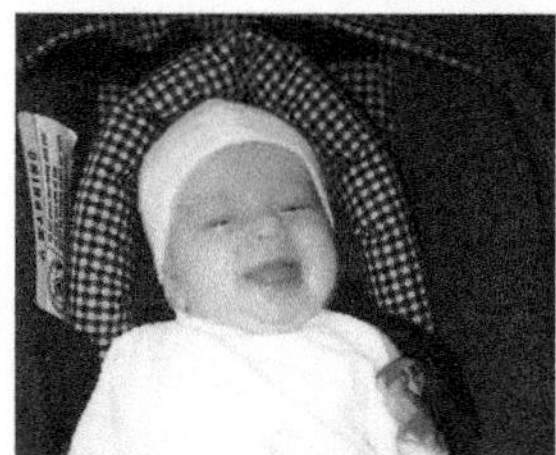

The smile of this 2-month-old delights parents.

3 MONTHS

Physical Development

Stares at hands. Reaches for objects but misses them. Carries hand to mouth. Can follow an object from right to left and up and down when it is placed in front of face. Supports head steadily. Holds rattle but will not reach for it.

Box 14.1 Physical Development, Social Behaviour, and Care and Guidance of Infants—cont'd

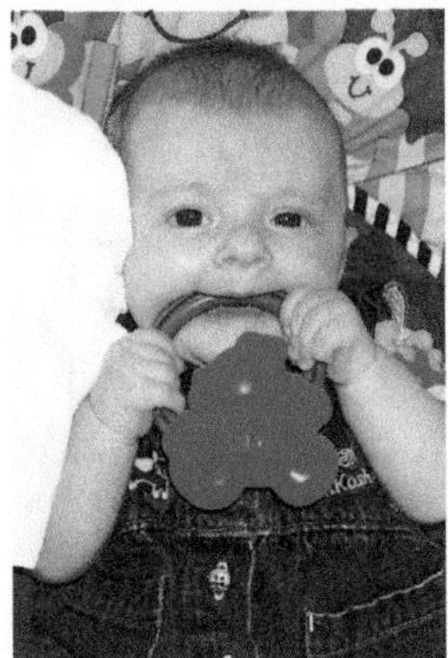

The 3-month-old will put hands or toys to their mouth.

Care and Guidance

Diet: Breastmilk or formula.

Exercise: May have short play period. Enjoys playing with hands.

Social Behaviour

Cries less. Can wait a few minutes for attention. Enjoys having people talk to them. Takes impromptu naps.

4 MONTHS

Physical Development

Drooling indicates appearance of saliva and beginning of teething. Lifts head and shoulders when on abdomen and looks around. Turns from back to side. Sits with support. Begins to reach for objects they see. Coordination between eye and body movements. Moves head, arms, and shoulders when excited. Extends legs and partly sustains weight when held upright. Rooting, Moro, extrusion, and tonic neck reflexes are no longer present.

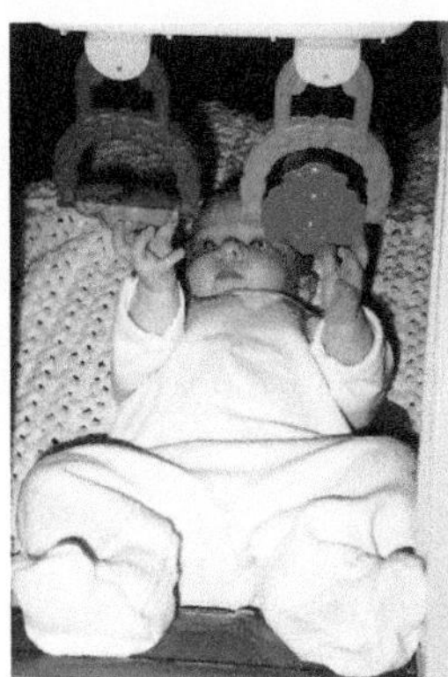

Visual stimulation is important to the growing infant.

Care and Guidance

Sleep: Stirs about in crib. Sleeps through ordinary household noises.

Diet: Breastmilk or formula.

Exercise: Plays with hand rattles and dangling toys. Place where infant can roll with safety.

Immunization: Second DTaP, IPV, and Hib (see Chapter 32).

Elimination: One or two bowel movements per day. May skip several days if breastfed.

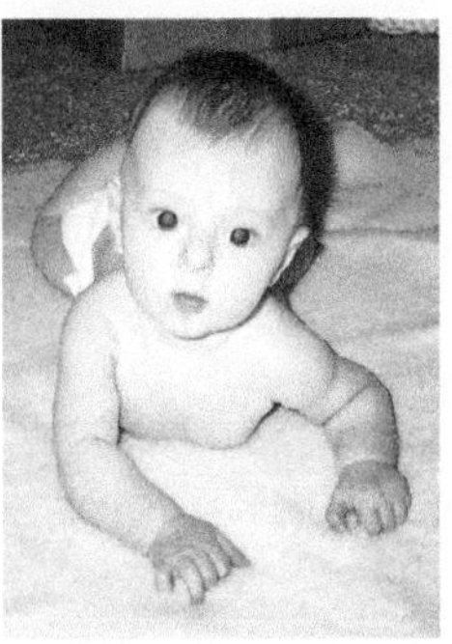

While on the abdomen the 4-month-old can lift the head and shoulders and look around.

5 MONTHS

Physical Development

Sits with support. Holds head well. Grasps objects offered. Puts everything into mouth. Plays with toes.

Social Behaviour

Talks to self. Seems to know whether persons are familiar or unfamiliar. May try to hold bottle if bottle fed.

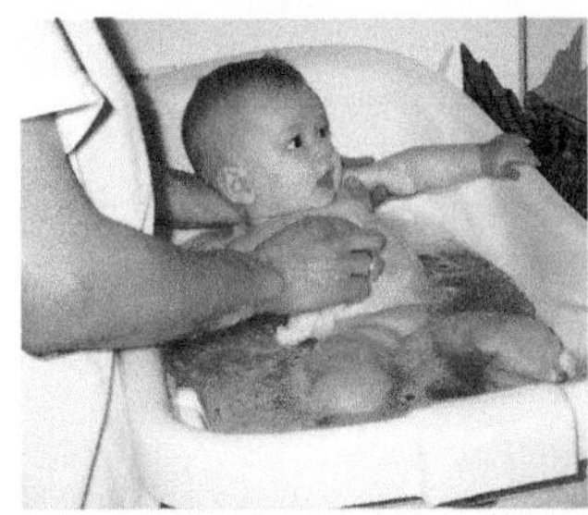

At 5 months the infant enjoys the bath. Firm head and shoulder support is essential for safety.

Care and Guidance

Sleep: Takes two or three naps daily.

Diet: Breastmilk or formula.

Exercise: Provide space to pivot around. Makes jumping motions when held upright in lap.

Safety: Check toys for loose buttons and rough edges before letting child play with them.

6 MONTHS

Physical Development

Birth weight has at least doubled (average weight 7.0 kg). Gains about 85 to 140 g per week during the next 6 months. Length grows about 1.25 cm per month. Sits alone momentarily. Springs up and down when sitting. Turns completely over. Hitches (moves backward when sitting). Bangs table with rattle. Pulls to a sitting position. Chewing is more mature. First solid food is introduced. Approximates lips to rim of cup.

Continued

Box 14.1 Physical Development, Social Behaviour, and Care and Guidance of Infants—cont'd

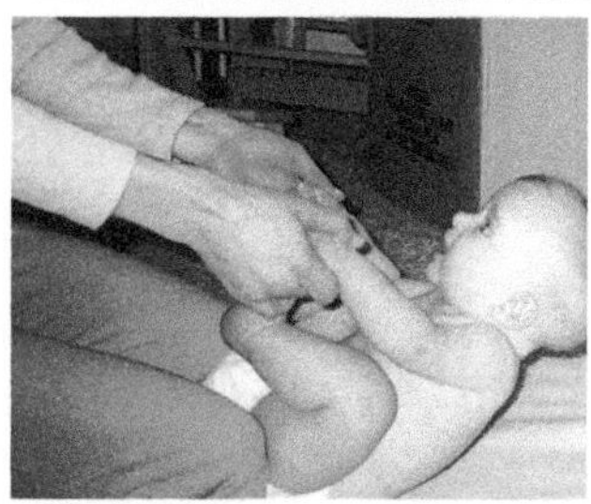

The infant can pull to a sitting position without head lag at 6 months.

Social Behaviour

Cries loudly when interrupted from play. Increased interest in world. Babbles and squeals. Sucks food from spoon. Awakens happy.

Care and Guidance

Diet: Introduced to first complementary food: First solids should be iron-rich meat, meat alternatives, and iron-fortified cereal.

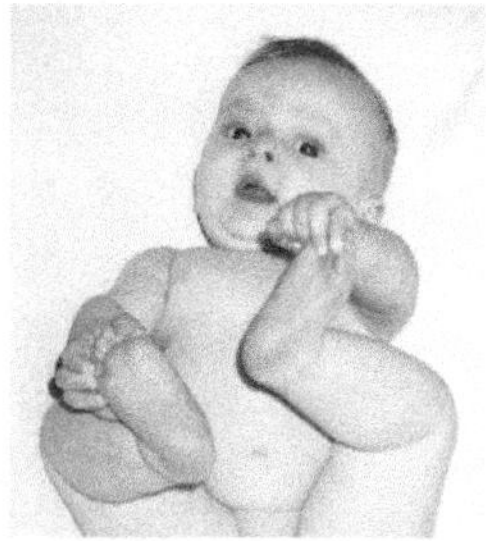

A 6-month-old discovers and plays with their feet.

7 MONTHS

Physical Development

Two lower teeth may appear (between 6 and 10 months). These are the first of the deciduous teeth—the central incisors. Can grasp objects more easily. Transfers objects from one hand to the other. Bears full weight on feet when held standing. Holds an adult's hands and bounces actively while standing. Struggles when being dressed.

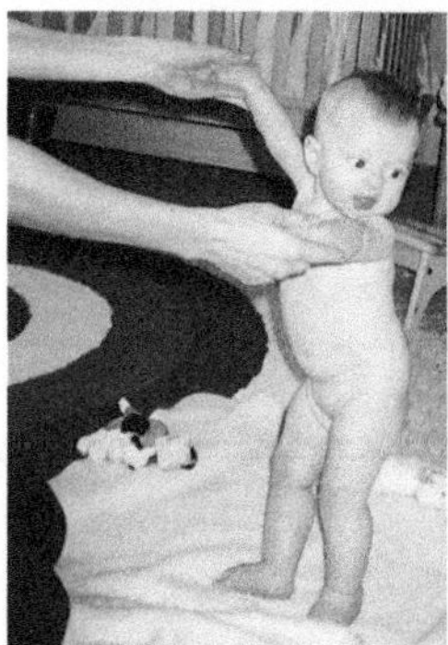

The infant enjoys standing position with assistance for a brief period.

Social Behaviour

Shifts moods easily—crying one minute, laughing the next. Shows fear of strangers. Anticipates spoon-feeding. Sleeps 14 hours per day with one to two naps.

Care and Guidance

Sleep: Fretfulness caused by teething may appear. This is generally evidenced by lack of appetite and wakefulness during the night.

Diet: Add finger foods, such as toast or cheese.

Exercise: Primitive locomotion.

8 MONTHS

Physical Development

Sits steadily alone. Uses index finger and thumb as pincers. Pokes at objects. Enjoys dropping article into a cup and emptying it. Begins to crawl. Moves forward, using chest, head, and arms; legs drag.

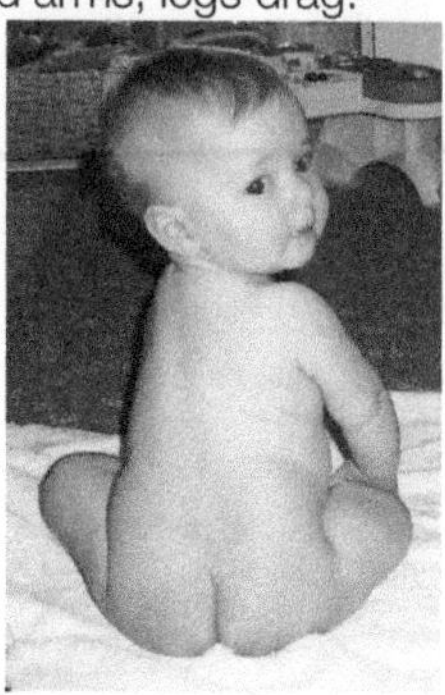

At 8 months, the infant is able to sit steady with back straight.

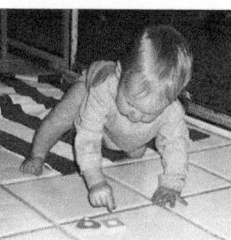

The pincer action is developed, and the infant can pick up small objects between the thumb and forefinger.

Social Behaviour

Plays pat-a-cake. Enjoys family life. Amuses self longer. Reserved with strangers. Indicates need for sleep by fussing and sucking thumb. Impatient especially when food is being prepared.

Care and Guidance

Sleep: Takes two naps a day.

Diet: Continue to introduce new foods with a variety of textures.

Exercise: Enjoys jump chair. Rides in stroller. Stuffed toys or those that squeak or rattle are appropriate.

Safety: Remain with infant at all times during bath in tub. Protect from chewing paint from windowsills or old furniture. Paint containing lead can be poisonous. Use safety-lock doors to ovens, dishwashers, washing machines, dryers, and refrigerators.

Box 14.1 Physical Development, Social Behaviour, and Care and Guidance of Infants—cont'd

9 MONTHS

Physical Development

Can raise self to a sitting position. Holds bottle. Creeps (carries trunk of body above floor but parallel to it; more advanced than crawling). When standing, may move while holding on to furniture (cruise).

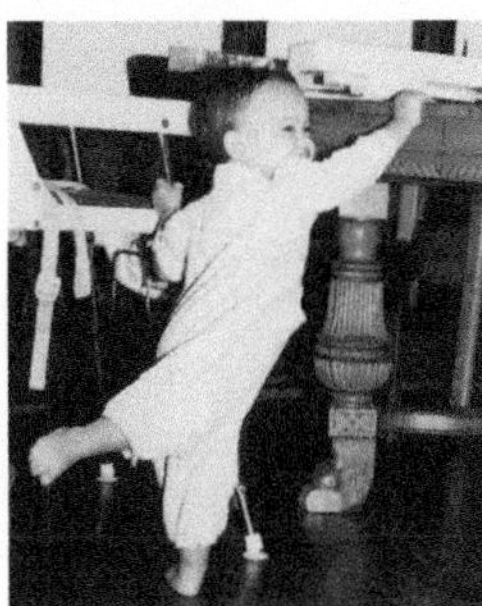

Infant cruises on furniture. Be sure it is stable!

Care and Guidance

Sleep: Has generally begun to sleep longer at night.

Diet: Should have a diet of various foods but still considered complementary to breastmilk or formula. Continue to add new foods to diet with a variety of textures. Allow infant to pick up pieces of food by hand and put them into mouth.

Safety: Know phone number of nearest poison control centre. Avoid using tablecloths with overhangs that infant could reach.

Exercise: Is busy most of the day exploring surroundings. Provide sufficient room and materials for safe play. Help infant to learn. Distract curious child from danger.

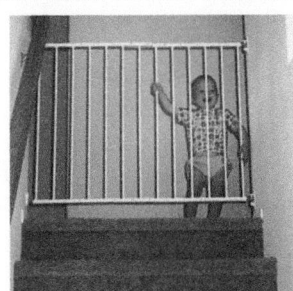

Stairway gates prevent falls. (Courtesy Pat Spier, RN-C.)

10 MONTHS

Physical Development

Pulls to a standing position. Throws toys to floor for parent to pick up. Cries when they are not returned. Walks around furniture while holding on to it.

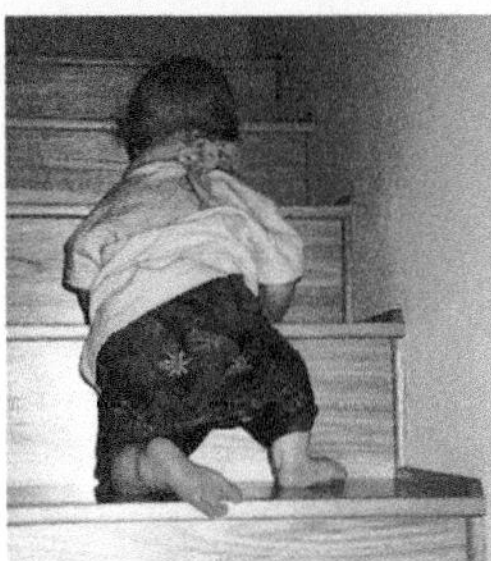

Infant is able to climb steps but needs supervision. (Courtesy Pat Spier, RN-C.)

Social Behaviour

Knows name. Plays simple games such as peek-a-boo. Feeds self a cookie. May cry out in sleep without waking.

Care and Guidance

Sleep: Avoid strenuous play before bedtime.

Diet: Takes water from cup. In general, solid foods are taken well.

Exercise: Tours around room holding adult's hands. Daytime clothing should be loose so as not to interfere with movement.

11 MONTHS

Physical Development

Stands upright holding on to an adult's hand.

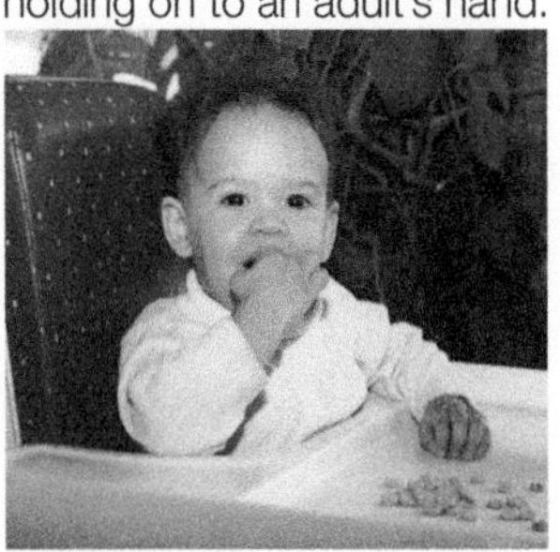

The 11-month-old can feed herself finger foods and drink from a "sippy cup."

Social Behaviour

Understands simple directions. Impatient when held. Enjoys playing with empty dish and spoon after meals.

Care and Guidance

Sleep: Greets parents in morning with excited jargon.

Diet: Still spills from cup. Enjoys blowing bubbles.

Exercise: Plays with toys in tub. Enjoys gross motor activity. Kicks, pulls self up.

Safety: Cover electrical outlets. Put household cleaners and medicines out of reach if not previously done.

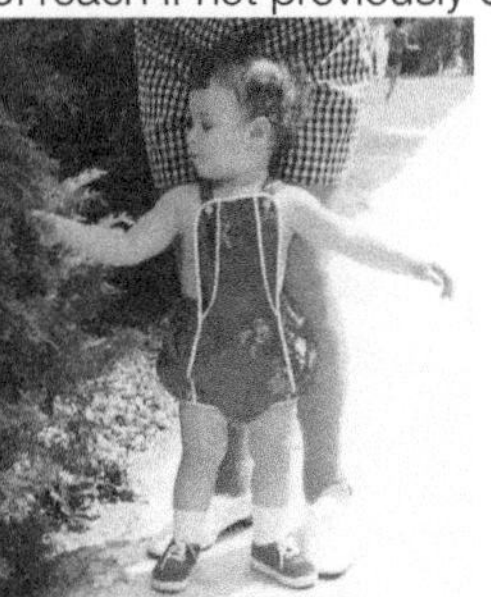

The 11-month-old is alert to surroundings and touches the leaves.

12 MONTHS

Physical Development

Triples birth weight (average 9.75 kg). Average height is about 74 cm. Stands alone for short periods. May walk. Puts arm through sleeve as an aid to being dressed. Six teeth (four above and two below). Drinks from a cup; eats with a spoon with supervision. Pincer grasp is well established. Handedness (the preference for the use of one hand), although not fully established, may be evidenced.

Continued

Box 14.1 Physical Development, Social Behaviour, and Care and Guidance of Infants—cont'd

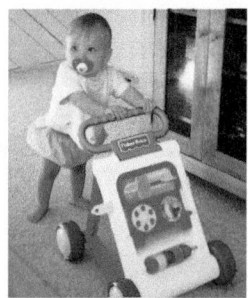

At 12 months the infant can stand alone and walk with assistance.

Social Behaviour

Friendly. Repeats acts that elicit a response. Recognizes "no-no." Verbalization slows because of increased concentration about ambulation. Enjoys rhythmic music. Shows emotions such as fear, anger, and jealousy. Reacts to these emotions from adults. Plays with food and removes it from mouth.

Care and Guidance

Sleep: May take one long nap daily.

Diet: Eating all food. Should have a regular schedule of meals and snacks.

Exercise: Enjoys putting objects in a basket and then removing them. Places objects on head. Distraction is an effective way to handle the infant's determination to do what they want regardless of outcome.

These services are provided in a variety of health care facilities. Ideally, the infant is seen by a health care provider at least five times during the first year, after the first month, and then at specific intervals (2 months, 4 months, 6 months, 9 months, and 1 year).

These visits are as important for the parents as they are for the infant. They provide caregiver support and reassurance as well as information and anticipatory guidance for the many developmental changes and health issues of the infant's first year. More serious physical or psychological concerns can be discussed with the health care provider and referral offered as appropriate.

A careful health history is obtained during routine clinic visits. Growth charts during infancy include measures of weight, length, and head circumference. The reading and recording of growth charts is described in Chapter 13. There are numerous developmental screening tests. Most pediatric health care providers initiate their assessment at birth to enable early intervention when needed. General screening tools are available to identify children in need of referral and further care.

Routine assessment of hearing is completed soon after birth in most provinces and territories (see Chapter 11 for more discussion of newborn hearing assessment). Vision is also an integral part of the examination. The Canadian Paediatric Society (CPS) recommends that eyes be assessed from birth. Initially assessment of the structures of the eye and red reflex are done between 1 and 3 months. Between 6 and 12 months the eyes should be checked for strabismus; corneal light reflex and fixation on a target are also assessed (Amit, & CPS Community Paediatrics Committee, 2009/2018). Laboratory tests may include urinalysis and measurement of hemoglobin or hematocrit levels to detect anemia, but only if determined to be necessary.

COMMUNITY CARE

The prevention of disease during infancy is important and involves a variety of health providers from different disciplines as well as resources within the community. There are many community resources for the health promotion of infants, including the following:

- The Canada Prenatal Nutrition Program (CPNP) is a community-based program that provides support to pregnant women, new mothers, and babies facing challenging life circumstances. The goals of CPNP are to improve maternal–infant health, increase the rates of healthy birth weights, and promote and support breastfeeding mothers.
- The Aboriginal Head Start on Reserve Program (AHSOR) is funded by the federal government and provides activities that support early intervention strategies to address the learning and developmental needs of young children living in Indigenous communities. The program is centred around six components: education; health promotion; culture and language; nutrition; social support; and parental and family involvement.
- Public health departments and hospital clinics provide follow-up care.

A prime responsibility of the nurse in the community-based clinic is to guide the parents and assist in the development of the skills necessary to ensure the proper growth and development of their child. The nurse can provide encouragement and explanations of strategies that will enable parents to be successful in coping with various infant behaviours.

The nurse is the important link in the initiation of referral to the multidisciplinary health care team, follow-up of progress, and maintenance of communication between the family and members of the health care team. Some new parents may have difficulty parenting, which is often due to circumstances of their own lives, such as socioeconomic factors or physical and emotional problems. Nurses need to provide support to families to enhance child development and work with the families to identify their strengths and resources. A social worker and community health nurse are valuable links to community-based care resources.

SPECIFIC CONCERNS OF PARENTS

Diaper Rash

A common concern is diaper rash, which can cause discomfort to the infant. The parents should be taught the importance of frequent diaper changes, how to wipe from front to back, and the importance of exposing the skin in the diaper area to the air for periods of time. Some commercial diaper wipes may contain fragrance or other ingredients that can further irritate a diaper rash. Soiled areas can be washed with water and mild soap if needed. To prevent skin breakdown, unscented barrier ointments such as petroleum jelly or a cream with zinc oxide can be applied when the skin in the diaper area appears reddened and irritated.

Coping With the Irritable Infant

One of the goals of early parent–infant interaction is that the infant be able to respond to their parents and the environment. Success in this area promotes a feeling of competence in the parent, which can ultimately enhance parenting skills. Some infants cannot tolerate environmental stimulation and handling and start to cry during diaper changes, feeding, and rocking. Lights, sound, and movement cause some infants to become irritable. Techniques that nurses can teach parents to cope with these problems include the following:

- Shield the infant's eyes from bright light.
- Sit quietly with the infant without talking or singing.
- Eliminate noise from radio, television, and computer.
- Talk in a soft voice.
- Change the infant's position slowly.
- Recognize and respond to pre-cry cues in a calm manner.
- Stop the interaction and reduce environmental stimuli if the infant turns away, squirms, grimaces, or puts their hands in front of their face.
- Place the infant skin-to-skin.
- Swaddle the infant snugly in a lightweight blanket with extremities flexed and hands near the face.
- Provide non-nutritive sucking.
- Rock the infant slowly and gently.
- Avoid sudden movements.

The nurse should reassure parents that an infants' irritability is normal and transient and usually resolves by 3 months (Feigelman, 2016).

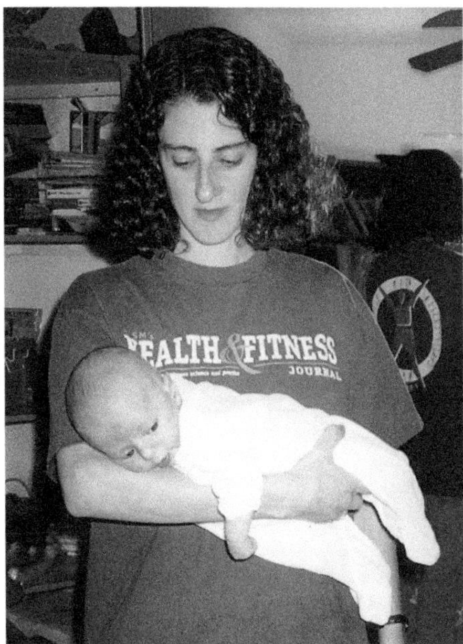

Fig. 14.4 The colic carry.

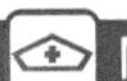 **Nursing Tip**

An infant's repetitious banging of toys on a table may be perceived by the parent as an irritating type of behaviour. Parents should be taught that this is a normal developmental phase of motor activity and should be encouraged!

Coping With Colic

Colic is characterized by periods of unexplained irritability and crying in a healthy, well-fed infant. The condition is generally described as paroxysmal abdominal pain or cramping that is manifested by loud crying and drawing the legs up to the abdomen. Other definitions include variables such as duration of cry greater than 3 hours a day, occurring more than 3 days per week, and parental dissatisfaction with the child's behaviour (Breen-Reid, 2017). Although the exact cause is unknown, it is thought to be a combination of the infant feeding too rapidly, swallowing air, having a cow's milk allergy, disrupted sleep patterns, or emotional tension between child and parent (Breen-Reid, 2017). The treatment probably involves a combination of interventions given that there can be many causes for colic.

Colic can interfere with parent–infant interactions if the infant is not soothed by being held or carried, and parental fatigue and guilt can develop. Supporting parents as they cope with a colicky infant is important; they should be encouraged to get periods of rest and take breaks to decrease parental frustration. The colic carry (Fig. 14.4) is a position that can be used for infants when they are irritable, because the carry typically confers a calming effect. Holding the infant face down and close to the body while supporting the abdomen and providing a gentle rocking motion of the pelvis often soothes the colicky infant.

Nursing Care Plan 14.1 The Family Care Plan When the Infant Has Colic

PATIENT DATA

The parents of a 3-week-old infant state that they feel inadequate as parents because their infant is often fussy and irritable and does not respond to their efforts to calm him. They ask what they are doing wrong.

Selected Nursing Diagnosis Family stress as a result of a fussy infant

Goals	Nursing Interventions	Rationales
Parents will demonstrate increased coping behaviours by 1 week. Parents will verbalize feelings of increased confidence in caring for the infant.	Educate parents about common manifestations of colic.	No single cause has been established for colic. Infant appears otherwise healthy but demonstrates cramp-like pain, drawing legs to abdomen and producing irritable cry. It is time-limited to about 3 months.
	Determine whether health care provider has ruled out other causes.	Intestinal obstruction and infection may mimic symptoms of colic. Bowel movements are not abnormal with colic.
	Identify soothing measures used by parents and their effectiveness.	Environment may be overstimulating infant; parents may not know how to soothe the infant.
	Teach about the following interventions: abdominal massage, wind-up swing for short periods, and car rides, give smaller, more frequent feeds, avoid exposure to secondhand smoke.	These measures may help to relieve symptoms; burping before and after feedings and placing infant in an upright position after feedings may also decrease distress.
	Demonstrate "colic carry" (see Fig. 14.4).	Position may comfort infant by applying a little extra pressure on abdomen.
	Suggest periods of free time for parents.	Constant crying by infants produces a great deal of frustration in family members; caution against shaking infant, which can be harmful to the head and neck.
	Emphasize that colic is not a reflection on parenting skills.	First-time parents may feel anxious and incompetent. Nurse provides reassurance and support and builds on their strengths.

For a small number of infants colic is due to cow's milk allergy. For these infants a maternal hypoallergenic diet for breastfed infants and an extensively hydrolyzed formula for bottle-fed infants may result in resolution of colic (Critch & CPS Nutrition and Gastroenterology Committee, 2011/2018). See Nursing Care Plan 14.1 for care of the infant with colic.

Infants With Special Needs

All parents should be taught about normal growth and development and anticipated milestones for their children. When special needs are recognized, early intervention is essential to attain the best outcome.

Infants with special needs may require referral to community agencies for follow-up care. Specialized early childhood education programs can offer parents guidance concerning growth and development through infant stimulation programs. A psychologist can provide counselling, behaviour management techniques, and cognitive therapy. Neurodevelopmental therapy can be provided by a professional therapist or by an occupational therapist or physiotherapist. Speech therapy and auditory testing are also available within the community. The social worker can assist with social and environmental problems.

HEALTHY SLEEP PATTERNS

Most newborns sleep up to 18 hours a day for 2 to 4 hours at a time and wake up during the night to feed. By age 4 months babies sleep an average of 14 hours a day and usually nap three times a day. The number of naps decreases sometime between 6 and 12 months to two naps a day. Sometimes parents state that their baby does not sleep enough, which can indicate that they lack information about normal infant sleep patterns. There are a few things parents can do to encourage infants to learn to sleep at night and be awake during the day (CPS, 2017):

- Maintain a regular daytime and bedtime sleep schedule as much as possible.
- Provide a consistent bedtime routine. Many parents like to use the "3 Bs": bath, book, bed.
- Put the baby to bed without a bottle (bottle feeding in bed can lead to tooth decay).
- After 6 months, if the baby wakes at night and cries, parents should be encouraged to go and check to see if anything is wrong, such as being too cold or too warm, but not to take the child out of the crib. Comforting the infant by stroking the forehead or talking softly may help the infant learn how to self-soothe, an important step toward falling back to sleep on their own.

Helping the infant to achieve the ability to go back to sleep on their own will also make parents feel more confident in their parenting skills and less fatigued and frustrated. The Caring for Kids website from the Canadian Paediatric Society and Public Health Agency of Canada offer valuable information regarding healthy sleep patterns (see Online Resources at the end of this chapter).

Infants should be positioned for sleep on their backs on a firm, flat mattress in a crib, both for their safety and to lessen the risk of sudden infant death syndrome (SIDS). Overheating should be avoided. It is recommended that nothing be put into the crib, such as blankets, bumper pads, and stuffed animals. The use of pacifiers during sleep has a protective effect on preventing SIDS but is not recommended until breastfeeding is well established (Hunt & Hauck, 2016). Infants under 6 months should share a room with parents but not share the bed. See Chapter 11 (Prevention of Sudden Infant Death Syndrome) for more information.

When placing an infant in a car seat, care should be taken that the infant's chin does not rest on their chest as this can cause oxygen desaturation and hypoxia. For this reason, car seats should not be used as a prolonged sleeping arrangement for infants (Hagan & Duncan, 2016; Narvey & CPS Fetus and Newborn Committee, 2016).

Newborns must be put in the prone position at least daily for "tummy time." This should be done when the infant is awake and supervised. Tummy time will prevent plagiocephaly (flattening of head) and facilitates development of upper shoulder girdle strength. Babies should also have their position alternated in the crib so they can have the opportunity to move their head to different sides.

Safety Alert!

The Public Health Agency of Canada, Canadian Paediatric Society, Canadian Foundation for Study of Infant Deaths, Canadian Institute for Child Health, and Health Canada (2018) recommend a supine or back-lying position on a firm mattress for infants to avoid occurrence of sudden infant death syndrome (SIDS). Pillows, bumper pads, blankets, and stuffed animals should not be put into cribs.

IMMUNIZATIONS

Immunization schedules differ slightly between the provinces and territories, so it is important for nurses to aware of the schedule for their specific province. See the Government of Canada link at the end of the chapter for the provincial and territorial routines. Health personnel should stress to parents the importance of immunizations. A delay can lead to undue risks of serious illness, sometimes with fatal complications.

The nurse can teach working parents that an unprotected child may become sick, making it necessary for them to lose valuable working hours. Immunizations are also required before school entry. A delay or interruption in a series does not interfere with final immunity. It is not necessary to restart any series, regardless of the length of delay. Accurate records prevent confusion regarding immunizations. See Chapter 32 for a detailed discussion of immunizations and common childhood communicable diseases.

NUTRITION COUNSELLING

The nutritional needs of infants reflect rates of growth, energy expended in activity, basal metabolic needs, and the interaction of nutrients consumed (Mahan & Raymond, 2017). The infant is born with a rooting reflex, which aids in finding the nipple for breastfeeding. The sucking reflex is present at birth, with a forward and backward movement of the tongue. As the infant grows, neuromaturation of the cheeks and tongue enables advancement to a more mature sucking pattern that uses negative pressure to obtain milk. At about the third to fourth month, the **extrusion reflex** (protrusion of the tongue), which pushes food out of the mouth to prevent intake of inappropriate food, disappears.

The digestive system then continues to mature. By 6 months, it can handle more complex nutrients and is less susceptible to food allergens. The stomach capacity expands from 5 to 20 mL at birth to 200 mL by 12 months. This expansion enables the infant to consume more food at less frequent intervals. As the pincer grasp becomes more developed, the infant can pick up food with tiny fingers and place it in the mouth.

Taste cells develop during the eighth week of gestation, and the fetus begins to respond to flavours when swallowing amniotic fluid. At birth, the infant demonstrates a preference for certain tastes, preferring sweet and rejecting sour. Breastmilk may supply flavour experiences based on the mother's diet. Infants should be given an opportunity to develop their own personal tastes by being offered various foods when solids are introduced.

Parental Concerns

During the first year of the infant's life, parents have many concerns about feeding their infant. This is a period when readiness to receive nutrition education is usually high; therefore, the nurse should look for opportunities to provide accurate information. The nurse should assess parental knowledge; infant development, behaviour, and readiness; parent–child interactions; and cultural and ethnic practices. Teaching can focus on developmental levels and assisting parents in recognizing changes in feeding patterns. The components of a nutritional assessment are discussed in Chapter 13.

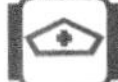 **Nursing Tip**

Human breast milk supplies adequate fluid and nutrition for the first 6 months of an infant's life.

Table 14.1 Common Milk Preparations for the First Year

MILK PREPARATION	ADVANTAGES	DISADVANTAGES
Human breastmilk	No preparation needed; nonallergenic; provides antibodies	No disadvantages
Prepared, ready-to-feed formula	No preparation needed; no refrigeration needed before opening bottle	Expensive. Not equivalent to breastmilk for nutritional value
Formula concentrate	Easy to prepare; can prepare one bottle at a time or a maximum of one day's feeding at a time	Must be refrigerated after preparation; open cans of formula must be covered and refrigerated immediately after opening. Must use accurate proportions; safe water supply necessary to dilute concentrate (water from a natural well may have a high nitrate concentration). Less expensive
Powdered formula	Least expensive formula; lasts up to 1 month after opening	Necessitates accurate measurement; requires safe water supply and must be shaken thoroughly to dissolve powder; powder is not sterile and has been linked to outbreaks in high-risk infants (not recommended for preterm infants)

A suggested parental guide to determine adequacy of the infant's diet includes the following:

- The infant has gained 140 to 200 g per week for the first 6 months.
- The infant has at least six wet diapers per day.
- The infant sleeps after feedings (how long the infant sleeps depends on the age of the infant).

Monitoring of weight, height, and head circumference determines if the diet is adequate; therefore, the value of periodic well-baby examinations should be stressed. Breastfed and formula-fed infants are fed on demand, although formula-fed babies usually have longer intervals between feedings because breastmilk is more easily digested. A flexible schedule that provides a rest period between feedings is best for the parent and the infant. The nurse should reassure parents that most children eat enough to grow normally, although intake is seldom constant and varies in quantity and quality. Forced feedings are not appropriate.

Infant Feeding

In proportion to their weight, infants require more calories, protein, minerals, and vitamins than adults. Their fluid requirements are also high. Exclusive breastfeeding is recommended for the first 6 months and is sustained for up to 2 years or longer with appropriate complementary feeding (Health Canada, CPS, Dietitians of Canada, and Breastfeeding Committee for Canada, 2015a). Infants who are breastfed longer than 6 months gain less weight by age 1 year than bottle-fed infants and are less apt to be obese in later life.

Breastfeeding is the normal and unequalled method of feeding infants. Human milk contains the ideal balance of nutrients in a readily digestible form. Breastfeeding soon after birth helps to promote bonding and stimulates milk production. Breastmilk has immunological properties that help to protect the infant from certain microorganisms, and allergic reactions are minimal. The only recognized contraindications to breastfeeding in the newborn are galactosemia or certain inborn errors of metabolism (such as phenylketonuria [PKU]). Maternal contraindications are a positive human immunodeficiency virus (HIV) status; herpes lesions on both breasts; active, untreated infectious pulmonary tuberculosis (TB); or a severe illness that prevents the mother from caring for her infant. Most medications are compatible with breastfeeding, although some medications, such as antimetabolites, chemotherapeutic agents, and radioactive isotope therapies, can cross over to the infant, and if substitutes cannot be found, a mother may need to at least temporarily avoid breastfeeding. Women should be cautioned against using illicit drugs and given support to abstain from use during pregnancy and breastfeeding. Illicit drugs can have harmful effects on breastfed infants and impair the mother's ability to care for her infant. If the mother is unable to stop use or chooses not to stop illicit drug use, she should be advised of the importance of breastfeeding and the risks the drug use poses, based on her circumstances (Health Canada, CPS, Dietitians of Canada, and Breastfeeding Committee for Canada, 2015a). Breastfeeding is discussed in Chapter 9.

Breastmilk

The foremilk at the beginning of a breastfeeding is thin and has a high lactose content that relieves the infant's thirst, then changes to a thicker form that contains more fat for satiety. To support optimal growth, the balance of nutrients in breastmilk changes during feedings and over time as the infant matures (Health Canada et al., 2015a).

Formula feeding

If parents make the informed decision to formula feed or must do so due to medical reasons, there are different options of commercially prepared infant formulas available (Table 14.1). Iron-fortified formulas are recommended until the child has an adequate iron intake in diet. Whole cow's milk or goat's milk is not recommended for infants because they are low in iron, essential fatty acids, and other essential nutrients; contain a less-digestible form of protein; and have a high renal solute load (Health Canada et al., 2015b).

Table 14.2 Development of Mealtime Behaviour and Implications for Caregivers

AGE	HUNGER BEHAVIOUR	COMMUNICATION	FEEDING BEHAVIOUR	SATIETY	PARENTAL GUIDANCE
Birth to 3 months	Cries; hands fisted; body tense	Roots in search of nipple	Strong suck reflex; needs to be burped	Falls asleep when full; hands relaxed; body relaxed; withdraws head from nipple	Burp frequently. Avoid overfeeding or underfeeding. Recognize signs of satiety.
3–5 months	Grasps and draws breast/bottle to mouth; tongue protrudes in anticipation of nipple; fusses; mouths hands	Reaches with open mouth to receive nipple	Strong suck; holds nipple firmly; preference for tastes; pats breast/bottle	Tosses head back; ejects nipple; distracted easily by surroundings; plays with nipple	Provide consistent eating routine.
6–9 months	Reacts to food preparation; reaches for breast/bottle	Vocalizes hunger; pulls spoon to mouth; holds bottle	Picks up small food with raking, then pincer action; draws food from spoon with lips; chewing begins	Changes posture; closes mouth; plays with utensils; shakes head "no"	Offer foods with a variety of textures. Finger foods should also be offered.
10–12 months	Vocalizes; grasps utensils; fussy	Feeds self; purses lips to cup's edge; can drink from open cup	Skilled pincer action to pick up pieces of food and place in mouth; drinks from cup; chews food	Shakes head "no"; sputters food; throws food to floor	Allow infant to assist with feeding. Offer liquids (water) in open cup. Avoid foods that can be aspirated.

Note: Parents who are alert to their infant's communication of hunger and satiety help the infant develop self-regulation and communication skills.

Parents are sometimes unsure of how much formula the infant needs at each feeding or when their infant has had enough formula. It is important to explain satiety (hunger satisfaction) behaviour at the various ages (Table 14.2). Coaxing infants to finish the last drop in a bottle is unnecessary.

Types of infant formula. It is not possible to produce an infant formula to be exactly like breastmilk, although the manufacture of commercial infant formula is highly regulated to meet national quality criteria. Any new ingredient change is monitored by Health Canada. There are many options for breastmilk substitutes; Health Canada et al. (2015a) have made the following recommendations:

- Use cow milk–based commercial infant formula for an infant who is not exclusively fed breastmilk. Soy-based infant formula is indicated only for those infants who have galactosemia or who cannot consume dairy-based products for cultural or religious reasons.
- Use infant formulas for special medical purposes only when it is suspected or determined that the formula-fed infant has the indicated condition.
- Use of homemade, evaporated milk formula is discouraged. Cow milk, goat milk, soy beverage, rice beverage, or any other beverages should not be given to young infants.
- Use proper preparation and storage to reduce the risk of bacteria-related illness.

The nurse must know the difference between various commercial formulas. Feeding an infant the wrong infant formula is considered a medication error and must be reported according to facility policy. The clinical decision about which formula is best for a specific infant should be made in partnership between the health care provider and the parent.

Safe bottle feeding. The nurse should teach parents the basic principles of safe bottle feeding to prevent problems that can result in illness or injury:

- Nurses should warn parents of the risk of an infant choking when left alone while feeding and should explain the dangers of propping a bottle.
- Always check the expiration date on the formula container; do not buy formula that has expired.
- Clean kitchen surfaces and wash hands thoroughly with soap and warm water.
- Thoroughly wash bottles, nipples, caps, tongs, measuring cups, or other containers.
- Sterilize the washed equipment by boiling in an open pot of clean water for 2 minutes and allow to air dry and cool (Government of Canada, 2012).

- Wash top of can with detergent and hot water before opening it.
- Use a clean can opener to open can and wash it between uses. Check the can opener for food or rust spots before using it again.
- Avoid cross-contamination from other foods prepared in the kitchen.
- Follow the product directions precisely when mixing formula.
- Heat bottle of formula by placing the bottle in a bottle warmer or hot water for no more than 15 minutes until it is between room and body temperature (depending on preference of infant).
- Test formula temperature by shaking a few drops on the inner wrist, not just feeling the bottle.
- Do not heat bottle in a microwave oven; the liquid often warms unevenly unless stirred. The container may remain cool, while the formula inside is hot enough to burn the newborn.
- Keep prepared bottles of formula refrigerated until ready to use.
- Opened containers of liquid formula should be tightly covered and stored in the refrigerator for no longer than is designated on the label.
- After a formula can is opened or a formula is mixed, use it right away or refrigerate it, because bacteria multiply rapidly at warm temperatures.
- Carry filled bottles away from home in an insulated bag or cooler with ice packs inside.
- Infant formula should be used within 2 hours from the start of a feeding and any leftovers should be discarded. Microorganisms will grow, and the newborn can develop diarrhea (infection).
- Note that older hard, clear plastic bottles made of polycarbonate may contain bisphenol A (BPA). Plastic bottles with the number 7 stamped inside a triangle on the bottom of the bottle do contain BPA.

Further information on formula feeding is in Chapter 9.

Nursing Tip

Whole cow's milk should not be given to infants until 9 to 12 months of age. Low-fat milk should not be given to infants under 2 years of age. Milk intake should be limited to no more than 750 mL per day

Adding Solid Foods

Parents often wonder when to begin adding solid foods. The addition of complementary solid food at 6 months is recommended because breastmilk or formula may not offer all of the nutrition the older infant needs at this point in life. Complementary foods should be energy dense and rich in nutrients such as iron (Health Canada et al., 2015b).

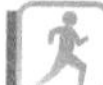

Health Promotion

Directions for Home Preparation of Infant Foods

- Select fresh, high-quality fruits, vegetables, and meats.
- Be sure all utensils, including cutting boards, grinder, and knives, are thoroughly clean.
- Wash hands before preparing the food.
- Clean, wash, and trim the food in as little water as possible.
- Cook the foods until tender in as little water as possible. Prevent overcooking, which may destroy heat-sensitive nutrients.
- Add little or no salt or sugar. Do not add honey to food for infants less than age 1 year. (Botulism spores have been reported in honey, and young infants do not have the immune capacity to resist this infection.)
- Strain or puree the food with an electric blender, food mill, baby food grinder, or kitchen strainer.
- Pour the food into an ice cube tray and freeze.
- When food is frozen hard, remove the cubes and store in freezer bags.
- In a serving container, unfreeze and heat (in water bath or microwave oven) the amount of food that will be consumed at a single feeding (Mahan & Raymond, 2017).

Around 6 months of age, sucking becomes more mature, and munching (up-and-down chopping motion) commences. Iron-rich food is introduced first (e.g., meat, meat alternatives, rice cereal). Fig. 14.5 illustrates how feeding skills develop in infants and toddlers.

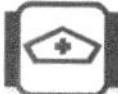

Nursing Tip

Cereal and baby food should *not* be mixed in a bottle with formula.

Aside from iron-rich foods being the first foods introduced, there is no particular order for the introduction of other foods or food groups (except cow's milk). Vegetables, fruit, and milk products such as cheese and yogurt can be introduced between 6 and 9 months, (Health Canada, 2015b). Only small amounts are offered at first (one to two teaspoonfuls). A small amount of food is placed on the back of the tongue. A different new solid can be introduced each day. If there is a family history of allergies, a new food that is allergenic can be offered every 2 days to determine if there is a reaction to that food. Cereal may be diluted with breastmilk, formula, or water. The consistency is thickened, and amounts of solid foods are gradually increased as the infant becomes more familiar with them. A small bowl and a spoon with a long, straight handle are suggested.

If the infant refuses a certain food, it should be temporarily omitted. Mealtime should be kept pleasant; it is ideal if the infant is fed during the family mealtime. The infant should be allowed to try new foods, even ones the parents dislike. The amount of food consumed varies with the child.

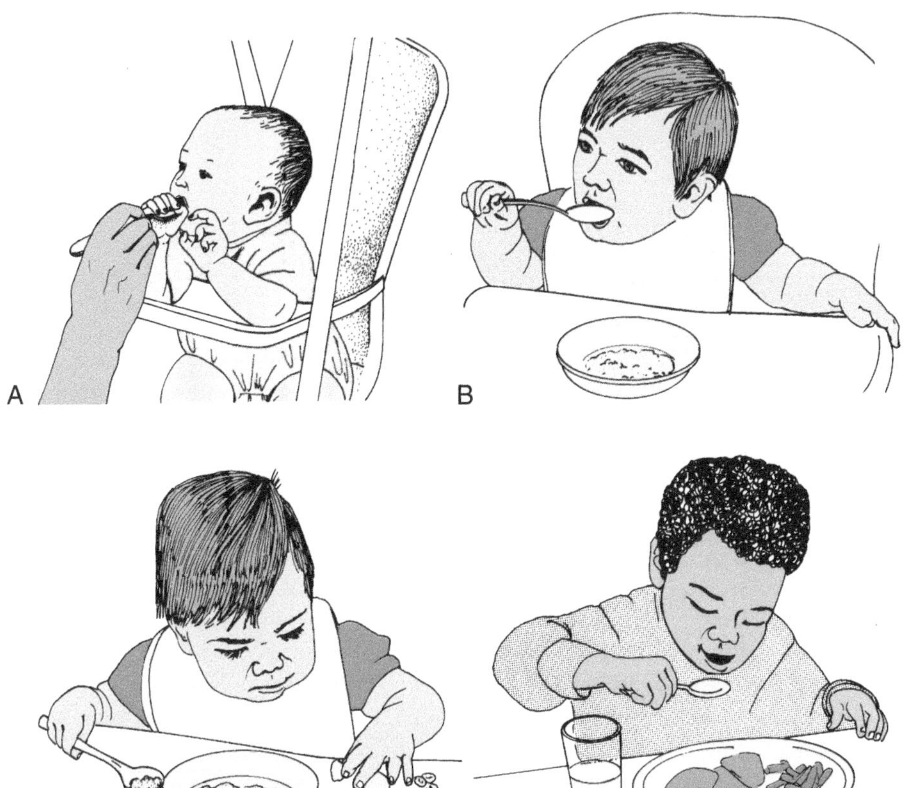

Fig. 14.5 Development of feeding skills in infants and toddlers. **A,** At 7 months, this child begins to reach for the spoon. **B,** At 9 months, the child begins to use a spoon independently, although they are not yet able to keep food on it. **C,** The 9-month-old shows a refined pincer grasp to pick up food. **D,** The 2-year-old is much more skilled at self-feeding and has the ability both to rotate the wrist and to elevate the elbow to keep food on the spoon. (Modified from Mahan, L. K. & Raymond, J. L. [2017]. *Krause's food and the nutrition process* [14th ed.]. Philadelphia: Elsevier.)

Fruit juices should be avoided until 2 years of age because drinking juice has been associated with dental decay. Juice fills up a child, and the child will not get the appropriate nutrients they need from solid food and breastmilk. It is important that parents and caregivers provide a variety of soft textures (such as lumpy, tender-cooked, and finely minced, pureed, mashed, or ground) and finger foods from 6 months of age. Safe finger foods include pieces of soft-cooked vegetables and fruits; soft, ripe fruit such as bananas; finely minced, ground, or mashed cooked meat, deboned fish, and poultry; grated cheese; and bread crusts or toast (Health Canada, 2015b). Foods that have a lumpy texture should be offered no later than 9 months of age. Infants need to be observed closely during meals in case they exhibit choking (Fig. 14.6).

When the infant is age 6 to 8 months, parents and caregivers should work toward offering complementary foods in two to three feedings and one to two snacks each day, depending on the infant's appetite. By age 9 months this should increase to three feedings a day with one to two snacks, depending, once again, on the infant's appetite. The frequency of feedings and the amount of food increase with age to accommodate higher energy requirements for development and growth (Health Canada et al., 2015b).

Sample menus are listed on the Health Canada website, found in the Online Resources at the end of the chapter.

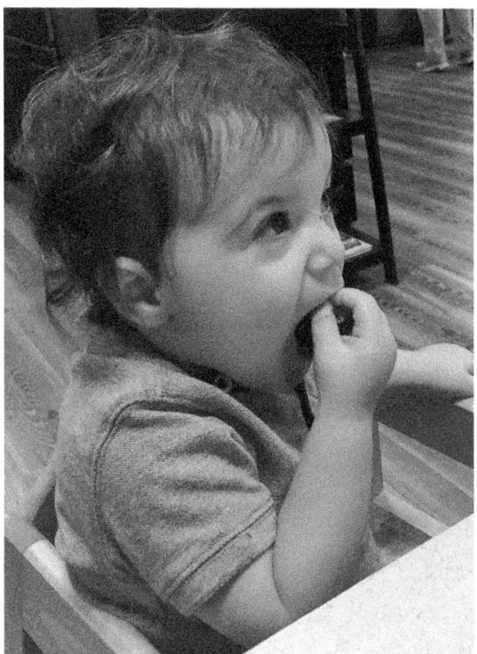

Fig. 14.6 When self-feeding starts, infants must be closely observed.

Nursing Tip

New solid foods should be introduced *after* the milk feedings to encourage the infant as solid foods are considered complementary to breastmilk or formula intake. Milk should be the major source of calories initially. The infant should decide how much they want to eat and not be forced to eat a specific quantity.

As liquids other than breastmilk or formula, such as water, are introduced, they should be offered in an open cup along with complementary foods. At first the child will need help with the cup from a caregiver, but they are able to learn to drink from a cup safely and easily. Encouraging use of an open cup for older infants can help avoid prolonged bottle-feeding (Health Canada et al., 2015b).

 Safety Alert!

To prevent development of botulism, honey should not be included in the diet of infants younger than 1 year.

Recommended Fat Intake During Infancy

Fat contains more calories than carbohydrates and proteins. Because infants have a limited stomach capacity and a high caloric need, fats in easily digestible forms are needed to meet their caloric needs for growth and development and for brain development. Infants have a high basal metabolic rate (BMR) and require almost three times more calories per kilogram of weight than adults do to maintain their rapid growth and development in the first year of life. In the young infant, breastmilk and infant formulas provide the necessary fats that the infant is able to digest. Feeding a low-fat diet to infants younger than 2 years will compromise their growth and development. There is no evidence that such restrictions provide any benefits during childhood. Nutritious foods that contain fat, such as breastmilk, homogenized (3.25% M.F.) cow's milk, cheese, avocado, and nut butters, provide a concentrated energy source during a life stage when requirements are particularly high. Similar to the advice in *Canada's Food Guide*, there is no need to restrict unsaturated fats such as vegetable oils, salad dressings, margarine, and mayonnaise during meal preparation for young children (Health Canada et al., 2015b).

The fat and cholesterol content may not be designated on the label of many baby foods. By age 6 months, amylase and lipase are present in the digestive tract to aid in digesting the fat present in solid foods. A well-balanced diet provides appropriate fat and cholesterol intake.

Buying, Storing, and Serving Foods

Commercial baby food is not recommended to given to infants because of high sugar and salt content. If used, parents should be taught to check safety seals before purchase. The expiration date of the product should be checked. Unopened jars of baby food and juices should be stored in a dry, cool place.

When a jar is opened, a definite "pop" is heard when the vacuum seal is broken. Food is then transferred to a serving dish. The infant should not be fed out of the jar, and leftovers should not be returned to the jar, because saliva may turn certain foods to liquid by digesting them in the jar. Unused portions may be stored in the refrigerator in the original jar. Special precautions should be taken when food is heated in the microwave because food sometimes heats unevenly.

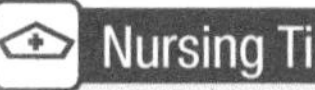

- Encourage breastfeeding.
- Discourage overfeeding.
- Teach recognition of satiety signs.
- Prevent early introduction of solid foods.

Weaning

Weaning is defined as substituting a cup for a bottle or breastfeeding. Because sucking is a major source of pleasure in the first year of life, weaning is a major step in growth and development. Signs of readiness to wean can be seen in the infant who eagerly looks forward to new tastes and textures. The approaching stage of autonomy provides the child with motivation to manipulate the cup. Imitation of older siblings or parents also contributes to readiness. Weaning should be very gradual and start with daytime feedings. Weaning is usually completed by 2 years of age but may continue longer for many children.

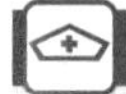 Nursing Tip

The nutritive value of the food and the nutritional needs of the infant should be the primary focus of food selection.

INFANT SAFETY

Car Safety

Infant seats should be used for all infants travelling in automobiles. A rear-facing infant seat should be used for infants until they weigh at least 10 kg. It is recommended they remain rear-facing as long as possible. They should not be in a forward-facing car seat until they are at least 12 months of age or have outgrown the rear-facing car seat. The car seat should be located in the centre of the rear seat of the automobile, if possible. Passenger-side safety air bags pose a danger to infants in infant seats that are placed in the front seat. The infant seat should be firmly anchored to the vehicle by the car seat belt (see Chapters 11 and 15). Infant car seats are not recommended for use other than for automobile safety.

Fall Prevention

An infant should never be left unattended on a flat surface, such as a changing table. Newborn infants have crawling reflexes that can cause them to fall off a changing table. Infants younger than 4 months have rounded backs and can accidentally roll off a flat surface. Infants older than 4 months can voluntarily roll over. In the hospital, crib rails should be raised and securely locked. Infants should be secured in high chairs or swings. An infant seat should not be placed on a table or high surface. Crawling infants should be protected from stairways, and neither heavy nor unsteady furniture should be available for them to use to pull themselves to a standing position. Given the increased risk of injuries, baby walkers are illegal in

Table 14.3 **Toys for the First Year**

AGE	VISUAL STIMULATION	AUDITORY STIMULATION	SENSORIMOTOR STIMULATION
0–2 months	Caregiver's face Black-and-white contrasting mobiles placed at midline of infant's vision	Talk Music Ticking clock	Cuddle, rock
3–5 months	Unbreakable mirrors Infant seat positioned to view room	Talk to infant, provide rattles	Cradle gym, infant swing
6–9 months	Peek-a-boo (teaches object permanence) Encouraging imitation of facial expression	Use appropriate names for objects Speak clearly	Introduce various textures for infant to touch Use teething toys
10–12 months	Large picture books Shopping trips Soft blocks Nested boxes	Reading, singing nursery rhymes Imitating sounds of animals	Push-pull toys Activity boxes

Note: Toys for each age group should be varied to stimulate vision, touch, hearing, and movement. Safety for age and diagnosis is of utmost importance in selection of a play activity or toy.

Canada. They may delay a child in walking and have the increased risk of falling down stairs. They also enable the child to reach for things that are higher than the child that could fall on them.

A safe environment for a crawling infant includes storage of poisonous items out of the infant's sight and reach. Cabinet locks are available for purchase and should be placed to protect infants from harm. Plants, batteries, pool areas, plugs, loose hanging wires, and pets can be hazardous to an infant. Close supervision at all times is essential to safety in any environment. Resource consultants are available in most communities for information concerning childproofing the home.

Toy Safety

While toys should be appropriate for the developmental level of the child, safety is the most important feature involved in toy selection. Infants put everything into their mouths; therefore, choking is a major problem if a toy has small or removable parts. When the pincer skill is developed, infants will be able to pick up small objects, such as pins, and put them into their mouths. Toys appropriate for older siblings can be dangerous to infants. For example, the glue from a model airplane that an older sibling is playing with can be deadly if an infant drinks it. Thus constant supervision is essential. Toys should nurture growth and development (Table 14.3). A child's response to a toy can indicate readiness to learn new skills. An infant who is able to reach for and pick up a toy shows readiness for communication.

DEVELOPMENTAL CHANGES IN THE FIRST YEAR

Following is a summary of the average findings for an infant, but it is important to remember that each child may be different:

- Weight doubles by age 6 months and triples by age 1 year.
- Height increases by 2.5 cm per month for the first 6 months and 1.25 cm in the 7- to 12-month period, to reach 74 cm by age 1 year (increase is mainly in the trunk of the body).
- Head circumference increases 1.5 cm each month for the first 6 months and 0.5 cm monthly for the second 6 months; average is 46 cm by age 12 months.
- Closure of the posterior fontanelle occurs by age 3 months.
- Closure of the anterior fontanelle occurs by age 18 months.
- Voluntary movements replace primitive reflexes.
- Maternal iron stores decrease by age 6 months.
- Digestive processes increase functioning by age 3 months. Amylase and lipase are deficient until age 4 to 6 months, which decreases the ability to digest the fats found in solid foods.
- Teething, which is evidenced by drooling, begins at 4 months of age. Tooth eruption begins at age 6 months, when biting activities start.
- Binocular vision is established by age 4 months.
- Depth perception begins to develop at age 9 months.
- Infants older than 4 months can voluntarily roll over.
- By age 1 year, infants can take some independent steps.
- *Separation* (of self from others), **object permanence** (objects exist even if they are out of visual field), and *symbols* (saying "bye-bye" means someone is leaving) are major aspects of cognitive development in the first year of life.

Get Ready for the Certification Examination!

Key Points

- The development of a sense of trust begins in infancy and is vital to a healthy personality.
- Sensory stimulation is essential for the development of the infant's thought processes and perceptual abilities.
- Health maintenance visits are essential during the first year to detect variations from normal growth patterns, provide immunizations, and educate and support parents.
- The most common cause of concern is an atypical-for-age slowing of any aspect of development.
- For safety and to prevent sudden infant death syndrome (SIDS), infants should be positioned for sleep on their backs on a firm mattress in the crib. The infant can be placed on their abdomen during playtime.
- The nurse must educate parents about the value of immunizations for infants and children.
- Breastmilk is the most desirable food for at least the first 6 months of the infant's life and can be continued for up to 2 years.
- Complementary solid food should be introduced after age 6 months when the child shows readiness for eating.
- Human milk or properly prepared formula supplies an adequate fluid intake for the infant under normal conditions.
- Whole cow's milk can be introduced after between 9 and 12 months of life.
- Seasonal fruits and vegetables provide the best nutritive value at the lowest cost.
- Feeding an infant a low-fat diet before age 2 years will compromise growth and development.
- An appropriate car seat should be used for automobile safety. The car seat should not be used as a prolonged sleeping arrangement outside of the automobile.
- Infants must be observed carefully when playing, to avoid accidents.

Additional Learning Resources

evolve Go to your Evolve website (http://evolve.elsevier.com/Canada/Leifer) for the following learning resources:

- Answer Key for Critical Thinking Questions
- Answer Key for Textbook Review Questions
- Audio Glossary
- Fluids & Electrolytes tutorial
- Interactive Review Questions
- Skills Performance Checklists
- Video clips and more

Online Resources

- Canadian Paediatric Society, Caring for Kids: https://www.caringforkids.cps.ca/
- Canadian Paediatric Society, *Feeding Your Baby in the First Year:* https://www.caringforkids.cps.ca/handouts/feeding_your_baby_in_the_first_year
- Government of Canada, *Canada's Provincial and Territorial Routine (and Catch-up) Vaccination Routine Schedule Programs for Infants and Children:* https://www.canada.ca/en/public-health/services/provincial-territorial-immunization-information/provincial-territorial-routine-vaccination-programs-infants-children.html
- Health Canada, *Infant Feeding* (includes sample menus): https://www.canada.ca/en/health-canada/services/food-nutrition/healthy-eating/infant-feeding.html
- Public Health Agency of Canada, *Safe Sleep:* https://www.canada.ca/en/public-health/services/health-promotion/childhood-adolescence/stages-childhood/infancy-birth-two-years/safe-sleep.html
- Unlockfood.ca, *Infant Feeding:* http://www.unlockfood.ca/en/Articles/Infant-feeding.aspx

Review Questions

1. A nurse teaching parents about car seat safety for an infant less than 10 kg should include which information?
   a. A car seat is not needed if the infant is held securely in the lap of an adult.
   b. The car seat should be placed close to the driver in the front passenger seat.
   c. The car seat should face the rear and be placed in the centre of the back seat.
   d. The car seat should face forward and be placed on the driver's side of the back seat.
2. The nurse is discussing home safety with the mother of a 3-month-old infant. Which of the following is a priority topic?
   a. Placing locks on cabinet doors that contain cleaning supplies
   b. Covering electrical outlets
   c. Putting the baby to sleep on back
   d. Encouraging reading and talking to the infant
3. A mother expresses concern that her 1-year-old infant is overweight. She states that her family has a tendency to be overweight and wishes to discontinue formula feedings and start the infant on low-fat milk. The nurse assesses that the present weight of the infant is 11 kg. The infant's birth weight was 3.7 kg. The best response of the nurse would be which of the following?
   a. Place the infant on a low-fat milk diet because the infant is slightly overweight at this time.
   b. Give the infant regular whole milk because the infant's weight is appropriate for his age.
   c. Indicate that the infant is underweight for his age and needs to have supplemental formula added to the diet.
   d. Note that infancy is a period of rapid growth and weight loss will occur as the infant becomes more active.

4. Which of the following is a developmental red flag for a 3-month-old infant that the nurse should record and report? *(Select all that apply.)*
   a. The infant does not attempt to raise their head when placed on the abdomen.
   b. The infant cannot sit without support.
   c. The infant exhibits stranger anxiety.
   d. The infant does not smile responsively.

Critical Thinking Question

1. A mother brings her 8-week-old infant to the clinic and states that the infant is fussy and acting as if he has colic. What information does the nurse need to obtain from the parent to develop a teaching plan?

REFERENCES

Amit, M., & Canadian Paediatric Society (CPS), Community Paediatrics Committee. (2009). Vision screening in infants, children, and youth. *Paediatric & Child Health, 14*(4), 246–248. Reaffirmed 2018. Retrieved from: https://www.cps.ca/en/documents/position/children-vision-screening.

Breen-Reid, K. M. (2017). The infant and family. In S. Perry, M. Hockenberry, D. Lowdermilk, et al. (Eds.), *Maternal child nursing care in Canada* (2nd ed.). Toronto, ON: Elsevier.

Canadian Paediatric Society. (2017). *Healthy bodies: Healthy sleep for your baby and child*. Retrieved from: http://www.caringforkids.cps.ca/handouts/healthy_sleep_for_your_baby_and_child.

Critch, N., & Canadian Paediatric Society (CPS), Nutrition and Gastroenterology Committee. (2011). Infantile colic: Is there a role for dietary interventions? *Paediatric & Child Health, 16*(1), 47–49. Reaffirmed 2018. Retrieved from: http://www.cps.ca/documents/position/infantile-colic-dietary-interventions.

Feigelman, S. (2016). The first year. In R. Kliegman, B. Stanton, J. St. Geme, et al. (Eds.), *Nelson textbook of pediatrics* (20th ed.). Philadelphia: Saunders.

Government of Canada. (2012). *Infant formula*. Retrieved from: https://www.canada.ca/en/health-canada/services/infant-care/infant-formula.html.

Hagan, J., & Duncan, P. (2016). Maximizing children's health: Screening; anticipatory guidance; and counseling. In R. Kliegman, B. Stanton, J. St. Geme, et al. (Eds.), *Nelson textbook of pediatrics* (20th ed.). Philadelphia: Saunders.

Health Canada, Canadian Paediatric Society (CPS), Dietitians of Canada, and Breastfeeding Committee for Canada. (2015a). *Nutrition for healthy term infants: Recommendations from birth to six months*. Retrieved from: https://www.canada.ca/en/health-canada/services/food-nutrition/healthy-eating/infant-feeding/nutrition-healthy--term-infants-recommendations-birth-six-months.html.

Health Canada, Canadian Paediatric Society (CPS), Dietitians of Canada, and Breastfeeding Committee for Canada. (2015b). *Nutrition for healthy term infants: Recommendations from six to 24 months*. Retrieved from: https://www.canada.ca/en/health-canada/services/food-nutrition/healthy-eating/infant-feeding/nutrition-healthy-term-infants-recommendations-birth-six-months/6-24-months.html.

Hunt, C., & Hauck, R. (2016). Sudden infant death syndrome. In R. Kliegman, B. Stanton, J. St, Geme, et al. (Eds.), *Nelson textbook of pediatrics* (20th ed.). Philadelphia: Saunders.

Mahan, L. K., & Raymond, J. L. (2017). *Krause's food and the nutrition process* (14th ed.). St. Louis: Saunders.

Narvey, M., & Canadian Paediatric Society (CPS), Fetus and Newborn Committee. (2016). Assessment of cardiorespiratory stability using the infant car seat challenge before discharge in preterm infants (<37 weeks' gestational age). *Paediatrics & Child Health, 21*(3), 155–158.

Public Health Agency of Canada (PHAC), Canadian Paediatric Society (CPS), Canadian Foundation for Study of Infant Deaths, Canadian Institute for Child Health, & Health Canada. (2018). *Joint statement on safe sleep: Preventing sudden infant deaths in Canada*. Retrieved from: http://www.phac-aspc.gc.ca/hp-ps/dca-dea/stages-etapes/childhood-enfance_0-2/sids/pdf/jsss-ecss2011-eng.pdf.

15 The Toddler

http://evolve.elsevier.com/Canada/Leifer

Lisa Keenan-Lindsay

Objectives

1. Define each key term listed.
2. Describe the physical, psychosocial, and cognitive development of children 1 to 3 years of age, listing age-specific events and guidance when appropriate.
3. Describe the task to be mastered by the toddler according to Erikson's stages of growth and development.
4. List two developmental tasks of the toddler period.
5. Discuss speech development in the toddler.
6. Discuss the principles of guidance and discipline for a toddler.
7. Discuss how adults can assist toddlers in overcoming their fears.
8. Identify the principles of toilet learning (bowel and bladder) that will help guide parents' efforts to provide toilet independence.
9. Describe the nutritional needs and self-feeding abilities of a toddler.
10. List two methods of preventing the following among toddlers: automobile accidents, burns, falls, suffocation and choking, poisoning, drowning, electric shock, and animal bites.
11. Describe the characteristic play and appropriate toys for a toddler.

Key Terms

autonomy
cooperative play
egocentric thinking
negativism
object permanence
parallel play
ritualism
separation anxiety
temper tantrums
time-out
toddlers

GENERAL CHARACTERISTICS

Children between 1 and 3 years of age are referred to as toddlers. They are able to get about by using their own powers and are no longer completely dependent persons. By 1 year of age, they have generally tripled their birth weight and gained control of their head, hands, and feet. The remarkably rapid growth and development that took place during infancy begins to slow down. The toddler period presents different challenges for the parents and the child.

The toddler is in Erikson's stage of autonomy versus shame and doubt, which is based on a continuum of trust established during infancy (see Chapter 14). Along with the toddler's increasing independence and curiosity to explore the widening environment come many challenging tasks to be mastered, including how to use the toilet, self-feeding, self-dressing, and speech development. One major parental responsibility is to maintain safety while allowing the toddler the opportunity for social and physical independence. Another major parental responsibility is to maintain a positive self-image and body image in the child whose behaviour is inconsistent and sometimes frustrating. Toddlers alternate between dependence and independence. They test their power by saying "no" frequently. This is called negativism. Offering limited choices and making use of distraction can be helpful strategies in handling toddlers (too many choices can cause confusion). Developing self-control and socially acceptable outlets for aggression and anger are important factors in the formation of personality and behaviour. Ritualism is another characteristic of toddler behaviour. Toddlers increase their sense of security by making compulsive routines of simple tasks, therefore, their rituals should be respected. Table 15.1 summarizes the toddler's physical development, social behaviour, and abilities at various ages.

PHYSICAL DEVELOPMENT

The toddler's body changes proportions (Fig. 15.1). The legs and arms lengthen through ossification and growth in the epiphyseal areas of the long bones. The trunk and head grow more slowly. The toddler gains 1.8 to 2.7 kg per year. The birth weight usually

Table 15.1 **Physical Development, Social Behaviour, and Abilities of Toddlers**

AGE	SOCIAL	FINE MOTOR	GROSS MOTOR	LANGUAGE	COGNITION
12–16 months	Imitates adults' activities Seeks alternate methods of achieving solitary play	Drinks from cup, holds spoon Builds tower of two blocks Prefers finger feeding	Begins to walk	Uses words Is activity oriented Follows simple commands	Classifies objects with function Object permanence begins to develop
16–18 months	Curious Parallel play	Places objects in appropriately shaped openings Improved self-feeding	Walks alone Can walk backward	Uses symbolic language ("bye-bye") Is able to point to familiar objects	Can imitate from memory Begins to realize cause and effect
24 months	Increased independence Egocentric—everything is "mine" Increased autonomy, often says "no"	Builds tower of six to seven blocks Turns pages of book Can undress self	Runs, throws ball Climbs steps Imitates oral hygiene Jumps with both feet	Uses plural words Uses words to tell story Names familiar objects	Continuous investigation and exploring Develops likes and dislikes
36 months	Establishes toilet independence Identifies sexual roles Begins to share May have imaginary playmate Ritualistic behaviour	Holds cup by handle and spoon with two fingers Copies a circle	Balances (hops) Jumps on one foot Uses tricycle Climbs stairs using alternate feet	Can hold a conversation Frequently asks why and how Says full name	Can understand one idea or concept at a time Knows two colours Imitates parental roles

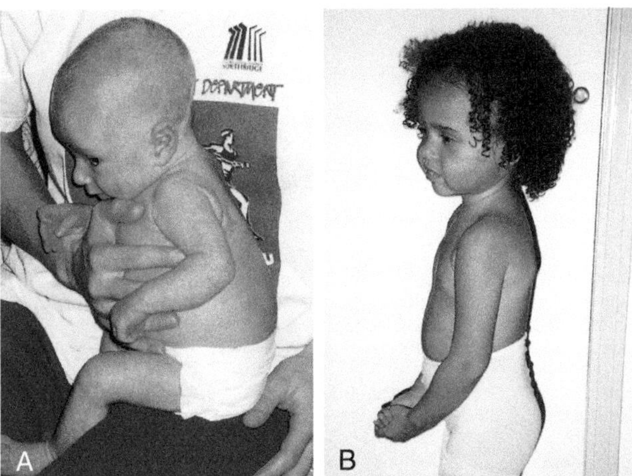

Fig. 15.1 Change in body contour. **A,** The back of the infant is rounded. **B,** In the toddler, the exaggerated lumbar lordosis makes the abdomen protrude.

quadruples by 2.5 years of age. The toddler grows approximately 7.5 cm per year in height. The height of a 2-year-old is thought to be one half of the potential adult height of that child. The height and weight are plotted carefully on a growth chart during each clinic visit to reflect what should be a steady pace of growth and development (see Appendix D).

The rate of brain growth decelerates. The increase in head circumference during infancy is 10 cm, whereas during the second year of life it is only 2.5 cm. Chest circumference continues to increase. After the second year, the child appears leaner because the chest circumference begins to exceed the abdominal circumference. The protuberant abdomen flattens when the muscle fibres increase in size and strength.

Myelination of the spinal cord is practically complete by 2 years of age, allowing for control of anal and urethral sphincters. Bowel and bladder control is usually complete by 2.5 to 3 years of age.

Respirations are still mainly abdominal but shift to thoracic as the child approaches school age. The toddler is more capable of maintaining a stable body temperature than is the infant. The shivering process, in which the capillaries constrict or dilate in response to body temperature, has matured.

The skin becomes tough as the epidermis and dermis bond more tightly, which protects the child from fluid loss, infection, and irritation. The defense mechanisms of the skin and blood, particularly phagocytosis, work more effectively than they did during infancy. The lymphatic tissues of the adenoids and tonsils enlarge during this period. The eustachian tubes continue to be shorter and straighter than in the adult. Tonsillitis, otitis media, and upper respiratory infections are common problems. Eruption of deciduous teeth continues until completion at about 2.5 years of age (see Fig. 13.12).

The blood pressure of a toddler may average 90/55 to 105/70 mm Hg; the respiratory rate slows to 20 to 30 breaths/min, and breathing continues to be abdominal. The pulse of a toddler slows to a range of 70 to 110 beats/min. Digestive processes and the volume capacity of the stomach increase to accommodate a three-meal-a-day schedule.

SENSORIMOTOR AND COGNITIVE DEVELOPMENT

The senses and motor abilities of the toddler do not function independently of one another. Two-year-old toddlers reach, grasp, inspect, smell, taste, and study objects with their eyes. Their attention becomes centred on characteristics of their surroundings that capture their interest. Binocular vision is well established by age 15 months. Visual acuity is about 20/40 by 2 years of age.

As memory strengthens, toddlers can compare present events with stored knowledge. They assimilate information through trial and error plus repetition. They try alternative methods of accomplishing a goal. Thought processes advance, preparing the way for more complex mental operations. The sensorimotor and preconceptual phase of development described by Piaget develops rapidly between 1 and 3 years of age, and the toddler's behaviour reflects this.

Separation anxiety, which consists of *protest, despair,* and *detachment,* develops in infancy and continues throughout toddlerhood. Separation anxiety peaks at 18 months and is mostly resolved at 24 months. For further discussion of separation anxiety see Chapter 19. Eventually, toddlers become aware of cause and effect. Often, they correlate a type of object with its function. For example, if their toys are stored in a paper bag, they will gleefully open any paper bag they see, expecting to find toys. If the bag contains garbage or drugs, they can be injured or may be punished. This can be confusing to the toddler and frustrating to the parents.

The concept of spatial relationships develops, and toddlers are able to fit square pegs in a square hole and round pegs in a round hole. Toys should be selected to promote this ability. **Object permanence** continues to develop, and the toddler becomes aware that there may be fun items behind closed doors and in closed drawers. The toddler's curiosity and ability to explore make it important to educate parents to keep dangerous objects out of their reach. The toddler begins to internalize standards of behaviour as evidenced by saying "no-no" when tempted to touch a forbidden object.

The toddler copies the words and the roles of the models seen in the home. The toddler may "help Mommy clean" or "help Daddy shave." By 2 years of age there is recognition of sexual differences.

Toddlers may confuse essential with nonessential body parts. Expelling feces and flushing them down the toilet can be upsetting to some toddlers, because they may feel they expelled a part of themselves that has disappeared. Toddlers' body image and self-esteem may be impaired if they are scolded in a way that makes them feel *they* are bad rather than their *behaviour* being bad. The nurse must help parents develop skills that will enable toddlers to feel they are loved even though the specific behaviour is unacceptable.

Table 15.2 Language Milestones

EXPRESSIVE LANGUAGE	AGE (MONTHS)	RECEPTIVE LANGUAGE	AGE (MONTHS)
Social smile	2	Becomes alert	1
Coos	3	Recognizes caregiver	2
Laughs	4	Orients to voice	4
Babbles	6	Understands "no"	9
"Dada," "mama"		Plays gesture games	9
Nonspecific	8	Follows one-step command:	
Specific	10	With gesture	12
First word	11	Without gesture	16
Second word	12	Knows one body part	18
Jargon	15	Points to one picture	18
Four to six words	16	Follows two-step command	24
Two-word phrases	21	Points to seven pictures	24
Two-word sentences	24	Follows prepositional commands	36
Pronouns	36		
Plurals	36		

Note: This table of language milestones is a guide to assessing normal language development, although not all children follow this exactly. While many children with developmental impairment are language delayed, not all language-delayed children are developmentally impaired. Some normal children also are late talkers.

Adapted from Canadian Paediatric Society. (2014). *Your child's development: What to expect*. Retrieved from https://www.caringforkids.cps.ca/handouts/your_childs_development; Simms, M. D. (2016). Language development and communication disorders. In R. Kliegman, B. Stanton, J. St. Geme, et al. (Eds.), *Nelson textbook of pediatrics* (20th ed.). Philadelphia: Saunders.

SPEECH DEVELOPMENT

Language development parallels cognitive growth. The increase in the level of comprehension is particularly striking and exceeds verbalization. By 3 years of age the child has a rather extensive vocabulary of about 900 words. Speech is more than 90% intelligible (Table 15.2). At about the end of the first year, the infant begins to make noises that sound like "bye-bye," "ma-ma," and "da-da." When toddlers see the happy response to these sounds, they repeat them. This is true throughout the toddler period. To want to learn to talk, small children must have an appreciative audience.

Children first refer to animals by the sounds the animals make. For example, before saying "dog," the toddler repeats "bow-bow." Soon the child can say short

Table 15.3 Symptoms of Possible Communication Disorder

AGE	BEHAVIOUR INDICATING HELP IS NEEDED
0–11 months	Before age 6 months the child does not startle, blink, or change immediate activity in response to sudden loud sounds. Before 6 months the child does not attend to the human voice and is not soothed by their caregiver's voice. By 6 months the child does not babble strings of consonant and vowel syllables or imitate gurgling or cooing sounds. By 10 months the child does not respond to their name. At 10 months the sounds the child makes are limited to shrieks, grunts, or sustained vowel production.
12–23 months	At 12 months the child's babbling or speech is limited to vowel sounds. By 15 months the child does not respond to "no," "bye-bye," or "bottle." By 15 months the child will not imitate sounds or words. By 18 months the child is not consistently using at least six words with appropriate meaning. By 18 months the child does not follow simple directions "Give me…," "Sit down," or "Come here," when spoken without gestural cues. By 23 months, two-word phrases have not emerged that are spoken as single units (e.g., "Whatzit," "Thank you," "All gone").
24–36 months	By 24 months, familiar listeners do not understand at least 50% of the child's speech. By 24 months the child does not point to body parts without gestural cues. By 24 months the child is not combining words into phrases ("Go bye-bye," "Go car," "Want cookie"). By 30 months the child does not demonstrate understanding of *on, in, under, front, back.* By 30 months the child is not using short sentences ("Daddy went bye-bye"). By 30 months the child has not begun to ask questions, using *where, what, why.* By 36 months unfamiliar listeners do not understand the child's speech.

Note: At any age, if the child is consistently dysfluent (not clear) with repetitions, hesitations, or blocks, or struggles to say words, the struggle may be accompanied by grimaces, eye blinks, or hand gestures, further medical follow up is advised.
Adapted from Moharir, M., Barnett, N., Taras, J., Cole, M., Ford-Jones, E. L., & Levin, L. (2014). Speech and language support: How physicians can identify and treat speech and language delays in the office setting. *Paediatric & Child Health, 19*(1), 13–18; Simms, M. D. (2016). Language development and communication disorders. In R. Kliegman, B. Stanton, J. St. Geme, et al. (Eds.), *Nelson textbook of pediatrics* (20th ed.). Philadelphia: Saunders

phrases, such as "Daddy gone car." Toddlers also respond to tone of voice and facial expression. If an adult sounds threatening, the toddler may answer "no" and then repeat it in a louder voice.

Sometimes adults scold the child merely for being too young to understand what is requested. However, imagine being punished in a foreign country because you could not speak or comprehend the language well enough to defend yourself. Adults who show empathy to the small child can help to minimize their frustrations.

Parents who are concerned about their child's delayed speech can discuss it with their health care provider during a routine physical examination so it can be evaluated in light of total physical growth and development (Table 15.3). Many late talkers are perfectly normal children who prefer listening rather than active participation. Lead poisoning and hearing deficits should be ruled out before screening for other developmental problems such as autism (Box 15.1) (autism spectrum disorder is discussed in Chapter 33). Some older homes may have lead paint and some soil has been contaminated by lead, which may be ingested by toddlers.

Box 15.1 Screening for Signs of Autism

- No pointing, gesturing (bye-bye) by 12 months
- No single words by 16 months
- No spontaneous two-word phrases by 24 months
- Loss of achieved language or social skills

Note: These are preliminary symptoms. Lead poisoning or hearing deficits should be ruled out.

Sources: American Psychiatric Association. (2013). *Diagnostic and statistical manual of mental disorders* (5th ed.) (DSM-5). Washington, DC: Author; Raviola, G., Trieu, M., Demaso, D., & Walter, H. (2016). Autism spectrum disorders. In R. M. Kliegman, B. F. Stanton, J. W. St. Geme, et al. (Eds.), *Nelson textbook of pediatrics* (20th ed.). Philadelphia: Saunders; Simms, M. D. (2016). Language development and communication disorders. In R. Kliegman, B. Stanton, J. St. Geme, et al. (Eds.), *Nelson textbook of pediatrics* (20th ed.). Philadelphia: Saunders.

GUIDANCE AND DISCIPLINE

Discipline for the toddler involves guidance. The goal is to teach, not to punish. Teaching the toddler self-control with positive self-esteem is more desirable than encouraging a completely submissive, "obedient" child. The toddler who scribbles on the wall must be given the opportunity to scribble on paper, a more socially acceptable outlet.

Nursing Tip

The toddler is beginning to exercise autonomy and independent functioning. Gentle guidance, positive discipline, and patience will help the toddler master the stage of autonomy and maintain a positive self-image.

Temper tantrums (uncontrolled anger reactions) often occur during the toddler years, and parent responses reinforce to the child either the desirability or the risks involved with such behaviour. Expectations must be commensurate with the child's physical and cognitive abilities. Toddlers get into many situations that are over their heads. When adults make firm decisions, the problem is resolved, at least for the time being. The child feels secure.

Setting limits should include praise for desired behaviour as well as disapproval for undesired behaviour. A time-out period in a safe place helps the child to develop the ability to tolerate delayed gratification and self-regulation. Timing should not begin until the child has settled down. The child is praised after they are calm. Timing for time-out is usually based on 1 minute per year of age.

Children, like adults, seek approval; it is effective and helps to increase their self-confidence. A positive approach should be taken as often as possible, which means one assumes that the toddler is going to be good rather than bad. "Thank you, Ruby, for giving me the matches" will make them arrive in your hand more quickly than "Give me those matches right now," said in a threatening tone. The use of fear or physical aggression should not be a part of discipline because it does not foster self-control and can lead to physical or emotional abuse of the child.

Fear is a valuable emotion to the child if it does not become too intense. Unfortunately, many children fear situations that are not in themselves dangerous, and this sometimes deprives them of activities that otherwise would be enjoyable. If the parent warns, "Be careful, don't fall," when a toddler begins to ride a tricycle, the toddler may develop a fear of taking risks that may be involved when experiencing new activities.

The physical and mental health of the child at the time of a fear-provoking experience affects the extent of the reaction. If the child is alone, fear may be greater than if someone such as a parent or nurse is present. After a fear has been learned, it is more difficult to eliminate. Clinging to favourite possessions and repetitive rituals are self-consoling behaviours for the toddler, particularly at bedtime and during separation from parents.

Stress increases fear of separation. Adults should attempt to control their own fears while in the presence of young children. Respect and understanding should always be accorded to children who are afraid. Making fun of the fear or shaming the child in front of others is detrimental to building self-esteem.

Many toddlers who independently explore the clinic examining room while waiting to be examined may cling to the parent when the stranger (the health care provider) enters the room and approaches the child. When talking to the toddler, the adult should be at eye level with the child so the adult seems less overwhelming. This is of particular importance when the child is in a fear-provoking environment, such as the hospital. The toddler who does not seek the parent during stressful situations or turns to a stranger for comfort reflects a need for closer evaluation of the parent–child relationship.

The "terrible twos," during which negative behaviour is predominant, begin the disciplinary pattern of the family that will continue throughout childhood and affect the child's personality. Corporal punishment (spanking) is not an effective method of discipline because regular spanking may reflect a desperate effort by the parent to gain control over a toddler who is exercising their beginning autonomy (independent functioning) and developing negativism. Potential injury, child abuse, and reciprocal aggressive behaviour by the child can be avoided with careful parental guidance concerning alternative techniques of discipline. Time-out, limit setting, clear communication, and frequent rewards and approval for positive behaviour are effective noncorporal techniques of discipline.

Communicating love and respect to the child with a clear message that it is the behaviour, not the child, that the adult disapproves of are the keys to effective discipline. Behaviour problems that can occur during early childhood are detailed in Table 15.4.

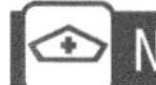 **Nursing Tip**

Caregivers must provide safe areas for the toddler to explore. They need to watch carefully before saying "no."

DAILY CARE

Toddlers' nutrition, dentition, and oral care are discussed in Chapter 13. A flexible schedule organized around the needs of the entire household is best for the toddler. The toddler needs a consistent routine, but it can differ for special occasions.

The clothing of toddlers should be simple and easy for them to put on and take off. Pants with elastic waists are convenient for them to pull down when they use the toilet. All clothing must be fairly loose to provide freedom of movement for jumping and other strenuous activities. Sunburn protection with clothing or sunscreen with an SPF 30 or higher is necessary to prevent skin damage (see Chapter 30).

The toddler wears shoes mainly for protection. They should fit the shape of the foot and be about a centimetre longer and half a centimetre wider than the foot. They must fit securely at the heel. Children should wear their usual shoes at their periodic checkups because this demonstrates how the shoes have been worn, which may indicate to the health care provider how the child is walking and using their body. The toddler may go barefoot whenever it is safe because this strengthens the foot muscles. Socks must be large enough that they do not flex the toes.

Good posture is the result of proper nutrition, plenty of fresh air and exercise, and sufficient rest. The toddler's mattress must be firm. The chair and play table should be adapted to size. In some cases, this can be easily accomplished by placing a rolled-up blanket or

Table 15.4 **Behaviour Concerns During Early Childhood, Normal Expectations, and Parental Guidance**

BEHAVIOUR	NORMAL EXPECTATIONS	FACTORS CONTRIBUTING TO PROBLEM	PARENTAL GUIDANCE
Sleep disorders	Occasional nightmares begin at about 36 months. Ritual bedtime routine begins; attempt to delay sleep peaks between 2 and 3 years. Head banging and rocking between 1 and 4 years provide a release of tension.	Excessive napping during the day Insufficient adult interaction during the day, leading to the use of bedtime as opportunity to gain adult attention Unusual fears related to darkness, being left alone Discomfort of wet diapers Illness	Provide one nap a day until end of second year, when naps may be eliminated. Use of bedtime rituals, such as a quiet activity or bedtime stories, is helpful. A favourite toy or blanket in the bed can ease insecurities involved in separation. Provide environment conducive to sleep. Avoid scary television shows. Restrict fluid intake before bedtime.
Temper tantrums	Tantrums peak at 2 years of age, decreasing in frequency and intensity until they rarely occur by about 4 years of age. Tantrums usually occur in response to the frustrated desires of a child, such as wanting a toy that cannot be purchased.	Used as a manipulative device to gain control of parental behaviour Insufficient positive interaction with adults, leading to use of tantrums to gain attention	Use simple explanations of behaviour expectations. Use "time-out" responses (1 minute per year of age). Maintain consistency of expectations from both parents. Reward good behaviour.
Toilet learning and bed wetting	Child has full physiological capacity for day control by age 3 years, night control by age 4 years. Daytime and nighttime "accidents" occur throughout early childhood, decreasing in frequency by age 4 years. Regression occurs with environmental or social changes, such as arrival of sibling, moving, or divorce.	Fears and anxiety in response to negative toilet independence Used as an attention-getting device if positive means of gaining attention are lacking May use constipation as a control mechanism Excessive fluid intake before bedtime	Use positive rewards for successful toileting and do not criticize child for accidents. Recognize signals of need to use toilet. Restrict fluid intake before bedtime. Use clothing that toddler can easily remove for self-toileting.
Aggressive or quarrelsome behaviour, sibling rivalry	Ability to play cooperatively begins to emerge at 3–5 years. Before this age, the child is seldom able to share toys and often wants toys that another child has. There is a predominant use of physical hitting and shoving to express displeasure; verbal abilities begin to emerge.	Insufficient positive adult attention, leading to deliberate use of aggression to gain adult attention May arise from actual or perceived adult preference for sibling or playmate	Prepare toddler for the separation and change involved in the arrival of a new sibling. Provide for any changes involved 1–2 months before arrival of sibling (e.g., change to a new bed or room). Provide toddler with doll to imitate parental behaviours. Provide for special individual time with toddler each day.
Inability to separate, excessive shyness	Child can separate easily by age 3 years if surroundings are consistent, predictable, and positive. Child continues to protest separation if environment changes or if confronted by total strangers. Child is shy in new and strange surroundings but relaxed and spontaneous in familiar surroundings.	Inadequate establishment of self-concept, leading to lack of confidence, even in familiar surroundings Uses protest of separation as a manipulative control device Fear of being abandoned	Prepare toddler for anticipated separation. Refer to time using concrete terms ("I will return after lunch" rather than "I will return at 1 PM"). Avoid radiating parental anxiety at the planned separation. Spend time with toddler and in new environment or with new caregiver before leaving.

pad in the seat of the chair. A small, sturdy stool placed in the bathroom will bring the child to the proper height for brushing the teeth. As in all areas of learning, the child's posture is greatly influenced by that of other members of the family. The toddler who is happy and is allowed to gradually increase independence develops a sense of security, which is reflected in the posture. Slouching is sometimes seen in children who are insecure and lack self-confidence.

TOILET INDEPENDENCE

There are many approaches to toilet learning (previously called *toilet training*). Much depends on the temperament of both the individual child and the person guiding the child. Readiness is important. Voluntary control of anal and urethral sphincters begins at about 18 to 24 months. If the child wakes up dry in the morning or after naptime, it is an indication of maturity. Children must be able to communicate in some fashion that they are wet or need to urinate or defecate. They must be willing to sit on the potty for several minutes at a time.

Toddlers seek approval and like to imitate the actions of parents. They wander into the bathroom and are curious about what is taking place there. If a parent feels that the child will respond to training at this time, the parent might first put the child in training pants or pull-up diapers. These can be removed quickly and easily, and the child becomes more aware of being wet.

The use of a child's potty chair or a device that attaches to an adult toilet seat is a matter of personal preference (Fig. 15.2). A potty chair may make the toddler feel more secure because it is small. It should support the back and arms of the child. The child's feet should touch the floor. If a potty chair is not available, the child can be placed on the standard-size toilet, facing the toilet tank. This method may increase feelings of security. The toddler can use a regular toilet with a bench to support the child's feet.

Bowel training is generally attempted first; however, some toddlers become bladder trained during the day because they enjoy listening to the "tinkle" in the potty. If toddlers have bowel movements at the same time each day, they may progress fairly rapidly in training. They should not be left on the potty chair for more than a few minutes at a time.

Bladder training is begun when the toddler stays dry for about 2 hours at a time. The parent may discover that the toddler has gone the entire night without wetting. It is then logical to put the child on the potty chair and to praise success. Bladder training varies widely, particularly during the night. Placing the half-asleep child on the potty chair accomplishes little in the training process.

Most children continue to have occasional accidents until age 4 years. If the toddler has a mishap, parents should accept it matter-of-factly and merely change the clothes. Children benefit when adults show continuous affection to them and accept both bad and good days.

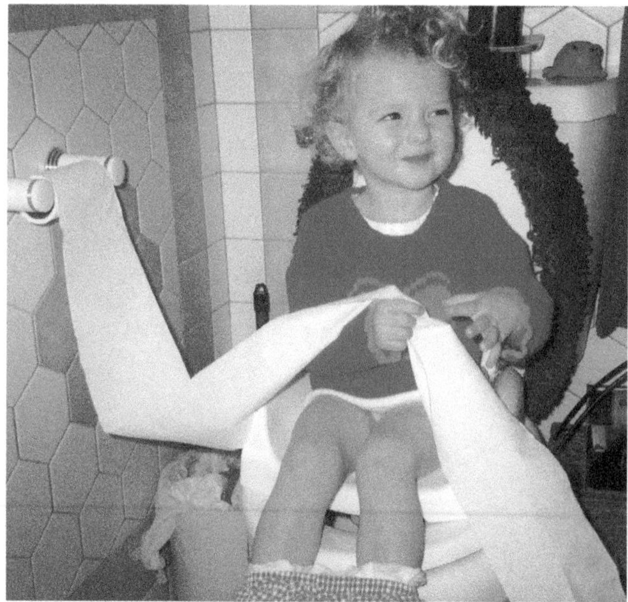

Fig. 15.2 Toilet learning. Toilet learning should be a nonstressful experience for the toddler. Nurses can help parents identify readiness for toilet independence. The nurse assesses the parents' expectations, family and cultural preferences, and developmental readiness of the child when instructing parents. Sitting on the potty too long without supervision may result in bathroom playtime!

The word that toddlers use to signal defecation or urination should be one that is recognized by others besides the immediate family. Sometimes a parent may forget to inform the babysitter or nursery school teacher of the word that the child uses. This can cause toddlers unnecessary frustration because those around them cannot understand what they are trying to say.

Toddlers who have learned to use the toilet at home should continue to use the potty chair in the hospital setting. Wetting the bed may acutely embarrass them. Although regression of bowel and bladder training is common during hospitalization, personnel often contribute to it by not taking time to investigate the child's needs. Nurses should regularly consult the child's nursing care plan to maintain continuity of care and to promote growth and development of the toddler.

Demands and threats do more damage than good. The process of toilet independence may be easier if the parent remains patient and keeps this new adventure pleasant. Training should not be undertaken when the family or child is under stress, such as during illness or a move to a new home.

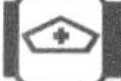 **Nursing Tip**

Nurses can help parents identify readiness for toilet independence.

NUTRITION COUNSELLING

Children need adequate protein intake and to have their energy requirements met to cover maintenance needs and provide for optimum growth. The Canadian Paediatric Society (CPS) recommends breastfeeding until

24 months of age. Dairy products provide the toddler with calcium and phosphorous. Daily consumption of more than 750 mL of milk limits the amount of solid foods that are eaten and can lead to dietary deficiencies of iron (Critch & CPS Nutrition and Gastroenterology Committee, 2014). Children between 1 and 3 years of age are high-risk candidates for anemia.

Canada's Food Guide can be used for children age 2 and over to help parents plan an adequate menu (see Appendix C). The toddler who is well nourished shows steady proportional gains on height and weight charts and has good bone and tooth development. The diet history should be adequate, avoiding excessive calories and large amounts of vitamins.

The toddler normally has a fluctuating appetite with strong food preferences. The nurse should remind parents that any nutritious food can be eaten at any meal; for example, soup for breakfast and cereal for dinner are acceptable. Families are encouraged to eat meals together and to eat "family-style" meals in which food is put into larger bowls or serving dishes on the table. The family members can then serve themselves based on hunger cues and food preferences (Government of Canada, 2019). Serving oneself also lets the child select what and how much they want on their plate and may encourage children to try new foods that they otherwise would have pushed aside (Government of Canada, 2019). A quiet time before meals provides an opportunity for the child to "wind down." The toddler's refusal to eat may result from fatigue or not being particularly hungry. The toddler might eat one food with vigour one week and refuse it the next. The individual family must work out a flexible schedule designed to meet the needs of the toddler and those of the rest of the family. Forcing toddlers to eat only creates further difficulties. They are quick to sense parents' frustration and may use mealtime to obtain attention by behaving poorly and refusing to eat. Discipline and arguments during mealtime only upset everyone's digestion.

Toddlers are fond of ritual. This is often seen at mealtime. They want a particular dish, glass, and bib. It is best to go along with their wishes as long as they do not become too pronounced. It gives them a sense of security and, in the long run, saves time and energy for the adult.

Toddlers have brief attention spans. They rarely sit at the table or stay in the high chair for long periods. They may try to stand in the high chair or may wander away from the table. They may be excused if they have eaten a fair amount of the meal; otherwise, distraction of some type may be necessary. Some restaurants that cater to families provide crayons and special place mats to keep the small child occupied until the adults finish their dinners. In the hospital, the toddler who is fed in a high chair wears an appropriate safety restraint, and the nurse remains with the child during the meal.

A variety of foods, with contrasts of colours and textures, should be offered to the toddler. A 2-year-old likes finger foods. Foods need to be served at moderate temperatures. Candy, cake, and juice between meals should be avoided.

Children like to eat from colourful dishes, which should be made of an unbreakable substance. Washable plastic bibs, place mats, and protection for the floor around the high chair are advisable. Eating utensils should be small enough that they can be handled easily. Seating equipment should be adjusted so the child is comfortable and maintains good posture.

THE PICKY EATER VERSUS A FEEDING DISORDER

A "picky eater" is one who is selective about foods and their colour, taste, texture, or smell but eats sufficient foods and fluids to maintain growth and development. It is normal for toddlers to be picky at different times when eating. See Table 13.7 for strategies of feeding the picky toddler. Meals should be eaten together as a family and the child should come to the table hungry.

A child who refuses to eat or drink a variety of foods or liquids to maintain adequate growth and development may have a feeding disorder. A feeding disorder results in weight loss for more than 1 month. A study of the gastrointestinal tract for anomalies should be performed before using strategies to increase appetite. Orexigenic medication to increase appetite, uniform feeding expectations and feeding environment, and gradually exposing the child to the smell, textures, and taste of new foods can increase the acceptance and intake of new foods (Kreipe & Palomaki, 2012).

DAY CARE

Many parents work outside the home and children may be cared for in a variety of different day care settings. It is ideal if parents can take an active role in ensuring high-quality care. Nurses need to be resource persons and family advocates because finding adequate day care can be stressful.

The decision to place a toddler in the care of others while parents work can be difficult and may produce feelings of guilt in the parent. Successful alternative child care arrangements depend on specific guidelines in selecting the facility (see Chapter 16), frequent visits to the facility, and close communication and conferences with the staff in the facility.

There are various types of child care. Unlicensed care is not regulated by the government and may be offered by relatives, friends, neighbours, or those who have advertised such services. In Ontario, unlicensed day care operators are not allowed to look after more than five children, including their own, under the age of 6. Most licensed day care centres are private businesses run for profit. They are subject to provincial regulations about physical layout, number of children per caretaker, education of personnel, and other factors. They are also inspected at least once a year. No matter what type of child care is chosen, parents must plan ahead for times when the child is sick and unable to attend. Employer-supported child care is a rapidly growing area, and these programs are very diverse. Some companies provide care at the place of work. Other employers assist parents through reimbursement, referral programs, or support of existing child care programs in the community.

The cost of child care can be difficult to afford for some families. There is some government assistance or private funding available; however, the parents must meet the qualifications to receive the funds. Inspection and monitoring of child care facilities to ensure compliance with health and safety standards are paramount. Ideally, all day care programs would include comprehensive health services and health education programs. Criteria for selecting a day care centre are similar to those discussed for nursery schools (see Chapter 16).

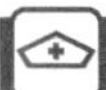
Nursing Tip

It is a major task for parents to "let go" and allow the toddler to interact with influences outside the family in day care centres or preschools.

PREVENTATIVE HEALTH CARE

The CPS recommends that all 18-month-old children have an enhanced well-baby visit (Williams, Clinton, & CPS Early Years Task Force, 2011). This visit should include the following:

- A developmental screening tool (e.g., the Nipissing District Developmental Screen [NDDS]), to stimulate discussion with parents about their child's development—both how they can support it and what concerns they may have
- Screening for parental morbidities (mental health problems, abuse, substance misuse, physical illness)
- Promotion of early literacy activities (reading, speaking, and singing to babies) for every family
- Information about community-based early childhood development resources for every family (parenting programs, parent and early learning resource centres, libraries, recreational and community centres)

INJURY PREVENTION

Accidents are the leading cause of death and injury in childhood. The best prevention is knowledge of age-appropriate risks and anticipatory guidelines. If parents understand their child's activities at certain ages, they can prevent many serious injuries by taking necessary precautions (see Health Promotion box).

Nurses have an important responsibility to review injury prevention with parents during each clinic visit. The normal behavioural characteristics of a toddler, including curiosity, mobility, and negativity, make the toddler prone to injuries that often occur in and around the home (Fig. 15.3). Car seat safety is discussed later in the chapter.

Nurses need to demonstrate safety measures to their patients and their families. Safety measures pertinent to the pediatric unit are discussed in Chapter 20. Nurses in the community can often contribute indirectly to the welfare of others by the example they set and by being aware of emergency medical facilities available in the community.

Health Promotion

How to Prevent Hazards Caused by the Behavioural Characteristics of Toddlers

BEHAVIOURAL CHARACTERISTICS	HAZARD PREVENTION STRATEGIES
TRAFFIC AND AUTOMOBILE	
Impulsive	Teach the child street safety rules.
Unable to delay gratification	Teach the child the meaning of red, yellow, and green traffic lights.
Increased mobility	Caution children not to run from behind parked cars or snow banks.
Egocentric	Use car seat restraints appropriately.
	Hold a toddler's hand when crossing the street.
	Supervise tricycle riding.
	Do not allow children to play in the car alone.
	Drivers must look carefully in front of and behind vehicles before accelerating.
	Teach children what areas are safe in and around the house.
	Supervise children under age 3 years at all times.

Continued

Health Promotion—cont'd

BEHAVIOURAL CHARACTERISTICS	HAZARD PREVENTION STRATEGIES
BURNS	
Fascination with fire Can reach articles by climbing Pokes fingers in holes and openings Can open doors and drawers Unaware of cause and effect	Teach the child the meaning of "hot" (an example of how to do this is by allowing the child to touch beach sand warmed by the sun). Put matches, cigarettes, candles, and incense out of reach and sight. Turn handles of cooking utensils toward the back of the stove. Be aware of hot liquids; avoid using tablecloths with overhang. Keep appliances such as coffee pots, electric frying pans, and food processors and their cords out of reach. Test food and fluids heated in microwave ovens to ensure that the centre is not too hot. Be aware of hot charcoal grills or gas barbecues. Use snugly fitting fireplace screens. Mark children's rooms to alert firefighters in an emergency. Keep a pressure-type fire extinguisher available, and teach all family members who are old enough how to use it. Practice what to do in case of fire in the home. Install smoke detectors. Cover electrical outlets with protective caps. Check bath water temperature before placing child in the water. Do not allow child to handle water faucets.
FALLS	
Likes to explore different parts of the house Can open doors and lean out open windows Has immature depth perception Capabilities change quickly May seem quite grown up at times but still requires constant supervision at home and on the playground	Teach children how to go up and come down stairs when they show readiness for this task. Use side rails on a large bed when child graduates from crib. Lock basement doors or use gates at top and bottom of stairs. Mop up spilled water on floor immediately. Use window guards. Use car seat restraints appropriately. Keep scissors and other pointed objects out of the toddler's reach. Use childproof doorknobs and drawer closures. Secure child in shopping cart at store. Supervise climbing child at playground. Keep clothing and shoelaces appropriate size and length to prevent tripping.
SUFFOCATION AND CHOKING	
Explores with senses; likes to bite on and taste things Eats on the run	Do not allow small children to play with any balloons; these can be sucked into the airway. Inspect toys for small or loose parts. Remove small objects such as coins, buttons, and pins from reach. Avoid popcorn, nuts, small hard candies, chewing gum, or large chunks of meat, such as hot dogs. Debone fish and chicken. Learn the Heimlich manoeuvre and cardiopulmonary resuscitation (CPR). Inspect width of crib and playpen slats. Keep plastic bags away from small children; do not use as mattress cover. If child is vomiting, turn them on their side. Do not use nightclothes with drawstring necks. Discard old refrigerators and appliances, or remove doors.
POISONING	
Ingenuity increases, can open most containers Increased mobility provides child access to cupboards, medicine cabinets, bedside stands, interior of closets Looks at and touches everything Learns by trial and error Puts objects in mouth	Store household detergents, laundry pods, and cleaning supplies out of reach and in a locked cabinet. Do not put chemicals or other potentially harmful substances into food or beverage containers. Keep medicines in a locked cabinet; put them away immediately after use. Use child-resistant caps and packaging. Expired medications should be disposed of in accordance with local laws. Follow health care provider's directions when administering medication. Do not refer to pills as "candy." Explain poison symbols to the child and parents. Keep telephone number of poison control centre available. When painting, use paint marked "for indoor use" or one that conforms to standards for use on surfaces that may be chewed on by children. Wash fruits and vegetables before eating. Obtain and record name of any new plant purchased. Alert family to location and appearance of poisonous plants on or around property or frequently encountered when camping. Use childproof locks on cabinets.

Health Promotion—cont'd

BEHAVIOURAL CHARACTERISTICS	HAZARD PREVENTION STRATEGIES
DROWNING	
Lacks depth perception Does not realize danger Loves water play	Watch child continuously while at the beach or near a pool. Empty wading pool when child has finished playing. Cover wells securely. Wear recommended life jackets in boats. Begin teaching water safety and swimming skills early. Lock fences surrounding swimming pools. Supervise tub baths; be aware that a young child can drown in a very small amount of water.
ELECTRIC SHOCK	
Pokes and probes with fingers	Cover electrical outlets. Cap unused sockets with safety plugs. Water conducts electricity; teach child not to touch electrical appliances when hands are wet; keep appliances out of reach. Keep electrical appliances away from tub and sink area.
ANIMAL BITES	
Has immature judgement	Teach child to avoid stray animals. Do not allow toddler to abuse household pets. Supervise closely. Teach child how to approach any pets.
SAFETY	
Easily distracted Trusting of others Falls frequently	Teach toddler stranger safety. Do not personalize clothes. Do not allow toddler to eat or suck lollipops while running or playing. Keep sharp-edged objects out of reach. Keep sharp-edged furniture out of play area.

Note: Keep first aid chart and emergency numbers handy. Know location of and how to get to the nearest emergency facility.

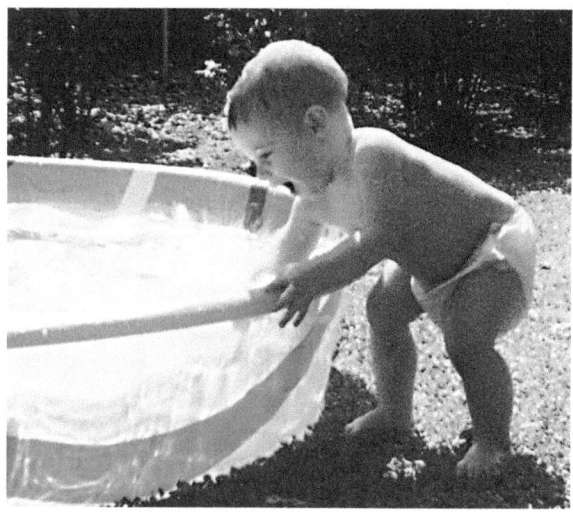

Fig. 15.3 The playful toddler needs close supervision during water play. Falling into a kiddie pool can result in serious injury.

CONSUMER EDUCATION

The federal government and concerned private agencies have attempted to regulate some of the variables that cause injuries. A few examples are ensuring the use of nonflammable material for children's sleepwear, mandating childproof caps on medicine bottles and certain household products, and establishing maximum temperatures for home hot-water heaters. Health Canada regulates the Consumer Product Safety Act and has established regulations for cribs, cradles, and bassinets. Safety warnings on the crib's carton advise buyers to use a snug mattress only. The nurse should reinforce this type of information.

Car safety is also important. The use of seat belts is effective if they are worn properly. In Canada, all provinces and territories have legislation that covers the use of car seats, although booster seats are not mandatory in all provinces and territories. Child seats, when used correctly, reduce the risk of fatal injury by 71%, and the risk of serious injury by 67%. Using a booster seat instead of a seat belt alone reduces the risk of injury by 59% (van Schaik & CPS Injury Prevention Committee, 2008). Car seats are safest in the middle of the rear seat of the car and should be rear facing at least until the child weighs 10 kg, is 1 year old, and is able to walk. It is recommended that children remain in rear-facing car seats as long as the child meets the weight and height limits in the manufacturer's instructions, even if they are beyond 1 year of age (Caring for Kids, 2019). A child seat placed in the front car seat close to the passenger air bag can be dangerous (Fig. 15.4). Ideally, children should be in a car seat until they weigh a minimum 22 kg. These restraints must follow standards established by Transport Canada. Unfortunately many car seats are not used correctly; misuse rates range from 44 to 81% for car seats, and 30 to 50% for booster seats (van Schaik & CPS Injury Prevention Committee, 2008). The top three errors in car seat use are as follows:

- Seat not tightly secured to the vehicle (moves more than 2.5 cm [1 inch] in any direction);

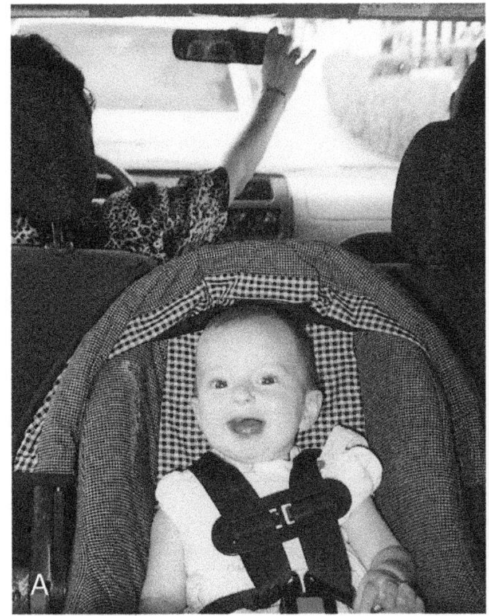

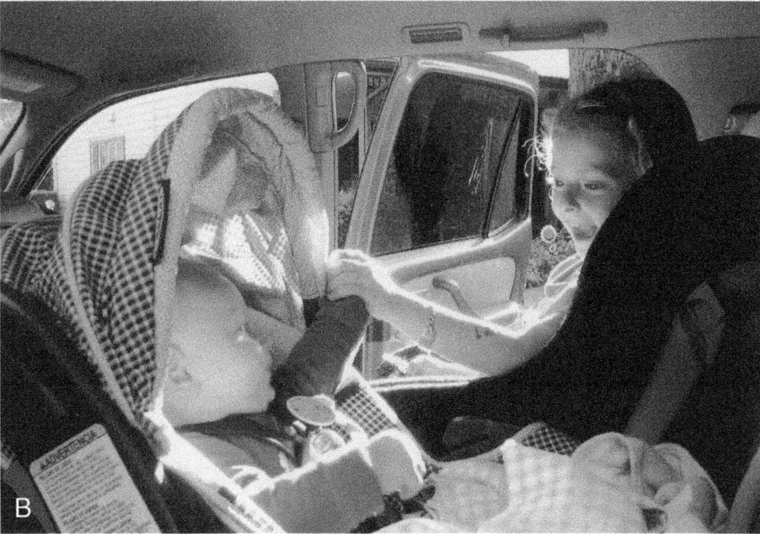

Fig. 15.4 **A,** The child under 10 kg sits in a car seat that faces the rear of the car to prevent the infant's large and heavy head from falling forward when the car stops suddenly or in case of an accident. Note that the metal clip or lock of the car seat belt is not under the chin of the infant, but rests firmly on the chest. **B,** The toddler's car seat can face front in the centre of the rear seat of the car and secured by the car's seat belt.

- Harness not snug (more than one finger width fits between the harness strap and the child); and
- Chest clip is not at armpit level.

All homes are required to have smoke detectors, and carbon monoxide detectors are recommended. Various other safety codes are mandatory for public buildings, with additional measures required for buildings specifically for the disabled. The education of parents is of monumental importance in decreasing death and disability of children.

TOYS AND PLAY

Children's toys and related products that are manufactured, imported, advertised, or sold in Canada are subject to the *Canadian Consumer Product Safety Act* and the *Toys Regulations*. In addition, parents must be taught to inspect toys routinely for damage and to buy toys suitable for the age, skills, and abilities of the individual child. Some labels now provide safety information and age guidelines for the intended user. In general, notification of recall for a specific toy is announced on radio and television, communicated via email, and is published in newspapers and consumer journals.

Toy boxes and toy chests are another potential hazard. The most serious injuries caused by a box or chest are the result of the lid falling on a child or a child being trapped inside. A parent can report a product hazard by emailing the Government of Canada, Consumer Product Safety Directorate.

Play is the work of a toddler. Through play, toddlers learn how to manipulate and understand their environment, socialize, and explore their world. High-priced toys are not necessary (Fig. 15.5). Toddlers prefer pots and pans from the kitchen, supervised water play, dancing to music, and crayons or finger paint and paper. A picture book reviewed while on the lap of a family member can often be enjoyed over and over again. Tricycles can be adapted to the size and ability of the toddler. Objects that can be pushed or pulled are preferred to wind-up toys for this age group because walking and running are the developmental tasks at hand. Providing materials such as fur, sandpaper, and felt can stimulate the sense of touch. Colours can be taught while having the toddler help sort the laundry. Pointing to familiar pictures in a book, newspaper, or magazine can stimulate memory. Counting can be

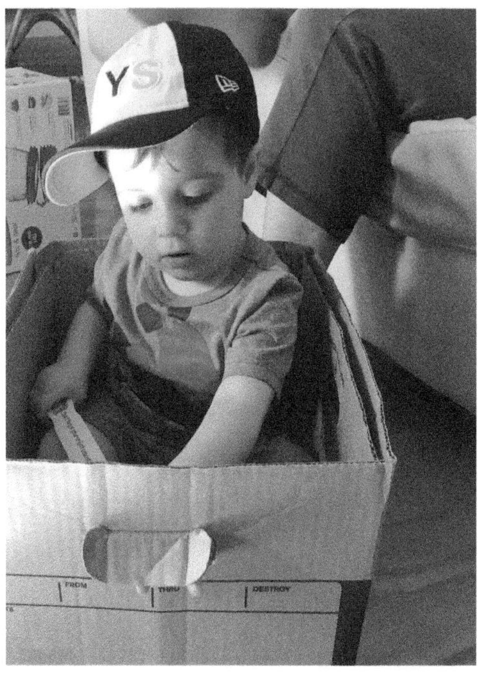

Fig. 15.5 Toddlers and preschoolers do not need expensive toys to spark their imagination in play activities. A simple box in which their toy was packed is often the preferred focus of play.

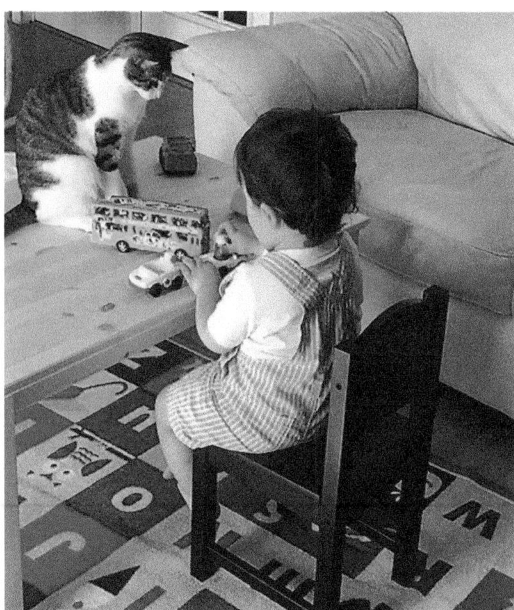

Fig. 15.6 Close supervision is necessary when a child plays in any home where there is a pet, whether large or small. Both the toddler and the pet have unpredictable behaviour.

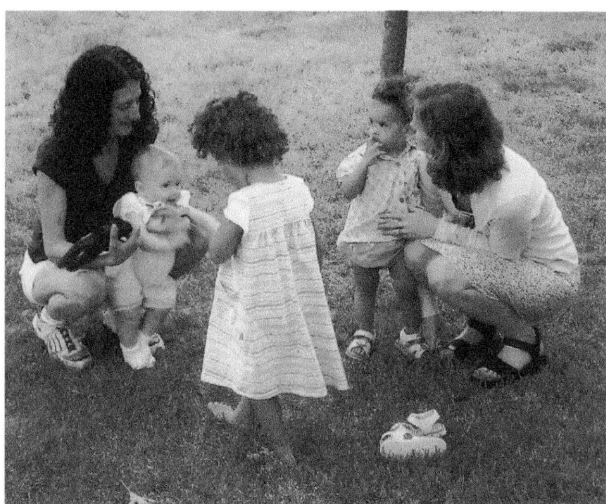

Fig. 15.7 Beginning social skills, parallel play, and short attention spans of toddlers require them to have close supervision in day care settings.

taught while climbing stairs. Supervision and maintenance of safety are key to a positive play experience for the toddler. Particular attention should be paid whenever a pet is part of the environment (Fig. 15.6).

As toddlers become aware of their expanding environment, their social development takes form. Egocentric thinking, in which children relate everything to themselves, predominates. They engage in parallel play, playing next to, but not with, their peers (Fig. 15.7). They gradually develop cooperative play, which involves imagination and sharing skills. Toddlers do not yet understand property rights and therefore believe all toys are theirs to play with. Frequent frustrations can lead to temper tantrums. It is important to calm and distract a child when they become frustrated rather than just removing them abruptly from the play area.

Nurses must closely assess children with special needs for safety precautions. Caregivers of children with disabilities require extended instruction according to the child's particular needs; these children include those with visual, motor, or intellectual impairments or with convulsive disorders. Immobile children must be protected from sunburn and wind or rainy weather. Adults must also guard these children from mosquitoes and other disease vectors. Injury prevention involves some of the methods mentioned in the discussion of consumer education: the use of items such as electric outlet covers, cabinet locks, drawer locks, and the creation of a hazard-free or "childproof" environment for the child (Fig. 15.8).

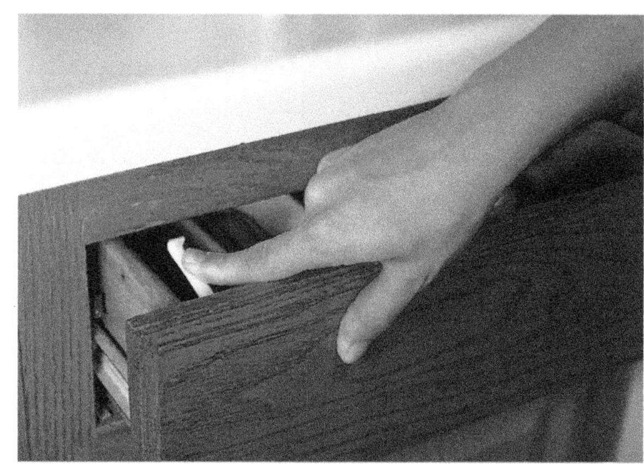

Fig. 15.8 Childproofing the home. A simple drawer or cabinet latch prevents access to the contents by the young child while the contents still remain accessible to the adult, who can press and release the latch with one finger. (From Harkreader, H., & Hogan, M. A. [2008]. *Fundamentals of nursing: Caring and clinical judgment* [3rd ed.]. Philadelphia: Saunders.)

Get Ready for the Certification Examination!

Key Points

- The birth weight for a toddler has quadrupled by age 2.5 years.
- Physical changes of the toddler include the acquisition of fine and gross motor skills, among which are increased mobility and increased eye–hand coordination.
- The digestive volume and processes of the toddler increase to accommodate a three-meal-a-day schedule.
- Complete bowel and bladder control is usually achieved by age 2.5 to 3 years.
- Erikson refers to the toddler stage as one in which the child's task is to acquire a sense of autonomy (self-control) while overcoming shame and doubt.

- The most evident cognitive achievements of the toddler involve language and comprehension.
- Some important self-regulatory functions mastered by the toddler include toilet independence, self-feeding, tolerating delayed gratification, separation from parents, and perfecting newfound physical skills and speech.
- Separation anxiety includes the stages of protest, despair, and detachment.
- Parental guidance is needed to handle the negativism, temper tantrums, and sibling rivalry that are characteristic of this age group.
- Discipline for the toddler should be designed to teach rather than punish.
- Some methods of dealing with the inconsistencies of the toddler include distraction, reward and praise, and time-out in a safe place.
- Accidents and poisoning are the leading causes of death in the toddler age group.
- Infants and young children should ride in a car safety seat for all car trips.

Additional Learning Resources

evolve Go to your Evolve website (http://evolve.elsevier.com/Canada/Leifer) for the following learning resources:

- Answer Key for Critical Thinking Questions
- Answer Key for Textbook Review Questions
- Audio Glossary
- Fluids & Electrolytes tutorial
- Interactive Review Questions
- Skills Performance Checklists
- Video clips and more!

Online Resources

- Canadian Paediatric Society–Caring for Kids: https://www.caringforkids.cps.ca/
- Canadian Paediatric Society–Caring for Kids, *Toilet Learning:* https://www.caringforkids.cps.ca/handouts/toilet_learning
- Canadian Paediatric Society–Caring for Kids, *Your Busy Toddler: Games, Toys and Play in the Second Year of Life:* https://www.caringforkids.cps.ca/handouts/your_busy_toddler
- Unlockfood.ca, *Nutri-eSTEP: Eating Habits Survey for Toddlers:* http://www.unlockfood.ca/en/Articles/Childrens-Nutrition/Nutri-eSTEP-Eating-Habits-Survey/Nutri-eSTEP-Eating-Habits-Survey-for-Toddlers.aspx

Review Questions

1. A parent states she is having a conflict with her toddler who seems to "always want to do things his way." He insists on putting on his right sock and shoe before his left and has a tantrum if the parent tries to put on the left sock and shoe first. The parent asks the nurse why the child is acting this way. What is the best response a nurse could give the parent?
   a. Explain to the child that it really doesn't matter which sock and shoe is donned first.
   b. Put the child in a "time-out" for the appropriate time.
   c. Explain that this is normal ritualistic behaviour at this age and should be respected.
   d. Let the child walk barefoot and take the shoes away.
2. A nurse assesses the vital signs of a 2-year-old and understands that a normal respiratory rate (per minute) would be which of the following?
   a. 18 to 20
   b. 20 to 30
   c. 35 to 40
   d. 40 to 50
3. Which statement by the parent would indicate a need for further guidance regarding car seat safety?
   a. "I use a car seat for my toddler whenever we are in the car, and he is right beside me as I drive so I can keep an eye on him."
   b. "I use a car seat for my toddler whenever we are in the car and secure it onto the rear seat of the car."
   c. "I use a car seat for my toddler that is designed to hold children up to 18 kg."
   d. "I use a car seat for my toddler that is designed to fasten with the seat belt.'
4. A mother tells a nurse that her 2-year-old toddler often has temper tantrums at the family dinner table and asks how to handle the behaviour. The best response of the nurse would be which of the following?
   a. Temper tantrums are normal for a 2-year-old, and the child will grow out of it.
   b. The toddler should be removed from the family dinner table until they are old enough to behave.
   c. Strict discipline and corporal punishment are appropriate to help the child gain self-control.
   d. Parents should agree on a method of discipline, such as time-out, and use it when the child misbehaves.
5. Which of the following is a developmental hallmark of the toddler that most frequently gives rise to safety hazards?
   a. Brief attention span
   b. Need for ritual
   c. Fluctuating appetite
   d. Need to explore
6. Which of the following observations of a 2-year old should be documented and reported to the health care provider? *(Select all that apply.)*
   a. He does not try to imitate sound or words.
   b. He does not respond to his name.
   c. He will not play with other children.
   d. He refuses to sit on the potty (toilet).
   e. He has temper tantrums.

Critical Thinking Question

1. The parents of a toddler discuss safety in the home with the nurse. The parents state that they will use a car seat as required by law and safety gates on the stairs to prevent accidental falls. However, they believe no other safety "childproofing" is necessary, because their child is a good child and they plan to teach him to be obedient so he will learn not to touch certain items. What is the best response of the nurse?

REFERENCES

Caring for Kids. (2019). *Car seat safety*. Retrieved from: https://www.caringforkids.cps.ca/handouts/car_seat_safety.

Critch, J. N., & Canadian Paediatric Society (CPS), Nutrition and Gastroenterology Committee. (2014). Nutrition for healthy term infants, six to 24 months: An overview. *Paediatrics & Child Health, 19*(10), 547–549.

Government of Canada. (2019). *Canada's Food Guide*. Retrieved from: https://food-guide.canada.ca/en/.

Kreipe, R., & Palomaki, A. (2012). Beyond picky eating. *Current Psychiatry Reports, 14*(4), 421–423.

van Schaik, C., & Canadian Paediatric Society (CPS), Injury Prevention Committee. (2008). Transportation of infants and children in motor vehicles. *Pediatrics & Child Health, 13*(4), 313–318.

Williams, R., Clinton, J., & Canadian Paediatric Society (CPS), Early Years Task Force. (2011). Getting it right at 18 months: In support of an enhanced well-baby visit. *Paediatrics & Child Health, 16*(10), 647–650.

The Preschool Child

16

Lisa Keenan-Lindsay

http://evolve.elsevier.com/Canada/Leifer

Objectives

1. Define each key term listed.
2. List the major developmental tasks of the preschool-age child.
3. Describe the physical, psychosocial, and spiritual development of children from age 3 to 5 years, listing age-specific events and guidance when appropriate.
4. Describe the development of the preschool child in relation to Piaget's, Erikson's, and Kohlberg's theories of development.
5. Describe the speech development of the preschool child.
6. Discuss the development of positive bedtime habits.
7. Discuss one method of introducing the concept of death to a preschool child.
8. Identify two toys suitable for the preschool child, and provide the rationale for each choice.
9. Discuss the value of the following: time-out periods, consistency, role modelling, and rewards.
10. Discuss the approach to concerns such as sexual curiosity, thumb sucking, and enuresis in the preschool child.
11. Discuss the characteristics that parents should look for in a preschool.
12. Describe the developmental characteristics that predispose the preschool child to certain accidents, and suggest methods of prevention for each type of accident.
13. Discuss the value of play in the life of a preschool child.
14. Explain the use of therapeutic play with a child who has a developmental delay.

Key Terms

animism
art therapy
artificialism
associative play
centring
echolalia (ĕk-ō-LĀ-lē-ă)
egocentrism
enuresis (ĕn-yū-RĒ-sĭs)
modelling
parallel play
play therapy
preconceptual stage
preoperational phase
sibling rivalry
symbolic functioning
therapeutic play
time-out

GENERAL CHARACTERISTICS

The child from age 3 to 5 years is often referred to as the *preschool child*. Slowing of the physical growth process and mastery and refinement of the motor, social, and cognitive abilities that mark this period will enable the child to be successful in their school years.

The major tasks of the preschool child include preparation to enter school, development of a cooperative type of play, control of body functions, acceptance of separation, and increase in communication skills, memory, and attention span.

PHYSICAL DEVELOPMENT

The infant, who tripled their birth weight at 1 year, has doubled the 1-year weight by the age of 5 years. For instance, the infant who weighs 9 kg on their first birthday will probably weigh about 18 kg by their fifth birthday. The preschooler grows taller and loses the chubbiness seen during the toddler period. Between 3 and 5 years of age, there will be an increase of 7.5 cm in height, mostly in the legs, which contributes to the development of an erect, slender appearance. Visual acuity is 20/40 at 3 years of age and 20/30 at 4 years of age. The achievement of 20/20 vision may be accomplished by school age. All 20 primary teeth have erupted. Hand preference develops by 3 years of age, and efforts to change a child's handedness from left to right can cause a high level of frustration. The child's appetite will fluctuate widely.

The normal pulse rate is 65 to 110 beats/min. The rate of respirations during relaxation is about 20 to 25 breaths/min. The systolic blood pressure is about 95 to 110 mm Hg, and the diastolic blood pressure is about 60 to 75 mm Hg.

Preschool children have good control of their muscles and participate in vigorous play; they become more adept at using already familiar skills as each year passes. They can swing and jump higher. Their gait resembles that of an adult. They are quicker and have more self-confidence than they did as toddlers.

COGNITIVE DEVELOPMENT

The thinking of the preschool child is unique. Piaget calls this period the **preoperational phase**. It comprises children from 2 to 7 years of age and is divided into two stages: the **preconceptual stage** (2 to 4 years of age) and the *intuitive thought stage* (4 to 7 years of age). Of importance in the preconceptual stage is the increasing development of language and symbolic functioning. **Symbolic functioning** is seen in the play of children who pretend that an empty box is a fort; they create a mental image to stand for something that is not there.

Another characteristic of this period is **egocentrism**, a type of thinking in which children have difficulty seeing any point of view other than their own. Because children's knowledge and understanding are restricted to their own limited experiences, misconceptions arise. One misconception is **animism**, the tendency to attribute life to inanimate objects. Another is **artificialism**, the idea that people created the world and everything in it.

The intuitive stage is one of prelogical thinking. Experience and logic are based on outside appearance (the child does not understand that a wide glass and a tall glass can both contain the same amount of juice). A distinctive characteristic of intuitive thinking is **centring**, the tendency to concentrate on a single outstanding characteristic of an object while excluding its other features.

More mature conceptual awareness is established with time and experience, and this process is highly complex. Table 16.1 summarizes some major theories of personality development in the preschooler.

EFFECTS OF CULTURAL PRACTICES

Cultural practices can influence the development of a child's sense of initiative, such as in families who practice authoritarian types of parenting styles that put a great value on obedience and conformity. Parents and older siblings are models for language development, and the mastery of sounds proceeds in the same order around the world. Some parents may speak two language in the home. Studies have shown that young children adapt quickly to a bilingual environment and cultural practices (Fig. 16.1). Cultural preferences related to dietary practices are discussed in Chapter 13.

LANGUAGE DEVELOPMENT

The development of language as a communication skill is essential for success in school (Fig. 16.2). Physiological, psychological, or environmental stressors can cause delays or problems in language expression. Typically, in the preschool period between 2 and 5 years of age, the number of words in the child's sentence should equal the child's age (e.g., two words at 2 years of age). By 2½ years of age, most children evidence possessiveness (*my* doll). By 4 years of age they can use the past tense, and by 5 years of age they can use the future tense. The development of language skills includes both the understanding of language and the expressing of oneself in language. Children who have difficulty expressing themselves in words often exhibit tantrums and other acting-out behaviours.

Table 16.2 lists the language, cognitive, and perceptual abilities required for success in school. Problems detected and treated during the preschool years can prevent many school problems in later years. Table 16.3 describes the clinical symptoms of typical language disorders. Evaluation of language development must be performed together with an assessment of problem-solving skills.

Normal development of speech and language is dependent on the infant's ability to see, hear, understand, remember, socially interact, and have oral motor skills. A disorder in the rhythm of speech known as *stuttering* can lead to anxiety and social phobia. Stuttering often improves by school age and improves while singing, talking to pets, or reading out loud. Preschool therapy with a speech-language pathologist is often helpful (Simms, 2016).

DEVELOPMENT OF PLAY

Play activities in the preschool child increase in complexity. At 2 to 3 years of age, the child imitates the activities of daily living of the parents (hammering, shaving, feeding the doll). By 4 years of age, the child may develop broader themes such as a trip to the zoo. By 5 years of age, a trip to the moon demonstrates the child's imaginary abilities. Play enables the child to experience multiple roles and emotional outlets, such as the aggressor, the victim, the superpower, or the acquisition of toys or friends they desire. Appealing to the child's magical thinking is the best approach to communication. Screen time should be limited to 1 hour per day of high-quality programs with parents present, if possible (Canadian Paediatric Society [CPS], 2017b) (Fig. 16.3).

SPIRITUAL DEVELOPMENT

Preschoolers learn about religious beliefs and practices from what they observe in the home. Preschoolers cannot yet understand abstract concepts; their concept of God or a higher being, sometimes treated as an invisible friend, is concrete. Preschool children can memorize Bible stories and related rituals, but their understanding of the concepts is limited. Observing religious traditions practiced in the home during a period of hospitalization (e.g., before-meal or bedtime prayers) can help the preschool child manage stressors.

Table 16.1 **Preschool Growth and Development**

AGE	INTELLIGENCE	EMOTIONAL ASPECTS	LANGUAGE	PLAY	PARENTAL GUIDANCE
3 years	Piaget's preoperational phase Understands time in relation to concrete activities Knows own sex Has attention span of approximately 15 minutes; is easily distracted	Freud's phallic stage Oedipus complex may develop in boys Erikson's stage of initiative vs. guilt Kohlberg: beginning moral development; wishes to please parents Ritualism provides security (see Chapter 15) Egocentric (unable to see viewpoint of others) Identifies with same-sex parent	Has vocabulary of approximately 300–800 words Uses plurals Forms three-word sentences Can repeat three numbers Understanding occurs before expressive ability	Develops understanding of good/bad Explains different emotions in pretend play Starts to engage in group play Is highly imaginative Establishes preference for hand use	Child usually wants to please parents. Guidance techniques are based on this principle. Overprotection during this stage of initiative can frustrate development of a coping mechanism in the child. Having the child "help" the parent will enhance self-esteem.
4 years	Can count to 5 Knows simple songs Sexual curiosity is high Has attention span of approximately 20 minutes Adds logic to thinking Understands that feelings are connected to actions	May use tantrums to relieve frustrations and, if successful, these may become a coping mechanism Has mood swings Is highly imaginative Asks many questions Likes to "show off" accomplishments Experiments with masturbation	Has vocabulary of 1500 words Uses four- to five-word sentences Experiments with language and words May use offensive words without understanding their meaning	Engages in rough-and-tumble play Learns how much they can control Demonstrates sibling rivalry	Minimize doing things for child such as puzzles. Repetition of words without comprehension (**echolalia**) should be referred for follow-up care. Teach self-control through setting limits. Guide parent in discipline techniques. Provide nutritious snacks. Answer questions truthfully.
5 years	Beginning concept of past, present, and future, although time is evidenced in activity rather than hours Knows days of the week Attention span reaches 30 minutes Can count to 10 Knows name and address Behaviours that result in rewards are considered right; behaviours that result in punishment are considered wrong	Is less egocentric and has beginning awareness of the outside world Enjoys activities with parent of the same sex	Has vocabulary of 2000 words Can name four colours Uses six- to eight-word sentences with pronouns	Wants to play "by the rules" but cannot accept losing Can copy sample shapes and print first name	Child can participate in own care. Teach front-to-back wiping after bowel movements. Provide information concerning vision assessment facilities in community. Review immunization status. Prepare parent for separation from child and their entrance into school.

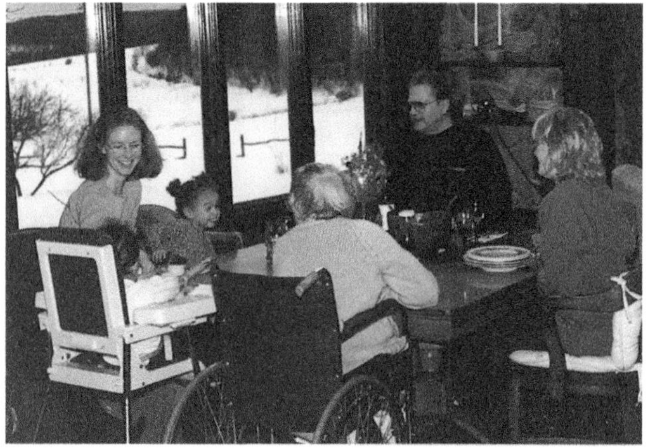

Fig. 16.1 The family meal. The multigenerational family enjoys a meal together. Cultural traditions and family bonding occur here.

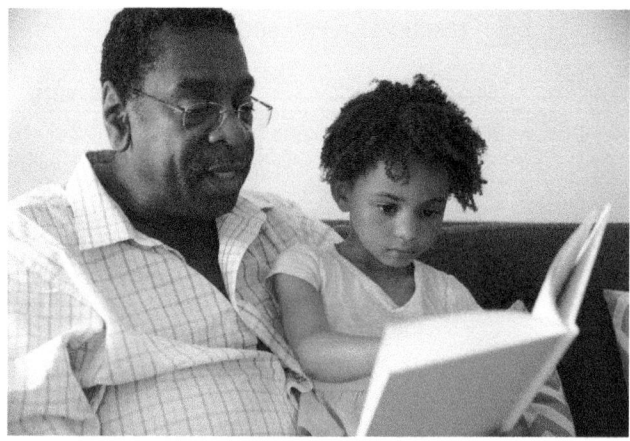

Fig. 16.2 Grandpa reads to his grandchild. Preschool language development depends on exposure to the written word and picture familiarity. In interactive reading, the child is asked questions about the pictures she sees and she receives immediate feedback. It is the ideal way to optimize the mastery of language. (istock.com/monkeybusinessimages)

Table 16.2 Selected Perceptual, Cognitive, and Language Processes Required for Elementary School Success

PROCESS	DESCRIPTION	ASSOCIATED PROBLEMS
Perceptual		
Visual analysis	Ability to break a complex figure into components and understand their spatial relationships	Persistent letter confusion (e.g., between *b, d,* and *g*); difficulty with basic reading and writing and limited "sight" vocabulary
Proprioception and motor control	Ability to obtain information about body position by feel and unconsciously program complex movements	Poor handwriting, requiring inordinate effort, often with overly tight pencil grasp; special difficulty with timed tasks
Phonological processing	Ability to perceive differences between similar-sounding words and to break down words into constituent sounds	Delayed receptive language skills; attention and behaviour problems secondary to not understanding directions; delayed acquisition of letter–sound correlations (phonetics)
Cognitive		
Long-term memory, both storage and recall	Ability to acquire skills that are "automatic" (i.e., accessible without conscious thought)	Delayed mastery of the alphabet (reading and writing letters); slow handwriting; inability to progress beyond basic mathematics
Selective attention	Ability to attend to important stimuli and ignore distractions	Difficulty following multistep instructions, completing assignments, and behaving well; peer interaction problems
Sequencing	Ability to remember things in order; skill with time concepts	Difficulty organizing assignments, planning, spelling, and telling time
Language		
Receptive language	Ability to comprehend complex constructions, function words (e.g., *if, when, only, except*), nuances of speech, and extended blocks of language (e.g., paragraphs)	Difficulty following directions; wandering attention during lessons and stories; problems with reading comprehension; problems with peer relationships
Expressive language	Ability to recall required words effortlessly (word finding), control meanings, and vary position and word endings to construct meaningful paragraphs and stories	Difficulty expressing feelings and using words for self-defense, with resulting frustration and physical acting out; struggling during "circle time" and in language-based subjects (e.g., English)

Adapted from Simms, M. D. (2016). Language development and communication disorders. In R. Kliegman, B. Stanton, J. St. Geme, et al. (Eds.), *Nelson textbook of pediatrics* (20th ed.). Philadelphia: Saunders.

Table 16.3 Not Talking: A Clinical Classification

WHEN PARENTS SAY	CLASSIFY THE SYMPTOMS AS
"I'm the only one who understands what she says."	Articulation disorder
"She'll do what I say, but when she wants something, she just points."	Expressive language delay
"He can't play 'show me your nose,' and the only word he says is 'mama.'"	Global language delay
"He never made those funny baby sounds or said 'mama' and 'dada,' and now he just repeats everything I say."	Language disorder
"He used to say things like 'Joey go bye-bye,' but now he doesn't talk at all."	Language loss

Adapted from Montgomery, T. (1994). When children do not talk. *Contemporary Pediatrics, 11*(9), 49, 1994; Simms, M. D. (2016). Language development and communication disorders. In R. Kliegman, B. Stanton, J. St. Geme, et al. (Eds.), *Nelson textbook of pediatrics* (20th ed.). Philadelphia: Saunders.

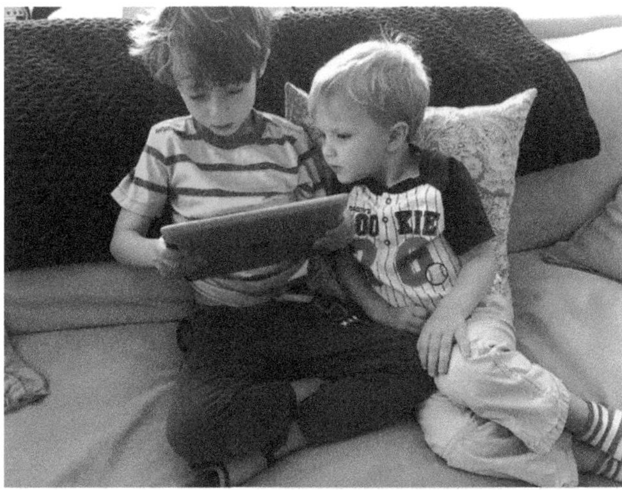

Fig. 16.3 The Canadian Paediatric Society recommends that children between 2 and 5 years of age have screen time limited to 1 hour per day. Children may be sitting next to each other, but they may not be interacting or communicating when using electronic devices.

SEXUAL CURIOSITY

When guiding parents concerning the sexual education of young children, the nurse should use the following common principles of teaching and learning:

- First assess the knowledge base of the child; then assess what specific information the child is seeking.
- Be honest and accurate in providing information at the child's level. Although the child may not understand completely at first, the child's repeated questions and explanations will form the basis of later learning and understanding.
- Use correct terminology so that misinformation or misinterpretation can be avoided.
- Provide sex education at the time the child asks the question. The asking of the question often indicates readiness to learn.
- Parents must understand that sexual curiosity starts as an inquiry into anatomical differences. Differences in how urination occurs may later become the focus. A general understanding of infants coming from "Mommy's tummy" precedes the more mature concept of sexual organs and functioning.

Preschool children are as matter-of-fact about sexual investigation as they are about any other learning experience.

Masturbation

Sexual curiosity displayed in the form of masturbation or "playing doctor" should be approached in a positive manner. Masturbation is common in both genders during the preschool years. The child experiences pleasurable sensations, which lead to a repetition of the behaviour. It is beneficial to rule out other causes of this activity, such as rashes or penile or vaginal irritation. Masturbation in the preschool child is considered harmless if the child is outgoing, sociable, and not preoccupied with the activity.

Education of the parents consists of assuring them that this behaviour is a form of sexual curiosity and is normal and not harmful to the child, who is merely curious about sexuality. Punitive reactions should be discouraged and the activity should not be treated as "bad" or "dirty." Parents are advised to ignore the behaviour and distract the child with some other activity. Teaching socially acceptable behaviour should be in the form of guidance rather than discipline. The child should know that masturbation is not acceptable in public, but this must be explained in a nonthreatening manner. Children who masturbate excessively and who have experienced a great deal of disruption in their lives benefit from ongoing counselling.

BEDTIME HABITS

The development and reinforcement of optimal bedtime habits are important in the preschool years. At this age, it is common for children to have some sleep problems and to resist going to bed. Parents should be guided to engage the child in quiet activities before bedtime, to maintain specific rituals that signal bedtime readiness (such as storytelling), and to verbally state "after this story, it will be bedtime." The use of a night light, a favourite bedtime toy, or a glass of water at the bedside are options. Avoiding screen time before bedtime may also improve the ability to fall asleep, as well as avoiding any food or drinks with caffeine.

Preschoolers may also wake up during the night from nighttime fears or nightmares (CPS, 2017a). It is important not to ignore bedtime fears. Nightmares can happen after a stressful physical or emotional event or can be caused by fever. If a child has nightmares, they need to be reassured and comforted (CPS, 2017a).

Some children experience night terrors which are different from nightmares. Children with night terrors scream uncontrollably, may breathe quickly, and seem to be awake. These children may be confused when awakened and may take longer to settle down and go back to sleep. Night terrors usually happen between the ages of 4 and 12, but can happen to children as young as 18 months old. While most children outgrow them, a health care provider should be consulted if they persist (CPS, 2017a).

The nurse should be aware that specific cultures encourage "family beds," where children regularly sleep with siblings and parents.

DEVELOPMENT THROUGH THE YEARS

THE 3-YEAR-OLD

Three-year-olds are usually a delight to their parents. They are helpful and can assist in simple household chores. They obtain articles when directed and return them to the proper place. Parents feel that the guidance provided during the trying 2-year-old period has been rewarded. Temper tantrums are less frequent, and in general the 3-year-old is less erratic. They are still individuals, but they seem better able to direct their primitive instincts than previously. They can help to dress and undress themselves, use the toilet, and wash their hands. They eat independently, and their table manners have improved.

Three-year-olds talk in longer sentences and can express thoughts and ask questions. They provide more company to their parents and to other adults because they can talk about their experiences. They are imaginative, talk to their toys, and imitate what they see about them. Soon they begin to make friends outside the immediate family. **Parallel play** (playing independently within a group) and **associative play** (playing in loosely associated groups) are both typical of this period. Because they can now converse with playmates, they find satisfaction in joining their activities. Three-year-olds play cooperatively for short periods. They can ask others to "come out and play." If 3-year-olds are placed in a strange situation with children they do not know, they commonly revert to parallel play because it is more comfortable.

Preschoolers begin to find enjoyment away from their parents, although they want them nearby when needed. They begin to lose some of their interest in their caregiving parent, who up to this time has been more or less their total world. The other parent's prestige begins to increase. Romantic attachment to the parent of the opposite sex may be seen during this period. A daughter wants "to marry Daddy" when she grows up. Children also begin to identify themselves with the parent of the same sex.

Preschool children have more fears than the infant or older child because of increased intelligence (which enables them to recognize potential dangers), memory development, and graded independence (which brings them into contact with many new situations). Toddlers are not afraid of walking in the street because they do not understand its danger. Preschool children realize that trucks can injure, and they worry about crossing the street. This fear is usually well founded, but many others are not.

The fear of bodily harm, particularly the loss of body parts, is unique to this stage. The little boy who discovers that his infant sister is made differently may worry that she has been injured. He wonders if this will happen to him. Other common fears include fear of animals, fear of the dark, and fear of strangers. Night wandering is typical of this age group.

Preschool children become angry when others attempt to take their possessions. They may grab, slap, and hang on to them for dear life. They become very distraught if toys do not work the way they should. They resent being disturbed from play. They are sensitive, and their feelings are easily hurt. Much of the unpleasant social behaviour seen during this time is normal and necessary to the child's total pattern of development.

THE 4-YEAR-OLD

Four-year-olds are more aggressive and like to show off newly refined motor skills. They are eager to let others know they are superior, and they are prone to pick on playmates. Four-year-olds are boisterous, tattle on others, and may begin to swear if they are around children or adults who use profanity. They recount personal family activities with amazing recall but forget where they left their tricycle. At this age, children become interested in how old they are and want to know the exact age of each playmate. It bolsters their ego to know that they are older than someone else in the group. They also become interested in the relationship of one person to another, such as Jacob is a brother but is also Daddy's son.

Four-year-olds can use scissors with success. They can lace their shoes. Their vocabulary has increased to about 1 500 words. They run simple errands and can play with others for longer periods. Many feats are done for a purpose. For instance, they no longer run just for the sake of running. Instead, they run to get someplace or see something. They are imaginative and like to pretend they are nurses or firefighters. They begin to prefer playing with friends of the same sex.

The preschool child enjoys simple toys and common objects. Raw materials are more appealing than toys that are ready-made. An old cardboard box that can be moved about and climbed into is more fun than a dollhouse with tiny furniture. A box of sand or coloured pebbles can be made into roads and mountains. Parents should avoid showering their children with ready-made toys. Instead, they can select materials that are absorbing and that stimulate the child's imagination.

Stories that interest young children depict their daily experiences. If the story has a simple plot, it must be related to what they understand to hold their interest. They also enjoy music they can march around to, enjoy music videos, and like simple instruments they can shake or bang. They often have great reactions to someone making up a song about their daily life.

The Concept of Death

Children between 3 and 4 years of age begin to wonder about death and dying. They may pretend to be the hero who shoots the intruder dead, or they may actually witness a situation in which an animal is killed. Their questions are direct. "What is 'dead'? Will I die?" The view of the family is important to the interpretation of this complex phenomenon.

Children may become acquainted with death through objects with no particular significance to them. For instance, the flower dies at the end of the summer and does not bloom anymore. It no longer needs sunshine or water, because it is not alive. Usually young children realize that others die, but they do not relate death to themselves. If they continue to pursue the question of whether or not they will die, parents should be casual and reassure them that people do not generally die until they have lived a long and happy life. Of course, as they grow older they will discover that sometimes children do die. The dying child is discussed in Chapter 22.

The underlying idea is to encourage questions as they appear and gradually help children to accept the truth without undue fear. There are many excellent books written especially for children about death that are available.

THE 5-YEAR-OLD

Five-year-old children are more responsible, enjoy doing what is expected of them, have more patience, and like to finish what they have started. Five-year-olds are serious about what they can and cannot do. They talk constantly and are inquisitive about their environment. They want to do things correctly and seek answers to their questions from those whom they consider to "know" the answers. Five-year-old children can play games governed by rules. They are less fearful because they believe that authorities control their environment. Their worries are less profound than at an earlier age.

The physical growth of 5-year-olds is not outstanding. Their height may increase by 5 to 7.5 cm, and they may gain 1.5 to 2.7 kg. They may begin to lose their deciduous teeth at this time. They can run and play games simultaneously, jump three or four steps at once, and distinguish a nickel from a dime. They can name the days of the week and understand what a weeklong vacation is. They usually can print their first name.

Five-year-olds can usually ride a tricycle around the playground with speed and dexterity. They can use a hammer to pound nails. Adults should encourage them to develop motor skills and should not continually remind them to "be careful." The practice children experience will enable them to compete with others during the school-age period and will increase confidence in their own abilities. As at any age, children should not be scorned for failure to meet adult standards. Overdirection by solicitous adults is damaging. Children must learn to do tasks themselves for the experience to be satisfying.

The number and type of television or computer programs that parents allow the preschool child to watch is an important topic to discuss with the family. Although children enjoyed television at age 3 or 4 years, it was usually for short periods. They could not understand much of what was occurring. The 5-year-old, however, has better comprehension and may want to spend a great deal of time watching television or playing computer games, however they should be limited to 1 hour per day or less of screen time. Television and computers should not be allowed to interfere with good health habits, sleep, meals, and physical activity. Most parents find that children do not insist on watching television if there is something better to do.

GUIDANCE

DISCIPLINE AND LIMIT SETTING

Much has been written on the subject of discipline, views of which have changed considerably over time. Today, authorities place much importance on the development of a continuous, warm relationship between children and their parents. They believe this helps prevent many problems. The following is a brief discussion that may help the nurse in guiding parents.

Children need limits for their behaviour. Setting limits makes them feel secure, protects them from danger, and relieves them from making decisions that they may be too young to formulate. Children who are taught acceptable behaviour may have more friends and develop good self-esteem. The manner in which discipline or limit setting is handled varies from culture to culture. Individual differences occur among families and between parents and vary according to the characteristics of each child.

The purpose of discipline is to teach and to gradually shift control from parents to the child—that is, to develop self-discipline or self-control. Positive reinforcement for appropriate behaviour has been cited as more effective than punishment for poor behaviour. Expectations must be appropriate to the age and understanding of the child. The nurse should encourage parents to try to be consistent, because mixed messages are confusing for the learner.

In order to be effective, discipline must be administered at the time the incident occurs. It should also be adapted to the seriousness of the infraction. The child's self-worth must always be considered and preserved. It may be helpful to warn the preschool child who appears to be getting into trouble. However, too many warnings without follow-up lead to ineffectiveness. For the most part, spankings are not productive and can be physically and psychologically damaging. The child associates the fury of the parents with the pain rather than with the wrong deed, because anger can be the predominant factor in the situation. Therefore, there is no real positive outcome in spanking children. Spanking in anger administered by parents as a release for their own pent-up emotions is totally inappropriate and can lead to child abuse charges. In addition, the parent serves as a role model of aggression. Whether a parent is affectionate, warm, or cold (uncaring) also plays a role in the effectiveness of child rearing and the development of personality responses in the child.

Time-out periods, usually lasting 1 minute per year of age, with the child sitting in a chair out of the way of activity is considered an effective discipline technique. There should be no interaction or eye contact during the time-out period, and a timer with a buzzer should be used to signal the end of the time-out. Often a child will attempt interaction during this period by asking, "How much more time is left?" The child should learn that any interaction restarts the timer at zero. Using the child's room or a soft comfortable chair for time-out is not effective, because the child may fall asleep or engage in another activity, and the objective of time-out is defeated. Time-out should be preceded by a short (no longer than 10-word) explanation of the reason and followed by a short (no more than 10 words) restatement of why it was necessary. Longer explanations are not effective for young children. If the child knows the rules and the behaviour that will precipitate a time-out and receives no more than one warning that there will be a time-out if the undesirable behaviour continues, they will learn self-control. Consistency is the key to helping the child learn acceptable behaviour. Parents must be taught to resist using power and authority for their own sake. As the child matures and understands more clearly, privileges can be withheld as a consequence for undesirable behaviour. The reasons for such actions need to be carefully explained.

Reward

Rewarding the child for good behaviour is a positive and effective method of discipline. This can be done with hugs, smiles, tone of voice, and praise. Praise can always be tied with the act, such as "Thank you, Sophia, for picking up your toys," or "Daniel, I appreciate your standing quietly like that." The encouragement of positive behaviour eliminates many of the undesirable effects of punishment.

Rewards should not be confused with bribes. The parent may offer a child a reward if they behave well in a specific situation *before* an incident occurs. For example, the parent may say, "You may pick out one small toy after we are finished shopping if you behave during this trip." If this agreement is not made *before* an incident and the child misbehaves and *then* is offered one small toy to behave, this is a bribe that serves to reinforce the bad behaviour and is not a desirable technique of behaviour management.

Consistency and Modelling

Being consistent is difficult for parents. Realistically, it is only an ideal for which to strive—no parent is consistent all the time. Consistency must exist *between* parents as well as within each parent. It is suggested that parents establish a general style for what, when, how, and to what degree punishment is appropriate for misconduct. Parents who are lax or erratic in discipline and who alternate it with punishment have children who experience increased behavioural difficulties.

Modelling, or setting a good example by parents, significantly influences children's education. Children identify and imitate adult behaviour, both verbal and nonverbal. Parents who are aggressive and repeatedly lose control demonstrate the power of action over words. Those who communicate well, show respect and encouragement, and set appropriate limits are more positive role models. Finally, parents may need assistance in reviewing parental discipline during their own childhood to recognize destructive patterns that they may be repeating. Modelling also involves teaching a child how to be self-sufficient and responsible. Asking children to do simple chores around the house is a good way to make them feel good about themselves; it gives them an opportunity to please the parent and to learn at the same time, as long as the chore is not expected to be performed with expertise. Some chores a preschooler can perform include setting the table, sorting coloured and white laundry, and picking up toys. If the chore is associated with a positive outcome, the concept of consequences can be learned. For example, "If we pick up the toys quickly, then we will have time to read a story before bedtime."

JEALOUSY

Jealousy is a normal response to actual, supposed, or threatened loss of affection. Both children and adults may feel insecure in their relationship with the person they love. The closer children are to their parents, the greater is their fear of losing them. Children may envy the newborn. They love the sibling but resent their presence; this is known as sibling rivalry. They cannot understand the turmoil within themselves (Fig. 16.4). Jealousy of a new sibling is strongest in children less than 5 years of age and is shown in various ways. Children may be aggressive and may bite or pinch, or they may be rather discreet and may hug and kiss the infant with a determined look on their face. Another common situation is children's attempts to identify with the infant. They revert to wetting the bed or may want to try the breast or bottle feed, but it is usually a big disappointment to them.

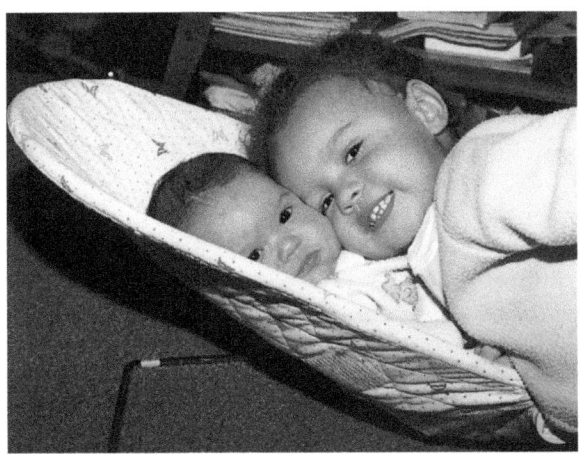

Fig. 16.4 A child and new sibling. A new sibling is welcomed into the home. Both children need attention to minimize the development of jealousy.

Preschool children may be jealous of the attention that their mother gives to their other parent. They may also envy the children they play with if they have bigger and better toys. There is less jealousy in an only child, who is the centre of attention and has a minimum number of rivals. Siblings of varied ages are apt to feel that the younger ones are "pets" or that the older ones have more special privileges.

Parents can help to reduce jealousy by the early management of individual occurrences. Preparing young children for the arrival of the new brother or sister assists with the adaptation. They should not be made to think that they are being crowded. If the newborn is going to occupy their crib, it is best to settle the older child happily in a large bed before the infant is born. Children should feel that they are helping with care of the infant. Parents can inflate their egos from time to time by reminding them of the many activities they can do that the infant cannot. Some hospitals offer sibling courses that assist parents in helping their children to overcome jealousy.

If the child tends to hit the infant or another child, both children must be separated. The child who has caused or is about to cause the injury needs as much attention as the victim, if not more. Similar aggressiveness is seen when the child is made to share toys. It is even more difficult to learn to share the primary caregiver, so the child must be given time to adjust to new situations. Children need to be assured that they are loved but also told that they cannot injure others.

THUMB SUCKING

Thumb sucking is an instinctual behavioural pattern and is considered normal. It is often seen by ultrasound about the twenty-ninth week of embryonic life. Although the cause is not fully understood, it satisfies and comforts the infant. Non-nutritive sucking in the form of thumb sucking or use of a pacifier has several documented benefits in the first year of life—when the infant is in the oral phase of development. Increased weight gain, decreased crying, the development of self-consoling ability, and increased behavioural organization have been documented in infants who have been allowed to suck unrestrained.

Finger or thumb sucking will not have a detrimental effect on the teeth as long as the habit is discontinued before 5 years of age. Most children give up the habit by the time they reach school age, although they may regress during periods of stress or fatigue. Education and support of the parents to relieve their anxiety about thumb sucking are important. The child who is trying to stop thumb sucking should be given praise and encouragement.

ENURESIS

Pathophysiology

Enuresis is involuntary urination after the age at which bladder control should have been established. The term *enuresis* is derived from the Greek word *enourein,* "to void urine." Bed-wetting has existed for generations and is found in many cultures. There are two types: primary and secondary. *Primary enuresis* refers to bed-wetting in the child who has never been dry. *Secondary enuresis* refers to a recurrence in a child who has been dry for a period of 1 year or more. *Diurnal,* or daytime, wetting is less common than *nocturnal,* or nighttime, episodes. It is more common in boys than in girls, and there may be a genetic influence involving chromosomes 12 and 13 (Elder, 2016). In some cases, organic causes of nocturnal enuresis include urinary tract infections, diabetes mellitus, diabetes insipidus, seizure disorders, obstructive uropathy, abnormalities of the urinary tract, and sleep disorders. Maturational delays of the nervous system and small bladder capacity have also been suggested as causes. Stressful events can also precipitate bed-wetting.

Approximately 92% of children achieve daytime dryness by 5 years of age (Elder, 2016). By 12 to 14 years of age, approximately 98% of children remain dry during the night. Sometimes enuresis is the result of inappropriate toilet learning. Parents who demand early toilet learning can cause a child to rebel and defy them by continuing to wet the bed. Parents who are not alert to the needs of the child may not recognize the readiness to become toilet independent and therefore frustrate the child's efforts to master this developmental task.

Treatment and Nursing Care

A detailed physical and psychological history is obtained. Factors such as the pattern of wetting, number of times per night or per week, number of daytime voidings, type of stream, dysuria, amount of fluid taken between dinner and bedtime, family history, stress, and reactions of parents and child are documented. The nurse also investigates any medications that the child may be taking and determines the extent to which the child's social life is inhibited by the problem, such as the inability to spend the night away from home. Developmental landmarks, including toilet training, are reviewed. If there appears to be an organic cause, appropriate blood and urine studies are undertaken. In most cases, the physical findings are negative.

Education of the family is crucial to prevent secondary emotional problems. Parents need to be reassured that many children experience enuresis and that it is self-limited. Power struggles, shame, and guilt are fruitless and destructive. Reassurance and support by the nurse are of great help, and children for whom enuresis is not distressing should not receive treatment (Feldman & CPS Community Pediatrics Committee, 2005/2016).

It is essential that the child be the centre of the management program. Liquids and caffeine-containing food after dinner should be limited, and the child should routinely void before going to bed. The child should also be included in morning clean-up in a nonpunitive manner.

The CPS (Feldman & CPS Community Pediatrics Committee, 2005/2016) recommends the following regarding treatment of enuresis:

- A conditioning alarm system is the most effective therapy, but it will be successful in the long term in less than 50% of children.
- Pharmacological therapy with desmopressin acetate has a place in special situations, such as at camp and sleepovers, or when the alarm system is impractical or not effective. Special care should be taken to avoid consuming fluids for 1 hour before and 8 hours after taking desmopressin. In difficult circumstances, imipramine hydrochloride may be used with caution but requires careful explanation to parents about the danger of overdose. Imipramine has a variety of adverse effects, including mood and sleep disturbances and gastrointestinal upsets. Overdose can lead to cardiac dysrhythmias, which may be life-threatening. Dosage and administration should be closely supervised. It is not recommended for children less than 6 years of age. Most children do not require imipramine hydrochloride.
- Treatment of primary nocturnal enuresis should be aimed at minimizing the emotional impact on the child. There is insufficient evidence about the good versus harm that behavioural therapies may exert in this regard. The response to various therapies is highly individual. Overzealous treatment is to be avoided. A nonpunitive, matter-of-fact attitude is most prudent.

PRESCHOOL

Attending preschool is a big step toward independence. At this age, children are adjusting to the outside world as well as to the family. Some children have the complicating factor of a new brother or sister in the house.

Many parents work outside the home and find it necessary to provide alternative care settings for their children. Some parents seek preschool experiences for their child to enhance growth and development by providing experience with playmates. Nurses can provide guidance to parents in selecting an appropriate preschool to meet their child's needs. Preschool programs provide structured activities that foster group cooperation and the development of coping skills. The child can gain self-confidence and positive self-esteem in a good preschool program. Qualified preschool teachers are objective in their interaction with the child and often can detect problems that can be followed up before the child enters kindergarten.

The following list of suggestions can guide the nurse in helping parents to select a facility appropriate for their child:

- The facility should be licensed by the province or territory.
- Teachers prepared in early childhood education should staff the preschool.
- The staff-to-student ratio should be reviewed; a one-to-eight staff-to-child ratio is the guideline.
- The philosophies of the facility, including discipline procedures, environmental safety, sanitary provisions, fee schedules, and facilities for snacks, meals, and rest time, should be reviewed.
- Schedules and facilities for active/passive and indoor/outdoor play should be reviewed.
- The school should routinely require a personal and health history of the child before admission to the program.
- The parent should visit the preschool and personally observe the environment. Talking with the parents of other children attending the school is helpful. There should be an open line of communication between staff and parents.
- Children usually start preschool between ages 2 and 5 years. Most sessions last about 3 hours.

DAILY CARE

The child between ages 3 and 6 years does not require the extensive physical care given to an infant but usually needs a bath every 1 to 2 days and a shampoo at least twice a week. Dental hygiene and nutrition are discussed in Chapter 13.

CLOTHING

Clothes should be loose enough so they don't restrict movement but allow for active play without hems getting stepped on or tripped over. Simple clothes make it easy for preschoolers to dress themselves. A place in the closet that is reachable for the child to easily hang up their clothes can help in this regard.

Preschool children should dress and undress themselves as much as they can. The child's parents can assist with dressing and undressing the child but should not take over.

Shoes should be sturdy and supportive. Protective gear such as helmets for bicycling must be a natural part of dressing for play activities. Dressing appropriately for the weather that will be encountered is essential. Flame-retardant sleepwear is available in most stores.

ACCIDENT PREVENTION

Accidents are still a major threat during the years from 3 to 5. At this age, children may suffer injuries from a bad fall. Preschool children hurry up and down stairs. They climb trees and stand up on swings. They play hard with their toys, particularly those they can mount. Stairways must be kept free of clutter. Shoes should have rubber soles, and new ones should be purchased when the tread of older shoes becomes smooth. When buying toys, parents must be sure they are sturdy and age appropriate. Preschool children should not be asked to do anything that is potentially dangerous, such as carrying a glass container or sharp knife to the kitchen sink.

Automobiles continue to be a threat. Children need to be taught where they can safely ride their tricycles and where they can play ball. They must not play in or around the car or be left alone in the car. The use of car seats continues to be important (see Chapter 15).

Burns that occur at this age often result from the child's experimentation with matches or lighters. Burns from hot coffee are also common. These items are common hazards for this age group; they should be kept well out of reach, and their dangers should be explained to the child.

Poisoning is still a danger for this age group. Children try to imitate adults and are apt to sample pills, especially if they are bright in colour. Their increased freedom brings them into contact with many interesting containers in the bathroom, garage, or basement.

Preschool children should also be taught the dangers of talking to or accepting rides from strangers. If a driver stops them, they should run to the house of people they know. Parents should make it clear to children in preschool that they will never send a stranger to pick them up. Preschools have strict guidelines regarding who can pick children up. Children must know the dangers of playing in lonely places and of accepting gifts from strangers. Children should always know where to go if the parents or babysitter cannot be found. Preschool children still require a good deal of indirect supervision to protect them from dangers that arise from their immature judgement or social environment (Fig. 16.5).

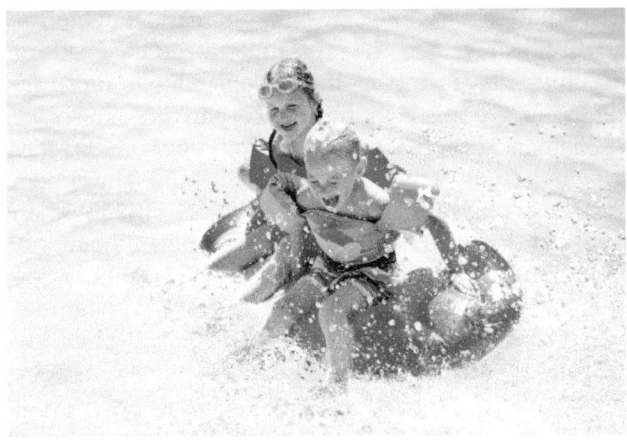

Fig. 16.5 Unsupervised water play can quickly lead to unexpected injuries. (istock.com/FamVeld)

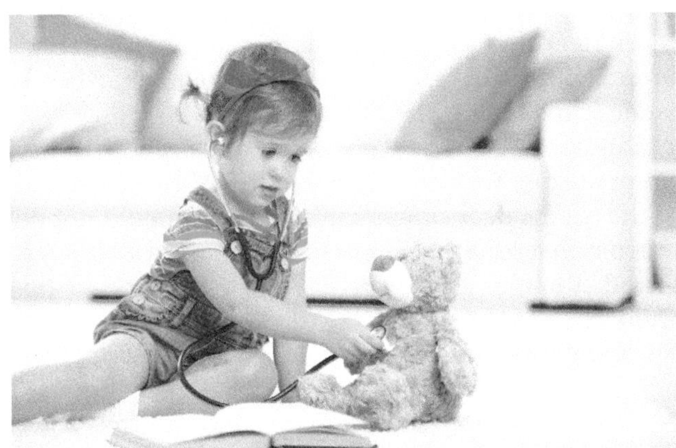

Fig. 16.6 A self-image begins to develop during the preschool years with imaginative play. (Evgeny Atamanenko/Shutterstock.com.)

PLAY DURING HEALTH AND ILLNESS

VALUE OF PLAY

Play is important to the physical, mental, emotional, and social development of both healthy and sick children (Fig. 16.6). Children climbing on a jungle gym develop muscles and coordination as they exercise all parts of their bodies. They use energy and develop self-confidence. Their imagination may take them to the jungle, where they swing from limb to limb. They may face imagined fears and solve problems that would be much more trying, if not impossible, in reality. They communicate with other children and take a further step in developing moral values, that is, taking one's turn and considering others. Other types of play help children learn colours, shapes, sizes, and textures and can enhance creativity. Nursing and health care personnel must be able to tap this natural and readily available outlet. Children may be unfamiliar with every facet of the hospital, but they know how to play, and playing is a good way for the nurse to establish rapport with children.

THE NURSE'S ROLE

Some hospitals have well-established playroom programs supervised by play therapists. Play therapy is an important part of every pediatric nursing care plan.

It is not necessary to be an expert in manual dexterity, art, or music; rather, one must understand the needs of the child. Play is not just the responsibility of those assigned to it, nor is it confined to certain times or shifts.

Many factors are involved in providing suitable play for children of various ages in the hospital. The child's state of health affects the amount of activity in which they can participate. The nurse can facilitate many activities that relieve stress and provide enjoyment for the child who has been prescribed bed rest. Overstimulation would be hazardous for some severely ill children. Nurses should always be on guard for signs of fatigue in patients and use their judgement accordingly.

The diagnosis of the hospitalized child should also be considered when choosing an appropriate toy. For example, a friction toy is inappropriate for a child in an oxygen-rich environment. Sparks from the toy could cause an explosion. A stuffed animal may not be an appropriate toy for a child with asthma, who may be allergic to the contents of the stuffing.

Safety must also be considered in selecting an appropriate toy. Toys should be safe, durable, and suited to the child's developmental level. Toys should not be sharp or have parts that are easily removed and swallowed. Providing too many toys at one time to the child can be confusing. Complicated toys are frustrating and disappointing. Well-selected toys such as crayons, blocks, and dolls are useful throughout the years. Boys and girls often enjoy playing with the same toys. A washable laundry bag tied to a hospitalized child's bed can be used to store the child's own toys neatly and safely. Toys may be taken home with the child or discarded after they are discharged from the hospital.

Each child needs sufficient time to complete an activity. In general, for both well and sick children quiet play should precede meals and bedtime. During routine procedures, the nurse can entertain the child with nursery rhymes, stories, nonsense games, songs, finger play, or puppets. Often the other children on the unit can be included in the game "I'm thinking of something blue, red, and green," and so forth. Simple crafts are fun. Scrapbooks are entertaining. Children may even enjoy making a storybook about their hospital experience. The nurse involved in enrichment programs for children can definitely make a positive contribution. Surprise boxes in which a gift is opened daily provide a sense of anticipation for the patient. Collections of scraps can be started consisting of bright ribbons, bits of string, pipe cleaners, paper bags, newspapers, or bits of cotton. Because the turnover of patients is rapid, many projects can be repeated with different children.

CDs, computers, electronic tablets, mp3 players, and instruments can provide music for the child to listen to. Older children enjoy sending emails and text messages to friends. Special children's recordings and films are available. The services of a music therapist are available in some institutions. Drawing materials, finger paints, and modelling clay foster expression and creativity. They require only a flat surface, such as the overbed table, and a particular medium. The bedridden child can participate in messy projects, too; the bed is simply protected with newspapers or plastic. Children in cribs require adequate back support for such projects, by using pillows. Simple computer games may be available in the hospital setting.

Playmates may be limited in the hospital setting if the child has a condition that is communicable. However, surgical and orthopedic patients can play together in a playroom with appropriate supervision. The nurse should guide the parents in how to play *for* a child who is fatigued or weakened by illness.

TYPES OF PLAY

Preschool children need playmates to promote social development. The play characteristics of each age group are shown in Table 13.9. The preschool-age child gradually moves from parallel and associative play to cooperative play with playmates.

The play of preschool children should be noncompetitive. The healthy preschool child requires active play activities that are supervised for safety. Large construction sets, number or alphabet games, crayons, play tools, housekeeping toys, musical toys, pop-up books, large puzzles, and clay are examples of suitable toys for the preschool-age child. Active play can involve simple climbing, sliding, and running activities (Fig. 16.7). Imaginary friends are common to the preschool-age child. They serve many purposes in helping the child adjust to an expanding world and increased independence. Parents can acknowledge the presence of the imaginary friend as part of pretend play, but the responsibilities of reality do not include the pretend

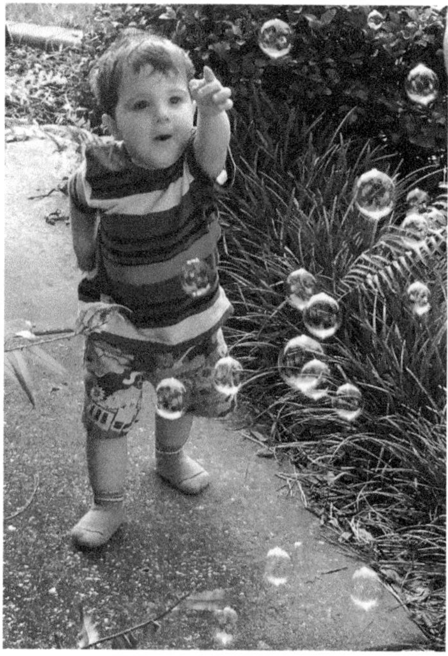

Fig. 16.7 Chasing bubbles can stimulate the imagination and promote physical exercise.

friend. Parents should not intervene in playgroups. Allowing the child to master frustration and develop social skills is essential to growth and development.

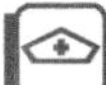 Nursing Tip

Imaginary playmates are common and normal during the preschool period and serve many purposes, such as relief from loneliness, mastery of feats, and provision of a "scapegoat."

Play and the Child With a Neurodevelopmental, Sensory, or Motor Disorder

The child with a neurodevelopmental, sensory, or motor disorder needs more stimulation through play than the child who is not challenged by these conditions. The nurse must consider the cognitive age and motor ability of the child rather than the chronological age when guiding parents about the selection of toys. The environment should be as colourful and bright as possible. The child may be introduced to objects of various sizes and textures. Play with other children must be supervised because the possible poor judgement of neurodevelopmentally impaired children may lead them into difficulty. They may be aggressive and unaware of their own strength. Adequate space is necessary in which the children can run. These children should be brought into group play gradually. Materials are presented one at a time.

Neurodevelopmentally or motor-impaired children may need to be taught how to play, because they may not have had the preschool play experience of the child without a disability. Repetition of play experiences is necessary. Equipment and play materials must be altered to accommodate the child's size and yet be suitable for the cognitive age. The nurse or teacher should improvise games and songs to meet the special needs of this group. (See Chapters 23 and 33 for a more complete discussion of the growth, development, and care of the neurodevelopmentally, sensory, or motor-impaired child.)

Therapeutic Play

Play and toys can be of therapeutic value in retraining muscles, improving eye–hand coordination, and helping children crawl and walk (push-pull toys). A musical instrument such as the clarinet promotes flexion and extension of the fingers. Blowing is an excellent prerequisite for speech therapy. Therapists supervise such activities. They leave specific instructions if they wish their work to be reinforced on the unit. Blowing out the light of a flashlight as if it were a candle is **therapeutic play** for a postoperative preschool child.

Play Therapy

Play therapy is a technique used for the child under stress. A well-equipped playroom is provided. Children are free to play with whatever articles they choose. A counsellor may be in the room observing and talking with the child, or the child may be observed through a one-way glass window. By using these as well as other methods, the therapist obtains a better understanding of the patient's struggles, fears, resentments, and feelings toward self and others. When children act out their feelings through "dramatic play," the feelings are externalized, which relieves tension. The interpretation of child behaviour is complex and should be done by a qualified therapist.

Art Therapy

Art therapy is useful in communicating with children. It is becoming more widely used. The art therapist is especially trained to assist children in expressing their feelings and communicating through drawings, clay, and other media. Some hospitals with inpatient mental health units have art therapy departments.

NURSING IMPLICATIONS OF PRESCHOOL GROWTH AND DEVELOPMENT

The nurse should anticipate parental concern with nutritional problems in the preschool child. Daily appetites may fluctuate widely, but the weekly pattern will probably show stability to meet the child's growth needs. During clinic visits the parents can be guided to provide age-appropriate foods at mealtimes in appropriate portions. The child's developing self-regulatory mechanism will determine how much they will eat based on feelings of hunger or satiety. Efforts to control the preschool child's intake may result in power struggles or patterns of overeating or undereating.

Safety is a high priority in this active age range. "Childproofing" the home and the need for adequate supervision and safety equipment during sports activities should be emphasized. Preschoolers, who will be given immunizations via a needle, can be calmed by giving pretend needles to their doll and having a parent present to comfort the doll. Explanations such as "the needle will hurt just a little but will prevent you from getting sick" are beyond the Piaget preoperational level of understanding of the preschool child. The ability to understand detailed explanations is not yet present in preschool-age children, even if verbal ability is high. The preschool-age child may have unfounded fears that respond best to reassurance and "protection" by parents, rather than reasoning about why the fear is unfounded.

The nurse should provide parental guidance concerning the changing behaviour patterns of the preschool-age child. The characteristic alternating dependence and independence can be frustrating for parents. Parents who do not volunteer any positive comments about their child during conversations may require further investigation and interview. Problems with day care and discipline must be discussed. The use of corporal punishment (spanking) as a major disciplinary technique can lead to child abuse. The use of time-out and alternative methods of discipline should be emphasized.

Hospitalization can be frightening to a preschool child who is egocentric and prone to magical thinking. Because the preschool child cannot fully understand cause and effect, they may perceive hospitalization as punishment for behaviour. The preschool child may feel abandoned by the parents and continues to be subject to separation anxiety. Separation anxiety (see Chapter 19) is manifested by the stages of *protest, despair,* and *detachment*, and *regression* to earlier behaviours may also occur. Bed-wetting is common in the hospitalized preschool-age child; parents should be encouraged to be patient and positive. Assigning a consistent caregiver and providing age-appropriate diversional activities are essential for a hospitalized preschool-age child.

The nurse who is with children daily can describe their behaviour. What is the child's approach to play? Does the child join in freely or linger outside the group? Does the child prefer active or quiet activities? Does the child seem to tolerate frustrations? Can the child talk with their playmates and convey ideas? What type of attention span does the child have? These observations and charting are meaningful and promote better understanding and appropriate interventions by nurses and other health care personnel.

Get Ready for the Certification Examination!

Key Points

- The child aged 3 to 5 years is often referred to as the *preschool child.* During this period, the child grows taller and loses the chubbiness of the toddler period.
- The major tasks of the preschool child include preparation to enter school, development of a cooperative type of play, control of body functions, acceptance of separation, and increase in communication skills, memory, and attention span.
- The Canadian Paediatric Society recommends that screen time for children 2 to 5 years of age be limited to 1 hour per day and that this should be supervised by parents.
- Gross and fine motor skills become more developed, as evidenced by participation in running, skipping, and drawing pictures.
- Piaget refers to the preschool period as one in which symbolic thought processes and language emerge.
- Erikson's preschool stage involves the development of initiative.
- Kohlberg's theory concerning preschoolers refers to moral development and the beginning awareness of the needs of others.
- Language ability develops rapidly, and the child is able to construct rather complicated sentences by the end of this period.
- The many questions of the preschool child must be listened to carefully and answered thoughtfully and truthfully.
- Play is the business of children. It contributes to physical and mental well-being by encouraging communication, socialization, and outlets for energy.
- Cooperative and highly imaginative play is characteristic of the preschool child.
- Social issues of the preschool period include learning to share and to control impulses.
- Common concerns of parents during this period include how to set limits, handle jealousy, and respond to the child's thumb sucking and masturbation.
- Corporal punishment of the preschool child can nurture rebellion and aggression. Appropriate discipline techniques can assist the child in developing self-control.
- Primary enuresis refers to bed-wetting in a child who has never been dry. Secondary enuresis refers to bed-wetting in a child who has been dry for a period of 1 year or more.
- Careful evaluation of preschool programs is important to ensure high-quality care.
- Accidents are still a major hazard for preschool children because of the child's immature judgement and increased locomotive skills.
- During the preschool years, the parents need guidance in understanding the developmental road map of physical, emotional, and cognitive growth to help the child meet life's challenges and goals and to enrich family interaction.

Additional Learning Resources

evolve Go to your Evolve website (http://evolve.elsevier.com/Canada/Leifer) for the following learning resources:

- Answer Key for Critical Thinking Questions
- Answer Key for Textbook Review Questions
- Audio Glossary
- Interactive Review Questions
- Skills Performance Checklists
- Video clips and more!

Online Resource

- Canadian Pediatric Society–Caring for Kids: https://www.caringforkids.cps.ca/

Review Questions

1. When selecting play activities for a healthy 4-year-old, a parent should be guided to understand that the 4-year-old enjoys doing which of the following?
   a. Solitary play, sitting next to a friend
   b. Cooperative play with friends
   c. Competitive play with teams
   d. Observing rather than participating

2. Which is an example of a therapeutic play activity for a preschool child who is recovering from an appendectomy?
   a. Wii game of bowling
   b. Blowing bubbles
   c. Reading a storybook
   d. Colouring with crayons
3. A nurse is guiding a parent to manage enuresis in their child. What would be the most appropriate suggestion by the nurse?
   a. Wake the child often during the night and take him to the bathroom to void.
   b. Limit liquids after dinner and have the child void before going to bed.
   c. Use a consistent technique of discipline whenever the bed is wet.
   d. Keep the child in diapers until bed-wetting is no longer a problem.
4. Which is the appropriate amount of time to use in a time-out period for a 3-year-old child?
   a. 1 minute
   b. 3 minutes
   c. 5 minutes
   d. 10 minutes
5. What does Erikson's stage for a 4-year-old child focus on?
   a. Autonomy
   b. Industry
   c. Initiative
   d. Identity
6. A parent asks a nurse if her preschool child can be allowed to have screen time since her older brother uses the electronic tablet. What would be an appropriate response of the nurse? *(Select all that apply.)*
   a. Screen time should be limited to 1 hour per day of quality programs.
   b. Parents should be present when the child is using the electronic tablet.
   c. Screen time should be balanced with active play during the day.
   d. Screen time can be allowed when the older sibling is using his tablet.
   e. Offering screen time is one way a parent can rest or get some work done in the home.

Critical Thinking Question

1. The parents of a preschool child discuss the typical play activities of their child. They express concern that they have seen their child choose to play the role of "the aggressive bad guy" in play scenarios and are concerned that he may be developing aggressive behaviour. They ask if they should stop him from assuming roles in play that are not acceptable behaviours. What is the best response of the nurse?

REFERENCES

Canadian Paediatric Society (CPS). (2017a). *Healthy sleep for your baby and child*. Retrieved from: https://www.caringforkids.cps.ca/handouts/healthy_sleep_for_your_baby_and_child.

Canadian Paediatric Society (CPS). (2017b). Screen time and young children: Promoting health and development in a digital world. *Paediatrics & Child Health, 22*(8), 461–468.

Elder, J. (2016). Enuresis and voiding dysfunction. In R. Kliegman, B. Stanton, J. St. Geme, et al. (Eds.), *Nelson textbook of pediatrics* (20th ed.). Philadelphia: Saunders.

Feldman, M., & Canadian Paediatric Society (CPS), Community Paediatrics Committee. (2005). Management of primary nocturnal enuresis. *Paediatrics & Child Health, 10*(10), 611–614. Updated 2013, Reaffirmed 2016.

Simms, M. D. (2016). Language development and communication disorders. In R. Kliegman, B. Stanton, J. St. Geme, et al. (Eds.), *Nelson textbook of pediatrics* (20th ed.). Philadelphia: Saunders.

17 The School-Age Child

http://evolve.elsevier.com/Canada/Leifer

Cheryl Dika

Objectives

1. Define each key term listed.
2. Contrast two major theoretical viewpoints regarding personality development during the school years.
3. Describe the physical and psychosocial development of children from 5 to 12 years of age, listing age-specific events and type of guidance where appropriate.
4. Discuss how to assist parents in preparing a child for school.
5. List two ways in which school life influences the growing child.
6. Discuss accident prevention in this age group.
7. Discuss the role of the nurse in providing guidance and health supervision for the school-age child.
8. Discuss the value of pet ownership for the healthy school-age child.

Key Terms

concrete operations
gender identity
latchkey children
preadolescent (prē-ăd-ō-LĔS-ĕnt)
sexual latency
stage of industry

GENERAL CHARACTERISTICS

School-age children (5 to 12 years of age) differ from preschool children in that they are more engrossed in fact than in fantasy and are capable of more sophisticated reasoning. School-age children develop their first close peer relationships outside the family group and their first affiliation with adults outside their family who will influence their lives in a significant way.

As a result of the increased contact with the outside world and increased cognitive abilities, school-age children begin to understand how others evaluate them. School-age children are often judged by their performance—through good grades or athletic feats. Their sense of industry and the development of positive self-esteem are directly influenced by their ability to become an accepted member of a peer group and meet the challenges in the environment.

The school-age child must be able to pay attention in class (with at least a 45-minute attention span), understand language, and progress from the *skill* of writing or reading to *understanding* what is written or read. To succeed in school, the child must work toward a delayed reward and must risk being unsuccessful in their efforts. However, parents must be guided to understand that multiple unsuccessful experiences for their child may lead to development of a fear of trying in the future. New experiences for the school-age child include the first night sleeping away from home at a friend's house or camp, successes that are formally celebrated, chores that are dependably performed, conflict resolution with peers, and the selection of adult role models.

School-age children have an ardent thirst for knowledge and accomplishment. They tend to admire their teachers and adult companions. They use the skill and knowledge they obtain to attempt to master the activities they enjoy, including music, sports, and art. Thus, Erikson refers to this phase as the **stage of industry**. Unsuccessful adaptations at this time can lead to a sense of inferiority. Participation in group activities heightens. Romantic love for the parent of the opposite sex diminishes, and children identify with the parent of the same sex. Freud refers to this period as a time of **sexual latency**. The type of acceptance that school-age children receive at home and at school will affect the attitudes they develop about themselves and their role in life. Piaget refers to the thought processes of this period as concrete operations. See Box 17.1 for further discussion of these theories.

Concrete operations involve logical thinking and an understanding of cause and effect. The egocentric view of the preschool child is replaced by the ability to understand the point of view of another person. The child can understand the origin or consequence of an event they are experiencing. By 10 years of age, the child understands that people do not always control events in life, such as death, spirituality, or the origin of the world.

Between 5 and 12 years of age, children prefer friends of their own sex and usually prefer the

Box 17.1 Features of Major Theories of Development During Later Childhood

SIGMUND FREUD

The child is in a period of sexual latency.

The child's repression of sexuality makes it possible to form same-sex friendships; the child assumes the role of leader or follower.

The child is heavily influenced by parents and teachers, who can bolster the child's self-image or more deeply repress sexuality.

ERIK ERIKSON

Other people heavily influence the child's development.

The child's leadership abilities and popularity depend on successfully controlling the environment.

By learning to be productive, self-directing, and accepted at school and in society, the child gains a positive self-concept.

JEAN PIAGET

The child can concentrate on more than one aspect of a situation at a time.

The child becomes capable of abstract reasoning, but thought is still limited to their own experience.

The child understands cause and effect.

company of their friends to that of their brothers and sisters. Outward displays of affection by adults may be embarrassing to them. Although they are now too big to cuddle on their parents' laps, they still require much love, support, and guidance.

Between 5 and 12 years of age, self-esteem becomes very important in the developmental process. Children are evaluated according to their social contribution, such as the ability to attain good grades, hit home runs, or earn a yellow belt in karate class (Fig. 17.1). Children's feelings about themselves are very important and should be assessed.

PHYSICAL GROWTH

Growth is slow until the spurt directly before puberty. Weight gains are more rapid than increases in height. The average gain in weight per year is about 2.5 to 3.2 kg (5.5 to 7 lb). The average increase in height is approximately 5.0 cm (2 inches). Growth in head circumference is slower than before, because myelinization within the brain is complete by 7 years of age. Head circumference increases from 51 to 53.5 cm between 5 and 12 years of age. At the end of this time, the brain has reached approximately adult size. (Dentition and nutrition are discussed in Chapter 13.)

Muscular coordination is improved, and the lymphatic tissues become highly developed. The skeletal bones continue to ossify, and the body has a lower centre of gravity. The body is supple, and skeletal growth is sometimes more rapid than growth of muscles and ligaments. The child may appear "gangling." There is a noticeable change in facial structures as the jaw lengthens. The sinuses are often sites of infection. The 6-year

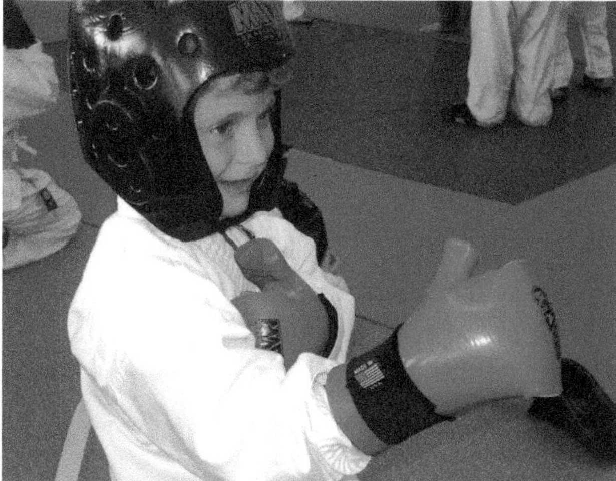

Fig. 17.1 School-age children are often evaluated by their peers according to their performance, such as achieving good grades or demonstrating their ability to spar by earning a yellow belt in karate.

molars (the first permanent teeth) erupt. The loss of primary teeth begins at about age 6 years, and about four permanent teeth erupt per year. The gastro-intestinal tract is more mature, and the stomach is upset less often. Stomach capacity increases, and caloric needs are less than in preschool years. The heart grows slowly and is now smaller in proportion to body size than at any other time of life.

The shape of the eye changes with growth. The age at which 20/20 vision occurs is probably sometime during the preschool years. The capabilities of the child's sense organs, including hearing, have an important bearing on learning abilities.

The vital signs of the child of school age are near those of the adult. See Appendix A for vital signs ranges. Boys are slightly taller and somewhat heavier than girls until changes indicating puberty appear. The differences among children are greater at the end of middle childhood than at the beginning.

The changes in body proportions help the child prepare for activities commonly enjoyed in school. However, size is not correlated with emotional maturity, and a problem is created when a child faces higher expectations because they are taller and heavier than their peers. Sedentary activities and habits in the school-age child are associated with a high risk of developing obesity and cardiovascular problems later in life.

SEXUAL DEVELOPMENT

Gender Identity

The sex organs remain immature during the school-age years, but interest in gender differences increases as the child progresses to puberty. Gender role development is greatly influenced by parents through differential treatment and identification. These two interdependent processes are at work in the family and in society. In infancy, boys and girls are often wrapped in blue or pink blankets. Later, their dress, the types of toys and games chosen for them, television, and the attitudes of family members may serve to fortify gender identity, although many families make an attempt to offer children gender-neutral activities and clothes.

The influence of the school environment is considerable. The teacher can have an impact on eliminating stereotyping through the assignment of schoolroom tasks, the choice of textbooks, and by not disapproving of behaviour that deviates from the child's gender role.

Gender identity is important starting at an early age. As early as 6 or 7 years old, a child may feel their sex assigned to them at birth differs from their gender identity. This can lead to social anxiety as they realize they do not feel the same as their peers, yet they want to be the same as them. Health care providers can play an important role in helping parents work through their questions regarding differences between sex, gender identity, gender expression, and sexual orientation (Canadian Paediatric Society [CPS], 2018). Providing an environment where parents and caregivers show love and acceptance to the child for who they are will help the child thrive.

Sex Education

Sex education is a lifelong process. Parents convey their attitudes and feelings about all aspects of life, including sexuality, to the growing child. Sex education is accomplished less by talking or formal instruction than by the whole climate of the home, particularly the respect shown to each family member.

Children's questions about sex should be answered simply and at their level of understanding. Correct names should be used to describe the genitalia. All people understand the hospitalized child who says, "My penis hurts." Private masturbation is normal and is practiced by both males and females at various times throughout their lives. It is not harmful. The young boy must be prepared for erections and nocturnal emissions ("wet dreams"), which are to be expected and are not necessarily the result of masturbation. The young girl needs to be prepared for menarche and provided with the necessary supplies. This is particularly important to the early maturer because an elementary school may not provide dispensing machines for supplies in the washrooms.

Both sexes are concerned during the school years with the disproportion of their bodies, and they may be self-conscious when undressing. They may compare themselves with their friends. They need reassurance about their awakening sexuality, which affects their thoughts and behaviour.

The initiation of sex education in schools varies across Canada. Some schools teach the anatomical names of body parts in kindergarten, while others report that sex education begins later in grade 5 or 6. Education including sexually transmitted infections (STIs) and their prevention is more consistent between grades 5 and 7. Topics such as sexual consent, Internet safety, and sexting vary among provinces and schools (Abortion Rights Coalition of Canada, 2017).

Factual knowledge concerning sex, alcohol, and drugs is an essential component of sex education, both in the home and at school. Nurses can assist in preparing sex education programs, used mainly in public settings, and the participation of parents is valuable. Sex education can be taught in the context of the normal process and function of the human body. Facts must be provided, and values clarification can be added, although this is also influenced by parents' views. If children realize that their parents are uncomfortable with discussing sex, they may turn to peers, who often supply erroneous and distorted information. The Sexuality Information and Education Council of Canada (SIECCAN) maintains that sex education programs should be accessible to all Canadians and be relevant for their needs—for example, those particular to sexual minorities, individuals with disabilities, and socioeconomically disadvantaged individuals (SIECCAN, 2008).

Regardless of the practice setting, nurses can help parents and children with sex education through careful listening and anticipatory guidance (Table 17.1). They can teach decision-making skills and responsibility. Nurses should review normal developmental behaviour and explain age-specific information. They can provide families with useful written information that stresses sexuality as a healthful rather than an illness-related concept. The nurse should always consider cultural differences when counselling families.

Sexually transmitted infections

Education concerning prevention of contracting an STI and human immunodeficiency virus (HIV) should be presented in simple terms. Audiovisual materials are available that are designed for the school-age child. Factual information about STIs and concrete information on how to say "no" to sexual intercourse and drugs are essential components in the sex education of the preadolescent. The nurse can help to implement educational programs in the school, the clinic, and community organizations. The facts concerning the harmful effects of drugs and unprotected sex should be communicated to the child without using scare tactics.

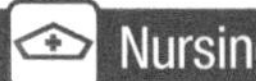

Nursing Tip

When discussing sexuality with school-age children, it is necessary to review slang or street terms. Most children hear the terms but may be confused about their meanings.

INFLUENCES FROM THE WIDER WORLD

SCHOOL-RELATED TASKS

The home, school, and neighbourhood each have an impact on the growth and development of the child. Schools have a profound influence on the socialization of children, who bring to school what they have learned and experienced in the home. Although many children come from healthy, intact, and financially secure families, many do not. The environment, family composition, and social determinants of health have an impact on the development of a child (see Chapter 1). Nurses must remember these factors, because they surface especially with this age group. Moral development occurs as they have experience with and understand rules and fairness. An understanding of what is right and wrong and the development of values occur as a result of their experience.

Children may be unable to verbalize their needs; therefore, caretakers must become particularly astute in their observations. Table 17.2 reviews the expected growth and developmental abilities related to required school tasks. Success in school requires an integration of cognitive, receptive, and expressive (language) skills. Repeating a grade in school can seriously impair self-image, thus it is important to identify deficits or health problems that affect learning as early as possible and provide opportunities to overcome these if possible.

A holistic attitude toward child care must focus not only on intellectual achievement and test scores but also on such qualities as artistic expression, creativity, joy, cooperation, responsibility, industry, love, and other attributes. The sensitive nurse can assist parents by affirming the individuality of children and by encouraging parents to share with their children the pride they experience as their children learn and progress through the elementary grades. The Patient Teaching box summarizes parental guidance that the nurse may find useful in helping them prepare their children for the beginning of school.

Table 17.1 Using the Nursing Process in Sex Education of the School-Age Child

INTERVENTION	OBSERVATION
Data collection, history taking	Readiness to learn is indicated by asking questions concerning sex, menstruation, "wet dreams," and pregnancy.
Analysis	Observe parent–child interactions and determine level of communication. Observe peer interaction to determine the child's self-image, self-confidence, and ability to communicate. Observe parent's knowledge and ability to discuss issues pertaining to sex education. Determine child's understanding of sexual development and body changes.
Planning and implementation	Discuss growth and development with the parent and the child. Reinforce teaching techniques and opportunities with parents.
Evaluation	With each clinic or home visit, evaluate the results of parent–child interaction concerning sex education.

Table 17.2 Growth and Development of the School-Age Child in School-Related Tasks

CHILD'S TASK	PARENT'S TASK	NURSING INTERVENTIONS
Adapt to differences in expectations of teachers.	Communicate with teacher to maintain consistency in expectations and discipline.	Nurse can facilitate age-appropriate expectations.
Compete with 30 or more peers for adult attention.	Praise child's accomplishments. Avoid making comparisons to other children.	Evaluate parent–teacher interactions, and provide guidance and positive support.
Learn to accept criticism from peers and teachers without losing self-esteem.	Supervise peer activities. Provide constructive activities.	Provide t–parent guidance.
Assimilate peer values, and integrate with family values.	Maintain open communication. Encourage peer activity. Introduce and accept other cultures in the community.	Provide anticipatory guidance in handling behaviour problems. Observe and respond to signs of prejudice.
Find satisfaction in achievements at school.	Allow children to achieve. Do not complete tasks for them.	
Participate in group activities.	Encourage child to join a group or club and actively participate as a member.	Refer to community agencies such as cultural affiliations, organizations, and club activities as needed.
Learn self-control. Handle prejudice from others in a positive way.	Encourage participation in activities away from home and with peers. Have faith in child's problem-solving abilities. Discuss coping with prejudices of others.	Encourage parents to "let go" and provide guidance while encouraging independence.

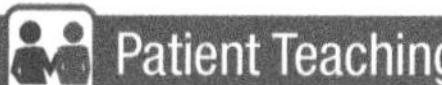

Patient Teaching

Parental Guidance for Children Starting School

Encourage parents to do the following:

- Review normal growth and development of 5- to 6-year-olds.
- Anticipate regression such as thumb sucking, clinging behaviour, and occasional soiling.
- Encourage children to express what they think school will be like.
- Arrange for children to meet others who will be entering school with them.
- Tour the school with the child.
- Introduce the child to the school crossing guard and the bus driver.
- Teach the child their family name and telephone number.
- Teach safety precautions about crossing the street and meeting strangers.
- Allow sufficient time in the morning to prepare for school.
- Encourage the child to take a special item from home (e.g., stuffed toy to provide comfort) if necessary.
- Provide a cheerful send-off.
- Walk with the child to school until the child understands the route, or designate a bus stop as appropriate for age.
- Listen to the child at the end of the day; take an interest in their school life.
- Get to know the child's teacher; take an interest in the school; attend information sessions.
- Inform the teacher of sudden or unusual stress in the child's life.
- Show interest in the child's learning.

Adapted from Ontario Ministry of Education. (2017). *Full-day kindergarten: Preparing your child*. Toronto, ON: Author. Retrieved from: http://www.edu.gov.on.ca/eng/multi/english/fdk_fs_preparing_your_child_en.pdf.

The nurse needs to observe patterns of communication between the parents and child and assist with specific behavioural issues. In general, the transition to junior high school or middle school means multiple classrooms, a series of teachers, and a change of buildings. The child is developing adult characteristics and has new feelings about their body, parents, teachers, and peers. The nurse's anticipatory guidance includes a review of normal physiology and how it changes with puberty. Information concerning sexuality is reviewed, and the child is encouraged to ask questions at the time they arise.

A warm, ongoing relationship between the parents and child helps to provide a safe atmosphere of caring. Adults should develop a heightened awareness for things such as school attendance problems, tardiness, bullying, and signs of loneliness or depression. They should continue to encourage children to discuss their school problems, feelings, and worries. Parents and children must set realistic goals. A good question for adults to contemplate periodically is "When was the last time this child had a success?" Homework should be the child's responsibility, with minimum assistance from the parents.

The nurse can guide the parents in determining health care requirements for the school-age child. Schools provide some health screening, but the financial resources of the family may prevent adequate follow-up care, clothing, or transportation. School lunch programs are available in most schools for children identified as being in need.

Safety is an important issue for the school-age child. The rules of the road should be taught before the child walks or rides a bike to school. Car safety and the use of seat belts must be a regular ritual. Caution in play is essential, but a child must not be made to feel afraid to try new activities or skills. The prevention of concussions is important, as are care postconcussion and safe return to play (See Chapter 23 for further discussion of concussions). Safe use of technology is important to teach to prevent exploitation or online bullying. (Box 17.2).

PLAY

Play activities for the school-age child involve increased physical and intellectual skills and some fantasy. The sense of belonging to a group is very important, and conformity to "being just like my friends" is of vital importance to the child. The culture of the school-age child involves membership in a group of some type.

Teams are important to growth and development, and competition is a new challenge. Participation in organized sports can develop skill, teamwork, and fitness, but excessive pressure and unrealistic expectations can have negative effects. High-stress and

Box 17.2 Internet Safety Tips for Children

- Discuss Internet expectations with your parent or caregiver.
- Keep your identity private.
- Never reveal personal information, including age or gender.
- Avoid posting pictures of yourself or friends on websites or in chat rooms.
- Assume any information posted will be available for anyone to see or read.
- First-time meetings with cyber buddies should be supervised.
- Let others know if you experience unwanted or hurtful material while online.
- People online may not be who they say they are.
- The Internet is unregulated; information found can be dangerous or illegal.

Sources: Canadian Paediatric Society. (2018). *Social media: What parents should know*. Retrieved from: https://www.caringforkids.cps.ca/handouts/social_media; Greig, A. A., Constantin, E., LeBlanc, C., Riverin, B., Tak-Sam, P., Cummings, C., & Canadian Paediatric Society, Community Paediatrics Committee. (2016). An update to the Greig health record: Preventive health care visits for children and adolescents aged 6 to 17 years—Technical report. *Paediatrics & Child Health, 21*(5), 265–268.

high-impact sports such as football are not desirable sports activities for the school-age child because of the risk of injury to the immature skeletal system.

Rituals such as collecting items and playing board games are enjoyable quiet activities for the school-age child. Television, computers, gaming consoles, smartphones, or electronic tablets are considered screen time and often considered to be a "babysitter" when overused, but many educational and exciting programs are offered during prime-time hours. Computer and video games challenge intellect and skill and are healthy outlets as long as they are educational, age appropriate, and interactive and do not completely replace active physical play. There should be a balance of physical activity and limited noneducational screen time activity. Meal times and bedrooms should be media free (CPS, 2017) (Fig. 17.2). The CPS recommends more than 60 minutes of moderate to vigorous physical activity at least three times a week, including activities that strengthen muscle and bone (Lipnowski, LeBlanc, & CPS Healthy Active Living Committee, 2012).

Play enables the child to feel powerful and in control. Mastering new skills helps the child to feel a sense of accomplishment, which is necessary to achieve Erikson's phase of industry successfully (Fig. 17.3).

Observing Play

Play is essential to a healthy lifestyle that includes a feeling of well-being and fitness. Play provides a link between the spontaneity of childhood and the disciplined activities of adulthood. Elements of play that should be assessed by care providers include the following:

- Motivation and intensity of engagement
- Whether the child initiated it or the child joined the group
- Relation to reality or creativity
- The element of choice in how to play
- Self-control
- Following or changing rules
- Sharing—giving and receiving cues from others
- Skills used in the play activity

Factors that may limit play effectiveness are adult intervention, limited space, and an older, dominant player or younger players that interfere with action.

LATCHKEY CHILDREN

latchkey children are those who are left unsupervised after school because parents are away from home or at work and extended family is not available to care for them. While many provinces have laws regarding the age of a child who can be left alone in the home, the decision should not be based solely on age (Ruiz-Casares & Radic, 2015). Children left home alone are subject to a higher rate of accidents and are at risk of feeling isolated and alone. Some children, however, enjoy the independence and become skilled in problem solving and self-care. A backup adult should be available to the child in case of emergencies.

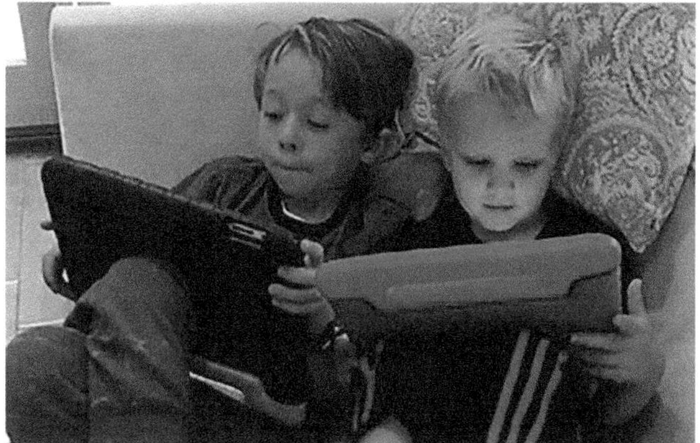

Fig. 17.2 The Canadian Paediatric Society recommends a limit of 2 hours per day of noneducational screen time for children ages 5 to 17.

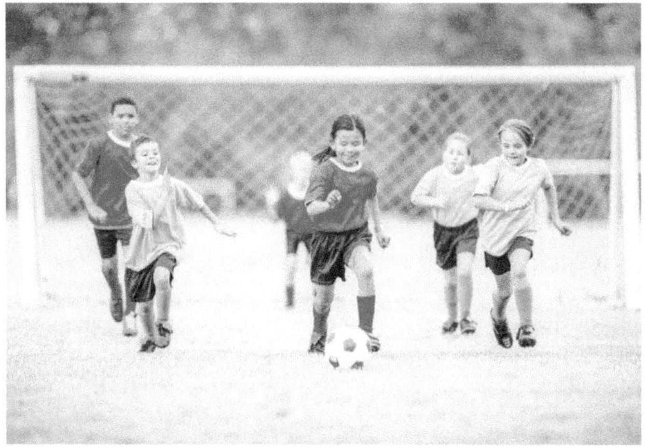

Fig. 17.3 Developing the skills of a team sport is important to the school-age child. (istock.com/FatCamera)

Local after-school programs and clubs have decreased the number of children left at home, but there are still many children who do not have these options available, and some families cannot afford a baby-sitter. Many latchkey children do not participate in after-school social and sports activities and may be slower to identify themselves as belonging to a group. The nurse can be a key resource for providing information about the needs of the school-age child and quality after-school care programs that may be available in the community.

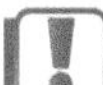

Safety Alert!

Caution parents about the safe storage of firearms. Many deaths caused by firearms occur in the home, not on the streets.

Nurses should be aware of local resources, such as Scouts Canada, Boys & Girls Club of Canada, and Young Men's Christian Association (YMCA) and Young Women's Christian Association (YWCA) after-school activities. Nurses can also assist in developing innovative programs such as cooperative babysitting, in which parents exchange child care services. Nurses should spend time with parents, lend support, and help them to explore their options (See Health Promotion box).

Health Promotion

Guidance for Children at Home Alone

CHILDREN SHOULD BE TAUGHT THE FOLLOWING SAFETY GUIDELINES:

Do not enter the house if the door is not locked or something does not look right.
Keep the door locked when at home.
Have a pre-arranged time to call parents when you get home.
Do not answer the door unless you know someone is visiting.
When answering the phone, do not say parents are not home. Develop an answer with parents (e.g., they are too busy to come to the phone).
Walk to and from school with friends.
Always use the same path to walk to and from school.
Do not accept a ride from anyone unless you have permission from your parents.
Have the phone number of parents and a trusted neighbour posted by the phone.
Know how to call 911 in an emergency.

PARENTAL CONSIDERATIONS

Consider getting child a cell phone that can be used for contact with parents..
Program all emergency numbers into cell phone.
Review child's path to and from school..
Notify a trusted neighbour that child is alone and ensure they can be called in an emergency.
Review fire safety plan.
Consider getting a pet for the child.
Praise the child for being successful at staying home alone.

CHORES AS TEACHING TOOLS

Chores help children do a job, take responsibility, feel that they are an important part of a family, and develop self-esteem. Age-appropriate chores for the school-age child may include loading the washer or dryer, taking out the garbage (Fig. 17.4), and caring for pets. The nurse can refer the parent to various websites for suggestions concerning age-appropriate chores.

PHYSICAL, MENTAL, EMOTIONAL, AND SOCIAL DEVELOPMENT

THE 5- AND 6-YEAR-OLD

At 5 and 6 years of age, children burst with energy and are on the go constantly. They soon become overtired, and it is necessary to limit their activities. They like to start tasks but do not always finish them because their attention span is fairly brief. They tend to be bossy, are sometimes rude, and experiment with language, but they are very sensitive to criticism. Their conscience is active, and they find it difficult to make decisions.

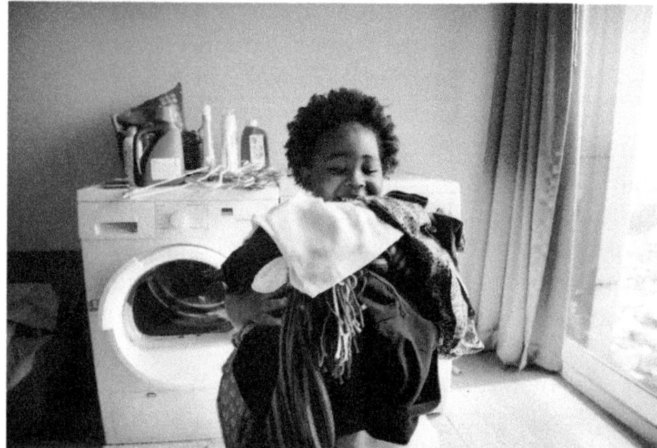

Fig. 17.4 Household chores. The school-age child contributes to the smooth running of the household by performing household chores. (istock.com/Rawpixel)

One of the most obvious physical changes at this age is the loss of the temporary teeth (Fig. 17.5). The important 6-year molars also erupt. Children can jump rope, throw and catch a ball, tie shoelaces, and perform numerous other feats that require muscle coordination. Their language differs from that of the preschool child. They use it for a purpose rather than for the pure joy of talking. Their vocabulary consists of about 2 500 words. They require 11 to 13 hours of sleep a night.

Boys and girls play together at this age, although they often begin to prefer to associate with children of their own gender. Most children enjoy collecting objects such as shells, leaves, or stones. Play at this time usually reflects events that occur in the immediate environment.

Five- and 6-year-old children need time and support to help them adjust to school. The transition may be more comfortable if they have preschool experience. Parents must observe children for signs of fatigue and stress. Not all children are ready for school merely because they reach the proper age. Even those who are ready need time and support from parents and teachers before they can settle down to the job at hand. Being in school exposes the child to infection more frequently than being at home, thus school-age immunizations and a physical examination are indicated (see Chapter 32).

THE 7-YEAR-OLD

The 7-year-old may be a quieter child, and some educators have noted that second-graders are the easiest children to teach. They set high standards for themselves and for their families. They have a good sense of humour, tend to be somewhat of a "tease" (e.g., wiggle loose teeth to annoy adults), and are a little more

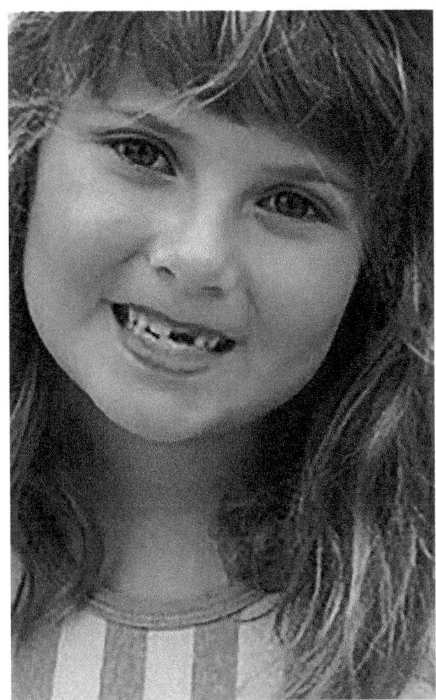

Fig. 17.5 One of the most obvious physical changes of the 6-year-old is the loss of primary teeth. The loss of primary teeth starts at 6 years of age, and about four permanent teeth erupt each year.

modest than at an earlier age. They enjoy being active but also appreciate periods of rest. The second-grader may have a "crush" on a friend of the opposite sex.

These children know the months and seasons of the year and begin to tell time. They have a beginning concept of mathematics, can count by twos and fives, and know that money is valuable. Their hands are steadier. Their interest in culture and religion is heightened during these years.

Active play is still important to both sexes. The boys are more apt to tease the girls than to participate in games such as jump rope or tag. Both sexes enjoy bike riding and table games. Realistic toys, such as dolls that can be bathed and fed and video games or radio-controlled cars, appeal to the 7-year-old. Graphic novels are also popular, especially if they can be read on an e-reader or tablet. Becoming increasingly independent, the children imagine themselves accomplishing feats more adventurous than those of their parents. They keep busy on their smartphones and they cannot understand how their parents ever chose to lead such "dull lives."

THE 8-YEAR-OLD

The 8-year-old wants to do everything and can play alone for a longer period than can the 7-year-old. The work of an 8-year-old is usually creative. These children enjoy group activities, such as Brownies and Cub Scouts, and prefer companions of the same sex. They become interested in group fads. Eight-year-olds like to be considered important, particularly by adults. They may behave better for company than for the family. Hero worship is evident.

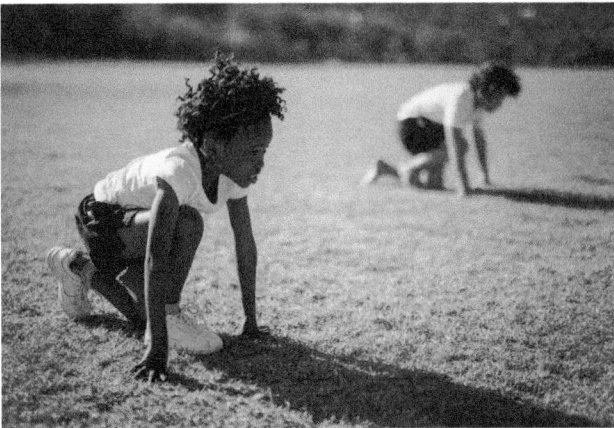

Fig. 17.6 Competitive sports. The 8-year-old is ready for competitive sports. (istock.com/Wavebreakmedia)

The arms and hands of the 8-year-old seem to grow faster than the rest of the body. The large and small muscles are better developed, and movements are smoother and more graceful. The child understands the number of days that must pass before special events such as Christmas, birthdays, and discharge from the hospital.

The 8-year-old enjoys competitive sports but is generally a poor loser (Fig. 17.6). Long, involved arguments often occur. A healthy way to teach a child to express anger is to have the child pound on a pillow (Fig. 17.7). Wrestling is common, and dramatic play is popular. Most children like to be the hero or heroine of their favourite program. Neighbourhood secret clubs are organized, and all members must strictly adhere to the rules.

THE 9-YEAR-OLD

Nine-year-olds are dependable, show more interest in family activities, assume more responsibility for personal belongings and for younger brothers and sisters, and are more likely to complete tasks. They resist adult authority if it does not coincide with the opinions or ideals of the group. However, they are more able to accept criticism for their actions. Individual differences are pronounced.

Worries and mild compulsions are common. Nervous habits, sometimes referred to as tics, may appear and may vary widely. Eye blinking, facial grimacing, and shoulder shrugging are but a few examples. The child cannot help such actions and should not be scolded for them because they are mainly caused by tension; they usually disappear when home and social life become more relaxed.

Hand and eye coordination is well developed, and manual activities are managed with skill. The child works and plays hard and can become overly tired. About 10 hours of sleep a night are needed. The permanent teeth are still erupting.

Competitive sports are still popular, as are reading, listening to music, watching television, playing online

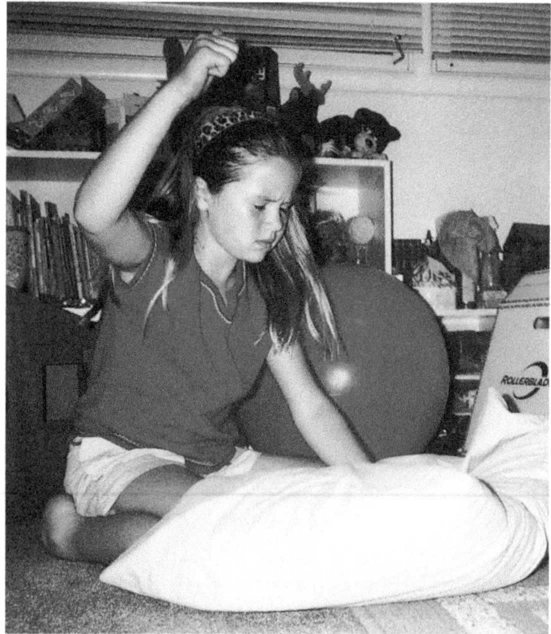

Fig. 17.7 A healthy outlet for feelings of anger is pounding on a pillow. (Courtesy Pat Spier, RN-C.)

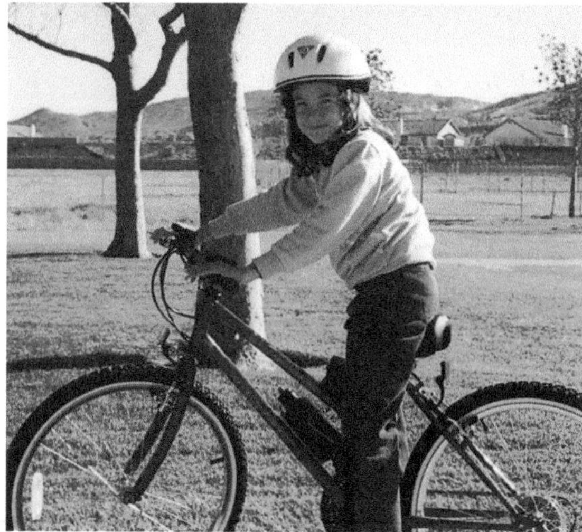

Fig. 17.8 Protective clothing is necessary for potentially hazardous play. Providing protective equipment appropriate for any sport the child plays is an important parental responsibility (e.g., helmets for bicycling, skateboarding, or ice hockey).

computer games, and texting. Sports programs that take into consideration the limitations of children at various ages should be encouraged. Teaching proper techniques and the use of adequate safety devices is essential (Fig. 17.8). Co-ed participation is not contraindicated at this age as motor skill, endurance, height, and weight are similar between boys and girls (Lipnowski et al., 2012).

These children may show an interest in music and they may wish to take lessons (Fig. 17.9). Children know the date, can repeat months of the year in order, can multiply and do simple division, and are ready for more complex math. They take care of their body needs, and by now their table manners have improved considerably.

THE 10-YEAR-OLD

Age 10 marks the beginning of the preadolescent years. Girls are more physically mature than boys. The 10-year-old begins to show self-direction, is courteous to adults, and thinks clearly about social problems and prejudices. These children want to be independent and resent being told what to do but are receptive to suggestions. The ideas of the group are more important than individual ideas. Interest in sex and sexual curiosity continue.

In general, girls are more poised than boys. Both sexes are fairly reliable about household duties (see Fig. 17.4). Slang terms are used. The 10-year-old can write for a relatively long period of time and maintains good writing speed. The child uses fractions and knows abstract numbers. Boys and girls begin to identify themselves with skills that pertain to their sex roles. They may be intolerant of the opposite sex. The play enjoyed by the 10-year-old is similar to that enjoyed by the 9-year-old. In addition, the child takes more interest in personal appearance. Sending texts to friends is important.

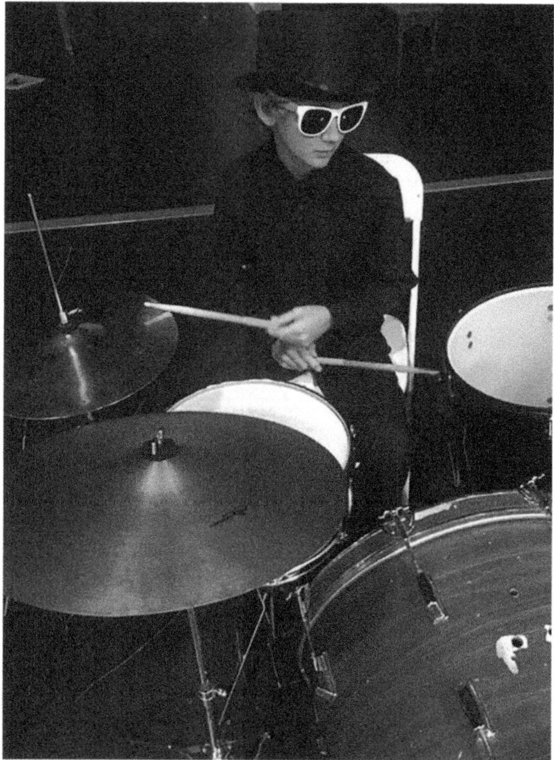

Fig. 17.9 Musical talent emerges and friends can form a band for healthy socialization.

11- AND 12-YEAR-OLDS

Adjectives that describe 11- and 12-year-olds include intense, observant, all-knowing, energetic, meddlesome, and argumentative. This period before the onset of puberty is one of complete disorganization. It begins earlier in some children; the onset and rate of physical maturity vary greatly. Before the end of this period the hormones of the body begin to influence physical growth. Posture may be poor. There are 24 to 26 permanent teeth.

The child has an overabundance of energy and is on the go every minute. Table manners may be a thing of the past, and the refrigerator may be constantly emptied. Children at this age are less concerned with their appearance. They often seem to be preoccupied, which, along with physical activities and numerous anxieties, accounts for some of the decline that may be seen in school grades. The ability to concentrate decreases, and parents state that the child "never hears anything." When asked to do a new task, these children moan and groan.

Group participation is still important. They enjoy being team players. Preadolescent children are not ready to stand alone, but they cannot bear the thought of depending on parents. They must overcome the problems they confront without parental help. Their attitude implies, "Can't you see that I'm not a child anymore?"

During preadolescence, children are interested in their bodies and watch for signs of growing up. Girls look forward to menstruation and wearing their first bra. Boys and girls tend to "ignore" those of opposite sex, but are very much aware of them. There is a tendency to tease one another. Their descriptions of each other are far from complimentary: "stupid," "crazy," and "nerd." At this age, words are often used without full understanding of their true meaning. Both genders enjoy earning money by obtaining odd jobs. The preadolescent often seeks an adult friend of the same sex to idolize.

Guiding preadolescents is not easy. They need freedom within limits and recognition that they are no longer young children. They should know why parents make a decision. They should not be expected to follow household rules blindly. Their conscience enables them to understand and accept reasonable discipline. They ignore constant verbal nagging. They should be provided constructive opportunities to release pent-up emotions and energy. One can more easily accept their irritating behaviour by realizing that much of it is indeed "just a phase." Texting friends occurs in regular spurts throughout the day.

Nursing Tip

Mutual respect involves accepting the child's feelings. When helping children to identify feelings, start with the words *mad, glad, sad,* or *scared.*

The CPS recommends sports that foster motor skills and fitness exercises in the school setting to promote positive attitudes toward exercise in later life. The focus should be on mastering the skill of the sport and enjoying the exercise rather than winning a game (Lipnowski et al., 2012). Selecting students for teams based on athletic prowess is inappropriate for the preadolescent child. Ceremonies should recognize all participants rather than just star players.

GUIDANCE AND HEALTH SUPERVISION

HEALTH EXAMINATIONS

A physical examination is done prior to school admission. This allows time to identify any concerns. Table 17.3 reviews the growth and development of the school-age child. A carefully obtained health history provides the nurse and health care provider with much-needed information regarding the child's health and development. Booster immunizations are given as needed (see Chapter 32). Also, the child's teeth are examined, and dental work may be completed. Good dental hygiene and regular professional dental care are essential as the permanent set of teeth erupts. Dental health and nutrition are discussed in Chapter 13.

The eating habits of school-age children should be basically sound, if a variety of nutritious foods are offered. Food preferences are common. A nutritious breakfast is important for healthy development and for preventing obesity; some provinces have school breakfast or lunch programs that provide nutritious meals, which help promote children's learning. Several provinces have banned junk food in school in response to concerns about childhood obesity (Dietitians of Canada, 2019).

Nursing Tip

Tips to help prevent obesity:

- Eliminate sugary drinks (pop and juice).
- Replace whole milk with skim milk.
- Eat breakfast every day.
- Encourage family meal times.
- Encourage "family-style" meals where children are allowed to serve themselves on the basis of hunger cues and food preferences.
- Parents should role model healthy eating and activity.
- Encourage 1 hour of physical activity or more per day.
- No more than 2 hours of screen time a day.

School health programs aimed at maintaining and promoting health are provided in most school systems. Nurses and other professional persons who take part in such programs can play an important role in counselling parents. They can also help meet the needs of children with disabilities who are enrolled in school. It is important that information be provided to children and parents in a culturally sensitive way.

Children who are inattentive at school should be screened for vision or hearing deficits and language or learning disabilities before being assessed for attention deficit–hyperactivity disorder (ADHD) (see Chapter 33

Table 17.3 **Summary of Growth and Development and Health Maintenance of School-Age Children**

AGE	PHYSICAL COMPETENCY	INTELLECTUAL COMPETENCY	EMOTIONAL-SOCIAL COMPETENCY	NUTRITION	PLAY	SAFETY
General: 5–12 years	Gains an average of 2.5–3.2 kg/year (5.0–7 lb/year) Has overall height gains of 5.0 cm/year (2 inches/year); growth occurs in spurts and mainly in the trunk and the extremities Loses deciduous teeth; most permanent teeth erupt Progressively more coordinated in both gross and fine-motor skills Caloric needs increase during growth spurts	Masters concrete operations Moves from egocentrism; learns that they are not always right Learns grammar and expression of emotions and thoughts Vocabulary increases to 3 000 words or more Handles complex sentences	Central crisis; industry versus inferiority; wants to do and make things Progressive sex education needed Wants to be like friends; competition is important Fears body mutilation, alterations in body image; earlier phobias may recur; nightmares; fears death Nervous habits are common	Fluctuations in appetite because of uneven growth pattern and tendency to become involved in activities Tendency to neglect breakfast in rush of getting to school Although school lunch is provided in most schools, child does not always eat it	Plays in groups, mostly of same gender; group activities predominate Books are important for all ages Bicycles are important Sports equipment, cards, board and computer games Most play consists of active games requiring little or no equipment	Enforce continued use of seat belts during car travel. Bicycle safety must be taught and enforced. Teach safety related to hobbies, handicrafts, and mechanical equipment.
5–7 years	Gross motor skill exceeds fine-motor coordination Has good balance and rhythm—runs, skips, jumps, climbs, gallops Throws and catches ball Dresses self with little or no help	Has vocabulary of 2 500 words Learning to read and print Begins concrete concepts of numbers, general classification of items Knows concepts of right and left; morning, afternoon, and evening; and coinage Has intuitive thought process Is verbally aggressive, bossy, opinionated, argumentative Likes simple games with basic rules	Boisterous, outgoing, and a know-it-all Whiny; parents should sidestep power struggles, offer choices Becomes quiet and reflective during seventh year; very sensitive Can use telephone Likes to make things; starts many projects, finishes few Give some responsibility for household duties	Persistence of preschool food likes and dislikes Tendency toward deficiencies in iron, vitamin A, and riboflavin; needs 100 mL/kg of water per day, 3 g/kg protein daily	Still enjoys dolls, cars, and trucks Plays well alone but enjoys small groups of both sexes; begins to prefer same-sex peers during seventh year Ready to learn how to ride a bicycle Prefers imaginary, dramatic play with real costumes Begins collecting for quantity, not quality Enjoys active games such as hide-and-seek, tag, jump rope, roller skating, kickball	Teach and reinforce traffic safety. Child needs adult supervision of play. Teach child to avoid strangers and never to take anything from strangers. Teach illness prevention and reinforce continued practice of other health habits. Restrict bicycle use to home grounds and no-traffic areas; teach bicycle safety. Child should wear helmet.

Continued

Table 17.3 Summary of Growth and Development and Health Maintenance of School-Age Children—cont'd

AGE	PHYSICAL COMPETENCY	INTELLECTUAL COMPETENCY	EMOTIONAL-SOCIAL COMPETENCY	NUTRITION	PLAY	SAFETY
8–10 years	Myopia may appear Secondary sex characteristics begin in girls Hand–eye coordination and fine-motor skills are well established Movements are graceful, coordinated Cares for own physical needs completely Is constantly on the move; plays and works hard	Learning correct grammar and expression of feelings in words Likes books they can read alone; will read funny papers and scan newspaper Enjoys making detailed drawings Mastering classification, seriation, spatial, temporal, and numerical concepts Uses language as a tool; likes riddles, jokes, chants, word games Rules are a guiding force in life Very interested in how things work and what and how weather, seasons, and the like are made	Strong preference for same-sex peers Antagonizes opposite-sex peers Self-assured and pragmatic at home; questions parental values and ideas Has a strong sense of humor Enjoys clubs, group projects, outings, large groups, camp Modesty about own body increases with time; sex-conscious Works diligently to perfect the skills they do best Happy, cooperative, relaxed, and casual in relationships Increasingly courteous and well mannered with adults Group stage is at a peak; secret codes and rituals prevail Responds better to suggestion than to authoritative approach	Needs about 2 100 calories/day; nutritious snacks Tends to be too busy to bother to eat Tendency toward deficiencies in calcium, iron, and thiamine Problem of obesity may begin now Has good table manners Able to help with food preparation	Ready for lessons in dancing, gymnastics, music Restrict television time to 1–2 hours each day Likes hiking, sports Enjoys cooking, woodworking, crafts Enjoys cards and computer games Likes radio and music Begins qualitative collecting	Stress safety with firearms; keep them out of reach, and allow their use only with adult supervision. Know who the child's friends are; parents should still have some control over friend selection. Teach water safety; an adult should supervise swimming. Enforce balance in rest and activity. Teach and set examples about harmful use of drugs, alcohol, and smoking
11–12 years	Vital signs approximate adult norms Growth spurt for girls Inequalities between sexes increasingly noticeable, with boys having greater physical strength Eruption of permanent teeth complete except for third molars Secondary sex characteristics begin in boys Menstruation may begin	Able to think about social problems and prejudices; sees others' points of view Enjoys reading mysteries, love stories Begins playing with abstract ideas Interested in whys of health measures and understands human reproduction Very moralistic; religious commitment often made during this time	Intense team loyalty; boys begin teasing girls, and hetero-sexual girls flirt with boys for attention Best-friend period Wants unreasonable independence; is rebellious about routines; has wide mood swings; needs some time daily for privacy Very critical of own work Hero worship prevails Facts-of-life chats with friends prevail Masturbation increases Appears under constant tension	Male needs 2 500 kcal/day; female needs 2 250 (70 calories/kg/day), both need 75 mL/kg of water/day and 2 g/kg protein daily	Enjoys projects and working with hands Likes to do errands and jobs to earn money Very involved in sports, dancing, talking on phone, texting Enjoys all aspects of acting and drama	Continue monitoring friends. Stress bicycle and roller blade safety on streets and in traffic and the use of helmets and other protective gear.

Data from Canadian Paediatric Society. (2016). *Greig HEALTH RECORD*. Retrieved from: https://www.cps.ca/en/tools-outils/greig-health-record; Dunn, W., & Craig, G. (2013). *Understanding growth and development* (3rd ed.). Englewood Cliffs, NJ: Pearson, Prentice-Hall.

for further discussion of ADHD). Increasing structure and decreasing distractions are the first steps in helping any child with a school problem. Emphasis should be placed on producing successful experiences and increasing complexity slowly. Realistic demands must be balanced by unconditional support during the successes and failures of the developing child. To help avert the development of behavioural issues, the nurse should be aware of parenting styles that demonstrate difficulty in "letting go" and those that demonstrate excessive pressure.

Active play with family members is important to the school-age child. Divorce, separation, domestic violence, and neighbourhood gangs can be an obstacle to such play and negatively affect the progress of development in the school-age child. The nurse can initiate appropriate referrals to community agencies.

Health supervision should include assessment of physical activity and school performance. Children who avoid activities that might reveal their physical appearance, such as changing into gym clothes or participating in health examinations, may have a negative perception of their own physical appearance. Parents need guidance to understand the difference between participation in sports activities that help to develop skill, teamwork, and fitness, and participation in high-stress activities that increase the risk of skeletal injury and focus on winning as a central theme. Often a 6-year-old with advanced athletic ability who is guided into early competition and who experiences outstanding commendations loses their self-esteem upon reaching 12 years of age—when the ability of peers reaches or exceeds their level and they no longer experience the spotlight.

The school-age child who is ill can understand simple explanations of their illness but sometimes can revert to believing illness is "punishment" for bad behaviour or thoughts. Nurses should work with parents to explain the feelings the child may have and the need for correct information regarding any illness.

School-age children need time and a place to study. They require a desk in their own room or at least a private area of the house where they can concentrate. Their furniture should be of the proper size; lighting should be adequate. They must learn to take responsibility for their assignments and school supplies. Parents can encourage school children by showing interest in what they are learning, by joining parent–teacher organizations, and by visiting periodically with the teacher. Parents should be encouraged to vote on civic matters that will benefit the school system in their community.

At this age, an allowance or at least a means of earning money provides children with opportunities to learn money's value. It takes time and encouragement for them to learn to spend money wisely. Such experiences aid in making the school-age child a more responsible person.

PET OWNERSHIP

Pet ownership is a common practice in families with children. After 7 years of age, children can be responsible for caring for the needs of a family pet. Studies have documented the positive influence of pet ownership on improving the medical and psycho-logical outcome after illness or surgery. Children with disabilities especially benefit from interacting with pets. The interaction with animals can lower blood pressure and heart rate, reduce loneliness and feelings of isolation, improve communication, foster trust, and motivate participation in physical therapy (Gadomski, Scribani, Krupa, et al., 2015). Pets allow the ill child who feels separated from other people to feel companionship and acceptance. Shy children often find pet ownership eases the path to socialization with others who initiate contact because of the pet.

The age of the child, the presence of allergies, and an immunocompromised family member are major factors that influence the desirability of pet ownership. Toddlers and young children may not understand the limitations in handling pets that can respond by biting or scratching. Also, parents should be aware that pets that have close contact with children have the potential of transmitting disease (Table 17.4).

Health Promotion

Guidelines for healthy living with animals:

- **WASH:** Make sure to immediately wash your hands after touching a pet, or anything in the area where they live, play, or touch.
- **DISINFECT:** Regularly clean any surfaces or objects your pet touches with soapy water followed by a household sanitizer.
- **SEPARATE:** Keep pets and all their supplies (e.g., food, containers, toys) away from the kitchen and other places where food is made or eaten.
- **SUPERVISE:** Always watch children when they touch or play with pets. Make sure they wash their hands afterward and do not let them put pets or pet supplies near their face or share their food or drinks with pets.
- **PROTECT:** Talk to your health care provider or veterinarian about the right pet if your family includes children under 5 years of age, people with a weakened immune system, pregnant women, or adults 65 years of age and older.

Sources: Health Canada. (2016). *Pets: Healthy ANIMALS, HEALTHY PEOPLE*. Ottawa, ON: Author. Retrieved from: https://www.canada.ca/en/public-health/services/publications/healthy-living/healthy-animals-healthy-people.html.

Immunocompromised children are at risk for contracting illness that is spread by some animals. Birds, rodents, turtles, and reptiles are not recommended as pets because they cannot be screened for potential pathogens, have few vaccines, and are most likely to transmit

Table 17.4 Diseases That Can Be Transmitted by Pets to Humans

VECTOR	DISEASE
Dog bites	Cellulitis, septicemia
Geckos, reptiles	Salmonella
Dogs, cats, birds, farm animals	*Campylobacter pylori* (gastroenteritis, Guillain-Barré syndrome)
Cats, dogs, ferrets, raccoons, skunks, bats, foxes, wolves	Rabies
Reptiles, rodents, cats, dogs	Cryptosporidiosis (gastroenteritis) and skin infections
Dogs, cats	Parasites, hypereosinophilia, toxocariasis, fungal skin infections, staph and strep infections
Dogs, cats, reptiles, turtles	Leptospirosis
Blood contact during birth of animals	Brucellosis, Q fever
Kitten	Cat scratch disease (lymphadenopathy)
Cats	Toxoplasmosis*
Birds, farm animals, cats	Q fever
Birds	Psittacosis, histoplasmosis, avian flu
Fish	Fish tank granuloma (related to *Mycobacterium marinum* organism that causes ulcerated skin lesions after cleaning the fish tank) and tularemia
Petting zoo	*E. coli, Giardia, Campylobacter,* and sensitivity to animal dander, scales, fur, and feathers

*Toxoplasmosis can cause congenital malformations in the fetus. Pregnant women are urged to avoid contact with litter boxes.
Data from Centers for Disease Control and Prevention. (2018). *Keeping PETS HEALTHY KEEPS PEOPLE HEALTHY TOO!* Retrieved from: https://www.cdc.gov/healthypets/index.html; Ginsburg, C., & Hunstad, D. (2016). Animals and human bites. In R. M. Kliegman, B. F. Stanton, J. W. St. Geme, et al. (Eds.), *Nelson textbook of pediatrics* (20th ed.).Philadelphia: Saunders.

disease. Infection can occur via contact with the pet's saliva, feces, or urine or by inhalation or skin contact with organisms. Risk factors in pet ownership of cats and dogs can be further reduced if children are cautioned not to kiss pets, if pets are not allowed to sleep in bed with the child, if exposure to animal feces is avoided, and if hand hygiene after handling a pet is encouraged.

Having an allergy to animal dander does not always rule out having a pet. Parent education concerning pet selection and hygiene can assist the family in making a decision that is best for all family members. Cats are most often the allergen offender because allergens are secreted in the saliva and by sebaceous glands onto the cat hair and skin.

If an allergenic pet is already part of the family, the risks can be minimized by frequent bathing and brushing, and by keeping the pet outdoors or at least out of the child's bedroom. Use of a HEPA filter when vacuuming or in the central heating and air conditioning systems can be helpful in reducing the spread of allergens. Desensitization of the child by an allergist is also an option. Education concerning the approach to and handling of pets is beneficial to children whether or not they own pets, because they are likely to come in contact with pets in their neighbourhood or at their friends' houses.

Get Ready for the Certification Examination!

Key Points

- School age (5 to 12 years of age) is a time of increased independence and a time when the child begins to incorporate, perfect, and process the skills and information gained in earlier years.
- Erikson calls this stage the *stage of industry* or *accomplishment.*
- Freud describes this period as the *sexual latency stage,* when the child's energy is directed toward cognitive and physical skills.
- Major changes occur in the child's cognitive-perceptual patterns. Piaget refers to this stage as the *concrete operations stage.*
- Growth is slow until the spurt that occurs directly before puberty.
- School has an important influence on the socialization of children.
- The child acquires a positive self-concept from the ability to be productive, self-directed, and accepted.
- Peers range from same-sex friends in the early years to opposite-sex friends around puberty.

- Group acceptance is important.
- Both sexes need accurate information and reassurance in advance about changes of puberty and reproduction.
- Meals may be sporadic because of the child's activities and the parents' working schedules.
- Accident prevention is still extremely important. School-age children are prone to injuries from motor vehicles, bicycles, skateboards, swimming, and their tendency to be overactive and distracted.
- Language development during the school-age years develops and expands the ability to communicate. The school-age child experiments with words without fully understanding their meanings.
- Moral development includes an understanding of rules, fairness, and values, and a knowledge of right and wrong.
- After-school day care and its relation to developmental needs is a concern for working parents.
- The nurse plays an important role in providing anticipatory guidance, health assessment, and community referral.
- Pet ownership can nurture a sense of responsibility and encourage socialization in a shy child.

Additional Learning Resources

evolve Go to your Evolve website (http://evolve.elsevier.com/Canada/Leifer) for the following learning resources:

- Answer Key for Critical Thinking Questions
- Answer Key for Textbook Review Questions
- Audio Glossary
- Interactive Review Questions
- Skills Performance Checklists
- Video clips and more!

Online Resources

- Boys & Girls Club of Canada: https://www.bgccan.com/en/
- Canadian Paediatric Society, *Active Kids, Healthy Kids:* https://www.cps.ca/en/active-actifs/how-much-for-school-age-children
- Centers for Disease Control and Prevention (CDC), *Keeping Pets Healthy Keeps People Healthy Too!:* www.cdc.gov/healthypets
- Gender Creative Kids: https://gendercreativekids.ca/
- Sexuality Information and Education Council of Canada (SIECCAN): http://sieccan.org/wp/

Review Questions

1. Which pulse rate is normal in a school-age child?
   - **a.** 100 to 120 beats/min
   - **b.** 95 to 100 beats/min
   - **c.** 85 to 100 beats/min
   - **d.** 60 to 95 beats/min
2. A parent asks a nurse if it is healthy to allow her school-age child to play computer games after school every day. The best response of the nurse would be which of the following? *(Select all that apply.)*
   - **a.** They will interest the school-age child and will keep the child off the streets.
   - **b.** They can challenge the intellect but should be balanced with active play activities with no more than 2 hours of screen time per day.
   - **c.** They should only be played on weekends and not on school days.
   - **d.** Some programs teach new skills and are appropriate for school-age children.
3. A parent of an 8-year-old child seeks advice from a nurse because the child is overweight. What would the nurse advise the parent to do?
   - **a.** Provide a reward for the child when he avoids between-meal snacks for a full week.
   - **b.** Limit privileges when the child eats sweets or junk food.
   - **c.** Include the child in meal planning and preparation.
   - **d.** Limit party-going activities where sweets will be served.
4. A 9-year-old practicing the piano continues to have difficulty in playing the theme song from a popular movie. The child starts to pound on the piano keys in frustration. A nurse would teach the parents that the best response would be to enter the room and say which of the following?
   - **a.** "Just what do you think you're doing? That piano cost money!"
   - **b.** "That's not difficult. Pull yourself together or you'll never amount to anything."
   - **c.** "That piece sounds hard. I can see how you could be discouraged."
   - **d.** "Here, let me show you how to play that."

Critical Thinking Question

1. Parents discuss their child's behaviour with the nurse. They state that they are anxious for their child to succeed in school so she can have all the advantages of a good education. However, the child does not seem to want their help, nor does she appreciate their efforts to help her. They give the example of a science project that was due for school last week. The child's father, an engineer, built the best-looking project for his child to take to school. "It earned an easy 'A' grade for him." However, the girl didn't appreciate the help given to her and didn't seem to care about the "A" grade received. They are worried that school may not have the same meaning for the child as it does for them. What is the best response of the nurse?

REFERENCES

Abortion Rights Coalition of Canada. (2017). *Position paper #39: Sex education in Canada*. Vancouver, BC: Author. Retrieved from http://www.arcc-cdac.ca/postionpapers/39-Sex-Education-in-Canada.pdf.

Canadian Paediatric Society (CPS). (2017). Screen time and young children: Promoting health and development in a digital world. *Paediatrics & Child Health, 22*(8), 461–468. Retrieved from https://www.cps.ca/en/documents/position/screen-time-and-young-children.

Canadian Paediatric Society (CPS). (2018). *Gender identity*. Retrieved from https://www.caringforkids.cps.ca/handouts/gender-identity.

Dieticians of Canada. (2019). *School nutrition*. Retrieved from https://www.dietitians.ca/Dietitians-Views/Children-and-Teens/School-Nutrition.aspx.

Gadomski, A., Scribani, M., Krupa, N., et al. (2015). Pet dogs and children's health: Opportunity for chronic disease prevention? *Prevention of Chronic Disease, 12*, E205.

Lipnowski, S., LeBlanc, C., & Canadian Paediatric Society (CPS), Healthy Active Living Committee. (2012). Position statement: Healthy active living: Physical activity guidelines for children and adolescents. *Paediatrics & Child Health, 17*(4), 209–210. Retrieved from https://www.cps.ca/en/documents/position/physical-activity-guidelines.

Ruiz-Casares, M., & Radic, I. (2015). *Legal age for leaving children unsupervised across Canada*. Canadian Child Welfare Research Portal. Retrieved from http://cwrp.ca/sites/default/files/publications/en/144e.pdf.

Sex Information & Education Council of Canada (SIECC). (2008). *Canadian guidelines for sexual health education*. Retrieved from http://sieccan.org/pdf/guidelines-eng.pdf.

18 The Adolescent

http://evolve.elsevier.com/Canada/Leifer

Cheryl Dika

Objectives

1. Define each key term listed.
2. Discuss three major theoretical viewpoints on the personality development of adolescents.
3. Discuss two main challenges during the adolescent years to which the adolescent must adjust.
4. List major physical changes that occur during adolescence.
5. Identify two major developmental tasks of adolescence.
6. Describe Tanner's stages of breast development.
7. List five life events that contribute to stress during adolescence.
8. Identify two ways in which a person's cultural background might contribute to their behaviour.
9. Discuss the importance of peer groups, cliques, and best friends in the developmental process of an adolescent.
10. Describe menstruation to an 11-year-old girl.
11. List a source for planning sex education programs for adolescents.
12. Summarize the nutritional requirements of the adolescent.
13. List two guidelines of importance for the adolescent participating in sports.
14. Discuss the common problems of adolescence and the nursing approach.

Key Terms

abstract reasoning
adolescence
asynchrony
cliques
epiphyseal closure (ĕp-ĭ-FĬZ-ē-ăl CLŌ-zhŭr)
formal operations
gay
growth spurt
intimacy
lesbian
menarche
puberty
self-concept
sexual maturity ratings (SMRs)

GENERAL CHARACTERISTICS

Adolescence is defined as the period of life beginning with the appearance of secondary sex characteristics and ending with cessation of growth and with emotional maturity. The term comes from the Latin word *adolescere*, meaning "to grow up." Adolescence is often divided into early, middle, and late periods, because the 13-year-old adolescent differs a great deal from the 18-year-old adolescent. Middle adolescence appears to be the time of greatest turmoil for most families. Perhaps one of the most characteristic features of adolescence is its uncertainty. It is a period of life that in our culture lasts a comparatively long time and involves a great number of adjustments. The major tasks of adolescence include establishing an identity, separating from family, initiating intimacy, and developing career choices. Some of the major theories of development are summarized in Box 18.1. The surge toward independence becomes more and more pronounced, sometimes making it difficult for adolescents to get along with their parents, who represent authority. When adolescents submit to parental wishes, they may feel humiliated and childish. If they revolt, conflicts arise within the family. Parents and adolescents must weather the storm together and try to discover solutions that are relatively satisfactory to all.

Numerous other factors account for the restlessness of adolescents. Their bodies are rapidly changing, and they may experience intense sexual drives. They want to be accepted by society, but they are not sure how to attain this goal. Adolescents question life and search to find what psychologists call their sense of identity; they ask, "Who am I?" "What do I want?" This is followed by the **intimacy** stage, in which adolescents must learn to avoid emotional isolation. They must face the fear of rejection in shared activities such as sports, in close friendships, and in sexual experiences. The older adolescent thinks about the future and is generally idealistic. Jean Piaget and other investigators indicate that during this time adolescents reach the final stages of **abstract reasoning**, logic, and other symbolic forms of thought, which increase sophistication in moral reasoning.

Box 18.1 Features of Major Theories of Development During Adolescence

SIGMUND FREUD

Adolescent is in the genital stage, the final stage of psychosexual development.

Self-love (narcissism) diminishes; love for others (altruism) develops.

Peers and parents are less influential than before but still provide love and support.

ERIK ERIKSON

The adolescent's main concerns are self-definition and self-esteem.

The adolescent experiences an identity crisis brought on by physical (including sexual) changes and conflict about future choices and expectations of others.

The adolescent must adapt to these changes and develop a new self-concept and appropriate vocational choices.

The adolescent learns to understand self in relation to others' perceptions and expectations.

JEAN PIAGET

The adolescent is in the stage of formal operations and therefore has the ability to reason logically and abstractly.

The adolescent is oriented toward problem solving.

These facts sound complicated in themselves, but they are intensified by a world that is constantly changing. Gender roles may be less defined in some households; some adolescents live in single-parent homes or with working relatives where there may be a lack of supervision.

Conformity is one of the strongest needs of the adolescent in society. Today, with electronic technology bringing common experiences to people all over the world via radio, television, computers, and smartphones, the combined pressure to conform often overrides cultural or traditional practices. Assimilation has begun to occur via technology.

The needs of the family often compete with the needs of the adolescent when parents try to push the adolescent into an activity or career that meets the parent's own personal need or dreams. Parents must be guided to enjoy the interests and activities of the adolescent without imposing their personal desires. The main challenges of the adolescent years include adjusting to rapid physical and physiological changes, maintaining privacy (Fig. 18.1), coping with social stresses (Fig. 18.2) and pressures, maintaining open communication, and developing positive health care practices and lifestyle choices.

GROWTH AND DEVELOPMENT

PHYSICAL DEVELOPMENT

Preadolescence is a short period immediately preceding adolescence. In girls, it comprises the ages

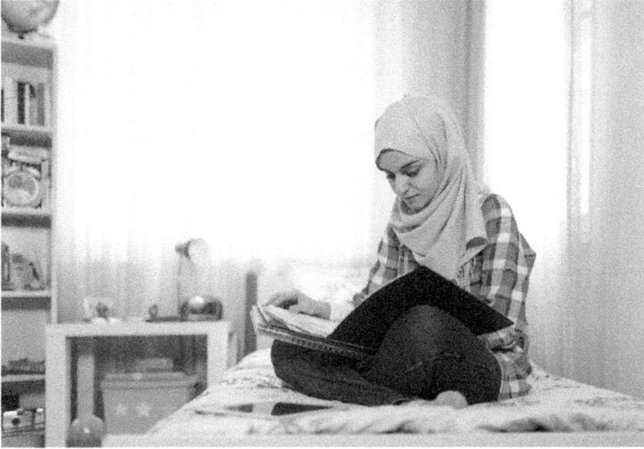

Fig. 18.1 Adolescents need privacy. (istock.com/Barcin)

of 10 to 13 years and is marked by rapid changes in the structure and function of various parts of the body. It is distinguished by **puberty**, the stage in which the reproductive organs become functional and secondary sex characteristics develop. Both sexes produce male hormones *(androgens)* and female hormones *(estrogens)* in comparatively equal amounts during childhood. During puberty, the hypothalamus of the brain signals the pituitary gland to stimulate other endocrine glands—the adrenals and the ovaries or testes—to secrete their hormones directly into the bloodstream in differing proportions (more androgens in the boy and more estrogens in the girl).

The age of puberty varies and is somewhat earlier for girls than for boys. The final 20% of mature height that is achieved during adolescence is called the **growth spurt** and usually occurs by 18 years of age. The major cause of weight gain is the increase in skeletal mass. The implications of growth and development for nursing assessments are illustrated in Fig. 18.3.

The general appearance of the adolescent tends to be awkward, that is, long-legged and gangling; this growth characteristic is termed **asynchrony**, because different body parts mature at different rates. The sweat glands are very active, and oily skin and acne are common. Both sexes mature earlier and grow taller and heavier than in past generations. Because of the gross motor development that occurs during adolescence, teenagers can gain satisfaction from sports. Table 18.1 outlines the growth and development of adolescents.

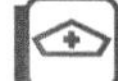 **Nursing Tip**

A *growth spurt* is a rapid period of growth in which the body reaches adult height and weight before age 18 years.

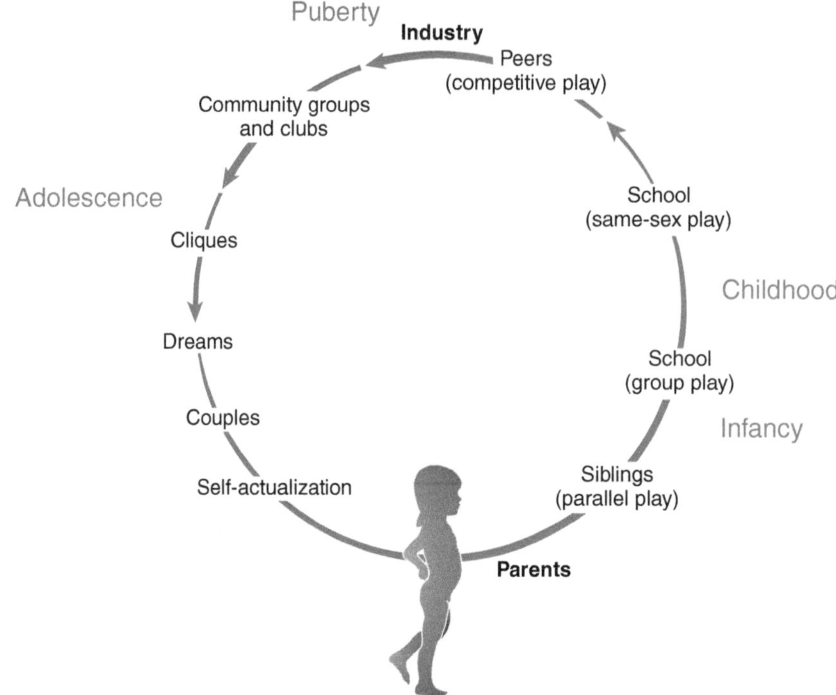

Fig. 18.2 Roadmap of social interaction. In infancy and early childhood, the child's focus is on parents. As the child grows, peers replace parents in importance. When adolescents mature, they return to the family with new respect, independence, and cooperation.

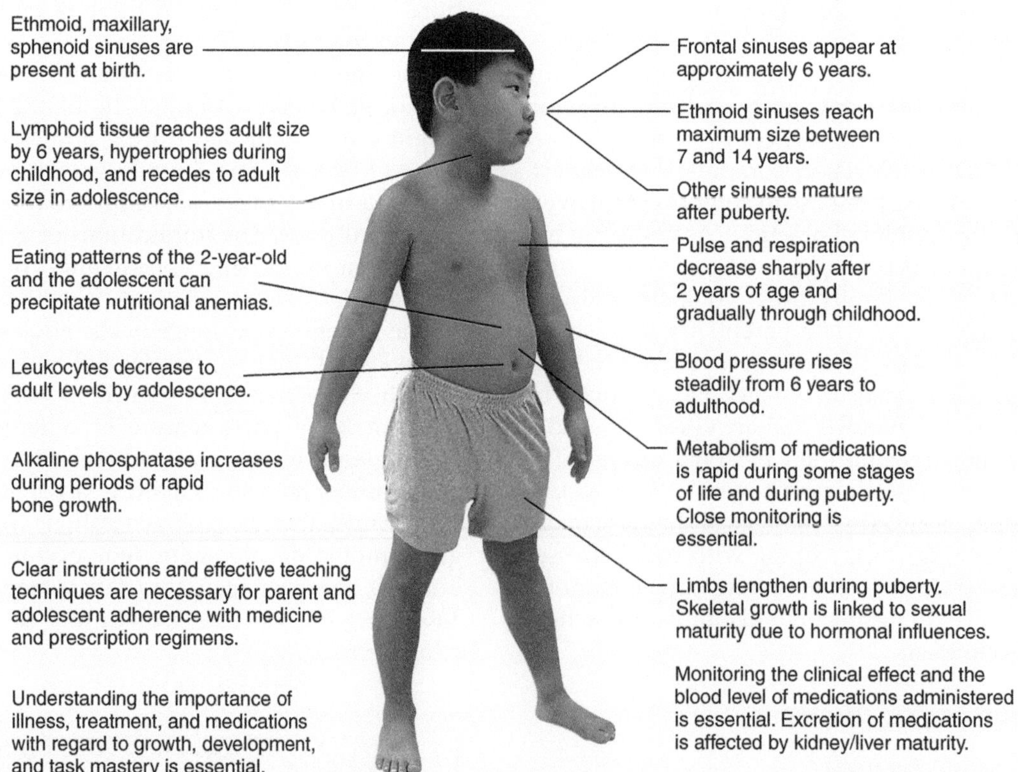

Fig. 18.3 Many developmental changes occur between infancy and adolescence. The nurse must understand the implications of growth and development for nursing assessments. (Art overlay courtesy Observatory Group, Cincinnati, Ohio.)

Table 18.1 **Growth and Development of the Adolescent**

	EARLY (11–14 YEARS)	MIDDLE (15–17 YEARS)	LATE (18–20 YEARS)
Physical growth	Appearance of secondary sex characteristics	Growth spurt in height	Growth slows
Body image	Self-conscious Adjusts to pubertal changes	Experiments with different "images" and "looks"	Accepts body image Personality emerges
Self-concept	Low self-esteem Denial of reality	Impulsive Impatient Identity confusion	Positive self-image Empathic Independent thinker
Behaviour	Behaves for rewards	Behaves to conform	Shows responsible behaviour
Sexual development	Sexual interest	Sexual experimentation	Sexual identity emerges Develops caring relationships
Peers	Cliques of unisex friends Has "best friend" Hero worship Has adult "crushes"	Begins dating Has need to please significant peer Develops heterosexual peer group	Values individual relationships Partner selection
Family	Is ambivalent to family Strives for independence	Struggles for autonomy and acceptance Rebels/withdraws Demands privacy	Achieves independence Re-establishes family relationships
Cognitive development	Concrete thinking Here-and-now is important	Early abstract thinking Daydreams, fantasizes Starts inductive and deductive reasoning	Abstract thinking Idealistic
Goals	Socializing is priority Goals are unrealistic	Identifies skills and interests	Identifies career goals Enters work or college (or both)
Health concerns	Concerned about normalcy	Concerned about experimenting with drugs or sex	Idealistic Decision making for lifestyle choice
Nursing interventions	Convey limits Encourage verbalization	Help them solve problems by providing choices Use peer group sessions Provide privacy	Discuss goals Allow participation in decisions Provide confidentiality

Nursing Tip

HEADSSS is a psychosocial history and development tool used for assessing adolescents

Interview questions regarding the following topics:

- **H** - Home & environment
- **E** - Education & employment
- **A** - Activities
- **D** - Drugs
- **S** - Sexuality
- **S** - Suicide/depression
- **S** – Safety/violence

Adapted from Norris, M. (2007). HEADSS up: Adolescents and the internet. *Paediatrics & Child Health, 12*(3), 211–216. Retrieved from https://doi.org/10.1093/pch/12.3.211.

Boys

During fetal life, the placental chorionic gonadotropin stimulates Leydig cells to secrete testosterone. Thus weeks 8 to 12 of fetal life are important in the sexual development of the male (XY) child. Luteinizing hormone (LH) maintains testosterone levels. Serum levels of LH increase during sleep 1 to 2 years before puberty. The secretion of gonadotropin stimulates gonad enlargement and the secretion of sex hormones. The interaction among the hypothalamus, pituitary, and gonads supports the development of puberty.

In boys, puberty begins with hormonal changes between 9½ and 14 years of age. The shoulders widen, the pectoral muscles enlarge, and the voice deepens. Hair begins to grow on the face, chest, axillae, and pubic areas (Fig. 18.4 and Box 18.2). Enlargement of the testicles and of internal structures and pigmentation of the scrotum are followed by enlargement of the penis. Erections and nocturnal emissions take place. The production of sperm begins between 13 and 14 years of age. An athletic scrotal support device (jockstrap) is necessary for boys participating in sporting events or for any activity in which support and protection of the genitalia are required. Good personal hygiene is necessary because heat and friction may lead to jock itch, a fungal infestation of the groin. Sharing athletic supporters is discouraged.

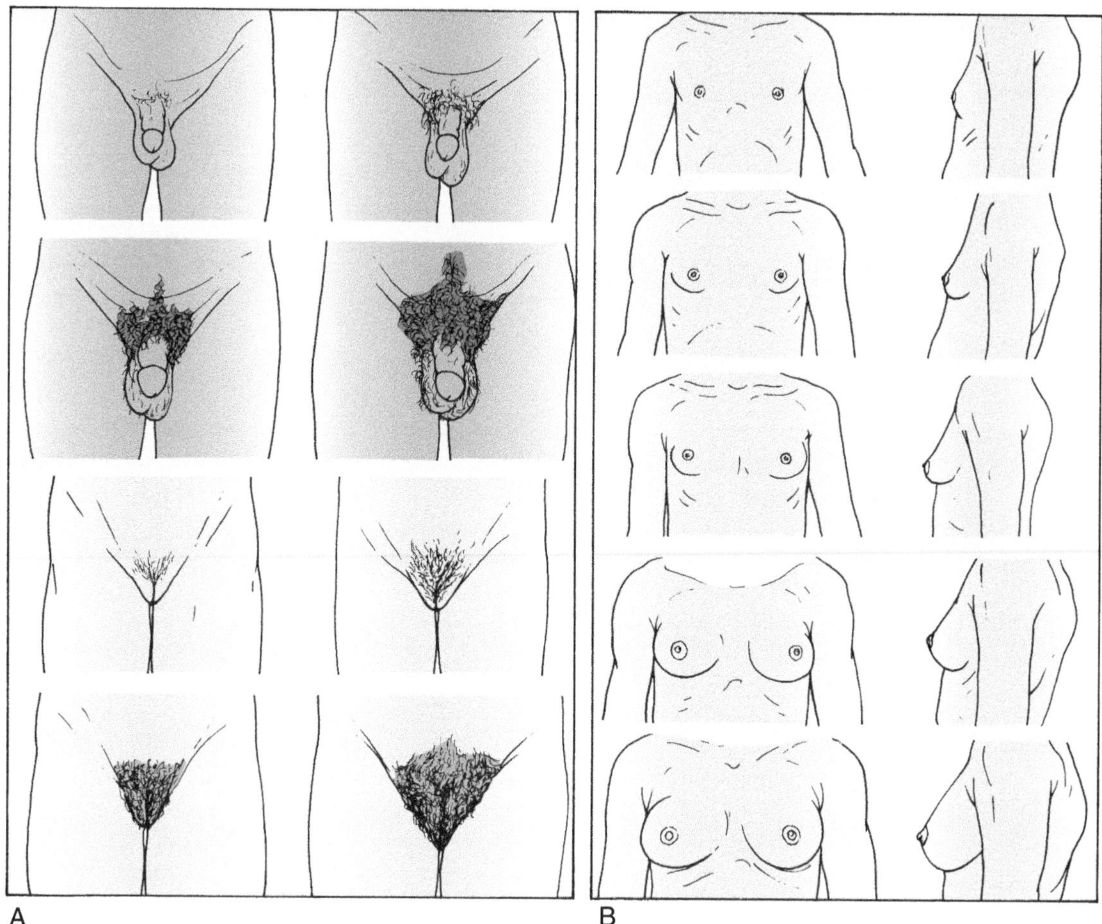

Fig. 18.4 **A,** Sexual maturity ratings (SMRs) of pubic hair changes in adolescent boys and girls. **B,** SMRs of breast changes in adolescent girls. Bone growth is closely correlated with SMR, because hormones control epiphyseal closure. (Redrawn from photographs of J. M. Tanner, MD, Institute of Child Health, Department of Growth and Development, University of London, London, England.)

Box 18.2 Tanner's Stages of Sexual Maturity

Sexual maturity ratings (SMRs) range from 1 to 5. A score of 1 represents the prepubertal child; 5 corresponds to adult status.

BOYS: GENITAL DEVELOPMENT

Stage 1: Preadolescent; testes, scrotum, and penis about the same size and proportion as in early childhood
Stage 2: Enlargement of scrotum and testes; skin of scrotum reddens and changes in texture; little or no enlargement of penis at this stage
Stage 3: Enlargement of penis, which occurs at first mainly in length; further growth of testes and scrotum
Stage 4: Increased size of penis with growth in breadth and development of glands; testes and scrotum larger; scrotal skin darkened
Stage 5: Genitalia adult in size and shape

GIRLS: BREAST DEVELOPMENT

Stage 1: Preadolescent: elevation of papilla only
Stage 2: Breast bud stage: elevation of breast and papilla as small mound; enlargement of areolar diameter
Stage 3: Further enlargement and elevation of breast and areola, with no separation of their contours
Stage 4: Projection of areola and papilla to form a secondary mound above the level of the breast
Stage 5: Mature stage; projection of papilla only because of recession of the areola to the general contour of the breast

BOTH SEXES: PUBIC HAIR

Stage 1: Preadolescent; vellus over the pubes is no further developed than that over the abdominal wall, that is, no pubic hair
Stage 2: Sparse growth of long, slightly pigmented, downy hair, straight or curled, chiefly at the base of the penis or along the labia
Stage 3: Considerably darker, coarser, and more curled hair; hair spreads sparsely over the junction of the pubes
Stage 4: Hair now adult in type, but area covered is considerably smaller than in the adult; no spread to the medial surface of thighs
Stage 5: Adult in quantity and type with distribution of the horizontal (or classically "feminine") pattern; spread to medial surface of thighs but not up linea alba or elsewhere above the base of the inverse triangle (spread up linea alba occurs and is rated stage 6)

Data from Tanner, J. M. (1962). *Growth of adolescence* (2nd ed.). Oxford: Blackwell Scientific; Holland-Hall, C., & Burstein, G. R. (2016). Adolescent physical and social development. In R. M. Kliegman, B. F. Stanton, J. W. St. Geme, et al. (Eds.), *Nelson textbook of pediatrics* (20th ed.). Philadelphia: Saunders.

After puberty, boys are encouraged to know what their testes feel like by occasionally examining them during or after a hot bath or shower. If a change is discovered, it should be reported immediately to a health care provider.

Girls

Pubertal changes in girls occur 6 months to 2 years before they occur in boys. Puberty is easily recognized in girls by the onset of menstruation (Fig. 18.5). The first menstrual period is called the menarche. Menarche may occur as early as age 10 years or as late as age 15 years. The average age of onset of menarche in Canadian girls is 12.72 years, with British Columbia having the lowest average age at less than 11.5 years (Al-Sahab, Ardern, Hamadeh, et al., 2010). Secondary sex characteristics become more apparent before the menarche. Fat is deposited in the hips, thighs, and breasts, causing them to enlarge (see Box 18.2). At this time, the adolescent girl may need to be fitted for a bra. Measurements must be ascertained and various styles tried on for comfort.

The external genitalia grow. Hair develops in the pubic area (see Fig. 18.4 and Box 18.2) and the underarms. It is important to note that in ballet dancers, runners, gymnasts, and adolescents engaged in other athletic activities that involve a lean body and high level of physical activity, the mechanisms affecting puberty can be altered and cause a delay in the onset of menarche. Energy balance, activity, and nutrition are important factors to evaluate when menstruation is delayed. Further growth can no longer take place when the ends of the long bones knit securely to their shafts (epiphyseal closure).

Menstrual health

Adjustment to the menarche is enhanced if information is provided over time to the premenstrual adolescent so that all questions can be answered and positive attitudes can be developed. The nurse should be aware of various cultural and religious practices that help form attitudes. The nurse who has contact with adolescent girls in the clinic or school setting should counsel them about the details of the menstrual cycle and menstrual health. Menstrual irregularities are discussed in Chapter 2.

There are two types of menstrual products available—internal, for example, tampons, and external, for example, adhesive stripped disposable mini and maxi pads. Many companies offer introductory packages for young girls with helpful educational materials. Products that contain deodorants can cause irritation and inflammation and the use of super-absorbent tampons have been associated with the development of toxic shock syndrome (see Chapter 2). Teens should be taught to wash their hands, avoid touching the tampon tip before inserting it, and change tampons at least every 4 hours. Tampons should not be worn for vaginal discharges between menstrual periods. A highly absorbent tampon that is hard to remove may cause vaginal irritation and infection, and the teen should be urged to use a less absorbent tampon or switch to a pad. Reusable menstrual cups and pads are also available for use.

The vagina is self-cleansing and normal vaginal secretions are odourless. An odour forms when the secretions mix with perspiration that is in the vaginal area. Regular bathing and hygiene with soap and water is important; the routine use of vaginal sprays or douches is not recommended. Sprays can cause irritation that could lead to infection, and douching can propel water and bacteria from the vagina toward the uterus. Removal of the normal mucus in the vagina can upset the vaginal flora and make the vagina more susceptible to infection. Toilet hygiene that includes wiping from front to back to avoid contamination of the vagina and urethra with fecal material is essential for vaginal health.

PSYCHOSOCIAL DEVELOPMENT

Sense of Identity

Physical growth and sexual interest correlate with sexual maturity. Cognitive growth and social changes correlate with chronological age and placement in school. Stress can increase when physical growth and cognitive growth occur at different rates in the same person. Although the early-maturing male often finds positive social adjustment and acceptance, early-maturing females may be embarrassed and develop low self-esteem. The adolescent's desire for freedom and independence is extremely important and necessary for developing individuality. To accomplish this, young persons must reject their childhood self and often the people most closely associated with it. Erikson identifies the major task of this group as *identity versus role confusion.*

Adolescents want to be people in their own right, and they "try on" different roles. Self-concept (one's view of oneself) fluctuates during this time and is moulded by the demands of and interactions with parents, peers, teachers, and others. This process is complicated by many factors, such as illness, broken homes, and the extent of formal education. Young persons who are unable to master confusion and establish an identity may become rigid in their actions, bewildered, or depressed, or they may cling to the conformity of peer groups long after the need should have passed. Some show an inordinate need for something "new and exciting." They may experience low self-esteem and alienation, and they may confront many other difficulties on entering the adult world.

While gender identity begins prior to adolescence, sexual orientation heightens during adolescence and can be a struggle for some teens. It is important that caregivers provide an inclusive and supportive environment for adolescents.

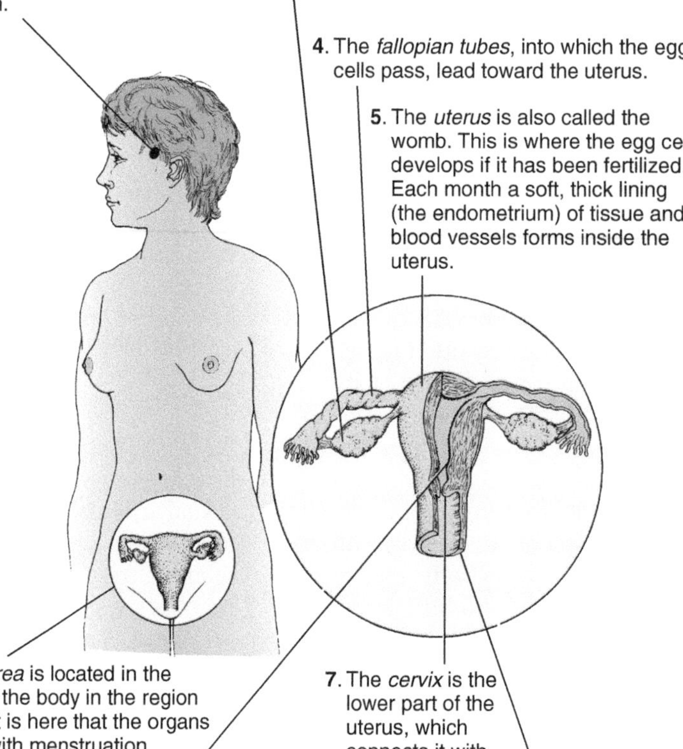

1. The *pituitary gland* is a small gland at the base of the brain. It sends chemical messengers through the blood to various parts of the body. These messengers, or hormones, are responsible for many steps of growth and change as one develops. When a girl reaches the age of puberty, the pituitary gland sends out a new hormone that affects the functions of a group of organs concerned with menstruation.
2. The *pelvic area* is located in the lower part of the body in the region of the hips. It is here that the organs associated with menstruation are located.
3. The *ovaries* are two small female organs that manufacture human egg cells. When a girl reaches the age of puberty, these cells receive a signal from the pituitary gland and begin to grow. Each month a cell escapes from an ovary and starts to travel along a passageway—one of the the fallopian tubes. This movement of the egg cell is called ovulation. If one of these cells becomes fertilized by a male cell, it can develop into a baby.
4. The *fallopian tubes*, into which the egg cells pass, lead toward the uterus.
5. The *uterus* is also called the womb. This is where the egg cell develops if it has been fertilized. Each month a soft, thick lining (the endometrium) of tissue and blood vessels forms inside the uterus.
6. The *endometrium*, or uterus lining, is where the fertilized egg implants and grows until it is ready to come into the world as a baby. But unless an egg cell has been fertilized and a baby started on its way toward birth, there is no need for the cell or for the blood and tissues of the endometrium. Therefore they are passed from the body.
7. The *cervix* is the lower part of the uterus, which connects it with the vagina.
8. The *vagina*, a passageway leading to the outside of the lower part of the body, carries away these materials in a flow of blood. This is called menstrual flow. When it occurs, it lasts for several days each month and is known as menstruation.

Fig. 18.5 Menstruation.

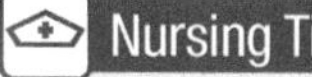 **Nursing Tip**

In adolescence, dependency creates hostility. Parents who foster dependence invite unavoidable resentment. Wise parents make themselves increasingly dispensable. Their language is sprinkled with such statements as "The choice is yours," "You decide about that," "If you want to," and "It's your decision."

Sense of Intimacy

Developing intimacy is closely entwined with the resolving of a person's sense of identity. As adolescents move toward young adulthood, they become ready to take the risks of close affiliations and friendships and to establish relationships with someone of the sex they find most interesting to them (Fig. 18.6). Avoidance of building these relationships may lead to a deep sense of isolation. Adolescence is a period of trying and testing. Disagreements with parents often revolve around dating, the family car, money, chores, school grades, choice of friends, smoking, sex, and the use of illicit drugs. The young person questions parental values and morals and is particularly sensitive to hypocrisy.

Adults who associate with adolescents should try to create an atmosphere of interest and understanding. Adolescents must know that adults care. Adolescents need practice in making decisions that must be respected even if they have made a mistake. Parents should set limits and expect them to be challenged but not exceeded. Parents and nurses who see other people's intrinsic

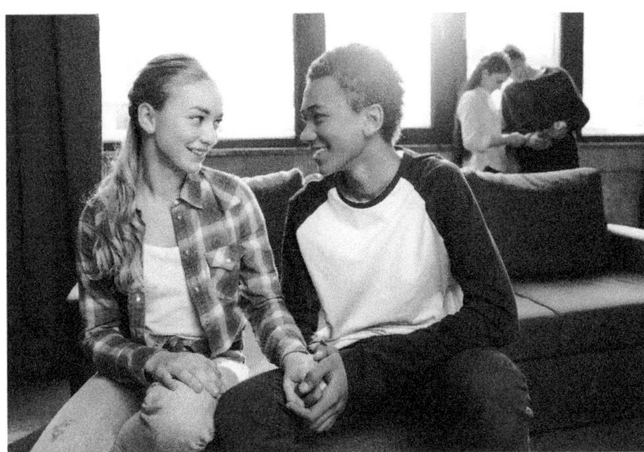

Fig. 18.6 As adolescents move toward young adulthood, they become ready to take the risks of close affiliations and friendship and to establish relationships with members of the sex they are attracted to. (istock.com/LightFieldStudios)

worth, feel good about themselves, and do not see the adolescent's behaviour as a reflection on their parenting or nursing provide a more secure environment for growth. Loving detachment is not easy, but it is an effective practice when interacting with adolescents.

Cultural and Spiritual Considerations

Canadians are multiethnic, multicultural, and multilingual. All may not adopt the value of independence as a goal of maturational and emotional development. Some immigrants come from societies that are patriarchal and highly structured and have distinct social roles. The good of the family takes precedence over personal goals. The protection of family image and neighbourhood reputation is essential.

As part of a search for their identity, adolescents focus on the values and ideals of the family and decide either to embrace them or to separate from them. Adolescents often perceive their feelings and thoughts as unique and therefore do not express their feelings freely. Adolescents can understand abstract concepts and symbols, and exposure to religion and religious practices other than those experienced within their own traditional family can help them stabilize their group identity (Fig. 18.7). This is key for the multicultural climate of Canada and the large Indigenous population. The nurse's awareness of these and other cultural influences on the adolescent's behaviour will help in the effort to provide holistic care.

Nursing Tip

Every culture is unique. Adolescent behaviours and expectations differ in other areas of the world and must be respected.

Body Image

In early adolescence, the young person must adjust to the dramatic changes of puberty. Focusing on body development during early and middle adolescence is

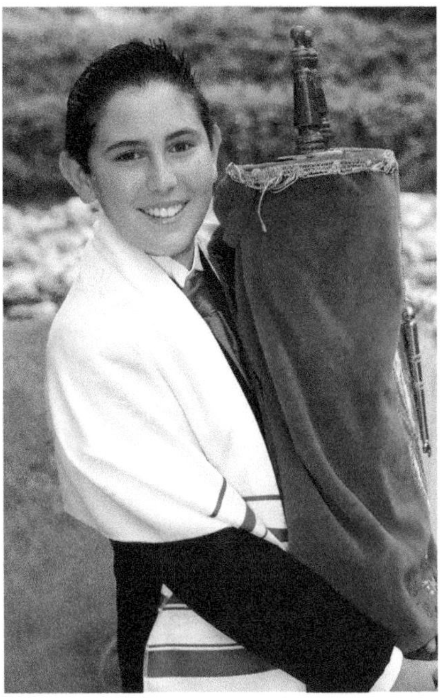

Fig. 18.7 Adolescents can understand abstract concepts and symbols, and religious traditions can help to stabilize identity. The bar mitzvah is a spiritual rite of passage into adulthood. (istock.com/CapturedNuance)

one factor that contributes to egocentrism, or self-centredness. Young persons create what has been termed an "imaginary audience." They believe that everyone is looking at them. This preoccupation with self is normal and accounts for the constant hair combing and makeup repairing often observed in a group of adolescents. Young adolescents may try to hide their changing body or may advertise it. They may take pride in their abilities or feel frustrated when their actual abilities do not match their perceived abilities.

In early adolescence, teens make every effort to be just like their peers. A pimple on the skin or a disability can be disastrous to the young adolescent. By late adolescence, most have completed their growth, are less self-conscious, and enjoy their individual skills, abilities, and interests. Chronic illness may complicate or exacerbate unresolved problems of body image.

Peer Relationships

Peer groups help adolescents feel that they "belong" and make it possible to experiment with social behaviours (Fig. 18.8). School assumes an important role in the psychological development of the adolescent by providing the focus for initiating social interaction. Small, exclusive groups form, which are called **cliques**. These often unisex groups are made up of adolescents with similar interests, values, and tastes. Belonging to the group is of utmost importance to the young adolescent.

Within the clique, the adolescent often develops a close personal relationship with one peer of the same sex. This best-friend interaction supports social development by enabling adolescents to experiment with behaviours together and listen to and care about each

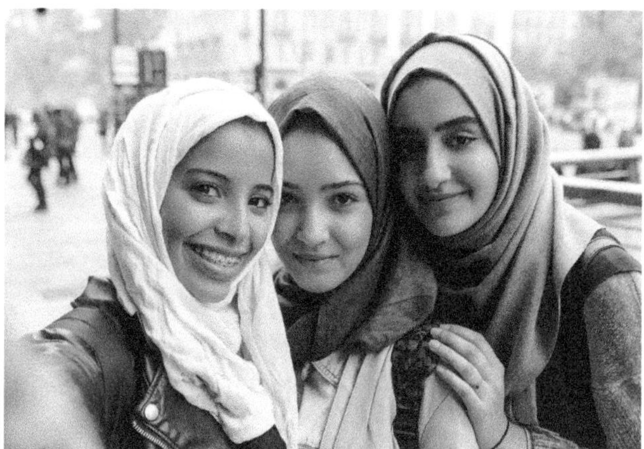

Fig. 18.8 Immersion into a peer group helps adolescents free themselves from childhood dependence. (istock.com/LeoPatrizi)

other (Fig. 18.9). Stable best-friend experiences often precede successful relationships in later life.

The peer group serves as a mirror for "normality" and helps to determine where one "fits in." It is vitally important in helping adolescents define themselves. Acceptance by one's friends helps to decrease the loneliness and sense of loss many adolescents experience on the road to adulthood.

The social norms and pressures exerted by the group may cause problems. The selection of friends and allegiance to them may bring about confrontations within the family. Parents need help in understanding that the adolescent's exaggerated conformity is necessary in moving away from dependence and obtaining approval from persons outside the nuclear family. Failure to develop social competence may produce feelings of inadequacy and low self-esteem.

Peer relationships are developed in person and through technology. Bullying can also take place in school, home, the community, or online. It is important to support adolescents through these challenges, for those being bullied as well as for those initiating bullying behaviour.

Nurses can assist the family by supporting and educating them in the dynamics of this age group. Parents can be directed to groups such as peer helpers (for the adolescent) and community educational programs sponsored by various agencies.

Career Plans

Some adolescents graduate from high school with a definite idea of what they would like to do as a working adult. Many, however, are unsure of what they want. To choose a career that is best suited for them, adolescents must first know themselves. What particularly interests them? What are they good at? What are their shortcomings?

By this time, many adolescents have already taken some definite steps toward a goal. Choice of high school curriculum and grades determine eligibility for college or preparation for a specific vocation. Parents

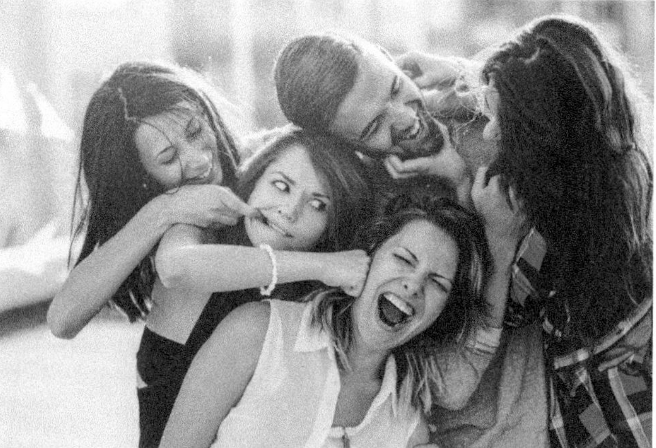

Fig. 18.9 Adolescents practice facial expressions. "Best friend" interaction supports social development by enabling the adolescent to experiment with behaviour and to care about others. (istock.com/filadendron)

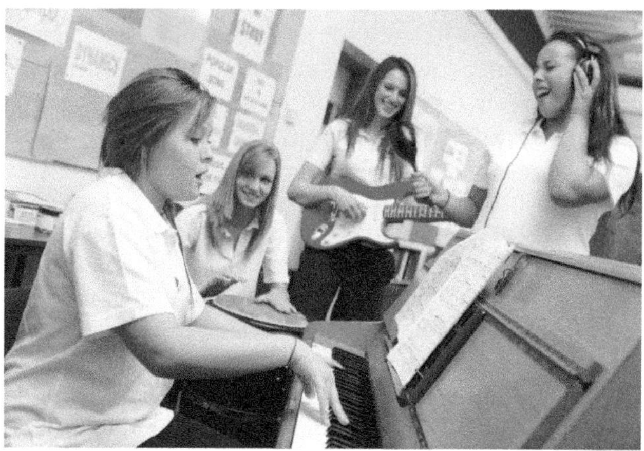

Fig. 18.10 Singing, playing a musical instrument, or developing mechanical skills is part of adolescent life. (istock.com/monkeybusinessimages)

should observe the interests of their children and encourage them to take advantage of their talents (Fig. 18.10). Whenever possible, an adolescent should investigate various fields by talking to people who are involved in those areas of interest.

Graduation and career goals may be a challenge for some adolescents to obtain. Although the rate of high school diploma completion has increased in Canada over the past 10 years, the rate is still significantly less for Indigenous teens than for non-Indigenous populations across Canada. It is important for the nurse to understand the unique challenges faced by Indigenous adolescents, whether they live on reservations or in an urban setting.

Valuable information can also be obtained by career exploration, which is available at most colleges, and from professional organizations, Internet sites, and other sources. The school guidance counsellor can administer aptitude tests as an additional guide and can work with adolescents to expose them to as wide a selection of careers as possible. The adolescent must make the final decision. To be happy in a career, the adolescent must choose it of their own free will and not because parents expect their child to follow in their footsteps.

The job market today is extremely competitive and almost nonexistent for some people without skills or higher education. Productive employment must fit young people's life framework and offer an opportunity for personal growth. Some positive aspects of employment include building self-esteem, promoting responsibility, testing new skills, constructively channelling energies, providing money for increased independence, engaging the young person in interactions with adults, and allowing the adolescent to assume an active rather than a passive role. In contrast, when adolescents are forced to take a job because of economic or personal pressures, they may need to drop out of school. With few skills and no experience, they may remain locked into low-level employment. This pattern may be perpetuated from one generation to another.

Responsibility

Adolescents look forward to challenges. Parents must encourage their children to take on new responsibilities. The adolescent is often humiliated by being placed in a dependent role, such as when a parent or sibling drives them to school. Driving a car, riding a bicycle, or walking provides a sense of independence and responsibility. Even routine jobs can be made more inspiring if youths are taught to see them in relation to a longer-term objective.

Young adolescents must also be taught the value of money. An allowance helps them to learn financial management. If money is simply handed out as requested, it is more difficult to develop responsibility for finances. Allowances should be increased from time to time to comply with the age and needs of the adolescent.

Middle and older adolescents who have jobs can be taught how to save money for special purchases. Many find satisfaction in purchasing their own clothes. An adolescent who buys an old car soon discovers that it takes money to insure, run, and repair it. Such experiences provide valuable lessons in finance. Babysitting is a common means of earning money among younger adolescents. Many boys and girls begin to assist with babysitting at about 12 or 13 years of age. Babysitting courses are valuable because young people need to be prepared for this important responsibility.

COGNITIVE DEVELOPMENT

Piaget's theory of cognitive development states that development is systematic, sequential, and orderly. Young adolescents are still in the *concrete phase* of thinking. They take words literally. A young adolescent girl, if asked by the nurse, "Have you ever slept with anyone?" may not connect the question with a vaginal infection or sexual intercourse. By middle adolescence the ability to think abstractly has increased. Piaget calls this the stage of **formal operations**. Older adolescents can see a situation from many viewpoints and can imagine or organize unseen or unexperienced possibilities. *Abstract thinking* and reasoning emerge. Therefore, when teaching early adolescents about menstruation, for example, the nurse should focus on concrete issues and concerns. When abstract thinking emerges in later adolescence, the abstract meaning of menstruation relating to womanhood or motherhood can be discussed. Empowering young adolescent girls by educating them according to their intellectual and emotional developmental level can improve their self-image.

Adolescents are able to sympathize and empathize. They can understand their own values and actions and can also understand and accept the differing values and actions of people from other cultures.

Daydreams

Adolescents spend a lot of time daydreaming in the solitude of their rooms or during a class lecture. Most of this behaviour is normal and natural for this age group. Daydreaming is usually considered harmless if the young person continues the usual active pursuits. It also serves several purposes. Adolescence is a lonely, in-between age; daydreaming helps to fill the void. Imaginatively acting out what will be said or done in various situations prepares adolescents to interact with others so they can better cope with real situations. Daydreams are also a valuable safety valve for the expression of strong feelings.

SEXUAL DEVELOPMENT

Sexual Behaviour

Adolescents meet and become acquainted with members of the sex they are attracted to. This may begin in preadolescence with admiration from afar, which is accompanied by daydreams as the young person attempts to attract the other's attention.

Group dates during structured school or community functions are often followed by double dating and then single-couple dating. Dancing provides an opportunity for the symbolic expression of sexual urges without physical contact. When adolescents are at home or feeling alone, long telephone or text messaging conversations link the adolescent to peers. "Crushes"—feelings of attachment to a person of the same or opposite sex who is popular or possesses qualities important to the adolescent—are a common occurrence. Competition and rivalry may be keen, but long-term commitment and deep romantic attachments are not often present.

Sexual experimentation often occurs as a response to peer pressure, as a means for momentary pleasure, as a learning experience to satisfy curiosity, or as a means of gaining a feeling of being loved and cared about. Sexual behaviour can affect the growth and development of the adolescent. Unplanned pregnancies or sexually transmitted infections (STIs) are two major complications of adolescent sexual interaction; adolescents may not realize the importance of using protection or know how to use it (Jatlaoui & Burstein, 2016).

The adolescent's cultural background influences patterns of dating. Conflict often arises when the adolescent wants to be independent and quickly adopts Canadian norms of dating while parents are insisting on strict traditional values. This is particularly noticeable with daughters.

Dating is one of the early social aspects of growing up and it may become a battleground for the struggle for independence. Parents' opposition is often based on their unspoken fears. Parents may also fear sexual experimentation, pregnancy, or infection with the human immunodeficiency virus (HIV). They may respond by imposing strict restrictions, such as curfews, chaperones, and limitations on use of the car. When these problems are not discussed openly, the adolescent may react by rebelling sexually or by other means to test general parental control, rather than for the sake of the prohibited act itself.

Sexual curiosity and masturbation are common among adolescents. There is also a need for the intimacy of close personal friendships. Seeking one person of the opposite or same sex to share confidences and feelings may lead to sexual intimacies. This may produce guilt feelings and can lead to isolation from friends and family. The breaking up of such romances is often a source of great emotional pain.

A wide variety of sexual behaviour is freely discussed and depicted in movies, in magazines, online, and on television. Music directed toward young people often centres on sexual themes. A variety of sexual activities occur during the teen years. According to Statistics Canada, 30% of teens aged 15 to 19 years old use oral contraception. Sexual activity rates vary across Canada, and it is a challenge to gather accurate information. A survey of children in British Columbia, in grades 7 to 12, reported three-quarters of youth had not engaged in oral sex or intercourse (McCreary Centre Society, 2015).

Sex Education

Sex education for the adolescent can be challenging. Nurses must put aside their own attitudes and biases; understand society, cultural, and moral values; and incorporate a broad understanding of physical and psychological growth and development to prepare an effective school or clinic program. Television, movies, magazines, and computer chat rooms or websites provide a source of information for sex education for the adolescent that may or may not be accurate and helpful to the young adult.

Sex education focuses on the physiology of sex, the reproductive systems, and STIs as well as personal values concerning sexuality, facts about contraception, safer sex, and peer pressure. Formal structured comprehensive sex education programs are available from the Sexuality Information and Education Council of Canada (SIECCAN) and other community agencies. These types of programs are geared toward kindergarten through grade 12 and present information about all aspects of health, such as nutrition, dental care, avoidance of drugs, and STIs. These courses should be presented as age appropriate. The physiology of the reproductive systems can be taught at about grade 5. By grade 8, topics such as coping skills for dating and sexuality, pregnancy, and giving birth can be reviewed. Abstinence, contraception, healthy relationships, and how to say "no" may also be discussed.

Decision making is also emphasized. Flowcharts should show the possible consequences of certain actions. The high school curriculum can include how to handle adolescent pregnancy, prenatal and postnatal care, and effective parenting techniques. A unit on intimate relationships can be presented as a series of discussions and activities designed to help students think about the nature of love. It can cover ideas such as compromise, problem solving, and communication skills. It should emphasize the many reasons why adolescents should say "no" to casual sex.

Factual and sensitive information provided by concerned parents is, of course, the ideal. However, too often peers provide erroneous material, or parents postpone education until a crisis arrives. Children must be told what body changes to expect and why these changes occur. Parents who have answered their children's questions truthfully throughout childhood offer a secure and natural foundation on which to build. Contrary to popular belief, adolescents who obtain early sex education information from caring parents or well-informed adults do *not* have a higher rate of sexual activity.

Concerns About Being "Different"

Adolescents have certain concerns that are specific to puberty. The girl who begins to experience physical changes at about 10 years of age may feel self-conscious because she towers over her friends or needs to wear a bra. She may be teased because she is different. The other extreme is the latecomer who feels abnormal and unattractive because her friends look more feminine.

Such problems are not limited to girls. Of particular concern is the boy on a slow schedule of development. Still short at 15 years of age, he is unable to compete for placement on school teams because of his size. He sees his male friends being admired for their height and strength, and this can be a threat to him. Such fears are natural and usually are alleviated by reassurances that, although boys begin to grow later than girls, their growth spurt lasts longer. When performing an assessment, the nurse has an opportunity to support the adolescent who is concerned about normal growth and development.

Traditional gender stereotypes define being "male" by activity and achievement and being "female" by sensitivity and interpersonal competence. Society's current trends toward equality of the sexes may affect these roles. Nevertheless, few adolescents escape the social pressures that dictate acceptable sexual attitudes and behaviour for each gender.

Sexual Orientation

When a person has an attraction for a person of their own sex, that person is referred to as homosexual. A lesbian is a female who prefers other females as sexual partners. A male is referred to as gay when he prefers another male as his sexual partner. Same-sex sexual behaviour in adolescence is not uncommon. Experimentation with this sexuality is not a positive predictor of adult sexual preference; it may merely indicate a desire to explore alternative lifestyles. It is thought that a combination of cultural, biological, and psychological factors contributes to sexual orientation and development. The nursing role is to support the parents during this time and create a safe environment for the adolescent to ask questions and seek help. It is also important to understand the differences between sex, gender identity, gender expression, and sexual orientation. The Canadian Paediatric Society (CPS) has resources for health care providers and parents that are listed in the Additional Learning Resources section at the end of this chapter.

Nurses must be sensitive to these issues when obtaining histories and working with young adolescents. They must also be aware of their own personal biases to determine their potential effectiveness with this population. Asking questions that are not gender specific, such as "Do you have sex with men, women, both, or people who identify in other ways?" can help to create a neutral environment for the teen. Support groups for parents and friends of gays, lesbians, bisexual, and transgender adolescents are available. Those who question their sexual orientation may be referred to counsellors and health agencies that can respond to their needs.

Table 18.2 provides an example of the use of the nursing process in planning sex education for the adolescent.

Table 18.2 Using the Nursing Process in Planning Sex Education for the Adolescent

NURSING PROCESS STEP	NURSING ACTIONS
Data collection	Determine the level of knowledge concerning puberty and body changes. Discuss peer acceptance. Determine sexual practices and sexual orientation.
Analysis	Review body image and understanding concerning body changes. Observe for signs of abuse. Determine risk factors involving sexual behaviour and substance use. Clarify sexual practices, including contraception.
Planning and implementation	Provide a private area and nonjudgemental environment for teaching. Discuss safer sex practices and personal views and values of the adolescent. Discuss contraceptive choices, if appropriate. Discuss the use of drugs, alcohol, and cigarettes. Teach the need for regular follow-up health care.
Evaluation	Follow-up during scheduled home or clinic visits concerning problems identified or teaching is completed.

PARENTING THE ADOLESCENT

The media have an increasing influence on the growth and development of the adolescent. Many high school students have a television in their bedroom and a computer in their house, and most frequent the Internet by computer, electronic tablet, or smartphone. Social networking is the norm. Parenting an adolescent requires major adaptations on the part of the parents. At times, it is difficult for parents to cope with adolescents. Parenting philosophies can range from the rigid rules of discipline, to permissiveness, to a middle-of-the-road position. Negotiation is a more successful strategy in managing adolescents than an authoritarian approach. Some parents are unsure of their own opinions and may hesitate to exert authority. Others refuse to "let go" or to change any of their beliefs to accommodate the world of today's youth. Issues of privacy and trust abound, and conflict occurs as the adolescent desires more adult liberties. Adolescents may need time alone to separate themselves from family and search for their identity.

Adolescents need to talk about their fears, such as school examinations or how they will look with a certain haircut. They need assistance in sorting out confused feelings. A confidential, accepting atmosphere will promote quality communications (Fig. 18.11). Physical symptoms, such as stomachaches, insomnia, and headaches, surface in relation to anxiety. Bizarre behaviour may be a call for long-overdue help.

Nursing Tip

Adolescent warning signs indicating need for psychosocial intervention and follow-up:

- Spends time on computer in early hours of the morning
- Changes screen on computer when parent enters room
- Has pornographic material on the computer
- Makes frequent international calls

Some approaches to such problems are presented in the Health Promotion box that follows. As adolescents try to separate themselves from their family, they may reject some family traditions such as family outings or dress codes. When parents respond to this behaviour negatively, the separation widens and tension grows. Often adolescents search for adults outside of the family as role models and confidants. Coaches or scout leaders can fulfill this role and serve as positive outlets for gaining a sense of belonging when there are conflicts at home.

Health Promotion

Effective Approaches to Problems

APPROACH	PURPOSE	EXAMPLE
Our values are our values, but not necessarily theirs	Allow adolescent to express their values (Some values, such as school, are non-negotiable but explore the clash of opinion.)	"What is it about that way of thinking that you like?"
"I" message	Communicating your feelings about how adolescent's behaviour affects you; used when you own the problem	"When I'm ill and the dishes are left for me to do, I feel disrespected because it seems no one cares about me." "When you borrow tools and don't return them, I feel discouraged because I don't have the tools I need when there's a job to do."
Model mature problem-solving; exploring alternatives	Role modelling behaviour	"What are some ways you could solve this problem?"
	Helping adolescents decide how to solve problems they own	"Which idea appeals to you most?" "Are you willing to do this until…?"
	Negotiating agreements with adolescent when you own the problem	"What can we do to settle this conflict between us?" "Are we in agreement on that idea?" "What would be a fair consequence if the agreement is broken?"
Maintain healthy boundaries and limits	Permitting adolescents, within limits, to decide how they will behave and allowing them to experience consequences	Adolescent who forgets coat on cold days becomes cold; adolescent who skips lunch becomes hungry. Adolescent who spends allowance quickly will not receive any more money until next allowance day; adolescent who neglects to study for a test receives low grade.

Adapted from Public Health Agency of Canada. (2012). *Overview Paper: Raising Today's Teens why Parents Matter*. Ottawa, ON: Author. Retrieved from: https://www.canada.ca/content/dam/phac-aspc/migration/phac-aspc/sfv-avf/sources/nfnts/nfnts-raise-ado/assets/pdf/HP20-13-2008E.pdf; NOAA Workforce Management Office. (2011). *Positive Parenting Strategies for the Teenage Years*. Retrieved from: http://www.wfm.noaa.gov/pdfs/ParentingYourTeen_Handout1.pdf.

Nurses should help parents keep the lines of communication open, promote respect and trust, and provide confidentiality and a sense of privacy. Despite the problems parents face with their adolescents, the family continues to play a major role in socialization.

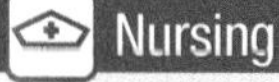

Nursing Tip

Privacy and confidentiality are essential when communicating with adolescents.

HEALTH PROMOTION AND GUIDANCE

NUTRITION

Adolescents grow rapidly; therefore, they need foods that provide for their increase in height, body cell mass, and maturation. Adolescents appear to be "always hungry" because their stomach capacity is too small to meet the increased caloric and protein requirements of their rapid growth spurt. Frequent meals are needed. Dietary deficiencies are more likely to occur at this age because of this growth acceleration and because eating patterns may become more irregular. In addition, foods and eating fads are often a source of conflict between adolescents and their parents. Nutritional requirements are more strongly correlated with **sexual maturity ratings (SMRs)** (see Box 18.2) than with age. For example, girls at SMR 2 and boys at SMR 3 are close to their peak growth velocities. They require adequate intake of nutrients and calories, regardless of their chronological age.

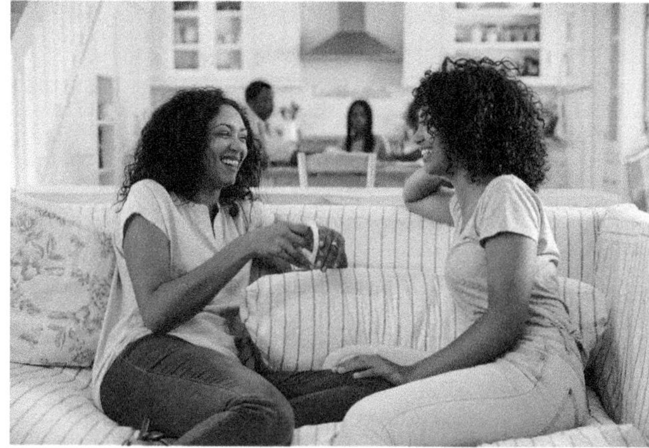

Fig. 18.11 Listening is an important practice for establishing rapport. A confidential, accepting atmosphere will promote good communication. (istock.com/monkeybusinessimages)

The most noticeable changes in the adolescent's eating habits are skipped meals, more between-meal snacks, and eating out more often. Breakfast and lunch are often omitted. Teens need to be taught to plan meals so meals are not skipped; the importance of not skipping breakfast should be emphasized. Part-time jobs, school activities, and socialization may result in the adolescent eating little or nothing during the day

Box 18.3 Preventing Obesity in Adolescents

- Discourage dieting and skipping meals.
- Encourage family meals.
- Discuss healthy eating.
- Focus on healthy food instead of weight.

From Golden, N., Schneider, M., Wood, C., & Committee on Nutrition, Committee on Adolescence, Section on Obesity. (2016). Preventing obesity and eating disorders in adolescents. *Pediatrics*, 138(3) e20161649; https://doi.org/10.1542/peds.2016-1649.

and then "catching up" in the evening. Fast-food restaurants are inexpensive and provide food quickly for the busy adolescent. These foods tend to be high in calories, fat, protein, sugar, and sodium and low in fibre and contribute to the development of obesity (Box 18.3). Most food chains have added salads and other healthier foods. Carbonated drinks often replace milk, resulting in low intakes of calcium, riboflavin, and vitamins A and D.

Foods should be selected from *Canada's Food Guide* (see Appendix C). In estimating food requirements, variables such as physical activity and sex must also be considered. The elements most likely to be inadequately supplied in the adolescent's diet are calcium, iron, and vitamin B_{12}. Zinc is known to be essential for growth and sexual maturation and is therefore of great importance in adolescence. Teens should be counselled to choose health foods that have little or no added sodium, sugars, or saturated fat (Government of Canada, 2019). Sports drinks and caffeinated energy drinks are not recommended for adolescents to consume as they contain high amounts of sugar and caffeine (Blair & Canadian Paediatric Society [CPS], Nutrition and Gastroenterology Committee, 2017).

Vegetarian Diets

Adolescents are now a growing segment of the vegetarian population. Ninety percent of adolescent vegetarian diets include eggs and milk. Iron-rich foods include fortified grain products. However, a high intake of whole grains, bran, and foods rich in oxalic acid (e.g., spinach) can impair the absorption of iron. Tofu, nuts, wheat germ, and legumes can provide the zinc necessary for cognitive development. If animal products are totally excluded from the diet, a vitamin B_{12} supplement may be necessary. The nursing role is to understand the eating pattern, identify fad diets, and understand the reason the diet was selected, and then evaluate and discuss any deficiencies or needs within that diet. Developing a partnership with the adolescent in meeting growth needs and allowing the adolescent to take responsibility for meeting their own health needs are the cornerstones for success in nutritional education.

Vegetarians who eat no animal protein, eggs, or dairy products (vegans) are at particular risk of developing deficiencies in protein, vitamin B_{12}, calcium, iron, iodine, and possibly zinc. A total vegetarian diet is adequate only if it is carefully planned. Referral to a dietitian for further education might be recommended. For discussion of a gluten-free diet, see Chapter 28, Celiac Disease.

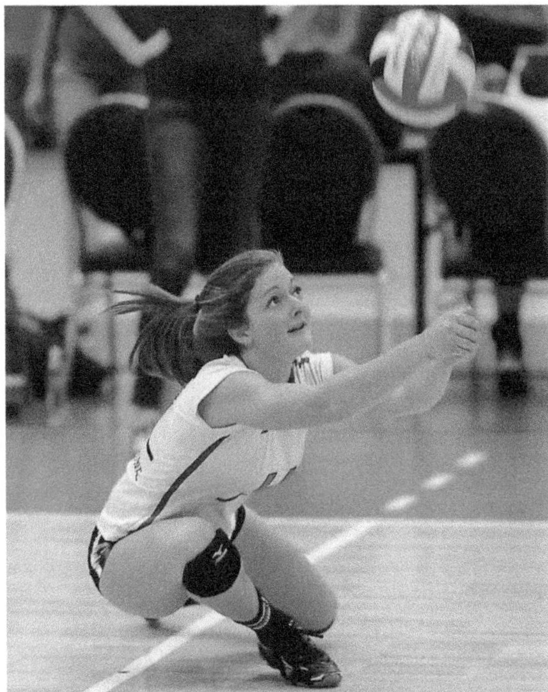

Fig. 18.12 Adequate nutrition and the choice and timing of food ingestion influence health and the athlete's performance.

Sports and Nutrition

The best training diet is one that contains a variety of healthy foods in sufficient quantities to meet energy demands and nutrient requirements. What to eat and when to eat it in relation to muscle exercise are vital to successful athletic performance (Fig. 18.12). Athletes exhaust reserves of muscle glycogen. Carbohydrates that can be rapidly converted to blood glucose and transported to muscles will provide the rapid recovery of muscle glycogen necessary for maintaining prolonged intense muscle activity. Eating a slowly absorbed glucose source will prevent the development of chronically low muscle energy stores. To hasten muscle energy recovery, the young athlete should consume protein and carbohydrates within 30 minutes of exercise, and again within 1 to 2 hours of exercise, to help reload muscles with glycogen and allow for proper recovery (Purcell & CPS Paediatric Sports and Exercise Medicine Section, 2013). Foods high in fat and protein will prolong carbohydrate metabolism.

Carbohydrates that provide both energy and other nutrients are best for athletes. Therefore, fruits and fruit juices are a better choice than sugar-rich soft drinks and candy. Some foods that provide a rapid supply of carbohydrates to muscles include corn flakes, bagels, raisins, maple syrup, potatoes, and rice. Some foods that supply a slow release of carbohydrates to muscles include apples, pears, green peas, chickpeas, skim milk, and plain yogurt.

Fluids lost by sweat must be replaced by drinking fluids during a workout. Before activity, athletes should consume 400 to 600 mL of cold water, 2 to 3 hours before their event. During sporting activities, athletes should consume 150 to 300 mL of fluid every 15 to 20 minutes. For events lasting less than 1 hour, water is sufficient. For events lasting longer than 60 minutes or taking place in hot, humid weather, sports drinks are recommended to replace energy stores and fluid and electrolyte losses (Purcell et al., 2013). Caffeine and alcohol deplete body water and are to be avoided.

Anabolic steroids, used by some athletes to gain weight and increase strength, are detrimental to bone growth. Iron is particularly necessary for female athletes, who may be borderline or deficient in their intake of this mineral.

Nutrition and School Examinations

Studies have shown that foods can affect behaviour, moods, and alertness. For the adolescent who is scheduled to take an important school examination, the nurse can offer nutritional guidance as part of the examination preparation. Carbohydrates such as pancakes and syrup, breakfast pastries, or a muffin and jelly increase serotonin in the brain, resulting in a soothing, sleepy response. Bacon and eggs are high in fat and cholesterol and are therefore slow to digest, diverting blood from the brain during the digestion process and causing decreased alertness. Drinking a caffeine-containing beverage such as coffee can cause overstimulation and nervousness. However, protein-rich meals increase amino acids and tyrosine, which will break down into norepinephrine in the brain and result in increased alertness. Fish, soy, peanuts, and rice increase choline and acetylcholine in the brain, which results in increased memory. Therefore a "proper" meal before a big school test may help the adolescent's achievement as well as their health.

PERSONAL CARE

Hygiene

The adolescent needs personal hygiene information, because body changes require more frequent bathing and the use of deodorants. The nurse can help the young person sort out the various claims of reliability for hair removal, menstrual hygiene, and cosmetic products and procedures. Body piercing, a popular adolescent fad, should be performed only by an experienced person using sterile instruments. The skin around the point of insertion of the body ring should be regularly inspected for signs of infection. Swapping body rings is discouraged. Adolescents should be warned not to use another's razor or toothbrush, particularly in light of the risk of HIV infection. Body tattoos and piercings are discussed in Chapter 20.

Dental Health

The prevalence of tooth decay has substantially decreased, as a result of the widespread use of fluorides, including community fluoridation, dental sealants, and dental products containing fluorides. Adolescents are nonetheless at risk for dental caries because of possible inadequate dental maintenance and frequent snacking on sucrose-containing candies and beverages. When dental hygiene is neglected, the period of greatest tooth decay in the permanent teeth is from ages 12 to 18 years. Lack of oral hygiene (inadequate brushing, flossing, and rinsing, particularly after meals) fosters the accumulation of plaque and food debris. Missing, aching, or decayed teeth contribute to poor nutrition. Young people with unattractive teeth may suffer from low self-esteem. Corrective orthodontic appliances are often worn during adolescence, and meticulous oral hygiene is essential to prevent discoloration of tooth enamel and other complications. Regular dental visits during adolescence must be maintained as a priority in the health care teaching of adolescents and their families. See Chapter 13 for a detailed discussion of dental health.

Tanning

Adolescents respond to movie and magazine pictures of the ideal "healthy suntanned body" as an attractive aspect of a body image. The young adult looks forward to sunbathing on the beach or at the pool during summer vacations and often prepares their body by trying to obtain a tanned appearance using artificial means. The nurse can play a vital role in educating the adolescent concerning the danger of the sun's rays and the need for skin protection with a sun protective factor (SPF) of at least 30. Protection of the eyes from the sun is also essential. Excessive sunlight and the use of artificial tanning machines can cause serious long-term reactions such as early aging of the skin or skin cancer (see Chapter 30). Teenagers are frequent visitors to tanning parlors, with girls being more frequent and sustained users. The Canadian Paediatric Society (CPS) recommends a ban on the use of commercial tanning facilities by Canadian children and youth under the age of 18 years and this has become legislation in some provinces (Taddeo, Stanwick, & CPS, Adolescent Health Committee, 2012/2018).

SAFETY

The chief hazard to the adolescent is the automobile (Fig. 18.13). Road and off-road vehicle accidents kill and cause serious injuries to adolescents at alarming rates. Some schools offer driver-training courses as an integral part of the educational program. Students learn how to drive and learn the accompanying responsibilities; however, this does not ensure that they follow through with the recommendations. Preventing motor vehicle accidents is of utmost importance to every community. Adolescents who ride motorcycles, motor scooters, or motorbikes should know the rules of the road and should wear special safety equipment, such as helmets.

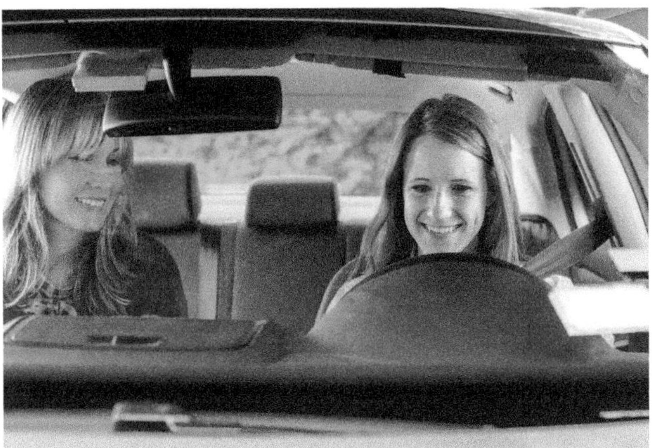

Fig. 18.13 Adolescents look forward to obtaining their driver's license. The search for independence also brings responsibilities. (istock.com/XiXinXing)

Young people should learn how to swim and practice swimming safety. Accidents result from diving into unsafe areas, from using alcohol or drugs while swimming, and from unsafe use of jet skis. If adolescents are interested in hunting or similar sports that require a gun, they must be instructed in the proper safeguards and take the appropriate courses for safe handling of firearms.

Sports Injuries

Sports involving body contact can be hazardous to the adolescent. Sports teams separated by age only are a special problem, because adolescents of one specific age group can vary in size, weight, and muscle strength. Protective gear should be worn by all team players in any contact sport. The feeling of strength and the need to show off can motivate the adolescent to participate in risky behaviour. Assessment of the female athlete in training should include identification of the "female athlete triad," which includes an eating disorder, amenorrhea, and osteoporosis. Coaches, parents, and health care providers must be vigilant in recognizing this condition as it has serious long-term complications.

Student athletes should be encouraged to have a comprehensive physical examination before participating in competitive sports activities. Each year, many high school athletes die in nontraumatic sports-related deaths. Most deaths result from cardiac problems that were not obvious. Guidelines for medical clearance for sports activities are available, although this is not mandatory or enforced in most provinces (Mirabelli, Devine, Singh, et al., 2015). The nurse can play a key role in safety education by working closely with school coaches and parents.

Nursing Tip

Obtaining a driver's license, graduating from high school, and reaching the legal drinking age are Canadian rites of passage through adolescence. Other cultures offer specific ceremonies to mark phases of development.

COMMON PROBLEMS OF ADOLESCENCE

School-age children begin an exposure to the outside world, where peers gradually become more important to them than their family contacts and they begin to spend more time in outside experiences and less time with family activities. During adolescence, more complex social tasks include entering high school where new friendships are formed, interacting with multiple teachers in one day, mastering increasing academic rigour, and experiencing romantic encounters. Social anxiety disorders affect many adolescents, although some are never recognized or treated. Many adolescents are shy, and basic shyness is a normal characteristic for an adolescent and should not be confused with a social anxiety disorder, which most often involves distress that impairs functioning. However, the adolescent that has few personal friends and displays impaired social skills may be at risk and may drop out of high school. The at-risk adolescent should be referred for professional care where diagnostic tools and therapy are available. The child with an emotional or behavioral condition is discussed in more detail in Chapter 33.

SMOKING AND VAPING

The regulation of tobacco use and education concerning the health risks to children and adults have decreased smoking of tobacco cigarettes. Many adult smokers now report using e-cigarettes, most of whom use e-cigarettes to quit or reduce smoking. However, substantial proportions of youth also report using e-cigarettes. In Canada, about 20% of youth aged 15 to 19 years report "ever trying" e-cigarettes (Hammond, Reid, Cole, et al., 2017). The easy access and flavouring make it especially enticing to adolescents and young adults and can lead to nicotine poisoning. *Vaping* is the inhalation and exhalation of vapour through a device such as an e-cigarette or Hookah pipe. The vapour does not contain tobacco. Most e-cigarettes contain tobacco-derived nicotine (Stanwick, 2015). In addition, the e-cigarette is powered by a battery and produces a vapour by heating a substance such as propylene glycol mixed with a flavouring and nicotine that activates when the user inhales. Little research on the glycol and other additives have been done, but the nicotine addiction is a continuing problem. Hammond et al. (2017) found that using e-cigarettes was associated with an increase in the initiation of using. The World Health Organization (WHO) and the CPS support stringent regulations until the safety of this product is known (Hua & Talbot, 2016; Stanwick, 2015). It is important to note that many vaping products may contain some form of sugar, and those who are diabetic should be warned about the effects these products may have in their ability to control elevated blood sugar levels.

DRUG USE

Drugs are often readily accessible to adolescents, in many communities and in schools. Because this age group faces many challenges as they explore their own value system and growing responsibilities, they may be more vulnerable to the influences of drug use. Although cannabis use is now legal in Canada, the legal age of being able to use cannabis depends on the province and is either 18 or 19 years.

Inhalants

Inhalants are common household products whose vapours can be inhaled to produce a psychoactive response. Inhalant use is a worldwide problem that is especially common among individuals from minority and marginalized populations and is strongly correlated with the social determinants of health. It often affects younger children more than do other forms of substance use and crosses social and ethnic boundaries (Baydala & CPS First Nations, Inuit and Métis Health Committee, 2010). Use of inhalants is popular among teens who do not have the money for street drugs. Higher rates of inhalant use are present in some Indigenous populations, possibly owing to health disparities, reduced access to services, and socioeconomic factors. The unique social and health contexts, as well as the widespread nature of inhalant use in some Indigenous communities, has led to the development of culturally specific treatment programs (Baydala & CPS First Nations, Inuit & Métis Health Committee, 2010). Inhalants such as glue, spray paint, and shoe polish are popular. The practice of *huffing* is the inhaling via a paper bag filled with a rag that is soaked with the product. Some common products used as inhalants include the following:

- *Benzene:* Found in gasoline and can cause reproductive toxicity and bone marrow injury
- *Propane* or *butane*: Found in lighter fluid and hair sprays, can cause sudden death and high risk of burns
- *Freon*: Found in refrigerants and aerosols. Can cause sudden death by cold stress to respiratory tissues
- *Toluene:* Found in paint removers, paint thinners, and gasoline and can cause impaired cognition and loss of coordination
- *Trichlorethylene:* Found in spot removers and can cause hearing and vision damage and liver failure

Education and Assessment

Education concerning the dangers of drug experimentation and use is essential in the home and in the school. See Chapter 33 for a detailed discussion of substance use.

Adolescents may be prone to mood swings as they try to adjust to the many physical and psychological changes occurring in their lives. The CPS recommends the CRAFFT screening interview as a highly sensitive tool for drug and alcohol problems in adolescents, and it is included in the Greig Health Record (Greig, Constantin, LeBlanc, et al., 2016).

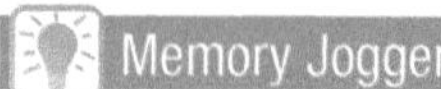
Memory Jogger

CRAFFT Screening Tool

C Have you ever ridden in a **c**ar driven by someone (including yourself) who was "high" or had been using alcohol or drugs?
R Do you ever use alcohol or drugs to **r**elax, feel better about yourself, or fit in?
A Do you ever use alcohol or drugs while you are by yourself, **a**lone?
F Do you ever **f**orget things you did while using alcohol or drugs?
F Do your **f**amily members or **f**riends ever tell you that you should cut down on your drinking or drug use?
T Have you ever gotten into **t**rouble while you were using alcohol or drugs? (Greig et al., 2016)

If two or more of the CRAFFT letters are problem areas, the adolescent may be at high risk for substance use and require a professional referral. Early referrals to treatment programs have resulted in significant improvements in the physical, mental, and social conditions of those affected (Baydala et al., 2010).

DEPRESSION

Sometimes an adolescent who appears to be adjusted and performing well in school may become depressed. Working parents and busy teachers can easily overlook behaviours that are slowly changing. A change in school performance, in appearance, or in behaviour can be a warning sign of depression, which can lead to suicide if left untreated. A threat of suicide is a call for help that must be addressed without delay. Suicide is the second leading cause of death in the adolescent group age 15 to 19 years, second only to accidental deaths (Statistics Canada, 2017). The nurse can help the adolescent by recognizing the depression, encouraging open communication, posting the numbers of available hotlines, identifying appropriate coping mechanisms, and providing professional referrals. See Chapter 33 for details concerning suicide and other behavioural problems. Suicide among Indigenous youth (aged 15 to 24 years) across Canada is five to six times higher than among non-Indigenous peoples. These elevated rates are seen for males and females, although they are higher among males (Crawford, 2016).

ADOLESCENT PREGNANCY

Adolescent pregnancy continues to be a social and health concern in Canada, although the rate of teenage pregnancy is continuing to decrease. Nurses must be familiar with the tasks of the adolescent years and recognize that adolescent pregnancy occurs while the adolescent is still struggling to manage developmental issues. There are many psychosocial factors that influence sexual activity during the adolescent years. The developmental and physiological impact of pregnancy on the adolescent, the tasks and adolescent responses,

Table 18.3 **Developmental and Physiological Impact of Pregnancy on the Adolescent**

FACTOR	RISK	EFFECT
Age at which pregnancy occurs	At menarche, the first menstrual cycles are irregular and anovulatory.	"Natural" methods of birth control are ineffective in young adolescents.
	Young adolescents have immature vascular development in the uterus.	Condition may lead to gestational hypertension and fetal perfusion problems that result in poor pregnancy outcome, such as prematurity and low birth weight.
	Long bone growth is incomplete until 2 years after menses start.	Pregnancy before long bone growth is complete can cause early closure of epiphysis because of increase in estrogen levels.
	Pelvis does not reach adult size and dimensions until 3 years after menarche.	A small pelvis increases problems during labour and birth and increases need for Caesarean birth.
Nutritional intake	Dietary intake often contains "empty" calories and consists of fad diets; eating disorders may be present; dieting to control weight and meet media definition of a beautiful body is common.	Inadequate nutrition, especially in early months of pregnancy, results in negative pregnancy outcome and birth defects. Poor nutrition can result in gestational hypertension, low-birth-weight newborn, and prematurity.
Sexual activity	Multiple partners or unprotected sex can result in sexually transmitted infections (STIs).	STIs increase risk of problems for fetus and newborn.
Limited access to health care	Adolescent may fear revealing pregnancy to parents.	Delayed prenatal care can result in problems for mother and fetus.

From Leifer, G. (2012). *Maternity nursing* (11 ed.). St. Louis: Saunders.

Table 18.4 **Nursing Care and the Effect of Adolescence on the Tasks of an Unplanned Pregnancy**

STATE OF PREGNANCY	TASK	ADOLESCENT RESPONSE	NURSING INTERVENTION
First trimester	Confirmation of pregnancy	Fear of disclosing pregnancy may result in delayed confirmation, hidden pregnancy, and delayed prenatal care	Educate concerning signs and symptoms of pregnancy so as not to confuse it with other conditions. Discuss health behaviours required for a healthy fetus.
Second trimester	Focus on newborn as real	Family chaos may result when parents, baby's father, and friends see reality of pregnancy; may try to maintain control by dieting and continuing to conceal pregnancy Egocentric phase may prevent full focus on baby as being real	Preserve adolescent image by her wearing appropriate clothes. Discuss disclosure to parents and friends. Discuss prenatal needs; show pictures of fetus at various gestational ages.
Third trimester	Preparation for newborn and birth process	Focuses on ending experience but may fear labour	Initiate discussions of child care; tour birthing facility and refer to community agencies as needed; provide education regarding birth process.

From Leifer, G. (2012). *Maternity nursing* (11th ed.). St. Louis: Saunders.

and the appropriate nursing interventions are described in Table 18.3 and Table 18.4. Nutritional needs and nursing care of the pregnant adolescent are discussed in Chapter 4, and nursing care during labour and birth is discussed in Chapters 6 and 7.

THE NURSING APPROACH TO ADOLESCENTS

The nurse must open the lines of communication with adolescents and enable them to feel at ease before initiating care or teaching. A sense of humour is helpful. Providing privacy and ensuring confidentiality and respect are basic to adolescent communication. The nurse must be careful not to behave like an adolescent, because the adolescent may perceive that behaviour as "phony." Adolescent hostility may be evidence of fear of the unknown, and rebellion may be an effort to grasp independence. The nurse should guide the parents concerning the need to listen, understand, and share with adolescents. Helping parents distinguish

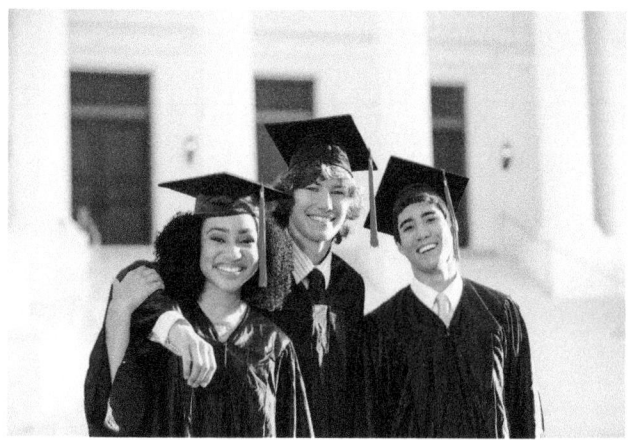

Fig. 18.14 Graduation from high school is the self-actualization of the adolescent. Peers and family share the joy with the new graduate. (istock.com/kali9)

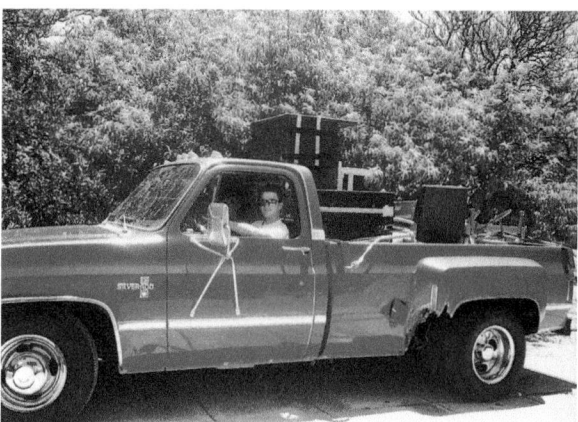

Fig. 18.15 Moving away from home and going away to college mark the entrance into adulthood.

between normal problems of adolescence and problems that need referral and follow-up is essential. For example, demands for privacy are normal, but overall withdrawal necessitates referral and follow-up care.

Health care teaching should include nutrition, dental care, personal care, body piercing, accident prevention, substance use, self-control, risk-taking behaviour, money, and time management. Open-ended questions concerning common problems of adolescence may encourage the discussion of a topic that adolescents may not initiate by themselves.

Graduation from high school is self-actualization for the adolescent (Fig. 18.14). Getting a job that will provide for self-support or going to college, which may involve leaving home, is the first step of entrance into independent adulthood (Fig. 18.15).

Get Ready for the Certification Examination!

Key Points

- Adolescence is defined as the period of life that begins with the appearance of secondary sex characteristics and ends with emotional maturity and the cessation of growth.
- According to Erikson, the major developmental task of adolescence is to establish a sense of identity. Other major tasks of adolescence include separating from family, initiating intimacy, and making career choices.
- Freud considered adolescence as the last stage of psychosexual development. He termed this the *genital stage.*
- Jean Piaget suggests that the cognitive development during adolescence reflects abstract reasoning and logic. He called this stage the *period of formal operations.*
- The physical development seen during this period is distinguished by puberty, the stage at which the reproductive organs become functional and secondary sex characteristics develop.
- Adolescents vary in their rate of physical and social maturation and their ability to resolve conflicts concerning self-esteem and autonomy.
- A nonjudgemental adult role model who can maintain confidentiality can help avoid a crisis for the adolescent.
- The Sexuality Information and Education Council of Canada (SIECCAN) is an example of a national organization that assists in the development and implementation of sex education programs.
- Some primary challenges of the adolescent years include adjusting to rapid physical changes, maintaining privacy, coping with stresses and pressures, maintaining open communication, and developing positive lifestyle choices.
- Peer groups help the adolescent to separate from the family and experiment with social behaviours.
- A clique affords the adolescent the opportunity to "belong" and to develop close personal relationships with others who have similar interests and values.
- The first menstrual period is called *menarche.*
- Menstrual health should be discussed with the teen.
- The adolescent may struggle with the development of a realistic body image.
- Accurate, safe, and timely sex education can help prevent STIs and HIV.

- Adolescence is a time of conflict with parental authority and values. The influence of peers and sexual relationships increases.
- Smoking tobacco, e-cigarettes, and vaping have health risks that should be discussed with the teen.
- Motor vehicle accidents, suicide, and drownings are the leading causes of mortality in the adolescent age group.
- A change in behaviour or decreased marks in school could indicate depression in the adolescent.

Additional Learning Resources

evolve Go to your Evolve website (http://evolve.elsevier.com/Canada/Leifer) for the following learning resources:

- Answer Key for Critical Thinking Questions
- Answer Key for Textbook Review Questions
- Audio Glossary
- Interactive Review Questions
- Skills Performance Checklists
- Video clips and more!

Online Resources

- Canadian Association for Suicide prevention: https://suicideprevention.ca/need-help/
- Canadian Paediatric Society, Adolescent Committee, *Position Statements:* https://www.cps.ca/en/documents/authors-auteurs/adolescent-health-committee
- Canadian Paediatric Society–Caring for Kids, *Your Teen's Sexual Orientation:* https://www.caringforkids.cps.ca/handouts/teens_sexual_orientation
- *Mandatory Bicycle Helmet Laws in Canada:* http://www.cycle-helmets.com/canada_helmets.html
- Participaction Canada, *Benefits & Guidelines: Canadian 24-Hour Movement Guidelines for Children and Youth: Ages 5–17:* https://www.participaction.com/en-ca/thought-leadership/benefits-and-guidelines/5-17
- Sexuality Information and Education Council of Canada (SIECCAN): www.sieccan.org

Review Questions

1. Which of the following is a task of adolescence as defined by Erikson?
   - **a.** Finding an identity
   - **b.** Sexual latency
   - **c.** Heterosexuality
   - **d.** Concrete operations
2. When communicating with an adolescent about safety concerns, which concept of adolescent behaviour should be considered?
   - **a.** The typical adolescent understands teaching and respects and usually follows the advice of adults.
   - **b.** Growth and development are complete in the adolescent, and muscle coordination and skills lessen the risks for injury.
   - **c.** Safety concerns at this age mostly focus on sports injuries.
   - **d.** Adolescents are risk takers and tend to experiment with potentially dangerous outcomes.
3. Puberty can most accurately be defined as the period of life characterized by which of the following?
   - **a.** Occurrence of sexual maturity and appearance of secondary sex characteristics
   - **b.** Substitution of adult interests and value systems for child interests
   - **c.** Most rapid rate of physical and mental growth and development
   - **d.** Awakening of sexual feelings and the initiation of sexual experience
4. A 16-year-old female towers over her companions, which bothers her. She confides to the nurse, saying, "I just hate school—everyone is always staring at me." The nurse's best response would be which of the following?
   - **a.** "Don't pay any attention to it."
   - **b.** "You just don't know how lucky you are to be tall."
   - **c.** "This will resolve itself in time. Don't worry."
   - **d.** "Tell me more about how this embarrasses you."
5. Which action is most important when planning nutrition management for the adolescent?
   - **a.** Planning a low-calorie diet
   - **b.** Incorporating favourite or fad foods into the diet
   - **c.** Encouraging a positive attitude toward obesity
   - **d.** Skipping a meal to reduce caloric intake

Critical Thinking Question

1. A grade 12 student expresses her concern to the nurse about taking her college entrance examination. The examination is given early in the morning, which is when she often feels sleepy and less alert and has trouble concentrating. She states that she usually studies hard the night before an examination and tries to eat a good breakfast on the day of the test. The breakfast usually consists of bacon and eggs, a muffin, and chocolate milk. What is the appropriate response of the nurse?

REFERENCES

Al-Sahab, B., Ardern, C., Hamadeh, M., et al. (2010). Age at menarche in Canada: Results from the National Longitudinal Survey of Children and Youth. *BMC Public Health, 10*, 736. https://doi.org/10.1186/1471-2458-10-736.

Baydala, L., & Canadian Paediatric Society (CPS), First Nations, Inuit and Métis Health Committee. (2010). Inhalant abuse. *Paediatrics & Child Health, 15*(7), 443–448.

Blair, B., & Canadian Paediatric Society (CPS), Nutrition and Gastroenterology Committee. (2017). Energy and sports drinks in children and adolescents. *Paediatrics & Child Health, 22*(7), 406–410.

Crawford, A. (2016). *Suicide among Indigenous peoples in Canada*. Retrieved from: https://www.thecanadianencyclopedia.ca/-en/article/suicide-among-indigenous-peoples-in-canada/.

Government of Canada. (2019). *Canada's food guide*. Retrieved from https://food-guide.canada.ca/en/.

Greig, A. A., Constantin, E., LeBlanc, C., et al. (2016). An update to the Greig health record: Preventive health care visits for children and adolescents aged 6 to 17 years—Technical report. *Paediatrics & Child Health, 21*(5), 265–268.

Hammond, D., Reid, J. L., Cole, A. G., et al. (2017). Electronic cigarette use and smoking initiation among youth: A longitudinal cohort study. *Canadian Medical Association Journal, 189*(43), E1328–E1336. https://doi.org/10.1503/cmaj.161002.

Hua, M., & Talbot, P. (2016). Potential health effects of e-cigarettes: A systematic review of case reports. *Preventative Medicine Report, 4*, 169–178.

Jatlaoui, T., & Burstein, R. (2016). Contraception. In R. M. Kliegman & B. Stanton (Eds.), *Nelson textbook of pediatrics* (20th ed.). Philadelphia: Elsevier.

McCreary Centre Society. (2015). *Sexual health of youth in BC*. Retrieved from: http://www.mcs.bc.ca/pdf/AHSV_sexual_health.pdf.

Mirabelli, M., Devine, M., Singh, J., et al. (2015). The preparticipation sports evaluation. *American Family Physician, 92*(5), 371–376. Retrieved from: http://www.aafp.org/afp/2015/0901/p371.htm.

Purcell, L., & Canadian Paediatric Society (CPS), & Paediatric Sports and Exercise Medicine. (2013). Sport nutrition for young athletes. *Paediatrics & Child Health, 18*(4), 200–202.

Stanwick, R. (2015). E-cigarettes: Are we renormalizing public smoking? Reversing five decades of tobacco control and revitalizing nicotine dependency in children and youth in Canada. *Paediatrics & Child Health, 20*(2), 101–105.

Statistics Canada. (2017). *Suicide rates: An overview*. Ottawa, ON: Author. Retrieved from: https://www150.statcan.gc.ca/n1/pub/82-624-x/2012001/article/11696-eng.htm.

Taddeo, E., Stanwick, R., & Canadian Paediatric Society (CPS), Adolescent Health Committee. (2012). Banning children and youth under the age of 18 years from commercial tanning facilities. *Pediatrics & Child Health, 17*(2), 89. Reaffirmed 2018.

The Child's Experience of Hospitalization

19

Lisa Keenan-Lindsay

http://evolve.elsevier.com/Canada/Leifer

Objectives

1. Define each key term listed.
2. Identify various health care delivery settings.
3. Describe three phases of separation anxiety.
4. List two ways in which the nurse can lessen the stress of hospitalization for the child's parents.
5. Describe two milestones in the physical and psychosocial development of a child of any age that contribute either positively or negatively to the adjustment to hospitalization.
6. Discuss the management of pain in infants and children.
7. Discuss the importance of using a language interpreter in the delivery of health care.
8. Identify two problems confronting the siblings of the hospitalized child.
9. Interpret a clinical pathway for a hospitalized child.
10. Contrast the problems of the preschool child and the school-age child facing hospitalization.
11. List three strengths of the adolescent that the nurse might use when formulating nursing care plans.
12. Recognize the steps in discharge planning for infants, children, and adolescents.

Key Terms

clinical pathway
conscious sedation
emancipated minor (ē-MĂN-sĭ-pā-ĭd MĪ-nŭr)
narcissistic (năhr-sĭ-SĬS-tĭk)
personal space
regression
respite care (RĔS-pĭt kār)
separation anxiety
transitional object

HEALTH CARE DELIVERY SETTINGS

OUTPATIENT CARE

Many hospitals today have well-organized outpatient facilities, satellite clinics for preventive medicine, and urgent care centres for the care of the child who is ill. Within clinics, there may be specialty areas (particularly at children's facilities) such as well-child clinics, asthma clinics, cardiac clinics, and orthopedic clinics. In some institutions, information is distributed about medical conditions and brief classes are held for waiting caregivers.

In many private medical offices, family doctors, pediatricians, or nurse practitioners provide care to children. The pediatric nurse practitioner is often the primary contact person for children in the health care system. The pediatric nurse practitioner may visit patients in the home, give routine physical examinations at the clinic, work with another health care provider, or work individually.

Another area of outpatient care is the pediatric research centre, such as Sick Kids in Toronto, Ontario. This type of institution offers highly specialized care for patients with particular disorders. In the outpatient clinic, as in all other settings, documentation and record review are important parts of data collection.

For patients with uncomplicated conditions, elective surgery (e.g., herniorrhaphy or tonsillectomy) at an outpatient surgery clinic offers the advantage of reduced incidence of health care–associated infection (HAI) and of recuperating at home in familiar surroundings. These outpatient clinics eliminate the need to separate the child from the family and reduce the extent of treatment and the emotional impact of the illness. Careful preparation must be provided to the child and family.

Promoting a Positive Experience

The attitude of nurses, receptionists, and other personnel in the clinic, office, or hospital unit is of the utmost importance. It can make the difference between an atmosphere that is warm and friendly and one in which the child is made to feel dehumanized. As more and more medical care is offered in outpatient clinics, there will be an even greater reduction in the number of children who require hospitalization. For many, the only exposure to medical personnel is through brief clinic appointments. Therefore, it is very important that these encounters are positive ones for children and their families.

Preparing the child for a treatment or procedure

Whenever possible, the caregivers should be involved in the preparation for and initiation of a treatment or procedure, and the child should be prepared according to their developmental level (Box 19.1 and see Chapter 13). For example, for infants, a familiar object is kept with the infant and the caregivers should cuddle and hug the infant following the procedure. For a toddler, the caregivers can model the behaviour desired (e.g., opening the mouth), tell the child it is okay to yell if the treatment or procedure is uncomfortable, and use distractions. For a preschooler, the treatment or procedure must be explained in simple terms. The child should be allowed to handle some of the equipment, and other equipment is kept out of sight. For a school-age child, one should explain in advance what the treatment or procedure is and the reason it is needed, and allow the child responsibility for simple tasks, such as applying tape. For adolescents, the treatment or procedure can be described in more detail and questioning encouraged. They should be involved in decision making and planning, such as who should be in the room. Proper preparation decreases anxiety, increases the child's ability to work with the team, and assists the child in coping with the experience.

Box 19.1 Preparing a Child for Treatments or Procedures

The developmental stage of the child guides the type of preparation needed.

INFANTS

Involve parents
Include familiar object
Soothe, distract, and hug after treatment or procedure

TODDLERS AND PRESCHOOLERS

Involve parents
Offer simple explanations
Give permission to express discomfort
Offer one direction at a time
Allow for choices, when possible
Use distraction
Hug after treatment or procedure

SCHOOL-AGE CHILD

All of the aforementioned, plus the following:
- Let child examine equipment
- Encourage verbalization of fears
- Offer small reward after treatment or procedure, for example, a sticker

ADOLESCENT

Provide privacy
Involve adolescent in treatment or procedure
Explain treatment or procedure and equipment
Suggest coping techniques

HOME

For many children care is provided in the home. Technical advancements and research in specific disease entities are also helping to advance the movement to home care (e.g., cryoprecipitate for hemophiliacs, Broviac catheters for chemotherapy, heparin or saline locks for intravenous [IV] access). However, home care is not merely a matter of supplying appliances and nursing care; it also includes assessment of the total needs of children and their families. Families need to be linked to a wide variety of network services. This ideally involves a multidisciplinary approach, often spearheaded by the nurse.

Local and national support groups for specific problems afford opportunities for families to share and support one another and to learn from others' successes and failures. Special groups and camps for children with chronic illnesses (e.g., diabetes camp) are also resources for families in the community. These programs have the potential for improving life for the child and family.

There have been dramatic changes in the delivery of health care to children and families. These changes affect the role and responsibilities of the nurse working both in wellness centres providing preventive care and in hospitals or homes treating illnesses.

PEDIATRIC HOSPITAL UNIT

The children's hospital unit differs in many respects from adult divisions. The pediatric unit or hospital is designed to meet the needs of children and their families. A cheerful, casual atmosphere helps to bridge the gap between home and hospital and is in keeping with the child's emotional, developmental, and physical needs. Nurses often wear colourful uniforms, and children often have coloured bedspreads and wagons, or strollers for transportation to provide a more homelike atmosphere.

The physical structure of the unit includes furniture of the proper height for the child, soundproof ceilings, and colour schemes with eye appeal. There is often a special treatment room for the health care provider to examine or treat the child. In this way, the other children do not become disturbed by the proceedings and the sick child is reassured that painful procedures will not happen in the child's bed.

Most pediatric departments include a playroom. It is generally large and light in colour. Bulletin boards and whiteboards are within reach of the patients. Mobiles may be suspended from the ceiling. Some playrooms are equipped with an aquarium of fish because children love living things. Various toys suitable for different age groups are available. This room may be under the supervision of a child-life specialist or a play therapist. Parents usually enjoy taking their children to the playroom and observing the various activities. The playroom is considered an "ouch-free" area, or a safe haven from painful treatments.

When the child cannot be taken to the playroom because of the diagnosis or physical condition, bedside play activities appropriate to the developmental level and diagnosis of the child should be provided. The daily routine of the pediatric unit emphasizes parent rooming-in, the provision of consistent caregivers, and flexible schedules designed to meet the needs of growing children.

THE CHILD'S REACTION TO HOSPITALIZATION

The child's reaction to hospitalization depends on many factors such as age, amount of preparation given, security of home life, previous hospitalizations, support of family and hospital personnel, and the child's emotional health. Some children may not understand what is going to happen to them even though they have been well prepared. At a time when children need their parents most, they may be separated from them, placed in the hands of strangers, and perhaps fed different foods. Add to this a totally new environment and physical discomfort, and the result can be a frightened and unhappy child.

Each child reacts differently to hospitalization. One may be demanding and exhibit temper tantrums, whereas another may become withdrawn. The "good" child on the unit may be going through greater torment than the one who cries and shows feelings outwardly. The best-prepared nurse cannot replace the child's parents. However, hospitalization can be a period of growth rather than just an unpleasant interlude. Children may see the nurse as someone who cares for them physically, as their parents would, and as a source of security and comfort (Fig. 19.1).

Often the major causes of stress for children of all ages are separation, pain, and fear of body intrusion. This may be influenced by the child's developmental age, cultural and economic factors, religious background, past experiences, state of health on admission, and other factors.

 **Nursing Tip**

Familiar rituals and routines must be incorporated into the plan of care for a hospitalized child.

SEPARATION ANXIETY

Separation anxiety normally occurs in infants and children from 6 to 30 months but is most pronounced at the toddler age. There are three stages of separation anxiety: protest, despair, and denial or detachment. Unless infants are extremely ill, their sense of abandonment is expressed by a loud *protest.* Toddlers may watch and listen for their parents. Their cry is continuous until they fall asleep in exhaustion. Toddlers may call out for a loved one repeatedly, and the approach of a stranger only causes increased screaming. The crying gradually stops, and the second stage of *despair* sets in. Children appear sad and depressed. They move about less and withdraw from strangers who approach. They do not play actively with toys. In the third stage, *denial* or *detachment,* children appear to deny their need for the parent and become detached or disinterested in their visits. They become more interested in their surroundings, their toys, and their playmates. On the surface, it appears the child has adjusted to the separation. However, it is important for the nurse to understand that the child is using a coping mechanism to detach and reduce the emotional pain.

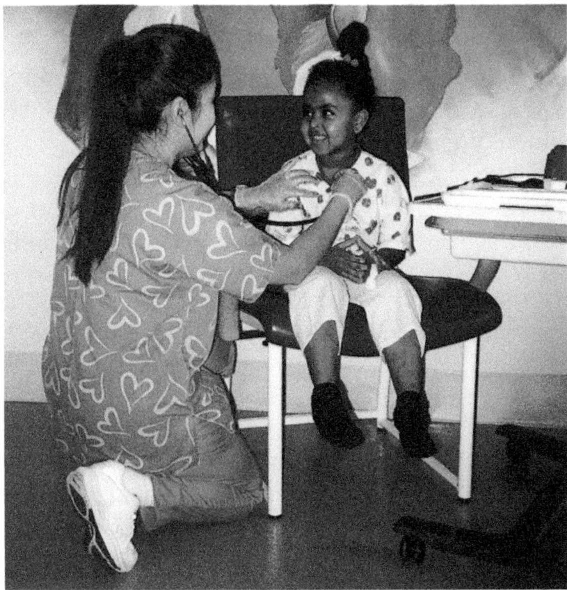

Fig. 19.1 The nurse greets the child at eye level in a nonthreatening manner. This child views the nurse as a person who cares for her physically and is a source of security and comfort. (Courtesy Pat Spier, RN-C.)

If the detachment stage is prolonged, an irreversible disruption of parent–infant bonding may occur. Nurses who do not understand the stages of separation anxiety may label the crying, protesting child as "bad," the withdrawn depressed child in despair as "adjusting," and the child who is in the detachment phase as a "well-adjusted" child. This misinterpretation can prevent nurses from providing desperately needed assistance and guidance to the child and family.

The nurse must understand that the child who is in despair reverts back to the protest stage when the parent arrives for a visit. Rather than showing joy, the child cries loudly when the parent appears at the door. This is a good sign. The child who has reached the detached phase appears unmoved and uninterested in the parent's arrival. Nursing interventions are needed in this case to preserve and heal parent–child relationships. Optimally the nurse helps the parents to understand they should not deceive the child into believing they will stay and then "sneak out" while the child is distracted. This may impact the bond of trust between the child and parent. In most hospitals today, parents or close adult relatives are encouraged to room in with the child during hospitalization to avoid separation anxiety. If a parent is unable to room in because of family commitments or distance from the hospital, the nurse must help support the parent to visit whenever possible and not make them feel guilty. Providing opportunities for the parent and child to communicate via the Internet or phone may help the older child cope better with the separation.

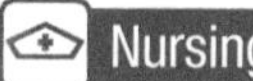
Nursing Tip

The stages of separation anxiety include protest, despair, and detachment or denial.

PAIN

Pain is defined as whatever the experiencing person says it is, existing whenever the experiencing person says it does. This includes verbal and nonverbal expressions of pain. Freedom from pain is a basic need and right of the infant and child. To increase awareness of pain during patient assessment, pain has come to be considered a "fifth vital sign." An assessment for pain is recorded with routine vital sign documentation.

The negative physical and psychological consequences of pain are well documented. Patients in pain secrete higher levels of cortisol, have compromised immune systems, experience more infections, and show delayed wound healing. Nurses must maintain a high level of suspicion for pain when caring for children. Infants cannot show the nurse where it hurts, and often a child's report of pain is not given the credibility of an adult's report. In addition, children may not realize they are supposed to report pain to the nurse.

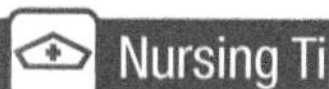
Nursing Tip

The nurse must be an advocate for adequate pain relief in children.

Pain Assessment

The nurse should ask the child who is old enough to express themselves about pain, using a pain rating scale. Fig. 19.2 shows some sample pain assessment tools. Children may sometimes refrain from saying they have pain if they believe they will receive an injection to relieve the pain. In infants, pain may be assessed according to a behaviour scale that includes tightly closed eyes, clenched fists, and a furrowed brow (see Fig. 11.11). An example of a pain assessment tool for preverbal children is the Neonatal/Infant Pain Scale (NIPS), which can be used for infants under 1 year of age (Fig. 19.2, *D*). In toddlers, crying may be caused by anxiety and fear rather than by the degree of pain. On the other hand, chronically ill children may not grimace or cry when in pain, but withdraw from interacting with their surroundings.

A pain indicator for communicatively impaired children (PICIC) has been developed and includes observations rated on a 4-point scale (1 = not at all, 2 = a little, 3 = often, 4 = all the time) including the following:

- Crying with or without tears
- Screaming or groaning
- Distressed facial expression
- Tense body
- Irritability to touch
- Difficulty in being comforted or consoled

The FLACC scale is a pain indicator that can be used with nonverbal children and is rated on a 0 to 2 scale for each observation, with 10 being the highest level of pain; it includes the following:

- **F**ace: grimace
- **L**egs: restless → kicking
- **A**ctivity: quiet → arched
- **C**ry: moan → scream
- **C**onsolability: touch → inconsolable

All factors relating to pain assessment should be considered. Family members also experience emotional pain when they see their child in pain.

Cultural aspects of pain assessment

Many cultures may interpret and show pain differently than the "expected" Western approach. Nurses need to be aware of cultural differences and provide care that is appropriate.

Latimer, Simandl, Finley, et al. (2014) explain that Indigenous children may have increased vulnerabilities related to pain and pain management due to the high prevalence of painful conditions among these children, potential cultural differences in how they express pain, the lack of culturally relevant validated pain assessments, inadequate pain care resulting in persistent pain, and the long-term impact on well-being of children with untreated childhood pain. Westernized pain assessment tools may not be appropriate for Indigenous children, resulting in inaccurate pain assessment and inadequate pain management. Further research is required to develop more accurate pain measurement tools that have a "two-eyed lens approach" that blends Westernized concepts with Indigenous concepts of pain (Latimer et al., 2014).

Nonpharmacological Management of Pain

Comfort measures and distractions are the initial interventions for mild or temporary pain.

Nonpharmacological techniques such as drawing, distraction, imagery, relaxation, and cognitive strategies may enhance analgesia to provide necessary relief from pain symptoms. The child may draw "how the pain feels" and where it is located. Distractions such as storytelling, quiet conversation, listening to music, reading, visiting with friends, and playing games are effective. Imagery techniques, such as having children imagine themselves in a safe place, relieves anxiety. Slowing down breathing and listening to relaxation tapes are effective in reducing pain in adolescents. Cognitive (thinking) techniques such

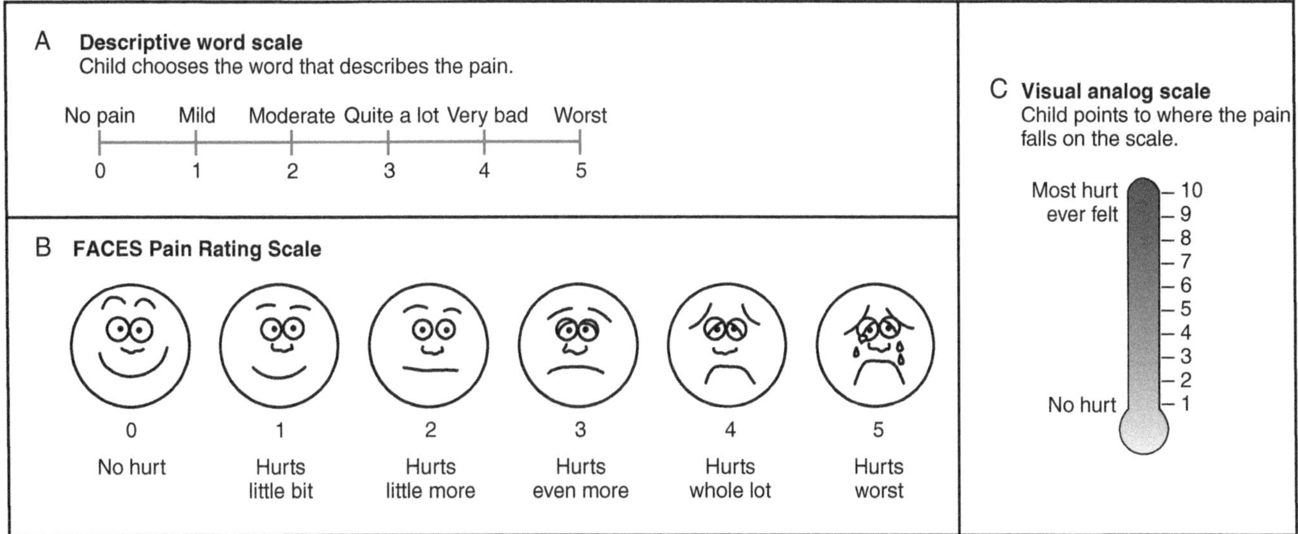

D Neonatal/Infant Pain Scale (NIPS)

(Recommended for children less than 1 year old)—A score greater than 3 indicates pain

Pain Assessment		Score
Facial Expression		
0 – Relaxed muscles	Restful face, neutral expression	
1 – Grimace	Tight facial muscles; furrowed brow, chin, jaw (negative facial expression—nose, mouth and brow)	
Cry		
0 – No Cry	Quiet, not crying	
1 – Whimper	Mild moaning, intermittent	
2 – Vigorous Cry	Loud scream; rising, shrill, continuous (Note: Silent cry may be scored if baby is intubated as evidenced by obvious mouth and facial movement)	
Breathing Patterns		
0 – Relaxed	Usual pattern for this infant	
1 – Change in Breathing	Indrawing, irregular, faster than usual; gagging; breath holding	
Arms		
0 – Relaxed/Restrained	No muscular rigidity; occasional random movements of arms	
1 – Flexed/Extended	Tense, straight legs; rigid and/or rapid extension, flexion	
Legs		
0 – Relaxed/Restrained	No muscular rigidity; occasional random leg movement	
1 – Flexed/Extended	Tense, straight legs; rigid and/or rapid extension, flexion	
State of Arousal		
0 – Sleeping/Awake	Quiet, peaceful, sleeping or alert, random leg movement	
1 – Fussy	Alert, restless, and thrashing	

Fig. 19.2 Pain assessment tools for children. (**A,** Data from Tesler, M. D., Savedra, M. C., & Holzemer, W. L. [1991]. The word-graphic rating scale as a measure of children's and adolescents' pain intensity. *Research in Nursing & Health*, *14*, 361–371. **B,** ©1983 Wong-Baker FACES Foundation. www.WongBakerFACES.org. Used with permission. Originally published in *Whaley & Wong's nursing care of infants and children*. © Elsevier Inc. **C,** Data from Cline, M. E., Herman, J., & Shaw, E. R. [1992]. Standardization of the visual analogue scale. *Nursing Research*, *41*[6], 378–380. **D,** From Lawrence, J., Alcock, D., McGrath, P., Kay, J., MacMurray, B., & Dulberg, C. [1993]. The development of a tool to assess neonatal pain. *Neonatal Network, 12*[6], 59–66. Copyright 1989, Children's Hospital of Eastern Ontario, Ottawa, Ontario, Canada.)

as "thought stopping" are also helpful in older patients. In this technique, the patient is instructed to identify positive facts about the painful event (e.g., it does not last long) or thinking about something else during the painful procedure. A backrub or hand massage is also relaxing, depending on the child's age and diagnosis. In newborns and infants undergoing brief painful procedures, skin-to-skin contact, breastfeeding, or oral sucrose can provide analgesia. Administering concentrated sucrose or glucose with or without non-nutritive sucking has been shown to have calming and analgesic effects for painful invasive procedures in newborns. A small volume (0.1 mL up to 2 mL) of glucose solutions (minimum 20%), given prior to and throughout the procedure, consistently reduces crying time, facial expression scores, and pain scores during a heel lance, venipuncture, or intramuscular injection (Bueno, Yamada, Harrison, et al., 2013; Stevens, Yamada, Ohlsson, et al., 2016) (see Chapter 11 for further discussion of newborn pain management).

Several types of complementary and alternative health modalities (CAHM), such as relaxation, hypnotherapy, biofeedback, yoga, massage, drumming, singing, and art therapy, are effective for pain control (see Chapter 21).

Pharmacological Management of Pain

Infants and children respond to medications differently than adults. Elimination of the medication from the body may be prolonged because of an immature liver enzyme system. However, the renal clearance of medications may be greater in toddlers than in adults. A decreased protein-binding capacity in the blood of small newborns may allow a greater proportion of free unbound medication to remain in the body of the small infant. Dosages are influenced by weight and differences in expected absorption, metabolism, and clearance. The nurse must calculate every medication to determine the safety of the dose before the medication is administered. See the dosage calculation technique in Chapter 20.

The World Health Organization (WHO) (2012) emphasizes the importance of pain management in children and focuses on the following key concepts:

- Using a two-step strategy
- Dosing at regular intervals
- Using the appropriate route of administration
- Adapting treatment to the individual child

This two-step strategy consists of a choice of category of analgesic medicines according to the child's level of pain severity: for children assessed as having mild to moderate pain, acetaminophen or ibuprofen should be considered as first options, and in children assessed as being in moderate to severe pain, administration of an opioid should be considered (WHO, 2012).

Acetaminophen is commonly used for the relief of mild to moderate pain in infants and children. The dose is 10–15 mg/kg/dose every 4 to 6 hours, for infants and children, with a maximum of five doses in 24 hours (or 65 mg/kg/day). Liver failure can be the result of toxicity.

Nonsteroidal anti-inflammatory drugs (NSAIDs), such as ibuprofen (Motrin), are given in a dosage of 5 to 10 mg/kg every 6 to 8 hours (not to exceed 40 mg/kg/day). Ketorolac (Toradol), another NSAID, is given orally or parenterally for a maximum of 5 days.

Opioids are used for moderate to severe pain, such as postoperative pain, sickle-cell crises, and cancer, and should be administered with stool softeners to prevent constipation. Morphine is considered the best opioid to use for children but if not suitable, fentanyl (Sublimaze) or hydromorphone (Dilaudid) is also effective. *Fentanyl* is a potent analgesic given for short surgical procedures. It has a rapid onset with a short duration of action. Codeine and tramadol are no longer recommended for children.

If opioids are used for long periods, tolerance to the pain-relieving effect can develop. Tolerance occurs because the body adapts to the use of the medication and therefore increasing amounts are required in order to achieve pain relief. The right dose of an opioid medication is the amount that relieves pain with a margin of safety for the child. The dose should be repeated before the pain recurs. Addiction is rare in children receiving opioids for acute pain (Zeltzer, Crane, & Palermo, 2016). *Naloxone* should be available for use in case of opioid overdose.

Administering NSAIDs and opioids together may enhance pain relief without increasing adverse effects. Providing adequate pain relief enables patients to focus on their surroundings and other activities, whereas inadequate pain relief causes the patient to focus on the pain and the time when more medication will be given to stop the pain.

Local anaesthetics are used with safety and effectiveness in children. *Topical anaesthetics* are used for skin sutures, IV catheter placement, and lumbar punctures. *EMLA cream* is a mixture of lidocaine and prilocaine (eutectic mixture of local anaesthetics) that is applied topically to the intact skin (Fig. 19.3) and can be used with children. "Numby Stuff" uses a mild electrical current (iontophoresis) to push a topical preparation of lidocaine and epinephrine into the skin, providing local anaesthesia within 10 minutes of the application of the patch. It is imperative to remove all metals from the injection site to avoid burns. A vapocoolant spray can provide superficial skin anaesthesia for short periods of time. Preoperative and postoperative care are discussed in Chapter 20.

Patient-controlled analgesia (PCA) allows the patient to press a button attached to an IV analgesic infusion to self-administer a bolus of medication. Parents and children as young as 5 or 6 years old can be taught to use PCA. A built-in lockout interval prevents accidental overdosing. Any child receiving opioid analgesic medications should be observed closely for adverse effects, such as respiratory depression.

More effective pain relief at lower dosages may be achieved when a low-dose analgesic is administered around-the-clock on a regular schedule rather than as needed (PRN). However, "breakthrough pain" can occur, and additional doses of an analgesic may have to be administered. This type of pain management is called *preventive pain control*. Unconventional pain medications include medications that were developed to treat specific conditions that have been found to also have analgesic properties such as select antidepressants, antiepileptics, and neurotropic medications (Zeltzer et al., 2016). The nurse must provide detailed observation of the child's responses to the medications and note, record, and report any adverse effects.

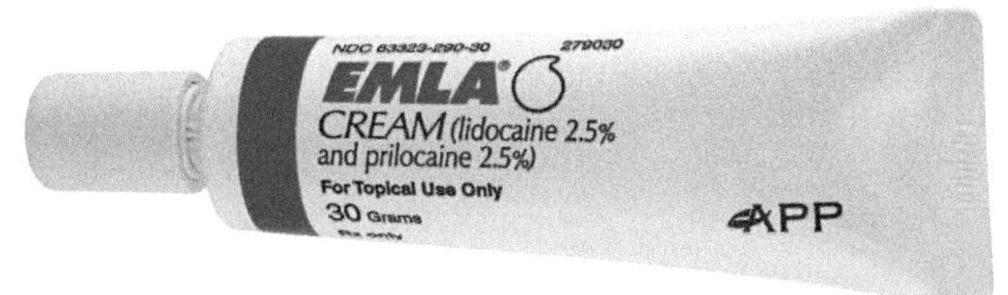

Fig. 19.3 EMLA cream, a topical anaesthetic used before performing an invasive procedure, to reduce pain involved in piercing the skin. (Courtesy APP Pharmaceuticals, Schaumburg, IL.)

Conscious sedation

Conscious sedation, also known as *procedural sedation,* is the administration of IV medications to a patient to impair consciousness but retain protective reflexes, the ability to maintain a patent airway, and often the ability to respond to physical and verbal stimuli. Conscious sedation is used to perform therapeutic or diagnostic procedures outside the traditional operating room setting. A registered nurse is required to continuously monitor the patient in an area where emergency equipment and medications are accessible for resuscitation.

A one-to-one nurse–patient ratio is continued until there are stable vital signs, age-appropriate motor and verbal abilities, adequate hydration, and a presedation level of responsiveness and orientation. Parents are instructed concerning diet, home care, and follow-up visits.

FEAR

Intrusive procedures, such as placing IV lines and performing blood tests, can be fear provoking for children. They disrupt the child's trust level and threaten self-esteem and self-control. They also may make it necessary to restrict activity. Care must be taken to respect the modesty, integrity, and privacy of each child. Hospital personnel can provide an environment that supports the child's need for mastery and control. These interventions are discussed according to age in this chapter and throughout the text. A selected nursing diagnosis for the hospitalized child and family is presented in Nursing Care Plan 19.1.

 **Nursing Care Plan 19.1 The Hospitalized Child and Family**

PATIENT DATA

A 3-year-old girl is admitted to the hospital with a diagnosis of a compound fracture of the right tibia. She cries whenever her parents leave or return to her room, and she has had episodes of bed-wetting since admission.

Selected Nursing Diagnosis Apprehension (restlessness, facial tension, insomnia, crying, clinging behaviour, regression to previous stage of growth and development) resulting from separation from parents and admission to hospital

Goals	Nursing Interventions	Rationales
Child and family will experience decreased apprehension as demonstrated by ability to relax, present a calm demeanor, and effectively participate in child's care.	Determine the child's and family's knowledge regarding reason for hospitalization.	Provides information to the nurse as to which areas need clarification and which need reinforcement of correct information.
	Explain routines usually followed on unit and orient the child and parent to the unit, including playroom.	Helps to decrease level of anxiety for the child and parents.
	Suggest that parents or family members bring in a photograph, favourite toy, or favourite DVD or CD for the child.	These items help to provide a link to home and help to promote a sense of security in the child.
	Recognize and teach the parent about age-appropriate separation anxiety.	The age of the child is a major factor to consider in the adjustment to separation from familiar people and surroundings.
	Instruct parents to explain to the child when they will return in an age-appropriate manner (e.g., "after your TV program is over" or "after lunch" or "before dinner").	Establishes a sense of trust that the child has not been abandoned. Also, toddlers and young children do not fully understand the concept of time. Using a favourite show or a mealtime as a marker helps to lessen the degree of anxiety the child may feel.
	Provide for consistency in personnel assigned to child as much as possible.	Consistency is necessary to develop a sense of trust. Maladaptive behaviours may be normal in unfamiliar circumstances. However, if consistency and support are not provided, coping abilities decrease.
	Support parents by showing a willingness to be available to listen to them and to answer questions.	The nurse's availability to answer questions provides family-centred care by showing interest for parents' concerns, prevents the potential for misunderstanding of prescribed treatments, and helps to lessen the anxiety of family members.
	Maintain child's contact with family; involve family in child's care when appropriate.	Increases a sense of security in the child and provides a sense of purpose for the family.

REGRESSION

Regression of growth and development during hospitalization can be expected. **Regression** is the loss of an achieved level of functioning to a past level of behaviour that was successful during earlier stages of development. Examples of regression include a child demanding a bottle when they usually drink from a cup, refusal to use a potty chair after bowel and bladder control has been achieved, or a child who had been walking independently demands to be carried. An accurate nursing assessment of the child's abilities and the planning of care to support and maintain growth and development can minimize regression. However, regression should not be punished. Nurses can guide parents to praise appropriate behaviour and ignore regressions. When the child is free of the stress that caused the regression, praise will motivate the achievement of appropriate behaviour.

CULTURAL RESPONSES AND THE USE OF LANGUAGE INTERPRETERS

Providing culturally sensitive care to families with hospitalized children decreases their anxiety. Flexibility and careful listening are necessary to understand cultural needs. Nurses must also be aware of their own cultural biases and how these might affect their assessments. The nurse must create a bridge between the Canadian health care system and the diverse people that the system serves. Effective use of health care services and the ability to complete a treatment plan is enhanced when the nurse's approach is sensitive to cultural needs and beliefs.

Teaching will be effective only if the parents and child understand the language used. In some cases, a translator may be required. While French and English are the main languages spoken in Canada, there are many other languages spoken. Having bilingual or multilingual staff is helpful but does not guarantee meeting the needs of all children and families. The nurse must be aware of available telephone language lines as well as mobile telephone apps and computer technologies that can be utilized to communicate effectively with patients and families. Printed material is often available in multiple languages, and these resources are an excellent supplement to translators. Such materials are often useful for parents to take home and read at a later time when they may be less overwhelmed. See Online Resources at the end of this chapter for resources from Sinai Health Services that are available in multiple languages. Nurses must take the time to use the services and avoid miscommunication to ensure that appropriate health care decisions are made between the health care provider, the patient, and the family. If at all possible, family members should not be used as interpreters as there is a risk of information being lost in translation, especially if technical language is not fully understood by the interpreter. Also in some cultures, it is not appropriate for a younger family member to tell an older family member bad news, so the information may not be accurate.

Nonverbal cues and body language are important in intercultural communication. Nurses should take the time to learn what their gestures and movements mean to the family from another culture.

In some developing countries the energy of parents may be focused on survival, and these practices become ingrained in the child-rearing practices handed down from generation to generation. For example, within these cultures, parents may believe that an ill infant must be near the caregiver's body at all times. Therefore, in the Western hospital, the nurse may find it a challenge to coax parents to allow the infant to remain in the crib, under an oxygen hood and separated from them. Crying may be interpreted by some cultures as a signal of an organic upset or illness. Because diarrhea is a common cause of infant death in developing countries, frequent feeding in response to crying is a survival response. Protective amulets or charms placed on the wrists or clothing of infants must be respected. Respecting cultural and religious beliefs will enhance collaboration between the family and the health care team. The nurse must assess the family through the eyes of its culture to ensure that the care provided is appropriate.

Intercultural Communication: Responses to Hospitalization

Personal space

Personal space is defined as an imaginary space that surrounds us. The size of that space and how securely it is guarded is largely determined by culture. We can observe the space by watching two friends of the same culture talk to each other. Some people stand close to each other. Nurses, who often must invade that personal space in carrying out their duties, can be perceived as "pushy" or suspect, and the parent who retreats to protect it can be thought of by the nurse as "cold."

Smiling

A smiling nurse may not be received in all cultures as a "friendly" nurse. In some cultures, a smile can indicate happiness and it would be inappropriate in a serious or sad situation. Nurses may interpret a nonsmiling person as "unfriendly" if they are unaware of this cultural difference. Members of some other cultures, however, smile in all circumstances. Their smile is a show of respect. When they are reprimanded, they smile to show they did not mind being reprimanded.

Eye contact

In Canada, establishing eye-to-eye contact with the person with whom one is communicating is usually considered a show of respect and attention. In some Asian cultures, however, eye-to-eye-contact is seen as disrespectful. Some Indigenous people consider it rude to stare at a speaker. Eye contact is acceptable for short periods only.

Touch

In North America, touch is often considered a gesture of friendliness. However, touch can give misleading messages. A pat on the head may imply superiority of the person touching the head. Nurses must touch patients frequently and often do so without thought about the implications of touching the person. It is important that a nurse ask for permission prior to touching any patient.

Focus

Some cultures are receptive to communication or teaching if the focus is on the problem. Some cultures deal with the problem by focusing on its future impact on the family or the life of the child. Teaching strategies must be designed to approach the topic from the perspective appropriate to the family.

When teaching infant and child care, the nurse must always determine the values of the cultural practice of the family before imposing a standardized process. Cultural humility is important to practise with patients to avoid any barriers and to ensure successful parent and child teaching. While culture evolves and is not static, most families from various cultures strive to maintain their cultural identity while adapting to Western practices. The nurse should support maintaining the individual cultural identity of each family. Providing culturally appropriate health care is also discussed in Chapter 1.

THE PARENTS' REACTIONS TO THE CHILD'S HOSPITALIZATION

When children are hospitalized, the entire family is affected. The parents of the hospitalized child need others to show interest in their physical and emotional needs. If they are frightened and tense, the child soon senses it.

Parents may believe they are to blame for the child's illness; they may believe they should have recognized the symptoms earlier or could have prevented an accident by using closer supervision. Immunizations and other types of preventive care may also have been missed. These feelings can cause a sense of guilt, helplessness, and anxiety.

Parents seldom are the direct cause for hospital admission of a child. Even in cases of child abuse or neglect, nothing is gained by blaming the parents. The nurse must remain objective and empathic. The nurse needs to listen carefully to parental concerns and acknowledge the legitimacy of their feelings; for example, "It is understandable that you feel this way; everything happened so fast." Parents also commonly express feelings of helplessness at the loss of the parental role as protector. The nurse should encourage and support parents and other family members, stress their importance to the child's recovery, and encourage their participation in the care of the child. The admission of a child to the hospital produces anxiety. The uncertainty of the situation can become overwhelming, causing feelings of panic. However, these feelings are usually temporary. The nurse should remain relaxed, reassure the parents, and reinforce positive parenting. The nurse should also provide information about the child's condition and the treatment plan. Needs are assessed, and interventions are planned to meet specific needs. Parents should be advised that pain-control techniques are available and will be used to minimize painful experiences for their ill child.

> **Nursing Tip**
>
> Many hospitals allow parents to be with their child during painful or stressful procedures and during the recovery phase postoperatively.

Family-centred care represents a philosophy that respects the important role that family members play in a child's care. It involves recognizing family members and health care providers as partners in caring for the child (Wright & Krug, 2016). Poor communication results in unnecessary fears. The nurse should explain in simple terms some of the equipment being used and facilities available on the unit. Siblings should be included in discussions if they are old enough to participate. The nurse needs to listen attentively and try to clear up any misconceptions. Rooming-in may alleviate some anxieties of parents. However, the nurse must continue promptly to tend to the needs of the child to indicate to the parents that their child is in good hands. Parental involvement in a child's care offers the nurse the opportunity to assess the relationship and to provide guidance and teaching as needed.

Parents may need to take time away from work, especially if treatment involves travel to special centres. Ronald McDonald House or Roger Neilson House offers lodging and other homelike amenities for parents of patients with life-threatening illnesses, as well as palliative care for children who are dying (see Online Resources at the end of this chapter). The availability of these facilities should be discussed with the family. The social worker may be of help in such instances. The care and welfare of other children at home while one parent is at work and the other is rooming in with the ill child should be discussed.

Parents may be faced with a disrupted home life throughout the child's hospitalization. Parents may have trouble coping with everyday tasks when they are worried about their children. The frequent trips to the hospital interfere with the daily routine, and other children in the family may resent the ill child. Contact with the health care provider is needed. Parents have a legal and ethical right to be informed of the benefits and risks of therapy and to be included in the decision-making process. Parents need the kind support of hospital personnel to enable them to make informed decisions and to handle these added strains.

Parents may ventilate their feelings and stresses through anger, crying, or body language. Behaviour may not only be a response to the current situation but often involve attitudes resulting from early childhood experiences. The nurse must not pass judgement on individuals whose behaviour may seem demanding or unreasonable. An understanding and acceptance of people and their problems is essential for the pediatric nurse to work successfully with parents.

Siblings are also affected when a brother or sister is hospitalized. They may be afraid or feel left out, guilty, or resentful of the attention focused on the ill child. Suitable interventions by the nurse include directing some attention to the siblings, supporting their efforts to comfort the family member, and engaging them in play or drawing pictures, such as "How it feels to have an ill brother or sister." They may also make cards and pictures for the patient. It is important to encourage a sibling to visit an ill brother or sister in the hospital. The child at home may have worries about exactly what is happening to their sibling and need to see the brother or sister in order to decrease their fears.

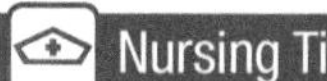 Nursing Tip

When a child is admitted to the hospital, every family member is affected.

THE NURSE'S ROLE IN THE CHILD'S HOSPITALIZATION

ADMISSION

Nurses are responsible for admitting new patients to the hospital unit. Besides performing the procedure skillfully, they must be prepared to meet the emotional needs of those involved. The impression the nurse gives can affect the child's adjustment. Empathy in responding to the fears of the child and family members makes the admission procedure stimulating and educational—a positive experience for all.

A child should be prepared for hospitalization, when possible. Ideally, the child and parents should tour the pediatric unit before admission. This enables the parents to meet some of the people who will care for their child. Children and their families may be overwhelmed by the size of the institution and the fear of becoming lost.

Between 1 and 3 years of age, children are worried about being separated from their caregivers. After 3 years of age, children may become more fearful about what is going to happen to them. Parents should try to be as matter-of-fact as possible about this new experience. Unless they have been hospitalized before, children can only try to imagine what will happen to them. It is not necessary to go into much detail; the child's imagination is great, and giving information that is beyond comprehension may create unnecessary fears. It is logical to dwell on the more pleasant aspects, but not to the extent of saying that hospitalization involves no discomforts. For example, one might mention that meals will be served on a tray, that baths will be taken from a basin at the bedside, and that the child will be with other children. The fact that there is a buzzer for calling the nurse may add to the child's sense of security. The parents may plan with the child what favourite toy or book to bring.

Listening to how the child feels and encouraging questions are more important than explaining certain occurrences. Parents should prepare children for a few days, but not weeks, in advance. Parents should never lure children to the hospital by pretending that it is some other place. In emergency situations, there is little time for preparation. In such cases the entire medical team must try to give added emotional support to the child. The initial greeting should show warmth and friendliness—staff need to smile and introduce themselves.

It is important that nurses use the child's name when speaking with them or their parents. It creates a much warmer feeling to speak of "Ahmad" or "Isabelle" rather than "your little boy" or "your daughter."

The parent is encouraged to do as much for the child as possible, for example, removing clothes. The nurse should try not to appear rushed. A soft voice and quiet approach are less frightening to the child. A nurse who looks anxious can cause unnecessary worry for everyone concerned. The nurse should remain available to answer questions that might arise. When there is a good relationship between the caregivers and nurse, the child benefits from receiving care that is based on input from the caregivers.

When children are hospitalized, the nurse should be aware of their developmental history as well as the medical history. A developmental history includes the following:

- Family relationships and support systems
- Cultural needs that may affect care and hospital routine
- Nicknames, rituals, routines
- Developmental level and abilities
- Communication skills
- Personality, adaptability, coping skills
- Past experiences, divorce, new siblings, extended family
- Previous separation experiences—vacations or hospitalizations
- Impact of current health problem on growth and development
- Preparation given to the child
- Previous contact with health care personnel

FALLS ASSESSMENT

When children are admitted to the hospital they should be assessed for the risk for falls. There are several tools developed to assess fall risk in pediatric patients; one such tool is called the *Humpty Dumpty Falls*

Scale (HDFS). This tool is a seven-item assessment scale used to document age, gender, diagnosis, cognitive impairments, environmental factors, response to surgery/sedation, and medication usage (Pauley, Houston, Cheng, et al., 2014). If a child scores greater than 12 they are at high risk for a fall and nurses must ensure that fall prevention strategies are developed for each individual child.

CHILDREN IN ISOLATION

When children have an illness that requires isolation, they need to be prepared for this and what to expect. If everyone who enters the child's room is required to wear a gown, mask, and gloves (personal protective equipment [PPE]), it can be frightening for the child and cause them to feel a loss of control. Children need an explanation that is age appropriate as to why others are wearing PPE. Older children can usually understand the concept of germs, but preschoolers may not understand the reason and feel they are being punished. They should be allowed to play with the PPE so it does not seem so scary to them. Nurses need to be aware that children may find them scary when they approach the child and need to take their time and talk to the child about everything they are doing.

When children are in isolation, the environment can be altered to increase sensory freedom, such as moving the bed toward the window; opening window shades; or providing musical, visual, or tactile activities (Sams, 2017).

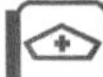 **Nursing Tip**

When explaining procedures to children, it is helpful to identify the child's role in the procedure, for example, "You will be asked to step on the scale."

DEVELOPING A PEDIATRIC NURSING CARE PLAN

Developing the pediatric nursing care plan is similar to developing an adult care plan. The care plan is the result of the nursing process. It states specifically what is to be done for each child and keeps the focus on the child—not on the condition or the therapy. A nursing diagnosis for a pediatric patient may require some modification. A survey of the child includes knowledge of growth and developmental processes. It also includes assessing the primary caregiver, who has a direct role in the safety and maintenance of the child's health. Nursing care plans are guides, and continual evaluation and re-evaluation are called for to determine whether the goals for the individual child are being met. Fig. 19.4 shows a nurse entering data in the unit computer, which may be located at the nursing desk or at the individual patient's bedside.

 **Nursing Tip**

Play is an important part of a nursing care plan for children.

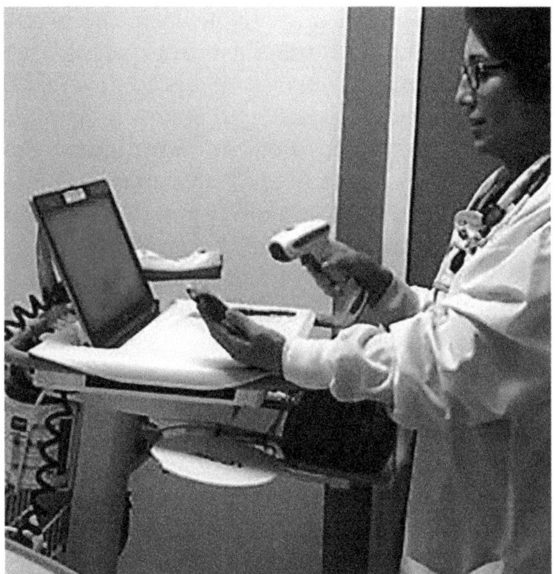

Fig. 19.4 The nurse scans the medication and correlates the information with the medical administration record (MAR) on the computer monitor prior to scanning the patient's ID band and administering the medication.

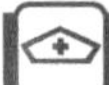 **Nursing Tip**

The achievement of developmental tasks should be part of the plan of care for the hospitalized child.

CLINICAL PATHWAYS

Clinical pathways are used in acute care settings as well as in alternate care settings. The **clinical pathway** is an interdisciplinary plan of care that displays the progress of the entire treatment plan for the patient. The main difference between a clinical pathway and a nursing care plan is that the nursing care plan focuses on the nurse's role in the care of the patient, whereas the clinical pathway focuses on the broader view of the entire multidisciplinary health care team and general outcome goals of care with specific timelines. Understanding the nursing process and the nursing care plan is essential to understanding the nurse's role in the clinical pathway. See Chapter 1 for details and an example of a clinical pathway.

Clinical pathways for children with specific conditions are presented in various chapters of this text.

MEETING THE NEEDS OF THE HOSPITALIZED CHILD

The Hospitalized Infant

During infancy, rapid physical and emotional development takes place. Infants are accustomed to receiving what they want when they want it, and hospitalization can be frustrating for them. Infants miss the continuous affection and physical contact of their caregivers. Their daily schedule is upset. The infant who drinks well from a cup at home may refuse it entirely at the hospital.

Nursing personnel must try to meet the needs of these patients by protecting them from excess frustration. It is not wise to expect infants to develop new habits when they need energy to cope with their illness and the strange environment. One of the nurse's major goals during this period is to assist with the parent–infant attachment process and to promote sensorimotor activities. This can be fostered by providing a means for the infant and primary caregiver to interact and by attempting to ease the tension of the parents. The nurse can serve as a role model by performing activities with the infant, such as cuddling, rocking, talking, and singing. A swing, a bath with squeeze toys, a pacifier, and a hanging mobile are also appropriate as the infant's condition permits.

Because the infant cannot understand explanations, the nurse must administer uncomfortable procedures as gently as possible and return the infant to the caregivers for consolation. Open visiting hours are essential (Fig. 19.5). When parents are not available, soothing support and gentle touch are provided; otherwise, the infant may learn to associate only pain with nursing care. Consistency in caregivers is also important at this stage of development.

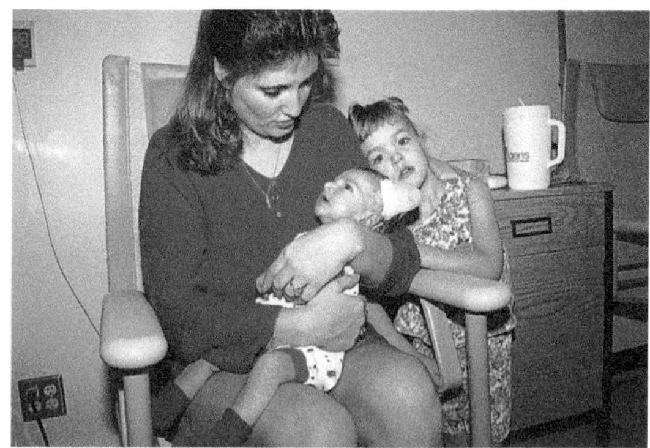

Fig. 19.5 Open visiting hours enable the parent to meet the needs of the hospitalized infant. Family-centred hospital care allows the sibling to maintain contact with the parent while visiting in the hospital. (Courtesy Children's Medical Center, Dallas, Texas.)

The Hospitalized Toddler

The toddler's world revolves around the parents, particularly the primary caregiver. Hospitalization can be a painful experience for toddlers. They cannot understand why they are separated from their parents, and they become very distressed. Toddlers who have a continuous, secure relationship with their parents react more violently to separation because they have more to lose. Nursing goals in the care of the hospitalized toddler are presented in Box 19.2.

Box 19.2 Nursing Goals in the Care of Hospitalized Toddlers

- Reassure parents, particularly the child's primary caregiver.
- Maintain the toddler's sense of trust.
- Incorporate home habits of the child into nursing care plans, for example, transitional objects.
- Allow the child to work through or master threatening experiences through soothing techniques and play.
- Provide individualized, flexible nursing care plans in accordance with the child's development and diagnosis.

Separation anxiety is at its peak in the toddler (see discussion earlier in chapter). The nurse who comprehends the various separation stages sees parental visits as necessary, even though the process of separation after reunion is painful. A cohesive staff is essential to meet the needs of the children and their parents. Educating parents helps to promote their continued visits and to decrease feelings of inadequacy. Ritualistic patterns of care create a sense of structure and are appropriate for children in this age group.

Repetitive games involving disappearance and return are helpful. Peek-a-boo and hide-and-seek serve such purposes. The use of a **transitional object**, such as a blanket or a favourite toy from home, promotes security. Pictures of the family and recordings of favourite stories are other tools that can help the child remain connected with the family. Older toddlers may be able to understand time by experience, so when the nurse or parent leaves, they need to explain when they will return in terms that the toddler can understand (e.g., after naptime or lunch) and then return promptly at that time. A loving hug, good-bye, and prompt exit are then necessary. The continued reappearance of the parents as promised is of value in reducing the child's anxiety and re-establishing their sense of trust. The parent should not wait until a child falls asleep to depart. This prevents confrontation, but it disturbs the child's sense of trust. The nurse can assure the parents that he or she will remain with the child for comfort.

Rooming-in is highly desirable. When rooming-in is impossible, consistent caregivers should be assigned to care for the child and the parent. Nurses can indicate through their approach that they consider the parent's contributions extremely important to the child's well-being. The nurse needs to interpret the stages of separation anxiety (Fig. 19.6) to the parent. The nurse must also realize that parents are under stress and should not be asked to assume responsibilities beyond their capabilities. The nurse should observe parents for signs of fatigue and suggest appropriate interventions.

The home habits of the toddler are recorded and used as a basis for everyday routine. The opportunity to use the potty should be provided if the child is trained. Some regression in behaviour is to be expected. If the toddler still prefers bottles to cups, there should be no attempt to change this in the hospital. Familiar toys and books are important. A steady, calm voice communicates safety. Toddlers are in the stage of

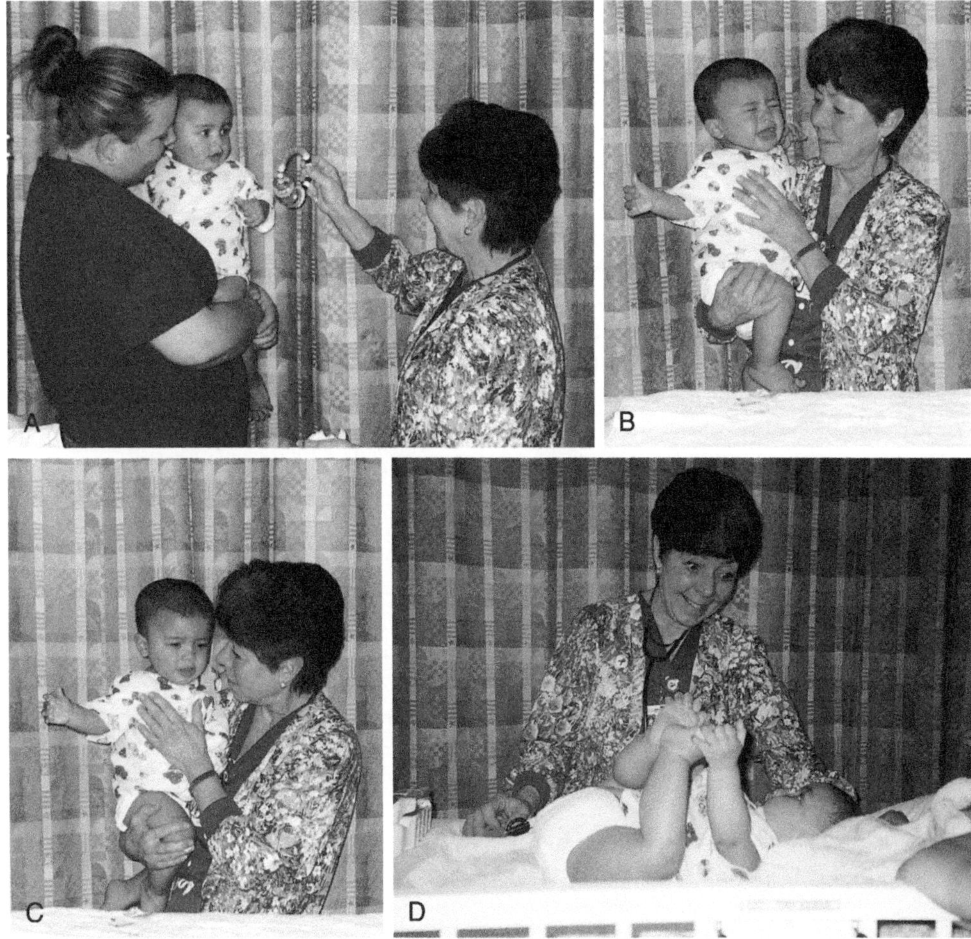

Fig. 19.6 **A,** The nurse approaches the small child calmly, slowly, at eye level, and with the parent present. **B,** The infant shows apprehension and anxiety when carried by the nurse. **C,** Beginning trust is established. **D,** After trust is established, general assessment can begin. (Courtesy Pat Spier, RN-C.)

autonomy. Loss of a small amount of the self-control they have achieved usually results in resistance and negativism.

Children should be forewarned about any unpleasant or new experiences that they may need to undergo while in the hospital. These are communicated in keeping with their level of understanding. Being truthful about things that may hurt prevents the child from feeling betrayed. Preparation and explanation are provided immediately before a procedure so that the child does not worry needlessly for an extended period. Crying and protesting when told about certain procedures are healthy expressions of feelings and relieve tension. Distractions such as blowing bubbles, looking through a kaleidoscope, and playing with pop-up toys may help to reduce anxiety and pain.

Supervised playroom activity contributes to intellectual, social, and motor development. Treatments in the playroom should be avoided. Toddlers can be encouraged to play with safe equipment used in their care, such as bandages, tongue blades, and stethoscopes. Whenever possible, they should be allowed out of their cribs, because confinement is frustrating for young children who have just begun to enjoy walking. Playtime establishes rapport and is an important part of the nursing care of toddlers.

When limitation of movement is required, it must be accompanied by increased emotional support such as rooming-in, additional attention from nurses, and suitable diversion.

It is common for children to experience changes in behaviour on their return home. They may be demanding and may cling to the parent every minute. "He just won't let me out of his sight" is a common description. The parent should be reassured that this is normal and to give the toddler extra attention and reassurance until trust is regained.

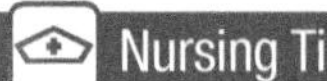

Nursing Tip

Toddlers experience some degree of separation anxiety any time their primary caregiver leaves, such as when the child is left with day care personnel, babysitters, or relatives.

The Hospitalized Preschooler

The experience of hospitalization may be easier for preschool children who have already had outside contact (e.g., preschool and kindergarten) than for those who have never been separated from their caregivers. Because children of this age operate with concrete thinking, they can understand more and they can be better prepared for hospitalization. Explanations must be made in realistic terms, because preschool children cannot understand abstract explanations. A preschooler may interpret a "needle-stick" as a stick in the arm, literally (Fig. 19.7). When explaining procedures, the nurse should be careful to use nonthreatening words (Table 19.1). Children should be made to realize that hospitalization is not a punishment for something they have done wrong. Children may feel guilty, particularly if an accident happened because of some mischief on their part, such as in the case of burns or falls.

Preschool children are distressed when their parents prepare to leave them; they can understand time relationships through activities—at breakfast, after lunch, and the like. The nurse and parents must not tell the child that they will return unless they truly intend to do so.

At this age, the child is afraid of bodily harm, particularly invasive procedures. The surgical patient must be shown the part of the body that requires surgery. The nurse can sketch a body outline and draw a circle around the operative site, giving simple information about the system that will be affected. The nurse should stress that only this area of the body will be involved. Children in this age group engage in magical thinking and fantasy. Fantasizing about the unknown can be frightening to a young child. The preschooler needs clear, understandable, and truthful explanations. Children who ask questions should be complimented and listened to; any misinterpretations should be corrected. Praise helps to increase the child's self-esteem. The child can attempt to relieve tension through role-playing. The sick preschool child likes to play with tongue depressors, adhesive bandages, and other materials related to everyday hospital life.

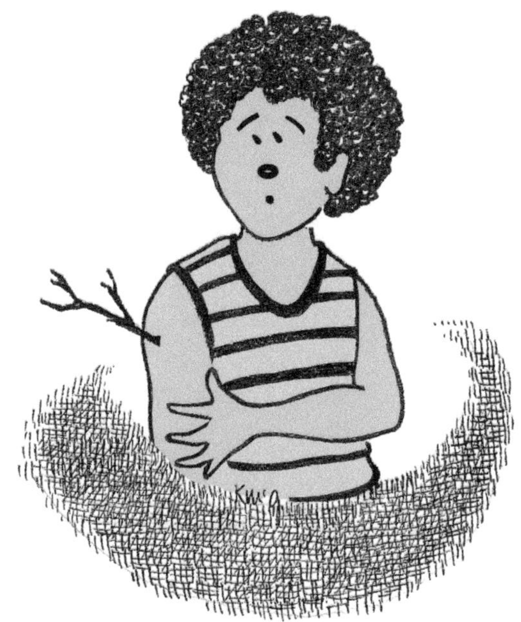

Fig. 19.7 The nurse is careful of the words used with a preschooler as they may interpret explanations literally.

Table 19.1 Words to Avoid and Words to Use

AVOID	USE INSTEAD
Shot	Medicine under the skin
Incision	Special opening
Put to sleep, anaesthesia	Special sleep
Electrodes	Stickers
X-ray	Special picture
Stretcher, gurney	Rolling bed
Catheter	Tube
Take "your temperature"	Check "your temperature"

The Hospitalized School-Age Child

Children of school age can endure separation from their parents if it is not prolonged. Children who have been cherished from birth can tolerate brief interruptions in their lives more easily than can those who have been denied a secure environment. The school-age child is in a stage of industry and independence. Forced dependency in the hospital (such as immobilization) can result in a feeling of loss of control and loss of security. School-age children need to feel "grown up." They can participate in their care and be offered simple choices to foster their feeling of independence. They can choose their menus within appropriate restrictions, "help the nurse" in various activities, and keep busy with age-appropriate toys.

Knowledge of growth and development in the school-age child helps the nurse provide anticipatory guidance. Nurses can also enlist parents to determine what, if any, successful approaches they use in guiding the child. Behavioural problems may be addressed by a team conference. Positive direction and consistency are practices of particular importance to the pediatric nurse.

The education of the school-age child must continue throughout any illness. This gives the child a sense of continuity with the outside world, provides periods of socialization, and reassures the child that they can return to their peers after discharge. The parents may act as liaisons between the school and hospital. To be effective at their job, the teacher must be informed of the child's physical and emotional health. The nurse should provide children with opportunities to study undisturbed so that they will be prepared for classes. Diagnostic tests and treatments should be scheduled around established school routines whenever possible. Some school districts have individual tutors for homebound or hospitalized school-age children and some large pediatric hospitals have teachers on staff.

It is common for school-age children to be "brave" and to show little, if any, fear in situations that actually upset them a good deal. Observation of body language may provide some clues to emotional states. The nurse's presence during unfamiliar procedures is comforting. Following treatments, the nurse should encourage children to draw and to talk about their drawings or to act out their feelings through puppet play.

> **Safety Alert!**
> Observation of nonverbal clues such as facial grimaces, bodily squirming, and finger tapping is important in determining the need for pain relief and support for the child.

The Hospitalized Adolescent

Adolescents in particular experience feelings of loss of control during hospitalization. Daily routines are disrupted, and dependence–independence issues come to the foreground. When feelings of independence, self-assertion, and identity are threatened, the adolescent may respond by withdrawing, by not following through with care, or with anger. Care plans must be designed to incorporate choice, privacy, and understanding.

Early adolescence

Nursing care plans must be oriented to the adolescent's age. Illness during early adolescence, or approximately 11 to 14 years of age, is seen mainly as a threat to body image. There may be a narcissistic concern about height, weight, and sexual development. Patients are aware of heightened body sensations and often have numerous physical concerns. Intense relationships with members of one's own sex can be prevalent. Patients in this age group are anxious about how the illness will affect their physical appearance, functioning, and mobility; however, they are not usually overwhelmed by forced dependence. Self-portrait drawings are effective at this time. Maintaining privacy and same-sex room assignments are essential.

Middle adolescence

During middle adolescence (approximately 15 to 17 years of age), adolescents may be anxious about their ability to appeal to people of the sex they are drawn to and to meet gender role expectations. Physical growth is practically complete. The peer group assumes greater importance in determining acceptability and behaviour. During middle adolescence they may struggle with thoughts of emancipation from the family, which, although erratic, are at their peak. It may be disturbing not only to the adolescent but also to parents, who must relinquish much of their control to hospital personnel. Incorporating choice, privacy, appropriate hair and cosmetic appearance, and the opportunity for peer visitors is important during hospitalization.

Late adolescence

Late adolescents, approximately 18 to 20 years of age, are usually mainly concerned with the tasks of education, career, marriage, children, community, and lifestyle. The dating partner becomes the person of primary importance. Hospitalization may pose the threat of postponement of career and future plans. Contact with school personnel, counselors, and teachers is important to prevent long-term impact on the education and development of the adolescent.

Sexuality

Adolescence is the time when children start to have a specific sexual orientation. They may be attracted to someone from the same sex. They may also have concerns with their gender identity and may identify with the opposite sex (transsexuals). It is important that nurses provide support to the teenager, no matter what their sexual orientation. When asking questions, the nurse should avoid making the assumption of heterosexuality, with questions about romantic and sexual partners asked in a nongendered way (Kaufman & Canadian Pediatric Society [CPS] Adolescent Health Committee, 2008/2016).

Adjustment to illness

The adolescent has many intellectual strengths, including the ability to think abstractly and to solve problems. Adolescents can understand the implications of their disease both in the present and in the future, and they are capable of participating in decisions related to treatment and care. The nurse who recognizes these skills and encourages their practice helps patients gain confidence in their intellectual abilities, thus increasing patients' sense of independence and self-esteem.

Roommate selection

Roommate selection, though often overlooked, is extremely important for this age group. Adolescents usually do better with one or more roommates than in a single room. Because few community hospitals have adolescent wings, it is helpful when patients participate in the decision regarding whether the adolescent is admitted to the pediatric or the adult unit. A few adjoining rooms at the ends of these units will suffice for adolescents. Placing the teenager next to a senile, dying, or severely debilitated patient in the adult unit or an infant in the pediatric unit should be avoided.

CONFIDENTIALITY AND LEGALITY

Respecting the confidentiality of children is important in establishing trust. In general, information should not be divulged or shared without consent. Many problems can be avoided if the confidentiality of the relationship is clearly defined during initial meetings. The nurse must avoid giving private information about a patient to telephone callers or visitors. Appointment books and computer screens in an office are concealed rather than kept open at the desk to view.

In Canada the adolescent may receive medical assistance without parental consent. The age of consent is considered when the patient is able to understand and make decisions regarding their own health and treatment. Two general requirements and conditions for obtaining consent to medical treatment are that the patient must have capacity for the treatment decision and that the consent must be informed. Many pediatric centres have an ethicist who can be contacted to determine age of consent if there is uncertainty and the child's and parents' wishes are not congruent. Quebec is the only province that has an age of consent—14 years—and if the medical treatment requires a hospital stay of more than 12 hours, parental notification of the stay is required if the child is over 14 years of age (Canadian Medical Protective Association, 2016).

The term **emancipated minor** generally refers to an adolescent younger than 18 years of age who is no longer dependent on their parents or legal guardians.

DISCHARGE PLANNING

Preparation for the patient's discharge ideally begins on admission, because the goal of hospitalization is to return a healthier child to the parents. An approach directed only toward good physical care of the patient's disease is not sufficient. The nurse must also consider the emotional growth of the child and the education of the patient and family. This focus will provide a positive learning experience for all involved.

If a patient requires specific home treatment, such as hyperalimentation, ostomy care, crutches, special diet, or insulin therapy, instructions are given to the parents gradually throughout their child's hospitalization. The instructions are written so they can be referred to as needed. If the older child is to administer any self-treatment, careful explanations and supervision are required until both patient and parents are confident they can carry out the procedure safely at home. This may require the participation of home health services.

Parents also must be prepared for behavioural problems that may arise after hospitalization. Guidance includes the following suggestions:

- Anticipate behaviours such as clinging, regression in bowel and bladder control, aggression, manipulation, and nightmares.
- Allow the child to become a participating family member as soon as possible.
- Take the focus off the illness; praise accomplishments unrelated to it.
- Be kind, firm, and consistent regarding misbehaviour.
- Build trust by being truthful.
- Provide suitable materials for play, such as clay, paints, and doctor and nurse kits.
- Allow time for free play.
- Listen to and clarify misconceptions about the illness.
- Prevent long periods of separation until a sense of security is regained.
- Allow the child to visit hospital staff during routine clinic visits if desired.

The services of a children's counselor may be helpful if nightmares and regression occur.

Whenever possible, parents are provided at least 1 days' notice of their child's discharge from the hospital so they can make the necessary arrangements. This is particularly important if both parents work or if transportation is a problem. The health care provider writes the discharge order. The approximate hour of dismissal is relayed to the parents. Parents are given a written return clinic appointment card when indicated.

The nurse may accompany the child and parents to the hospital exit to say good-bye. According to their condition, the child may be placed in a hospital wagon, wheelchair, or stretcher for transport. The nurse needs to ensure the use of a car seat or seatbelt, depending on the child's age, to secure the child safely into the vehicle.

> **Legal and Ethical Considerations**
>
> **Discharge Documentation**
>
> Discharge documentation should include who accompanied the child (and identification given), time of discharge, condition of the child, vital signs and weight, medications, and instructions given to parents or caregiver.

HOME CARE

Many children with acute and chronic conditions are cared for in the home. Home health care and other community agencies work together to provide holistic care. **Respite care** provides trained workers who come into the home for brief periods to provide support and help relieve parents of some the responsibilities, such as direct care. This enables the parents to shop, do business transactions, or simply take time for much needed self-care. The school system also shares in the responsibility for care, which is crucial if a family is to be successful in home care. The health care worker assisting in the home should do the following:

- Listen to the parents and observe how they attend to the physical needs of the youngster.
- Ask questions or discuss apprehensions the parents may have about their ability to care for the child.
- Be attuned to the needs of other children in the home.
- Be creative in exploring avenues for socialization, because these children may not often be invited to slumber parties or community activities.
- Post signs above the bed denoting special considerations, such as "Never position on left side" and "Do not feed with plastic spoon."
- Explore community facilities or support groups that might benefit the family.

Get Ready for the Certification Examination!

Key Points

- The care of sick children can take place in a variety of settings.
- Play is an important part of a nursing care plan for children.
- Nursing care plans for hospitalized children should include measures to minimize negative impact on growth and development.
- Pain is the "fifth vital sign" and should be assessed and treated in infants and children.
- There are various pain scales available to help the nurse determine the pain level in a nonverbal child.
- Nurses caring for children must maintain a high level of suspicion for pain, because children are often unable to verbalize discomfort.
- Techniques such as drawing, distraction, imagery, and relaxation; cognitive strategies; and analgesia provide relief from pain.
- Children require appropriate pain medication on an around-the-clock basis if necessary.
- Three major causes of stress for children of all ages are separation, pain, and fear of bodily harm.
- Separation anxiety is most pronounced in the toddler.
- The three stages of separation anxiety are protest, despair, and detachment.
- Culturally sensitive care toward families with hospitalized children decreases anxiety.
- Treatments should not be performed in the playroom.
- The surgical patient should be shown the part of the body where the operation will be performed. Children are assured that this is the only area of the body that will be involved.
- When a school-age child requires hospitalization, a school, home, or hospital teacher can be requested by the nurse to ensure that the child is able to keep up with schoolwork.
- Respecting the confidentiality of the adolescent is important to establishing trust.
- The pediatric nursing care plan is a product of the nursing process as applied to the child.
- Clinical pathways are a multidisciplinary plan of care with outcome goals that involve timelines.
- The developmental level of the child influences specific needs during the hospitalization experience.
- The child's age, sex, developmental level, and diagnosis are factors that influence placement on a unit.
- Discharge planning begins on the day of admission.

Additional Learning Resources

evolve Go to your Evolve website (http://evolve.elsevier.com/Canada/Leifer) for the following learning resources:

- Answer Key for Critical Thinking Questions
- Answer Key for Textbook Review Questions
- Audio Glossary
- Interactive Review Questions
- Skills Performance Checklists
- Video clips and more!

Online Resources

- About Kids Health—A health education website for children, youth and their caregivers: https://www.aboutkidshealth.ca/
- McGrath, Finley, Ritchie, & Dowden, *Pain, Pain Go Away: Helping Children With Pain* (a book for parents): http://pediatric-pain.ca/wp-content/uploads/2013/04/PPGA2003.pdf
- Roger Neilson House: https://rogerneilsonhouse.ca/
- Ronald McDonald House: https://www.rmhccanada.ca/
- Sinai Health System Library Services, *Multilingual Resources:* https://guides.hsict.library.utoronto.ca/multilingual

Review Questions

1. What are the stages of separation anxiety in the toddler?
   - **a.** Protest, despair, and detachment
   - **b.** Denial, dependence, and submission
   - **c.** Protest, sadness, and despair
   - **d.** Despair, anxiety, and regression
2. Assessment of pain is considered a fifth vital sign to be documented by the nurse. The nurse understands which of the following about pain in infants?
   - **a.** It cannot be reliably assessed.
   - **b.** It will not be remembered by the infant.
   - **c.** It can be assessed through observation of behaviour.
   - **d.** It is usually caused by fear and anxiety.
3. What is the best way to minimize separation anxiety in a hospitalized toddler?
   - **a.** Explain routines carefully.
   - **b.** Encourage parent to room in.
   - **c.** Provide age-appropriate roommates.
   - **d.** Provide an age-appropriate toy.
4. Which statement by the parent of a hospitalized 4-year-old child indicates an understanding of the child's needs?
   - **a.** "I am going to buy him a box of new toys to keep him busy while in the hospital."
   - **b.** "I am going to bring some of his favourite toys from home for him to play with while in the hospital."
   - **c.** "I'm glad there is a television in the room for him to watch all day."
   - **d.** "I will stay every day until he falls asleep and then I will go home."
5. A 4-year-old hospitalized child wets his bed. The parents tell the nurse that the child was completely toilet trained. What should the nurse understand?
   - **a.** The parents are denying a problem exists.
   - **b.** The child may be developmentally delayed.
   - **c.** The child may be experiencing regression.
   - **d.** The child is probably "punishing" the parents.

6. A nurse would have which medication available to administer in case of a reaction or overdose to a narcotic or sedative medication in children?
   a. Naloxone (Narcan)
   b. EMLA
   c. Flumazenil (Romazicon)
   d. Diazepam (Valium)

Critical Thinking Question

1. A 3-year-old child has been hospitalized for 2 days. She is watching the television mounted above her bed. She is expressionless but does not cry or appear to be in distress. Her mother calls on the telephone and states that because her child seems to be adjusted, she may not come in today to visit because she does not want to "upset her." How should the nurse interpret the child's behaviour? How should the nurse respond to the mother?

REFERENCES

Bueno, M., Yamada, J., Harrison, D., et al. (2013). A systematic review and meta-analyses of non-sucrose sweet solutions for pain relief in neonates. *Pain Research & Management, 18*(3), 153–161.

Canadian Medical Protective Association. (2016). *Can a child provide consent?* Retrieved from: https://www.cmpa-acpm.ca/en/advice-publications/browse-articles/2014/can-a-child-provide-consent.

Kaufman, M., & Canadian Paediatric Society (CPS), Adolescent Health Committee. (2008). Adolescent sexual orientation. *Paediatrics & Child Health, 13*(7), 619–623. Updated 2016.

Latimer, M., Simandl, D., Finley, A. F., et al. (2014). Understanding the impact of the pain experience on Aboriginal children's wellbeing: Viewing through a two-eyed seeing lens. *First Peoples Child & Family Review, 9*(1), 22–37.

Pauley, B. J., Houston, L. S., Cheng, D., et al. (2014). Clinical relevance of the Humpty Dumpty Falls Scale in a pediatric specialty hospital. *Pediatric Nursing, 40*(3), 137–142.

Sams, C. (2017). Reaction to illness and hospitalization. In S. Perry, M. Hockenberry, D. Lowdermilk, et al. (Eds.), *Maternal child nursing care in Canada* (2nd ed.). Toronto, ON: Elsevier.

Stevens, B., Yamada, J., Ohlsson, A., et al. (2016). Sucrose for analgesia in newborn infants undergoing painful procedures. *Cochrane Database of Systematic Reviews* (7), CD001069. https://doi.org/10.1002/14651858.CD001069.pub5.

World Health Organization (WHO). (2012). *Persisting pain in children package: WHO guidelines on the pharmacological treatment of persisting pain in children with medical illnesses.* Geneva: Author. Retrieved from: http://apps.who.int/iris/bitstream/10665/44540/1/9789241548120_Guidelines.pdf.

Wright, J., & Krug, S. (2016). Emergency medical services for children. In R. Kliegman, B. Stanton, J. St. Geme, et al. (Eds.), *Nelson textbook of pediatrics* (20th ed.). Philadelphia: Saunders.

Zeltzer, L., Krane, E., & Palermo, T. (2016). Pediatric pain management. In R. Kliegman, B. Stanton, J. St. Geme, et al. (Eds.), *Nelson textbook of pediatrics* (20th ed.). Philadelphia: Saunders.

Health Care Adaptations for the Child and Family

20

Angela Thable

http://evolve.elsevier.com/Canada/Leifer

Objectives

1. Define each key term listed.
2. List five safety measures applicable to the care of the hospitalized child.
3. Illustrate techniques of transporting infants and children.
4. Plan the daily data collection for hospitalized infants and children.
5. Demonstrate proper techniques of assessing vital signs in infants and children.
6. Identify the normal vital signs of infants and children at various ages.
7. Devise a nursing care plan for a child with a fever.
8. Discuss the techniques of obtaining urine and stool specimens from children.
9. Describe the positioning for a child undergoing a lumbar puncture.
10. Demonstrate techniques for administering oral, eye, and ear medications to infants and children.
11. Compare the preferred sites for intramuscular injection for infants and children.
12. Discuss two nursing responsibilities necessary when a child is receiving parenteral fluids and the rationale for each.
13. Calculate the safe dosage of a medicine that is in liquid form.
14. Demonstrate the appropriate technique for gastrostomy tube feeding.
15. Summarize the care of a child receiving supplemental oxygen.
16. Discuss the principles of tracheostomy care.
17. List the adaptations necessary when preparing a pediatric patient for surgery.

Key Terms

auscultation (ăw-skŭl-TĀ-shŭn)
body surface area (BSA)
dimensional analysis
fever
gastrostomy (găs-TRŎS-tŏ-mē)
hyperthermia
informed consent
intramuscular (IM) injection (ĭn-tră-MŬS-kyū-lăr ĭn-JĔK-shŭn)
low-flow oxygen
lumbar puncture (LŬM-băhr PŬNK-chŭr)
mummy restraint
parenteral (pă-RĔN-tŭr-ŭl)
phototoxicity (fō-tō-tŏk-SĬS-ĭ-tē)
saline lock
subcutaneous (subcut) injection (sŭb-kyū-TĀ-nē-ŭs ĭn-JĔK-shŭn)
total parenteral nutrition (TPN) (TŌT-ŭl pă-RĔN-tŭr-ŭl nū-TRĬ-shŭn)
tracheostomy (trā-kē-ŎS-tō-mē)

ADMISSION TO THE PEDIATRIC UNIT

INFORMED CONSENT

When the child is admitted to the pediatric unit, an informed consent is obtained for treatments that are provided. An **informed consent** implies that the parent or legal guardian or child is capable of understanding information given to them, including the purpose and risks of the procedure, and that they voluntarily agree to that procedure. Surgical procedures require written consent, and this must be signed by the parent or child, the health care provider who provides the information, and a witness. The nurse acts as a patient advocate by ensuring that the proper consent has been obtained *before* a procedure and that the child is also given age-appropriate information concerning the procedure and its possible outcomes. See Chapter 19 (Confidentiality and Legality) for discussion of what is considered age of consent for a minor in Canada.

IDENTIFICATION

Every child admitted to the pediatric unit must have an identification (ID) bracelet applied. The ID bracelet of the patient as well as one other identifier (e.g., asking the child their name or using addressograph) should always be checked before medications are administered or treatments are administered. If a bracelet applied on admission is taken off by the child or if it falls off, identification should be verified and a new bracelet applied (Fig. 20.1). The bracelet should be snug enough to prevent voluntary

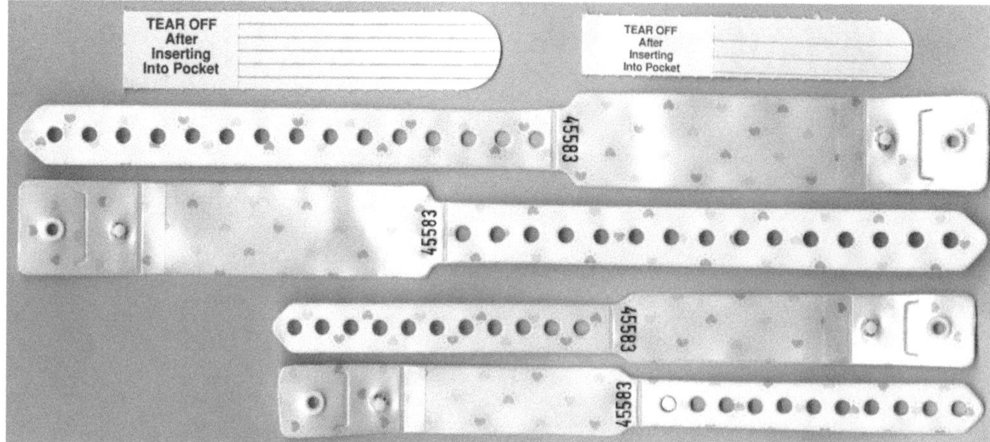

Fig. 20.1 Identification (ID) bracelets. All hospitalized children must have an ID bracelet that is checked before the nurse administers medications or provides care. Some ID bracelets have a computer chip sensor attached, compatible with the electronic medication administration system and also to alert staff if the child leaves the unit. (Courtesy Prosec Protection Systems Inc., Lakewood, NJ)

removal by the child. Many hospitals attach a security chip to the identification band that will activate an alarm if the child leaves the unit, and the chip may also be integrated with the electronic medication administration system of the facility. Documentation that the security chip is secured on the child should be reviewed at the time of patient hand-off and shift report.

ESSENTIAL SAFETY MEASURES IN THE HOSPITAL SETTING

The nurse must be especially conscious of safety measures in the children's unit of the hospital. Accidents are a major cause of death among infants and children. By demonstrating concern about safety regulations, the nurse not only reduces unnecessary accidents but is also able to teach parents about safety. Although personnel cannot alter the physical layout of each institution, many simple safety measures can be performed by the entire hospital team. The following lists of positive (Do's) and negative (Do Not's) measures are applicable to the children's unit:

Do's

- Keep crib sides up and locked in place at all times when the child is unattended in bed (Fig. 20.2).
- Identify a child by ID bracelet, not room number, along with one other identifier.
- Use a "bubble-top" or plastic-top crib for infants and children capable of climbing over the crib rails (Fig. 20.3).
- Place cribs so that children cannot reach sockets and appliances.
- Inspect toys for sharp edges and removable parts.
- Keep medications and solutions out of reach of the child.
- Identify the child properly before giving medications.

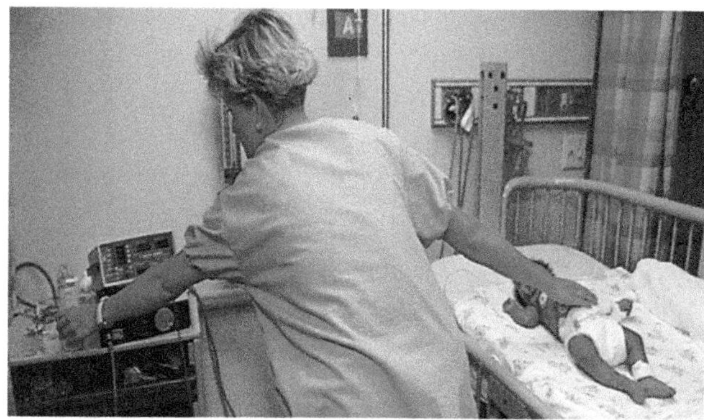

Fig. 20.2 The nurse should maintain hand contact if it is necessary to turn away from the infant or toddler. The side of the crib should be raised before leaving the infant or child to retrieve equipment that is out of reach or to fulfill any other purpose. (Courtesy Pat Spier, RN-C.)

- Document the infant or child's weight in kilograms in a prominent place on the medical record and review during each hand-off report.
- Keep items such as lotions, tissues, baby wipes, disposable diapers, and safety pins out of the infant's reach.
- Prevent cross-infection. Diapers, toys, and materials that belong in one patient's unit should not be borrowed for another patient's use.
- Remain with the child who uses the bathtub or shower.
- Apply a safety belt to the child in a high chair.
- Take proper precautions when oxygen is in use.
- Locate fire exits and extinguishers on the unit and learn how to use them properly.
- Become familiar with the hospital's fire procedure.

Do Not's

- Do not prop nursing bottles or force-feed small children. There is a danger of choking, dental caries, and reflux into the ears causing ear infections (otitis media) with bottle propping

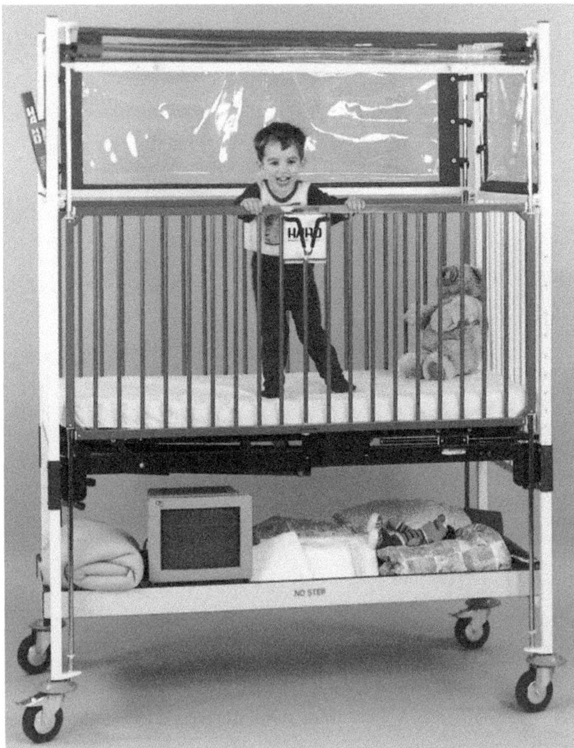

Fig. 20.3 A hard plastic "bubble top" or a soft plastic crib extender must be in place on the crib if the child is capable of climbing over the side rails. The extender stays in place when the side rails are lowered. (Courtesy Hard Manufacturing Co., Buffalo, NY)

- Do not allow ambulatory patients to use wheelchairs or stretchers as toys.
- Do not leave an active child in a baby swing, feeding table, or high chair unattended.
- Do not leave a small child unattended when out of the crib.

Many other safety measures must be implemented as the nurse becomes more familiar with the hazards of individual units. Nurses must continuously assess for any safety concerns and then take the necessary precautions.

Safety Alert!

Crib Safety

- The mattress must fit securely into the crib.
- Blankets should not be tucked in.
- Pillows should not be placed in cribs.
- The distance between crib slats should be no more than 6 cm (2⅜ inches).
- Decorative extensions on the corners of cribs can become caught on clothing and strangle the child.
- A bubble top or extension should be in place if the child is capable of climbing over the crib side.

PREPARATION STEPS FOR PERFORMING PROCEDURES

Nurses must take specific steps to prepare for performing any procedure on any patient. A simple explanation and discussion with the parent or an age-appropriate explanation to the child should precede any nursing intervention. The parent can be allowed to assist whenever possible, and the child should be familiarized with the equipment to be used or even allowed to assist in the simple aspects of the procedure when appropriate. Common nursing actions before the actual skill is performed include checking the written order of the health care provider, gathering equipment, identifying the patient, explaining the procedure to the parent and the child, providing privacy, performing hand hygiene, and using routine precautions or additional precautions (transmission-based precautions) as needed. These preparatory steps appear as icons within each skill as appropriate. Some specific pediatric skills can be found in the chapters that discuss related diagnoses or conditions.

TRANSPORTING, POSITIONING, AND THERAPEUTIC HOLDING

The means by which the child is transported within the unit and to other parts of the hospital depend on age, level of consciousness, and how far the child must travel. Older children are transported in the same way as adults. Younger children are often transported in their cribs, in a wagon or wheelchair, or on a stretcher. The side rails on a stretcher are raised during transport. The nurse needs to ensure that the child's ID band is secured before leaving the unit. A notation is made describing where the child is being taken, for what purpose, and who is accompanying the child.

Fig. 20.4 depicts three safe methods for holding an infant. Head and back support are necessary for young infants. The movements of small children are often random and uncoordinated; therefore, the children must be held securely. The *football hold* is useful when one hand needs to be free, such as for bathing the infant's head.

Therapeutic holding refers to the use of a secure, comfortable, temporary holding position that provides close physical contact with the parent or caregiver for 30 minutes or less. The use of restraints can often be avoided with adequate preparation of the child, parental or staff supervision of the child, or adequate protection of a vulnerable site such as an infusion device (Sams, 2017). The **mummy restraint** is a short-term restraint that might be necessary for examination or treatments such as a venipuncture or placement of a nasogastric tube. This restraint effectively controls the child's movements and can be modified to expose an arm, a leg, or the chest as needed. *Swaddling* of the newborn infant is accomplished by the same technique, although it must be done safely. See Chapter 11 for more information on safe swaddling. Skill 20.1 describes the application of a mummy restraint (swaddling) for infants and children.

Restraints may be used for infants and children to facilitate examinations or treatments and to maintain safety. The reason for the restraint must be explained to

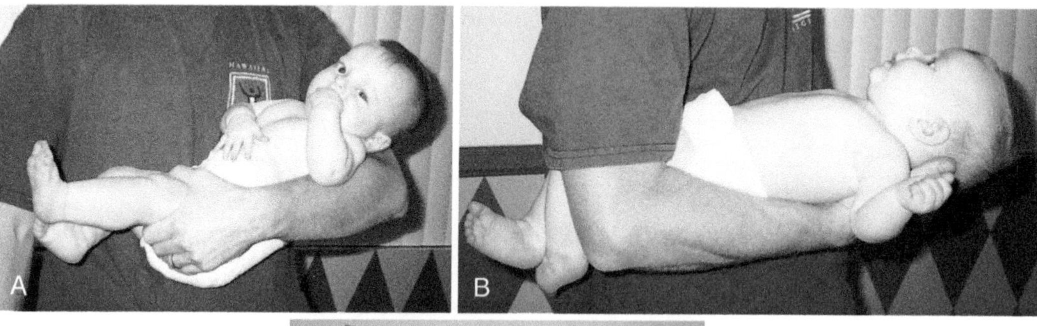

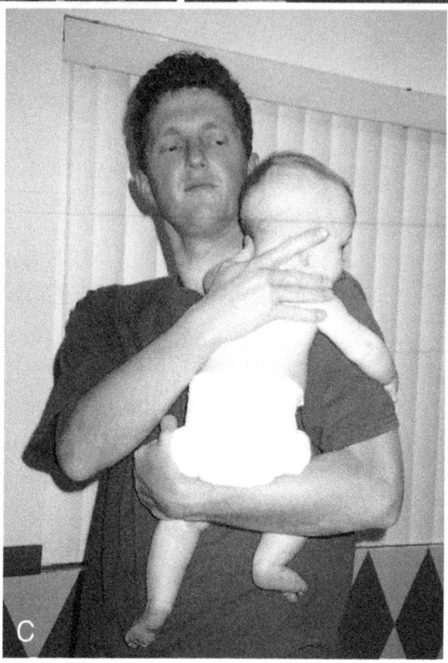

Fig. 20.4 **A,** The cradle position. **B,** The football position. **C,** The upright position.

Skill 20.1 The Mummy Restraint (Swaddling)

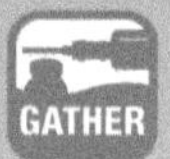

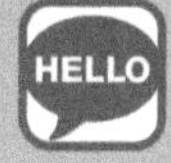

PURPOSE

To promote comfort or confine movements for procedure

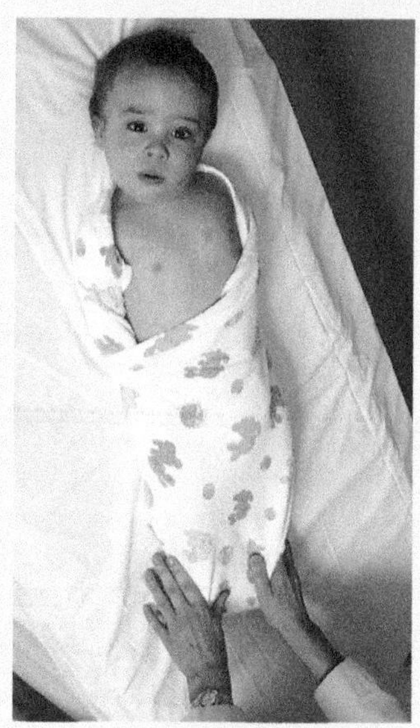

STEPS

1. Place a small, light blanket flat on the bed with the top at the infant's shoulders.
2. Fold the blanket over the body and under the arm at the opposite side, tucking in the excess under the infant.
3. Place the other arm at the side and fold the blanket over the body, tucking the excess under the infant. The weight of the infant holds the restraint in place.
4. Separate the bottom of the blanket and fold upward toward the shoulder, tucking the sides under the infant's body.
5. The arms should be in anatomical position. This restraint provides a feeling of snug security for the infant. It may be used for jugular venipunctures, nasogastric tube insertion, and other procedures.

the parents and the child. Restraints are used only when necessary. They are not a substitute for close observation and should involve the fewest joints possible in order to enable free movement, which is necessary for growth and development. Excessive restraints can result in the infant or child fighting the restraint, thereby wasting energy and increasing oxygen consumption needs. Parents should be taught the importance of fastening safety straps on infants who are in high chairs, shopping carts, and infant seats. The *colic carry* (see Fig. 14.4) is a position that can be used for infants when they are irritable, because the carry typically confers a calming effect.

DATA COLLECTION, OBSERVATION, AND RECORDING

Children are different from adults both anatomically and physiologically. Basic data collection is done to determine the level of wellness, the response to medication or treatment, and any need for referral.

ORGANIZING INFANT DATA COLLECTION

To obtain accurate results, the organization of the infant observation is important:

1. Select an area or room that is warm and not stimulating for the infant.
2. To prevent heat loss, expose only those areas of the body to be examined.
3. Without touching the infant, observe the following:
   - Position
   - Flexion
   - Colour
   - Respiratory rate
   - Ability to focus
4. Using minimal touch:
   - Auscultate lung sounds
   - Auscultate heart sounds
   - Auscultate bowel sounds
   - Measure head, chest, and length
5. Using invasive touch last:
   - Assess reflexes and blood pressure
6. Talk softly.
7. Use a pacifier to comfort the infant if this is appropriate and consent from the parent or guardian is received.
8. Hold the child closely (preferably by parents) after data collection is complete.
9. Use parent-teaching opportunities.
10. Document findings.

BASIC DATA COLLECTION

Basic data collection involves casual observation without touching the child and interviewing the parent. The child's general appearance will indicate if their condition is serious or within normal limits. In general, serious illness may be suspected if the child is not alert and responsive to the environment. If the child is lethargic, prompt intervention by a health care provider is essential. Applying knowledge of basic growth and development will enable the nurse to determine whether the activities and behaviour of the child are age appropriate. A child who has not mastered age-appropriate milestones should be referred for follow-up care (Rourke Baby Record, 2017). The presence of bruises on the body of the child that may be in different stages of healing, the lack of body cleanliness or appropriate dress, and the interaction or lack of interaction between parent and child are also areas that may require prompt referral for follow-up care. Is the child tipping the head or rubbing the ears? Is the child maintaining a rigid body position to breathe? If stridor or grunting sounds are heard during respiration, prompt referral should be made (Ducharme, Dell, Radhakrishnan, et al., 2015).

THE HISTORY SURVEY

The *personal history survey* provides the nurse the opportunity to teach parents about the child's needs and prevention of injury and illness as well as obtain the necessary information. Encouraging safe environments, such as the use of car seats and use of protective gear for sports activities, should be part of every teaching plan (Canadian Paediatric Society [CPS], 2016). The admission history should include information concerning the child's usual health habits and practices regarding eating, sleeping, toileting, activity patterns, and use of special words or gestures. Information concerning coping patterns, siblings, and family values is helpful. Questions concerning the use of complementary and alternative health modalities (CAHM) and over-the-counter medications should be included in every history data collection. This information can be used to formulate nursing diagnoses that are individualized for each child. The immunization record should be reviewed and plans for future immunizations discussed (Government of Canada, 2018).

THE PHYSICAL SURVEY

The physical survey includes a head-to-toe review that should be completed, at minimum, once each shift or once each clinic visit, even if the clinic visit is for a specific problem. Ear examinations should be done by holding the child in a position that will enable safe and quick collection of data (Fig. 20.5). Obtaining vital signs is a priority. Often the first sign of shock or body stress in infants or children is *tachycardia* (a rapid heartbeat). However, a drop in blood pressure may be a late sign of shock in children because of a compensatory mechanism that is activated early. Therefore, hypotension in an infant or child is considered an acute emergency. Extreme irritability or pupils that are unequal in response to light should be reported immediately. The anterior fontanelle, which is usually open until age 18 months, should be palpated. A sunken fontanelle may indicate dehydration, whereas a bulging fontanelle indicates increased intracranial pressure (ICP). A fontanelle that feels flat to the contour of the

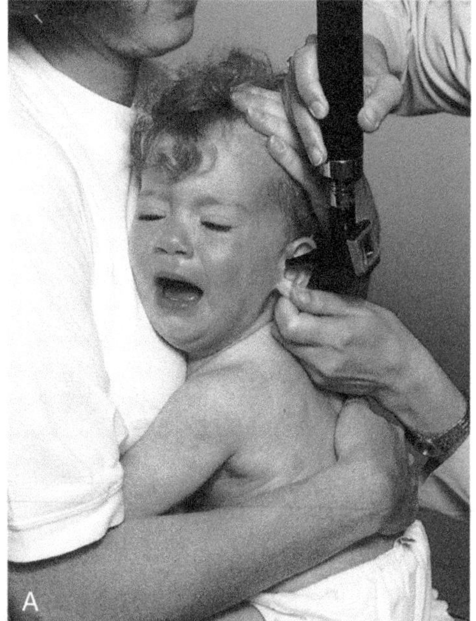

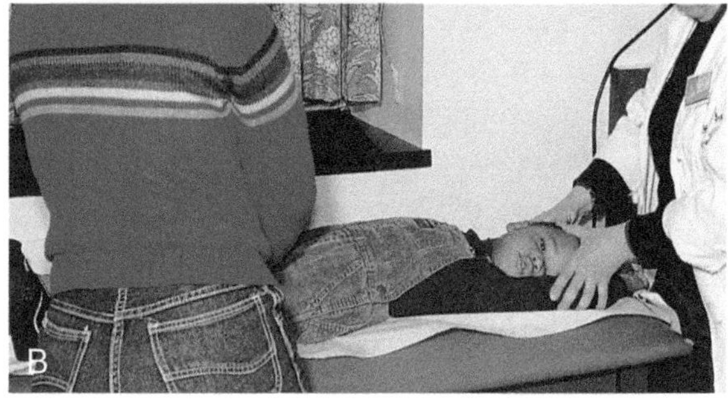

Fig. 20.5 Positioning the child for an ear examination. **A,** The parent or nurse can hold the infant close with one hand immobilizing the head. **B,** The nurse holds the arms above the child's head and prevents movement of the head with the thumbs. The parent or assistant can hold the hips or thighs. (**A,** from Hockenberry, M., & Wilson, D. [2015]. *Wong's nursing care of infants and children* [10th ed.]. St. Louis: Mosby; **B,** from Zitelli, B., et al. [2018]. *Atlas of pediatric physical diagnosis* [7th ed.]. St. Louis: Saunders.)

head is normal. Increased ICP in the older child and adult is manifested by an increase in systolic blood pressure and a widening pulse pressure, irregular respirations, and bradycardia. In the infant, however, the open fontanelles allow brain swelling to occur without these classic signs, and a decreased level of consciousness may be the only manifestation of increased ICP.

Bradycardia (a slow heartbeat) is always treated as a medical emergency in infants and young children. Unlike adults, infants and children cannot increase the stroke volume of their heart for a more effective cardiac output when the heart slows; instead, they must rely on increased heart rate alone to increase output. Therefore, fatigue and heart failure may result. Mottling of the skin of the extremities may be normal in young infants because of their immature temperature control mechanisms. Maintaining warmth during observation is essential for infants. Because of their large body surface area and high metabolic rate, they are prone to fluid loss and hypothermia as well as to cold stress.

An accurate kilogram weight should be recorded because the dosage of medications for infants and children is based on milligrams per kilogram of body weight. The weight should be updated each day for infants and at least twice a week for children. Infants in the recovery stage can incur rapid weight gain, which can change medication doses. The temperature would be assessed (See discussion below). The lungs should be clear to auscultation, and the chest should move symmetrically. Bowel sounds should be active in all four quadrants, and the abdomen should not be distended or tender to palpation. The skin should be observed for rashes or lesions.

Pulse and Respirations

The pulse of the older child is taken just like that of an adult. Apical pulses are advised for children younger than 5 years of age (see Fig. 11.2). The apical pulse is heard through a stethoscope at the apex of the heart. The nurse counts the rate for 1 full minute. The following are the most common sites to assess for a pulse: radial (thumb side of wrist), temporal (just in front of the ear), mandibular (on the lower jawbone), femoral (in the groin), and carotid (on each side of the front of the neck). The carotid pulse may not be appropriate to use in infants with chubby necks. Another common site to assess for a pulse in infants is the bracheoradialis artery, located near the inner junction of the elbow.

The pulse rate varies considerably in different children of the same age and size. The pulse rate and respiratory rate of the newborn are higher than the adult rates. Both pulse rate and respiratory rate gradually decelerate with age until adult values are reached. (See Appendix A for normal heart and respiratory rates at various ages.)

The child's respirations are counted in the same way as for an adult. For infants the nurse should auscultate the chest at the same time as noting the number of times the chest or abdomen rises and falls for 1 minute. The rate and character of respirations are important in determining the patient's general condition. The relationship of the pulse rate to the temperature and the respiratory rate should be assessed; the pulse rate will increase as the temperature increases because of the increased cardiac output and increased oxygen consumption needs that occur with an elevated temperature. When taking vital signs in infants, the respirations are often taken first because they are the least invasive, and after the infant cries, it is difficult to obtain an accurate respiratory rate.

Blood Pressure

Blood pressure (BP) is defined as the pressure of the blood on the walls of the arteries. It is an index of elasticity of arterial walls, peripheral vascular resistance, efficiency of the heart as a pump, and blood volume. Common sites for measuring BP in children are the brachial artery, popliteal artery, and posterior tibial artery.

Skill 20.2 Blood Pressure Measurement in Children

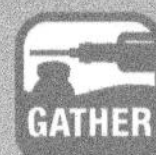

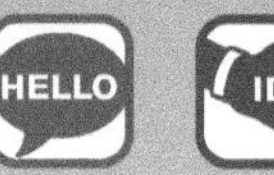

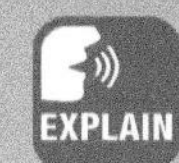

Common sites for measuring blood pressure in children are the brachial artery, popliteal artery, and posterior tibial artery. Blood pressure may be taken with a manometer and stethoscope or by an electronic machine that has been calibrated for use in children.

PURPOSE

To assess blood pressure

STEPS

Brachial Artery

1. Position limb at level of heart.
2. Place appropriate-size cuff on upper arm. The lower end of the cuff should be 2–3 cm above the antecubital fossa.
3. Auscultate brachial artery.

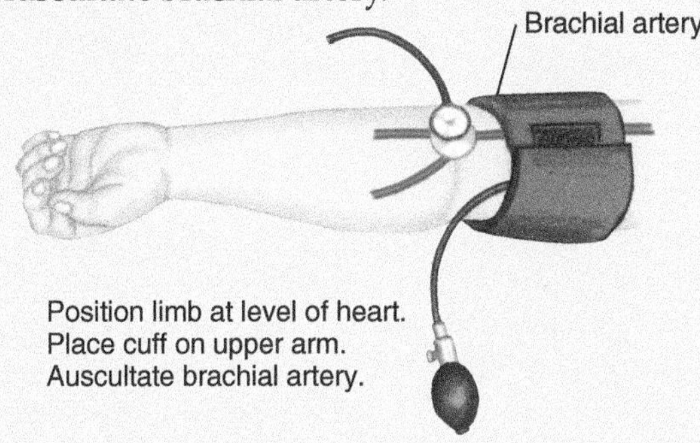

Brachial artery
Position limb at level of heart.
Place cuff on upper arm.
Auscultate brachial artery.

Posterior Tibial Artery

1. Place appropriate-size cuff above malleoli or at midcalf.
2. Auscultate either the posterior tibial artery or the dorsal pedal artery.

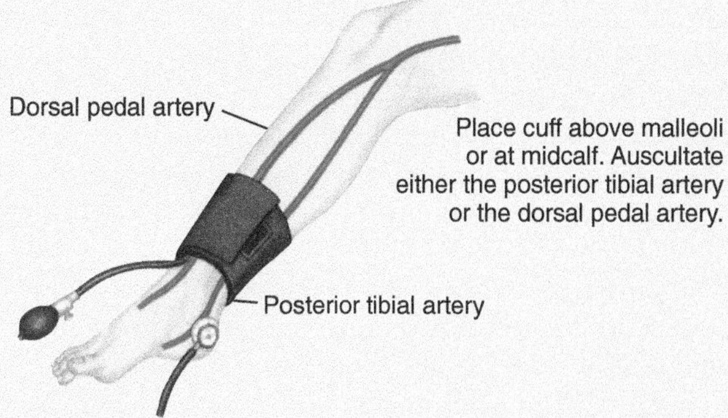

Popliteal Artery

1. Place appropriate-size cuff above knee at midthigh.
2. Auscultate the popliteal artery.

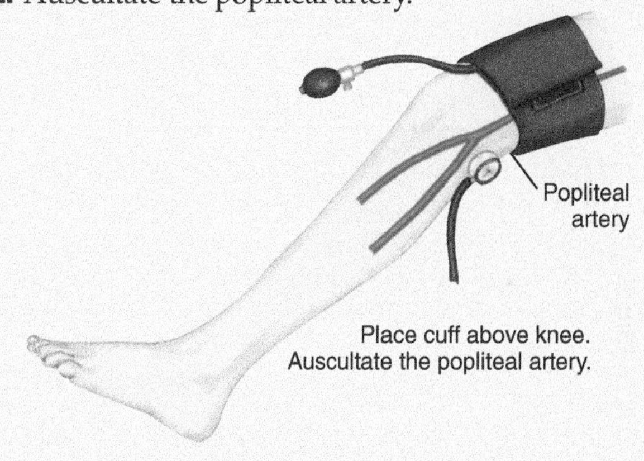

Figures from McKinney, E. S., James, S. R., Murray, S. S., & Ashwill, J. W. (2005). *Maternal-child nursing* (2nd ed.). Philadelphia: Saunders.

Hypertension in children and adolescents is defined as having a systolic or diastolic BP that consistently falls at or over the ninety-fifth percentile. Hypertension is further defined as follows:

- *Stage 1* is defined by BP between the ninety-fifth and ninety-ninth percentiles plus 5 mm Hg.
- *Stage 2* is defined by BP greater than the ninety-ninth percentile plus 5 mm Hg (Dionne, Harris, Benoit, et al., 2017). See Appendix A for normal BP values and Chapter 26 for further discussion of hypertension.

An abnormal BP reading on three different visits is cause for a diagnosis of hypertension. Routine BP screening is not recommended for children less than 3 years of age, but all other children should have their BP checked annually. Children should have their BP checked and recorded using an appropriately sized BP cuff. The wrist and forearm BP cuff technique should not be used for pediatric patients (Flynn, Kaelber, Baker-Smith, et al., 2017).

Auscultation

Auscultation of BP is done the same way as for an adult but with a pediatric stethoscope and pediatric BP cuff (Skill 20.2). The cuff bladder length should be 80 to 100% of the circumference of the arm and the width at least 40% (Flynn et al., 2017). For a child with a heart condition, the BP should be taken in both the arm and leg and compared. If the BP in the leg is not higher than the BP in the arm, the health care provider should be notified to rule out coarctation of the aorta (see Chapter 26). Pressure readings in the lower extremities are normally 10 to 20% higher than the brachial artery pressure. Once the cuff is inflated to 30 mm Hg above the last Kortokoff sound, air is slowly released from the cuff at approximately 2–3 mm Hg per second. The systolic BP reading is the first Korotkoff sound heard as the cuff deflates, and the sudden muffled tone that is heard is the most accurate index of diastolic pressure. To determine *pulse pressure,* the diastolic reading is subtracted from the systolic reading. This usually varies from 20 to 50 mm Hg. Widening pulse pressure may be a sign of increased ICP, overwhelming infection such as sepsis, or cardiac anomalies including patent ductus arteriosus (PDA) and should be reported to the health care provider. Mercury manometers are no longer used when taking the BP of patients. Aneroid and digital manometers are environmentally safer.

Palpation

Palpation is one of the oldest methods of measuring BP. The cuff is applied and inflated above the expected pressure. The fingers are placed over the brachial or radial artery. The systolic pressure is recorded at the point when the pulse reappears. Diastolic pressure is unobtainable. This method is useful in newborns if an electronic machine is not available.

Electronic or oscillometric measurement

This is a noninvasive type of BP monitoring that ultrasonically detects motion of the arterial wall. A transducer with an attached cuff is secured over an artery in the arm or leg. The cuff is inflated above systolic pressure and is then gradually deflated. The transducer transmits vascular sounds, and the measurement appears on a digital readout. Both systolic and diastolic pressures are recorded. Electronic BP machines do not require auscultation with a stethoscope. Electronic BP machines that are used for children must be calibrated and validated for use in the pediatric population (Flynn et al., 2017). An appropriate-sized cuff is applied, the machine is turned on, and a digital reading is obtained, usually in less than 1 minute.

The nurse should explain what is about to happen; for example, "This will hug your arm and feel tight for a few seconds." The child should be allowed to examine the sphygmomanometer and cuff.

Blood pressure is lower in children than in adults. If a patient needs BP measurements throughout hospitalization, the nurse reviews the previous readings before obtaining the current one. Significant changes from the previous readings and the current reading should be reported and documented. Many factors account for variations in BP measurements, including time of day, sex, age, exercise, pain, and emotion. A BP reading taken when a child is frightened or crying is not accurate. If a significant change is observed, the BP should be rechecked. Abnormal readings are charted and reported to the health care provider. When an abnormal BP reading is obtained by the oscillometric method, it should be verified via auscultation technique (Flynn et al., 2017; Nerenberg, Zarnke, Leung, et al., 2018).

Temperature

Pathogenesis of fever and the use of antipyretics

An infection from bacteria or other toxins stimulates immune substances to work along with prostaglandins in the body to stimulate the hypothalamus to raise the body temperature. This triggers a body response of

Skill 20.3 Axillary Temperature Technique

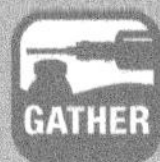

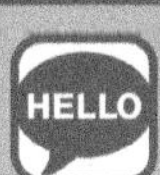

PURPOSE

To assess body temperature

STEPS

1. Place the thermometer well into centre of the axilla. Be sure there is skin-to-skin contact when the arm is placed firmly down to the side. Hold the thermometer in the axilla with the infant's arm pressed against the side until the temperature does not rise anymore (approximately 1 minute) or the thermometer beeps, indicating the reading is ready.
2. A paper or plastic strip digital thermometer can be used to measure the axillary temperature.
3. Perform hand hygiene.
4. Document the temperature and route used in the medical record.

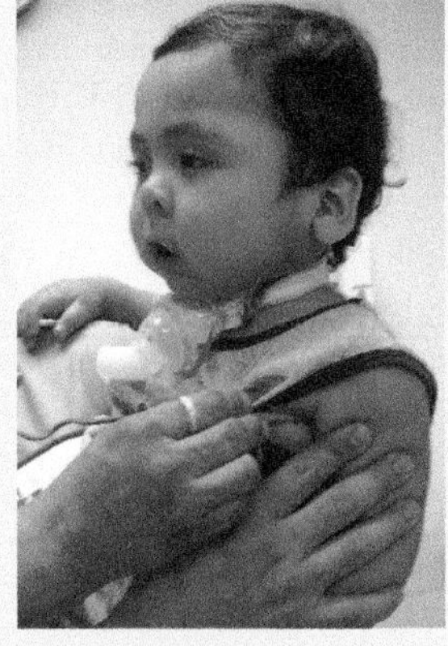

A skin sensor thermometer. (Courtesy Medical Indicators, Carlsbad, CA.)

vasoconstriction, shivering, and decreased peripheral perfusion that decreases body heat loss while maintaining homeostasis, and therefore the body temperature rises. Antipyretic medications such as ibuprofen or acetaminophen inhibit prostaglandin production, thereby preventing shivering, vasoconstriction, and alteration in perfusion, resulting in heat loss and lowering of body temperature.

Fever differs from hyperthermia. **Hyperthermia** is an increase in core body temperature occurring with central nervous system (CNS) impairment. Prostaglandins are not involved, and the homeostasis mechanism is bypassed. Hyperthermia can result from a medication reaction, trauma, or environmental overheating, such as when a baby is bundled and left in a hot automobile. Treatment of hyperthermia involves vigorous cooling measures such as cold blankets and intravenous (IV) fluids.

Fever results in an increased metabolic demand on the heart and lungs, and children with cardiopulmonary disease require antipyretics to minimize the increase in oxygen consumption that causes an increased demand on the heart. Antipyretics also provide comfort and may aid in enabling the child to consume fluids, lessening the risk of dehydration. Antipyretics may also be recommended for children with a history of febrile seizures to prevent a second seizure. Excessive use of antipyretics should be avoided because these medications can burden the kidneys and liver. Fever is thought to be a protective mechanism that aids in the recovery from infection. Nursing Care Plan 20.1 reviews the care of a child with a fever.

Temperature measurement

The pediatric body temperature can be measured via the skin; oral; axillary (underarm); tympanic (ear); or temporal (forehead) methods to determine if fever is present. Although rectal temperature measurement is the most accurate, it is no longer recommended for use in infants and children because of the risk of perforation in infants and discomfort and embarrassment for children. A table of Celsius and Fahrenheit temperature equivalents appears in Appendix A.

Fever is most often compared to a standard of the rectal temperature and is defined as at or above 38°C (100.4°F) (Leduc, Wood, CPS Community Paediatrics Committee, 2000/2017).

When evaluating the degree of illness in a febrile child, the response of the child to cuddling, alertness, hydration, sociability, and quality of cry should be assessed and recorded. A quiet, lethargic child who does not respond readily to the environment may be acutely ill. Because dehydration is a common problem in infants and children, skin turgor should be assessed (see Fig. 11.13). Measures to reduce fever may promote comfort for the child.

There are several types of thermometers available to measure body temperature. Glass thermometers containing mercury are no longer used. The documentation of the patient's temperature should indicate the method used, such as "O" for oral; "Ax" for axillary; "T" for tympanic, or "TA" for temporal artery.

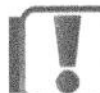

Safety Alert

Glass mercury containing thermometers are no longer used because of risks associated with breakage and mercury contamination (Leduc et al., 2000/2017).

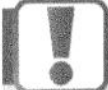

Safety Alert

A temperature reading below 36.0°C requires a report to the primary health care provider. A temperature reading above 38°C (100.4°F) must be reported promptly and follow-up care given.

Oral temperature. The procedure is the same as for adults and may be appropriate for older children or adolescents. An oral temperature technique can be used for a child over 5 years of age if they can keep their mouth closed and have not ingested a hot or cold beverage before measurement.

Axillary temperature. Axillary temperatures can be taken for newborns and young children in the home or in hospitals or clinics according to policy. See Skill 20.3.

Tympanic infrared thermometer. A tympanic infrared thermometer uses the tympanic membrane as the site of temperature measurement because it shares the blood supply with the hypothalamus, which is the thermal regulatory centre of the body. However, the small size of the ear canal in infants and children and inadequate straightening of the ear canal, by pulling the pinna of the ear properly (pulling up for infants or pulling up and back for children) before inserting the thermometer probe, may result in obtaining the temperature of the ear canal rather than the tympanic membrane. Therefore, an inaccurate reading may be obtained due to poor technique and should not be used in children under 2 years of age (Leduc et al., 2000/2017).

Temporal artery thermometer. The temporal artery thermometer uses the temporal branch of the temporal artery as the site for temperature measurement. The core body temperature is about 0.5°C (1°F) higher than thermometers available for home use. For infants under 2 months of age, a touch by the thermometer behind the ear, in the soft depression behind the earlobe, is all that is necessary to obtain a valid temperature as vasodilation is more widespread at that age. In cases where the head is bandaged or inaccessible, using the femoral site or a "zig-zag" motion in the upper chest area is all that is needed for an accurate reading. See Skill 20.4.

Pacifier thermometers. Pacifier thermometers may be used as a screening device in the home but are not considered reliable or accurate and their use should be avoided (Leduc et al., 2000/2017).

 Nursing Care Plan 20.1 **The Child With a Fever**

PATIENT DATA

A 6-year-old child is admitted with a diagnosis of dehydration and a fever of 39.6°C (103.3°F) and is unable to retain food because of nausea and vomiting

Selected Nursing Diagnosis: Potential for dehydration as a result of increased metabolic rate and inability to eat or drink

Goals	Nursing Interventions	Rationales
The child will not become dehydrated as evidenced by good skin turgor, moist mucous membranes, and no weight loss.	Increase fluid intake; offer juice, water, popsicles, and yogurt, as age appropriate.	Body's metabolic rate increases with fever. Children have a higher proportion of body water; therefore, more water can be lost rapidly. Body systems such as the kidneys are immature at some ages.
Child's temperature will be between 36.5° and 37.4°C (97.7° and 99.3°F).	Determine vital signs and reassess every 30 to 60 minutes.	Provides baseline data, and comparison of vital signs will show whether fever is decreasing.
	Expose skin to air; reduce room temperature; increase air circulation; wearing minimum clothing; prevent shivering.	Promotes cooling of skin. Need to prevent shivering as it can increase metabolic requirements. Tepid sponge baths are no longer recommended as they can cause discomfort and shivering.
	Administer antipyretic medications according to health care provider's instructions.	Frequently, child with a fever also has a headache and painful joints; antipyretic medications will relieve these discomforts and reduce fever.
	Apply moist compresses to forehead, neck, axilla, hands, femoral and feet area, preferably 1 hour after administration of antipyretics.	Compresses are more effective if given after antipyretic.
Injury during treatments will be prevented.	Keep side rails raised.	Side rails provide safety and prevent falls.
	Observe child frequently.	Frequent observation will allow subtle changes to be detected and possibly reduce complications.
Parent will understand and verbalize nature and treatment of fever.	Explain nature of fever (not always bad); control that is too vigorous may mask signs of illness.	Potential benefits of fever have been cited; it is thought to enhance the body's defense mechanisms and to increase antibody activity.
	Call health care provider if child looks sick or acts in a way different from normal. Children under 6 months should see a health care provider if fever occurs; over age 6 months it may be treated at home if they are drinking fluids and seem otherwise well.	Degree of fever does not always reflect the severity of disease.
Parent will verbalize understanding of how to read a thermometer.	Demonstrate how to read a thermometer.	This gives parents a sense of control; accuracy of fever detection will be ensured on discharge.
Parent will verbalize understanding of potential for convulsion.	Discuss with parent potential for convulsion.	Only a small number of children convulse with fever; however, teaching is advisable.
Parent will understand how to give appropriate care during a convulsion.	Review management of a convulsion.	Knowledge allays anxiety.
	Discourage use of tepid sponge baths.	Sponge baths may still be suggested by older relatives.

CRITICAL THINKING QUESTION

1. A mother states that her child has developed a fever after receiving an immunization, and she requests antibiotic treatment. What data collection and parent teaching are indicated?

Source: Canadian Paediatric Society. (2015). *Fever and temperature taking*. Retrieved from http://www.caringforkids.cps.ca/handouts/fever_and_temperature_taking

Skill 20.4 Temporal Artery Temperature Technique

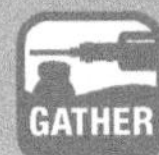

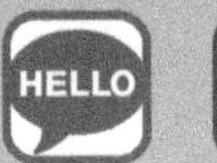

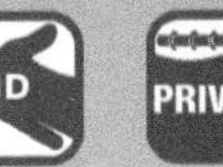

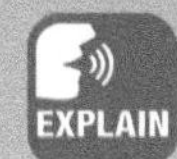

WASH

PURPOSE

To assess body temperature

STEPS

1. Place the probe flush on the centre of the exposed forehead. Depress the button and hold the button depressed.
2. Slide the probe in a *straight line* across the forehead to the hairline.
3. Lift the probe from the forehead and place it in the little soft depression on the neck behind the earlobe.
4. Release the button and read the temperature.
5. Perform hand hygiene
6. Record the temperature on the patient's record, indicating the technique used.

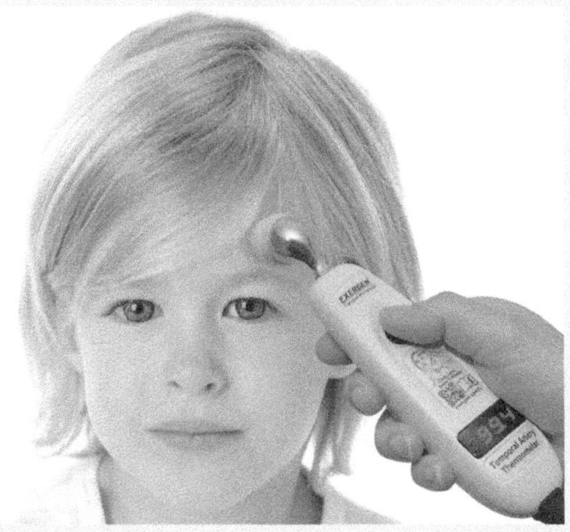

An alcohol swab must be used to wipe the probe head of the thermometer between patients. A full instrument sheath is available for isolation patients. (Courtesy Exergen Corporation).

Skin temperature (plastic strip). A plastic strip is pressed firmly against a dry forehead or axilla. Hold the strip in place for the required amount of time. Read the temperature on the strip before removing the strip. The plastic strips are usually disposable after use. An underarm long-term wearable plastic strip may be left in place for several days. These types of plastic strips may be used as a screening tool at home but are not considered reliable or accurate.

Pain

Pain is a fifth vital sign that must be addressed in the plan of care. See Chapter 11 for evaluation of pain in the newborn and Chapter 19 for evaluation of pain in the child or adolescent.

Weight

Weight must be accurately recorded in *kilograms* on admission. The weight of a patient provides a means of determining progress and is necessary for determining the dosage of medications. The way in which the nurse weighs the child depends on the child's age.

The infant is weighed completely naked in a warm room. A fresh absorbent pad or scale paper is placed on the scale. This prevents cross-contamination (the spread of germs from one infant to another). The scale is balanced to compensate for the weight of the pad. The infant is placed gently on the scale. The nurse's hand is held slightly above the infant to prevent them from falling (see Fig. 11.3). After the exact weight appears on the digital readout, the infant is removed from the scale, wrapped in a blanket, and soothed. The weight is immediately recorded. The scale paper is disposed of in the proper receptacle and the scale is cleaned.

The older child is weighed in the same manner as an adult (see Skill 13.1). A paper towel is placed on the scale for the patient to stand on. The patient is generally weighed in a hospital gown. The shoes are removed. If the child is unable to stand on the scale, it may be necessary for the nurse to hold the child and read the combined weights. The nurse is then weighed and that number subtracted from the combined weight to obtain the patient's weight. Occasionally a child is weighed while wearing a cast. The nurse records this, for example, "weight 15.4 kg (34 lb) with cast on right arm."

A critical care crib can be used for infants who cannot be moved out of their crib but require daily weight assessment for calculating safe medication doses and evaluating clinical progress. This crib has automatic mattress height and position controls, and all four sides of the crib can be lowered for complete access. The infant can be accurately weighed in the crib by a push of a button (Fig. 20.6).

Height

The child's height is measured along with weight. The infant's height must be measured while the infant is lying on a flat surface alongside a tape measure or yardstick. The knees should be pressed flat on the table. The measurement is taken from the top of the head to the heels and recorded (see Skill 13.1).

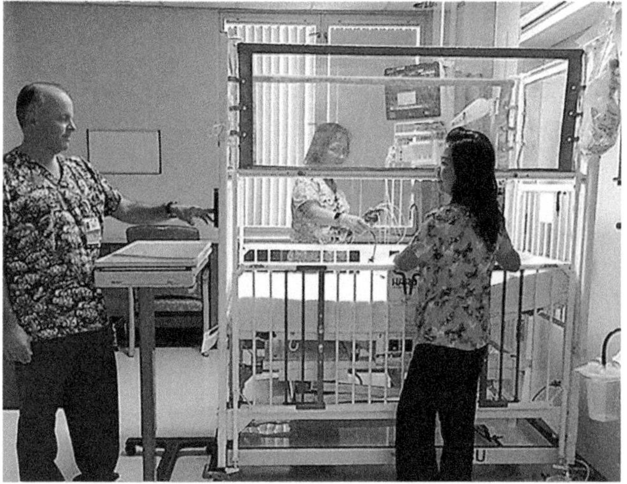

Fig. 20.6 Weighing the infant in a critical care crib. The nurse gently lifts the infant a few inches above the mattress to enable the weight of the crib contents (linen, pads, etc) to be "zeroed out" by pressing a button at the foot of the crib. The infant is gently replaced in the crib, and pressing the same button provides an accurate infant weight in kilograms (kg) while the infant is lying in the crib.

Head Circumference

Head circumference increases rapidly during infancy as a result of brain growth. It is generally measured on infants and toddlers and on all children with neurological defects. The tape measure is placed around the head slightly above the eyebrows and ears and around the occipital prominence of the skull (see Skill 11.1). The measurement is recorded.

Skin Assessment

Skin assessments are important in children, especially if there are any mobility issues. The Braden Q scale is a pediatric scale used to determine the risk for pressure injuries in children (see Table 20.1). Assessment for pressure injury risk is the first step in preventing skin breakdown. If a child is determined to be at risk for developing a pressure injury, nursing interventions must be implemented to decrease this risk. See Chapter 24 for further discussion of immobility.

SPECIMEN COLLECTION

Urine Specimens

A urine specimen is usually obtained from the newly admitted patient. There are certain general principles of collecting specimens:

- Explain the procedure to the child (as age appropriate).
- Use a clean container or urine collection device.
- Label all specimens clearly and attach the proper laboratory slip.
- Send specimen to the laboratory according to hospital policy.
- Record in nurses' notes and on intake and output (I&O) sheet. Check frequently for results.

The procedure for collecting a "bagged" urine specimen from an infant is described in Skill 20.5. The bagged urine specimen can be used for urinalysis but not for urine culture (Robinson, Finlay, Lang, et al., 2014). A sterile catheter collection is preferred for children who have not achieved toilet independence (Robinson et al., 2014).

Urine collected directly from ultra-absorbent disposable diapers may yield inaccurate protein, pH, and specific gravity measurements because of the chemicals in the diaper.

Obtaining a clean-catch specimen

Special sterile containers are available for clean-catch specimens; the manufacturer's directions should be followed. The procedure necessitates cleansing of the perineum with an antiseptic. Rinsing and drying the perineum are important to prevent contamination of urine from the antiseptic. Wiping is done from front to back. After the urine stream has started, the midstream specimen is caught in the sterile container. The nurse's participation is either direct or supervisory depending on the child's age or the availability of a parent. Adolescents, who may be embarrassed by carrying a urine specimen through the halls, may be given a bag or other suitable camouflage. The specimen should be sent to the laboratory promptly.

Obtaining a 24-hour specimen

At times, a 24-hour urine specimen may be requested to determine the rate of urine production and measure the excretion of specific chemicals from the body. The nurses on each shift must closely supervise this test to maintain its accuracy, because lost specimens necessitate restarting the test. Problems can arise if the collection device does not adhere to the skin properly; therefore, the nurse must be alert for this occurrence. Diversions suitable to the child's age are used. A sign is attached to the infant's crib to alert personnel of a 24-hour urine collection. The average daily amount of urine excreted, by age, is shown in Table 20.2.

Testing for albumin

The nurse working in a health care provider's office or clinic may also be requested to test urine for albumin (protein). Normally, little or no albumin is found in the urine of a healthy child. Reagent strips especially intended for this purpose are available. The nurse dips the end of the strip into urine and compares the strip with a special colour chart. Specific instructions accompany test materials.

Stool Specimens

Stool specimens are obtained from older children in the same manner as from adults. This is embarrassing for most children, who are "turned off" by the suggestion. The ambulatory child can use a bedpan placed beneath a toilet seat. It may be difficult for a child to tell the nurse that the sample has been collected. The

Table 20.1 **The Braden Q Scale for Predicting Pediatric Pressure Ulcer Risk**

INTENSITY AND DURATION OF PRESSURE					
					SCORE
Mobility: The ability to change and control body position.	**1. Completely Immobile:** Does not make even slight changes in body or extremity position without assistance.	**2. Very Limited:** Makes occasional slight changes in body or extremity position but unable to completely turn self independently.	**3. Slightly Limited:** Makes frequent though slight changes in body or extremity position independently.	**4. No Limitations:** Makes major and frequent changes in position without assistance.	
Activity The degree of physical activity.	**1. Bedfast:** Confined to bed.	**2. Chair fast:** Ability to walk severely limited or non-existent. Cannot bear own weight and/or must be assisted into chair or wheelchair.	**3. Walks Occasionally:** Walks occasionally during day, but very short distances with or without assistance. Spends majority of each shift in bed/chair	**4. All patients too young to ambulate OR walks frequently:** Walks outside the room at least twice and inside room at least once every 2 hours during day.	
Sensory Perception The ability to respond in a developmentally appropriate way to pressure-related discomfort.	**1. Completely Limited:** Unresponsive (does not moan, flinch or grasp) to painful stimuli due to diminished level of consciousness or sedation OR has limited ability to feel pain over most of the body surface.	**2. Very Limited:** Responds only to painful stimuli. Cannot communicate discomfort except by moaning or restlessness OR has sensory impairment which limits the ability to feel pain or discomfort over half the body.	**3. Slightly Limited:** Responds to verbal commands but cannot always communicate discomfort or need to be turned. OR has some sensory impairment which limits ability to feel pain or discomfort in 1 or 2 extremities	**4. No Impairment:** Responds to verbal commands. Has no sensory deficit which limits ability to feel or communicate pain or discomfort.	
TOLERANCE OF THE SKIN AND SUPPORTING STRUCTURE					
Moisture Degree to which skin is exposed to moisture.	**1. Constantly Moist** Skin is kept moist almost constantly by perspiration, urine, drainage etc. Dampness is detected every time the patient is moved or turned.	**2. Very Moist:** Skin is often but not always moist. Linen must be changed at least every 8 hours.	**3. Occasionally Moist:** Skin is occasionally moist requiring a linen change every 12 hours.	**4. Rarely Moist:** Skin is usually dry; requires routine diaper changes. Linen only requires changing every 24 hours.	
Friction / Shear *Friction* occurs when skin moves against support surfaces. *Shear* occurs when skin & adjacent body surfaces slide across one another.	**1. Significant Problem:** Spasticity, contracture, itching or agitation leads to almost constant thrashing and friction.	**2. Problem:** Requires moderate to maximum assistance in moving. Complete lifting without sliding against sheets is impossible. Frequently slides down in bed or chair requiring frequent repositioning with maximum assistance.	**3. Potential Problem:** Moves feebly or requires minimum assistance. During a move skin slides to some extent against sheets, chair, restraints or other devices. Usually maintains good position in chair but occasionally slides down.	**4. No Apparent Problem:** Able to completely lift patient during position change. Moves in bed and chair independently & has sufficient muscle strength to lift up completely during move. Always maintains good position in chair or bed.	

Continued

Table 20.1 The Braden Q Scale for Predicting Pediatric Pressure Ulcer Risk—cont'd

					SCORE
Nutrition Usual food intake pattern.	1. **Very Poor:** NPO and/or maintained on clear liquids or IVs for more than 5 days OR Never eats a complete meal. Rarely eats more than half of any food offered. Protein intake includes only 2 servings of meat or dairy per day. Takes fluids poorly. Does not take a liquid dietary supplement.	2. **Inadequate:** On liquid diet or tube feed / TPN which provides inadequate calories & minerals for age OR albumin less than 3 mg/dL OR rarely eats a complete meal & usually only eats half of any food offered. Protein intake includes only 3 servings of meat or dairy per day. Occasionally takes a dietary supplement.	3. **Adequate:** On tube feeds or TPN which provides adequate calories and minerals for age OR eats over half of most meals. Eats a total of 4 servings of meat & dairy each day. Occasionally refuses a meal but usually takes a supplement if offered.	4. **Excellent:** On a normal diet providing adequate calories for age. Eats & drinks most of every meal. Never refuses a meal. Usually eats 4 or more servings of dairy & meat daily. Occasionally eats between meals. Does not require a supplement.	
Tissue Perfusion and Oxygenation	1. **Extremely Compromised:** Hypotensive (MAP less than 50 mmHg; less than 40 in newborn) **OR** does not physiologically tolerate position changes.	2. **Compromised:** Normotensive; O2 saturation may be less than 95% OR Hgb may be less than 100 g/L **OR** capillary refill may be greater than 2 seconds. Serum pH is less than 7.40.	3. **Adequate:** Normotensive; O2 saturation may be less than 95% **OR** Hgb may be less than 100 g/L **OR** capillary refill may be greater than 2 seconds. Serum pH is normal.	4. **Excellent:** Normotensive; O2 saturation greater than 95%; normal Hgb. capillary refill less than 2 seconds.	
				Total Score	

TPN, total parenteral nutrition; *Hgb*, hemoglobin; *MAP*, mean arterial pressure; *NPO*, nothing by mouth

From Quigley, S., & Curley, M. (1996). Skin integrity in the pediatric population; Preventing and managing pressure ulcers. *Journal for Specialists in Pediatric Nursing, 1*(1), 7–18. Retrieved from https://www.clwk.ca/buddydrive/file/guideline-braden-risk-assessment/

Skill 20.5 Collecting a Routine Urine Specimen in Infants

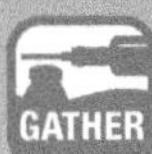

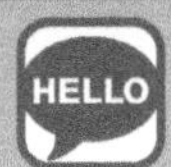

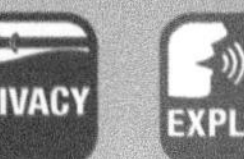

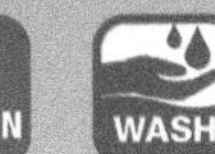

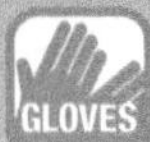

GLOVES

PURPOSE

To obtain a specimen for clinical laboratory assessment

STEPS

1. Clean and dry the infant's skin, avoiding use of oil, baby powder, or lotion soap, which may leave a residue on the skin and interfere with the ability of the adhesive to stick.

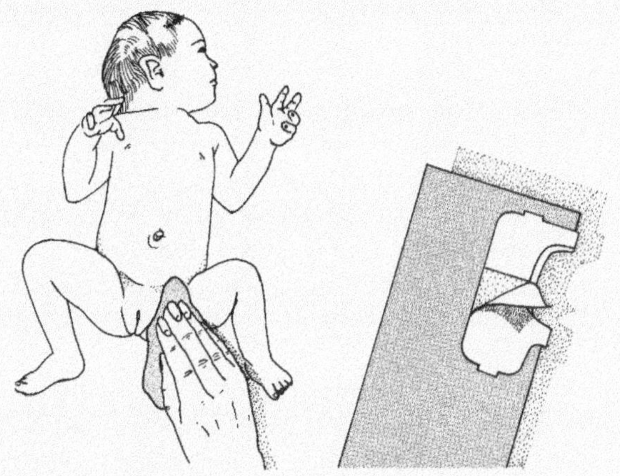

2. Begin by applying the urine collector to the tiny area of skin between the anus and the perineum. The narrow "bridge" on the adhesive patch keeps feces from contaminating the specimen and helps to position the collector correctly. After applying the adhesive section between the anus and perineum, the remainder of the urine collector is fitted to the rest of the genital area.
3. Placing a cold, damp gauze or washcloth on the suprapubic area of the infant may stimulate voiding within minutes (Morris, 2018).

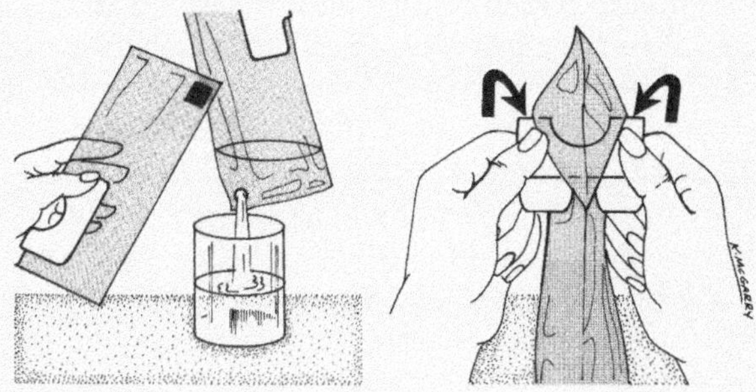

4. Recover the specimen. Drain the urine bag collector into a clean specimen container by removing the tab in the lower corner, or seal the specimen inside the collector itself by folding the sticky adhesive sides together.
5. Place the collector with specimen into a plastic bag.
6. Replace infant's clean diaper, position child in crib, and raise side rails.
7. Remove gloves and perform hand hygiene.
8. Label specimen container for transport to laboratory according to hospital protocol.
9. Document in medical record the amount of urine collected and time sent to laboratory.

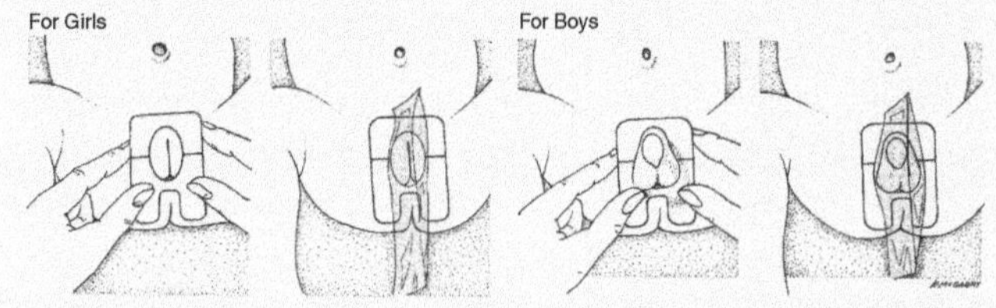

Table 20.2 Average Daily Excretion of Urine

AGE	MILLILITRES (ML)	FLUID OUNCES (OZ)
Days 1–2	30–60	1–2
Days 3–10	90–300	3–10
Day 10–2 months	270–450	9–15
2 months–1 year	420–510	14–17
1–3 years	510–600	17–20
3–5 years	600–720	20–24
5–8 years	660–1020	22–34
8–14 years	810–1410	27–47

nurse can acknowledge these feelings by giving the child permission to express them without being critical; for example, the nurse could say, "I know this must be embarrassing for you. It is for grown-ups, too, but we need this specimen." An infant's stool specimen can be obtained from the infant by scraping the specimen from the diaper with a tongue depressor and placing it in the specimen container. Some specimen containers contain a portion of liquid. The label indicates a "fill line." The amount of infant stool needed for a specimen is the amount which, when placed into the container, results in the fluid level rising to the fill line.

Some specimens must be sent to the laboratory while they are warm. The specimen container is labelled properly and placed in a plastic bag, and the laboratory slip is attached. The nurse charts the time; colour, amount, and consistency of the stool; the purpose for which it was collected (e.g., blood, ova, parasites, or bacteria); and any related information.

Blood Specimens

Positioning the child for drawing blood is extremely important. The nurse is often asked to assist in these procedures. The most common site for blood specimens are the arms and hands. Holding a child for this procedure is best done by being placed in a nurse's (or parent's) lap, facing the holder so the child can be gently hugged, while the arm is outstretched and held by the person collecting the specimen. Occasionally the femoral or jugular veins are used when all other areas have been exhausted. Fig. 20.7 depicts how to position the patient for a femoral venipuncture. Both the jugular and the femoral veins are large; therefore, the patient is frequently checked to ensure that there is no bleeding afterward. The infant is soothed, because crying and thrashing may precipitate oozing. Distraction and simple pain relief techniques should be used during any painful procedure. The nurse charts the site used, the name of the blood test, and any untoward developments.

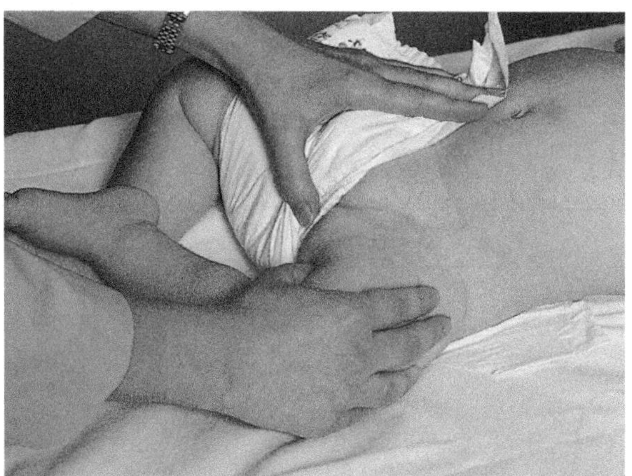

Fig. 20.7 An infant positioned for femoral venipuncture. This position exposes the groin area. (From Hockenberry, M., & Wilson, D. [2015]. *Wong's nursing care of infants and children* [10th ed.]. St. Louis: Mosby.)

Lumbar Puncture

The nurse often assists the health care provider with a lumbar puncture, which is also referred to as a *spinal tap*. It is done to obtain spinal fluid for examination or to reduce pressure within the brain in conditions such as hydrocephalus or meningitis.

Normal spinal fluid is clear like water. The opening pressure ranges from 60 to 180 mm Hg. It is somewhat lower in infants. The procedure for children is essentially the same as that for adults. The main difference lies in the patient's ability to assist with positioning. The nurse needs to explain to the child that they must lie quietly and that they will be helped to do this. Sensations during a lumbar puncture include a cool feeling when the skin is cleansed and a feeling of pressure when the needle is inserted. The way in which the child is held can directly affect the success of the procedure.

The child lies on the side with the back parallel to the side of the treatment table. The knees are flexed, and the head is brought down close to the flexed knees. The nurse can keep the child in this position by placing the child's head in the crook of one arm and the knees in the crook of the other arm. The nurse's hands are then clasped together or placed as shown in Fig. 20.8. The nurse leans forward, gently placing the chest against the patient.

After the child is positioned, the health care provider prepares the lower back using sterile technique. A vial of local anaesthetic may be necessary unless this is provided in the sterile setup. The top of the vial is cleansed according to hospital protocol. After the area has been locally anaesthetized, the health care provider inserts a special hollow needle into the patient's lower back and collects the spinal fluid in two or three test tubes. Pain relief techniques, such as allowing an infant to suck on a sucrose-sweetened nipple, or distraction techniques should be used during any painful procedure (see Chapter 11 for pain management in infants and Chapter 19 for children of other ages). When the procedure is completed, a sterile bandage is placed over the injection site, and the child is comforted. Specimens are labelled and taken to the laboratory with the appropriate requisition form.

The child may avoid post–lumbar puncture headache by lying flat for some time. The nurse charts the date and time of the lumbar puncture and the name of the attending health care provider. Also charted are the amount of fluid obtained and its character (e.g., cloudy or bloody), whether or not specimens were sent to the laboratory, and the patient's reaction to the procedure.

PHYSIOLOGICAL RESPONSES TO MEDICATIONS TO INFANTS AND CHILDREN

Medication administration is a primary responsibility of the nurse. It is important for the nurse to understand

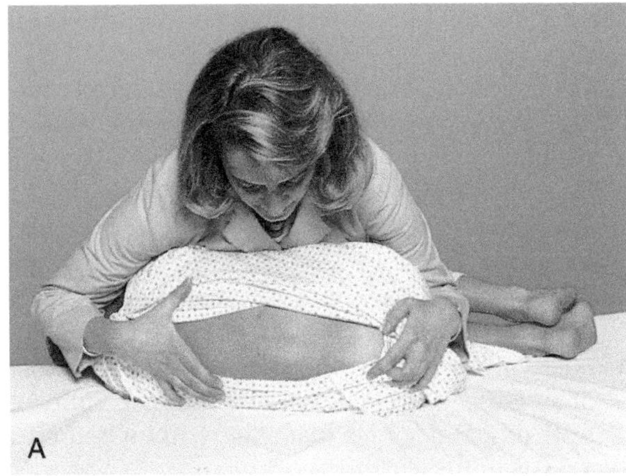

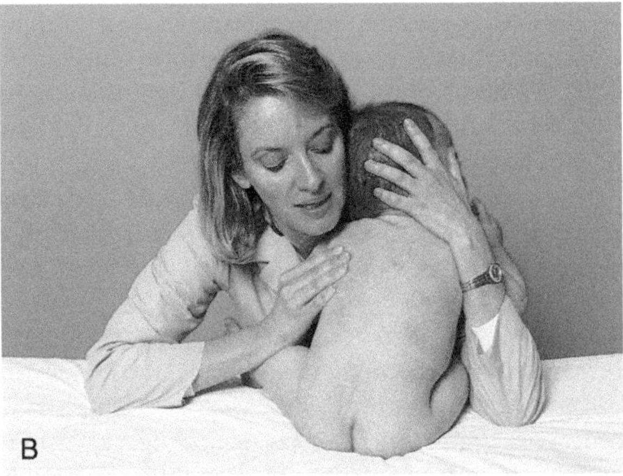

Fig. 20.8 A child positioned for a lumbar puncture. **A,** An older child may be placed in a side-lying fetal position and held firmly by the nurse. **B,** Placing an infant in a sitting position allows for flexion of the lumbar spine. The nurse hugs the child for support and security. (From Hockenberry, M., & Wilson, D. [2015]. *Wong's nursing care of infants and children* [10th ed.]. St. Louis: Mosby.)

that the responses of infants differ from those of children and that the responses of infants and children differ from those of adults. These concepts must also be communicated to the parents, who often administer over-the-counter medications to their growing child. The most common over-the-counter medication administered by parents to infants and children is acetaminophen (Tylenol). The toxic effects of Tylenol overdose are discussed in Chapter 28.

Understanding the differences in medication absorption, distribution, metabolism, and excretion between children and adults is essential to providing safe pediatric medication administration. Age is the most important variable in predicting response to any medication therapy. The functions of various organs in the body mature as the child grows and develops.

ABSORPTION OF MEDICATIONS IN INFANTS AND CHILDREN

Gastric Influences

In the newborn, there is an absence of free hydrochloric acid in the stomach. The acid content of the stomach reaches adult levels by age 2 years. Therefore, medications that require an acid medium in the stomach for absorption may not be completely absorbed if the child is less than 2 years of age. The administration of such medications near the time of feedings will further decrease the acid content of the stomach. After 2 years of age, the ingestion of orange juice increases gastric acidity, causing more effective absorption of medication that requires an acid medium to absorb.

Intestinal Influences

Children less than 5 years of age have a more rapid intestinal transit time than adults. Medication may move out of the small intestines before it is completely absorbed. Therefore, delayed or timed-release oral medication may not be fully absorbed by children younger than 5 years of age. There may be a low amount of pancreatic enzymes for infants less than 1 year of age. Some medications depend on pancreatic enzymes to help absorb the medication.

Topical Medications (Ointments)

Pediatric patients have a thin stratum corneum that allows topical medications to be absorbed. The larger skin surface area also increases the amount of absorption of topical medication as compared to that of adults. The use of a plastic diaper can also cause increased absorption of a topically applied medication in the diaper area of the skin. Hydrocortisone and hexachlorophene may produce adverse systemic responses when applied to the buttocks and covered with a plastic diaper or dressing.

Parenteral Medications

Poor peripheral perfusion in the young infant will slow intramuscular (IM) medication absorption. IM medications administered to infants and children less than 4 years of age should be water soluble to prevent precipitation. In newborns, medication may pass through the blood–brain barrier more easily than in older children and adults. Therefore, medications that depress respiration may have a more powerful effect on newborns than in adults.

METABOLISM AND MEDICATIONS IN INFANTS AND CHILDREN

Most medications are metabolized in the liver. Because the liver and its enzymes do not function at a mature level until 2 to 4 years of age, medications generally metabolize more slowly in the infant and young child than in the adult. Medications given at frequent intervals to infants and children may result in toxic levels and responses. An example would be the administration of meperidine (Demerol), which is rarely used in pediatrics because of CNS adverse effects such as seizures or agitation. Codeine is converted to morphine by the liver and requires a specific enzyme to achieve its pain-relief effect. Some ethnic groups are deficient in this enzyme and obtain poor pain relief while other ethnic groups who have this enzyme rapidly metabolize the medication, resulting in symptoms of medication overdose. The use of codeine is not recommended for pain management in children (Government of Canada, 2016; Tobias, Green, & Coté, 2016). Morphine is recommended for moderate to severe pain after surgery, and nonopioid analgesics should be used for mild to moderate pain (World Health Organization [WHO], 2012). See Chapter 19, Pharmacological management of pain, for further discussion. Careful calculations of safe doses and close monitoring are essential.

EXCRETION OF MEDICATIONS IN INFANTS AND CHILDREN

Many medications such as penicillin and digoxin depend on the kidneys for excretion. The immature kidney function prevents effective excretion of medications from the body in infants less than 1 year of age.

The combination of slow stomach emptying (delays medication from being absorbed), rapid intestinal transit time (may prevent the full amount of medication from being absorbed), unpredictable liver function (may impair metabolism of the medication), and inability to excrete medications effectively via the kidneys can result in altered responses to medication and a high risk for toxicity.

NURSING RESPONSIBILITIES IN ADMINISTERING MEDICATIONS TO INFANTS AND CHILDREN

It is a legal and ethical responsibility of the nurse to understand that children who are growing differ in their ability to respond to medications. Nurses must observe for toxic symptoms whenever medications are administered and must document positive and negative responses. Close attention must be paid to pediatric dose calculations. Every medication administered should have the safety of the prescribed dose calculated and confirmed by the nurse before administration. The manufacturer's pocket insert, the *Compendium of Pharmaceuticals and Specialties: The Canadian Drug Reference for Health Professionals (CPS),* or other current drug reference books provide safe dosage levels for various age groups.

Parent Teaching

Parent teaching is essential to ensure they are able to follow through with medication administration when the child is sent home. Instructions should cover the following six areas:

1. The importance of administering the medicine.
2. The importance of completing the prescribed course of treatment.
3. Techniques for measuring the amount of medication to administer in each dose. The use of the teaspoon in the home is not advisable when administering medication to infants and children. Inexpensive and accurate measuring devices are available in pharmacies.
4. Techniques for administering medications to the infant or child:
   - Using a dropper, a syringe, or a measured cup
   - Not mixing medication with formula, food, or water
   - Shaking medication before administering
   - Refrigerating unused portions of medication if indicated
5. Techniques for encouraging child to take the medication:
   - Allowing toddlers and young children autonomy of assisting with taking their own medication by squirting the contents into their own mouth or drinking it from the cup
   - Providing praise for completing the task and perhaps a chart of stars or stickers for reward
   - Providing a good-tasting liquid or a popsicle following administration of a medication that has a bad taste
6. The importance of writing a schedule and documenting the administration to avoid forgetting or double dosing.

Administering Oral Medications

The administration of medication by mouth is preferred in children but is not always possible because of vomiting, malabsorption, or refusal. Children younger than 5 years of age cannot safely swallow tablets or capsules. Most pediatric medications are available in liquid, suspension, or chewable tablets. Only scored tablets should be divided. Extended-release tablets should not be chewed or crushed. Gel tablets should not be cut or dissolved. Suspensions must be fully shaken before use and are often refrigerated.

Medications should not be diluted in formula or water because medications should be given in the smallest amount possible to ensure the complete dose is consumed. If the medication is placed in the bottle and the infant does not finish all the milk in the bottle, the complete dose of the medication will not have been administered. The use of important sources of nutrients, foods, or liquids (e.g., orange juice) for disguising the taste of the medication is discouraged because the child may develop distaste for these foods. The medication is never referred to as "candy." Medication is administered slowly, especially if the child is crying. The child's head and shoulders are elevated to prevent aspiration. Toddlers may attempt to push away the medicine cup. In anticipation of this response, the nurse or parent holds the child in a "hug" position in their lap in a semi-sitting position (Skill 20.6).

If a nasogastric tube is in place, the nurse tests for proper placement of the tube *before* pouring medication into the funnel. A small amount of water is administered afterward to flush (cleanse) the tube. The procedure is recorded on the I&O sheet.

For infants, an oral syringe is an excellent device for measuring small quantities. It is easily transported, and medication can be provided directly from the syringe. The syringe is placed midway back at the side of the mouth. The medication can also be administered via the syringe while the infant is sucking on a pacifier. A Medibottle, a device that consists of a syringe attached to a nipple, can be used for infants who will suck the medication from the nipple while the plunger of the syringe is slowly depressed (Fig. 20.9).

A plastic medicine dropper is useful, and the drug manufacturer may provide one with the medication. It is used only for the medication specified; it is not intended for measuring other liquids. A medication ordered in teaspoons should be measured in millilitres to ensure accuracy (5 mL = 1 teaspoon). The nurse administering medications on the pediatric unit must keep the medicine tray or cart in sight at all times. This prevents other patients from upsetting or ingesting the contents.

Administering Parenteral Medications

Nose drops, ear drops, and eye drops

Except for a few differences, the principles for administering nose drops, ear drops, and eyedrops to children are essentially the same as for adults. Infants and small children may need to be held using therapeutic holding (see discussion above).

Nose drops. The procedure for administering nose drops to a small child is detailed in Skill 20.7.

Ear drops. The health care provider may prescribe a medication to be instilled into the ear to relieve pain. If the drops were refrigerated, they should be allowed to warm to room temperature before administration (Skill 20.8).

Eye drops and creams. Ophthalmic medication is administered to a child in the same manner as for the adult. The child is informed of the need for the medication. The patient is identified, and the orders and the label on the bottle are checked for correct medication and concentration. The nurse ascertains which eye requires treatment. Hand hygiene is performed before and after the procedure. With the thumb and index finger, gentle pressure is applied in opposite directions to open the eye. The older child is instructed to "look up." Supporting the hand on the patient's forehead, the medication is instilled into the centre of the lower lid (conjunctival sac) (see Skill 6.5 and accompanying illustration). The child is instructed to close the eye but not to squeeze it, because this could expel some of the solution.

Ointment is applied to the same conjunctival sac as eye drops. Occasionally, children refuse to open their

Skill 20.6 Administering Oral Medications

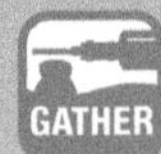

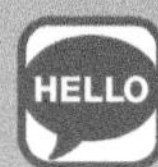

PURPOSE

To safely administer oral medications

STEPS

1. Verify medication orders and assemble supplies.
2. Place the infant's legs between your knees to maintain control of them.
3. Place one of the infant's arms behind your back and "hug" the infant with the other arm (this helps to prevent the child from tipping the medication cup).
4. Give the medication slowly by cup or syringe to allow the child time to swallow. An older child may be given the choice to self-administer the medication by cup or syringe.
5. Provide "chasers" of water, fruit juice, or frozen popsicles to help lessen the residual taste of the medicine. The patient's age and diet prescription are considered when choosing a chaser.
6. Perform hand hygiene.
7. Document in the medication administration record (MAR) the medication, route, time, and dose given.

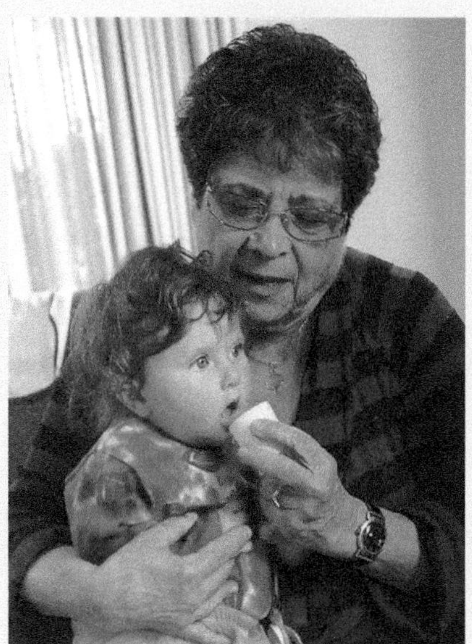

The syringe or cup method of administering oral medications to infants or children. The infant's arms can be placed behind the nurse's back while the nurse holds the other. The legs of the infant can be held between the knees of the nurse for better control during medication administration.

Skill 20.7 Administering Nose Drops

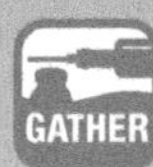
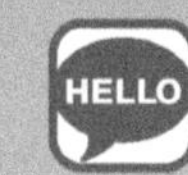

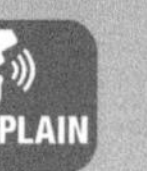

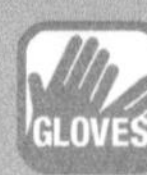

PURPOSE

To administer medication by nasal route

STEPS

1. It may be necessary to have another nurse assist with holding an infant.
2. Wipe excess mucus from nose with a tissue.
3. Place the infant on their back, with the head over the side of the mattress or the neck extended over a pillow.
4. Encircle the infant's cheeks and chin with the left arm and hand to steady.
5. Instill drops with the right hand.
6. Keep infant in this position for 30 seconds to 1 minute to allow the drops to reach the proper area.
7. Make the infant comfortable.
8. Remove gloves and perform hand hygiene.
9. Chart the following: time, name of nose drops, strength, and number of drops instilled, how the patient tolerated the procedure, and any untoward reactions.

Skill 20.8 Administering Ear Drops

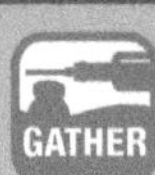
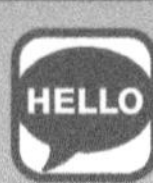

PURPOSE

To administer medications into the ear canal

STEPS

1. Place child in supine position with unaffected ear down.
2. Instill the ordered number of drops:
   a. In children less than 7 years of age, pull the pinna (earlobe) of the affected ear down and back to straighten the canal.
   b. In older children, pull the upper pinna (auricle) up and back to straighten the canal.
3. Gently massage the area in front of the ear to facilitate entry of the drops.
4. Keep the patient in a supine position for a few minutes to permit the fluid to be absorbed.
5. Perform hand hygiene.
6. Document the time, name of medication, number of drops administered, area (right or left ear), any untoward reactions, and whether or not the patient obtained relief.

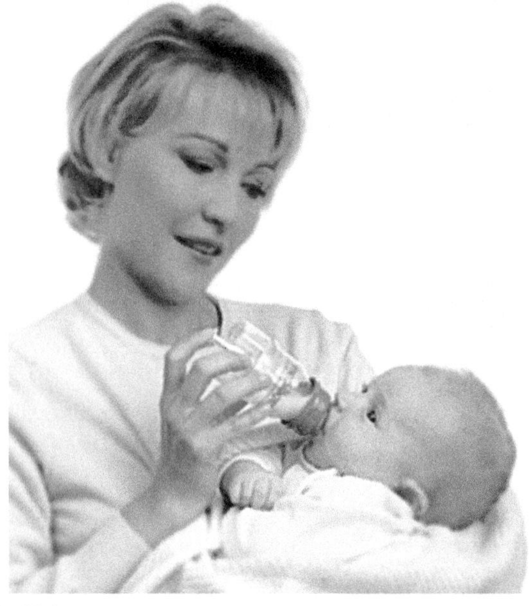

Fig. 20.9 The Medibottle is attached to the syringe so the infant can suck on the nipple to consume the medication. The nurse controls the flow with gentle pressure on the syringe barrel. (Courtesy, The Medicine Bottle Co., Inc.)

eyes. The nurse must use ingenuity to coax reluctant children. It may help to involve the parents.

Rectal medications

Some medication, such as sedatives and antiemetics, come in the form of suppositories. Children's suppositories are long and thin in comparison with the cone-shaped types administered to adults. Wearing a glove, the nurse inserts the lubricated suppository well beyond the anal sphincter, about half as far as the forefinger will reach. The nurse applies pressure to the anus by gently holding the buttocks together until the child's desire to expel the suppository subsides.

Subcutaneous and intramuscular injections

Most medications are given to infants and children by the oral or IV route. However, some medications must be given by the subcutaneous route, such as insulin for diabetic children. Some medications must be administered via the IM route, such as immunizations or vitamin K to newborn infants. The site and technique of injection can affect the absorption rate and the effect of the medication on the child. Needles should not be recapped, and the syringe must be disposed of in the appropriate container after use. See Skill 6.6 for how to give injections to newborns.

The subcutaneous route. In subcutaneous (subcut) injections, absorption occurs by slow diffusion into the capillaries. If a medication such as epinephrine is given IM instead of subcutaneously, a life-threatening cardiac dysrhythmia could occur. If the extremity in which the subcutaneous medication was given is exercised immediately before or after an injection, the absorption rate is increased. (If insulin is the medication injected, hypoglycemia could occur because of the rapid absorption.) Sites should be rotated. Irritating solutions should not be injected subcutaneously. A 23- to 25-gauge needle, with 1.5 cm (5/8 inch) needle length is used for infants and children greater than 1 month of age (Government of Canada, 2017).

The intramuscular route. An intramuscular (IM) injection places medication into the skeletal muscle below the subcutaneous tissue. The medication spreads among the muscle's elastic fibres and absorbs rapidly. Aspirating the plunger after insertion and observing for a flashback of blood serves to prolong a painful procedure and is not necessary when the needle is inserted appropriately at a 90-degree angle (Government of Canada, 2017). Because there are no large vessels in the recommended injection sites for infants and children, aspiration is not necessary. The IM route is only used when necessary and IV or subcutaneous routes are preferred.

Medication Safety Alert!

Maximum volume for IM administration can vary depending on institution policy.

IM injections are administered into the thickest part of the *vastus lateralis* muscle of the anterolateral thigh in all infants (Fig. 20.10, *A*). The site is free of major nerves and blood vessels, but small nerve endings can cause the injection to be painful. The *ventrogluteal* site places the medication into the gluteus medius and gluteus minimus muscles, which are free of major nerves and blood vessels (Fig. 20.10, *B*).

The *dorsogluteal* site involves a high risk for sciatic nerve injury or piercing of a major blood vessel *and should never be used for any IM injections in any patients unless no other sites are available.* The *deltoid* site in the upper arm has a small muscle mass that limits the amount of medication that can be injected at one time. Immunizations are often administered via the deltoid site (Fig. 20.10, *B*).

Reducing the pain of injections. Nurses can take the time to reduce the discomfort associated with injections. *Positioning* the patient properly can minimize muscle tenseness and ease the procedure. The infant or child can be held in the "hug" position on the lap of the parent or coworker Fig. 20.11. Administering an injection while the infant is restrained and lying down on a bed or a table is a traumatic experience for the infant or child. Infants should be put to the breast or skin-to-skin with the parent or offered a sucrose-sweetened nipple to suck on during the procedure. See Chapter 11, Pain, for more information on pain management in newborns. The older child should be distracted. For an injection into the deltoid area, the child can be held in the "hug" position with the elbow flexed and the arm supported and held. A *topical anaesthetic* such as a eutectic mixture of local anaesthetics (EMLA) (see Fig. 19.3) can be used when the time of injection can be planned in advance. The needle should be inserted rapidly. The medication is injected rapidly, unless the package insert states that slow injection is preferred. Rapid removal of the needle and mild massage or exercise of the extremity will increase absorption and comfort.

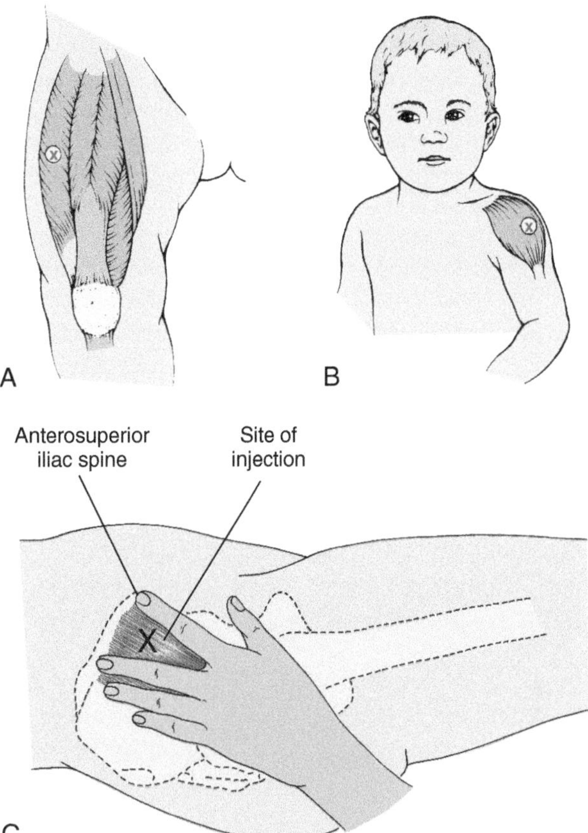

Fig. 20.10 Appropriate sites for intramuscular (IM) injection in children. **A,** The thigh (Vastus lateralis). **B,** Deltoid. **C,** Ventrogluteal the thigh is preferred in children less than 3 years of age.

The sizes of the syringe and needle vary with the size of the child, the volume of medication prescribed, the amount and general condition of the muscle tissue, the frequency of injections, and the viscosity (thickness) of the medication. A small needle, such as 25-gauge with a length of 1.3 to 2.5 cm (½ to 1 inch), is commonly used for infants. As a general rule, 1 mL is the maximum volume to be given in one site to infants and small children. Small or premature infants may tolerate even less. For volumes less than 1 mL, a tuberculin syringe or low-dose syringe is preferred. Although a change of needle may be recommended after drawing up a medication from a glass ampule before injecting the infant, a change of needle is not necessary when drawing up medication from a vial.

The nurse should anticipate some protest from children about injections. The child's first injection is particularly important because it establishes the pattern for future reactions. The school-age child may assist in selecting the site, if possible. This helps to increase feelings of mastery and control. Injections are more of a threat to toddlers and preschool children, who are too young to understand their necessity. The nurse should be careful not to shame the child who has difficulty with the procedure. Fortunately, the necessity for administering IM injections to children is decreasing, because most medications can now be administered orally, rectally, or intravenously.

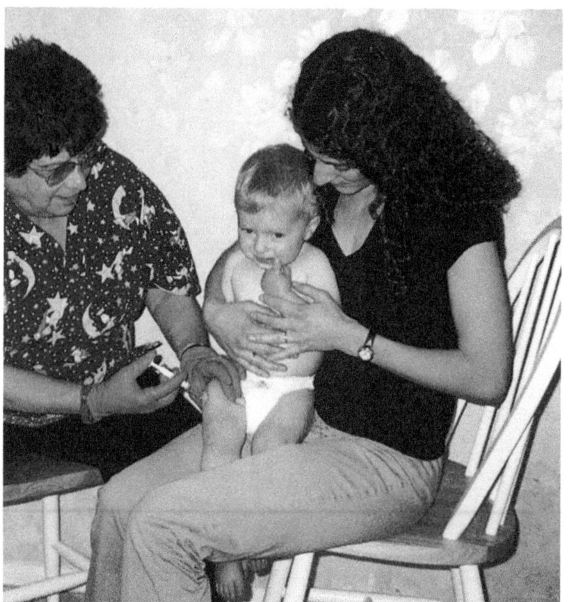

Fig. 20.11 The "hug" restraining position for administration of intramuscular injections. Note that the mother holds the arms, and that the child's legs are held between the mother's knees. The mother comforts the child during the procedure and may breastfeed during the procedure. The site for intramuscular injections in infants is vastus lateralis, and the nurse wears a protective glove.

Intravenous medications

An IV injection places the medication directly into the bloodstream in a faster, more predictable time frame.

Medications provided by the IV route are being administered routinely in pediatric patients. In some cases, this prevents repeated IM injections. Other medications are effective only if given by this method. The medication is also absorbed more rapidly.

IV medications can cause phlebitis, and the nurse must observe the child's IV site closely for reddened areas or signs of inflammation. Infiltration is also a risk for children who are active. The IV site should be observed hourly, because infants cannot communicate the burning or pain that may accompany infiltration or inflammation. Leakage at the IV site, tense tissue turgor, and cool, blanched skin around the IV site may indicate infiltration; this should be reported. Because the medication reaches the heart and brain within seconds, adverse reactions can occur quickly. The nurse must be aware of the adverse effects associated with each medication administered. A rapid rate of flow of IV solution can cause fluid overload (manifested by increased pulse rate or BP, distended neck veins, and puffy eyes), or a slow rate of infusion can result in clot formation that obstructs the patency of the IV line. The nurse should monitor the rate of the IV flow, observe condition of the IV site hourly, identify the responses of the child, and document findings. IV pumps may be set to alarm hourly so that the nurse will be reminded to observe the IV site and the responses of the infant or child and to document findings.

Sites for IV infusion in children are illustrated in Fig. 20.12. A pediatric arm board may be used (Fig. 20.13) to restrain the extremity used for IV access, and the insertion site is secured and covered to prevent tampering by the child. The child with an IV in the extremity or in the scalp will benefit from being held and rocked. Infusion pumps and syringe pumps are used in pediatrics to control the administration of small volumes of fluid and to prevent changes in rate resulting from changes in position or activity in the infant or child. When the health care provider orders IV access discontinued before discharge from the hospital, the nurse will remove the IV catheter (Skill 20.9).

Long-term peripheral venous access devices

Saline lock. A saline lock is a long-term peripheral venous access device also known as an intermittent infusion device which keeps a vein open for long-term intermittent medication administration. It allows children to be more ambulatory because they are freed from IV tubing. Repeated "sticks" can be avoided when a patient has a saline lock in place. The apparatus consists of an IV catheter attached to an 8.3-cm (3¼ -inch) plastic tube plugged by a resealable rubber insert. This rubber top allows the insertion of a needle so that blood can be drawn or medications administered. The original catheter remains in place and is flushed routinely according to specific hospital policy with sterile saline solution to prevent clotting. Each catheter flushing should be documented.

Central venous access devices (CVAD). A peripherally inserted central catheter (PICC) is a type of CVAD that is inserted for moderate-length therapy. The tip of the catheter usually terminates in the superior vena cava. Specially trained registered nurses may insert the PICC line. Dressings are changed per established protocol, the insertion site is assessed, and care is taken to prevent dislodgement during this procedure. PICC flushing with sterile saline solution is done according to hospital policy. Time between flushes is dependent on whether the PICC line is in use or not.

Total parenteral nutrition. Total parenteral nutrition (TPN), also known as *hyperalimentation*, provides the total nutritional needs for infants and children who cannot use the gastrointestinal tract for nourishment for a prolonged period. It allows highly concentrated solutions of proteins, glucose, and other nutrients to infuse directly into a large vessel such as the superior vena cava via a CVAD. In general, these concentrated solutions are not administered through peripheral veins. The nursing responsibilities are similar to those for other IV infusions. The solution is sterile and prepared in the pharmacy. Monitoring vital signs, recording I&O, and tracking laboratory reports are essential nursing responsibilities.

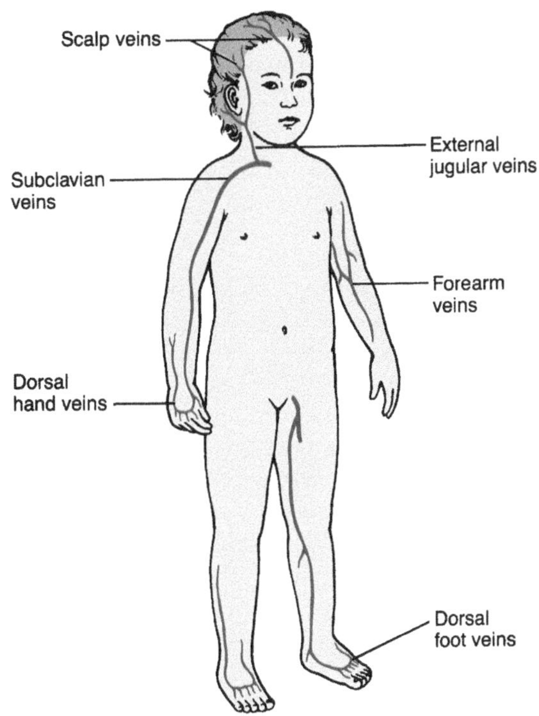

Fig. 20.12 Sites for intravenous (IV) infusion in children.

Hypoglycemia, hyperglycemia, and electrolyte imbalances can occur. Before discontinuing TPN therapy, the rate is *gradually* decreased, and the child is monitored for adverse responses. Parents may need extensive teaching and return demonstrations if they are expected to care for their child who is to receive TPN treatment at home. Community agencies should be contacted to aid and support the family.

Nursing care of a child receiving parenteral fluids

Parenteral (*para,* "beside or apart from," and *enteron,* "intestine") fluids are those given by some route other than the digestive tract. They are necessary when vomiting or loss of consciousness accompanies sickness, or when the gastrointestinal system requires rest. The insertion site is secured and covered and the extremity is usually put on an arm board. A pacifier should be provided for infants who are given nothing by mouth (NPO status) to fulfill their developmental need for sucking, if the parents agree. Diversional therapy will prevent the child from focusing on the IV tubing and using it as a toy. The infant should be picked up, rocked, and played with.

IV pumps prevent a change in IV infusion rate when position or activity changes. The IV pump allows the administration of microdrops of IV solution so that a slow rate of infusion can be maintained. Adult IV sets administer 15 drops per 1 mL. Pediatric IV sets administer 60 drops per 1 mL.

The nurse observes the child hourly for the following:

- Low volume in the bag
- The rate of flow of the solution
- Pain, redness, or swelling at the catheter insertion site
- Moisture at or around the catheter insertion site

An accurate I&O record is kept for all children receiving IV fluids. Nursing guidelines for IV therapy at

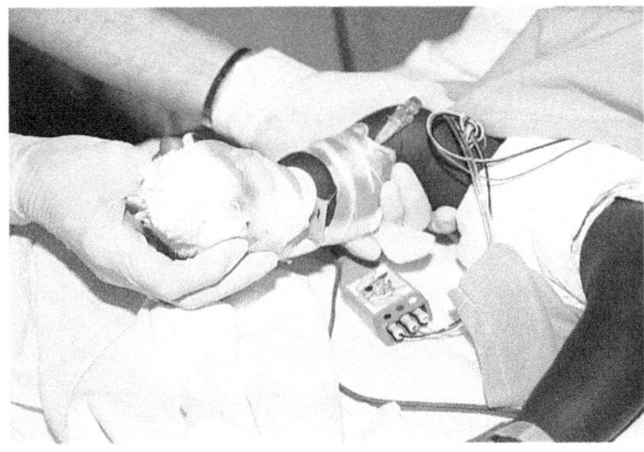

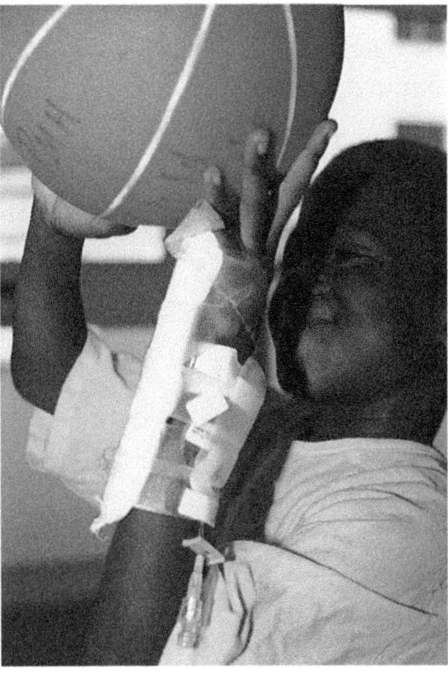

Fig. 20.13 The arm board immobilizes the arm during intravenous (IV) therapy and permits movement. (From McKinney, E. S., James, S. R., Courtesy Parkland Health and Hospital System, Dallas, TX.)

Skill 20.9 Removal of a Peripheral Intravenous Catheter

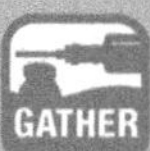

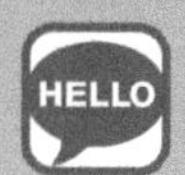

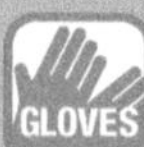

PURPOSE

To safely remove the peripheral intravenous (IV) catheter

STEPS

1. Turn off the infusion pump and clamp the IV tubing.
2. Perform hand hygiene and don clean gloves.
3. Remove the tape:
   a. To remove the Tegaderm or Opsite, pull the opposing edges parallel to the skin to loosen the bond.
   b. To remove sticky adhesive, use an adhesive removal pad and wash the skin afterward. This should not be used on preterm infants.
4. When all tape is removed and the catheter is movable and free, pull the catheter out of the vessel (in the opposite direction to that of insertion), keeping a straight line and not pulling upward or downward.
5. Exert firm pressure at the site with dry, sterile gauze.
6. Apply dry dressing or adhesive bandage at the insertion site.
7. Inspect catheter tip to ensure it is intact.
8. Remove gloves and perform hand hygiene.
9. Document on chart.

Note: Encourage the child's participation when appropriate (for example, when removing the tape).

various stages of development are described in Table 20.3. Selected tips for providing medication to children of various ages are offered in Box 20.1.

Preventing Medication Errors

Each provincial regulatory body has medication administration guidelines that are important to adhere to, although this is not always a guarantee of error-proofing medication administration to children.

Medication Safety Alert!

The fact that the medication dose is ordered by the health care provider is not in itself a guarantee of safety, and the nurse has a responsibility to double-check the medication dosage with the recommended dosage published in a current recognized drug source.

Prescribing medication in a tense emergency setting increases the challenge of maintaining safety of the dosage prescribed for the small infant or young child.

Medication Safety Alert!

Some of the rights of medication administration include the following (although these will be different depending on provincial jurisdiction):

1. Right patient
2. Right drug
3. Right dose
4. Right time
5. Right route
6. Right patient education
7. Right documentation
8. Right to refuse
9. Right assessment
10. Right evaluation

There have been many efforts to reduce the number of medication errors through the design of charts and the use of colour-coding systems, and nurses must be familiar with those used at their hospital or clinic. A Broselow pediatric emergency tape is used to determine the length of the child and serves as a guide in the administering of emergency medications by correlating dosage calculation and equipment sizes for emergency use. Based on the successful use of Brose-low tape for many years, a system of colour-coded ID bracelets for each child admitted to a hospital unit, based on the child's weight, correlates to reference guides for each weight group and provides an extra check point for the nurse to monitor the safety of the dose for that individual child before administering it (Broselow, Luten, & Schuman, 2008).

Medication Safety Alert!

For each pediatric patient, the right dose involves calculating the recommended dose in milligrams per kilogram (mg/kg), comparing with the dose ordered, and checking with the pharmacist or health care provider if there is any question or discrepancy. A second nurse must check insulins, hypoglycemics, opioids, digoxin, inotropic drugs, anticoagulants, potassium, and calcium salts before these are administered.

Calculating pediatric medication dosages

Body surface area. Most pediatric medications are prescribed in milligrams per kilogram of body weight per 24 hours. A hospital drug reference is usually available on the unit to enable the nurse to determine the safety of a particular dose. If there is any question, one should consult the charge nurse, the health care provider who wrote the order, or the hospital pharmacist.

Table 20.3 Nursing Guidelines for Pediatric Intravenous (IV) Lines at Various Stages of Development

DEVELOPMENTAL CHARACTERISTICS	IV PLACEMENT (IDEAL SITES)	PREPARATION OF CHILD	FAMILY INVOLVEMENT	RELATED NURSING ACTIONS	PROTECTION OF IV SITE	MOBILITY CONSIDERATIONS	SAFETY NEEDS
Infant (First Year)							
Infant is dependent on others for all needs. Infant needs to feel physically safe through close relationship with one caregiving person. Trust develops through needs being met consistently. Mistrust and anxiety develop when needs are met inconsistently. Stranger anxiety begins at approximately 6 months.	Hand, forearm, foot, scalp vein	It is best not to feed infant immediately before IV insertion if possible (vomiting and aspiration are possible).	Prepare family about need for IV therapy, insertion procedure, appearance of infant with IV, and fluid needs. Encourage family to continue providing infant with tactile and verbal stimulation and tender, loving care. Demonstrate safe ways to hold an infant with IV.* Encourage questions and clarify misconceptions.	Hold infant during insertion. Comfort and cuddle during and after insertion. Observe carefully during insertion for problems such as vomiting and aspiration. Firmly immobilize extremity with IV (see next column). Use of pacifier may diminish stress, especially for infants who are NPO.	IV may be secured with tape and is wrapped. Extremity may be protected by using small arm board.	Allow for motion. Use minimal restraint, such as elbow restraint or arm board. Use mitten hands with cotton and stockinette to prohibit infant from grasping IV. Restraining all extremities should not be done. Remember infant's need for sensory stimulation.	Maintain strict intake and output (I&O) record. Secure IV tubing out of range of kicking legs and flailing arms. Check armboards frequently for effectiveness and presence of adequate circulation. Check IV pump pressure settings and administration rate.
Toddler (Age 1–3 Years)							
Discovers and explores self and surrounding world. Enjoys new mobility skills. Develops egocentric thinking and need for parallel play. Tolerates short separations from parent. Transitional objects (security blanket, special toy) provide some comfort. Child is in oppositional syndrome ("no" stage).	Hand, arm, foot Important: for this age group and older, the less dominant extremity should be used for IV whenever possible Determine handedness before IV insertion	Prepare child immediately before procedure (child has limited attention span and is likely to become more anxious if prepared sooner). Give very simple explanation in concrete terms. Show equipment to be used. Do not offer choice. See discussion of preparation for preschool age and assess ability of each child to understand.†	Prepare family about need for IV therapy, insertion procedure, and appearance of child with IV. Whether parents remain with child during procedure varies. If they stay with child, their role should be to comfort rather than to assist with holding. Demonstrate to parents how to handle child with IV safely.	Holding a toddler for an IV usually requires more than one person. Reassure child through verbal and tactile stimulation during procedure. Provide toys such as pegs to hammer for therapeutic and distraction techniques. Many hospitals have child-life specialists who help provide atraumatic care.	See Infant (above). A securely anchored IV is essential for the normally active toddler. Even the best site of protection will not remain effective unless it is coupled with close nursing supervision and distracting activities for child.	Toddlers cope with the world and learn about it through action. Therefore, minimal restraints should be used. Parental presence during waking hours permits child to be constantly supervised. Appropriate play and distraction can be effective.	Child is unaware of danger at this age and will not know that movement of IV causes pain. Constant supervision is needed when child is out of bed. Frequently remind child not to touch IV, but do not expect the ability to cooperate. Distracting activities accomplish much more than does a scolding. Tape IV securely.

Preschool (Age 3-5 Years)							
Magical thinking, based on what child would like to believe. Child cannot always distinguish fantasy from reality. Fears intrusive procedures. Castration fears are common. Develops conscience (guilt), while asserting independence and mastering new skills. Child is learning to share.	Hand, forearm (less dominant)	Prepare child just before procedure. Using small bottle, tubing, and doll or stuffed animal, explain in literal terms the need for IV and insertion procedure. Allow child to see and touch equipment. Explain how child can help with procedure by cleaning site, opening packages, and taping, for example. Allow child some control in the situation. State that you will help child to hold still and that it is OK to cry.	As with toddlers, parents may or may not stay with child during procedure. If they stay, they should provide comfort and support, but they should not be asked to hold child for IV insertion. Reinforce child's need for honest, simple explanations. Reassure parents that child can still play and be active, even with IV.	Tell child purpose of IV in simple terms. *Never* bribe or threaten with IVs (e.g., "Drink, or you'll get another IV"). Praise for ability to cooperate or any efforts in that direction. Maintain patient privacy. Do not start an IV in the sight of other patients, visitors, or staff. Child needs support to cope with intrusiveness of this procedure. Show understanding.	See Infant (above). As with toddlers, securely anchored IVs are essential but inadequate unless coupled with close supervision and age-appropriate activities.	Preschoolers need maximum mobility to master surroundings. Provide a range of out-of-bed activities whenever possible.	Child will be curious about IV. Child is capable of understanding instructions not to touch it but needs frequent reminders and distraction. IV clamps should be out of reach or taped over. Constant supervision is needed when child is out of bed. Child is likely to take off running down the hall, heedless of the IV bag, for example. Short attention span limits duration of ability to follow instructions.
School-Age Child (Age 5-12 Years)							
Struggles between mastery of new skills and failure. Enjoys school, learning skills, and games with rules. Needs to succeed. Fears body mutilation. May feel need to be brave. Can understand hospital rules. World is now expanding beyond family. Peer group becomes important. Child is competitive.	Hand, forearm (less dominant)	Prepare child ahead of time but on same day of insertion. Carefully explain and demonstrate equipment and reasons for IV therapy, letting patient watch or help set up equipment. Ask child for questions about need for IV and procedure. Give child choices and let child help in procedure whenever possible. Tell child crying is OK because needles hurt; child can help by remaining still.	Whenever possible, family and child should be prepared together so that family can reinforce what child has been told. Stress to family the child's need for some independence in activities of daily living, even with an IV. Parental presence or participation in IV insertion may be appropriate, but child's preference should be considered primary.	Approach child expecting the child to assist (this age group likes to please adults), but expect that child will need help remaining still. Allow child to clean site with alcohol swab and to cut tape before insertion. Praise cooperative efforts. Give child step-by-step explanation of procedure as it progresses. Child may like to take some responsibility in keeping I&O record.	Child will need less protection than younger children owing to interest in making IV work correctly. May naturally protect extremity with IV. Some children appreciate a warning sign, "Hands Off," on a piece of tape over IV as a reminder. Use child's natural curiosity and interest in learning. Tell child the rules of safe IV handling.	Show patient and family how to manipulate IV safely for out-of-bed activities (e.g., walking in hall with IV bag, keeping tubing out of wheelchair wheels).	Remind patient periodically about necessary caution with IV. Show patient clamps and caution against handling them. Teach patient signs of IV problems. Enlist child's help but do not entirely depend on it. Tape tubing connections. Child may forget about IV. Emphasize need for caution in some activities, especially if play includes other children.

Continued

Table 20.3 Nursing Guidelines for Pediatric Intravenous (IV) Lines at Various Stages of Development—cont'd

DEVELOPMENTAL CHARACTERISTICS	IV PLACEMENT (IDEAL SITES)	PREPARATION OF CHILD	FAMILY INVOLVEMENT	RELATED NURSING ACTIONS	PROTECTION OF IV SITE	MOBILITY CONSIDERATIONS	SAFETY NEEDS
Adolescent (Age 12–18 Years)							
Vacillates between needs for independence and dependence. Has adult cognitive abilities, deductive reasoning. Coping mechanisms: rationalization, intellectualization. Peer acceptance is very important. Egocentric, rebellious at times, especially against parents and authority figures. Very concerned with body image, body changes, sexuality, and role. Searching for "who I am."	Hand, forearm (less dominant)	Prepare patient several hours to a day before procedure, if possible. Needs time between preparation and insertion to absorb explanations and ask questions. For most adolescents, approach discussions on an adult level. Explain need for IV therapy and expected duration, and show equipment. Patient may need much support for acceptance of therapy.	Explain therapy needs and duration as with patient. Decision regarding parental presence during procedure should be patient's, not parents'. Stress that patient's participation in decisions affecting care is important.	Be aware of IV adding to patient's dependency status and need for some control. Encourage child to keep own I&O sheet and to help in counting drip rate, for example.	See School-Age Child (above). If patient is very active, will need well-protected, well-anchored IV, because movements may be more forceful and strength may be greater than that of younger patients.	See School-Age Child (above). Encourage child being mobile as much as possible as a means of independence for adolescent.	Be aware of possibility of adolescent rebellion, showing itself by lack of assistance with therapy. These patients may rebel if feeling threatened and may be manipulative in testing behaviours. Consistent limits, clearly communicated to patient, parents, and staff, are needed. Instruct patient about signs of infiltration and phlebitis, for example.

Age-appropriate pain relief measures should be implemented for every infant or child. Appropriate distraction will enhance pain relief measures.

*No child should be restricted to bed simply because they have an IV! † Each stage builds on the earlier ones, and during hospitalization many children regress to behaviours appropriate to earlier levels of development.

Modified from Guhlow, L. J., & Kolb, J. (1979). Pediatric IVs: Special measures you should take. *RN, 42,* 40. Reprinted by permission.

Box 20.1 Selected Age-Appropriate Techniques for Giving Medications to Children

INFANT

Support and elevate head and shoulders.
A plastic disposable oral syringe is accurate and safe for administering oral medications.
Depress chin with thumb to open mouth.
Slowly insert medication along the side of the infant's mouth; this helps to prevent gagging.
Allow time for swallowing. The syringe may be placed at the corner of the mouth while the infant is sucking on the pacifier.
The recommended site for intramuscular (IM) injections is the vastus lateralis muscle.
The buttocks are never used for any IM injections.
As a rule of thumb, provide no more than 1 mL of solution in a single site; if in doubt, confer with the charge nurse or health care provider.
Soothe infant after procedure is completed.
Provide nonpharmacological pain-relief methods, such as sucrose solution, skin-to-skin contact, or breastfeeding.

TODDLER

Place the child in the "hug position".
Let child explore an empty medicine cup.
Explain reasons for the medication.
Crush tablets if they are not chewable. *Do NOT crush enteric-coated tablets.*
If child is able, they may hold the medicine cup.
Allow the child to drink at their own pace.
When administering IM medications, perform the injection quickly and gently.
Be prepared to find that resistive behaviour is at its peak, particularly kicking, crying, and thrashing about.
Be prepared to be surprised, because some toddlers are able to assist.

PRESCHOOL

Chewable tablets and liquids are preferred.
Regression in pill taking may be seen.
Watch for loose teeth that may be swallowed.
Avoid prolonged reasoning.
Involve parents whenever possible.
Have child make choices when appropriate.
Whenever possible, follow bad-tasting medicine with good-tasting fluid.
Provide puppet play to help child express frustrations concerning injections.
Praise child after the procedure.

SCHOOL AGE

Child can take pills and capsules; instruct the child to place pill near the back of the tongue and immediately swallow water.
Emphasize swallowing of fluid to distract the child when swallowing the pill.
Some children continue to have a difficult time swallowing pills, and other forms of the medication should be explored (many come in suspensions); never ridicule the child.
Child can be unpredictable from day to day regarding being able to assist; allow more time for giving pediatric medication.
Allow child to make realistic choices before, during, and after procedures. Child can choose if they want to self-administer liquid medication via syringe or cup.
Whenever possible, follow bad-tasting medicine with good-tasting fluid.
Always ascertain that the child is fully awake (particularly after nap time and during the night shift).
Always inform child of what you are about to do.
Remain with the fearful child after the procedure until they regain composure.

ADOLESCENT

An adolescent needs more time to process information and needs to know the results of blood studies and other tests.
Prepare the adolescent with explanations suitable to their level of understanding.
Always ensure privacy.
Teach the adolescent what adverse effects to report.
Identify adolescents on contraceptives to prevent medication interactions (they may have been too embarrassed to provide information during history-taking or may be attempting to keep this a secret from significant others).
Remain with patient until medication is consumed.
Anticipate mood swings affecting ability to collaborate.
Consider possibility of adolescent addiction (e.g., drugs, alcohol) even though this may not be a presenting problem; metabolism of many medications is altered by such conditions.

The nurse should not be interrupted when preparing medications.

The health care provider calculates a particular dosage of a medication for each child. One method, calculation by **body surface area (BSA)**, is considered to be the most accurate. BSA is determined using the following formula:

$$BSA = SQR\ [BW\ (kg) \times Ht(cm)\ /3600]$$

Kilograms (kg) and centimetres (cm) must be used for this calculation. See Additional Learning Resources for a BSA calculator.

Calculating the safe medication dose

Milligrams per kilogram (mg/kg). For adults, most medications have an "average dose." There is no average dose in pediatrics, because the weight of the child can vary from 1 kg (2.2 lb) to 68 kg (150 lb), and at different ages the ability to metabolize and excrete drugs may be limited. Therefore, it is necessary for the nurse to calculate whether the ordered dose is safe. The nurse can use the mg/kg protocol when calculating safe doses for an infant or child. For example, the health care provider orders 25 mg of a medication to be administered. The nurse checks the *CPS* or other current drug reference books or resources and finds that the safe dose for that medication is 2 to 4 mg/kg. This child weighs 7 kg. Using the highest safe dose, the nurse inserts the actual weight of the child in kilograms (kg) into the formula so that the formula now reads as follows: the safe dose of *this* medication for *this* child is 4 mg × 7 kg, or 28 mg. The health care provider's order does not exceed 28 mg, and therefore the dose ordered is safe to give. If the health care provider's order had exceeded the computed safe dose, the nurse would have needed to contact the health care provider.

If a child weighs more than 68 kg, the ordered dose should once again be verified according to the mg/kg protocol and compared to the *CPS* or current drug resources to ensure the dose is safe for that child, as heavier children can often be underdosed when adult doses are reached. If this is the case, the health care provider should be notified.

Dimensional analysis. Dimensional analysis is one method of calculating dosages using basic arithmetic and algebra (Box 20.2). Some examples are provided in this section.

Example: A health care provider orders 0.025 g of a medication. Each tablet is 12.5 mg. How many tablets will you give?

You know that 1 000 mg = 1 g. Therefore:

$$\left(\frac{1000\text{ mg}}{1\text{ g}} \times \frac{0.025\text{ g}}{?\text{ mg}} = 1000 \times 0.025 = 25\ mg\right)$$

You will give 25 mg. Remember that each tablet is 12.5 mg:

$$\textit{What you have}:\textit{What you want to give}:$$

$$\frac{1\text{ tablet}}{12.5\text{ mg}} \times \frac{25\text{ mg}}{?\text{ tablets}} = 2\ \textit{tablets}$$

You would give two tablets.

Example: A health care provider orders 5 mg of a medication. The label reads "10 mg/2 mL." How many mL do you administer?

$$\frac{\text{Unit}}{\text{Dose}} = \frac{2\text{ mL}}{10\text{ mg}} \times \frac{5\text{ mg}}{?\text{ mL}} = \frac{10}{10} = 1\text{ mL}$$

You will give 1 mL.

Determining whether a dose is safe for an infant. A health care provider orders 200 mg q6h. The *CPS* states that a 40-mg/kg dose is a safe dose for infants. The infant weighs 5.5 kg.

$$\begin{matrix}\textit{Dose} & \textit{Weight} & \textit{What infant}\\ \textit{ordered} & \textit{of infant} & \textit{is receiving}\end{matrix}$$

$$\frac{200\ mg}{\text{Dose}} \times \frac{1}{5.5\text{ kg}} = 36.3\text{ mg/kg/dose}$$

Box 20.2 Formula for Dimensional Analysis

$$\frac{\text{Unit}}{\text{Dosage on hand}} \times \frac{\text{Dosage wanted}}{\text{Unit to give}}$$

Because 36.3 mg/kg does not exceed the stated safe dose of 40 mg/kg, the dose ordered is safe for this child.

In addition to knowing the correct amount and route of a medication, the nurse must also be aware of the adverse effects that might occur. The absorption, distribution, metabolism, and excretion of drugs differ substantially in children, who also react more quickly and violently to medication. Medication reactions are therefore not as predictable as they are in adult patients. The medication's impact on normal growth and development must be considered. Drug inserts must be read carefully to determine the suitability of a particular medication for children. **Medications should be administered only by the route indicated.**

Double-checking with another nurse is required for medications that are labelled high-risk medications by the Institute of Safe Medication Practices (ISMP). Medications such as digoxin (Lanoxin), insulin, or heparin are on this list as well as many other medications. See the resources at the end of the chapter for a link to ISMP. Two identifiers on the hospital ID band should be used to correctly identify the child. The child's assigned nurse must always know what medications the patient is receiving, whether or not the nurse personally administers them.

Preventing Medication Interactions

Selected medication–environment interactions

Some medications can cause skin reactions when the child is exposed to the sun (phototoxicity). Parents should be advised to keep their child protected from the sun while the child is taking these medications. Medications that decompose when exposed to the air or light are dispensed in darkened bottles. These medications should not be purchased in the large economy size because some tablets may deteriorate before all are used. Table 20.4 lists some examples of medication–environment interactions.

Selected medication–medication interactions

The nurse should be alert to possible interactions between medications prescribed and between prescription and over-the-counter medications. Table 20.5 includes a partial list of some common medication–medication interactions.

Selected medication–food interactions

The nurse should be aware that food and nutrients can influence the absorption, metabolism, and excretion of certain medications. Foods that influence gastrointestinal motility or the pH of gastric secretions can affect absorption, thus lessening the medication's therapeutic value. Table 20.6 lists some medication–food interactions.

Table 20.4 Selected Medication–Environment Interactions

MEDICATION	INTERACTS WITH	RESULT OF INTERACTION
Imipramine (Tofranil), phenothiazines, griseofulvin, tetracyclines, chlorothiazide (Diuril)	Sun	Skin rash when child is exposed to sun
Vitamin C	Air	Decomposes when exposed to air

SELECTED PROCEDURES AND THEIR ADAPTATION TO CHILDREN

NUTRITION, DIGESTION, AND ELIMINATION

Gavage Feedings

A gavage feeding may be ordered when a child cannot take food or fluids by mouth but the gastrointestinal tract is functioning. A gavage feeding places nutrients directly into the stomach so that natural digestion can occur. This can be accomplished by placing a nasogastric tube into the stomach via the nose, securing it in place with tape or by using the oral route, and reinserting a new tube with each feeding. When long-term feeding is required, a gastrostomy may be performed and a tube inserted directly into the stomach.

Gastrostomy

A **gastrostomy** (*gastro,* "stomach," and *stoma,* "opening") is designed to introduce food directly into the stomach through the abdominal wall by means of a surgically placed tube or button (see Skill 20.10). It is used in infants or children who cannot have food by mouth because of anomalies or strictures of the esophagus or who are severely debilitated or in a coma. Cleansing of the skin around the tube prevents irritation from formula or gastric secretions. The nurse needs to observe for and report vomiting or abdominal distention. Brown or green drainage may indicate that the tube has slipped through the pylorus into the duodenum. This could cause an obstruction and must be reported immediately.

Enema

Administering an enema to a child is essentially the same as for adults; however, the type, the amount, and the distance for inserting the tube require modifications. In addition, a child's bowel is more easily perforated under pressure. An isotonic solution (saline) is used in children. Tap water enemas are contraindicated because plain tap water is hypotonic to the blood and could cause rapid fluid shift and overload if absorbed through the intestinal wall. The type of solution intended is always confirmed. The amount of fluid varies somewhat in procedure recommendations. The smaller the child, the less solution is used. The exact amount for infants should be prescribed by the health care provider's order. Guidelines range from a low of 50 mL for infants to a high of 500 to 750 mL for the adolescent. The nurse needs to consult the procedure manual for the institution's guidelines.

The tube is inserted from 0.4 to 1.6 cm (1 to 4 inches) according to the size and age of the child. Infants and small children may be unable to retain the solution; therefore, it may be necessary to hold the buttocks together for a short time.

Commercial enemas specific for the child may be used; however, some are not recommended for infants and children. The Fleet Enema contains sodium biphosphate and sodium phosphate and has an osmotic action that can result in metabolic acidosis. Other commercially prepared enemas can cause complications in a dehydrated child. An oral polyethylene-glycol lavage solution, GoLytely or NuLytely, can be used to cleanse the bowel, as can a solution of magnesium citrate, without causing a risk for an electrolyte imbalance.

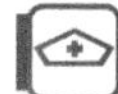
Nursing Tip

Saline enemas may be made by combining 5 mL of table salt with 500 mL of tap water.

RESPIRATION

Tracheostomy Care

A **tracheostomy** is a surgical procedure in which an opening is made in the trachea to enable the patient to breathe. This artificial airway may be necessary in emergency situations, may be an elective procedure, and may be combined with mechanical ventilation. Some of the childhood conditions that may require tracheostomy are acute epiglottitis, head injury, and burns. Nursing care is indispensable to the survival of the child, because blockage of the tube by mucus or other secretions can lead to suffocation. In many hospitals, the child is placed in the critical care unit immediately after surgery because this is a critical period that requires frequent suctioning and close observation. The child is placed on heart and respiratory monitors. When the child's condition stabilizes, the child is usually transferred to a general unit.

The child is placed in an area of high visibility. This is important because small children communicate their needs by crying and the tracheostomy prohibits vocalization. Whenever possible, one nurse is assigned to the child and to work with the parents. Parents may be fearful and will need reassurance and guidance from the nurse when managing the child with a tracheostomy. The nurse reinforces preoperative teaching and explains what happened; for example, "You were having a lot of trouble breathing. This operation is called a tracheostomy and helps you to breathe more easily. A small

Table 20.5 **Selected Medication–Medication Interactions**

MEDICATION	INTERACTS WITH	RESULT OF INTERACTION
Antacids	Steroids Digoxin NSAIDs Tetracycline Theophylline	Decreased absorption Decreased absorption Decreased absorption Decreased absorption Increased toxicity
Barbiturates	Oral contraceptives Steroids Influenza vaccine Theophylline	Decreased protection Decreased steroid effectiveness Barbiturate toxicity Decreased theophylline effect
Bleomycin	Oxygen	Increased lung toxicity
Erythromycin	Phenytoin Theophylline	Decreased phenytoin effect Increased theophylline toxicity
Isoniazid	Antacid Phenytoin Valproate	Decreased absorption Increased phenytoin toxicity Hepatic and central nervous system toxicity
Phenytoin (Dilantin)	Alcohol Antacid Antidepressants (tricyclic) Contraceptives Steroids Digoxin Folic acid Isoniazid Theophylline Valproate	Acute toxicity Decreased phenytoin effect Increased phenytoin toxicity Decreased protection Decreased steroid effectiveness Decreased digoxin effect Decreased phenytoin effect Increased phenytoin toxicity Decreased effect of both medications Increased phenytoin toxicity

NSAIDs, Nonsteroidal anti-inflammatory drugs.

Table 20.6 **Selected Medication–Food Interactions**

MEDICATION	INTERACTS WITH	RESULT OF INTERACTION
Aminoglycosides Gentamicin Penicillin Tetracycline	Any food	Decreased absorption rate
Theophylline (Theolair)	High-protein foods Low-carbohydrate diet	Decreased time of medication activity in body
Monoamine oxidase inhibitors (MAOIs) (phenelzine [Nardil], tranylcypromine [Parnate], isocarboxazid [Marplan])	Tyramine-containing foods such as yogurt, processed meats, beer	Possible hypertensive crises
Iron supplements	Starch, egg yolks	Decreased iron absorption
Antihypertensives	Licorice or natural licorice extract	Can counteract effect of antihypertensive medications
Vitamin C	Foods high in vitamin B_{12}	Decreased absorption of vitamin B_{12} if both vitamins are taken together

opening has been made in your neck. A hollow tube was inserted to keep the area open. It is frightening not to be able to speak. When you are better, the hole will close by itself and your voice will return." An explanation of suction might be, "We have to keep the area in your neck open. This tube goes into the throat and clears it." The use of suction can be shown with a glass of water. The child is then prepared for the unfamiliar sound. "You might feel like gagging, but afterward you will feel better. I know this is difficult for you and I'm sorry."

The nursing care of the child with a tracheostomy is a significant responsibility. The anatomical differences between children and adults and the small child's inability to communicate through writing increase the need for close observation. In addition, toddlers often have short, stubby necks that become easily irritated. It

Skill 20.10 Gastrostomy Tube Feeding

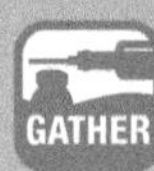

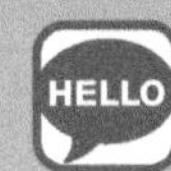

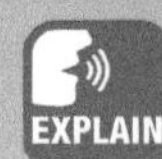

PURPOSE

To introduce nutrition directly into the stomach

STEPS

1. Verify order for type and amount of feeding.
2. Position child comfortably either flat or with head slightly elevated if not contraindicated, or hold child. Provide pacifier to relax infant if appropriate and agreed to by parents. Place absorbent pad under gastrostomy tube extender to protect bed linens.
3. Check residual stomach contents by attaching syringe to gastrostomy tube and aspirating. If amount of residual is large (10–25 mL for newborns, more than 50 mL for older children), replace residual and decrease present formula by equal amount, or delay feeding for a short time. (This may vary according to the health care provider's protocol.) Overloading the stomach can cause reflux and increases the danger of aspiration. If residual continues or increases, report this to the health care provider. If no residual is obtained, inject 2 to 5 mL of water into the tubing to clear tubing and test residual again. (Verification of tube placement is usually obtained via X-ray after initial insertion and when any question of placement occurs.)
4. Attach the syringe barrel (if not already present for continuous infusion) to the gastrostomy tube. If the tube has more than one lumen, be sure to use the port labelled for *food or formula*. Fill with formula. Remove clamp. This prevents air from entering the stomach and causing distention. (**Note:** When administering medication via gastric tube, first flush the tubing so medication will not mix with the milk or formula and flush between each medication administered. Flushing after giving a medication ensures that all the medication has entered the body and none is left in the tubing.)
5. Elevate the receptacle. Allow the formula to flow slowly by gravity—force should not be used. (**Note:** Medications and feedings should flow by gravity and be followed with enough fluid as a flush to ensure the medication or feeding is in the stomach and does not remain in the tubing.)
6. Continue to add formula to the syringe before it empties completely (to prevent excess air from entering the tubing).
7. Clamp the tube as the final formula or water is passing through the lower part of the syringe. The gastrostomy tube extender may remain in place and be clamped or it may be removed from the gastrostomy button and the button closed and locked. (**Note:** With infants, some health care providers may prefer that the gastrostomy tube remain open at all times to produce a safety valve in the event that the infant vomits. In such cases, the tube is elevated above the patient's body.)
8. Whenever possible, hold the patient quietly during and after feeding. Reposition in Fowler's position or on the right side to promote gastric emptying.
9. Perform hand hygiene.
10. Record in the medical record the type (gastrostomy feeding), the amount given, the amount and characteristics of residual, and how the child tolerated the procedure.
11. Record the intake on the intake & output record.
12. An increase in gastric residual, abdominal distention, vomiting, or bradycardia should be reported to the health care provider promptly.

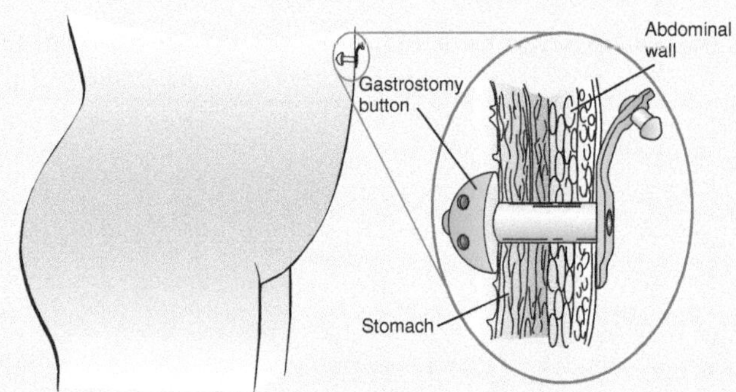

The gastrostomy button allows feedings to be administered directly into the stomach through the abdominal wall. (From Hockenberry, M., Wilson, D., et al [2003]. *Wong's nursing care of infants and children* [7th ed.]. St. Louis: Mosby.)

may be helpful to place a reminder on the intercom at the clerk's desk or in other suitable areas indicating that this patient cannot cry or speak. The nurse's touch and quiet voice and the presence of family help to make the child feel secure. Repeating familiar stories incorporates calming routines. The child should be encouraged to keep a favourite article, such as a blanket or toy nearby. A supply of teaching aids and of dramatic play material should also be made available. Puppets are particularly valuable.

Tracheostomy tube

Maintaining patency of the tracheostomy tube is of utmost importance. Plastic or Silastic tubes are generally used because they are flexible and reduce crust formation. They are lightweight and disposable, and most do not have inner cannulas. Cuffed tubes are not usually necessary in infants and small children, because their air passages are smaller and the tracheostomy tube provides a sufficient seal. The surgeon chooses a tracheostomy tube that is appropriate for the patient's neck size and condition. Administering oxygen by manual resuscitator ("bagging") before or after the procedure may be done to prevent hypoxia. It is vital for the nurse to have extra tracheostomy supplies and emergency equipment available at the bedside should an emergency ensue.

Suctioning

It is important for the nurse to select a suction catheter that does not block the tube during suctioning. The diameter should be about half the size of the tracheostomy tube. The nurse first performs hand hygiene and then may use sterile gloves for the procedure depending on patient status and hospital protocol. Suction is applied as the catheter is *withdrawn*. The tube is rotated to allow the removal of secretions on all sides. With Y-tube technique, suction is achieved by closing the port with the thumb. A drop of saline solution may be inserted before suctioning to aid in loosening secretions. Because variations in this procedure exist and modifications are often required, the nurse must understand what is intended for the particular patient and must ask for clarification of specific procedures of the institution. Administering oxygen by manual resuscitator ("bagging") before or after the procedure can help prevent hypoxia.

Suctioning is done periodically and when necessary. Indications for suctioning include noisy breathing, bubbling of mucus, and moist cough or respirations. Patients can rapidly become hypoxic during suctioning, thus it is limited to no more than 5 seconds for pediatric patients. Two or three breaths for reoxygenation are allowed between suctioning with no more than three passes done at any given time. The depth of suctioning is important to bear in mind: In general, suctioning is limited to the length of the tracheostomy tube or slightly beyond to stimulate coughing. The catheter is cleared with sterile water between insertions. Unnecessary suctioning should be avoided. The suction catheter is discarded after each use. Disposing of water after suctioning prevents the growth of opportunistic organisms.

Tracheal stoma

The tracheal stoma is treated as a surgical wound. The area is kept free of secretions and exudate to minimize the risk of infection. Cotton-tipped applicators dipped in half-strength hydrogen peroxide and saline solution may be used to remove crusted mucus. Tapes around the child's neck should be loose enough to allow one finger to be easily inserted between tape and neck. The knot is placed to the side of the neck (Fig. 20.14). The condition of the skin beneath the tape is assessed, and the tape is changed as necessary. Two people are required for this procedure—one to hold the outer cannula and the other to change the tape. When feeding the infant, the nurse covers the tracheostomy with a bib or a moist piece of gauze to prevent aspiration of food particles.

Observing for complications

The nurse must observe the patient for symptoms such as restlessness, rising pulse rate, fatigue, apathy, dyspnea, sternal retractions, pallor, cyanosis, and inflammation or drainage around the incision. Possible complications include tracheoesophageal fistula, stenosis, tracheal ischemia, infection, atelectasis, cannula occlusion, and accidental extubation. Baseline monitoring of the patient is done on each shift and before suctioning. The patient's mental status, respirations, pulse rate and rhythm, and chest sounds are of particular importance. Accurate recording of observations is essential to evaluation. The time and frequency of suctioning, the character of secretions, the relief the patient receives from the procedure, the behaviour of the patient, the appearance of the wound, and other pertinent data are recorded.

A sterile hemostat is kept at the bedside for emergency use. Accidental *extubation*, or expulsion of the tube, is uncommon but can occur as a result of severe coughing if the tapes are too loose. Patency of the airway is maintained by spreading the edges of the wound with the sterile clamp until a duplicate sterile tube is inserted. An extra tracheostomy tube and the equipment needed for its replacement are always kept in a visible, easily reached area at the bedside for use in such emergencies. As the child's condition improves, they are weaned from the tube. The opening gradually closes by granulation. Children whose tubes must remain in place for a longer time may require periodic tube changes.

Additional nursing measures

Additional nursing measures include frequent changes of position, oral feedings (unless contraindicated), and careful bathing to prevent water from entering the tube. The health care provider orders the diet. Although patients may initially be NPO, they progress to a soft or normal diet as the condition improves. The Fowler's

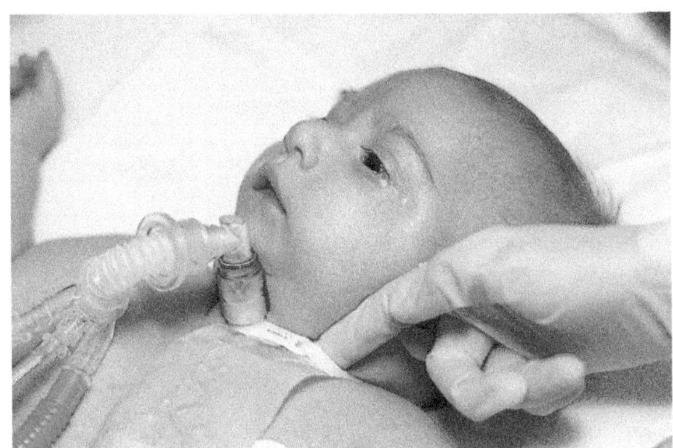

Fig. 20.14 Tracheostomy. The tracheostomy ties should be snug but should allow one finger to be inserted between ties and neck to ensure that it is not too tight. (From Hockenberry, M., & Wilson, D. [2015]. *Wong's nursing care of infants and children* [10th ed.]. St. Louis: Mosby.)

position is preferred during feedings. The older child can help by holding the head flexed with the chin down. This position decreases swallowing difficulties because the esophagus opens and the airway narrows.

Discharge

Certain patients are discharged with a tracheostomy. This situation is anticipated, and instruction and demonstration for the parents begin early. Parents who are comfortable with the procedure during hospitalization will feel more secure when the child returns home. Information about parent support groups, visiting home nurses, and other referrals is provided before discharge.

Oxygen Therapy

Box 20.3 shows a review of selected considerations for the child receiving oxygen. See Chapter 12 for care of a child in an isolette.

Safety considerations

All equipment used for oxygen therapy must be inspected periodically. Combustible materials and potential sources of fire are kept away from oxygen equipment. These materials are essentially the same as for adults; for the child, however, friction toys are also to be avoided, because the sparks the toys can create could ignite the oxygen. Nylon or wool blankets are not to be used. One should know where the nearest fire extinguisher is located. Parents should be alerted to the precautions and to the presence of "no smoking" signs.

Following infection prevention and control guidelines is extremely important. It is imperative that cross-infection via unclean equipment be prevented. Humidifiers and nebulizers, which are warm and moist, serve as an excellent medium for the growth of disease-producing organisms. Although most masks, tents, and cannulas that come into direct contact with the child are disposable, other pieces of mechanical equipment

Box 20.3 Selected Considerations for the Child Receiving Oxygen

GENERAL CONSIDERATIONS

Signs of respiratory distress include an increase in pulse rate and respirations, restlessness, flaring nares, intercostal and substernal retractions, and cyanosis. In addition, children with dyspnea may vomit, which increases the danger of aspiration. Maintain a clear airway by suctioning if needed.

Organize nursing care so that interruptions are kept at a minimum.

NEWBORN

Oxygen may be provided via hood, which may be used in an isolette.

Oxygen may be provided via isolette; keep sleeves closed to decrease oxygen loss.

Oxygen must be warmed to prevent newborn cold stress.

Analyze oxygen concentration carefully.

Parents are the primary focus of preparations; help them to develop self-confidence in their ability to care for the newborn who is ill.

INFANT

Nose may need to be suctioned by bulb syringe to remove mucus.

Make sure crib sides are up.

Avoid the use of baby oil, A + D ointment, petroleum jelly (Vaseline), or other oil-based or alcohol-based substances around nares.

Anticipate stranger anxiety at around 6 to 8 months of age; infant clings to parents and turns away from nurse.

An extremely irritable infant may benefit from comforting in parent's lap; clarify at report time.

Nasal catheters often are well tolerated and allow in-bed activity of infant.

TODDLER

A nasal catheter is tolerated best.

Anticipate regression.

When toddlers are restless and fussy, they may pull at oxygen tubing.

Toddler may be comforted by a transitional object, such as a blanket.

PRESCHOOL

Nasal catheters are better tolerated.

Because thought processes are immature in preschool children, reality and fantasy are inseparable.

To decrease fear, prepare child for all procedures.

Anticipate that child will feel lonely and isolated.

Child will enjoy stories, puppets, and dramatic play.

If extremely restless and anxious, the child may benefit from holding the parent's hand.

Do not allow child to play with toys that could set off a spark.

SCHOOL AGE

Nasal catheters are tolerated best.

Preparatory information continues to focus on what the child will see, hear, feel, and be expected to do.

Child may benefit from writing a story about the experience; nurse can review story with child and clarify misconceptions; posting story on unit affirms child's self-esteem and mastery (*always* ask permission to post).

Allow child to make realistic choices before, during, and after procedures.

Encourage child to draw "what it feels like to have an oxygen tent" and discuss this.

ADOLESCENT

Nurse remains available to the patient to answer questions as they arise.

Trust is extremely important as the adolescent attempts to move beyond the nuclear family.

Anticipate problems of being restricted by apparatus. A nasal catheter is tolerated best.

Adolescent may feel weird when visited by peers; may waver between feeling self-confident and feeling ineffective.

Reiterate no smoking and other safety precautions with patient and peers.

Include patient in therapy; they may be able to manage their own oxygen needs.

For comfort and survival, review safe use of oxygen in the home, if required.

cannot be discarded. They require periodic cleansing if therapy is extended and terminal cleansing according to product direction. The respiratory therapy department should be contacted as necessary.

Prolonged exposure to high oxygen concentrations can be toxic to some body tissues (e.g., the retina in preterm infants and the lungs in the general population), but particularly in children with pulmonary diseases such as asthma or cystic fibrosis. The amount of oxygen administered depends on the child's arterial oxygen concentration. Blood gas determinations (oxygen and carbon dioxide pressures, or Po_2 and Pco_2, respectively) ensure safe and accurate therapy. Noninvasive pulse oximeters that measure blood oxygen saturation via the skin are used whenever oxygen is administered to patients (see Skill 12.1). Saturation rates displayed on the pulse oximeter should be frequently documented on the medical record.

Oxygen is a dry gas and requires the addition of moisture to prevent irritation of the respiratory tract. High-humidity concentrations may be achieved by the use of jet humidifiers on several oxygen units. Compressed air, rather than oxygen, may also be used for this purpose. **Oxygen therapy is terminated gradually.** This allows the patient to adjust to *ambient* (environmental) oxygen. The nurse slowly reduces litre flow or opens air vents in the isolette. The child's response is closely monitored via a pulse oximeter. An increase in restlessness and in pulse rate and respirations indicates that the child is not tolerating withdrawal from the oxygen-enriched environment.

! Safety Alert!

The nurse should inspect all toys when a child is undergoing oxygen therapy. Mechanical or battery toys as well as stuffed toys can create a spark that can be dangerous in high-oxygen environments.

Methods of administration

Oxygen (O_2) is administered to children as appropriate for age via an isolette, nasal cannula, mask, hood, or tracheostomy. Regardless of the method used, the child is observed frequently to determine the effectiveness of the oxygen therapy. The desired goals include decreased restlessness and improved breathing, vital signs, and colour. High concentrations of oxygen can be delivered by way of a plastic hood. Warmed, humidified oxygen is delivered directly over the child's head. It may be used in a radiant warmer.

A health care provider's order often reads, "Keep O_2 saturation at 93%." This means that if the O_2 saturation on the pulse oximeter reads above 93%, the oxygen litre flow can be lowered and the child carefully monitored. If the O_2 saturation level reads below 93%, the litre flow can be gradually increased and the child closely monitored until the reading reaches 93% (see Chapter 12 for discussion of pulse oximeters).

Low-flow oxygen. Low-flow oxygen is a method of oxygen delivery used for children with chronic lung disease (e.g., cystic fibrosis) who are oxygen dependent for prolonged periods. These children react poorly to high oxygen concentrations. Approximately 1 or 2 L/min of oxygen is administered via nasal cannula or a "blow-by" catheter that is placed on the upper lip just below the nostrils (Fig. 20.15). Because this type of oxygen delivery is used for prolonged periods, parent teaching concerning home management is a nursing responsibility.

Management of Airway Obstruction

Emergency abdominal thrusts and back blows are recommended to dislodge food or foreign bodies from the airway. These techniques work on the principle that forcing the diaphragm upward causes residual air in the lung to be forcefully expelled, resulting in popping the obstruction out of the airway.

Older child standing or sitting

The nurse stands behind the standing or sitting victim and wraps the arms around the victim's waist, with one hand made into a fist (Fig. 20.16, C). The thumb side rests against the victim's abdomen, slightly above the navel and well below the tip of the sternum (xiphoid process). The fist is grasped with the other hand and is pressed into the victim's abdomen with a quick upward thrust. From 6 to 10 thrusts may be necessary to dislodge the object. Each thrust should be a separate and distinct movement. The child may be placed in a side-lying position for the recovery phase.

Older child lying down (conscious or unconscious)

The child is positioned on their back. The nurse kneels at the child's feet if the child is on the floor or stands at the child's feet if the child is on a table. The heel of one hand is placed on the child's abdomen in the midline, slightly above the navel and well below the rib cage. The fist is grasped with the other hand and pressed into the victim's abdomen with a quick upward thrust. The 6 to 10 thrusts are repeated as needed. Thrusts are directed upward into the midline and not to either side of the abdomen. The smaller the child, the gentler the procedure.

Infant

The nurse should determine airway obstruction. If the object is visualized, it is removed, trying not to push the object deeper into the throat. If this approach is unsuccessful, the infant is positioned prone with the head lower than the trunk. The nurse supports the head and neck with one hand and straddles the infant face down over the forearm, which is supported on the nurse's thigh (see Fig. 20.16, *A, B*). Resting the infant on the thigh, the nurse performs five forceful back blows between the shoulder blades with the heel of one hand. After delivering the back blows, the free hand is placed on the infant's back so that they are sandwiched between the two hands; the infant is then turned on their back, with the head still lower than the trunk. Five thrusts are delivered in the midsternal region in the same manner as for external chest compressions, but at a slower rate (3 to 5 seconds) (see Fig. 20.16, C). This is repeated until the foreign body is expelled. The nurse should not perform abdominal thrusts, because this may cause injury to the infant's abdominal organs. Conventional cardiopulmonary resuscitation (CPR) can be initiated when the airway is cleared. Because all nurses are required to have basic CPR certification, the technique is not reviewed in the context of this chapter.

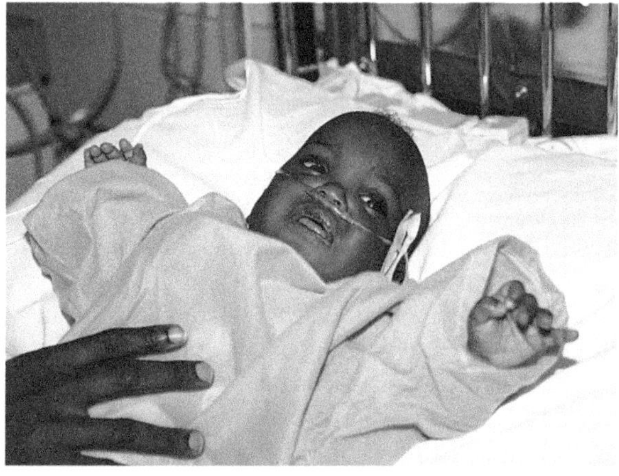

Fig. 20.15 Child receiving blow-by oxygen therapy via nasal catheter. The prongs may be placed below (blow-by) or in the nares, and the loop is slipped over the ears to stabilize the position. The cannula can be taped to the side of the child's face to prevent slippage. (From James, S. R., Nelson, K., & Ashwill, J. W. [2013]. *Nursing care of children: Principles and practice* [4th ed.]. Philadelphia: Saunders.)

Safety Alert!

Blind finger sweeps in the mouths of infants and children should be avoided, as foreign bodies may be pushed further into the throat and aspirated.

PREOPERATIVE AND POSTOPERATIVE CARE

Children are particularly fearful of surgery and require both physical and psychological preparation at the child's level of understanding. Listening to the child is especially valuable to clarify misunderstandings. The child is asked to point to the operative site on a body outline. "Show me what they are going to fix." Anaesthesia is explained, and the child is allowed to play with a mask. Children and their caregivers need reassurance.

Nursing interventions after surgery are aimed at assisting the child in mastering a threatening situation and minimizing physical and psychological complications. Table 20.7 and Table 20.8 summarize preparation for surgery and postoperative care. Parents are included in all aspects of preoperative and postoperative care (Fig. 20.17).

When adults are prepared for surgery, they are usually kept NPO from midnight before the scheduled surgery date. The surgery may be done in the morning or afternoon. Infants should not be maintained NPO for longer than 4 to 6 hours because of the high risk for dehydration. It is a nursing responsibility to check that the test procedure or surgery is scheduled as early as possible in the morning to avoid a prolonged wait. If parents consent, pacifiers should be provided to infants who are NPO, to meet their developmental need for sucking.

Surgery and Body Piercing, Body Jewelry, and Tattoos

Body piercing jewellery and tattoos are very common today among teens at every socioeconomic level.

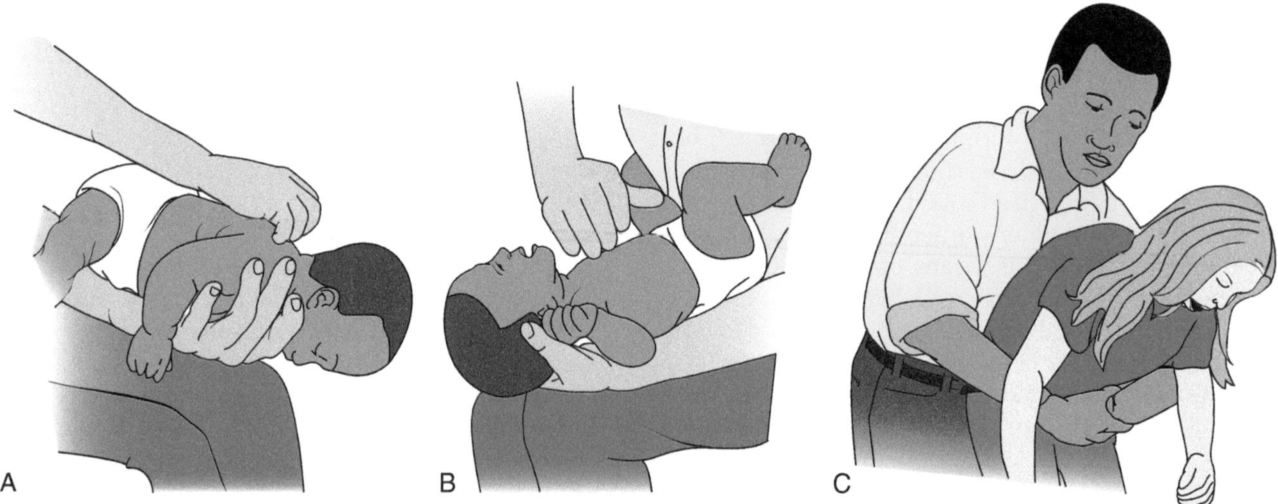

Fig. 20.16 Procedures for clearing an airway obstruction. **A,** Back blow on an infant. **B,** Chest thrust on an infant. **C,** Abdominal thrust on a child. (From Hockenberry, M. J., & Wilson, D. [2017]. *Wong's essentials of pediatric nursing* [10th ed.]. St. Louis: Mosby.)

Most body jewellery is designed to stay in place and can be covered with an occlusive dressing during surgery without being removed, as long as it is not in the operative area. If removed, the teen should supply a flexible plastic retainer to preserve the opening. Although nipple rings need to be removed before mammography, most body jewellery is made of titanium, niobium, or stainless steel and is not ferromagnetic and thus can safely remain in place during magnetic resonance imaging (MRI). Patients with tattoos or permanent cosmetics are at a slight risk for developing edema or burning during MRI. Tattoo pigments may interfere with the quality of the MRI results; therefore, the radiologist should be made aware of the tattoo through accurate documentation. Appropriate equipment such as ring-opening pliers should be used to remove body jewellery when necessary to avoid skin trauma. The nurse needs to know policies and best practices when the teen with body art is hospitalized.

Table 20.7 Comparative Summary of Surgery Preparation of the Adult and Child

PROCEDURE	ADULT	CHILD	MODIFICATION
Consent	Yes	Yes	Parent, legal guardian, or child (depending on level of understanding)
Blood work	Yes	Yes	Age-appropriate collection
Urinalysis	Yes	Yes	Age-appropriate collection Assist school child Age-appropriate instructions
Evaluate for respiratory infection, nutritional status	Yes	Yes	Use more objective observations in infants and toddlers because of child's limited verbal skills
Allergies	Yes	Yes	Indicate clearly on chart
Nothing by mouth (NPO)	Yes	Yes	Increase fluids before NPO Length of time may vary with age and type of surgery (4–6 hours) for clear fluids, breastmilk, or formula. If surgery is late, place appropriate notice on child: "Do not feed me" Remove "goodies" from bedside stand No gum or hard candy Supervise hungry ambulatory patients carefully
Vital signs	Yes	Yes	Approach child carefully, explain, demonstrate Allow more time
Void before surgery	Yes	Preferred	Not always possible in infants and toddlers
Clothing	Yes	Yes	Hospital gown; may wear underwear or pajama bottoms depending on age, type of surgery
Identification	Yes	Yes	ID bracelet
Teeth	Yes	Yes	Check for loose teeth, orthodontic appliance
Skin preparation	Yes	Possible	May be done in operating room
Glasses or contact lenses	Yes	Yes	Have children and adolescents remove glasses or contact lenses
Enemas	Possible	Possible	Not routine
Transportation	Yes	Yes	Crib or stretcher Parents may accompany to operating room
Emotional or psychosocial preparation	Yes	Yes	Preoperative tour Group and individual puppet play Body drawings of parts involved Play selected by child as mode of expression Support parents during surgery A child life specialist, if available, can be called on to help child work through feelings and fears via games and drawings
Sedation	Yes	Yes	Usually 20 minutes before surgery
Record all pertinent data	Yes	Yes	Essentially the same with pediatric modifications as indicated previously

Table 20.8 Comparative Summary of Postoperative Care of the Adult and Child

PROCEDURE	ADULT	CHILD	MODIFICATION
Return from recovery room	Yes	Yes	Notify parents, often allowed to visit in recovery room Younger patients generally in crib Age-appropriate safety precautions
Note general condition, alertness	Yes	Yes	Infant and toddler cannot verbalize fear or pain
Vital signs	Yes	Yes	Every 15–30 minutes until stable Blood pressure is sometimes omitted for infant
Evaluate for shock	Yes	Yes	Essentially the same
Assess operative site for bleeding, condition of dressing	Yes	Yes	Essentially the same Elevate casted extremities Circle drainage on dressing
Restraints	Possible	Possible	May be necessary to protect intravenous line (IV), use of restraints is not recommended unless absolutely necessary Remove periodically for range of motion
Connect dependent drainage (urinary catheter, nasogastric tubes)	Yes	Yes	Prepare child for sight and noises of equipment; draw pictures to clarify purpose
Intravenous line (IV)	Yes	Yes	Should have pediatric adapting device and infusion pump with appropriate pressure Monitor rate meticulously, because infants and small children respond quickly to fluid shifts Measure and record intake and output
Assess elimination	Yes	Yes	Bowel and bladder
Relief of pain	Yes	Yes	Hold, comfort young children unless contraindicated Be sensitive to behavioural changes such as increase in irritability, crying, regression, nail biting, passivity, withdrawal Administer pain relievers Involve parents in care Provide transitional object such as blanket, favourite toy, pacifier Be aware of cultural considerations that provide familiarity and comfort
Nothing by mouth (NPO)	Yes	Yes	Until fully awake Infants are breastfed or given bottle of water if formula fed unless contraindicated Avoid brown or red liquids, which may be confused with old or fresh blood Monitor bowel sounds
Consider diet	Yes	Yes	Advance from clear to full liquids to soft to regular diet
Observe for complications	Yes	Yes	Turn, cough, deep breathe; dangle feet; ambulate early; less of a problem in children Hold operative site with hands as a splint when child coughs
Psychosocial adjustment			A child life specialist, if available, can be called on to assist child in adjusting to postoperative self-image or other issues through therapeutic play

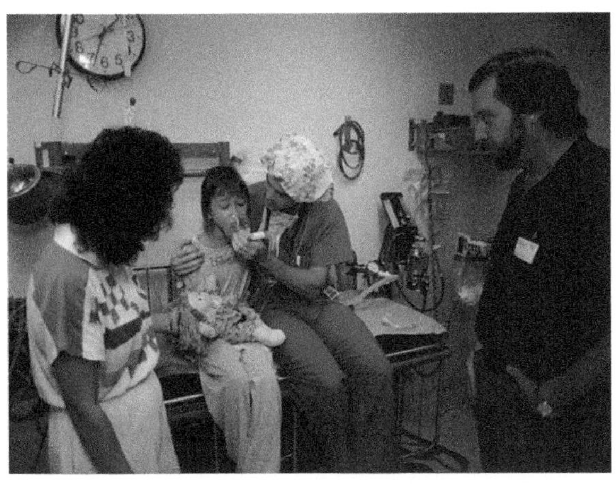

Fig. 20.17 Preparing the child for the sights and sounds of surgery. The parents may be present during early induction of anaesthesia to relieve anxiety during the preoperative period. (From Hockenberry, M., & Wilson, D. [2015]. *Wong's nursing care of infants and children* [10th ed.]. St. Louis: Mosby.)

Get Ready for Certification Examination!

Key Points

- The nurse must be especially conscious of safety measures on the children's unit, particularly the following: keeping crib sides up when the child is unattended, safe transport, and proper identification of the child.
- The parents are included in both the planning and implementing of care. Children are prepared for and encouraged to express their feelings about treatments.
- The nurse must report the body temperature of an infant or child that is below 36°C (97°F) or above 38°C (100.4°F) and institute nursing interventions promptly.
- Weight measurements must be accurately recorded in kilograms because medication is calculated according to the child's weight as mg/kg per day or per dose.
- The child's weight in kilograms is part of the mandatory nursing data collection and must be prominently recorded on the medical record and reviewed on each shift hand-off report.
- The correctly sized blood pressure cuff must be used for children to obtain an accurate reading. It should cover two-thirds of the upper arm.
- Special urine collection bags are used for newborns and infants.
- Proper positioning of the child for jugular and femoral puncture is important. Because these are large veins, the infant is frequently checked for bleeding after these procedures.
- Medications for children must be adapted to size, age, and body surface. The absorption, distribution, metabolism, and excretion of medications differ substantially in children. Their reactions to medications are less predictable than those of adults.
- The nurse should be familiar with tools and techniques that decrease medication errors in pediatric patients.
- The recommended IM injection site for children is the vastus lateralis or ventrogluteal.
- Careful observation of the child receiving IV fluids is necessary because overload of fluids in an infant can lead to cardiac failure. IV pumps are used to ensure accurate rate and safe administration of IV fluid. Intake and output sheets must be accurate.
- The nurse must monitor the rate of the IV flow, observe the condition of the IV site, and document hourly the response of the child.
- When administering ear drops to children younger than 7 years old, the pinna of the ear is pulled down and back to straighten the ear canal. In the older child, the pinna of the ear is pulled up and back.
- Children who are receiving oxygen therapy should not play with toys that can make a spark. A pacifier should be offered to infants whose status is NPO (nothing by mouth) if parents provide consent for this.
- Preoperative and postoperative care assists the child in mastering threatening situations and minimizing physical and psychological complications.
- Most body jewellery made of titanium or surgical stainless steel is not ferromagnetic and may not need to be removed before MRI or surgery.

Additional Learning Resources

evolve Go to your Evolve website (http://evolve.elsevier.com/Canada/Leifer) for the following learning resources:

- Answer Key for Critical Thinking Questions
- Answer Key for Textbook Review Questions
- Audio Glossary
- Fluids & Electrolytes tutorial
- Interactive Review Questions
- Skills Performance Checklists
- Video clips and more!

Online Resources

- *Body Surface Area Calculator:* https://www.calculator.net/body-surface-area-calculator.html
- Institute for Safe Medication Practices (ISMP), *List of High-Alert Medications in Acute Care Settings:* https://www.ismp.org/tools/institutionalhighAlert.asp

Review Questions

1. Which approach is best when administering an oral medication to a young child?
   a. "Would you please take your medicine now, David?"
   b. "Look how good Johnny took his medication. Can you do that too, David?"
   c. "You must take your medicine now if you want to get better."
   d. "It's time for your medication, David. Would you like water or juice after it?"
2. Which of the following are the appropriate sites for an intramuscular injection for a 6-month old? *(Select all that apply.)*
   a. Dorsogluteal
   b. Ventrogluteal
   c. Vastus lateralis
   d. Deltoid
3. The health care provider orders 1.0 mg of morphine for a patient after surgery. If the label reads 5 mg/mL, how much would the nurse administer?
   a. 2.0 mL
   b. 0.8 mL
   c. 0.5 mL
   d. 0.2 mL
4. The temporal artery thermometer may give an inaccurate reading in which of the following situations? *(Select all that apply.)*
   a. The lens is dirty.
   b. The side of the forehead measured has been resting on a pillow.
   c. The patient had just finished drinking iced cold water.
   d. The patient is hypothermic.
5. Which medication can be crushed when administered to a pediatric patient?
   a. Potassium chloride (Slo-K) capsule
   b. Colace gel tablet (Docusate)
   c. Ditropan XL tablet (oxybutynin)
   d. Simethicone tablet
6. During the administration of medications, a 17-year-old patient tells the nurse that he has never had that particular pill before. The best nursing actions would be which of the following? *(Select all that apply.)*
   a. Check the patient's ID band again.
   b. Assure the patient that the medication packet has his name on it.
   c. Ask the patient to take the medication since the ID band and the medication administration record match.
   d. Check the health care provider's written orders to confirm if this medication is newly prescribed.

REFERENCES

Broselow, J., Luten, A., & Schuman, A. (2008). Preventing death by a decimal point. *Contemporary Pediatrics, 25*(7), 38.

Canadian Paediatric Society (CPS). (2016). *The Greig health record.* Retrieved from https://www.cps.ca/en/tools-outils/greig-health-record.

Dionne, J. M., Harris, K. C., Benoit, G., et al. (2017). Hypertension. Canada's 2017 guidelines for the diagnosis, assessment, prevention, and treatment of pediatric hypertension. *Canadian Journal of Cardiology, 33*(5), 577–585.

Ducharme, F., Dell, S., Radhakrishnan, D., et al. (2015). Diagnosis and management of asthma in preschoolers: A Canadian Thoracic Society and Canadian Paediatric Society position statement. *Canadian Respiratory Journal, 22*(3), 135–143.

Flynn, T., Kaelber, D., Baker-Smith, C., et al. (2017). Clinical practice guideline for screening and management of high blood pressure in children and adolescents. *Pediatrics, 140*(3), 1–74.

Government of Canada. (2016). *New safety measures for prescription codeine and hydrocodone to further restrict use in children and adolescents.* Retrieved from http://healthycanadians.gc.ca/recall-alert-rappel-avis/hc-sc/2016/59584a-eng.php?_ga=2.13210928.687398953.1516646959-2095975037.1509475806.

Government of Canada. (2017). *Canadian immunization guide: Part 1—Key immunization information.* Retrieved from https://www.canada.ca/en/public-health/services/publications/healthy-living/canadian-immunization-guide-part-1-key-immunization-information/page-8-vaccine-administration-practices.html.

Government of Canada. (2018). *Provincial and territorial immunization information.* Retrieved from https://www.canada.ca/en/public-health/services/provincial-territorial-immunization-information.html.

Leduc, D., Woods, S., & Canadian Paediatric Society (CPS), Community Paediatrics Committee. (2000). *Temperature measurement in paediatrics.* Reaffirmed in 2017. Retrieved from http://www.cps.ca/documents/position/temperature-measurement#ref38.

Morris, L. (2018). PURLs: An easy approach to obtaining clean-catch urine from infants. *The Journal of Family Practice, 67*(3), 166–169.

Nerenberg, K. A., Zarnke, K. B., Leung, A. A., & for Hypertension Canada., et al. (2018). Hypertension Canada's 2018 guidelines for diagnosis, risk assessment, prevention, and treatment of hypertension in adults and children. *Canadian Journal of Cardiology, 34*(5), 506–525. https://doi.org/10.1016/j.cjca.2018.02.022.

Robinson, J., Finlay, J., Lang, M., et al. (2014). Urinary tract infections in infants and children: Diagnosis and management. *Paediatrics & Child Health, 19*(6), 315–319.

Rourke Baby Record. (2017). *The Rourke baby record.* Retrieved from http://www.rourkebabyrecord.ca/default.asp.

Sams, C. (2017). Pediatric variations of nursing interventions. In S. Perry, M. Hockenberry, D. Lowdermilk, et al. (Eds.), *Maternal child nursing care in Canada* (2nd ed.). Toronto, ON: Elsevier.

Tobias, I., Green, T. P., & Coté, C. J. (2016). Codeine: A time to say no. *Pediatrics, 138*(4), e1–e7. Retrieved from http://pediatrics.aappublications.org/content/early/2016/09/15/peds.2016-2396.

World Health Organization (WHO). (2012). *Persisting pain in children package: WHO guidelines on the pharmacological treatment of persisting pain in children with medical illnesses.* Geneva: Author. Retrieved from http://apps.who.int/iris/bitstream/10665/44540/1/9789241548120_Guidelines.pdf.

Complementary and Alternative Health Modalities in Pediatric Nursing

21

Cheryl A. Sams

http://evolve.elsevier.com/Canada/Leifer

Objectives

1. Define each key term listed.
2. Define complementary and alternative health modalities (CAHM) therapy.
3. Describe the involvement of the federal government in CAHM therapy.
4. Discuss the role of the nurse in CAHM therapy.
5. Discuss the integration of CAHM therapy into nursing practice.
6. Discuss the role of CAHM therapy in Indigenous health care.
7. State three herbs that should be discontinued 2 weeks before surgery.
8. Discuss the use of meridians, dermatomes, and reflexology lines in CAHM therapy.
9. Describe five types of CAHM therapy in common use.
10. Identify three herbal products commonly used in pediatrics.
11. Discuss the use of hyperbaric oxygen therapy in the care of carbon monoxide poisoning and necrotic ulcers.

Key Terms

alternative therapy
aromatherapy
coin-rubbing
complementary and alternative health modalities (CAHM)
complementary therapy
dermatomes (DŬR-mă-tōmz)
herbal medicine
hyperbaric oxygen therapy (HBOT)
meridians (mĕ-RĬD-ē-ănz)
reflexology
rolfing (RŎL-fĭng)
shiatsu (shē-ĂHT-sū)

COMPLEMENTARY AND ALTERNATIVE HEALTH MODALITIES

Complementary and alternative health modalities (CAHM) comprise a broad domain that includes all health systems, modalities, and practices and their accompanying theories and beliefs other than those usually used in the mainstream medical care of a particular culture (Vohra, Clifford, & Canadian Paediatric Society [CPS], Drug Therapy and Hazardous Substances Committee, 2005/2019). Across the world, traditional medicine (TM) is either the mainstay of health care delivery or serves as a complement to it (World Health Organization [WHO], 2013). **Complementary therapy** refers to traditional medicine or nonconventional, non-Western medical therapy that is used *with* conventional (Western medical) therapy. An example would be the treatment of hypertension with medication *plus* relaxation or biofeedback techniques. **Alternative therapy** refers to nonconventional or traditional therapy that *replaces* conventional therapy. CAHM are also known as *integrative therapy, integrative healing,* or *holistic healing*. The World Health Organization (WHO) states that CAHM are widely used around the world (unlike Western medicine) and has developed a TM strategy that aims to harness the potential contribution of TM to health, wellness, and people-centred health care and to promote the safe and effective use of TM by regulating, researching, and integrating TM products, practitioners, and practice into health systems, where appropriate (WHO, 2013).

More than three quarters of Canadians have used at least one complementary or alternative therapy sometime in their life. Massage is the most common type of therapy that Canadians have used over their lifetime, with 44% having tried it (Esmail, 2017). The most quickly growing therapies over the past two decades are massage, yoga, acupuncture, chiropractic care, osteopathy, and naturopathy. High-dose or mega-vitamins, herbal therapies, and folk remedies appear to be declining in use (Esmail, 2017).

Natural health products (NHPs) is a term used to describe herbs and other supplements made from natural sources. They are sold to prevent illness or promote health (CPS, 2018). Canadians may receive NHPs from a health care provider, seek NHPs on the recommendation of a care provider, or opt for self-care by purchasing NHPs over the counter, either from a pharmacy or from other commercial establishments (Vohra et al., 2005/2019).

FEDERAL REGULATIONS

In Canada, Health Canada regulates and monitors NHPs through the Natural and Non-prescription Health Products Directorate (NNHPD). This Directorate was created to ensure that Canadians have ready access to NHPs that are safe, effective, and of high quality, while respecting freedom of choice and philosophical and cultural diversity (Health Canada, 2013). All NHPs now have either a Natural Product Number (NPN) or a Homeopathic Medicine Number (DIN-HM). Over 20 000 NHPs now have product licenses (Health Canada, 2018).

PEDIATRIC USE

Canada is a country made up of many different cultures and views on health traditions, thus CAHM treatments and NHPs are increasingly being used and sometimes effectively integrated into conventional Western medicine treatments. This growing trend has created new challenges and opportunities for pediatric health care providers. Parents may want to include CAHM into their children's health care, without discussing it with their health care providers. It is important for the health care community to have an open discussion and explore their patients' perspectives and provide resources for them.

Because infants' and children's physiological development is less mature than that of adults, younger patients may experience responses to CAHM that are different from those in adults. Some adverse effects can be dangerous for children. Yet many parents are influenced by testimonials that often do not provide evidence-based information. There is a lack of research and evidence on how CAHM and NHPs affect the pediatric population (Vohra et al., 2005/2019).

THE NURSE'S ROLE

Nurses have long used complementary therapies such as imagery, journalling, therapeutic touch, humour, and support groups as part of patient care and thus have an integral role in the development and assessment of CAHM therapy. The greater acceptance of CAHM therapies by many people has resulted in the need for nurses to better understand CAHM therapies, how they can be used, and how they may interact with or enhance traditional medical or nursing care. For example, Table 21.1 lists herbs that patients should stop using 2 weeks before undergoing surgery, because of potential adverse effects and it is important that nurses are aware of these.

Because nurses are partners in the decision-making process regarding patient care and treatment, they are responsible for ensuring that patients and their families have the appropriate information they need to make informed choices. Knowledge concerning CAHM therapy can also expand the nurse's knowledge about health care practices used in many cultures. Healing is best achieved by giving consideration to the cultural and environmental influences that affect the overall health and wellness of the patient and family.

Families may want to incorporate CAHM as well as cultural beliefs and traditions into their care. Along with accepting treatment prescribed by a conventional health care provider, the patient or family may also be consulting other healing authorities such as holistic practitioners, naturopaths, and nutritional consultants (Fig. 21.1). Food therapy, vitamin and mineral

Table 21.1 Herbs That Should Be Discontinued 2 Weeks Before Surgery

HERB	ADVERSE EFFECTS	PROBLEM DURING SURGERY
Echinacea	Unpleasant taste sensation, potential liver toxicity	May potentiate barbiturate toxicity
Garlic	Increased bleeding time, hypotension	Increased risk of intraoperative hemodynamic instability
Ginger	Increased bleeding time	Increased risk of intraoperative hemodynamic instability
Ginkgo biloba	Platelet dysfunction	Increased intraoperative and postoperative bleeding tendencies; may decrease effectiveness of intravenous barbiturates
St. John's wort	Dry mouth, dizziness, constipation, nausea	Increases risk of bleeding and increases metabolism of select medications, including altering effects of anaesthetic agents
Ginseng	Hypertension, insomnia, headache, vomiting, epistaxis, prolonged bleeding time, hypoglycemia	Increased risk of intraoperative hemodynamic instability
Kava kava	Characteristic scaling of the skin	Increases level of sedation; can lead to coma; interacts with other medications and can cause liver failure
Feverfew	Mouth ulcers, gastrointestinal irritability, headache	Increased risk of intraoperative hemodynamic instability
Ephedra (ma huang)	Hypertension, tachycardia, stroke, dysrhythmias	May interact with volatile anaesthetic agents (e.g., halothane) to cause fatal cardiac dysrhythmias; profound intraoperative hypotension

supplements, herbal therapy, and acupressure are common forms of alternative therapies practiced by many people.

It is essential to note that not all alternative therapists are licensed, and evidenced-based information is not always available to support the use of the therapy. This may mean the consumer has knowledge of the use of herbal medications but at the same time needs increased understanding of possible adverse interactions and effects. Box 21.1 lists some cautions concerning the use of CAHM therapy.

Some insurance companies provide coverage for selected CAHM therapy practices, and some CAHM practices are part of nursing practice (e.g., massage, imagery, acupressure, and aromatherapy). Therefore, it is essential that nurses understand basic underlying philosophies and beliefs concerning CAHM interventions. The nurse's role is not to promote the acceptance of CAHM therapy but to recognize and respect its use by patients and to use critical thinking skills to determine interactions with traditional therapy. When documenting a patient's health history, nurses should ask questions concerning the family's use of CAHM therapies.

When nurses provide CAHM therapies, they must ask themselves the following questions:

- Is the therapy appropriate and do I have the necessary knowledge regarding the therapy?
- Do I have the knowledge, skill, and judgement to administer the therapy?
- Do I understand, and can I manage, the outcomes?

In deciding to provide a complementary therapy, nurses must understand that they are accountable for determining the appropriateness of the therapy, given the patient's status, and for competently providing that therapy.

The provincial and territorial regulatory bodies for the practical nurse may vary in scope of practice in terms of CAHM and NPH therapies. However, all nurses must demonstrate the knowledge, skill, and judgement to use certain therapies. Some therapies require further certification. Each nurse needs to have knowledge of the CAHM and NPH for their specific jurisprudence. The use of these therapies also depends on employer policies.

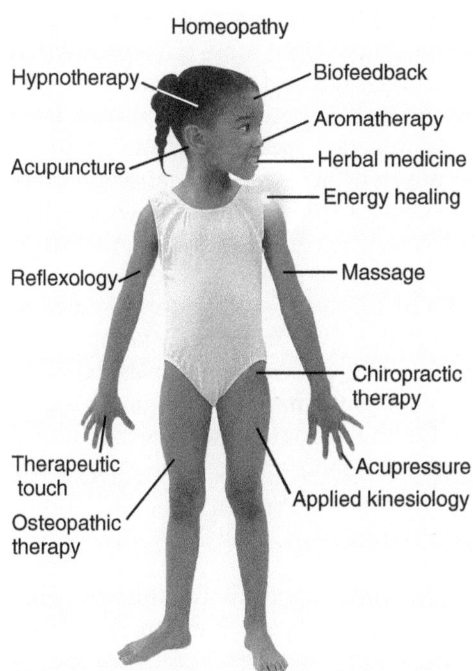

Fig. 21.1 Types of alternative health care. (Art overlay courtesy Observatory Group, Cincinnati, Ohio.)

COMMON ALTERNATIVE HEALTH CARE PRACTICES

Indigenous Traditional Healing

Nurses must be knowledgeable in the CAHM therapies that may be used by Indigenous people. Health care providers must work with traditional healers in a respectful manner and advocate for the support of Indigenous traditional medicine approaches to healing (Aboriginal Nurses Association, 2009; HealthCareCAN, 2016). While minimal research has been done on the effectiveness of Indigenous CAHM, such modalities may provide emotional, mental, and spiritual support during an illness. People who are part of traditional healing rituals and ceremonies may feel a powerful connection with their community and the earth. Stress, anxiety, and depression can be eased with feelings of support and acceptance (Canadian Cancer Society [CCS], 2019).

Many traditional healers are elders who know the traditions and values of their particular group and serve as guides and teachers. Healing is seen as a journey, and there is as much focus on spiritual and emotional healing as there is on the physical aspects of healing (CCS, 2019).

One important icon in Indigenous healing is the medicine wheel (Fig. 21.2). The number 4 is considered sacred by many Indigenous peoples, and there are four parts to the medicine wheel. The four parts of the medicine wheel represent the four directions, the four seasons, and the four aspects of health (spiritual, mental, physical, and emotional). *Four* also represents

Box 21.1 Cautions in Complementary and Alternative Medicine Therapy

- Herbs can interact with cardiac medications.
- Herbs can affect glucose control in patients with diabetes.
- Herbs can lower the concentration of some synthetic medications.
- Herbs can lower the blood level of some medications used for human immunodeficiency virus (HIV) and/or acquired immunodeficiency syndrome (AIDS).
- Polypharmacy (the use of many medicines) should be avoided; the use of some medications in tandem with herbal remedies may be dangerous.

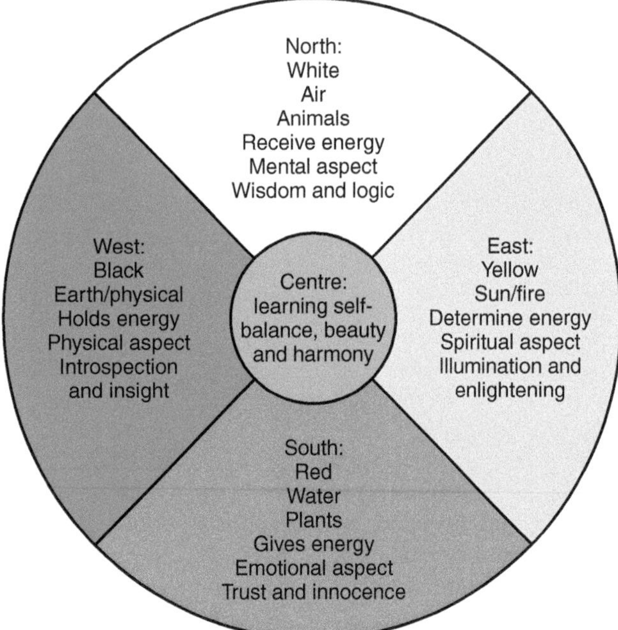

Fig. 21.2 Indigenous medicine wheel. The medicine wheel symbolizes the interconnection of all life, the various cycles of nature, and how life represents a circular journey to the Indigenous peoples of North America. (From UOttawa. [2017]. *Introduction to Indigenous peoples in Canada*. Retrieved from http://www.med.uottawa.ca/SIM/data/Vul_Indigenous_e.htm. Also found here: http://traditionalnativehealing.com/native-american-medicine-wheel.)

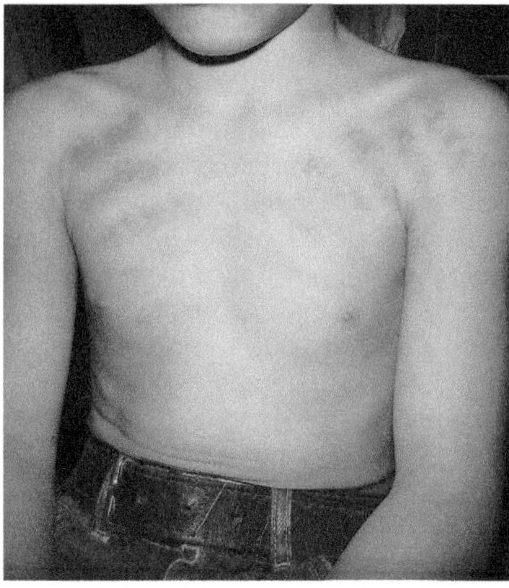

Fig. 21.3 "Cao-gio" (coin-rubbing) is a form of fascial manipulation believed to bring the body in alignment with gravity. (From Shah, B. R., & Laude, T. A. [2000]. *Atlas of pediatric clinical diagnosis.* Philadelphia: Saunders.)

four sacred herbs considered to be medicines that are important to Indigenous cultures and traditional healing practices (CCS, 2019). These four medicines are tobacco, sweetgrass, cedar, and sage, all of which are used in a variety of ways.

Some methods of healing that Indigenous healers use include the following (CCS, 2019):

- Sweats comprise a cleansing and healing ritual. They are most often done in a sweat lodge. Sacred medicines may be added to the smoke and steam during the ceremony.
- Smudging involves burning sacred medicines. A person puts their hands into the sacred smoke and carries it to their body, especially to areas that need healing.
- Healing circles are groups of people who gather together in the shape of a circle with the clear purpose of healing. The circle gives a voice to everyone.
- Ceremonies may include dancing, drumming, and singing.
- Traditional diets with emphasis on game, fish, and wild nuts and berries may be recommended.
- Herbal medicines may be used in various forms, such as teas, powders, or ointment.

Massage

An underlying premise of some alternative healing techniques is that the symptoms are the result of a problem in the body that may not be related to the specific symptom manifested. The body is thought to have a self-healing ability that can be aided by spinal or energy manipulation. Soft-tissue massage is thought to bolster the immune response. Fascia pressure, stretching, and manipulation, known as **rolfing**, are thought to improve muscle and bone function. "Cao-gio," or **coin-rubbing**, is a form of skin manipulation thought to help bring the body into healthy alignment (Fig. 21.3). Coin-rubbing is a form of CAHM therapy that can easily be mistaken for child abuse because of the lingering marks on the skin after treatment. Neuromuscular massage helps to relieve muscle tension and the trigger points of pain and generally improves circulation.

Massage therapy is often used for children with asthma, arthritis, and eating disorders. Gentle touch massage therapy has had positive effects on premature infants—they gain weight more quickly after receiving the therapy. Massage and manipulative therapy may be contraindicated in patients with cancer, osteoporosis, localized infection, and cardiac and circulatory disorders because of the increase it causes in blood flow to affected areas. Children with Down syndrome are particularly prone to cervical spine anomalies and may be injured by manual manipulative therapy. Children who have a history of sexual abuse may not respond well to touch therapy; prior to initiating the therapy they, like any other patient, must be asked permission to be touched. Gentle massage and gentle touch therapy are used in the neonatal intensive care unit (NICU) to calm preterm infants and to promote bonding (Kassity-Kritch & Jones, 2013).

Osteopathy

Osteopaths combine manipulative therapy with traditional (allopathic) medicine. Pressure point therapy is based on the theory that certain areas of the body are connected to specific identified pressure points such as the feet, the hands, and the ears. It is believed that channels conduct vital energy through the body. Many osteopaths currently practice in the mainstream of Western medicine.

Energy Healing

Energy healing involves the belief that an electromagnetic flow emerges from the therapist's hands and can funnel energy into the patient. Some believe that repatterning a patient's own energy field can aid in healing. The body, mind, spirit, and emotions are usually involved in this type of therapy.

A wristband that uses transcutaneous electrical nerve stimulation (TENS) placed on identified trigger points can prevent nausea and vomiting during chemotherapy and pregnancy-induced nausea and vomiting. TENS, shen, reiki, and the use of magnets are other forms of energy therapy.

Light therapy or sunlight is an ancient form of healing therapy. Light therapy is used in treating persons with seasonal affective disorder.

Acupuncture and Acupressure

Acupuncture is an ancient Chinese practice that works on the principle that the body has complex **meridians**, which are imaginary lines that are thought to be pathways carrying energy to specific organs or parts of the body (Fig. 21.4, *A*). These meridians surface at specific locations called *acupuncture points.* It is at these 150 points on the 12 meridian sites that positive or negative energy can be realigned through stimulation. *Chi* energy is thought to regulate proper body function, and acupuncture or acupressure is applied to restore a balance of chi energy. In acupuncture, hair-thin needles are applied to specific meridians and may stimulate nerve cells to release endorphins.

A **dermatome** is a specific area of the skin that is supplied by a sensory neuron that originates from a specific, single spinal nerve root (see Fig. 21.4, *B*). The general dermatome pattern is similar for all people, although the specific area of innervation within that pattern might be unique to the individual. Obstructing the dermatome line can anaesthetize that area of the skin.

Acupressure involves finger pressure and massage on the meridian sites rather than use of needles. Acupuncture and acupressure have achieved popularity in the Western world and can be used to control nausea, backache, and pain. Acupressure wristbands are available for use to prevent nausea and vomiting during travel or pregnancy. These techniques have also been useful for minor problems such as constipation.

Shiatsu is a finger pressure used with an emphasis on preventing disease rather than treating symptoms. Pressure is applied to achieve a level of sensation between pain and pleasure in the individual.

Traditional Chinese medicine practitioners or registered acupuncturists are regulated in some provinces and territories to provide acupuncture. In most Canadian provinces and territories, health care practitioners must be trained in acupuncture in order to practice it as a complement to their own professional training.

Reflexology

Reflexology deals with reflex points in the hands and feet that are thought to correspond to every organ or part of the body. *Reflexology lines* divide the body into 10 zones of longitudinal lines. Blockage of the lines is thought to obstruct vital energy pathways. The foot or hand represents a map of the entire body linked by energy pathways (see Fig. 21.4, C). Massaging these reflex points can relieve specific problems.

Ayurveda

Ayurveda is an ancient Hindu healing regimen that deals with the biological rhythms of nature and can include music, herbs, massage, aromatherapy, and a diet tailored to the specific body type.

Aromatherapy

Aromatherapy is an ancient practice that involves concentrated fluid or the essence of specific aromatic plants that are combined with steams or baths to inhale or bathe the skin. Essential oils are concentrated and, if undiluted, are usually used in 2- to 5-drop doses. Often a few drops of the herbal oil are added to soaps or regular lotions immediately before use. Concentrated oils are volatile and must be freshly prepared and stored properly. Compounds that may be antibacterial, antiviral, antifungal, and anti-inflammatory are used in health care to provide physical, emotional, and spiritual health and well-being (Allard & Katseres, 2016). Aromatherapy with oils such as jasmine, citrus, clary sage, lavender, and peppermint has been shown to relieve anxiety, reduce nausea, and improve the general feeling of well-being. Peppermint has been used as a respiratory stimulant; chamomile is used to regulate circadian rhythm (Kassity-Kritch & Jones, 2013).

Some essential oils are contraindicated for use during pregnancy because of the effect on the mother or fetus; these include anise, juniper, thyme, wintergreen, nutmeg, pennyroyal, and mugwort.

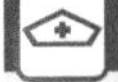 **Nursing Tip**

Lavender, chamomile, and sandalwood essential oils are useful in aromatherapy for children with persistent pain.

Hypnotherapy

In *hypnotherapy*, the patient enters a hypnotic state of induced sleep. Under the guidance of the practitioner, specific and potentially long-lasting suggestions are given to the patient. Smoking cessation and pain control have been successfully achieved using this method. Some patients resist the trance state and are not candidates for hypnotherapy.

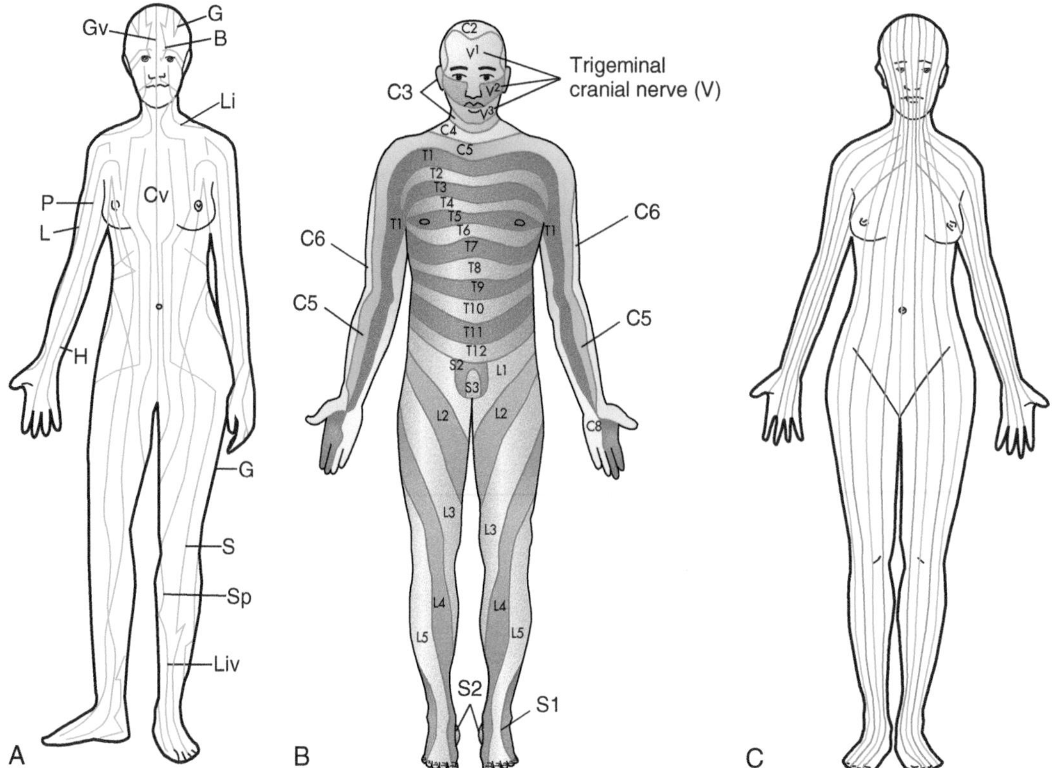

Fig. 21.4 **A,** Meridians. Acupuncture is based on the belief that the correct flow of energy through meridians (invisible tracks running through the body) controls the health of all vital organs. Stimulating any of the 12 meridians with heat, electricity, needles, or pressure can affect corresponding parts of the body. **B,** Dermatomes. These are areas of the skin innervated by the dorsal roots of the spinal cord. Obstructing one dermatome line can anaesthetize that segment of the skin and adjacent structures (although some dermatome lines from adjacent dorsal roots of the spine can overlap). **C,** Reflexology lines. (**A** and **C,** from Moore, S. [1997]. *Understanding pain and its relief in labour.* London: Churchill Livingstone. **B,** from Patton. K. T., & Thibodeau, G. A. [2018]. *Anatomy & physiology* [9th ed.]. St. Louis: Mosby.)

Hydrotherapy

Hydrotherapy is the therapeutic use of water to promote relaxation. It is often used during labour in the form of a bath or shower (see Box 7.1).

Guided Imagery

Guided imagery is based on the ancient Greek belief that the mind can influence the body. Asking the patient to focus on a specific image can result in reduction of stress and increased performance. This technique, when combined with breathing and relaxation techniques, may be used to manage pain.

Biofeedback

Biofeedback is a type of relaxation therapy that enables the patient to recognize tension in the muscles via responses on an electronic machine and visual electromyography responses. Traditional health care providers also use the process for conditions such as substance use and persistent-pain control. Biofeedback is an experimental treatment for attention- deficit/hyperactivity disorder (ADHD) (McClafferty & Kemper, 2016).

Sauna/Heat Therapy

Overheating the body has long been used to speed up metabolism and inhibit the replication of viruses and bacteria. The sweating that results from the sauna is thought to help eliminate body waste. Patients should monitor their pulse during treatment. Some medical conditions can inhibit the ability to perspire, and heat can adversely affect the cardiac status of some patients. Therefore, medical guidance should be sought before using this type of therapy.

Chiropractic Care

Chiropractic care concerns the relationship between the spinal column and the nervous system and involves nerve energy thought responsible for restoring and maintaining health. Some chiropractors also use massage, diet, and nutrition for a more comprehensive approach. Chiropractors may offer well-child care with preventive manipulation.

The Canadian Paediatric Society (CPS) suggests that all parents be asked if their child is using any CAHM therapies, and if they disclose that the child is being treated by a chiropractor to then question whether neck manipulations or forceful thrusts have been used and if herbal or homeopathic preparations have been given. It is important to know the conditions for which the parent has used chiropractic care for the child (Spigelblatt & CPS Community Paediatrics Committee, 2002/2018). Chiropractors are the only CAHM therapists that are regulated across Canada.

Homeopathy

Homeopathy is one of the more popular alternative therapies used in children (Spigelblatt & CPS Community Paediatrics Committee, 2005/2018). In homeopathy, plants, herbs, and earth minerals thought to stimulate the body's immune system are used to manage specific health problems. Homeopathic philosophy involves the belief that disease is an energy imbalance and that prescribed remedies assist the body to re-establish correct balance. Homeopathic remedies are taken sublingually and should not be combined with caffeine, alcohol, or some Western medications. Some homeopathic medicines are alcohol based, and some contain mercury or arsenic bases that can cause toxicity or allergic responses in children. Only one remedy is administered at a time, and minimum dosage is the principle of most practitioners.

The most common use of homeopathy in pediatrics is in children with conditions of the ear, nose, and throat or respiratory symptoms. There is limited research showing possible benefits of homeopathy when prescribed by trained practitioners for a selected number of specific conditions in children. Therefore, more rigorous studies showing efficacy need to be completed before it can be recommended as a credible CAHM therapy for the pediatric population (Spigelblatt, & CPS Community Paediatrics Committee, 2005/2018).

Herbal Remedies

The use of herbal medicinal products and supplements has increased over the past three decades, with no less than 80% of people worldwide relying on them for some part of primary health care (Ekor, 2014). **Herbal medicine** has been used for thousands of years in many countries. Herbs come from plants and most are safe to ingest. Many current medications are related to herbal remedies. Digitalis originates from foxglove, opiates originate from poppy flowers, and quinine originates from the cinchona tree.

Occasionally an allergic type of reaction to herbal products is encountered, possibly because of differences in processing or storing of the products. In addition, dietary supplement labels may not accurately reveal the contents of the ingredients, and some may be unintentionally contaminated with pesticides, mercury, or other harmful ingredients. The processes of growth, processing, storage, and contents are regulated by Health Canada through the NNHPD. Herbal products are sold in stores and online.

Some herbs have proven their effectiveness for certain health problems. For example, fennel, chamomile, licorice, and baby mint are used for colic. Ginger has been shown to be effective for nausea, and probiotics have been an effective treatment for antibiotic-associated diarrhea and constipation. Aloe vera is used to treat mild burns, and *Echinacea* is used for prevention of upper respiratory infections. Tea tree oil is an antibacterial for treating acne and is a pediculicide.

However, some herbs, such as ephedra, can be fatal to children. Herbal remedies consumed during pregnancy can cross the placenta and reach the fetus. Breastfeeding mothers who use herbal remedies can pass the substance to their infants. Home-grown herbs, such as chamomile used for tea, can be contaminated with botulism. It is important to take time to elicit an accurate history from parents to reveal any practice of using herbal remedies in the family.

Medication–herbal interactions can also occur. Herbs that are apparently safe for adults may be harmful for infants and young children, especially when combined with some prescription medications. For example, peppermint, commonly contained in dinner mints, relaxes gastrointestinal spasms but can exacerbate gastroesophageal reflux. St. John's wort may enhance elimination of many medications, such as oral contraceptives and antibiotics, causing them to be ineffective.

Herbal capsules are about four times stronger than herbal teas, and *herbal extracts* are about four to eight times stronger than capsules. *Herbal tinctures* contain a high amount of alcohol and are not often recommended. *Herbal baths* are relaxing and soothing, and herbal salves, oils, compresses, and poultices use the skin as the body's organ of ingestion. Most practitioners emphasize that herbal dosage is determined by body weight and that megadoses can be harmful.

Herbs and pediatrics

The use of CAHM therapy has increased for children with various chronic illnesses. Table 21.2 reviews herbs commonly used for children. Parents sometimes prefer "natural remedies" such as herbs to prescription medicines for their children diagnosed with, for example, ADHD. Herbal treatments for ADHD focus on improving cognition, producing sedation, or alleviating anxiety. These herbs are obtained without a prescription, and their use is often not supported by scientific studies concerning their effectiveness or safety. Parents often do not discuss CAHM therapy they used for their children unless directly asked about it by the nurse or health care provider.

Cannabis

Cannabis is the most common illicit drug used worldwide, and it is used frequently by Canadian teenagers. In 2018, cannabis became a legal substance in Canada, although users must be 18 or 19 years of age, depending on the province or territory in which they reside. In 2010, Canadian youth ranked first for cannabis use among 43 countries and regions across Europe and North America (WHO, 2012). Researchers have shown that Indigenous youth are particularly at risk; nearly two thirds of 15- to 19-year-old Inuit participants in Nunavik, Quebec, self-reported past-year use (Brunelle, Plourde, Landry, et al., 2010). The CPS has the following concerns about the potential impact of youth exposure to cannabis:

- Cannabis can cause functional and structural changes to the developing brain during adolescence, leading to impaired neurological development, cognitive decline, and diminished school performance.

Table 21.2 Herbs Commonly Used in Pediatrics

HERB	USE	TOXICITY OR CAUTIONS
Blue-green algae *(Cyanobacteria spirulina)*	Stimulates tumour necrosis Anti-inflammatory Antiviral Antifungal Used in children with ADHD	There are no clinical studies supporting cognitive improvement in children. Contaminated source of collection can cause toxicity, liver failure, and cholera. Should not be used in children with phenylketonuria. Nutritional value is limited in humans.
Chamomile *(Matricaria recutita)*	Used to calm infants with colic Used as an antispasmodic, reduces anxiety	Use with caution if allergic to ragweed.
Ephedra (ma huang)	Used for asthma; decongestant; central nervous system stimulant	Often used by adolescents as a stimulant. Can cause hypertension, anxiety, and toxic psychosis. Overdose can be deadly.
Echinacea	Thought to be an immune enhancer	Increases barbiturate toxicity. Do not use with immunosuppressant therapy.
Evening primrose oil *(Oenothera biennis)*	Relieves eczema, asthma, and diabetic retinopathy	Nausea, diarrhea, and headache can occur.
Fennel seed oil	Reduces stomach spasms and increases colon motility	Do not use if allergic to carrots or celery.
Feverfew *(Tanacetum parthenium)*	Migraine relief	Contraindicated during pregnancy and lactation, and in children less than 2 years of age. Can cause mouth ulcers; may interact with antithrombotic medications.
Fish oil	Improves visual processing and coordination Reduces asthma risk	Flatus, bad breath can occur. Do not use with anticoagulants or in bleeding disorders.
Ginger *(Zingiber officinale)*	Used for nausea and motion sickness	In large doses can cause heartburn and diarrhea.
Ginkgo biloba	Thought to improve alertness and memory Possibly decreases hypoxia damage to brain	Headache, dizziness can occur. Decreases the effectiveness of barbiturates. Do not use with aspirin or in persons with bleeding disorders.
Siberian ginseng *(Eleutherococcus senticosus)*	Stimulant Aids resistance to stress Used in ADHD	Potentiates the effect of caffeine and other stimulants. Not to be taken with steroids or hormones.
Kava kava *(Piper methysticum)*	Thought to reduce anxiety	Scaly skin rash can occur. Enhances barbiturate levels. Can cause oculomotor problems. Do not use with sedatives or anticoagulants. Increases high-density lipoproteins (HDLs).
Lemon balm *(Melissa officinalis)*	Used for nervous stomach discomforts, nausea, and sleep disorders	May inhibit thyroid hormones.
Licorice *(Glycyrrhiza glabra)*	Treatment of asthma and stomach problems	Contraindicated for use in persons with hypertension or kidney and heart disease.
Melatonin (*N*-acetyl-5-methoxytryptamine)	Antioxidant Sleep-cycle disorders	Reduced alertness, headache, irritability, possible suppression of puberty can occur. Use with caution in children with seizures.
Peppermint *(Mentha piperita)*	Used for newborn colic, flatulence, nausea, indigestion Slows colon motility	Should not be used in persons with gastroesophageal reflux disease (GERD).
Probiotics (*Lactobacillus* species, *Saccharomyces boulardii, Bifidobacterium* species) (found in yogurt, buttermilk, kefir, miso, sauerkraut)	Used for antibiotic-induced diarrhea or traveller's diarrhea, irritable bowel syndrome, and viral gastroenteritis	
Prebiotics	A nondigestible food ingredient that stimulates the growth of probiotic bacteria, such as *Bifidobacterium*	

Continued

Table 21.2 **Herbs Commonly Used in Pediatrics—cont'd**

HERB	USE	TOXICITY OR CAUTIONS
Psyllium *(Plantago ovata)*	Used for constipation	Inadequate fluid intake can lead to intestinal obstruction or fecal impaction.
Pycnogenol (oligomeric proanthocyanidin [OPC])	Antioxidant Improves behaviour in ADHD	Avoid use in bleeding disorders. Do not use with anticoagulants.
Siete Jarabes (commercial syrup)	Used as expectorant and laxative Relieves asthma and congestion	Is a combination of sweet almond, castor oil, licorice, honey, and other products. May cause diarrhea or hypertension.
St. John's wort *(Hypericum perforatum)*	Antidepressant	Can cause photosensitivity. Do not use with nasal decongestants, asthma medications, MAOIs, or medications with phenylalanine content. Can cause high blood pressure.
Valerian *(Valeriana officinalis)*	Sleep disorders Used for anxiety	Gastrointestinal upset, headache can occur. Do not use with other sedatives.

ADHD, Attention deficit/hyperactivity disorder; *MAOIs,* monoamine oxidase inhibitors.
Data from Thompson Healthcare. (2010). *PDR for herbal medicines* (4th ed.). Montvale, NJ: Author; Gardiner, P., & Kemper, K. (2005). For GI complaints: Which herbs and supplements spell relief? *Contemporary Pediatrics, 22*(8), 50–55; Rakel, D. (2018). *Integrative medicine* (4th ed.). Philadelphia: Elsevier.

- Marijuana use in adolescence is strongly linked to cannabis dependence and other substance use disorders.
- Cannabis use may lead to the initiation of tobacco smoking and long-term smoking.
- Cannabis use may be associated with an increased presence of mental illness, including depression, anxiety, and psychosis.
- There may be an increased risk for motor vehicle accidents when youth are driving under the influence of cannabis.
- Younger children who have ingested cannabis unintentionally will likely require acute medical care and hospitalization (Grant, Bélanger, CPS Adolescent Health Committee, 2017).

The CPS states that there is insufficient evidence to support either the efficacy or safety of medical cannabis use for any indication in children. In addition, an increasing body of data points toward possible harm in specific conditions. Thus the potential for cannabis as a therapeutic agent must be evaluated carefully for its efficacy and safety. Also, smoking is not an acceptable way to deliver this medication in children (Rieder & CPS Drug Therapy and Hazardous Substances Committee, 2016).

Hyperbaric Oxygen Therapy

In **hyperbaric oxygen therapy (HBOT)**, an airtight enclosure is used to provide compressed air or oxygen under increased pressure. HBOT is used to revive patients with carbon monoxide poisoning, to aid wound healing, and to treat the diving syndrome known as decompression illness. Many hospitals currently use HBOT as standard treatment for diabetic wound healing and other specific problems. HBOT is also used as CAHM therapy in private centres. HBOT is contraindicated during pregnancy because the increased oxygen saturation can cause the ductus arteriosus to close, resulting in fetal death. Research concerning the use and the effects of HBOT is ongoing.

Get Ready for the Certification Examination!

Key Points

- To promote positive outcomes, nurses must be well informed about the use and validity of complementary and alternative health modalities (CAHM) practices and understand the potential interactions with prescribed medications and treatments.
- Complementary therapies are treatments used *in conjunction with* conventional medicine.
- Alternative therapies are treatments that *replace* conventional medical therapy.
- Many herbal preparations do not have research-based data to guide determination of safe dosage and use.
- Many CAHM therapies are used effectively and integrated with conventional Western medicine.
- Nurses have successfully used some CAHM therapies, such as guided imagery, massage, and therapeutic touch, for many years.
- It is likely that nurses will encounter some form of CAHM therapy as part of the health care delivery system.
- Nurses must use critical thinking skills to determine the interactions between CAHM therapy and conventional prescribed Western treatments.
- As part of routine history data collection, nurses should ask all patients if they use a form of CAHM therapy; this information should be recorded on the chart.

- It is important to be aware of Indigenous traditional healing practices and to incorporate them into the care provided.
- Transcutaneous electrical nerve stimulation (TENS) is a form of energy therapy used to prevent nausea.
- Coin-rubbing is a type of CAHM therapy that can be mistaken for child abuse because of the lingering skin marks after treatment.
- Meridians are invisible (imaginary) lines running through the body that are thought to control the health of vital organs. Stimulation of any of the 150 pressure points on the 12 meridian sites is the basis of acupressure and acupuncture.
- Dermatomes are areas of the skin that are innervated by the dorsal roots of the spinal cord and affect specific segments of the skin and adjacent structures.
- Reflexology lines divide the body into 10 zones of longitudinal lines. Blockage is thought to obstruct energy pathways; this is the basic concept of reflexology.

Additional Learning Resources

evolve Go to your Evolve website (http://evolve.elsevier.com/Canada/Leifer) for the following learning resources:

- Answer Key for Critical Thinking Questions
- Answer Key for Textbook Review Questions
- Audio Glossary
- Interactive Review Questions
- Skills Performance Checklists
- Video clips and more!

Online Resources

- Public Health Agency of Canada, *Complementary and Alternative Health:* http://www.phac-aspc.gc.ca/chn-rcs/cah-acps-eng.php
- World Health Organization, *Traditional, Complementary and Integrative Medicine:* http://www.who.int/traditional-complementary-integrative-medicine/publications/en/

Review Questions

1. What should a nurse communicate to parents about herbal medicines sold over the counter?
   a. They are harmless to children.
   b. They are effective substitutes for traditional medication.
   c. They can interact with prescribed medications and produce adverse effects.
   d. They should never be given to children.
2. What instruction would a nurse give a patient who is using an herbal product?
   a. Take high doses of a single herb to maximize effectiveness.
   b. Depend on the label for claims of benefits of use.
   c. Buy the least expensive brand of the product.
   d. Inform the health care provider of all herbal products used.
3. A patient in a pediatric clinic asks a nurse about the use of alternative or complementary therapies for her 3-year-old child. What would be the most appropriate response of the nurse?
   a. Discussing CAHM therapy is not within the scope of practice of the practical nurse (LPN/RPN).
   b. All CAHM therapies should be stopped until the child is an adult.
   c. Many complementary therapy techniques are taught in pediatric clinics.
   d. Only those herbs approved by Health Canada should be used during childhood.
4. What is the branch of the federal government that regulates the safety and efficacy of specific CAHM therapies?
   a. Natural and Non-prescription Health Products Directorate (NNHPD)
   b. National Center for Complementary and Alternative Medicine (NCCAM)
   c. Food and Drug Administration (FDA)
   d. Drug Enforcement Agency (DEA)
5. What roles does a nurse play in CAHM therapy? *(Select all that apply.)*
   a. Encourage the use of CAHM therapy in pediatric patients.
   b. Discourage the use of CAHM therapy in pediatric patients.
   c. Discuss the impact or interaction of the CAHM therapy with prescribed therapy.
   d. Provide a resource of certified CAHM therapists for pediatric patients.
   e. Obtain a history of CAHM practices in the family during health and illness.
6. The advantages of CAHM therapy include which of the following?
   a. It offers time-tested effectiveness.
   b. It incorporates cultural practices and beliefs.
   c. "Natural" therapies are safer than chemical-containing medications.
   d. All of the above.
7. The mother and grandmother of a child are at the bedside, rubbing the skin of the child. When a nurse enters the room, the visitors are startled and drop the item they were using to rub the child's skin. The nurse picks up the item realizes it is a coin. The best response of the nurse would be which of the following?
   a. Ask, "What are you doing to that child with this coin?"
   b. Give the coin back to the mother and leave the room to give them their privacy.
   c. Tell the family they could hurt the child with the coin and there are many germs on coins.
   d. Return the coin to the mother and open a dialogue about the practice they are using.

Critical Thinking Questions

1. Explain the ways in which complementary and alternative therapies can be used in adolescence.
2. Identify complementary and alternative techniques that could be taught to school-age children to use.

REFERENCES

Aboriginal Nurses Association. (2009). *Cultural competence and cultural safety in nursing education*. Retrieved from: https://www.cna-aiic.ca/~/media/cna/page-content/pdf-en/first_nations_framework_e.pdf?la=en.

Allard, M. E., & Katseres, J. (2016). Using essential oils to enhance nursing practice and for self-Care. *American Journal of Nursing, 116*(2), 42–49, quiz 50–51. https://doi.org/10.1097/01.NAJ.0000480495.18104.db.

Brunelle, N., Plourde, C., Landry, M., et al. (2010). Patterns of psychoactive substance use among youths in Nunavik. *Inditera, 2*, 15–27.

Canadian Cancer Society (CCS). (2019). *Aboriginal traditional healing*. Retrieved from: http://www.cancer.ca/en/cancer-information/diagnosis-and-treatment/complementary-therapies/aboriginal-traditional-healing/?region=on.

Canadian Paediatric Society (CPS). (2018). *Natural health products and children*. Retrieved from: https://www.caringforkids.cps.ca/handouts/natural_health_products_and_children.

Ekor, M. (2014). The growing use of herbal medicines: Issues relating to adverse reactions and challenges in monitoring safety. *Frontiers in Pharmacology, 4*, 177. https://.org/10.3389/fphar.2013.00177. Retrieved from: https://www.frontiersin.org/articles/10.3389/fphar.2013.00177/full.

Esmail, N. (2017). *Complementary and alternative medicine: Use and public attitudes 1997, 2006, and 2016*. Fraser Institute. Retrieved from: https://www.fraserinstitute.org/studies/complementary-and-alternative-medicine-use-and-public-attitudes-1997-2006-and-2016.

Grant, C. N., Bélanger, R. E., & Canadian Paediatric Society (CPS), Adolescent Health Committee. (2017). Cannabis and Canada's children and youth. *Paediatrics & Child Health, 22*(2), 98–102. Retrieved from: https://www.cps.ca/en/documents/position/cannabis-children-and-youth.

Health Canada. (2013). *The approach to natural health products*. Retrieved from: https://www.canada.ca/content/dam/hc-sc/migration/hc-sc/dhp-mps/alt_formats/pdf/prodnatur/nhp-psn-eng.pdf.

Health Canada. (2018). *General questions—Regulation of natural health products*. Retrieved from: http://www.hc-sc.gc.ca/dhp-mps/prodnatur/faq/question_general-eng.php#a2.

HealthCareCAN. (2016). *The Truth and Reconciliation Commission of Canada: Health-related recommendations*. Ottawa, ON: Author. Retrieved from: http://www.healthcarecan.ca/wp-content/themes/camyno/assets/document/IssueBriefs/2016/EN/TRCC_EN.pdf.

Kassity-Kritch, N., & Jones, J. (2013). Complementary and integrative therapies. In C. Kenner & W. J. Lott (Eds.), *Comprehensive neonatal care* (5th ed.). St. Louis: Saunders.

McClafferty, H. H., & Kemper, K. J. (2016). Integrative medicine. In I. L. Rubin, J. Merrick, G. E. Greydanus, et al. (Eds.), *Health care for people with intellectual and developmental disabilities across the lifespan*. New York: Springer.

Rieder, M. J., & Canadian Paediatric Society (CPS), Drug Therapy and Hazardous Substances Committee. (2016). Is the medical use of cannabis a therapeutic option for children? *Paediatrics & Child Health, 21*(1), 31–34. Retrieved from: https://www.cps.ca/en/documents/position/medical-use-of-cannabis.

Spigelblatt, L., & Canadian Paediatric Society (CPS), Community Paediatrics Committee. (2002). Chiropractic care for children: Controversies and issues. *Paediatrics & Child Health, 7*(2), 85–89. Reaffirmed 2018. Retrieved from: https://www.-cps.ca/en/documents/position/chiropractic-care-children.

Spigelblatt, L., & Canadian Paediatric Society (CPS), Community Paediatrics Committee. (2005). Homeopathy in the paediatric population. *Paediatrics & Child Health, 10*(3), 173–1777. Reaffirmed 2018. Retrieved from: https://www.cps.ca/en/documents/position/homeopathy.

Vohra, S., Clifford, T., & Canadian Paediatric Society (CPS), Drug Therapy and Hazardous Substances Committee. (2005). Children and natural health products: What a clinician should know. *Paediatrics & Child Health, 10*(4), 227–232. Reaffirmed 2019. Retrieved from: https://www.cps.ca/en/documents/position/natural-health-products.

World Health Organization (WHO). (2012). *Social determinants of health and well-being among young people. Health behaviour in school-aged children (HBSC) study: International report from the 2009/2010 survey*. Retrieved from: http://www.hbsc.unito.it/it/images/pdf/hbsc/prelims-part1.pdf.

World Health Organization (WHO). (2013). *WHO traditional medicine strategy: 2014–2023*. Retrieved from: http://apps.who.int/iris/bitstream/handle/10665/92455/9789241506090_eng.pdf;jsessionid=44D73E081EF66AD2CFFC7BFF22242359?sequence=1.

22 Chronic Conditions and Palliative Care: Caring for the Child and Family

http://evolve.elsevier.com/Canada/Leifer

Tanya Heuver

Objectives

1. Define each key term listed.
2. Discuss the broad spectrum of disorders that can be defined as chronic conditions.
3. Discuss the impact of having a chronic condition on the child or adolescent.
4. Discuss the effects of chronic illness on the growth and development of children.
5. Discuss family issues related to having a child with a chronic condition.
6. Understand how to carry out interventions to promote health and normalization for children with chronic conditions and their families.
7. Discuss nursing interventions and strategies to assist the child in gaining independence.
8. Discuss one chronic illness in children and how to provide nursing care to the child and family.
9. Discuss the nurse's role in helping families cope with a child who is dying.
10. Discuss the role of palliative care in the care of a child with a life-threatening condition.
11. Formulate techniques the nurse can use to facilitate the grieving process.
12. Contrast age-appropriate responses to a sibling's death and the nursing interventions required.
13. Define the stages of dying.
14. Discuss pain assessment and management for the dying child.

Key Terms

athetosis
cerebral palsy (CP)
chronic condition
congenital
developmental delay
developmental disability
disability
exacerbation
impairment
palliative care
remission
respite care (RĔS-pĭt kăr)
sibling rivalry

CHRONIC CONDITIONS

Chronic conditions are the leading cause of death and **disability** internationally. The terms *chronic illness* and *chronic condition* are interchangeable and can be defined as a condition that persists for a minimum of 6 months and requires supportive management and care to control the symptoms. Chronic conditions may include physical, cognitive, psychological, and social **impairment** that can range from mild to substantial deficiencies (van der Lee, Mokkink, Grootenhuis, et al., 2007). The incidence of chronic conditions is increasing worldwide (World Health Organization [WHO], 2018a).

Children with chronic conditions are living longer, largely due to advances in technology and treatment (Cohen, Lacombe-Duncan, Spalding, et al., 2012). In Canada, the percentage of children between the ages of 5 and 14 years estimated to be living with a cognitive or physical disability is 4%, and the four significant chronic conditions most commonly affecting Canadian children are asthma, obesity, cancer, and diabetes (Statistics Canada, 2008). In 2012, the Chronic Disease Indicator Framework was developed to increase access to current surveillance data by providing current, reliable information on chronic disease (Public Health Agency of Canada [PHAC], 2017). Some of the terms used to refer to children with chronic conditions include children with complex chronic conditions; children with special health care needs; and children who are disabled, medically fragile, medically complicated, challenged, handicapped, impaired, or technology dependent (Bowden & Smith Greenberg, 2010; Cohen, Kuo, Agrawal, et al., 2011).

In children and adolescents, chronic conditions take many forms, some being **congenital** (congenital heart defect), some acquired (diabetes), and some with no known cause (e.g., attention-deficit/hyperactivity disorder [ADHD]). Some chronic conditions remain fixed (cerebral palsy) whereas others alternate between periods of **remission** and **exacerbation** (ulcerative colitis, asthma). Some chronic conditions advance throughout childhood, sometimes resulting in a shortened lifespan (cystic fibrosis) or death during childhood (muscular dystrophy) (Bowden & Smith Greenberg, 2010). For some of these children and their families, their chronic conditions may result in significant lifestyle changes and numerous hospitalizations, while for others their chronic condition may result in minimal impact.

Having a chronic condition often affects the quality of life of the individual affected and the well-being of the family (Berglund, 2014; Tétreault, Blais-Michaud, Marier Deschênes, et al., 2014). The child and family need time to adjust to the demands of life and those of the chronic condition (Berglund, 2014; Petersson, Simeonsson, Enskar, et al., 2013).

THE CHRONICALLY ILL CHILD AS A FAMILY MEMBER

Families living with a child with a chronic condition are faced with many opportunities and challenges. They learn to care for the needs of their child in the hospital and in their own home, as well as to manage their child's condition within the community. Relationships between families and children can have a considerable impact on how they cope with living with a family member with a chronic illness. Families with positive relationships have better health outcomes, whereas strained family relationships may contribute to deterioration of their children's health.

Children with chronic health conditions learn how to manage their conditions through everyday life experiences with their families, peers, health providers, and others in their communities (Beacham & Deatrick, 2015). Children have indicated that the way their families learned about and accepted their chronic condition and incorporated condition management into family life helped them frame the condition for themselves (Beacham & Deatrick, 2015; Knafl, Deatrick, & Havill, 2012).

Management of Chronic Conditions

Children with chronic health conditions have diverse medical needs that often conflict with the regular day-to-day function of the family. These children and their families need to learn to coordinate this care into the daily life routines of the family (Kelo, Eriksson, & Eriksson, 2013). In order to support their children's special health needs, families create new routines. Families have acknowledged the importance of routines and rituals in adjusting to their children's care, as less emphasis is placed on the chronic condition and the care becomes integrated into the family's daily routine (Kelo et al., 2013; Knafl, Deatrick, Knafl, et al., 2013; Santos, Crespo, Silva, et al., 2012). The required changes to the family's routines and lifestyle can result in significant stress for children and their families if these changes are not managed successfully (Drutchas & Anandarajah, 2014; Fayed, Kraus de Camargo, Elahi, et al., 2014).

The chronically ill child is a contributing member to the family unit. The child must be treated normally, and overprotection and excessive restriction should be avoided. Focusing on what the child can do and providing successful experiences are more effective than focusing on the disability.

Involvement of the entire family with the care of the chronically ill child aids in normal family interaction. The child should be integrated into, rather than isolated from, the community and society. Nurses can assist the child and the family in developing strategies to cope with chronic illness and to promote optimal growth and development. The wellness of the child should be the centre of the child's life, rather than the disability.

Caring for a child with chronic health challenges can be stressful and exhausting at times for families. Parents may feel conflicted in trying to balance the needs and wishes of every member of the family while ensuring that the complex needs of their child with chronic health issues are being met. In order to care for their families, parents need to take care of themselves. One approach in this regard is **respite care**. This short-term relief from caregiving responsibilities allows caregivers the opportunity to have a break, relax, and re-energize (Sherman, 1995). Respite care can be provided within the family's own home or in various locations in the community. This important break has the potential to provide positive social experiences for the child and family, thereby benefitting the entire family. Respite care can provide parents the opportunity to connect as partners and can serve to strengthen the spousal relationship.

Nursing Tip

When caring for a child who has a chronic condition, explain to the child what to expect, include the child in decision making and treatment, and allow the child some control whenever possible. Promote the normality of routines.

THE IMPACT OF CHRONIC CONDITIONS ON THE CHILD

Chronic conditions during childhood often affect these children's growth and development (see Chapter 19 and Table 22.1). Specific programs that foster feelings of security and independence within the limits of the situation are essential. Behaviour problems are lessened when children can verbalize specific concerns with persons sensitive to their problems. To be in school and to be considered a member of their peer group are very important to children. If they feel rejected by and different from their peers, they may be prone to depression. Hospital school programs can provide familiarity and enable patients to keep pace with their classmates. The recreational therapist may also be helpful in preventing boredom and providing outlets for tension.

Table 22.1 **The Effects of Chronic Illness on Growth and Development***

AGE	FEATURE	EFFECT
Infancy	Trust	A visible defect can delay bonding. Prolonged illness may separate child from the family. Irritability promotes parental negativity.
Toddler	Autonomy	Physical restrictions impede development of motor and language skills. Toilet training may be delayed. Fear may erode self-confidence. Separation anxiety occurs.
Preschooler	Initiative	Impaired ability to experience world outside of family impedes social skills. Overprotective parents delay teaching self-discipline. Child may develop negative body image. Child develops sense of guilt at their inability to master tasks.
School age	Industry	Loss of grade level in school because of illness and inability to participate or compete can lead to a sense of inferiority. Sense of independence and accomplishment can be lost. Being different from peers may impede child's sense of belonging.
Adolescent	Identity	Adolescent feels loss of control and inability to conform to peers. The developing self-concept may become negative. Adolescent may grieve for a lost ability. Enforced dependence may impair plans for future goals. Rebellion results in decreased adherence to treatment.

*Chronic illness can impede growth and development. The nurse should reinforce teaching concerning the developmental needs of chronically ill children at different age levels to promote self-acceptance and positive self-esteem.

When caring for adolescents with a chronic condition, nurses must help these teenagers to accept their body with all its strengths and imperfections. They must develop an awareness of the adolescent's fears of forced dependence, body invasion, mutilation, rejection, and loss of face, especially within peer groups. The nurse can anticipate a certain amount of reluctance to adhere to hospital regulations, which reflects the adolescent's need for self-determination. Recognizing this as an asset rather than a liability enables the nurse to respond creatively.

Promoting Normal Development

Children with chronic health conditions experience the same developmental stages as their healthy peers (see Chapter 13). Many studies have shown that children with chronic conditions find living a regular life difficult; they talk about their active involvement in everyday life as a balancing act, alternating between limitations and modifications related to living with a chronic condition (Freeborn, Dyches, Roper, et al., 2013; Lewis & Parsons, 2008). They find managing their conditions to be complicated, onerous, boring, and ill-timed, causing disruptions to their daily life and leaving them feeling very different from their peers and others (Beacham & Deatrick, 2015; Lambert & Keogh, 2015). Some children have discussed the support provided by their friends and how this helps make them feel normal (Beacham & Deatrick, 2015).

Restrictions are often imposed on children with chronic conditions, by the condition itself, by the environment, or by others, including parents, health care providers, and teachers. These restrictions may lead to children feeling rejected, lonely, different, and constantly reminded of their conditions as they are prevented from participating in regular, age-appropriate activities.

Infancy

As discussed in Chapter 13, the first stage of Erikson's theory of psychosocial development, trust versus mistrust, occurs between birth and 1 year of age, when infants are completely dependent on adults for survival. During this time, infants rely on adults to meet their needs for love, food, safety, and nurturing. The infant's ability to trust during this stage is dependent on their needs being met consistently and lovingly. If infants learn to trust the adult caregivers in their lives, they feel safe. Infants whose needs are not met consistently or whose caregivers are emotionally or physically unavailable develop feelings of mistrust.

For infants with chronic conditions, there are factors that can negatively affect the caregiver's ability to meet the infants' needs consistently. For example, infants born with significant congenital anomalies often require care in a neonatal intensive care unit (NICU) or require surgery immediately after birth. Both of these experiences can delay bonding with parents, as infants and families might be separated because of prolonged illness. At times, when infants are born with significant health or medical challenges, parents are afraid to touch or hold them for fear of interfering with medical treatment or tubes and monitors.

Toddlers

The second stage of Erikson's theory of psychosocial development, autonomy versus shame and doubt, occurs during the toddler years. During this developmental stage, toddlers are just beginning to gain a little independence as they learn to achieve basic activities on their own. Toddlers can be encouraged to make choices and gain control while making simple decisions about their preferences. For example, when toddlers are given the choice between two shirts to wear, they develop autonomy and a greater sense of personal control over their environment.

As toddlers learn to exert control over their environment, they often exude this control by saying "no" and refusing to do what is being requested of them. This can be especially frustrating and challenging for parents and health care providers caring for a child with a chronic condition, as there are many aspects of the condition's management that are not optional. By continuing to offer toddlers choices as often as possible however, many of them will be better able to assist with the components of management and care that are not optional. For example, when administering medication to a toddler, they could be offered the choice of drinking the medicine from a cup or a syringe, or the choice of chasing the medicine with water or juice. This way, taking the medication is the non-negotiable part of the management, but how the toddler chooses to take the medicine is within their control. Other challenges that toddlers with chronic conditions may face are physical or emotional restrictions that may impede the development of motor and language skills.

Preschool

Erikson's third stage of psychosocial development, initiative versus guilt, takes place during the preschool years. During this stage, children begin to influence their control through guiding play and other social exchanges. When an ideal balance of personal initiative and readiness to collaborate with others emerges, children feel a sense of purpose, leading them to feel capable, resourceful, and able to lead others. Children without this sense of resolution may be left with feelings of uncertainty, shame, and doubt. Often, in the care of children with chronic conditions, clinical management decisions are made by adults—health care providers and parents. A recent study advocates that children be included in these discussions and decisions at a much younger age than they have in the past (Beacham & Deatrick, 2015). Nurses can help foster this sense of purpose in preschool-age children by including them in conversations and offering them choices and control as much as possible.

School age

Erikson's fourth psychosocial stage, industry versus inferiority, occurs during the early school years, from approximately age 5 to 12. During this time, children develop a sense of pride in their abilities and accomplishments. As children are praised and encouraged, their self-confidence and feelings of competence build. Those children who receive little or no praise and reinforcement will doubt their ability to succeed. For school-age children with chronic conditions, their opportunities to achieve this sense of industry might be limited by their inability to participate in certain activities or events due to their condition. Some children might miss school more frequently because of factors related to their condition such as appointments, treatments, and illness. School-age children with chronic health conditions often do learn how to cope with life and their conditions in and outside their homes (Beacham & Deatrick, 2015).

School-age children with chronic illness often find ways to help them manage their chronic conditions and help decrease their symptoms. These may include, when away from home, having a plan for expected treatments and unexpected occurrences, along with having access to parents. This ultimately allows the child to increase their confidence.

Since family is the main source of information and support for school-age children, including and encouraging children to be involved in discussions with the health care team will help facilitate healthy growth and development for those with chronic conditions. These children will better understand their condition and have the confidence to ask questions and manage their care more independently, as well as build competence (Kirk, Beatty, Caller, et al., 2012). Despite continually striving for a normal life, children with chronic health conditions often report feeling different from their peers (Spencer, Cooper, & Milton, 2013). To avoid being perceived as unusual by their peers, school-age children may withdraw socially, avoid certain activities or interactions, and not follow the management required for their condition (Gauntlett-Gilbert & Connell, 2012). As these school-age children near their teens, they may worry or have questions about their health that they want to discuss with the health care team alone, without the presence of their parents. Nurses play a pivotal role in advocating for and supporting the developmental needs and growth of school-age children with chronic conditions.

Adolescence

Erikson's fifth psychosocial stage, identity versus confusion, takes place during adolescence. This stage is crucial to youths' development as they discover their independence and personal identity. This identity is continually shaped by new experiences and information obtained during day-to-day interactions with others. These new experiences will continue to influence the adolescents' behaviour and may support or impede their sense of self throughout life. Adolescents whose positive choices are encouraged and praised will develop a healthy sense of self accompanied by feelings of increasing independence. Adolescents who are not encouraged or commended for their affirmative decisions are often left feeling insecure about themselves and their future. For adolescents faced with chronic conditions, this stage can be very challenging for them, as it is a time of self-discovery. Some teens feel a loss of control, as they are unable to do what their peers are capable of. For some adolescents with chronic conditions, this situation may lead to a negative self-concept and feelings of worthlessness. Their ongoing dependence on routines or treatment to manage their chronic condition may impair their future dreams or plans.

There are a number of factors that can be challenging for parents and youth living with chronic conditions as adolescents move toward increasing independence and more separation from parents. Some of these considerations include the adolescent's need for ongoing treatment and follow-up and parenteral reluctance and fear of letting the adolescent have more control over their condition. Nurses and other health care providers can help support adolescents by using the following strategies (Pinzon, Harvey, & Canadian Paediatric Society [CPS] Adolescent Health Committee, 2006/2018):

- Adolescents need to be aware of treatment choices and should be encouraged to be assertive when discussing and participating in this decision making.
- Providing choices for adolescents as much as possible will encourage independence and support collaboration with condition management.
- Support families in balancing the need for parental guidance and the adolescent's need for more control over their life.

THE IMPACT OF A CHILD'S CHRONIC ILLNESS ON PARENTS

Having a child diagnosed with a chronic health condition has a significant impact on parents. The time of diagnosis can be marked by multiple losses for parents, which may include the loss of their previously healthy child, their independence, and their own self-confidence (Marshall, Carter, Rose, et al., 2009). For some, these feelings of loss can be long-lasting.

Caring for children with chronic conditions involves myriad biological, physical, and psychosocial components. Parents may feel stressed about their child's health, caregiving responsibilities, finances, and available support and services. Since parents are primarily responsible for their children they need to be constantly vigilant in their care; this constant care and devotion can have a lasting impact on the lives of all involved (Rifshana, Breheny, Taylor, et al., 2017). Many parents describe facing challenges within the health, social services, and education systems (Ray, 2002). Parents often spend considerable periods of time trying to search for information, find appropriate services, and advocate for the needs of their child and family. In spending significant amounts of time trying to navigate the system, parents are often left feeling exhausted, frustrated, and with a sense of hopelessness and despair. It is essential that nurses and other professionals involved with children with chronic conditions and their families help alleviate some of this stress by being empathetic and compassionate when providing information, and helping them navigate a complex health care system and find reliable respite options (Coughlin & Sethares, 2017). Table 22.2 lists strategies to support some of the normal responses of parents of children with chronic illness.

With respite care, trained workers come into the home for periods of time to relieve parents of the responsibility of caring for the child. This enables the parents to shop, take care of business transactions, or simply take a much-needed break or vacation. It is important that nurses spend time discussing with families the importance of respite care. Parents sometimes feel guilty for considering respite or think they are abandoning their child or that they should be the ones caring for their child all the time. For parents to appreciate the importance and necessity of respite, nurses need to spend time discussing the benefits of respite and strategies that families can use to help care for each other.

THE IMPACT OF CHRONIC ILLNESS ON SIBLINGS

Most siblings of children with chronic health conditions have either emotional scars or develop protective coping mechanisms to handle their experiences. Siblings of children with long-term illness are at risk of developing poor self-esteem and problems with their own peer relationships. Some siblings, however, are resilient and develop strength and positive coping mechanisms. **Sibling rivalry**, a competition between siblings for the attention or love of parents, is a normal part of growth and development, but feelings of guilt in other siblings can enter the picture when one sibling becomes ill. Sibling rivalry teaches interactive social skills that will be used with friends and at work later in life. A child who is left at home with a babysitter while the parents tend to an ill sibling in the hospital or are continually at appointments may feel abandoned and often is burdened with extra household responsibilities that may add to the stress. Some children may react negatively to the stress of making dinner for the rest of the family, whereas other children react positively and develop positive self-esteem, knowing they are trusted with this task.

The nurse can provide support for the family system, identify available resources, and collaborate with the health care team to meet total family needs.

FAMILY-CENTRED CARE

Children with chronic conditions and their families have many needs and require support from numerous individuals in the health care system and community. In order to partner collaboratively, a family-centred care approach is used. In a family-centred care approach, a collaborative partnership is vitally important, where each individual is treated with respect and dignity and the health care system is responsive to the choices, wishes, and strengths of the family. By partnering with families, the well-being of parents and children is promoted to encourage a positive environment for the whole family (King & Chiarello, 2014).

TRANSITIONS—HOSPITAL TO HOME

Children with complex chronic conditions often have significant and specialized needs, and their care is frequently provided in their own home. The transition

Table 22.2 **Supporting the Emotional Responses of Parents**

EMOTION	EXAMPLES	PROBLEMATIC EXAMPLES	NURSING CARE	EXPECTED OUTCOMES
Grief	Despair, remorse	Withdrawal; unrelenting sadness	Validate feelings. Offer support. Help parents re-establish structure in their lives.	Parents begin to integrate fact that child has chronic condition into how they view the child in a positive way.
Denial	Forgetting Overcompensation Disbelief	Interference with treatment Distrust	Reflect back statements. Clarify feelings. Offer feedback. Help parents recognize that responses are normal.	Parents begin to make appropriate plans for the future.
Guilt	Self-blame	Spousal blame Continual self-recrimination	Give information. Explore ideas about why child has the condition.	Self-blame comments decrease. Projection of blame onto others decreases. Coping with realistic guilt.
Anger	Aggression Hostility	Acts helpless Interferes with treatment plan	Include parents when developing treatment plan. Remain nondefensive.	Parents begin to actively participate in planning care. Parents accurately and constructively direct anger.
Fear	Anxiety Self-doubt Disoriented	Hypochondriacal Panic attacks Avoidance	Have parents participate in development and implementation of treatment plan. Point out parental competence. Repeat instructions, if needed.	Parent initiates discussion of new treatment approaches. Parent carries out needed treatments.
Loneliness	Quiet Isolated	Marital discord Job difficulties	Assist in establishing contact with potential support person/groups. Help family re-establish or develop social connections.	Family contacts support group and goes to meetings. Family reports social activities that give them enjoyment.

Adapted from Johnston, C. E., & Marder, L. R. (1994). Parenting the child with a chronic condition: An emotional experience. *Pediatric Nursing, 20*(6), 611–614.

from hospital to home-based care can be challenging because of numerous specialized needs and medical complexity that can increase the risk of adverse outcomes and readmission to hospital (Breneol, Belliveau, Cassidy, et al., 2017).

In order to plan for, anticipate, and support the needs of these children and their families, a multifaceted, interdisciplinary approach is fundamental to making the transition in care from hospital to home. Nurses are well positioned to function in a coordinator role to facilitate discussions with the children, families, and members of the interdisciplinary team to plan for a positive transition from hospital to home for these children and their families (Breneol et al., 2017; Carter, Bray, Sanders, et al., 2016).

Home health care and other community agencies work together to provide holistic care. Box 22.1 discusses strategies that are useful for in-home caregivers. The school system also shares some responsibility in providing positive school-related activities, which is crucial to a family being successful in implementing home care.

CEREBRAL PALSY

Cerebral palsy is one example of a chronic condition in children that will be discussed further in the next sections.

Box 22.1 **Strategies for Home Health Care Workers Caring for Children**

- Observe how the family interacts with the child.
- Do not wait for the child to cry out for attention, because the child may be unable to communicate in this way.
- Watch for facial expressions and body language.
- Post signs above the bed denoting special considerations, such as "Never position on left side" and "Do not feed with plastic spoon."
- Listen to the parents and observe how they attend to the physical needs of the child.
- Do not be afraid to ask questions or discuss apprehensions you may feel about your ability to care for the child.
- Be attuned to the needs of other children in the home.
- Be creative in exploring avenues for socialization.
- Explore community facilities or support groups that might benefit the family.

PATHOPHYSIOLOGY

Cerebral palsy (CP) is a term used to describe a group of nonprogressive motor disorders caused by a lesion in the various motor centres of the developing fetal brain. It also involves problems with sensation and communication secondary to the musculoskeletal problems. It

Table 22.3 Types of Cerebral Palsy

TYPE	CHARACTERISTICS
Spastic	Involves damage to the cortex of the brain Spasms occur with movement Related to cerebral asphyxia
Athetoid (dyskinetic)	Involves damage to the basal nuclei ganglion Continuous involuntary writhing movements Often associated with hyperbilirubinemia
Ataxic	Uncoordinated movements and ataxia from a lesion in the cerebellum
Mixed	Usually a combination of spastic and athetoid

is now believed that CP results most often from existing prenatal brain abnormalities, exposure to maternal chorioamnionitis in utero, prematurity, hypoxic brain injury, or severe hypoglycemia (Johnston, 2016). While CP is not fatal in itself, currently there is no cure. It is one of the most common disabling conditions seen in children and occurs in as many as 3.6 per 1 000 live births, with males being more affected (Johnston, 2016).

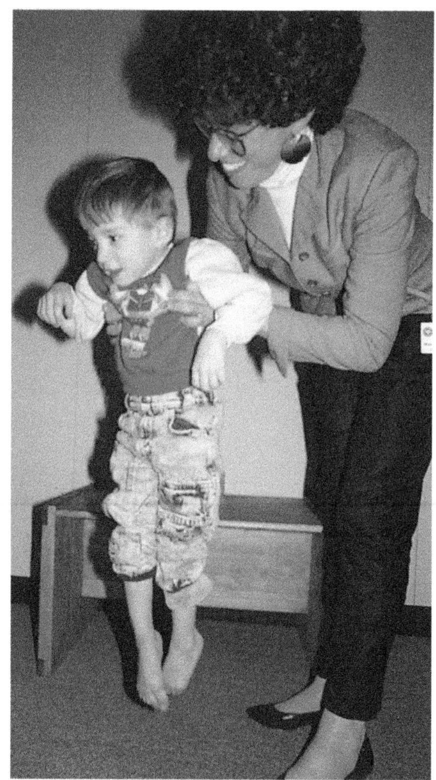

Fig. 22.1 Child with cerebral palsy with spasticity. Note the legs crossing in a scissorlike pattern when the child is supported in vertical suspension.

MANIFESTATIONS

The symptoms of CP vary with each child and may range from mild to severe. Some children with CP have developmental delays, but many children with severe, spastic quadriplegia have average intelligence. Developmental milestones are not achieved at the expected age levels. Persistence of primitive reflexes such as the Moro and tonic neck reflexes may be seen. Diagnostic tests may include metabolic and genetic testing and magnetic resonance imaging (MRI). Early recognition is important for appropriate referrals.

There are four types of CP (Table 22.3). Two of the more common types are marked by spasticity (Fig. 22.1) and athetosis. These conditions occur in about 70% of cases. *Spasticity* is characterized by tension in certain muscle groups. The stretch reflex is present in the involved muscles. When the child tries to move the voluntary muscles, jerky motions result. Eating, walking, and other coordinated movements are difficult to accomplish. The lower extremities are usually involved. The legs cross and the toes point inward. The arms and trunk may also be affected. In **athetosis** the child has involuntary, purposeless movements that interfere with normal motion. Speech, sight, and hearing defects or seizures may be complications.

TREATMENT AND NURSING CARE

The goal of treatment of children with CP is to assist them in making the most of their abilities and to guide them in becoming adults who are able to perform at their maximum ability. Both short- and long-term goals must be realistic. Parents may need help in accepting the child's limitations. Early diagnosis can result in fewer physical and emotional problems.

The specific treatment of CP is highly individualized and depends on the severity of the disability. Parents of children with CP are the experts in caring for their children and should be included as an integral part of the health care team.

Botulinum toxin has been used successfully to manage spasticity problems and reduce drooling, and levodopa has helped control some athetoid symptoms. An implanted pump that delivers baclofen directly into the intrathecal space around the spinal cord can reduce spasticity. This type of medication delivery produces less acute adverse effects than oral baclofen. Antiepileptic drugs such as carbamazepine (Tegetrol) and valproic acid (Depakene) may be prescribed if seizures are present. Pain management is important for children with CP. Medication for gastroesophageal reflux may also be prescribed. Dental hygiene is important because phenytoin, often prescribed for seizures, causes gum hyperplasia. Good skin care is essential for the child with CP. The nurse needs to observe the skin for redness and other evidence of pressure sores.

All precautions must be taken to prevent the formation of *contractures* (degeneration or shortening of the muscles because of lack of use), which could result in permanent loss of function of the part involved (e.g., leg, arm, or finger). Physical therapy is essential to prevent contractures and deformities. Other measures necessary to prevent contractures include frequent changes of position, the use of splints, and the performance of passive, range-of-motion, and stretching exercises. The nurse should encourage children to do as much as they can for themselves. When they bathe, they should try to put their muscles and joints through the normal range of motion. The nurse must use judgement in assessing their capabilities and assist only in those areas where they are lacking. The nurse must also ensure that the child maintains good posture while in bed, through the use of footboards and the proper positioning of pillows and other comfort devices.

Braces are often used to treat contractures. A *brace* is a mechanical aid that supports weakened muscles or limbs. All braces are routinely checked for correct alignment, loose or missing parts, and the condition of straps and buckles. It may take the child some time to adjust to the use of a brace. Wheelchairs and crutches are designed to fit the child.

Orthopedic surgery may be indicated and may be followed by an extensive period of rehabilitation. The nurse must remember that the child is in a continuous state of psychological and physical growth during this period. Maintaining interest and efforts in achieving developmental milestones whenever possible may have an impact on the child's future development.

Feeding problems can lead to nutritional deficiencies. Vitamin, mineral, or protein supplements may be indicated for some children. Gastrostomy tube feedings may be required to augment nutritional intake. Swallowing and sucking may be difficult. Vomiting is common because the gag reflex is overactive. It is important to be especially careful to feed the child slowly to prevent aspiration. It is often difficult for these infants to adjust to solid foods, and it takes a great deal of patience on the part of parents and nurses to help the child adapt to this new experience (see Skill 22.1 and Fig. 22.2). As the children grow, they can be taught to manage special feeding equipment so they are able to eat independently. They are also taught such activities as dressing and combing their hair. Dental care is discussed in Chapter 13.

The child with a physical challenge needs opportunities to play alone and with other children. Games suited to ability, such as finger painting, are fun and allow freedom of expression. Activities that require fine muscular movements of the hand cause frustration in the child whose arms and hands are affected by the disease. Computerized toys that are customized to the child aid in developing hand–eye coordination. The nurse can learn a great deal from the parents about the types of play the child enjoys.

Communication can be enhanced through technology that uses text-to-speech or eye-tracking devices or a voice synthesizer (speech-generating system) to augment language expression or manage a wheelchair. Augmented and alternative communication can enable the child's communication and aid in achieving optimum growth and development (Box 22.2).

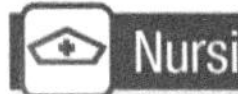

Nursing Tip

The use of technology is an effective form of communication in the child with CP.

Children with CP tire easily but may find it difficult to relax. They use a great deal of energy to accomplish the simplest of tasks, and they do not respond well to being hurried or overly stimulated.

Educational opportunities geared toward the child's abilities are essential. Canadian provinces have

Skill 22.1 General Modifications and Precautions in Pediatric Feeding Techniques for Children With Difficulty Swallowing

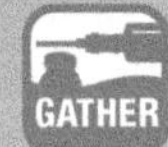

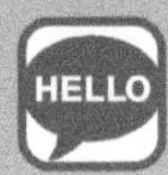

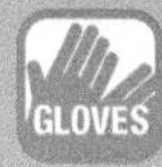

PURPOSE

To facilitate safe feeding and prevent aspiration

STEPS

1. Ensure proper positioning and support of the head and back before feeding solid foods.
2. Place small amounts of food on a spoon to prevent choking.
3. Avoid tilting the head back during feeding of solid foods, because this will place the swallowing mechanisms out of alignment.
4. Do not touch the tip of the child's tongue with the spoon, because this can activate the tongue extrusion reflex.
5. Use rubber-coated spoons for children with hyperactive bite reflex to protect the teeth from injury.
6. Gently stroke the angle of the jaw below the ears to relax the bite of a child who has clamped down on a spoon.
7. Gently stroke the area under the chin in a circular motion to stimulate chewing when food is held in the mouth.
8. Gently press upward under the chin to stimulate swallowing when fluid is held in the mouth.
9. To help a child with a disability drink from a cup, cut the top portion of the paper or plastic cup away to provide space for the nose. This will enable the cup to be tilted without the child's head being tilted back.
10. Avoid excessive pressure on the back of the head when positioning a child with a disability for feeding to prevent reflex responses in the body or torso position.

education laws which ensure that all students receive free and appropriate education. However, the definitions of "appropriate education" vary by province, and clear definitions do not exist (Kohen, Uppal, Khan, et al., 2010). Many children are integrated into regular classes and a small majority require special education classes. The child's mental capacity is determined not just in light of the intelligence quotient (IQ) itself but also by the demonstrated potential of the individual. Preschools and summer camps for exceptional children are available. These programs vary in quality and extent of services. Parents are also referred to Cerebral Palsy Canada, a national organization that provides education and support services. The expanding role of nurses in the home and schools may further assist in mainstreaming these children into educational and social situations.

Successful experiences help to improve a child's self-concept; repeated failures are demoralizing and may lower self-esteem. The health care team must work to bring satisfaction to these children by making it possible for them to succeed. The amount of confidence and self-respect that a child with a disability has depends a great deal on a supportive environment.

Parents must be informed of community resources available to them. The family's religious affiliation should not be overlooked because it can be a source of support and help during times of stress. The long course of this disability can place a financial burden on the family. Caregivers need respite care from time to time to enhance their coping skills. Respite care offers family members the opportunity to focus on themselves and other family members and allows them to take a break from the constant need to provide care for the child with the chronic illness.

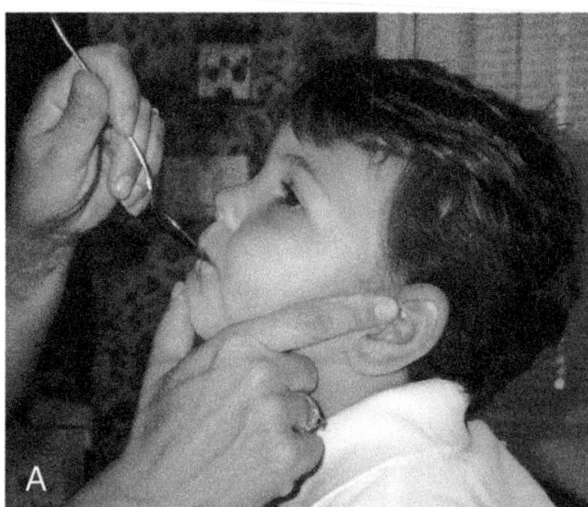

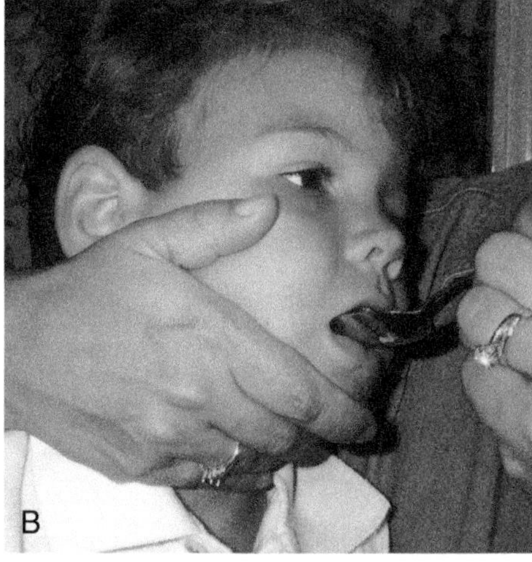

Fig. 22.2 Feeding the child with a disability. **A,** Manual jaw control is supplied anteriorly. **B,** Manual jaw control is provided from the side. (From Hockenberry, M., & Wilson, D. [2015]. *Wong's nursing care of infants and children* [10th ed.]. St. Louis: Mosby.)

Box 22.2 Treatment Protocol for Cerebral Palsy

1. Establish communication.
2. Establish locomotion.
3. Use and optimize existing motor functions.
4. Provide intellectual stimulation.
5. Promote socialization.
6. Provide technology to encourage self-care and promote growth and development.
7. Provide multidisciplinary approach to care.

MENTAL HEALTH NEEDS OF THE PHYSICALLY CHALLENGED CHILD

The requirements for good mental health in the physically challenged child do not differ from those of other children. They need to have their basic human requirements satisfied and they need people who are genuinely interested in them. Children and adolescents with neuromotor disorders have more mental health symptoms than the general population, including difficulties with social skills, self-esteem, behaviour, anxiety, mood, and attention (Klein & CPS Mental Health and Developmental Disabilities Committee, 2016).

The child with a disability should be encouraged to participate to the fullest extent possible in family, school, and community activities. Friendships with other non–able-bodied and able-bodied peers are encouraged. Extended family and the community are important resources. Educational programs are integrating the disabled more fully into the community. Barrier-free buildings and modifications that improve accessibility contribute positively to these efforts.

DEVELOPMENTAL DISABILITES

Children who have a **developmental disability** that affects their intellect or ability to cope face some unique difficulties. They may often be overprotected, unable to break away from supervision, and deprived of necessary peer relationships. The pubertal process, with its emerging sexuality, is a concern to parents and may precipitate a family crisis.

INTELLCTUAL DISABILITY

Intellectual disability or *impairment* is often used to describe a type of developmental disability characterized

Box 22.3 Identifying Adaptive Behaviour Deficits

Intellectual functioning below IQ of 75
Limitations in at least 2 of the following 10 areas of adaptive behaviours:

1. Communication
2. Self-care
3. Home living
4. Social skills
5. Community use
6. Self-direction
7. Health and safety
8. Functional academics
9. Leisure
10. Work

Box 22.4 Elements Involved in Mental Functioning

LEVEL OF CONSCIOUSNESS
Attention
Short- and long-term memory
Perceptions

THOUGHT PROCESSES
Insight
Judgement
Affect
Mood

EXPRESSIVE LANGUAGE
Vocabulary
Abstract thinking
Intelligence

by a mental impairment. Intellectual impairment or disability has been defined as below-average mental functioning (IQ below 70) and a deficit in adaptive behaviour, conceptual skills, or social skills manifested during the developmental period (before 18 years of age) (Box 22.3). The definition of intellectual disability has shifted away from IQ alone and toward a relationship-oriented concept of adaptive behaviour within the environment. Intellectual disability involves impairment of mental abilities that affect functioning related to everyday tasks and includes language, reading, math, reasoning, memory, social skills, judgement, communication skills, and self-management abilities.

When a child is diagnosed as intellectually impaired, it is important to correlate growth and development with mental functioning. For example, abstract thinking does not begin to appear before 12 years of age. A child classified as intellectually impaired is not necessarily impaired in all areas of mental functioning (Box 22.4). There is a variability in the pattern of strengths and weaknesses (Shapiro, Kilburn, & Hardin, 2014).

Numerous tests are available to measure intelligence. Intelligence in children is difficult to evaluate and is best tested on an individual basis. All such tests have their limitations, and their accuracy is subject to the abilities of the person interpreting them. Nonetheless, the tests are of value when used in conjunction with a thorough study of the child's physical, mental, emotional, and social development.

There are many causes of intellectual impairment. Some conditions that can be detected during the newborn period are phenylketonuria, hypothyroidism, fetal alcohol spectrum disorder, Down syndrome, malformations of the brain (e.g., microcephaly, hydrocephalus, craniosynostosis), and maternal infections such as cytomegalovirus (CMV). Injuries or anoxia during or shortly after birth may also cause intellectual impairment. Conditions such as meningitis, lead poisoning, neoplasms, and encephalitis can cause intellectual impairment in a child or adult of any age. Heredity is a factor in intellectual impairment. Lack of appropriate stimulation may also lead to intellectual impairment. In certain cases, early recognition and intervention can lessen or prevent intellectual impairment. The child may be classified as having a **developmental delay** before a diagnosis of cognitive impairment is made.

Other symptoms of intellectual impairment are associated with milestones of the growth process. Children who do not achieve milestones at the expected age may be cognitively impaired. Unusual clumsiness and failure to respond to stimuli are also early indications. Sometimes this disorder is not discovered until the child enters school.

The education system uses various criteria for classroom placement and eligibility for available resources. It is ideal to provide the least restrictive environment possible for learning and mainstreaming with nonimpaired students whenever possible.

There are many tests for assessing adaptive behaviours. Each case must be frequently re-evaluated according to the child's individual progress. The goal of care is to normalize the opportunities for the child and family as much as possible. Specific behavioural disorders are discussed in Chapter 33.

Nursing Tip

Children with cognitive or intellectual impairment have the same psychosocial needs as all other children, but they cannot express themselves or respond as other children do.

The pediatric nurse must help the parents to understand that providing experiences in which the child can be successful and concentrating on their strengths rather than weaknesses are key to helping a child who is developmentally different. A child who experiences consistent failure can become angry, which may cause behaviour difficulties that can affect the therapy.

Nursing Tip

The child with an intellectual impairment needs to develop a sense of accomplishment. Do not "take over" projects because of your own need to assist or speed up the process.

Treatment and Nursing Care

The Canadian Charter of Rights and Freedoms is a part of the Canadian Constitution. Every individual in Canada is to be considered equal regardless of physical or mental disability (Government of Canada, 2018). As nurses caring for and supporting children with disabilities, it is essential to advocate for these rights and freedoms as recognized by this Charter.

An individualized plan of care with goals and objectives is vital to providing care for children with intellectual impairment and helping their families. Children with intellectual disabilities have higher rates of vision, hearing, behavioural, and emotional disorders. The initial step is to present the findings to the family and to provide the emotional support necessary to help parents and siblings learn to provide care for a child with a disability. The child's competence and adaptive behaviours should be discussed along with the deficiencies. Introduction to the multidisciplinary team for long-term care is important. Play therapy should be prescribed to nurture growth and development. Receptive and expressive communication skills are developed with professional help.

Nurses must be familiar with the resources of the community so that they can direct the family to them. Summer camps, such as those run by the Easter Seals Society, provide stimulation and opportunities for socialization to children with intellectual and developmental disabilities. The child guidance clinic or the psychological services of a nearby hospital may provide support. Arrangements for proper dental care must be made because some children may be unable to cope with the necessary procedures. The Special Olympics introduces healthy competition to the cognitively and physically impaired child.

The nurse caring for the intellectually impaired child in the hospital must know the child's stage of maturation and ability. A detailed history, including a habit and care sheet, is completed by the family. Self-help activities are documented. Home routines are to be followed as closely as possible to avoid the reversal of gains already made. Good communication between the parents and the nurse can aid in make the transition from home to hospital as smooth as possible for the child. A positive approach is recommended when obtaining information about the child from the parents. A request such as "Tell me about Carla's eating habits" is preferable to "Does she feed herself?" and the former is likely to yield more helpful information.

> **Nursing Tip**
>
> Nursing responsibilities for children with disabilities include the following:
> - Emphasizing the *strengths* present
> - Maintaining communication with the family
> - Avoiding labels
> - Using simple terms
> - Contacting the school and planning for school needs
> - Providing daily experiences in which the child can succeed
> - Referring family to local, provincial, and national support groups

Prevention

The outlook is good for continued success in the prevention of intellectual impairment. Nurses can contribute to this effort by promoting genetic counselling, immunizations, newborn screening, and regular prenatal care (Table 22.4). Comprehensive programs for early assessment and treatment of children with intellectual impairment must also be promoted. The nurse can serve as an advocate for the child and adolescent to help ensure that their rights are upheld.

THE CHILD WHO IS DYING

Some children with chronic illnesses will not recover and may eventually die from their condition. **Palliative care** for children is an approach that improves the quality of life of children and their families who are facing problems associated with life-threatening illnesses. It prevents and relieves suffering through the early identification, correct assessment, and treatment of pain and other problems, whether physical, psychosocial, or spiritual (WHO, 2018b). Addressing suffering involves taking care of issues beyond physical symptoms. Palliative care uses a team approach to support patients and their caregivers. This includes addressing practical needs and providing bereavement counselling. It offers a support system to help patients live as actively as possible until death (WHO, 2018b). Optimally, this care begins when a life-threatening illness or condition is diagnosed and continues regardless of whether or not a child receives treatment directed at the underlying illness.

ADVANCE CARE PLANNING

Children and their families should have discussions regarding advance care planning early in the course of a disease for which there may be no cure. The primary goal of this discussion is to make decisions to optimize the quality of life and perhaps to forgo selected life-sustaining treatments. All health care providers should be aware of their own potential feelings of failure when a child has a terminal illness, which may contribute to reluctance to initiate discussion. It may be helpful during discussions to ensure families understand that one is not "giving up" on the child but rather accepting or "giving in" to the reality of the disease process (Tsai & CPS Bioethics Committee, 2008/2018).

FACING DEATH

Facing death is often a difficult personal issue for the nurse. The nurse must understand the grieving process, personal and cultural views concerning that process, the views of a parent losing a child, and the perceptions of the child facing death. Integrating these understandings and helping all involved to cope successfully involve a multidisciplinary approach. The response to a child's death is influenced by whether there was a long period of uncertainty before the death or whether it was a sudden, unexpected event. Sensitive,

Table 22.4 **Interventions Currently Available to Prevent Intellectual and Developmental Disabilities**

FACTOR	INTERVENTION
Nearly Total Elimination	
Congenital rubella	Early immunization, antibody screening
Phenylketonuria, galactosemia, congenital hypothyroidism	Newborn screening, dietary management, replacement therapy
Kernicterus	Reduction of sensitization (RH negative/ABO incompatibility)
Major Reduction	
Tay-Sachs disease	Carrier screening, prenatal diagnosis in high-risk persons
Measles encephalitis	Early vaccination
Significant Reduction	
Morbidity from prematurity	Newborn intensive care nurseries
Neural tube defects	Prenatal folic acid supplements
Lead intoxication	Early screening for lead levels when risk factors present, improvement in environment, chelation when necessary
Fetal alcohol spectrum disorder	Public education
Morbidity from head injury	Automobile child restraints, safety helmets and equipment; education
Child neglect and abuse	Parenting classes and family life education through the schools
Special Assistance and Relief	
Multiple disabilities, hearing, speech, Down syndrome	Early identification, support for families, genetic counselling of special risks

Modified from Carey, W., Crocker, A., Elias, E., Feldman, H., & Coleman, W. (2009). *Developmental-behavioral pediatrics* (4th ed.). Philadelphia: Saunders.

competent care can result if the nurse is aware of the personal and cultural practices of the family. The nurse can facilitate the grief process by anticipating psychological and somatic responses and maintaining open communication. The family's efforts to cope, to adapt, and to grieve must be supported.

The response of the family to the death of the child may initially be manifested by somatic distress such as weakness, anguish, or shortness of breath. A family member may feel detached from the world and have a sense of unreality or disbelief. A sense of guilt and blame may follow ("I should have" or "I could have"). Hostility is a normal response and may drive away those who do not understand its normality in the acute grieving process. A restlessness and general irritability or inability to function may follow. Assistance in the care of other children or household responsibilities may be necessary. Nursing priorities include being a patient and family advocate, providing support, and facilitating the grieving process. Palliative care may be available in the community, either at home or in a hospice, and can play an important role in the care of the child and the family before and after the death.

SELF-EXPLORATION

One important, if not the most important, task to prepare for in working with the dying patient is self-exploration. Our attitudes about life and death affect our nursing practice. Emotions buried deep within can form barriers to effective communication unless they are recognized and released. How nurses have or have not handled their own losses affects the ability to relate to patients. At times, nurses need compassionate detachment from patients and their families to become revitalized and often must find constructive outlets, such as exercise and music, to maintain equilibrium. An active support system consisting of nonjudgemental people who are not threatened by natural expressions of feelings is crucial. Proper channelling of these emotions can be a valuable part of the empathetic response to others. It is vital that nurses support one another in the work environment.

THE CHILD'S REACTION TO DEATH

Each child, like each adult, approaches death in an individual way, drawing on limited experience. Nurses must become well acquainted with patients and view them within the context of the family and social culture. Their anxiety often centres on symptoms. They fear that treatments may be painful. Nurses must be honest and inform patients about the upcoming procedures in terms the child will understand. Expressing feelings is encouraged by statements such as "You seem angry." Sufficient time should be given for a response. Children should be allowed to have as much control as possible regarding what happens to them; including them in decisions concerning their welfare fosters this control. However, the child should not be offered a choice when there is none. Children often communicate symbolically. The nurse needs to listen to what they say to adults, to their toys, and to other children. Crayons and paper can be provided for self-expression.

Although age is a factor, the child's level of cognitive development, rather than chronological age, affects the response to death. Children younger than 5 years of age are mainly concerned with separation from their parents and abandonment. Preschool children respond to questions about death by relying on their experience and by turning to fantasy. They may believe death is reversible or that they are in some way responsible. Children usually do not develop a realistic concept of death as a permanent biological process until 9 or 10 years of age.

Nursing Tip

Brothers and sisters often feel neglected and lonely when a sibling is dying. They are frustrated because they are unable to comfort their parents and loved ones. They need to be included in the plan of care.

Health Promotion

A Child's Response to a Sibling's Death

AGE	RESPONSE OR UNDERSTANDING	PARENTAL GUIDANCE
Infant	Does not understand concept of death; reacts on emotional level to anxiety of parents	Maintain normal routine. Use a support network to assist in care.
Preschooler	Thinks death is temporary; may blame self for sibling's death	Use accurate terms and simple explanations. Reassure child and *listen*.
School age	Realizes death is final; may be interested in details of death; may fear parents will die; may try to "take care of" parents	Respond to child's need for reassurance and security. Refer to death using accurate terms. Allow child to participate in funeral and feel useful.
Adolescent	Can understand abstract concept of death but has feelings of own immortality; may express anger at death of sibling	Accept adolescent's behaviour. Encourage communication and discussion.

Dying adolescents face conflicts between their treatment regimens and their need to establish independence from their parents and conformity with their peers. This combination can lead to anger and resentment, which are often displaced onto hospital staff members. An atmosphere of acceptance and nonjudgemental listening allows adolescents the freedom to vent their hostility in a nonthreatening environment. Nursing Care Plan 22.1 specifies nursing interventions for the dying child.

Box 22.5 Nurse's Role in Helping the Family Cope With the Dying Child

Listen. Giving advice is a reflection of the nurse's need to "solve the problem."
Provide privacy. Family members need to express their emotions and comfort one another without being embarrassed.
Provide therapeutic intervention. Assess coping behaviours and work with clergy and social workers to meet immediate needs for patient comfort and family coping.
Provide information. Avoid the tenseness of waiting for test results. Be truthful to the child and family.
Use appropriate phrases and open-ended questions and concrete statements. When speaking with a sibling of a child who has died, avoid using phrases such as "He isn't hurting anymore," "He is living with God," or "He has passed away." These terms are confusing to children; explanations should be short, direct, and truthful.

The Child's Awareness of Their Condition

Surprising as it may seem, many investigators have shown that terminally ill children are generally aware of their condition, even when it is carefully concealed. This is reflected in their drawings and play and can be detected through psychological testing. Failure to be honest with children leaves them to suffer alone, unable to express their fears and sadness, or even to say good-bye. The family should be referred as needed for support and social services.

STAGES OF DYING

The stages of dying as detailed by Kübler-Ross (1969)—*denial, anger, bargaining, depression, acceptance,* and *reaching out to help others*—can be applied to parents and siblings as well as to the sick child. It is important to accept and support each participant at whatever stage has been reached and to refrain from directing progress. Nurses should make themselves available for children and families, (Box 22.5).

Parents are encouraged to assist in the care of their child; hospice care and the movement toward home care can facilitate this assistance. It is therapeutic for children to be in their own surroundings whenever possible. Siblings involved in patient care feel less neglected, and the sacrifices they must make become more meaningful. Discussions before death allow them to make amends for their hostilities toward the sick child. The family's religious and spiritual philosophy can be a source of strength and support, as can caring neighbours and friends.

Nurses must observe signs of tension between parents so that suitable intervention may be implemented, as there is an increased rate of divorce of couples after the death of a child. Each parent grieves in an individual time and way, often making it difficult for spouses to be supportive of each other. The suppression of

Nursing Care Plan 22.1 The Dying Child

PATIENT DATA

The parents of a terminally ill school-age child sit stoic and silent at the bedside of their child. The child appears cranky and withdrawn and states he wants to go home and see his friends.

Selected Nursing Diagnosis Apprehension resulting from the potential death of child

Goals	Nursing Interventions	Rationales
Parents will express anxieties to the nurse on an ongoing basis.	Remain available to family as child grows weaker.	Nurse's presence provides support.
Communication among parents, other children, the patient, and nurse remain open.	Give parents permission to talk and grieve about the upcoming death and to think about funeral arrangements if they choose.	Helps to prepare family for the inevitable; sorts out and identifies actual sources of feelings.
	Involve siblings in plans for and progress of brother or sister.	Siblings will feel less isolated.
	Provide permission for laughter, play, friends (make every day count).	Laughter and play reduce tension.
	Suggest that overprotection and inordinate attention, even when provided out of love, can be detrimental to the dying child.	Child will feel more in control if not overprotected.
	Encourage family to maintain as normal a lifestyle as possible and encourage each member to take time for their own needs.	When all members are taking care of themselves, they will have more energy to cope with crises.
	Facilitate honesty about child's imminent death among family members and patient.	Information helps to relieve anxiety.
	Explain that family members often cannot support one another because each grieves in their own way.	Explaining this to the family helps to relieve the guilt stemming from irritability or anger.
	Recognize that grief is often expressed as anger.	Anger is a natural emotion; it does not provoke fear in itself, although its expression may. Family has a right to all feelings.
	Provide for ventilation of guilt (e.g., "If only I had taken her to the health care provider sooner").	Prevents accumulation or repression of guilt.
	Suggest meditation, progressive relaxation, and/or guided imagery.	Helps to reduce stress.

Selected Nursing Diagnosis Worry in the dying child as a result of pain, isolation, and lack of information

Goals	Nursing Interventions	Rationales
Child will verbalize feelings of comfort; if nonverbal, child rests comfortably, with no crying.	Administer pain relievers regularly. Do not wait until the child has pain.	Child may deny pain because of fear of treatment. Waiting until the child has pain is not an effective way to manage pain.
Child is not isolated.	Encourage parents to hold, cuddle, and touch their child as much as possible.	Reduces anxiety, thereby reducing pain.
	Encourage visits from friends and siblings as age appropriate.	Provides emotional support and distraction from the disease.
Child will verbalize understanding of treatment, procedures, and outcome as age appropriate.	Decorate hospital room with cards, pictures, mementos; provide telephone or electronic tablet as age appropriate.	Attractive environment promotes mental health.
	Investigate possibility of home or hospice care.	Familiar and stable environment may facilitate child's emotional healing.
	Explain all procedures.	Information relieves anxiety.
	Determine child's knowledge about impending death.	Nurse can determine level of understanding as age appropriate; this aids in communication.
	Answer all questions about death honestly; use open-ended questions to assist patient in the expression of feelings.	Conveys that all feelings are acceptable.
	Listen to what child says during play.	Children work through many fears in play.
	Assist child in drawing "a wish," "yesterday, today, tomorrow."	Drawings promote release of feelings and provide a means of communication.
	Allow the child to grieve (behaviour may be sulky, cranky, withdrawn).	Therapeutic grieving prevents depression.

Nursing Care Plan 22.1 The Dying Child—cont'd

Selected Nursing Diagnosis Grieving among family members as a result of death of child

Goals	Nursing Interventions	Rationales
Family members will have an opportunity to say good-bye. Family members will express feelings of grief, fear, anger, loss, and guilt.	Provide time for family to be alone with the dead child as desired. Remain available; express your own loss and grief. Assist parents in making decisions. Offer a beverage. Determine spiritual need; refer to pastoral counselling if desired. Respect family's beliefs, worldview, and philosophy. Listen to expressions of grief.	Family needs to say good-bye. Parents derive comfort from knowing others loved their child. Even a simple decision such as when to telephone relatives becomes monumental at this stage. Denotes concern. A belief in a higher being provides strength for many persons; pastoral counsellors are effective. Supporting beliefs keeps the lines of communication open and provides a supportive relationship. Family needs to repeat story to work through grief.

CRITICAL THINKING QUESTION

1. The parents of a child dying from a terminal illness stay in the corner of the child's room, hugging each other and crying. What would be the best nursing intervention?

strong feelings of guilt, helplessness, and outrage can be devastating. Feelings left unexpressed can cause depression, physical illness, or both.

Maintaining hope and helping patients to live until they die is the real challenge. While it is not appropriate to offer false hope, it is important to provide the child and family something to live for each day, whether it is a visit from a special friend or the absence of pain.

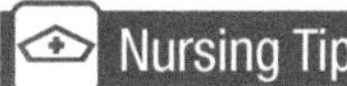

Nursing Tip

Grandparents, teachers, and friends are also grieving. Be alert for the emotional responses of all the significant others.

TREATMENT AND NURSING CARE

The nurse who provides palliative care to the child must ensure that symptoms are managed. Alleviation of symptoms reduces suffering of the child and family and allows them to focus on other concerns and participate in meaningful experiences (Ulrich, Duncan, Joselow, et al., 2016). Symptoms that are priorities for care include pain, fatigue, dyspnea, and skin care.

Pain

Effective pain relief is essential. See Chapter 19 for more discussion on pediatric pain management. The use of a nonopioid together with opioid analgesics may be required for more severe pain. Medications should be administered via the simplest, most effective, and least distressing route. Parents may require teaching regarding medication: The use of strong medications is not just for extreme situations or the very end of life; opioids do not have a "ceiling effect"; escalating symptoms may be treated with an increase in dose; and there are differences between tolerance, physical dependence, and addiction (Ulrich et al., 2016). Around-the-clock pain management is important to carry out, rather than waiting until symptoms get worse.

Fatigue

Fatigue is a common symptom in children with advanced illness and is a priority for nursing care. Some nonpharmacological methods to decrease fatigue include the following (Ulrich et al., 2016):

- Sleep hygiene (establish a routine, promote habits for restorative sleep)
- Regular, gentle exercise; prioritize or modify activities
- Address potentially contributing factors (e.g., anemia, depression, adverse effects of medications)
- Use of aromatherapy (peppermint, rosemary, basil)

Dyspnea

Dyspnea, or the feeling of shortness of breath, may have multiple causes in the dying child. Dyspnea can be relieved with the use of regularly scheduled and as-needed doses of opioids. Opioids work directly on the brainstem to reduce the sensation of respiratory distress, as opposed to relieving dyspnea via sedation (Ulrich et al., 2016).

Skin Care

Good skin care is important when caring for the dying child. Frequent skin assessments and turning and repositioning help to alleviate pressure wherever possible.

Pruritus may be secondary to systemic disorders or medication therapy. Treatment includes avoiding excessive use of drying soaps, using moisturizers, trimming fingernails, and wearing loose-fitting clothing, in addition to administering topical or systemic steroids (Ulrich et al., 2016).

Physical Changes of Impending Death

The physical changes that occur with impending death include cool, mottled, cyanotic skin and the slowing of all body processes. There may be a loss of consciousness, but hearing is intact. Rales in the chest may be heard, which result from increased secretions pooling in the lungs. Movement and neurological signs lessen. If thrashing or groaning occurs, the patient is assessed for pain, and pain relief should be provided. Family members need to have these changes explained to them so they understand what is occurring.

Get Ready for the Certification Examination!

Key Points

- Children who are chronically ill must be aided in mastering developmental tasks.
- Care for the chronically ill child requires an interdisciplinary approach where the child and the family are the experts in the care.
- The family of a child with a chronic illness must be supported and provided with information to help them cope.
- Respite care for families who have a child with a chronic illness is important to help the family have time to focus on other things besides the ill child.
- Cerebral palsy is a nonprogressive muscular weakness that can have a significant impact on the life of the child and family.
- The four types of cerebral palsy are spastic, athetoid, ataxic, and mixed.
- Many children with spastic quadriplegia have average intelligence.
- Computer technology can help the physically impaired child communicate and achieve mobility.
- Intellectual disability involves three components: intelligence, adaptive behaviour, and failure to meet developmental milestones, with onset before 18 years of age.
- Palliative care is an interdisciplinary approach that should be initiated early in the care of a child with a life-threatening illness.
- The stages of dying according to Kübler-Ross include denial, anger, bargaining, depression, acceptance, and reaching out to help others.
- The nurse can help the family of a dying child by listening and assessing their needs, reinforcing information, providing privacy, and using appropriate phrases and open-ended, concrete questions and statements.

Additional Learning Resources

evolve Go to your Evolve website (http://evolve.elsevier.com/Canada/Leifer) for the following learning resources:

- Answer Key for Critical Thinking Questions
- Answer Key for Textbook Review Questions
- Audio Glossary
- Interactive Review Questions
- Skills Performance Checklists
- Video clips and more!

Online Resources

- Canadian Hospice Palliative Care Association, *Pediatric Hospice Palliative Care: Guiding Principles and Norms of Practice:* http://www.chpca.net/media/7841/Pediatric_Norms_of_Practice_March_31_2006_English.pdf
- Canadian Network of Palliative Care for Children: http://www.cnpcc.ca
- Canuck Place: Children's Hospice in BC: www.canuckplace.org
- Chronic Disease Prevention Alliance of Canada: http://www.cdpac.ca/
- Darling Home for Kids: A Children's Hospice/Respite Experience: https://www.darlinghomeforkids.ca
- Easter Seals Canada: https://easterseals.ca/english/
- Emily's House: A Special Place for Kids: www.emilyshouse.ca
- Government of Canada, *Child Disability Benefit:* https://www.canada.ca/en/revenue-agency/services/child-family-benefits/child-disability-benefit.html
- Life & Death Matters: https://www.lifeanddeathmatters.ca
- Provincial Health Services Authority, *Living Well With Chronic Illness:* http://www.phsa.ca/health-info/living-with-illness
- Roger Neilson house (pediatric palliative care services in Eastern Ontario): https://rogerneilsonhouse.ca/
- Ronald McDonald House (homes where families of sick children can stay while their children are hospitalized): https://www.rmhccanada.ca/what-we-do

Review Questions

1. Which of the following is a positive example of support for a family with a child diagnosed with a chronic condition?
   a. Encourage the family to always be cheerful.
   b. Transfer care of the child to a group home indefinitely.

Get Ready for the Certification Examination!—Cont'd

c. Insist that the parents use respite supports daily.
d. Encourage friends to deliver meals to the home of the family.

2. At the local public health clinic, a community health nurse leads a support group for adolescents with chronic conditions. Discussions often focus on peer relationships and which directions the adolescents want to take in school and in life. The community health nurse knows that these adolescents are in which phase of Erikson's psychosocial development?
   a. Identity versus role confusion
   b. Relationship experimentation
   c. Adolescent rebellion
   d. Intimacy versus solidarity
3. While speaking with the parents of a child with a chronic condition, what should a nurse identify as an appropriate goal of care for the child?
   a. Encourage the child to participate in self-care activities as possible.
   b. Teach the child something new every day.
   c. Encourage more lenient behaviour limits for the child.
   d. Achieve age-appropriate social skills.
4. Which nursing interventions will facilitate self-care in the child with a chronic illness who requires repeated hospitalizations? *(Select all that apply.)*
   a. Teach the school-age child how to use an inhaler.
   b. Teach the preschool-age child a simple task, such as hand hygiene.
   c. Encourage the adolescent to assume more responsibility for their daily care.
   d. Ask the toddler to select a site for insulin injections.
   e. Encourage parents to join support groups to facilitate coping.

Critical Thinking Questions

1. If parents approached a nurse asking if they should take their dying child home from the hospital, what would an appropriate response of the nurse be? What factors need to be considered?
2. What factors should be considered when assessing the growth and development of children with chronic conditions?
3. What are some activities that a parent can do with a school-age child with a chronic condition at home that could contribute to a sense of industry?

REFERENCES

Beacham, B. L., & Deatrick, J. A. (2015). Children with chronic conditions: Perspectives on condition management. *Journal of Pediatric Nursing, 30*(1), 25–35. http://doi.org/10.1016/j.pedn.2014.10.011.

Berglund, M. (2014). Learning turning points—in life with long-term illness—visualized with the help of the life-world philosophy. *International Journal of Qualitative Studies on Health and Well-being, 21*(9). https://doi.org/10.3402/qhw.v9.22842.

Bowden, V., & Smith Greenberg, C. (2010). *Children and their families; The continuum of care* (2nd ed.). Philadelphia: Wolters Kluwer Lippincott Williams & Wilkins.

Breneol, S., Belliveau, J., Cassidy, C., et al. (2017). Strategies to support transitions from hospital to home for children with medical complexity: A scoping review. *International Journal of Nursing Studies, 72*, 91–104. https://doi.org/10.1016/j.ijnurstu.2017.04.01.

Carter, B., Bray, L., Sanders, C., et al. (2016). "Knowing the places of care": How nurses facilitate transition of children with complex health care needs from hospital to home. *Comprehensive Child and Adolescent Nursing, 39*(2), 139–153. https://doi.org/10.3109/01460862.2015.1134721.

Cohen, E., Kuo, D., Agrawal, R., et al. (2011). Children with medical complexity: An emerging population for clinical and research initiatives. *Pediatrics, 127*(3), e1463–e1470. https://doi.org/10.1542/peds.2012-0175.

Cohen, E., Lacombe-Duncan, A., Spalding, K., et al. (2012). Integrated complex care coordination for children with medical complexity: A mixed-methods evaluation of tertiary care-community collaboration. *BMC Health Services Research, 12*(366). https://doi.org/10.1186/1472-6963-12-366.

Coughlin, M. B., & Sethares, K. A. (2017). Chronic sorrow in parents of children with a chronic illness or disability: An integrative literature review. *Journal of Pediatric Nursing, 37*, 108–116.

Drutchas, A., & Anandarajah, G. (2014). Spirituality and coping with chronic disease in pediatrics. *Rhode Island Medical Journal, 97*(3), 26–30.

Fayed, N., Kraus de Camargo, O., Elahi, I., et al. (2014). Patient-important activity and participation outcomes in clinical trials involving children with chronic conditions. *Quality of Life Research, 23*(3), 751–757. https://doi.org/10.1007/s11136-013-0483-9.

Freeborn, D., Dyches, T., Roper, S., et al. (2013). Identifying challenges of living with type 1 diabetes: Child and youth perspectives. *Journal of Clinical Nursing, 22*(13-14), 1890–1898. https://doi.org/10.1111/jocn.12046.

Gauntlett-Gilbert, J., & Connell, H. (2012). Coping and acceptance in chronic childhood conditions. *Psychologist, 25*, 198–201.

Government of Canada. (2018). *Rights of people with disabilities*. Retrieved from: https://www.canada.ca/en/canadian-heritage/services/rights-people-disabilities.html.

Johnston, M. (2016). Cerebral palsy. In R. M. Kliegman, B. F. Stanton, J. W. St. Geme, et al. (Eds.), *Nelson textbook of pediatrics* (20th ed.). Philadelphia: Saunders.

Kelo, M., Eriksson, E., & Eriksson, I. (2013). Perceptions of patient education during hospital visit—described by school-age children with a chronic illness and their parents. *Scandinavian Journal of Caring Sciences, 27*(4), 894–904. https://doi.org/10.1111/scs.12001.

King, G., & Chiarello, L. (2014). Family-centered care for children with cerebral palsy: Conceptual and practical considerations to advance care and practice. *Journal of Child Neurology, 29*(8), 1046–1054. https://doi.org/10.1177/0883073814533009.

Kirk, S., Beatty, S., Callery, P., et al. (2012). Perceptions of effective self-care support for children and young people with long-term conditions. *Journal of Clinical Nursing, 21*, 1974–1987. https://doi.org/10.1111/j.1365-2702.2011.04027.x.

Klein, B., & Canadian Paediatric Society (CPS), Mental Health and Developmental Disabilities Committee. (2016). Mental health problems in children with neuromotor disabilities. *Paediatrics & Child Health, 21*(2), 93–96.

Knafl, K., Deatrick, J., & Havill, N. (2012). Continued development of the family management style framework. *Journal of Family Nursing, 18,* 11–34. https://doi.org/10.1177/1074840711427294.

Knafl, K., Deatrick, J., Knafl, G., et al. (2013). Patterns of family management of childhood chronic conditions and their relationship to child and family functioning. *Journal of Pediatric Nursing, 28,* 523–535. https://doi.org/10.1016/j.pedn.2013.03.006.

Kohen, D., Uppal, S., Khan, S., et al. (2010). *Access and barriers to educational services for Canadian children with disabilities.* Ottawa: Canadian Council on Learning. Retrieved from: http://en.copian.ca/library/research/ccl/access_barriers/access_barriers.pdf.

Kübler-Ross, E. (1969). *On death and dying.* New York: Routledge.

Lambert, V., & Keogh, D. (2015). Striving to live a normal life: A review of children and young people's experience of feeling different when living with a long-term condition. *Journal of Pediatric Nursing: Nursing Care of Children and Families, 30*(1), 63–77.

Lewis, A., & Parsons, S. (2008). Understanding of epilepsy by children and young people with epilepsy. *European Journal of Special Needs Education, 23*(4), 321–335. https://doi.org/10.1080/08856250802387273.

Marshall, M., Carter, B., Rose, K., et al. (2009). Living with type 1 diabetes: Perceptions of children and their parents. *Journal of Clinical Nursing, 18*(12), 1703–1710.

Petersson, C., Simeonsson, R., Enskar, K., et al. (2013). Comparing children's self-report instruments for health-related quality of life using the International Classification of Functioning, Disability and Health for Children and Youth (ICF-CY). *Health and Quality of Life Outcomes, 11,* 75. https://doi.org/10.1186/1477-7525-11-75.

Pinzon, J., Harvey, J., & Canadian Paediatric Society (CPS), Adolescent Health Committee. (2006). Care of adolescents with chronic conditions. *Paediatrics & Child Health, 11*(1), 43–48. Reaffirmed 2018.

Public Health Agency of Canada (PHAC). (2017). The 2017 Canadian chronic disease indicators. *Health Promotion and Chronic Disease Prevention in Canada, 37*(8), 248–251 https://doi.org/10.24095/hpcdp.37.8.03.

Ray, L. D. (2002). Parenting and childhood chronicity: Making visible the invisible work. *Journal of Pediatric Nursing, 17*(6), 424–438.

Rifshana, F., Breheny, M., Taylor, J., et al. (2017). The parental experience of caring for a child with type 1 diabetes. *Journal of Child and Family Studies, 26*(11), 3226–3236. https://doi.org/10.1007/s10826-017-0806-5.

Santos, S., Crespo, C., Silva, N., et al. (2012). Quality of life and adjustment in youths with asthma: The contributions of family rituals and the family environment. *Family Process, 51*(4), 557–569. https://doi.org/10.1111/j.1545-5300.2012.01416.x.

Shapiro, C., Kilburn, J., & Hardin, J. (2014). Prevention of behavior problems in a selected population: Stepping Stones Triple P for parents of young children with disabilities. *Research in Developmental Disabilities, 35*(11), 2958–2975. https://doi.org/10.1016/j.ridd.2014.07.036.

Sherman, B. R. (1995). Impact of home-based respite care on families of children with chronic illnesses. *Children's Health Care, 24*(1), 33–45.

Spencer, J., Cooper, H., & Milton, B. (2013). The lived experiences of young people (13–16 years) with type 1 diabetes mellitus and their parents—A qualitative phenomenological study. *Diabetic Medicine, 30*(1), e17–e24. https://doi.org/10.1111/dme.12021.

Statistics Canada. (2008). *Educational services and the disabled child.* Retrieved from: http://www.statcan.gc.ca/pub/81-004-x/2006005/9588-eng.htm.

Tétreault, S., Blais-Michaud, S., Marier Deschênes, P., et al. (2014). Support to families of children with disabilities. *Child & Family Social Work, 19,* 272–281. https://doi.org/10.1111/j.1365-2206.2012.00898.x.

Tsai, E., Canadian Paediatric Society (CPS), & Bioethics Committee. (2008). Advance care planning for paediatric patients. *Paediatrics & Child Health, 13*(9), 791–796. Reaffirmed in 2018. Retrieved from: https://www.cps.ca/en/documents/position/advance-care-planning.

Ulrich, C., Duncan, J., Joselow, M., et al. (2016). Pediatric palliative care. In R. M. Kliegman, B. F. Stanton, J. W. St. Geme, et al. (Eds.), *Nelson textbook of pediatrics* (20th ed.). Philadelphia: Saunders.

van der Lee, J., Mokkink, L., Grootenhuis, M., et al. (2007). Definitions and measurement of chronic health conditions in childhood: A systematic review. *JAMA: Journal of the American Medical Association, 297*(24), 2741–2751.

World Health Organization (WHO). (2018a). *Global forum on chronic diseases prevention and control.* Retrieved from: http://www.who.int/chp/about/global_forum/en/.

World Health Organization (WHO). (2018b). *Palliative care.* Retrieved from: http://www.who.int/news-room/fact-sheets/detail/palliative-care.

23 The Child With an Eye, Ear, or Neurological Condition

http://evolve.elsevier.com/Canada/Leifer

Ivanna Yau

Objectives

1. Define each key term listed.
2. Discuss the cause and treatment of external eye and periorbital disorders.
3. Compare the treatment of paralytic and nonparalytic strabismus.
4. Review eye disorders that require immediate medical attention.
5. Discuss the prevention and treatment of external and middle ear infections.
6. Outline the nursing approach to serving the hearing-impaired child.
7. Provide an overview of the nervous system.
8. Describe the components of a neurological assessment.
9. Discuss neurological monitoring specific to infants and children.
10. Outline the approach to altered mental status and the approach to spinal assessment.
11. Describe the symptoms and management of spina bifida in a child.
12. Describe signs of meningitis and encephalitis in a child.
13. Describe the management of care of a child with hydrocephalus.
14. Discuss the classification of seizures and potential triggers.
15. Prepare a plan for seizure first aid and seizure safety.
16. Describe conditions that can mimic seizures in children.
17. Discuss the management of acute head injury and submersion injuries.

Key Terms

amblyopia (ăm-blē-Ō-pē-ă)
barotrauma
blepharitis
clonic movement
concussion
conjunctivitis
encephalitis
enucleation (ē-nū-klē-Ā-shŭn)
epicanthal folds
extensor posturing
flexor posturing
habilitation
hydrocephalus
hyperopia (hī-pŭr-Ō-pē-ă)
intracranial pressure (ICP)
ketogenic diet
meningitis
meningocele
meningomyelocele
myopia
myringotomy (mĭr-ĭng-GŎT-ŏ-mē)
neurological assessment
nystagmus (nĭs-TĂG-mŭs)
opisthotonos (ō-pĭs-THŎT-ō-nŏs)
papilledema (păp-ĭl-ă-DĒ-mă)
postictal (pōst-ĬK-tăl)
posturing
proptsis
sepsis (SĔP-sĭs)
shaken baby syndrome
shunt
sign language
spina bifida
status epilepticus
strabismus (stră-BĬZ-mŭs)
stye
tonic movement

THE EYES

The eye is the organ of vision. The anatomy of the eyeball is depicted in Fig. 23.1. Vision is a complex process beginning with receptors in both eyes, a lens system that focuses light on those receptors, and a network of nerves for conducting impulses from the receptors to the brain. Visual dysfunction can be caused by abnormal ocular movements or alterations in visual acuity, lens refraction, colour vision or accommodation, or secondary to neurological insult.

The eyes begin to develop as an outgrowth of the forebrain in the 4-week-old embryo. The retinal vessels vascularize (develop) at 40 weeks of gestation; therefore, infants born prematurely often have vision problems throughout their lives. At birth, the eye is 65% of adult size. The newborn's sight is not mature, but the newborn can see. Visual acuity is estimated to be in the range of 20/400. This improves rapidly and may reach 20/40 to 20/30 by 2 or 3 years of age and 20/20 by 6 or 7 years of age. The shape of the newborn's eye is less spherical than the adult's eye. Newborns keep their eyes closed most of the day, can focus and fixate on objects 12 to 30 cm (8 to 12 inches) away for only a few seconds at a time, and cannot coordinate or follow

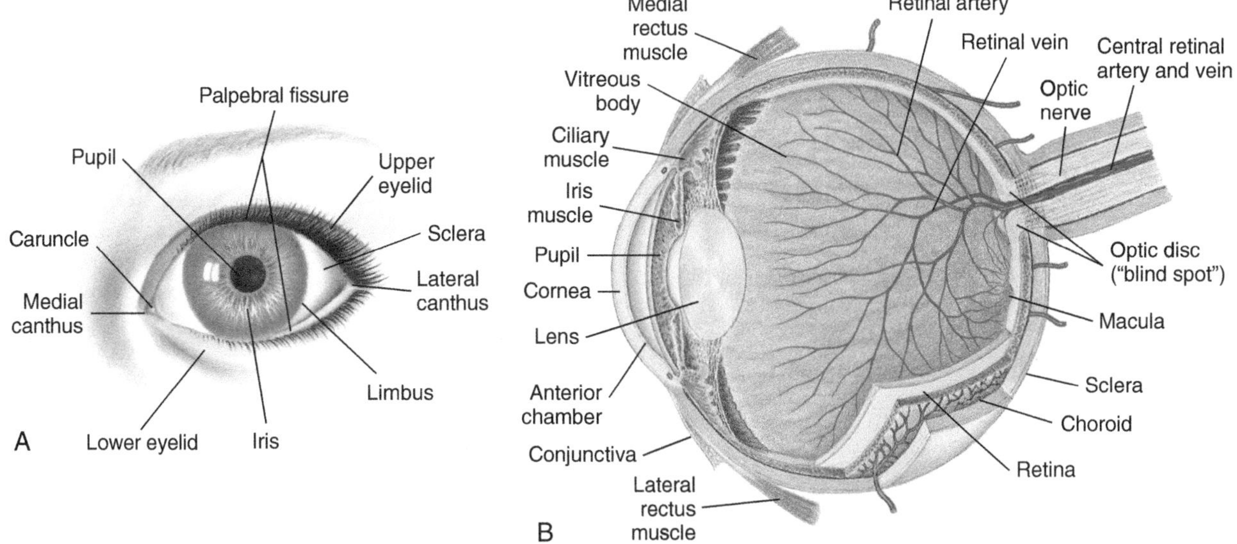

Fig. 23.1 The normal eye. **A,** External view. **B,** Internal view showing relationship of the optic nerve, eye muscles, and chambers of the eye. (**A,** from Hockenberry, M., & Wilson, D. [2011]. *Wong's nursing care of infants and children* [9th ed.]. St. Louis: Mosby. **B,** from Seidel, H. M., Ball, J. W., Dains, J. E., & Benedict, G. W. [2003]. *Mosby's guide to physical examination* [5th ed.]. St. Louis: Mosby.)

without turning their heads. By 2 to 4 months of age infants can move their eyes to follow people or objects that may be 2 metres away. By 4 to 5 months their eyes are open most of the day, and the tears, when the infant is crying, can be seen to overflow onto the face (visible tears). Eye–hand coordination also develops. The nurse should document this, because the ability to transfer objects from one hand to another is partially dependent on the ability to see the object. Depth perception is not developed until 9 months of age. When the child walks or runs, visual depth perception influences the child's ability to run without falling.

The Canadian Paediatric Society (CPS) recommends that all children between 3 and 5 years of age undergo preschool visual screening during well-child visits and whenever concerns arise (Amit & CPS Community Paediatrics Committee, 2009/2018). Risk factors for visual problems may include familial blindness, genetic syndromes, maternal infection in pregnancy, prematurity, structural abnormalities of the orbit or central nervous system, systemic disease such as diabetes, inflammatory diseases, eye and head trauma, or acquired brain injury.

Nursing Tip

At birth, the quiet, alert infant will respond to visual stimuli by ceasing to move. Visual responsiveness to the mother during feeding is noted. The infant's ability to focus and follow objects in the first months of life should be documented. Coordination of eye movements should be achieved by 3 to 6 months of age.

Behaviours that may indicate visual problems in children include the following:

- Lack of fixation or hand regard
- Holding objects closely
- Covering or shutting one eye
- Tilting one's head
- Excessive blinking or rubbing of eyes

On physical examination, the nurse observes the eyes to see if they are symmetrical and are an equal distance from the nose. **Epicanthal folds** (*epi*, "upon," and *canthus*, "angle") are folds of skin that extend on either side of the bridge of the nose and cover the inner eye canthus. Some folds are broad and cover a large portion of the inner eye, causing the eye to appear crossed. Large epicanthal folds occur as part of some chromosomal factors (e.g., Down syndrome). Pupils are observed for size, shape, and movement. By shining a penlight into the eye and then quickly removing it the nurse can observe the eyes' reaction to light. The healthy pupil constricts (gets smaller) as the light approaches and dilates (gets larger) as it disappears (Fig. 23.2). Older children should be given explanations concerning the examination. The nurse should assess and document the general appearance of the child as well as achievement of developmental milestones. Assessment includes observing for symmetry of the eye orbit and eyelids, excessive tearing, squeezing of the eyelids, and strabismus (crossed eyes).

Nursing Tip

The achievement of developmental milestones such as transferring objects from hand to hand is partially dependent on seeing the object. Therefore, assessment of visual ability is part of assessment of growth and development.

CONDITIONS OF THE EYE

Table 23.1 lists conditions of the eye that require a referral to a health care provider. Retinopathy of prematurity (ROP) is discussed in Chapter 12.

External Eye Structures Conditions

External structures that protect the eye include the eyelids, conjunctivae, and the lacrimal apparatus.

Infection and inflammatory responses are the most common conditions affecting these supporting structures. Redness, edema, and itching are common symptoms related to inflammation of the eyelids known as **blepharitis**. This is typically caused by *Staphylococcus aureus* or seborrheic dermatitis. A **stye** (hordeolum) is an infection of the sebaceous glands of the eyelids (see Fig. 30.2). These are usually treated symptomatically with warm compresses.

Conjunctivitis

Conjunctivitis (*conjungere,* "to join together," and *itis,* "inflammation") is an inflammation of the conjunctiva, which is the mucous membrane that lines the eyelids (Fig. 23.3). A wide range of bacterial and viral agents, allergens, irritants, toxins, and systemic diseases can cause conjunctivitis. Conjunctivitis that occurs with viral exanthems such as measles is usually self-limiting. It is common in childhood and may be infectious or noninfectious. The acute, infectious form is commonly referred to as *pinkeye.* Pinkeye is no longer considered contagious after 24 hours of appropriate antimicrobial therapy. Conjunctivitis can also result from an obstruction of the lacrimal duct.

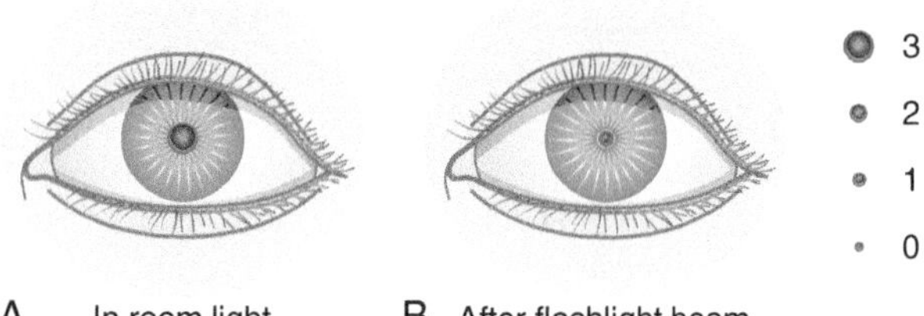

Fig. 23.2 The response of the pupil of the eye to a flashlight beam. **A,** The pupil of the eye is a *3* in room light. **B,** The pupil of the eye is a *1* after a flashlight beam is directed at the eye. The letters *B, S,* and *N* may be used to denote brisk movement, slow movement, or nonmovement of the pupil response, respectively. This illustration would be recorded "3/1 B." The other eye should respond symmetrically. Sluggish movement, nonmovement, or asymmetrical response should be reported immediately.

Table 23.1 Conditions of the Eye That Require Immediate Referral

SIGNS AND SYMPTOMS	POSSIBLE CONDITIONS
Irregular/ nonreactive pupils	Cranial nerve or brainstem dysfunction
White red reflex (leukocoria)	Retinoblastoma
Proptosis	Blunt trauma, penetrating injury, foreign body
Acute nystagmus	Central nervous system (CNS) disorder
Severe eye pain	Unresolved conjunctivitis, orbital cellulitis, or CNS disorder
Double or blurred vision	Orbital cellulitis or CNS disorder
Acute vision loss	Orbital cellulitis or CNS disorder

In general, the common forms of conjunctivitis respond to warm compresses and topical antibiotic eyedrops or eye ointments. Ointments blur vision and are not generally used during daytime hours in the ambulatory child. The nurse should instruct the parents to administer the eye medication for the prescribed time to prevent recurrence. Parents and older children are taught to wipe secretions from the *inner canthus downward and away from the opposite eye.* Because conjunctivitis spreads easily, affected children should use separate towels and be instructed to wash their hands frequently.

Ophthalmia neonatorum, an acute conjunctivitis in the newborn, is discussed in Chapter 6. Allergic conjunctivitis is often associated with allergic rhinitis (*rhin,* "nose," and *itis,* "inflammation") in children with hay fever. Symptoms include itching, tearing of one or both eyes, and edema of the eyelids and periorbital tissues. The child may appear distracted and irritable.

Dacryostenosis

Dacryostenosis is blockage of tear ducts that occurs in infants, typically owing to residual epithelial membranes that have not fully opened. This happens in 5 to 7% of newborns. Parents usually report excessive tearing with frequent mucous discharge in the medial canthal area. Lacrimal sac massage (gentle downward pressure to express contents of sac) is a traditional method used to unblock the tear ducts, although the dacryostenosis may resolve spontaneously. Referral to an ophthalmologist is indicated if there is no resolution by 12 months or repeated infections occur.

Periorbital Cellulitis

An infection of the eyelid and tissues surrounding the eye sometimes occurs in school-age children as a complication of bacterial sinusitis (inflammation of the sinus). Pain and swelling around the eye are common symptoms of periorbital cellulitis. Intravenous antibiotics may be required to prevent spread of the infection to the brain.

Hyphema

Hyphema, the presence of blood in the anterior chamber of the eye, is one of the most common ocular injuries. It can occur from either a blunt or perforating

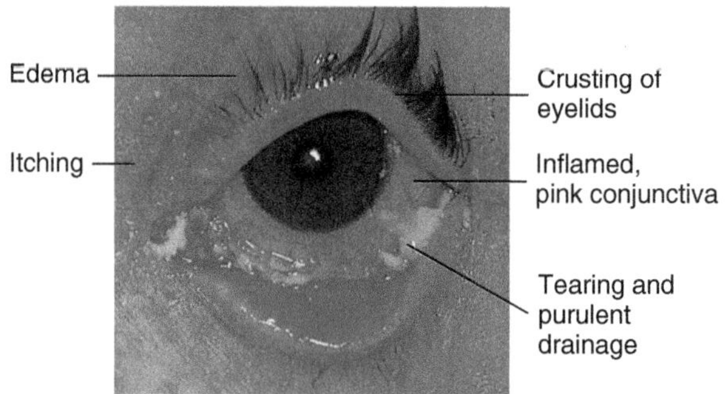

Fig. 23.3 Acute bacterial conjunctivitis. Signs of conjunctivitis are evident in this highly contagious infection. (From Newell, F. W. [1992]. *Ophthalmology: Principles and concepts* [7th ed.]. St. Louis: Mosby.)

injury. Blows from flying objects (e.g., baseballs, snowballs) and forceful coughing or sneezing can cause this condition. These accidents are common among active school-age children. Hyphema appears as a bright red or dark red spot in front of the lower portion of the iris.

Treatment includes bed rest and topical medication. The head of the bed is elevated 30 to 45 degrees to decrease intraocular pressure and decrease intracranial pressure if there is an associated head injury. The use of nonsteroidal anti-inflammatory medications (NSAIDs) is contraindicated (Olitsky, Hug, Plummer, et al., 2016). The condition generally resolves itself without residual problems.

VISUAL ACUITY TESTS

The ability of an infant to fixate and focus on an object can be demonstrated by 6 weeks of age. The object should not emit a sound so it can be determined that the infant is turning toward a sight stimulus rather than a sound stimulus.

There are a variety of visual acuity charts (Fig. 23.4, *A*). The Snellen alphabet chart and the Snellen E version for preschoolers who have not learned the alphabet are commonly used to assess the ability of young children to see near and far objects. Picture cards are also useful for children who do not know letters. Visual acuity can be tested by 2½ to 3 years of age (see Fig. 23.4, *B*).

The Titmus machine is often used for school-age children and adolescents. Directions for testing are standardized and must be carefully adhered to for proper results. Computerized tests, such as the random-dot stereogram, are also useful in the visual

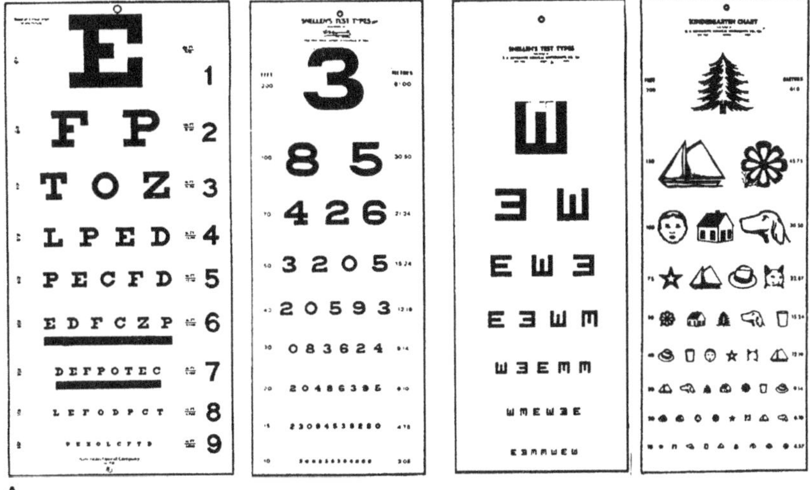

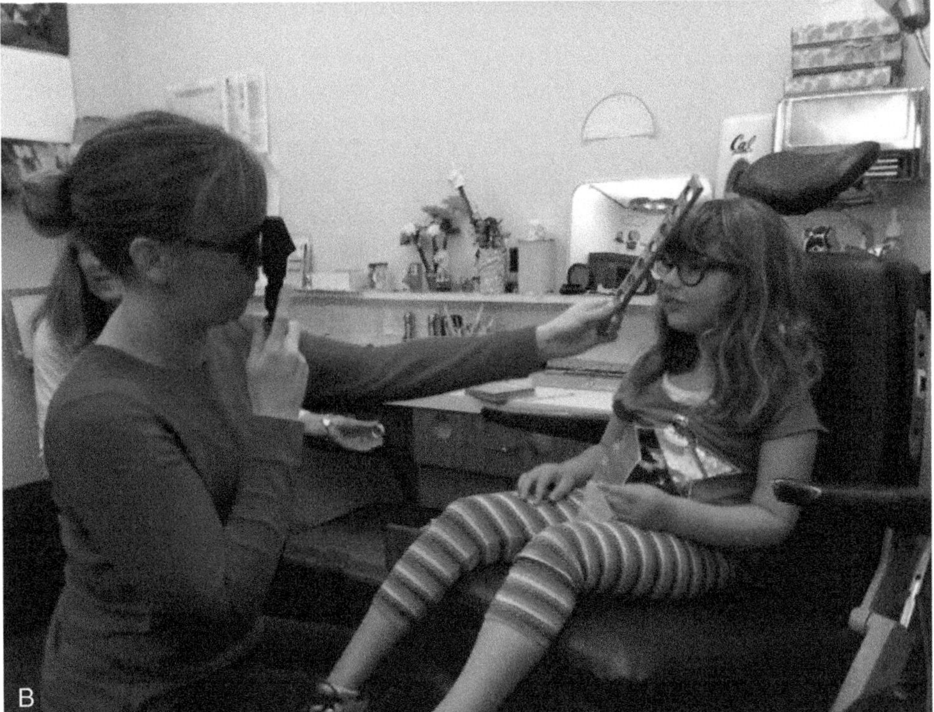

Fig. 23.4 **A,** Various types of visual acuity charts. The "E" chart is often used for young children who can "show which way the fingers of the *E* are pointing." **B,** A 3-year-old child responds to a detailed vision assessment.

screening of children. Visual acuity is important in the learning process.

Treatment and Nursing Care

Early detection and prompt treatment of visual disturbances are essential. The goal of treatment is to obtain normal and equal vision in each eye. Treatment consists of eyeglasses for significant refractive errors such as hyperopia (farsightedness) and myopia (nearsightedness), and patching (occlusion) of the *good eye.* The good eye is patched to force the use of the affected eye. Daytime patching may be tried first, since part-time occlusion is sufficient in some cases. Occlusion therapy is often difficult to maintain. The nurse can help by explaining to the child and parents the importance of the procedure. In some cases atropine eye drops are given to blur the vision in the better eye (Olitsky et al., 2016). The nurse also needs to provide the child emotional support, as some children may be subject to teasing by peers.

VISUAL DYSFUNCTION

Strabismus

Strabismus (cross eyes) is the deviation of one eye from the other when looking directly at something. Strabismus is caused by hypertonic or weak muscles in one of the eyes. The deviation can be inward, outward, upward, or downward, causing misalignment. Although strabismus is common in the newborn, if it continues to persist after 9 months of age, early intervention is required to prevent amblyopia (also known as "lazy eye"), which causes reduction or loss of visual acuity. This results as misaligned eyes project two images to the brain instead of one. The brain responds by favouring one vision and shutting down the other, which, if left untreated, can become permanent.

Pathophysiology

There are two types of strabismus. *Nonparalytic strabismus* (concomitant) is most common and involves a constant deviation in the gaze. Here the extraocular muscles are generally weak but not isolated to one muscle in particular. *Paralytic strabismus* (incomitant) involves a paralysis or weakness of an extraocular muscle (Scott, 2015). Double vision is experienced. Deviation of the gaze occurs with movement, when the eye attempts to focus. To prevent double vision *(diplopia)* the child will tilt their head or squint when focusing on an object. Visual exercises or surgery may be required to restore muscle balance. Strabismus may be present at birth or may manifest after a disease or injury. Acute strabismus that occurs after a head trauma may indicate cranial nerve damage.

Early intervention is associated with improved outcomes. One commonly accepted diagnostic sign is that vision in the normal eye is at least two Snellen lines (on E charts) better than that in the affected eye. Symptom onset may be present from birth or develop later; 50% by 1 year, or 80% by age 4 years for nonparalytic strabismus (Govindan, Mohney, Diehl, et al., 2005).

Nursing Tip

Symptoms of strabismus include the following:
- Eye "squinting" or frowning to focus
- Reaching for objects and missing them
- Covering one eye to see
- Tilting the head to see
- Dizziness and/or headache

Treatment

In nonparalytic strabismus, the refractory error is usually corrected with eyeglasses. When paralytic strabismus is seen during early infancy, the health care provider may recommend that a patch cover the unaffected eye until the infant is old enough to wear glasses. The affected eye may improve through use of the patch and often becomes normal. Eye exercises and glasses are effective ways of treating the condition medically. If they do not help, surgery is considered. It is generally performed when the child is 3 or 4 years of age.

Nursing care

The child undergoing surgery for strabismus might be hospitalized for only a brief period. The surgery involves structures outside the eyeball; therefore, the child is allowed to be up and about postoperatively. Eye dressings are kept at a minimum, and the child is encouraged to not touch the dressings.

Retinoblastoma

Retinoblastoma is a malignant tumour of the retina of the eye.

Pathophysiology

There are hereditary and spontaneous forms of retinoblastoma. The average ages at diagnosis are 15 months for bilateral tumours and 27 months for unilateral tumours (Olitsky et al., 2016). Gene-mapping techniques have shown chromosome 13 to be affected in hereditary forms. Chromosome 13 is known to cause other congenital defects as well.

Manifestations

A yellowish white reflex is seen in the pupil because of a tumour behind the lens. This is called the *cat's eye reflex* or *leukokoria* (*leuk,* "white," and *kore,* "pupil"). This may be accompanied by loss of vision, strabismus, hyphema, and, in advanced tumours, pain. Metastasis to the unaffected eye is common in unilateral tumours. When retinoblastoma is suspected in children, an examination is performed using an anaesthetic so the pediatric ophthalmologist may carefully examine the fundus of the eye.

Treatment and nursing care

The standard treatment for unilateral disease is enucleation (removal) of the eye if there is no possibility of saving the vision. Small tumours are treated with laser photocoagulation to destroy the blood vessels supplying the tumour. Larger tumours can be treated with systemic chemotherapy followed by laser therapy, cryotherapy, and brachytherapy (Olitsky et al., 2016).

On return from enucleation surgery, the child has a large pressure dressing on the eye. Elbow immobilizers may be necessary to prevent removal of the dressing. The bandage is observed for bleeding, and the vital signs are assessed. After a few days, the surgeon removes the dressing and applies an eye patch. Other structures of the eye, such as the lids, lashes, and tear glands, are not affected. An eye prosthesis is fitted when the socket has healed. Instructions for care of the prosthesis are provided at the time of final fitting. Providing education and emotional support for the child and family and referral to the multidisciplinary health care team is essential (Canadian Retinoblastoma Society, 2009).

THE EARS

Fig. 23.5 summarizes ear, eye, and neurological differences between children and adults. The three divisions of the ear are the external ear, the middle ear, and the inner ear (the latter is involved in both hearing and equilibrium) (Fig. 23.6). The fetus can hear at 20 weeks' gestation and the auditory nerve function has matured by 5 months of age. In the newborn, the tympanic membrane is almost horizontal and is more vascular than in the adult. It has a dull and opaque appearance and an inconsistent light reflex. The eustachian tube is shorter and straighter in the infant than in the adult. Three functions of the eustachian tube are *ventilation* of the middle ear, *protection* from nasopharyngeal secretions and sound pressure, and *drainage*. Middle-ear infections are common during early childhood.

To examine the ear, the nurse observes both its exterior and interior. Ear alignment should be observed. The top of the ear should cross an imaginary line drawn from the outer canthus of the eye to the occiput (see Fig. 11.9). Low-set ears may be associated with genetic disorders and intellectual or developmental disabilities. The outer ear and the area around it are inspected for drainage. The inside of the outer ear is examined with an otoscope.

One method of holding the child when assisting with examination of the ear is to lay the child on a table with the arms held alongside the head, which is turned to the side. Another method of positioning a child for an ear examination is to place the child in the lap of the adult and immobilize the child's head (see Fig. 20.5, *A*).

DISORDERS AND DYSFUNCTION OF THE EAR

Excessive or Impacted Cerumen

Cerumen (ear wax) is a protective substance that coats the ear canal. Overzealous cleaning with cotton-tipped applicators is the most common cause of impaction. This can obscure visualization of the tympanic membrane during acute infection. Placing a few drops of

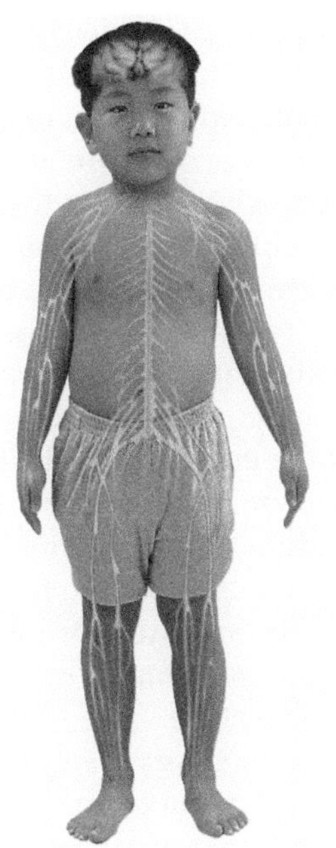

EARS

- The eustachian tube in infants is shorter, wider, and straighter than in older children and adults, and this may contribute to infections.
- In newborns and young infants, the walls of the ear canal are pliable because of underdeveloped cartilage and bony structures.

EYES

- Infants' eyes may occasionally cross until about 6 weeks of life.
- Tears are scant or absent for the first 2 to 4 weeks of life.

NERVOUS SYSTEM

- Brain and nerve cell growth and specialization are most rapid from birth until about 4 years of age.
- The suture lines and fontanelles of the infant allow for moulding during birth and also help compensate for increases in intracranial pressure.
- By the end of the first year, the brain has increased in weight about 2½ times. Brain growth is almost complete by 2 years of age. Measuring head circumference in infants helps determine neurological growth.
- Myelinization of nerve tracts in the central nervous system accelerates after birth and follows the cephalocaudal and proximodistal sequence. This allows for progressively more complex neurological and motor functions.

Fig. 23.5 Summary of the ear, eye, and neurological differences between the child and adult. (Art overlay courtesy Observatory Group, Cincinnati, Ohio.)

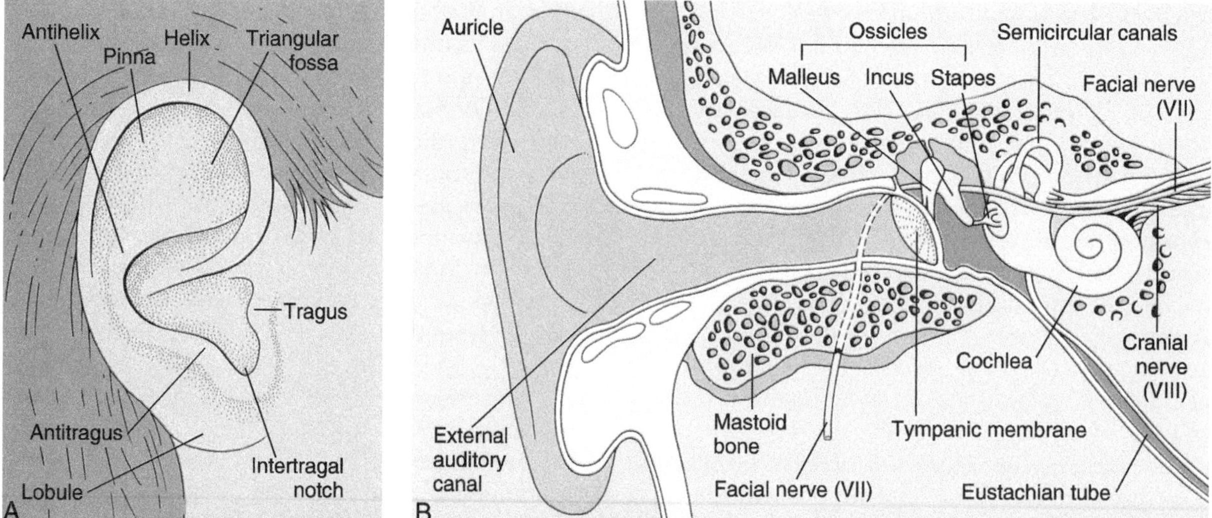

Fig. 23.6 Anatomy of the ear. **A,** The normal external ear—the auricle (pinna) and tragus—is shown with common landmarks labelled. **B,** There are three divisions of the ear: outer ear, middle ear, and inner ear. In the newborn, the mastoid process and the bony part of the external canal are not fully developed, leaving the tympanic membrane vulnerable to injury. The eustachian tube connects the middle ear and the pharynx, and it serves to vent the middle ear. (From Zitelli, B. J., McIntire, S., & Nowalk, A. [Eds.]. [2012]. *Atlas of pediatric physical diagnosis* [6th ed.]. St. Louis: Saunders.)

mineral oil in the canal for 20 minutes can help soften the wax for removal. Parents should be cautioned not to put anything into the ear canal.

Otitis Externa

An acute infection of the external ear canal is called *otitis externa* and is often referred to as *swimmer's ear,* because prolonged exposure to moisture is often the precipitating factor. Pain and tenderness on manipulating the pinna or tragus of the ear are specific signs of this type of infection. The ear canal may be erythematous, but the tympanic membrane is normal. A foreign body, cellulitis, diabetes mellitus, and herpes zoster should be ruled out. Irrigation and topical antibiotics or antivirals are the treatments of choice. The health care provider may insert a loose cotton gauze (wick) into the outer third of the ear canal. The wick is kept moist with frequent drops of the appropriate medicated solution.

Acute Otitis Media

Pathophysiology

Otitis media (OM) (*ot,* "ear," *itis,* "inflammation of," and *media,* "middle") is an inflammation of the middle ear. The middle ear is a tiny cavity in the temporal bone. Its entrance is guarded by the sensitive *tympanic membrane,* or *eardrum,* which transmits sound waves through the "oval window" to the inner ear, which contains the organs of hearing and balance. The middle ear opens into air spaces, or *sinuses,* in the mastoid process of the temporal bone. It is also connected to the throat by a channel called the *eustachian tube.* These structures—the mastoid sinuses, the middle ear, and the eustachian tube—are lined by mucous membranes. As a result, an infection of the throat can easily spread to the middle ear and can lead to mastoiditis. The eustachian tube also protects the middle ear from nasopharyngeal secretions, provides drainage of middle ear secretions into the nasopharynx, and equalizes air pressure between the middle ear and the outside atmosphere. These protective functions are diminished when the tubes are blocked. Unequalized air pressure within the ear creates a negative pressure that allows organisms to be swept up into the eustachian tube.

OM occurs most often after an upper respiratory tract infection and usually affects children between 6 and 36 months of age and in early childhood. It is caused by various organisms, of which *Streptococcus pneumoniae* and *Haemophilus influenzae* are the most common. Polyvalent pneumococcal polysaccharide vaccines have reduced the incidence of pneumococcal OM, but these vaccines are not effective in children less than 2 years of age because they are not capable of producing an antibody response.

Infants are more prone to middle ear infections than older children and adults because their eustachian tubes are shorter, wider, and straighter. When infants lie flat for long periods, microorganisms have easy access from the eustachian tube to the middle ear. Feeding methods may have a bearing on middle ear infection; for instance, the pooling of fluids such as milk in the throat of an infant who falls asleep with a bottle of milk provides a source for growth of organisms. The infant's humoral (*humor,* "body fluid") defense mechanisms are immature.

Children in passive smoking environments have more respiratory infections because of the effect of secondary smoke on the protective cilia that line the nose. Day care attendance can contribute to the risk of upper respiratory infections and OM because of increased exposure to ill children. Upper respiratory infections are discussed in detail in Chapter 25.

Nursing Tip

Signs and symptoms of ear infection can include the following:

- Fever
- Irritability
- Rubbing or pulling at the ear
- Rolling the head from side to side
- Hearing loss
- Loud speech
- Inattentive behaviour
- Articulation problems
- Speech development problems

Manifestations

The symptoms of OM are pain in the ear, which is often very severe; irritability; and diminished hearing. Fever, which may be as high as 40°C (104°F), headache, vomiting, diarrhea, and febrile seizures may also occur. Earaches in infants may be manifested by general irritability, frequent rubbing or pulling at the ear, and rolling of the head from side to side. The older child can point to the place that is tender. Visualization of the tympanic membrane via otoscope shows a reddened and bulging membrane.

If an abscess forms, a rupture of the eardrum may result, and drainage from the ear may be evident. When this happens, the pressure is relieved and the child is more comfortable. Some amount of hearing loss may result from the rupture. OM is considered chronic if the condition persists for more than 3 months. Recurrent attacks can lead to serious complications. Chronic OM can lead to cholesteatoma (*chole,* "bile," *steato,* "fat," and *oma,* "tumour"), a cyst-like sac filled with keratin debris. This may occlude the middle ear and erode adjacent ossicle bones, causing hearing loss. This condition is best treated by an otolaryngologist. Complications of repeated attacks of acute OM can include the development of chronic OM with effusion (fluid accumulation). Again, hearing loss can result. Treatment may be indicated because hearing loss may impair cognitive and language development that can hamper the education and communication abilities in developing children.

Treatment

OM caused by viruses or less virulent bacteria resolves equally quickly with or without antibiotics. A bulging tympanic membrane, especially if yellow or hemorrhagic, is likely to be bacterial in origin. Perforation of the tympanic membrane with purulent discharge similarly indicates a bacterial cause. Immediate antibiotic treatment is recommended for children who have a high fever (≥39°C [≥102°F]), are moderately to severely systemically ill or have very severe otalgia, or have already been significantly ill for 48 hours. For all other cases, either parents can be provided with a prescription for antibiotics to fill or the child can be reassessed if the child does not improve within 48 hours. Amoxicillin is the medication of choice. For children less than 2 years of age, 10 days of therapy is given, whereas older children can be treated for 5 days (Le Saux, Robinson, & CPS Infectious Diseases and Immunization Committee, 2016).

The nurse should teach the parents how to administer medications to their child. It is essential that the nurse have a knowledge and understanding of medications prescribed for the patient.

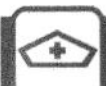
Nursing Tip

Instruct caregivers that the child's condition may improve dramatically after antibiotics are taken for a few days. To prevent recurrence, caregivers must continue to administer the medication until the prescribed amount has been completed.

Ototoxicity may develop with the use of certain antibiotics (aminoglycosides), particularly in the presence of tympanic membrane perforation or tympanostomy tubes. In this situation, alternative antimicrobial drops should be selected (Leis, Rutka, & Gold, 2015).

Surgical treatment

Surgical intervention may be necessary when medical treatment is unsuccessful. The health care provider may incise the tympanic membrane to relieve pressure and to prevent a tear by spontaneous rupture. This is called a **myringotomy** (*myringa,* "eardrum," and *otomy,* "incision of"). A tympanic membrane button or tympanostomy ventilating tube (pressure equalizer [PE]) may be inserted if the condition becomes chronic, lasts more than 3 months, or causes hearing difficulties that impair school performance. The PE tube may fall out spontaneously within 6 to 12 months. In some children, the tubes may have to be reinserted to continue ventilation. No routine precautions are necessary for water-related activities, such as the use of earplugs, headbands, or the avoidance of swimming or water sports (Rosenfeld, Schwartz, & Pynnonen, 2013). All children should be followed up to make sure that the condition is resolved and to evaluate any hearing loss that may have occurred.

Comfort measures

Antipyretics may be given to reduce fever, and a warm compress may be applied locally for comfort. If the eardrum has ruptured, the child is placed on the affected side. Cold may also be beneficial. An ice pack may be prescribed to reduce edema and pressure. The skin around the ears must be kept clean and protected from any drainage to prevent tissue breakdown. Parents are instructed not to insert cotton swabs into the ears.

Hearing Impairment

Hearing-impaired children present special challenges to the health care team. Hearing loss can affect speech, language, social and emotional development, and behaviour, as well as academic achievement. The nurse should have a basic understanding of how to approach and work with a child with a hearing impairment.

Pathophysiology

Permanent hearing loss is one of the most common congenital disorders of childhood, occurring in about 2 per 1 000 live births. Universal newborn hearing screening leads to earlier diagnosis and intervention, which means better outcomes for children with a hearing impairment (Patel, Feldman, & CPS Community Paediatrics Committee, 2011/2018). See Chapter 11 for further discussion of newborn hearing screening.

Hearing loss can be central or peripheral and is classified according to where the problem is. *Congenital hearing loss* in the newborn may be hereditary or occur as a result of in utero infection, low birth weight, prolonged resuscitative measures, or specific anomalies or syndromes.

Sensorineural hearing loss occurs when the hair cells along the cochlea and acoustic nerve are damaged, which can occur from exposure to environmental toxins, genetic anomalies, or exposure to loud noise. (Some rattles and squeaky toys can emit sounds exceeding 100 decibels and should not be placed near the ear of an infant.)

Conductive hearing loss occurs when the tympanic membrane prevents sound from entering the middle ear. Common causes of conductive hearing loss in older children include impacted cerumen (ear wax), perforation of the tympanic membrane, and some types of ear infections. Teens who use earphones or earbuds at high volumes or attend loud rock concerts, are near fireworks, or work with power equipment are at risk for developing conductive hearing loss.

Hearing loss is expressed in terms of *decibels (dB)*, which are units of loudness and are the basis for rating the severity of a hearing loss. A hearing loss above the 15-dB threshold requires some intervention to prevent developmental problems, and a hearing loss above 70 dB is considered legally deaf (Haddad & Keesecker, 2016). If hearing loss is complete, the child misses all the pleasures of sound and has difficulty communicating (children learn to talk by imitating what they hear). Behavioural issues may arise because these children do not understand verbal directions. They may become aggressive with other children in their attempt to communicate. If playmates ridicule them, personality development may be affected. Unless these children are helped early in life, they may become socially isolated.

Nursing Tip

When addressing a child with a hearing impairment, the nurse should do the following:

- Be at eye level with the child.
- Be face-to-face with the child.
- Establish eye contact.
- Talk in short sentences.
- Avoid using exaggerated lip or face movement.

Diagnosis and treatment

The CPS recommends that provinces and territories have an integrated program that provides newborn hearing screening for all babies by age 1 month so that any diagnoses can be confirmed by 3 months and interventions are in place by 6 months of age (Patel et al., 2011/2018).

The evoked otoacoustic emissions (OAE) test is a preferred method for newborn testing. Another test, the auditory brainstem response (ABR) test, records brain wave responses generated by the auditory system (see Fig. 11.10). These tests are easily administered to the newborn infant, and many hospitals routinely screen newborns for hearing ability before discharge. Lack of response by the infant to sounds or music or lack of the startle reflex in infants less than 4 months of age are the first signs that may alert the parents or nurse to the possibility of hearing impairment. Early diagnosis and prompt treatment are primary requisites, regardless of the child's age.

Tympanometry measures ear pressure but is difficult to perform adequately on an active infant or small child. A tuning fork is used to evaluate for air conduction (Rinne test) or bone conduction (Weber test). These types of tests require the child to be able to communicate what is heard or felt. Diagnosis of hearing loss can be confirmed by visual reinforcement audiometry (VRA), which identifies sensitivity to sounds in young infants.

Many hearing defects are amenable to medical or surgical treatment. Hearing aids can amplify sound waves and can be used with infants as young as 2 months of age; they are fitted by a pediatric audiologist. Surgically placed cochlear implants are used for some children as young as 2 years of age. All children with cochlear implants must be immunized with pneumococcal vaccine before surgery to avoid complications related to bacterial infection (Haddad & Keesecker, 2016). Children who have a severe loss of hearing need more extensive help from personnel at an auditory training centre. These children must begin treatment as soon as the hearing loss is discovered.

Nursing care

Various methods are used to bring the child into the world of sound. Lip reading, sign language, writing, visual aids, and amplified sound are but a few examples. Sign language is the use of hand signals that correspond to words and assist in communication with a deaf child. The parents need to be taught a means of communication that correspond with those used by the teachers.

The nurse must be aware of the symptoms of deafness in the child. Newborns should be observed for their responses to auditory stimuli. The Brazelton Neonatal Behavioural Assessment Scale is a tool that can be used to evaluate the infant's orientation response to the sound of a voice. When hearing impairment is found, the nurse should inquire about facilities that are available in the community for hearing-impaired children.

The child with a hearing impairment who is hospitalized needs the same opportunities to communicate as the child who does not have this disability. The nurse should smile when approaching the child. Body language communicates a lot, especially if there is a severe communication problem. The nurse needs to face the child when speaking and be positioned at eye level with the child. The nurse must ensure that the child sees them before touching the child, to avoid startling the child. Previously developed speech patterns may regress during hospitalization. Visual aids, writing, or drawing can be used to enhance communication.

The Hearing Foundation of Canada provides information and support to families as well as information regarding hearing-assistance devices. Hearing aids are designed to fit in the ear, behind the ear, on eyeglass frames, or on the body with wires to the ear.

The nurse should check ear hygiene and be sure hairs are not caught on the end of the hearing aid to ensure a proper fit and to minimize noise and whistling problems. Teaching safe battery handling and storage and promoting self-care are important nursing responsibilities.

Home care of the child with a hearing impairment should include speech therapy. Flashing lights should be installed in the home to alert the child to doorbells and other sound-based devices. Telecommunication devices for the deaf (TDD) are available to enable telephone communication. Closed captioning devices for television are available to the child who can read.

The nurse can help the family nurture the child's socialization skills. Some children with a hearing impairment attend special schools for the deaf, and some attend regular school. The multidisciplinary health care team should follow each child with a hearing impairment, along with their family, to provide individualized care.

Nursing Tip

Emphasize to parents the need to supervise the care and storage of hearing aid batteries to prevent accidental ingestion. When inserting the earpiece of a hearing aid, be sure that the ear canal is free of hair.

Barotrauma

Barotrauma occurs when there is a change in the atmospheric pressure between the internal body systems and the surrounding environment. An example of barotrauma is the painful obstruction of auditory tubes when in a pressurized cabin of an airplane. Many children travel with their families via airplane and may react to a change in altitude and barometric pressure. During airplane descent, children should be encouraged to yawn or chew gum, to promote swallowing. Infants should be breast or bottle fed to promote swallowing, which produces autoinflation and relief of symptoms. Systemic decongestants can be taken before air travel and timed so that their peak effectiveness occurs during airplane descent.

Adolescents participating in recreational underwater diving may experience barometric pressure stress to the ear that results in a severe earache and other serious problems. Underwater diving should be done slowly during the descent phase to minimize negative-pressure buildup. Sensory hearing loss and vertigo with nausea and vomiting may be early signs of decompression sickness when it occurs during the ascent phase of diving. The diver should be referred for medical care. Upper respiratory infections or tympanic membrane perforation are contraindications to diving because vertigo, nausea, vomiting, and disorientation can occur, with dangerous results.

THE NERVOUS SYSTEM

The nervous system is divided into three main anatomical divisions:

1. The central nervous system (CNS), comprising the brain and spinal cord
2. The peripheral nervous system (PNS), consisting of nerves that leave the brain and spinal cord to the rest of the body
3. The autonomic nervous system (ANS), which includes both the sympathetic and parasympathetic systems

The function of the nervous system is to smoothly integrate signals between the brain and the rest of the body in a coordinated fashion. The anatomy of the nervous system is depicted in Fig. 23.7 along with the 12 cranial nerves and their functions in Fig. 23.8.

Neural tube development occurs during the third to fourth weeks of fetal life. This eventually becomes the CNS. The fusing process of the neural tube is critical; its failure to fuse may lead to congenital conditions such as spina bifida. Most neurological disabilities in childhood result from congenital malformation (birth defects), brain injury, or infection.

NERVOUS SYSTEM ASSESSMENT

Skull X-ray films, electroencephalography (EEG), computed tomography (CT), magnetic resonance imaging (MRI), electromyography (EMG), and other

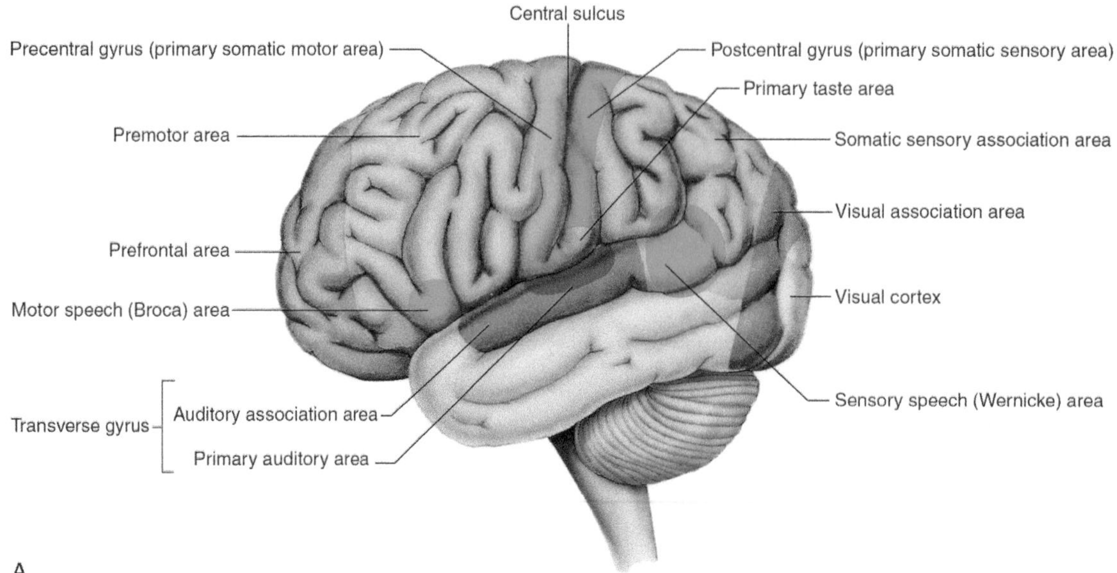

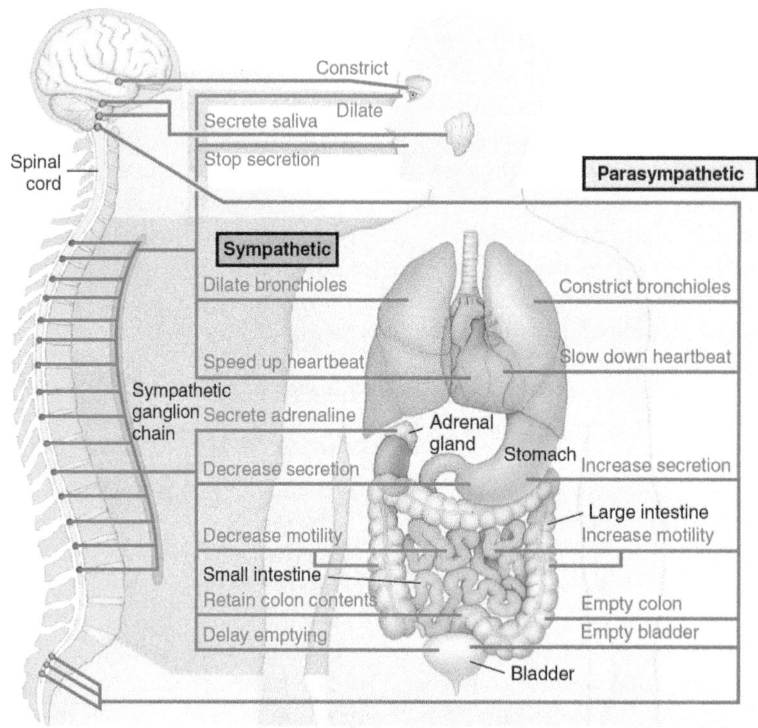

Fig. 23.7 **A,** Functional areas of the brain. Each area of the brain has a specific function. Damage to the local area can cause loss of that function. **B,** The nervous system, and the innervation of target organs by the autonomic nervous system. The sympathetic pathways are shown in orange, and the parasympathetic pathways are shown in green. (**A,** from Patton, K. T., & Thibodeau, G. A. [2015]. *Anatomy & physiology* [9th ed.]. St. Louis: Mosby. **B,** from Thibodeau, G. A., & Patton, K. T. [2016]. *Structure and function of the body* [15th ed.]. St. Louis: Mosby.)

methods, including a **neurological assessment**, may be used to detect CNS dysfunction or injury (Table 23.2). The neurological examination can also be used to detect decline or improvement in neurological status to determine the best care for the patient. Conducting this assessment in young children has its unique challenges that require adaptations, as one's approach and impressions are influenced by the child's age and developmental milestones. The child's ability will reflect the maturation of the nervous system, which matures from birth to early adulthood. Something that is normal at one developmental stage may not be normal at another stage. When making an assessment, nurses should ask themselves: What should a child of this age be able to do? And does it look the same on both sides?

Some examples are as follows: 2-year-old children are not able to hop on one foot, but they should be able

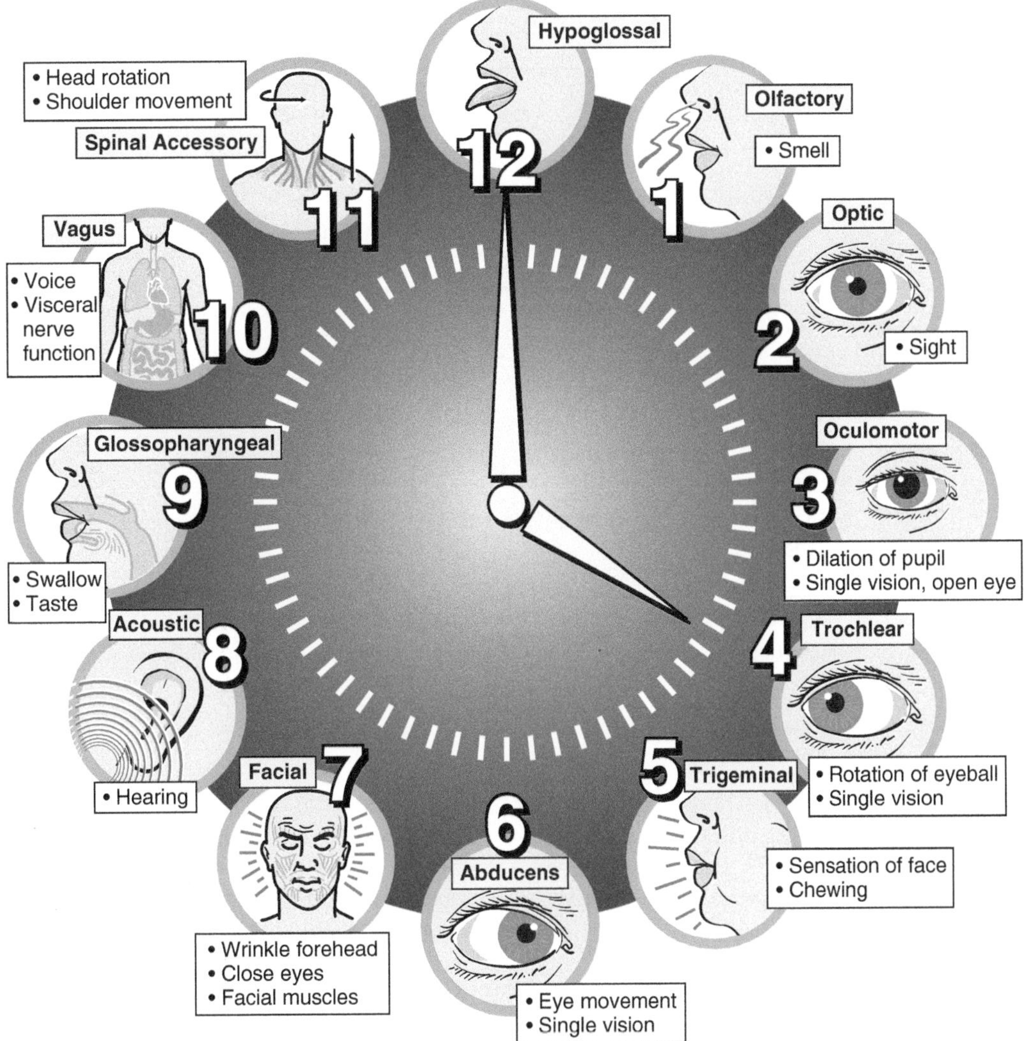

Fig. 23.8 The 12 cranial nerves and their functions.

to do so at 4 years. Having a wide-based gait is normal in a 1-year-old but abnormal in a 2-year-old. Primitive reflexes such as the Babinski should be present in children up to age 2 years.

Basic components to a neurological assessment include the following:

- A thorough birth, developmental, and health history
- Growth parameters and head circumference measurement
    - Assessment of mental state: level of consciousness, age-appropriate cognitive function, which may be extrapolated by a child's school performance
- Assessment of language and comprehension function
- Assessment of the 12 cranial nerves
- Motor assessment (symmetry, muscle tone, and power are assessed)
- Sensory assessment (light touch, vibration, temperature, and pain)
- Deep tendon reflexes
- Gait, balance, and coordination

Nursing Tip

- Early hand preference in a child under 1 year old should not be present and may indicate a deficit or weakness of the unfavoured hand or arm that should be evaluated.
- The persistence of primitive reflexes is indicative of delayed maturation or impaired CNS function.
- Asymmetrical motor or sensory findings and reflex responses can help localize the neurological deficit. If reflex responses are diminished or absent, this suggests upper motor neuron dysfunction, whereas asymmetry can be due to either upper or lower motor neuron dysfunction.

States of Consciousness

Consciousness is the awareness of environmental stimuli, the ability to react to stimuli, and the cognitive ability to respond to the stimuli either verbally or physically *in an age-appropriate manner.* Assessment of consciousness requires adaptations for infants and children less than 5 years of age. A pediatric Glasgow Coma Scale (GCS) is available for assessing consciousness in

Table 23.2 The 12 Cranial Nerves: Selected Dysfunctions and Nursing Interventions

CRANIAL NERVE	DYSFUNCTION	NURSING INTERVENTIONS
I Olfactory	Inability to smell	Appetite may be suppressed; present food attractively.
II Optic	Inability to control pupil reflex	Protect eyes from glaring lights.
III Oculomotor	Double vision	Cover eyes.
IV Trochlear	Inability to move eyes	When communicating, remain in child's view.
V Trigeminal	Difficulty in chewing	Provide soft foods.
VI Abducens	Inability to control corneal reflex	Have eye ointment or eye patch on hand to protect cornea.
VII Facial	Inability to close eye	Protect eyes with moist dressing.
VIII Acoustic	Inability to hear	Maintain body language for communication.
IX Glossopharyngeal	Inability to taste or to control gag and cough reflexes	Provide visually attractive food. Keep tracheotomy tray and suction at bedside.
X Vagus	Difficulty in talking or swallowing; visceral malfunction	Provide means of communication. Assess for aspiration. Assess body system functions and vital signs.
XI Spinal accessory	Controls head, turns, and shrugs shoulders	Provide position change and support.
XII Hypoglossal	Controls tongue movement, thick speech	Have suction ready; observe ability to chew and swallow. Provide method of communication.

children of these ages (Table 23.3). The pediatric GCS includes measures for eye opening and motor and verbal responses. Changes in the GCS score also reflect overall cortical and brainstem function. The lower the score, the deeper the level of unconsciousness or coma (Box 23.1).

Levels of consciousness include the following:

Confusion and disorientation to time, place, or person; the inability to answer simple or complex questions

Delirium: Disorientation involving fear, agitation

Lethargy: Sleepy, difficult to arouse

Stupor: Deep sleep, responding only to vigorous or pain stimuli

Coma: Unconscious, nonresponsive to any external stimuli and may include posturing (see Box 23.1)

Some causes of altered consciousness include infection, trauma, hypoxia, poisoning, electrolyte imbalance, metabolic disturbances, increased **intracranial pressure (ICP)**, or head injury (Box 23.2). The effect of head injuries on the state of consciousness and nursing care during altered levels of consciousness are discussed later in the chapter.

Nursing Tip

Infants with altered levels of consciousness may have signs of:

- Extreme and persistent irritability that is unexplained or inconsolable
- Floppy or decreased tone
- Difficulty to arouse and not responsive to stimuli
- Poor feeding
- Weak cry

Altered Mental Status

The child with *altered mental status* is unable to produce verbal or motor responses to stimulation at a level appropriate to their developmental stage. Changes in level of consciousness are particularly meaningful and necessitate immediate medical attention. After airway, breathing, and circulation are established, the child's alertness is recorded for use as baseline data. Parents are excellent resources for knowing when their child does not appear to be themselves. In general, children should be oriented to person, time, and place (according to developmental capabilities). The nurse should ask the child, "What is your name?" and "Do you know where you are?" Older children may know the day of the week. The child should recognize their parents. To assess this the nurse points to the mother and asks, "Who is this?" The child should also be able to follow simple commands, such as "Turn over."

When the child does not respond to verbal stimuli, the upper arm is gently pinched and the response is observed. The presence or absence of crying or speech should be noted. It is not unusual for children to fall asleep, but they should be easily aroused. The nurse needs to record changes in sleeping posture, movements of extremities, and any signs of tremors or restlessness. Children often cannot localize pain accurately and may not offer an accurate history. The *AVPU chart* can be used as a guide to rapidly document the altered mental status of a child (Hartman & Cheifetz, 2016):

A = Awake and responsive
V = Responds to verbal stimuli
P = Responds only to pain stimuli
U = Unresponsive

Table 23.3 **Pediatric Glasgow Coma Scale (PGCS)**

	>1 YEAR	<1 YEAR		SCORE
Eye opening	Spontaneously	Spontaneously		4
	To verbal command	To shout		3
	To pain	To pain		2
	No response	No response		1
Motor response	Obeys	Spontaneous		6
	Localizes pain	Localizes pain		5
	Flexion-withdrawal	Flexion-withdrawal		4
	Flexion-abnormal (decorticate rigidity)	Flexion-abnormal (decorticate rigidity)		3
	Extension (decerebrate rigidity)	Extension (decerebrate rigidity)		2
	No response	No response		1
	>5 YEARS	**2–5 YEARS**	**0–23 MONTHS**	**SCORE**
Verbal response	Oriented	Appropriate words/ phrases	Smiles/coos appropriately	5
	Disoriented/confused	Inappropriate words	Cries and is consolable	4
	Inappropriate words	Persistent cries and screams	Persistent inappropriate crying and or/ screaming	3
	Incomprehensible sounds	Grunts	Grunts, agitated, and restless	2
	No response	No response	No response	1
Total Pediatric Glasgow Coma Score (3–15):				

Merck Manual. (2018). *Modified Glasgow coma scale for infants and children*. Retrieved from https://www.merckmanuals.com-/professional/injuries-poisoning/traumatic-brain-injury-tbi/traumatic-brain-injury-tbi#CHDEHEFH.

Originally adapted from Davis, R. J., et al. (1987). Head and spinal cord injury. In M. C. Rogers (Ed.), *Textbook of pediatric intensive care*. Baltimore: Williams & Wilkins; James, H., Anas, N., & Perkin, R. M. (1985). *Brain insults in infants and children*. New York: Grune & Stratton; and Morray, J. P., et al. (1984). Coma scale for use in brain-injured children. *Critical Care Medicine, 12*, 1018.

Box 23.1 **Causes of Altered Level of Consciousness**

- A fall to 60 mm Hg or below of Pao_2
- A rise above 45 mm Hg of $Paco_2$
- Low blood pressure causing cerebral hypoxia
- Fever (1°C rise in fever increases oxygen need by 10%)
- Medications (sedatives, antiepileptics)
- Seizures (**postictal** state)
- Increased intracranial pressure (ICP)

The bladder is also observed for distention, which can contribute to irritability. Incontinence in the child who is toilet-trained is significant. The child's behaviour should be described in the nurse's notes.

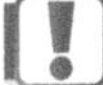 Safety Alert!

The sudden appearance of a fixed and dilated pupil is a neurological emergency.

Vital Signs

An increase in blood pressure and a decrease in pulse and respiration can be evidence of increased ICP. Temperature elevations may result from inflammation, systemic infection, or damage to the hypothalamus, which regulates body temperature. Mild elevations caused by trauma are not uncommon during the first 2 days after a head injury.

Spinal Assessment

Examination of the child's motor and sensory function along with their autonomic responses will help determine any pathology related to the spinal cord. The spinal cord is mapped out into myotomes (muscle) and dermatomes that are innervated by cervical, thoracic, lumbar, and sacral nerves. This system allows for localization of disease or injury (ASIA scale) (Fig. 23.9) and the Oxford Muscle scale is used to assess muscle strength (Table 23.4).

CONGENITAL DISORDERS OF NERVOUS SYSTEM

Spina Bifida

Spina bifida, also known as *myelodysplasia*, refers to a group of CNS disorders characterized by malformation of the spinal cord.

Pathophysiology

Spina bifida ("divided spine") is a congenital embryonic neural tube defect in which there is an imperfect closure of the spinal vertebrae. There are two forms: occulta (hidden) and cystica (sac or cyst) (Fig. 23.10).

Spina bifida occulta is a relatively minor variation of the disorder in which the opening is small and there is no associated protrusion of structures. It often goes undetected and occurs most commonly at the L5 and S1 levels. There may be a tuft of hair (Fig. 23.11), dimple, lipoma, or discoloration at the site. In general,

Box 23.2 Neurological Assessment of Infants and Children

Many subtle clues to a change in neurological status in infants and children can be missed unless the nurse performs a full neurological assessment. The lack of the child's ability to communicate and assist poses challenges in the neurological assessment of infants, but a knowledge of normal growth and development aids the nurse in evaluating the status of their patient. For example, an infant should turn their head toward the spoken word by age 6 months. However, assessing after a full feeding may cause a delayed response that may not be pathological.

PAIN STIMULI

There are two types of pain stimuli: *central,* a response of the brain; and *peripheral,* a response of the spinal cord. The pain stimulus should continue for a few seconds to determine the optimal function response.

Central pain stimulus:

Trapezius muscle: Firmly pinch large muscle mass at the angle where the neck and shoulder meet.

Suborbital pressure: Exert firm pressure on the "notch" that can be located under the centre of the eyebrow.

LEVEL OF CONSCIOUSNESS

In children and adolescents, one can determine the difference between arousal, awareness, orientation, and memory. In infants, the Glasgow Coma Scale is used (see Table 23.3).

AROUSAL AWARENESS

Child responds to their name, which is indicative of basic cerebral function. Child can interact with environment, indicating cerebral cortex functioning.

Orientation: Determine awareness of person, place, or time. Use open-ended or multiple-choice questions rather than questions that can be answered by "yes" or "no."

Attention span: Although attention span can differ with the age of child, the child would not normally fall asleep in the middle of a response requiring rearousal stimuli. This should be recorded if it occurs.

Language: Understanding the level of language development is essential in determining if the language pattern is normal or abnormal. Speaking clearly and recognizing familiar objects is a skill that is age related in the pediatric setting.

Irritability, lethargy, and vomiting: These are clinical symptoms of increased intracranial pressure (ICP) in infants, in addition to signs such as a bulging fontanelle.

Memory: A child's ability to recognize family members or repeat what he or she had for breakfast is a valid observation for memory.

CRANIAL NERVE RESPONSE

Cranial nerve responses are valuable in determining priority of need related to survival and safety.

I. Olfactory: A strong-smelling substance under the nose of an alert infant will elicit a grimace or a startle response.

II. Optic: Infant is able to fix eyes on object and follow a short distance. Pupils react equally to light.

III. Oculomotor: Pupils respond to light. In "doll's-eye test," eyes move away from direction head is rotated; infant is able to open eyes.

IV. Trochlear: Infant is able to move eyes and follow object.

V. Trigeminal: Infant turns head in response to stroking cheek.

VI. Abducens: Corneal reflex is present; eyes follow past midline.

VII. Facial: Wrinkles brow; facial movements symmetrical; closes eyes when crying.

VIII. Auditory: Tested via auditory screening machine; infant turns head toward sound source.

IX. Glossopharyngeal: Elicits a positive gag reflex, moves tongue in mouth.

X. Vagus: Infant has ability to swallow and a lusty cry and cough.

XI. Accessory: Turn infant's head to one side, and infant will return head to midline.

XII. Hypoglossal: Infant able to suck and swallow; tongue protrusion is present.

MOTOR RESPONSE

Symmetrical spontaneous body movements are an important observation to record. Asking the child to follow a simple motor request is more accurate than a hand grasp, because in some age groups a hand grasp is a reflex rather than a voluntary response. A purposeful voluntary motor response is a more valuable observation than a reflex response to remove irritants such as an attempt to pull out a nasogastric tube.

POSTURING

In children and adolescents, posturing can indicate a change in neurological status that necessitates immediate notification to the health care provider.

Decorticate (flexor): Flexion of the arms to centre of body and flexing of wrists indicate partial brain function (indicates injury to the cerebral cortex of the brain) (see Fig. 23.20, *A*).

Decerebrate (extensor): Arms are extended along the side of the body and the hands are pronated. This indicates brainstem function only (see Fig. 23.20, *B*).

Opisthotonos position: Hyperextension of the neck and arching of the spine are positions assumed by infants with pathologic cerebral disturbance (see Fig. 23.13).

EYES

The pupils of the eyes should be observed for size, equality, and response to light (see Fig. 23.2). It may be best to evaluate the eye in a slightly darkened room so the pupils may be somewhat dilated and the response to sudden light from a flashlight can be readily assessed.

Pupils that remain *pinpoint* can indicate damage to the pons or part of the brainstem or can indicate medication toxicity.

Bilateral dilated pupils can be indicative of hypoxia or intoxication with atropine-like medications.

Pupils that are *unequal* in size can signal brain herniation; *immediate action is required.*

Pupillary response to light can be brisk, sluggish, or absent. Recording should indicate the size of the pupil in normal light (e.g., 3), size of pupil after flashlight intervention (e.g., 1), and how fast the change occurred (*B,* brisk; *S,* sluggish or slow; *A,* absent). A normal recording for pupillary response would be as follows: R 3/1 B; L 3/1 B.

Keep in mind that infants and children who are blind will not have a meaningful light response test.

Box 23.2 Neurological Assessment of Infants and Children—cont'd

When the pupil constricts in response to light, be sure that constriction is maintained and that the eye does not dilate again before light is removed.

Glasgow Coma Scale eye opening responses may be recorded as follows: 4—spontaneous; 3—to sound; 2—to pain; 1—none.

FONTANELLE

A bulging anterior fontanelle is indicative of increased ICP.

SCALP VEIN DISTENSION

Scalp veins distend because of the obstruction of flow from the bridging veins of the scalp to the sagittal sinus.

ATAXIA: SPACTICITY OF LOWER EXTREMITIES

These occur with damage to the corticospinal pathways.

REFLEXES: MORO OR TONIC NECK WITH WITHDRAWAL

In infants, an absence of these reflexes can occur with increased ICP.

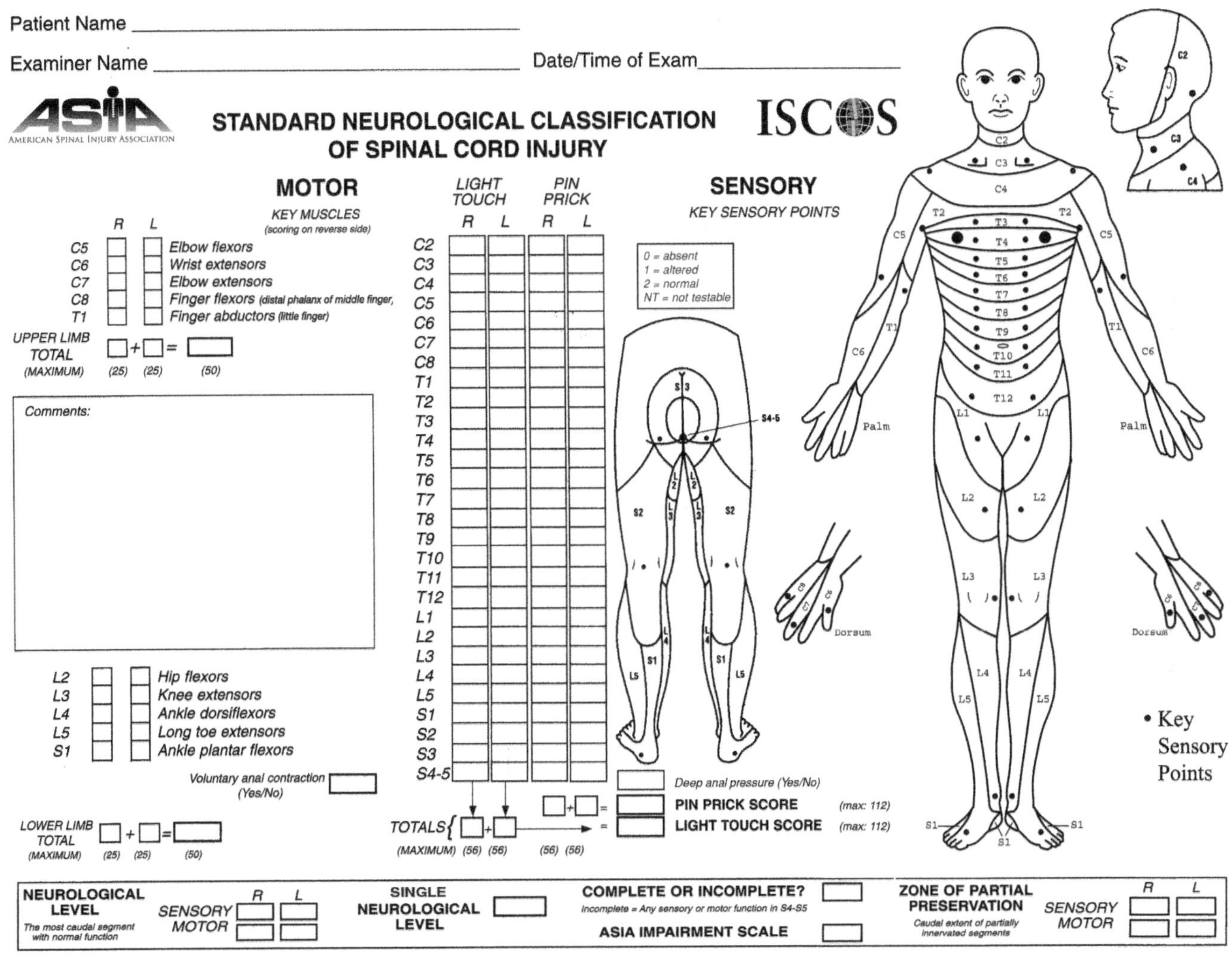

Patient Name ____________

Examiner Name ____________ Date/Time of Exam ____________

ASIA — AMERICAN SPINAL INJURY ASSOCIATION

STANDARD NEUROLOGICAL CLASSIFICATION OF SPINAL CORD INJURY

ISCOS

MOTOR

KEY MUSCLES (scoring on reverse side)

	R	L	
C5			Elbow flexors
C6			Wrist extensors
C7			Elbow extensors
C8			Finger flexors (distal phalanx of middle finger)
T1			Finger abductors (little finger)

UPPER LIMB TOTAL (MAXIMUM) □ + □ = □ (25) (25) (50)

Comments:

	R	L	
L2			Hip flexors
L3			Knee extensors
L4			Ankle dorsiflexors
L5			Long toe extensors
S1			Ankle plantar flexors

Voluntary anal contraction (Yes/No)

LOWER LIMB TOTAL (MAXIMUM) □ + □ = □ (25) (25) (50)

SENSORY

KEY SENSORY POINTS

	LIGHT TOUCH R	LIGHT TOUCH L	PIN PRICK R	PIN PRICK L
C2				
C3				
C4				
C5				
C6				
C7				
C8				
T1				
T2				
T3				
T4				
T5				
T6				
T7				
T8				
T9				
T10				
T11				
T12				
L1				
L2				
L3				
L4				
L5				
S1				
S2				
S3				
S4-5				
TOTALS (MAXIMUM)	(56)	(56)	(56)	(56)

0 = absent
1 = altered
2 = normal
NT = not testable

Deep anal pressure (Yes/No)

PIN PRICK SCORE (max: 112)

LIGHT TOUCH SCORE (max: 112)

NEUROLOGICAL LEVEL (The most caudal segment with normal function) — SENSORY R L; MOTOR R L

SINGLE NEUROLOGICAL LEVEL

COMPLETE OR INCOMPLETE? (Incomplete = Any sensory or motor function in S4-S5)

ASIA IMPAIRMENT SCALE

ZONE OF PARTIAL PRESERVATION (Caudal extent of partially innervated segments) — SENSORY R L; MOTOR R L

This form may be copied freely but should not be altered without permission from the American Spinal Injury Association.

REV 04/11

Fig. 23.9 Standard neurological classifcation of spinal cord injury. (From: International Standards for Neurological Classification of Spinal Cord Injury, revised 2011, published by the American Spinal Injury Association [ASIA]. Retrieved from https://www.ncbi.nlm.nih.gov/pmc/articles/PMC3232636/.)

treatment is not necessary unless neuromuscular symptoms appear. These symptoms consist of progressive disturbances of gait, such as footdrop, or disturbances of bowel and bladder sphincter function.

Spina bifida cystica involves the development of a cystic mass in the midline of the opening in the spine. Meningocele and meningomyelocele are two types of spina bifida cystica. A **meningocele** (*meningo*, "membrane," and *cele*, "tumour") contains portions of the membranes and cerebrospinal fluid (CSF). The size varies from that of a walnut to that of a newborn's head.

More serious is a protrusion of the membranes and spinal cord through this opening, which is a **meningomyelocele**. Although it resembles a meningocele, there may be associated paralysis of the legs and poor control of bowel and bladder functions. Hydrocephalus is a common complication. Prenatal detection is possible through ultrasound and prenatal screening (see Chapter 5).

Prevention

The specific cause of meningomyelocele is unknown. The use of medications during early pregnancy and poor nutrition may contribute to the development of a neural tube defect. *Canada's Food Guide* recommends that all women of childbearing age take a daily multivitamin that contains 0.4 mg of folic acid (see discussion on folic acid in Chapter 4). Studies have shown that the intake of folic acid before conception dramatically decreases the occurrence of neural tube defects such as spina bifida.

Nursing Tip

The intake of a daily multivitamin containing 0.4 mg of folic acid before conception can reduce the risk of neural tube defects such as spina bifida. A higher dose of folic acid may be prescribed if the mother has a previous history of giving birth to a child with a neural tube defect.

Treatment

The treatment for spina bifida is surgical closure. The prognosis for patients with these conditions depends on the extent of involvement. When a patient with meningocele has no weakness of the legs or sphincter involvement, surgical correction has excellent results. Surgery is also indicated for a patient with meningomyelocele for cosmetic purposes and to help prevent infection. A multidisciplinary approach is necessary, because, depending on the extent of the defect, the child may have difficulties associated with hydrocephalus, orthopedic problems, and impaired urinary and bowel function.

Habilitation is necessary after the operation because the legs remain paralyzed and the patient is incontinent

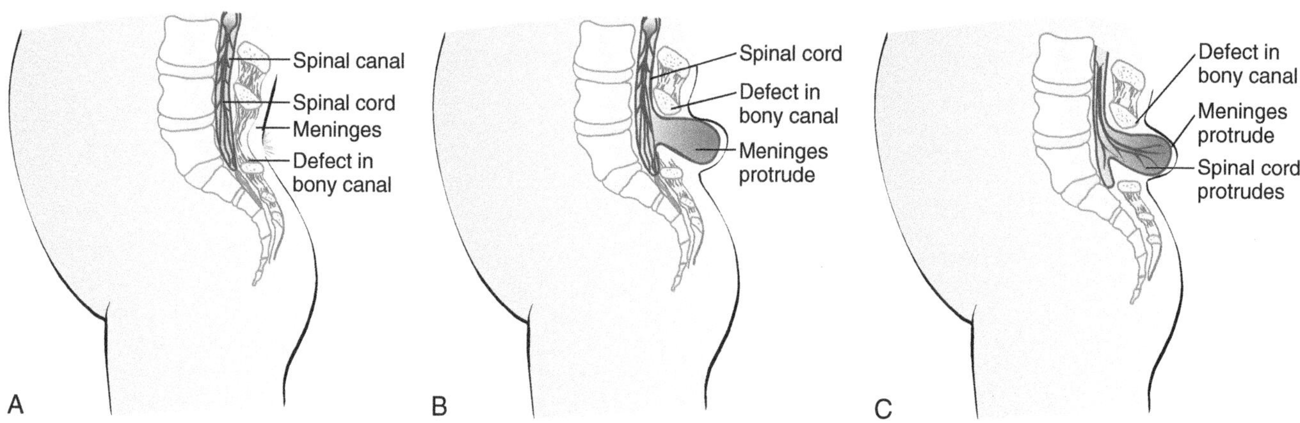

Fig. 23.10 Types of spina bifida. **A,** Spina bifida occulta. There is a defect in the bony canal. The meninges and spinal cord are normal. **B,** Spina bifida cystica meningocele. The spinal cord is normal, but there is a defect in the bony canal. The meninges protrude through this defect. **C,** Spina bifida cystica meningomyelocele. There is a defect in the bony canal. The meninges protrude, and the spinal cord protrudes through the defect.

Table 23.4 Oxford Muscle Scale: Grading of Muscle Strength

GRADE	ABILITY TO MOVE
5	The muscle can move the joint it crosses through a full range of motion, against gravity, and against full resistance applied by the examiner.
4	The muscle can move the joint it crosses through a full range of motion against moderate resistance.
3	The muscle can move the joint it crosses through a full range of motion against gravity but without any resistance.
2	The muscle can move the joint it crosses through a full range of motion only if the part is properly positioned so that the force of gravity is eliminated.
1	Muscle contraction is seen or identified with palpation, but it is insufficient to produce joint motion even with elimination of gravity.
0	No muscle contraction is seen or identified with palpation; paralysis.

Adapted from Wright, W. G. (1912). Muscle training in the treatment of infantile paralysis. *Boston Medical Surgery Journal, 167*, 567–574; Lovett, R. W., & Martin, E. G. (1916). Certain aspects of infantile paralysis and a description of a method of muscle testing. *JAMA*, 66, 729–733; Kendall, F. P., McCreary, E. K., & Provance, P. G. (1993). *Muscles: Testing and function*. Baltimore, MD: Williams & Wilkins.

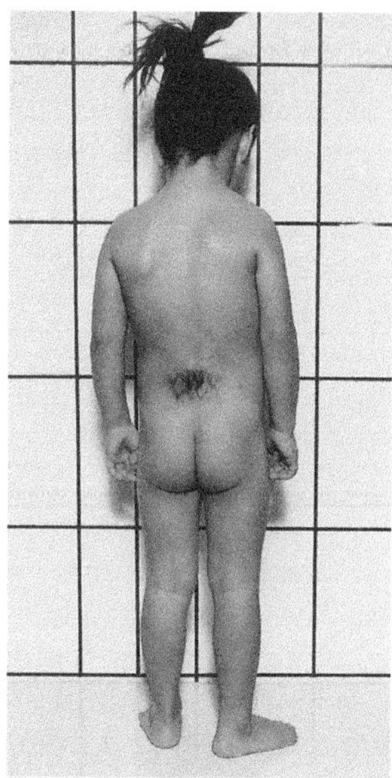

Fig. 23.11 A child with a hairy patch in the lumbosacral region, indicating the site of a spina bifida occulta. (Courtesy Dr. A. E. Chudley, Section of Genetics and Metabolism, Department of Pediatrics and Child Health, Children's Hospital and University of Manitoba, Winnipeg, Manitoba, Canada. From Moore, K. L., Persaud, T. V. N., & Torchia, M. G. [2013]. *The developing human: Clinically oriented embryology* [9th ed.]. Philadelphia: Saunders.)

of urine and feces. **Habilitation**, rather than *rehabilitation*, is the term used to describe this treatment because the patient has the condition from birth and therefore is learning rather than relearning. The aim of habilitation is to minimize the child's disability and put to constructive use the unaffected parts of the body. Every effort is made to help the child have a healthy development

Eventually the child can be taught to use a wheelchair and possibly to walk with braces, crutches, or other walking devices. The implantation of an artificial urinary sphincter in early childhood can help some children to become continent and prevent the complications associated with constant urinary dribble. Medications such as oxybutynin chloride are available to increase bladder storage. Children can also be "bowel trained" with the use of suppositories that promote timed bowel movements, helping the child avoid the social issues that can be caused by bowel incontinence.

Nursing care

The main objectives of nursing care include prevention of infection of or injury to the sac, correct positioning to prevent pressure on the sac and development of contractures, good skin care (particularly if the infant is incontinent of urine and feces), adequate nutrition, accurate observations and charting, education of the parents, continued medical supervision, and habilitation.

Immediate care of the sac is essentially the same regardless of whether the cord is involved. After birth, the newborn is placed in an isolette. Moist, sterile dressings of saline or an antibiotic solution may be ordered to prevent drying of the sac. Some method of protecting the mass is necessary if surgery is to be delayed. Protection from injury and maintenance of a sterile environment for the open lesion are essential.

Along with routine observations made for every newborn, other pertinent nursing observations must be made and recorded:

- The size and area of the sac are checked for any tears or leakage.
- The extremities are observed for deformities and movement. (There may be spasticity or paralysis of the limbs, or they may be normal, depending on the type and location of the cyst.)
- The head circumference is measured to determine the possibility of associated hydrocephalus.
- Fontanelles are observed to provide baseline data.
- The lack of anal sphincter control and dribbling of urine are significant in the differential diagnosis (Fig. 23.12). In general, the higher the defect on the spine, the greater the neurological deficit.

Positioning of the infant is important—the goal is to prevent pressure on the sac and to prevent postural deformities. When positioning infants with multiple deformities, the nurse must try to guard against aggravating existing problems. The infant is usually placed prone with a pad between the legs to maintain abduction and to counteract hip subluxation. A small roll is placed under the ankles to maintain foot position. Some infants may be supported in a side-lying posture to provide periods of relief. The disadvantage of this position is that it reduces movement of the arms and flexes the hips. The physiotherapy staff may provide helpful consultation. Surgery is generally done early.

Postoperative nursing care involves neurological assessment and prevention of infection. The status of the fontanelles and any signs of increased ICP, such as irritability or vomiting, are significant. Sometimes a shunt is performed shortly after closure of the spine, if hydrocephalus is present, to allow extra CSF to drain into the peritoneum (see discussion of hydrocephalus later in the chapter). Complications that can be life-threatening include meningitis, pneumonia, and urinary tract infection.

Urological monitoring is essential, because many of these infants have urinary incontinence. Medication to prevent urinary tract infection is routinely given. The Credé method of bladder emptying (applying pressure above the symphysis pubis) may be used for infants. Older children may be taught intermittent, clean self-catheterization. This technique can be performed by parents and learned by children.

Skin care can be a challenge. Constant dribbling of feces and urine irritates the perineal area and can infect the sac or the incision. Meticulous cleanliness is necessary. The bedding must be dry and free of wrinkles.

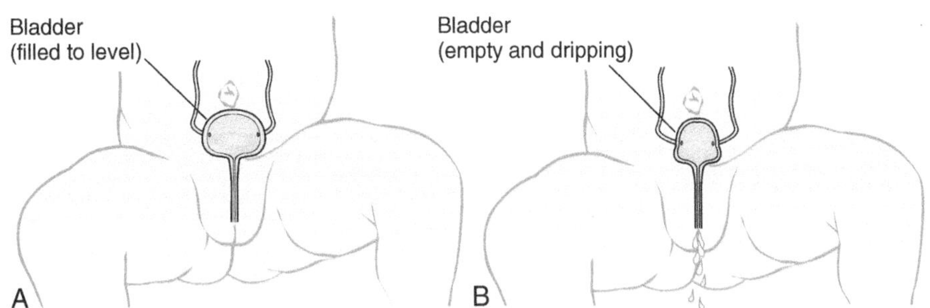

Fig. 23.12 Incontinence in the newborn. **A,** Normally, when the bladder fills to a certain level, a sensor stimulates contraction of the bladder, and expulsion of a volume of urine into the diaper occurs. A normal newborn has about six wet diapers a day. **B,** A newborn is considered incontinent when the sensor does not function and the bladder does not fill to its capacity before emptying. There is a constant dribble of urine into the diaper. The diaper is always wet.

Frequent cleansing, application of a prescribed ointment or lotion, and light massage help to maintain skin integrity. If range-of-motion exercises are ordered, they are performed gently.

Feeding is facilitated by early closure of the defect. In delayed cases, gavage feeding may be used. These patients need cuddling and sensory stimulation. An infant who cannot be held can be soothed by touch. The nurse should talk to the infant and, when possible, provide face-to-face (en face) communication. Mobiles should be placed appropriately. Periodically moving the isolette or crib provides diversity of view. Soft music is also soothing.

Many infants with spina bifida develop a latex allergy. A latex-free environment should be adopted whenever possible. Parents should be informed that latex products such as balloons, "koosh" balls, tennis balls, and adhesive strips can cause allergic reactions that may include rashes and wheezing. The parents should be informed about food sensitivities that are common in children with latex allergies. Foods to avoid include bananas, avocados, and kiwi. Other commonly used items to avoid include latex-based pacifiers, feeding nipples, and water toys. The child should wear a medical identification (ID) tag indicating the latex allergy. In some cases, antihistamines and steroids may be prescribed before and after surgery. Nurses should wear nitrile gloves instead of latex gloves while caring for these patients.

Special consideration must be given to the establishment of parent–infant relationships. This problem is complicated if the infant is transferred to a large medical centre. The parents need understanding and support, as they may be overwhelmed. It is not unusual for them to find it difficult to look at the cyst. Most experience a sense of loss for what was to have been their "perfect baby." The astute nurse may recognize steps of the grieving process. Information and education about this disorder can be obtained from the Spina Bifida and Hydrocephalus Association of Canada.

DISORDERS AND DYSFUNCTION OF THE NERVOUS SYSTEM

Meningitis

Meningitis is an inflammation of the meninges (the covering of the brain and spinal cord).

Pathophysiology

Various organisms can cause bacterial meningitis. Group B streptococcus is the main cause of the infection in newborn infants. Organisms may invade the meninges indirectly by way of the bloodstream (**sepsis**) from centres of infection such as the teeth, sinuses, tonsils, and lungs, or directly through the ear (otitis media), or from a fracture of the skull.

Bacterial meningitis is often referred to as *purulent,* that is, pus forming, because a thick exudate surrounds the meninges and adjacent structures. This can lead to certain sequelae such as subdural effusion and, less frequently, hydrocephalus. The peak incidence for bacterial meningitis is between 6 and 12 months of age. Meningococcal meningitis is readily transmitted to others. *H. influenzae* type B vaccine and pneumococcal vaccines PCV-13 and PCV-23 have decreased the incidence of bacterial meningitis. The approaches to nursing care for all types of meningitis are similar.

Manifestations

The symptoms of purulent meningitis result mainly from intracranial irritation. They may be preceded by an upper respiratory infection and several days of gastrointestinal symptoms such as poor feeding. Severe headache, drowsiness, delirium, irritability, restlessness, fever, vomiting, and stiffness of the neck (nuchal rigidity) are other significant symptoms. Often the infant is resistant to cuddling and rocking as they increase discomfort from the inflamed meninges. A characteristic high-pitched cry is noted in infants. Seizures are common. Coma may occur fairly early in the older child. In severe cases, involuntary arching of the back caused by muscle contractions is seen (Fig. 23.13). This condition is called **opisthotonos** (*opistho,* "backward," and *tonos,* "tension"). The presence of *petechiae* (small hemorrhages beneath the skin) suggests meningococcal infection. Diagnosis is confirmed by examination of the CSF.

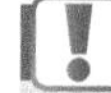

Safety Alert!

The acutely ill and lethargic child who develops a rash with petechiae must be referred for immediate follow-up care.

Treatment

At the first indication of meningitis, the health care provider performs a spinal tap (lumbar puncture, see Chapter 20) to obtain a specimen of CSF for laboratory

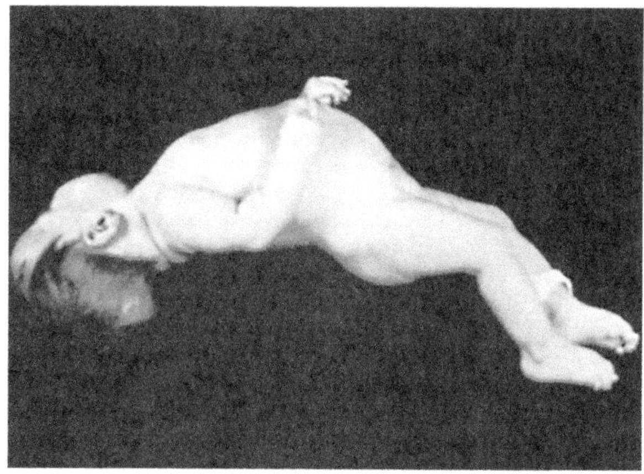

Fig. 23.13 The opisthotonos position. An involuntary arching of the back and extension of the neck are seen in children with brain injury or meningeal irritation. Note that the back is arched so that the head is on an even level with the heels. (From Lehman, R. K., & Schor, N. F. [2016]. Neurologic evaluation. In R. Kliegman, B. Stanton, J. St. Geme, et al. [Eds.], *Nelson textbook of pediatrics* [20th ed.]. Philadelphia: Saunders.)

testing. The spinal fluid may be clear in the early stages of the illness, but it rapidly becomes cloudy. The CSF pressure is increased, and further laboratory analysis indicates a high white cell count, an increase in protein, and a decrease in glucose.

The child is placed in isolation until 24 hours after antibiotic therapy has been initiated. An intravenous (IV) line is established for the administration of antibiotics and to restore fluid and electrolyte balance. Antibiotics are selected on the basis of culture and sensitivity laboratory results. Antibiotics are usually administered for a minimum of 10 to 21 days. A sedative may be provided to reduce the child's restlessness. An anticonvulsant such as phenytoin (Dilantin) may also be required to decrease the risk of seizure activity. Steroids such as dexamethasone reduce complications of bacterial meningitis but are not used in nonbacterial meningitis.

Nursing Tip

When a spinal tap is planned, the infant can be sedated and EMLA cream applied to the area to reduce discomfort during needle insertion.

Nursing care

The isolation room is prepared in accordance with hospital protocol and the child should be on droplet precautions. Nursing responsibilities include performing frequent neurological checks and maintaining an accurate recording of the child's vital signs and intake and output. The nurse should also organize care so that the child is disturbed as little as possible.

The child with meningitis may be overly sensitive to stimuli; therefore, the room should be dimly lit and noise kept to a minimum. The nurse should carefully raise and lower the sides of the crib to avoid jarring the bed. The nurse needs to avoid startling the child and so should use a soft voice and gentle touch. These precautions also need to be explained to the parents.

Frequent monitoring of the child's vital signs is necessary. A slowed pulse rate, irregular respirations, and increased blood pressure are reported immediately, because they could indicate increased ICP. Antipyretics or a hypothermia (cooling) mattress may help control fever. The nurse should observe the child for additional or subtle signs of increased ICP, especially a change in alertness or muscles twitching. The joints are also observed for swelling, pain, and immobility. Oxygen is given as needed.

The child's intake and output are carefully observed and recorded. Careful attention is given to maintaining the IV line. Good oral hygiene is essential during this stage when the child is receiving nothing by mouth (NPO). As the child's condition improves, the diet progresses from clear fluids to an age-appropriate diet. A special formula may be given when nasogastric feedings are necessary. During the convalescent period, oral fluids are encouraged unless contraindicated.

The nurse should promptly report a decrease in output of urine (oliguria), which could signal urinary retention. Bowel movements are recorded each day to detect constipation and prevent *fecal impaction* (an accumulation of feces in the rectum). The nurse needs to continue to monitor neurological status and record and report findings such as weakness of the limbs, speech difficulties, mental confusion, and behaviour concerns. The child should be assessed for developmental deficiencies.

When recovery is uneventful, the child may be discharged home. The parents are taught the principles of intermittent IV therapy that can be accomplished in the home setting with visits from a home health agency nurse. The nurse should discuss the concerns of the parents and help them meet the needs of their child in recovery.

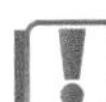 **Safety Alert!**

A child diagnosed with meningitis remains on additional droplet precautions until 24 hours after appropriate antimicrobial therapy has been started.

Encephalitis

Pathophysiology

Encephalitis (*encephalo,* "brain," and *itis,* "inflammation") is an inflammation of the brain. The condition is known as *encephalomyelitis* (*myelo,* "spinal cord") when the spinal cord is also infected. This condition can occur as a complication of disorders such as upper respiratory tract infections, German measles (rubella), or measles (rubeola), and it may also result from lead poisoning.

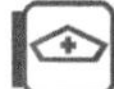 **Nursing Tip**

Encephalitis may occur as a complication of childhood diseases such as measles, mumps, or chicken pox. It is crucial that children receive the immunizations available for the diseases that are preventable.

Manifestations

The symptoms of encephalitis result from the CNS response to irritation. Characteristically, the history is that of a headache followed by drowsiness that may proceed to coma. Seizures are seen, particularly in infants. Fever, cramps, abdominal pain, vomiting, stiff neck (nuchal rigidity), delirium, muscle twitching, and abnormal eye movements are other manifestations of the disease.

Treatment and nursing care

The treatment is supportive and aimed at providing relief from specific symptoms. Sedatives and antipyretics may be prescribed. Seizure precautions are taken. Adequate nutrition and hydration are maintained. The nurse should provide a quiet environment, good oral hygiene, skin care, and frequent changes of position. Oxygen is administered as ordered, and the mouth and nose are kept free of mucus by gentle aspiration. Bowel movements are recorded daily, because the child may be constipated from the lack of activity. Preventing the secondary effects of immobilization is paramount.

The nurse needs to closely observe the child for neurological changes. Fatality rates and residual effects are higher among infants than among older children. Speech, mental processes, and motor abilities may be slowed, and permanent brain damage and intellectual or developmental disabilities can result. Growth and development and hearing evaluations should be monitored.

Parents are encouraged to help with the care of the child as soon as the condition is stable. They need to be instructed about the nursing procedures for home care and any required follow-up care.

Brain Tumours

Pathophysiology

Brain tumours are the second most common type of neoplasm in children (the first is leukemia). The majority of childhood tumours occur in the lower part of the brain (cerebellum or brainstem). The etiology of these tumours is unknown. They occur most commonly in school-age children.

Manifestations

The signs and symptoms are directly related to the location and size of the tumour. Most tumours create increased ICP with the hallmark symptoms of headache, vomiting, drowsiness, and seizures (Fig. 23.14). **Nystagmus** (constant jerky movements of the eyeball), strabismus, and decreased vision may be evident. **Papilledema** (edema of the optic nerve) may occur. Other symptoms include ataxia, head tilt, behavioural changes, and cerebral enlargement, particularly in infants. Deviations in vital signs are noticeable when the tumour presses on the brainstem.

Treatment and nursing care

Clinical manifestations, laboratory tests, and CT, MRI, and EEG findings confirm the diagnosis. Angiography is used to assist in the surgical approach by identifying the tumour's blood supply. Radiotherapy, chemotherapy, or surgery may be indicated.

Preoperative emphasis is placed on carefully explaining various procedures and on familiarizing the child and family with the recovery room, critical care unit, and hospital personnel. The nurse needs to explain that the child will have part or all of their head shaved. The size of the postoperative dressing should also be carefully described. Applying a similar dressing to a doll may be helpful to the child.

Postoperative care is usually provided in the critical care unit. Adjuncts to care may include use of a hypothermia (cooling) blanket or a mechanical respirator. Use of the Trendelenburg position is to be avoided because it increases ICP. Parents must be prepared for the appearance of the child after surgery. Empathic family support and appropriate referral should be offered.

Radiation treatment may be prescribed. The radiologist outlines the areas to be treated on the child's head. *These marks are not to be washed off.* Small doses of radiation are provided throughout a period of weeks. Chemotherapy may follow irradiation.

> **Nursing Tip**
>
> The timing of providing information is important when preparing the child for various procedures.

> **Safety Alert!**
>
> Sluggish, dilated, or unequal pupils may indicate increased ICP and must be reported promptly.

Hydrocephalus

Pathophysiology

Hydrocephalus (*hydro,* "water," and *cephalo,* "head") is a condition characterized by an increase of CSF within the ventricles of the brain, which causes pressure changes in the brain and an increase in head size. It results from an imbalance between the production and absorption of CSF or improper formation of the

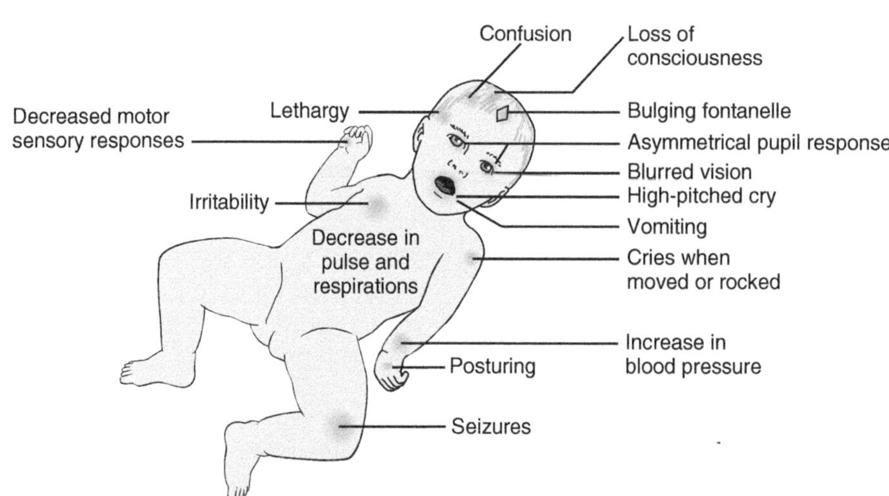

Fig. 23.14 Signs of increased intracranial pressure (ICP) in infants and children.

ventricles. Hydrocephalus may be congenital or acquired. It is most commonly acquired by an obstruction, such as a tumour, or as a sequela of infections (encephalitis or meningitis) or perinatal hemorrhage. The symptoms depend on the site of obstruction and the age at which it develops.

Hydrocephalus is classified as noncommunicating (obstructive) or communicating. *Noncommunicating hydrocephalus* results from the obstruction of CSF flow from the ventricles of the brain to the subarachnoid space. *Communicating hydrocephalus* results when CSF is not obstructed in the ventricles but is inadequately reabsorbed in the subarachnoid space (Fig. 23.15).

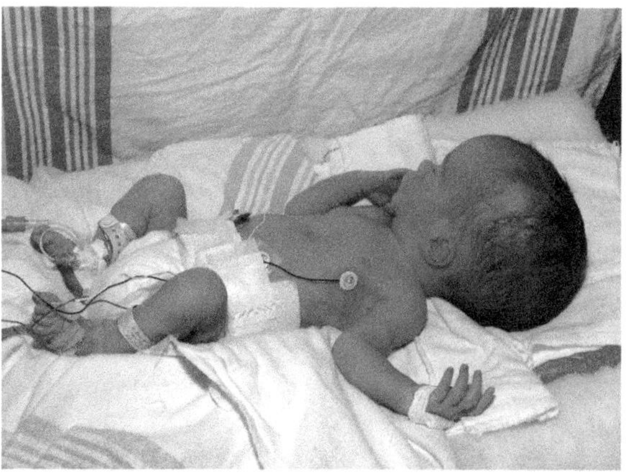

Fig. 23.16 Marked hydrocephalus. Note the characteristic large head, distended scalp veins, and full (enlarged) fontanelle. (Kleigman, R. M., Stanton, B. F., St. Geme, J. W., et al. [Eds.]. [2016]. *Nelson textbook of pediatrics* [20th ed.], Philadelphia: Elsevier.)

Manifestations

The signs and symptoms of hydrocephalus depend on the time of onset and the severity of the imbalance. The classic sign is an increase in head size (Fig. 23.16). If hydrocephalus occurs in utero, the enlarged head may necessitate a Caesarean birth. At birth, the head enlarges rapidly and the fontanelles bulge. The cranial sutures separate to accommodate the enlarging mass. The scalp is shiny, and the veins are dilated. In advanced cases, the pupils of the eyes may appear to be looking downward and the sclera may be seen above the pupils, much like the look of a setting sun. A foreshortened occiput suggests pathology of the fourth ventricle, with the brainstem protruding through the cervical canal. This is called the *Arnold-Chiari malformation* (Kinsman & Johnston, 2016). When the enlarged head involves a prominent occiput, the condition usually involves an atresia of the foramen of Lushka and the foramen of Magendie and is known as the *Dandy-Walker syndrome*. The infant is helpless and lethargic. The body becomes thin, and the muscle tone of the extremities is often poor. The cry is shrill and high-pitched. Irritability, vomiting, and anorexia are present, and convulsions may occur.

When hydrocephalus occurs in the older child, the head cannot enlarge because the cranial sutures are fused; therefore, headache is the predominant symptom, with cognitive slowing, personality changes, spasticity, and other neurological signs.

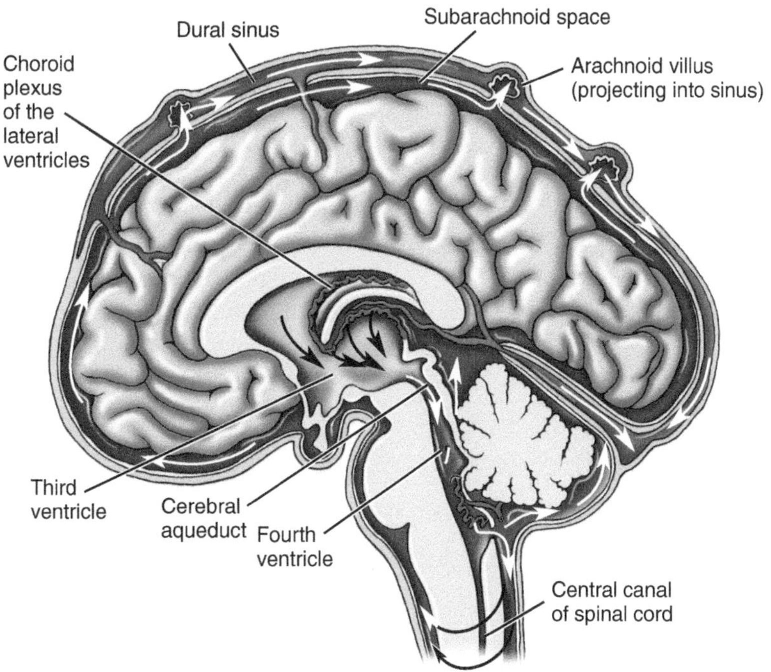

Fig. 23.15 Cerebrospinal fluid (CSF) circulation. The CSF is formed in the choroid plexus. The total volume of CSF is approximately 50 mL in the infant and 150 mL in the adult. It flows from the lateral ventricles through the foramen of Monro to the third ventricle. From the third ventricle, the CSF fluid flows through the aqueduct of Sylvius to the fourth ventricle, and then through the foramen of Luschka and the foramen of Magendie into the cisterns at the base of the brain. Flow continues to the spinal canal. The CSF is then absorbed by the arachnoid villi (which are also known as pacchionian bodies). Communicating, or nonobstructive, hydrocephalus occurs when the arachnoid villi are malformed or malfunction. Noncommunicating, or obstructive, hydrocephalus results when the tiny aqueduct of Sylvius is obstructed within the ventricles. When hydrocephalus occurs, excessive CSF causes the ventricles to enlarge and press the brain tissue against the bony skull. (From Herlihy, B., & Maebius, N. K. [2011]. *The human body in health and illness* [4th ed.], Philadelphia: Saunders.)

Diagnosis

Transillumination (*trans*, "across," and *illuminare*, "to enlighten")—the inspection of a cavity or organ by passing a light through its walls—is a simple diagnostic procedure useful in visualizing fluid. A flashlight with a sponge-rubber collar is held tightly against the infant's head in a dark room. The examiner observes for areas of increased luminosity. A small ring of light is normal, but a large halo effect is not. The child's head is measured daily. Echoencephalography, CT scanning, and MRI are used to visualize the enlarged ventricles and to identify the area of obstruction. A ventricular tap or puncture may be performed using a sterile technique to determine pressure and to drain CSF. The equipment needed is the same as that for a lumbar puncture. A specimen is labelled and sent to the laboratory for analysis.

Treatment

The use of acetazolamide (Diamox) and furosemide (Lasix) reduces the production of CSF and may provide some relief, but most often surgery is indicated (Kinsman & Johnston, 2016). The surgeon attempts to bypass, or **shunt**, the point of obstruction. The CSF may thus be carried to another area of the body, where it is absorbed and finally excreted. This is accomplished by inserting special tubing, which is replaced at intervals as the child grows. The procedure, known as a *ventriculoperitoneal shunt* (Fig. 23.17), allows the excess fluid to drain into the peritoneal cavity, where it is absorbed.

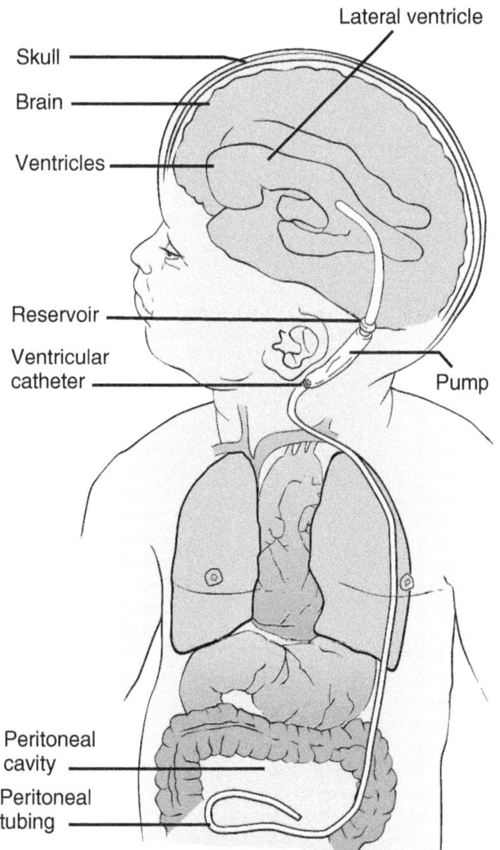

Fig. 23.17 Shunting procedure for hydrocephalus, in which a catheter drains the ventricular system into the peritoneal cavity. Note the pump behind the ear, which can be depressed intermittently to clear obstructions.

The prognosis for the child with hydrocephalus has improved with modern medications and surgical techniques. If the brain is not seriously damaged before the operation, mental function may be preserved. Motor development is sometimes slower if the child cannot lift the head, normally because of its increased weight. Complications of shunts are usually mechanical (kinking or plugging of tubing) or infection. The shunt acts as a focal spot for infection and may need to be removed if infection persists.

Nursing care

Preoperative care. Most often, surgical correction can be accomplished in utero via fetal surgery or shortly after birth to prevent brain damage caused by increased ICP. The immediate preoperative care is routine, involving assessment of vital signs and skin preparation, and emotional support of the parents. However, when the infant does not have access to corrective surgery, the general nursing care of an infant with hydrocephalus who has not undergone surgery presents several challenges. As the child grows, the child may be barely able to raise the head. Mental development is delayed. Lack of appetite, a tendency to vomit easily, and poor resistance to infections complicate management of these infants.

The position of the infant must be changed frequently to prevent hypostatic pneumonia and pressure sores. Hypostatic pneumonia occurs when the circulation of the blood in the lungs is poor and the infant remains in one position too long. It is particularly prevalent in infants who are poorly nourished or weak or who have a debilitating disease. When the nurse turns an infant who has hydrocephalus, the head must always be supported. To turn the infant in bed, the weight of the head is borne in the palm of one hand, and the head and body are rotated together to prevent a strain on the neck. When the infant is lifted from the crib, the head must be supported by the nurse's arm and chest.

The tissues of the head, ears, and bony prominences tend to break down. A pad of lamb's wool or sponge rubber placed under the head may help to prevent these lesions. If the skin becomes broken, it is given immediate attention to prevent infection. The infant must be kept dry, especially around the creases of the neck, where perspiration may collect.

In most cases, the nurse or parent may hold the infant for feedings. One needs to sit with the arm supported because the infant's head is heavy. A calm, unhurried manner is necessary. The room should be as quiet as possible. After the feeding, the infant is placed in a side-lying position. The infant should not be disturbed once settled, because vomiting occurs easily. The nurse must organize daily care so that it does not interfere with meals.

Observations to be recorded and reported include the type and amounts of food taken, any vomiting, the condition of the skin, motor abilities, restlessness, irritability, and changes in vital signs. Fontanelles are inspected for size and signs of bulging. Head circumference is measured around the occipitofrontal area and is recorded on the chart.

Symptoms of increased pressure within the head are an increase in blood pressure and a decrease in pulse rate and respirations. Signs of a cold or other infection need to be immediately reported to the nurse in charge and recorded.

Postoperative care. In addition to routine postoperative care and observations, the nurse should observe the patient for signs of increased ICP and of infection at the operative site or along the shunt line. As with any postoperative care, pain-control management is essential.

Bacterial infection is a life-threatening complication that sometimes necessitates shunt removal. Signs of infection include an increase in vital signs, poor feeding, vomiting, pupil dilation, decreased levels of consciousness, and seizures. The operative area must be observed for signs of inflammation. An internal flushing device may be used to ensure patency of the shunt tube when increased ICP is suspected. The surgeon may order the pump to be routinely depressed a certain number of times each day to facilitate drainage. This is accomplished by compressing the antechamber or reservoir that is under the skin behind the ear (see Fig. 23.17).

Positioning of the child depends on several factors and may vary with the child's progress. If the fontanelles are sunken, the infant is kept flat because too rapid a reduction of fluid may lead to seizures or cortical bleeding. If the fontanelles are bulging, the child is usually placed in the semi-Fowler's position to promote drainage of the ventricles through the shunt. The child is always positioned in a way that prevents pressure on the operative site. The surgeon will leave orders for the patient's position and activity. Assessment of skin remains a priority. Head and chest measurements are recorded. In patients with peritoneal shunts, the abdomen is measured or observed to detect malabsorption of fluid.

The child should be observed for signs of increased ICP. The development of a high-pitched cry, unequal pupil size or response to light, bulging fontanelles, irritability or lethargy, poor feeding, or abnormal vital signs should be reported and recorded. Evidence of increased ICP in the older child may be manifested by a change in personality, a change in level of consciousness, and headaches that are unrelieved by over-the-counter medications. The need for pain control should be assessed and medications given as needed. Intake and output need to be carefully recorded and the child observed closely for signs of fluid overload. The child is usually fed after active bowel sounds are heard. The surgical suture lines should be kept clean and dry and the diaper should be kept well below the abdominal suture line to prevent contamination.

Parent education, support, and guidance are essential. Parents should be taught signs that indicate shunt malfunction, how and when to "pump" the shunt by pressing against the valve behind the ear, and the need for multidisciplinary follow-up care. Signs of tube malfunction in the *older* child involve signs of increasing ICP, such as headache, lethargy, and changes in level of consciousness. Community resources, such as the National Hydrocephalus Foundation, and information concerning special car seats for children with special needs should be made known to the parents. There is approximately an 80% survival rate for infants treated early, and approximately one third of the cases result in normal physical and neurological functioning. Other survivors may have varying degrees of developmental disabilities.

Seizure and Epilepsy Disorders

Seizures are the most commonly observed neurological symptom in children. Seizures are sudden, unexpected events that may involve altered levels of consciousness, movement, sensation, perception, or behaviour. In Canada, it is estimated that 10% of the population will have at least one seizure in their lifetime (Canadian League Against Epilepsy, n.d.). A seizure may be in response to transient insult or loss of homeostasis of the brain. Typically, neurons in the cerebral cortex fire in small groups to accomplish a task and then cease to fire. In contrast, during a seizure, many neurons fire together to produce an abnormal sustained, synchronized burst of electrical activity similar to an "electrical storm."

This resultant burst of electrical activity produces observable or nonobservable changes, depending on the functional brain areas involved during the seizure.

Causes of seizures can be

1. Structural
2. Metabolic
3. Post-traumatic/infectious
4. Genetic
5. Cryptogenic (unknown)

The etiology varies (Box 23.3).

Box 23.3 Causes of Seizures in Children

INTRACRANIAL
Epilepsy
Congenital anomaly
Birth injury
Infection
Trauma
Degenerative diseases
Vascular disorder

EXTRACRANIAL
Fever
Heart disease
Metabolic disorders
Hypocalcemia
Hypoglycemia
Dehydration and malnutrition

TOXIC
Anaesthetics
Medications
Poisons

Febrile seizures

Febrile seizures are a transient condition common in children between 6 months and 5 years of age. There may be a genetic predisposition, which explains why children in the same family tend to have this problem. The seizure occurs in response to a rapid rise in temperature—often above a level of 38.8°C (102°F). Because the seizure lasts a short time and is no longer present when the child reaches a hospital, causes other than fever may have to be ruled out. Simple febrile seizures can be prevented by teaching the parent to control the fever through appropriate use of antipyretics (e.g., acetaminophen) and cooling measures (e.g., removing heavy blankets and clothing and providing fluids). Tepid sponge baths are not recommended to reduce fevers. Parents should be reassured that the condition is self-limiting. The use of phenobarbital is not effective and may decrease cognitive function. Antiseizure medications are not recommended for first-time treatment. Rectal or oral diazepam for the duration of a febrile illness may be prescribed if febrile seizures recur. Febrile seizures rarely develop into epilepsy, and the affected child has an excellent prognosis without residual problems.

Epilepsy

Pathophysiology. The term *epilepsy* (chronic recurrent seizures) derives from the Greek *epilēpsía,* which means "seizure." In the past, words such as *fit, spell,* and *blackout* were commonly used to describe this entity. *Epilepsy* is defined as having at least two or more unprovoked seizures, which are likely to be recurrent. In Canada, 1% of the population has epilepsy, with the majority having onset either in the first decade of life or over 60 years old, equivalent to 15 000 new diagnoses annually (Public Health Agency of Canada [PHAC], 2017).

The International League Against Epilepsy (ILAE) is the world's main scientific body that is devoted to the understanding of epilepsy. In 2017, a new classification of seizures was developed in order to help make diagnosis easier and more accurate with common terminology (Scheffer, Berkovic, Capovilla, et al., 2017) (Fig. 23.18). There are three basic features to this classification system:

1. Where does the seizure begin in the brain?
2. Is there preserved or loss of consciousness?
3. Describe other features of the seizure.

A **tonic movement** is a stiffening (contraction) of muscles. A **clonic movement** is an alternating contraction and relaxation of muscles.

Types of seizures. *Focal seizures:* Previously called *partial seizures,* these start in an area or network of cells on one side of the brain. The person maintains awareness even if unable to talk or respond during the seizure.

Generalized seizures: Previously called *primary generalized,* these engage or involve networks on both sides of the brain at the onset. There is presumed loss of awareness for all generalized seizures.

Unknown onset: If the onset of a seizure is not known, the seizure falls into the unknown onset category. Later on, the seizure type can be changed if the beginning of a person's seizures becomes clear.

Focal to bilateral seizure: A seizure that starts in one side or part of the brain and spreads to both sides has been called *secondary generalized seizures.* Now the term *generalized* refers only to the start of a seizure. The new term for secondary generalized seizure, *focal to bilateral seizure,* also replaces the term *complex partial seizures* (Scheffer et al., 2017) (see Fig. 23.18). Absence seizures often are recognized when an intelligent child is referred for medical evaluation because of unexplained failure to achieve in school. The reason for school failure is found to be absence seizures, which cause a temporary loss of awareness that results in a lack of continuity in the learning environment.

Epilepsy syndromes. The developing and immature brain is more susceptible to seizures and developmental or cognitive and behavioural comorbidities. Many etiologies in childhood (genetics, infections, metabolics, structural and head trauma) can contribute to the development of epilepsy, resulting in various syndromes.

Safety Alert!

Infantile spasm (West syndrome) is a unique seizure disorder that has onset typically in the first year of life, peaking at 2–6 months of age. They manifest as flexor or extensor spasms of the neck and trunk with jackknife appearance and occur in clusters usually before or after sleep that have a distinct EEG pattern called *hypsarrhythmia* because of its erratic appearance. This syndrome requires *immediate medical attention* as it is associated with developmental regression and poor outcome if not treated quickly.

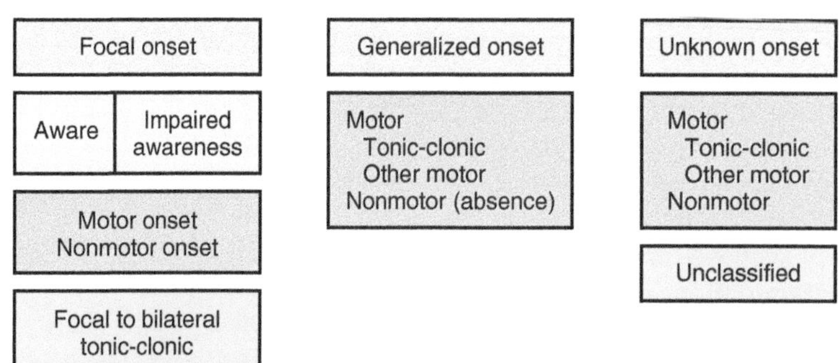

Fig. 23.18 Classification of seizure types. *ILAE,* International League Against Epilepsy. (From: Scheffer, I. E., Berkovic, S., Capovilla, G., et al. [2017]. ILAE classification of the epilepsies: Position paper of the ILAE Commission for Classification and Terminology. *Epilepsia, 58*[4], 512–521.)

Nursing assessment and care. The nurse observes and records the following: the child's activity immediately before the seizure; body movements; changes in colour, respiration, or muscle tone; any incontinence; and the parts of the body involved. When possible, the seizure is timed. The child's appearance, behaviour, and level of consciousness after the seizure are also documented. Table 23.5 describes the first aid response and nursing responsibilities during a seizure.

Safety Alert!

In general, if someone is having a seizure:

STAY CALM

- Seizures usually end on their own within seconds or a few minutes.

CREATE A SAFE SPACE

- Move sharp objects out of the way.
- If the person falls, place something soft under their head and roll them on their side as the seizure subsides.
- If the person wanders, stay by their side and gently steer them away from danger.

TIME IT

- Note the time the seizure begins and ends.

CALL 911 IF

- The seizure lasts more than 5 minutes.
- It repeats without full recovery between seizures.
- If consciousness or regular breathing does not return after the seizure ends.
- The person is pregnant, has diabetes, appears injured, or is in water.
- You are not sure the person has epilepsy or a seizure disorder.

PROVIDE REASSURANCE

- When the seizure ends, stay with the person until complete awareness returns.

DO NOT...

- Restrain the person.
- Put anything in their mouth.

From Epilepsy Ontario. (2018). First aid. Retrieved from http://epilepsyontario.org/about-epilepsy/first-aid/.

The following are some areas that require extra precautions for children with epilepsy.

Bathing. Water is especially dangerous for children with epilepsy, so children should bathe in low levels of water. Even when as little water as possible is used, drowning is a possibility if the child falls unconscious, which can occur without making a sound. The bathroom door should not be locked when the child bathes. Children with frequent seizures should take showers while sitting on a stool. Taking showers is safer than taking baths, but injuries may still occur. Even older children struggling to gain independence should ensure that someone else is home when they bathe or shower. They should not be permitted to bathe when there is no one else in the house.

Swimming. Children with epilepsy can swim under the watchful eye of lifeguards or responsible adults who are trained in lifesaving and ready to act in case of an emergency. Supervisors should be informed that the child has epilepsy so that they are ready to deal with a seizure, should one occur. While swimming, children with epilepsy should have a "buddy" who swims with them.

Head protection. When a child has a tonic (drop) seizures, the loss of posture may be so rapid that the child crashes violently to the ground. Because this type of seizures is difficult to control, the individual may be exposed to physical injury. Sometimes helmets are a necessity. Children with epilepsy should also wear a helmet whenever they will be participating in sports where there is a risk of head injury.

Driving. Provincial laws regulate that health care providers must report to the Ministry of Transport any health conditions that may impair one's ability to drive safely, which includes uncontrolled seizures. While each province and territory has its own laws, in most provinces, once a person with seizures has been seizure free for 6 months with a favourable recommendation from the health care provider, a driver's license may be reinstated.

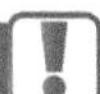

Safety Alert!

The nurse is responsible for maintaining seizure precautions for a child diagnosed with a seizure disorder.

In the hospital:

- Keep side rails up.
- Pad all sharp or hard objects around the bed.

In the community:

- Make sure the child wears a medical alert bracelet.
- Provide supervision during potentially hazardous play, such as swimming.
- Avoid triggering factors (lack of sleep, febrile events, and alcohol).
- Teach the importance of adhering to the medication regimen.

Treatment. Initially, treatment is aimed at determining the type, site, or cause of the seizure disorder. Diagnostic measures include a complete history and physical and neurological examinations. Skull radiography and CT or MRI scans are used to establish the presence or absence of tumours, skull abnormalities, hematomas, and intracranial calcifications. The EEG is also a valuable tool in diagnosing seizures. It is especially helpful in differentiating between focal and generalized seizures. Prolonged EEG monitoring (>24 hours) is another diagnostic technique.

Laboratory studies such as complete blood count (CBC), determinations of serum calcium and blood urea nitrogen (BUN), and tests to rule out lead poisoning or other metabolic disorders are performed. Anticonvulsant medications are prescribed when epilepsy is diagnosed (Table 23.6). The medication of choice depends on the type of seizure.

The duration of therapy is based on the individual child and the etiology and prognosis of the epilepsy syndrome. Initially, the health care provider prescribes the lowest dose of anticonvulsant medication likely to control the seizures. The goal is to control the seizures and minimize the toxic effects of the medication. Drowsiness, a common adverse effect of many anticonvulsants, may interfere with the child's activities. Careful recording of seizure activity and ability to follow the medication regimen are of particular importance in determining a suitable program. The medication is administered at the *same time each day,* generally with meals or at bedtime.

If it is necessary for the child to take medication during school hours, it is important that teachers are aware of this. The responses of the teacher, particularly during and after a seizure, will have a significant effect on the attitude of classmates toward the child.

Abrupt withdrawal of anticonvulsant medications is the most common cause of status epilepticus

Table 23.5 Seizure Recognition and First Aid Response

SEIZURE TYPE	WHAT IT LOOKS LIKE	OFTEN MISTAKEN FOR	WHAT TO DO	WHAT NOT TO DO
1. General Seizure				
Generalized tonic-clonic seizure (previously called *grand mal seizure*)	Sudden cry (or *aura*), fall, rigidity, followed by *muscle jerking;* shallow, irregular breathing; possible loss of bladder or bowel control; usually lasts seconds to minutes, followed by some confusion, a period of sleep (*postictal lethargy*), and then return to full consciousness	Heart attack, stroke	Look for medical identification. Protect from nearby hazards. Observe and record stages and manifestations. Following seizure, maintain patent airway, turn on side, loosen clothing, reassure person. If multiple seizures, or if one seizure lasts longer than 5 minutes, call ambulance (911). If person is pregnant, injured, or diabetic, call for aid at once.	**DO NOT** put any hard implement in the mouth. **DO NOT** try to hold tongue; it cannot be swallowed. **DO NOT** try to give liquids during or just after seizure. **DO NOT** restrain person.
2. Absence Seizure				
(previously called *petit mal* seizure)	A blank stare, beginning and ending abruptly, lasting only a few seconds; most common in children; may be accompanied by rapid blinking, some chewing movements of the mouth; person is unaware of what is going on during seizure but quickly returns to full awareness after it has stopped; may result in learning difficulties if not recognized and treated	Daydreaming, lack of attention, deliberate ignoring of adult instructions	No first aid necessary, but if this is first observation of seizure(s), medical evaluation should be recommended. Can be triggered by flashing lights or hyperventilation.	
3. Partial				
A. Aware focal seizure (previously called *simple partial*)	Jerking may begin in one area of body such as arm, leg, or face; cannot be stopped, but person stays awake and aware; jerking may proceed from one area of the body to another and sometimes spreads to become a generalized seizure	Acting-out, bizarre behaviour, hysteria, mental illness, psychosomatic illness, parapsychological or mystical experience, tics	No first aid necessary unless seizure becomes generalized, then give first aid as indicated. No immediate action is needed other than reassurance and emotional support. Medical evaluation should be recommended.	

Table 23.5 **Seizure Recognition and First Aid Response—cont'd**

SEIZURE TYPE	WHAT IT LOOKS LIKE	OFTEN MISTAKEN FOR	WHAT TO DO	WHAT NOT TO DO
B. Focal impaired awareness (previously known as *complex partial seizure*)	Usually starts with blank stare, followed by chewing, followed by random activity; person appears unaware of surroundings, may seem dazed and may mumble; is unresponsive; actions are clumsy, not directed; may pick at clothing, pick up objects, try to take off clothes; may run, appear afraid; may struggle or flail at restraint; after pattern established, same set of actions usually occurs with each seizure; can last 1 to 2 minutes; no memory of actions or behaviour	Disorderly conduct	Speak calmly and reassuringly to person and others. Guide person gently away from obvious hazards. Stay with person until completely aware of environment. Offer to help getting home.	**DO NOT** grab hold of person unless sudden danger threatens (such as a cliff edge or an approaching car). **DO NOT** try to restrain person. **DO NOT** shout. **DO NOT** expect verbal instructions to be obeyed.
4. Atonic Seizure				
Also called *drop attacks*	More frequent occurrence in the morning with jerking motions on awakening; suddenly collapses; after 10 seconds to 1 minute, person recovers and can stand and walk again	Clumsiness, normal childhood stage; lack of good walking skills; drunkenness	No first aid is needed (unless hurt during fall), but the person should be given a thorough medical evaluation.	

(prolonged seizures). In the hospital, the nurse needs to clarify with the health care provider whether anticonvulsants should be withheld if the child is to be NPO. When children are old enough, they can assume responsibility for their own medications. During puberty and adolescence, the dosages may have to be adjusted to meet growth needs and hormone changes, which may influence seizure recurrence. Anticonvulsant medications should be taken during pregnancy with caution and under medical supervision because birth defects can occur with certain of these medications. Children with focal epilepsy may be considered candidates for epilepsy surgery, which can be curative (Mikati & Hani, 2016). Eligibility of candidacy for surgery must be done at qualified epilepsy centres requiring multidisciplinary review and specialized testing. If surgery is successful, gradual medication weaning may be considered if the child has been seizure free for 2 years and has a normal EEG.

The **ketogenic diet** is sometimes prescribed for children who do not respond well to anticonvulsant therapy. As the diet is high in fats and low in carbohydrates, a specialized health care team is required to monitor for adequate protein for growth as well as supplementation of micronutrients. This diet produces ketoacidosis in the body, which appears to reduce convulsive episodes. Adherence to the ketogenic diet may be difficult and requires support from the whole family, as there is no room for "cheating." Long-term effects of this type of diet, such as hyperlipidemia, are unknown but may lead to heart attack or stroke (Epilepsy Foundation, 2018).

The greatest untapped resource for persons with epilepsy is often within themselves. A fundamental principle of comprehensive epilepsy management is that the child must become an active member of the health care team. In a comprehensive multidisciplinary treatment approach, team members help the child to mobilize their inner resources to handle lifelong treatment and to lead a fully productive, normal life. With a few safety guidelines, this is possible.

A family assessment is helpful in establishing rapport and setting realistic short- and long-term goals. Too much attention to seizures by well-meaning adults can make seizure control difficult. Teaching should include first aid treatment for seizures (see Table 23.5), the importance of adhering to a long-term medication regimen, and general reassurance that the child can lead a normal life.

Table 23.6 Properties of Selected Anticonvulsant Medications

MEDICATION	ADVERSE EFFECTS	COMMENTS
Carbamazepine (Tegretol)	Grapefruit juice may increase levels Increased levels with erythromycin can cause drowsiness, diplopia, dizziness Rarely liver and pancreatic complications	Few adverse effects, fewer sedative properties; used for focal seizures Give with food.
Phenobarbital	Drowsiness, irritability, hyperactivity, balance issues	Altered sleep patterns, often combined with other medications Provide vitamin D and folic acid supplements.
Phenytoin (Dilantin)	Ataxia, insomnia, nystagmus, gum overgrowth, hirsutism (hairiness), rash, nausea, vitamin D and folic acid deficiencies	Generally effective and safe; may cause cognitive impairment; regular massaging of gums decreases hyperplasia; used in combination with phenobarbital. Intravenous (IV) doses should not be mixed with glucose solutions. May discolour urine.
Valproic acid (Depakene), other derivatives (Divalproex Sodium have different doses)	Gastrointestinal upset, liver toxicity, amenorrhea, weight gain, platelet dysfunction	Take with food. Do not chew; potentiates action of phenobarbital and other medications. Do not administer with carbonated beverages. Should not be taken during pregnancy. Monitor complete blood count (CBC) and platelets, liver and pancreatic enzymes.
Primidone (Mysoline, Myidone, Apo-Primidone, Sertan)	Personality changes, anorexia, fatigue, dermatitis	May be used alone or in combination; adverse effects minimized by starting with small amounts. Provide folic acid supplements. Administer with foods.
Ethosuximide (Zarontin)	Anorexia, gastrointestinal upset	Often used for absence seizures Give with food. Monitor for anorexia and weight loss.
Topiramate (Topamax, Apo-Topiramate)	Slowed cognition, fatigue May cause psychomotor slowing	Used for focal or generalized seizures. Increase fluid intake to prevent nephrocalcinosis. Monitor for cognitive effect.
Gabapentin (pms-Gabapentin)	Weight gain and somnolence	Used in poorly controlled seizures. Do not give with antacid. Monitor vision and concentration.
Lamotrigine (Lamictal)	Ataxia, rash, photosensitivity, and drowsiness	Do not give with valproic acid. Observe for skin rash.
Keppra (Levetiracetam)	Sleepiness, incoordination, behaviour changes	Used with other medications for generalized and focal seizures. Monitor coordination.

Note: The health care provider determines the child's medication by the type of seizure and other factors. The goal is to achieve the best control with the minimum dosage and the least number of adverse effects. An important aspect of nursing intervention includes reinforcing the need for medication supervision and adherence.
Data from David, R. (2010). *Pediatric neurology*. New York: Demos Medical Publishing; Mikati, M., & Hani, A. (2016). Seizures in childhood. In R. Kliegman, B. Stanton, J. St. Geme, et al. (Eds.), *Nelson textbook of pediatrics* (20th ed.). Philadelphia: Saunders; Skidmore-Roth, L. (2017). *Mosby's 2017 nursing drug reference* (30th ed.). Philadelphia: Elsevier.

Nursing Tip

Common triggering factors for seizures include the following:

- Flashing of dark/light patterns
- Photosensitivity
- Poor sleep
- Febrile illness
- Alcohol intake
- Poor medication adherence

Medications used in the treatment of epilepsy are outlined in Table 23.6. The gum hypertrophy (Fig. 23.19) that occurs as an adverse effect of phenytoin (Dilantin) requires meticulous oral hygiene and special care, especially if orthodontic treatment is necessary.

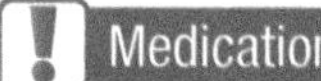

Medication Alert!

Children taking phenobarbital or phenytoin should receive vitamin D and folic acid supplementation. Phenytoin should not be given with milk. As with many medications, seizure medications should not be ingested with grapefruit juice, as this may compete with metabolizing liver enzymes that may cause diminished or toxic medication metabolites.

Sudden unexplained death in epilepsy. Although rare, children and adults with epilepsy are at greater risk for sudden unexplained death in epilepsy (SUDEP), which is threefold compared to the risk in the general population. The major risk factor is uncontrolled seizures with at least three generalized tonic-clonic

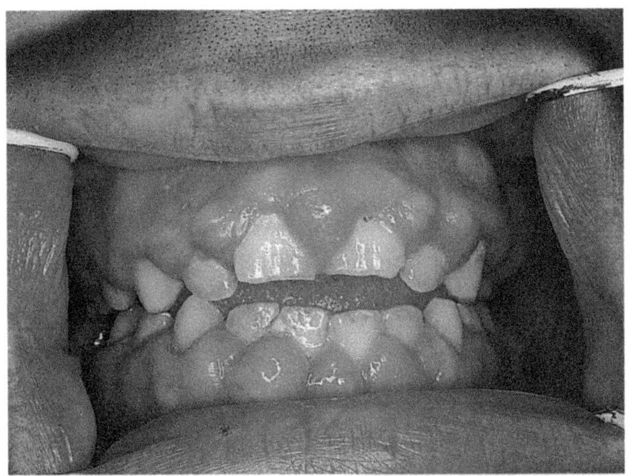

Fig. 23.19 Phenytoin-induced gum hyperplasia. (From Callen, J. P., Greer, K. E., Paller, A. S., et al. [2000]. *Color atlas of dermatology* [2nd ed.]. Philadelphia: Saunders.)

events per year. Adherence to the medication regimen and improved seizure control can decrease the risk of SUDEP (DeGiorgio, Markovic, Mazumder, et al., 2017).

Status epilepticus. A prolonged seizure that does not respond to treatment for 30 minutes or more is called **status epilepticus**; it can result in brain hypoxia. A common cause is sudden stopping of epilepsy medication or generalized infection. Treatment includes managing the airway, providing oxygen, observing and documenting details of the seizure, and providing IV therapy. Diazepam (Valium), lorazepam (Ativan), phenytoin (Dilantin), or a pentobarbital (Nembutal) medication may be given intravenously. Rectal diazepam or intranasal midazolam (Versed) are safe and effective approaches for treating status epilepticus. The child may need to be supported on a mechanical ventilator until seizures are controlled.

Other Conditions That Can Mimic Seizures

Several conditions are mistaken for epilepsy because they involve paroxysmal altered levels of consciousness. These conditions do not respond to antiepileptic medications.

Benign paroxysmal vertigo

This condition occurs in children less than 3 years of age, who often develop ataxia and fall. Nausea, vomiting, and symptoms of motion sickness and migraine headache follow. The condition responds to dimenhydrinate (Gravol) medication.

Breath-holding spells

Breath holding can result in cyanosis or extreme pallor. Episodes of breath holding are most common between 2 and 5 years of age and is often the result of immaturity of the autonomic system. The child loses consciousness, and the parents are frightened. Counselling parents to avoid reinforcing the behaviour by refusing to play with or hold the child after the episode is helpful. The parents should be counselled to prepare the child for any unpleasant experiences and avoid sudden surprises.

Prolonged QT syndrome

One type of sudden loss of consciousness is associated with vigorous exercise. It can be caused by a heart problem and reflected as a prolonged QT segment on the electrocardiogram (ECG), and it can result in loss of consciousness and death. It usually occurs during adolescence and arises from a defect in chromosome 11. Beta blockers may be lifesaving. Knowledge of cardiopulmonary resuscitation (CPR) and exercise restriction are essential.

Rage attacks or episodic dyscontrol syndrome

Rage attacks are sudden, recurrent attacks of violent physical behaviour. These attacks appear to be out of control and are followed by fatigue, remorse, and amnesia. The EEG is usually normal. This condition is often mistaken for focal seizures, previously known as complex partial seizures.

Head Injuries

Head injuries are the major cause of death and permanent injury in children older than 1 year of age. More physical force is needed to produce brain trauma when the head is in a fixed position than when it is freely moving—a fact that supports the use of infant car seats. Children have poorly developed neck muscles, thus participation in collision sports increases the risk of concussion and a second injury before the first one heals, resulting in prolonged cognitive changes. A **concussion** is a temporary disturbance of the brain that is usually followed by a period of unconsciousness. It jars the brainstem and is often accompanied by a loss of memory for events that occurred immediately before (retrograde amnesia), during, and after the accident. In a skull fracture the skull bone is broken or depressed. Bleeding may occur, resulting in pressure being exerted on the brain.

The response of the child to a head injury may differ from that of the adult. Loss of consciousness may not be evident, but changes in behaviour, sleep, cognition, and balance may occur. For example, the child may find it difficult to stand on one foot with the eyes closed. The location and type of skull fracture may not correlate with clinical findings. Careful clinical assessment is essential to determine the extent of brain injury. The surface area of a child's scalp is large and very vascular, thus significant blood loss can result from scalp lacerations.

 **Safety Alert!**

A concussion with resulting amnesia and confusion can be more serious than the presence of a fractured skull with no clinical symptoms.

Pathophysiology

A skull fracture, brain concussion, contusion, or intracranial hemorrhage may occur at the time of injury. Brain injury may occur at the point of impact, or on the opposite side of the brain *(coup-contre-coup)*. Therefore, a blow to the occiput can result in an injury to the temporal area as the brain hits the bony skull. Children are more susceptible to the effects of a concussion than adults because children have muscles that are not fully developed framing the CNS. The myelin sheath development is not yet mature, so conduction of impulses from the CNS to the rest of the body is not completely developed, making the signs and symptoms of concussion difficult to recognize by the untrained eye. Cognitive skills such as focusing, processing information, and recall are often the functions of the brain that are affected by a concussion. Concussion is not limited to a direct head injury and can be the result of a biomechanical impulsive force transmitted from a blow to another site of the body transmitted to the brain (Norton, Feltz, Brocker, et al., 2013). Hypoxia, increased ICP, cerebral edema, and infection can occur within a few days. Hypoxia causes the brain to need increased energy, which results in increased cerebral blood flow. This increased blood flow *(hyperemia)* increases cerebral edema. If the ICP rises too high, cerebral perfusion diminishes, and brain damage or death results. If the fontanelles are open, the tolerance for increased ICP is higher in infants. Older children and adults do not have this advantage.

A child who sustains a mild bump to the head, retains consciousness, and does not vomit may have a covered ice pack applied to the site. During the first night after a bump on the head, parents are advised to be sure that they can arouse the child at least once, because intracranial bleeding occasionally occurs from a minor injury. They should be advised to contact a health care provider if the child appears confused, has trouble seeing or speaking, or walks unsteadily. Confusion, cognitive changes, or amnesia after any head injury may indicate a concussion even if consciousness is not lost.

The second impact syndrome (SIS) results when a second blow to the head occurs before the first injury incident is fully healed. Even if the second impact is less severe than the first, the outcome can be devastating (Brown & Fishman, 2017).

The CPS recommends the use of the CATCH rule to determine the severity of a head injury (Farrell & CPS Acute Care Committee, 2013/2018) (Box 23.4). Children require a CT scan if they have any of the high risk or medium risk factors. High risk predicts the need for neurological intervention and medium risk predicts brain injury on CT scan.

Roughly shaking an infant can cause the brain to strike the inside of the skull (**shaken baby syndrome** or nonaccidental injury), causing tearing of blood vessels surrounding the brain and secondary torsion injury to the brain tissue. This can result in retinal, subarachnoid, and subdural hemorrhages as well as high-level cervical spine injuries and permanent disability or death. Teaching coping techniques to parents of children who cry inconsolably can help prevent this type of injury. Suspected shaken baby syndrome found in infants must be reported to local authorities.

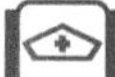 **Nursing Tip**

Nurses should stress to parents the dangers of shaking infants roughly, including jumping on a trampoline with an infant in their arms.

Management

A child who has suffered a blow to the head is often brought to the hospital for overnight observation to rule out or confirm the extent of injury. The child may experience all or some of the following symptoms:

- Headache (manifested by fussiness in the toddler)
- Drowsiness
- Blurred vision
- Vomiting

Box 23.4 Canadian Assessment of Tomography for Childhood Head Injury: The CATCH Rule

CT of the head is required for children with a minor head injury* *plus any one* of the following findings:

High risk (need for neurological intervention)

- Glasgow Coma Scale score <15 at 2 hours after injury
- Suspected open or depressed skull fracture
- History of worsening headache
- Irritability on examination

Medium risk (brain injury on CT scan)

- Any sign of basal skull fracture (e.g., hemotympanum, "raccoon" eyes, otorrhea or rhinorrhea of cerebrospinal fluid, Battle sign)
- Large, boggy hematoma of the scalp
- Dangerous mechanism of injury (e.g., motor vehicle collision, fall from a height >0.9 metre or down five stairs, falling from a bicycle without a helmet)

Minor head injury is injury in the past 24 hours with witnessed loss of consciousness, definite amnesia, witnessed disorientation, persistent vomiting or persistent irritability (in a child under 2 years of age) in a patient with a Glasgow Coma Scale of 13–15.

CT, Computerized tomography.

Source: Osmond, M. H., et al. (2010). CATCH: A clinical decision rule for the use of computed tomography in children with minor head injury. *Canadian Medical Association Journal, 182*(4), 341–348.

- Dyspnea

Management of children with mild head injury (GCS >14) includes the following:

- Children who are asymptomatic can be discharged home if caregivers are reliable with instructions to monitor for signs of worsening headache, vomiting, or change in level of consciousness, in which case immediate return to the hospital is advised.
- Children who are less than 2 years of age should be monitored with greater caution and require more careful assessment, owing to thinner skull bones that are not fully mature and fused, which may have increased risk of bleeding or injury.

In severe cases, the child may be completely unconscious. Decerebrate posturing (**extensor posturing**) or decorticate posturing (**flexor posturing**) may be evident (Fig. 23.20). In decerebrate (extensor) rigidity, all four limbs are extended and the hands are pronated. This may indicate brainstem injury. In decorticate (flexor) rigidity, the arms, wrists, and fingers are flexed. Plantar flexion occurs in the feet. This may indicate damage to the cortex of the brain. These pathological postures (**posturing**) are seen with severe brain injury.

A careful history is obtained to determine any preexisting conditions and to ascertain the exact circumstances of the accident. Of particular importance is the child's state of consciousness immediately after the accident.

The nurse needs to observe the child for signs of increasing ICP. There are four components of a cranial or neurological check:

1. Level of consciousness
2. Pupil and eye movement (see Fig. 23.2)
3. Vital signs
4. Motor activity (see Box 23.2)

Children should be handled gently and be inspected for injuries to other areas. They should be placed in a crib or bed in accordance with their age. Side rails should be raised, because seizures are not uncommon. The head of the bed is slightly elevated to decrease cerebral edema.

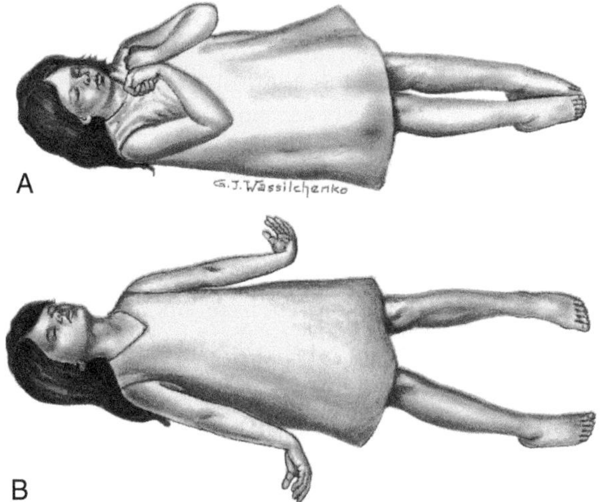

Fig. 23.20 Posturing. Pathological posturing that may occur in the children with severe brain damage. **A,** Decorticate (flexor) posturing. **B,** Decerebrate (extensor) posturing. (From Hockenberry, M., & Wilson, D. [2015]. *Wong's nursing care of infants and children* [10th ed.]. St. Louis: Mosby.)

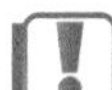

Safety Alert!

After a head injury, the presence of asymmetrical pupils is a medical emergency.

Nursing care

Nursing care of children with head injuries includes examination of wound swelling if a laceration of the head is present. The type and amount of drainage from the ears and nose are recorded. The nurse checks for *nuchal* (neck) rigidity, which might indicate an infection such as meningitis. Occipital-frontal circumference of the head is monitored in infants, as are tension of the fontanelles and the presence of a high-pitched cry. Fluids are carefully monitored to control *cerebral edema.* Feeding difficulties should be noted as the child's diet is increased. The child is observed for signs of shock, which can also occur.

Children whose condition has remained stable are discharged. Parents should be instructed about any additional observations and follow-up care. Most children are advised to decrease cognitive activities after a concussion, including texting, cellphone use, watching television, listening to loud music, and computer use, with a gradual return to full activity. Signs of postconcussion syndrome include headache, fatigue, photophobia, and disturbed thinking (Norton et al., 2013).

Nurses should teach parents and children the importance of using appropriate protective equipment when engaging in sports activities.

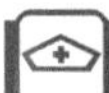

Nursing Tip

A positive glucose oxidase screening test can determine if watery nasal discharge is CSF or a concurrent cold (rhinorrhea).

Following even a slight head injury, the child should be assessed before continuing in sports activities. Mild traumatic brain injury can occur even without loss of consciousness and long-term effects can result. Complications of concussion can include postconcussion syndrome, which involves cognitive and emotional problems and chronic traumatic encephalopathy. Coaches are not qualified to assess head injuries, and baseline function should be established *before* entering into contact sports activities.

Submersion Injury

The term *submersion injury* has replaced the term *near-drowning* and should be used to describe injury occurring up until the time of drowning-related death. This term includes injury to any person who experiences distress from near-drowning submersion or immersion in liquid that results in death (*drowning*) or survival at least 24 hours after submersion (*near-drowning*) (Sams, 2017).

In Canada, drowning is the second leading cause of unintentional injury death in children 1 to 4 years of age, accounting for more than one fifth of deaths in this age group (Lifesaving Society, 2017). Infant and toddlers' drownings tend to occur in or around the home, with infants' drownings occurring mostly in bathtubs, and toddlers drowning after falling into swimming pools.

Proper supervision and environmental safety precautions are the best measures to prevent drowning. In adolescents, the use of illicit substances and alcohol during recreational swimming contributes to drowning incidents. The priorities in immediate response include immediate CPR and treatment of hypoxia, aspiration, and hypothermia.

Cardiorespiratory survival has increased with advances in emergency medical treatment by paramedics on site and with the technology available in critical care units in the hospital. However, CNS injury remains the major cause of death or long-term disability.

Safety Alert!

All children who experience a submersion injury should be admitted for a 24-hour observation period of close monitoring for the development of cerebral edema, which may be evidenced by an altered level of consciousness.

Submersion for more than 10 minutes with failure to regain consciousness at the scene or within 24 hours is an ominous sign and is predictive of severe neurological deficits if the child survives. Respiratory and cardiovascular support, controlled rewarming, and maintenance of adequate cerebral oxygenation are priorities of care (Nursing Care Plan 23.1). The parents need to be offered support, explanations of the therapy, and referral to social services, religious organizations, or community agencies for follow-up. Adult supervision and water safety and survival training can prevent most submersion injuries. Nurses should advocate for these safety measures in schools and communities.

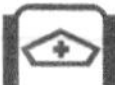

Nursing Tip

The Canadian Paediatric Society recommends that children over 4 years of age take swimming lessons. Children less than 4 years of age do not have the developmental ability to master independent water survival skills for swimming. Programs should be led by certified trainers, with a focus on building confidence and educating parents on water safety.

Nursing Care Plan 23.1 **The Child With Altered Level of Consciousness**

PATIENT DATA

A 4-year-old child fell into a pool while playing, hitting his head on the pool deck. Cardiopulmonary resuscitation re-established a heartbeat and spontaneous respirations. The child is admitted with signs of increased intracranial pressure, including a decreased level of consciousness and an absence of the gag reflex.

Selected Nursing Diagnosis Difficulty in maintaining patent airway as a result of altered level of consciousness

Goals	Nursing Interventions	Rationales
Child will demonstrate effective breathing pattern as evidenced by patent airway, age-appropriate respiratory rate (RR), lungs clear to auscultation, and ability to breathe on their own without mechanical assistance.	Observe airway for patency. Observe for: presence or absence of gag and swallow reflex, RR, rhythm, and effort; note any irregularities.	Diminished oxygenation can lead to cerebral anoxia and/or death. Inability to protect the airway can lead to aspiration pneumonia. A marked increase or decrease in respiratory pattern can be a sign of impending respiratory failure.
	Auscultate breath sounds, noting and reporting any adventitious breath sounds.	Adventitious breath sounds are indicative of accumulated respiratory secretions, thereby increasing the risk for pneumonia or atelectasis.
	Provide meticulous pulmonary care to prevent respiratory compromise.	Good oral hygiene, suctioning of oral secretions, cleaning of buccal cavity, and turning child every 2 hours will help prevent respiratory problems.

Selected Nursing Diagnosis Risk for adverse effects of immobility

Goals	Nursing Interventions	Rationales
Child will maintain intact skin without signs or symptoms of tissue breakdown or pressure ulcer formation.	Inspect all skin surfaces, noting areas of erythema, blanching, or edema. Pay particular attention to all bony prominences and areas in direct contact with the bed.	Lying in one position for extended periods increases the risk of tissue breakdown and pressure ulcer formation.

Nursing Care Plan 23.1 The Child With Altered Level of Consciousness—cont'd

Goals	Nursing Interventions	Rationales
	Reposition every 2 hours. Place child in prone position periodically (unless contraindicated by medical condition).	Repositioning helps to improve circulation and relieves pressure areas.
	Bathe the child daily and keep bedding free of wrinkles and crumbs.	Bathing increases circulation because of the massaging of the skin with the washcloth. Having a bed free of wrinkles and crumbs prevents additional areas of potential skin breakdown and decubitus ulcer formation.

Selected Nursing Diagnosis Family stress as a result of hospitalization of child

Goals	Nursing Interventions	Rationales
Parent and/or family will demonstrate management skills as evidenced by expressing a realistic understanding of child's illness and active participation in child's care.	Assess level of anxiety or concern of parent(s) and/or family members.	Provides data to determine type of assistance or support that is needed.
	Provide opportunities for instruction on how to care for the ill child.	Enhances feelings of control and involvement in the health care of the child.
	Reinforce or clarify medical explanation of child's condition and prognosis.	Ensures that parent and family have a clear understanding of information received.
	Identify community agencies and support services within the community available to the family.	Provides family with sources of emotional and spiritual support in times of crisis.

Get Ready for the Certification Examination!

Key Points

- In paralytic strabismus, the unaffected eye is patched.
- Infants are more prone to ear infections than older children because their eustachian tubes are shorter, wider, and straighter.
- Level of consciousness is the most important indicator of neurological health.
- The Glasgow Coma Scale (GCS) is used to determine level of consciousness in infants and children.
- Nursing care of the unconscious child includes assessing the child for increased intracranial pressure (ICP), maintaining an open airway, providing adequate nutrition and fluids, positioning, maintaining flexibility of joints, and preventing injury.
- A high-pitched cry may be indicative of increased ICP.
- Spina bifida is a congenital embryonic neural tube defect in which there is an imperfect closure of the spinal vertebrae.
- Folic acid supplementation during the early weeks of pregnancy can prevent neural tube anomalies.
- Meningitis is an inflammation of the meninges that cover the brain and spinal cord.
- Measuring head size is important in infants with hydrocephalus.
- A seizure is a symptom of an underlying pathological condition.
- Generalized tonic-clonic seizures involve an aura, muscle jerking, and postictal lethargy.
- Decerebrate, decorticate, or opisthotonos posturing indicates brain damage.
- The response of the pupils to light and ascertaining level of consciousness are essential assessments to determine brain injury.
- Shaken baby syndrome can result in subdural hematoma and death.
- Confusion and amnesia after a head injury may indicate concussion even if consciousness is not lost.
- The priority of care for a child who has experienced a submersion injury is to prevent hypoxia, aspiration, and hypothermia.

Additional Learning Resources

evolve Go to your Evolve website (http://evolve.elsevier.com/Canada/Leifer) for the following learning resources:

- Answer Key for Critical Thinking Questions
- Answer Key for Textbook Review Questions
- Audio Glossary
- Interactive Review Questions

Get Ready for the Certification Examination!—Cont'd

- Skills Performance Checklists
- Video clips and more!

Online Resources

- Brain Injury Canada: https://www.braininjurycanada.ca/
- Canadian Hearing Society: http://www.chs.ca/
- Epilepsy Canada: http://www.epilepsy.ca/
- Hydrocephalus Canada: http://mybrainwaves.ca/
- Learning Disabilities Association of Canada: https://www.ldac-acta.ca/

Review Questions

1. Which symptom would indicate an earache in an infant?
   a. External drainage, pain, and decrease in temperature
   b. Tugging at the ear and rolling head from side to side
   c. Crying and pointing to affected ear
   d. Redness of the cheeks and cyanosis of the ear
2. Which signs would indicate increased intracranial pressure in a 3-year-old child?
   a. Headache, lethargy
   b. High pitched cry, bulging fontanelles
   c. Apnea, crossed eyes
   d. Painful head movement, anorexia
3. Which is a priority nursing intervention when administering phenytoin to a patient diagnosed with epilepsy?
   a. Recording blood pressure
   b. Providing good oral hygiene
   c. Encouraging bed rest
   d. Administering it with milk
4. Distinct phases of a generalized tonic-clonic seizure include which of the following? *(Select all that apply.)*
   a. Aura
   b. Agitation
   c. Muscle jerking
   d. Postictal lethargy
5. A nursing responsibility when a child has a seizure would include which actions? *(Select all that apply.)*
   a. Time the seizure.
   b. Place the child in prone position.
   c. Move furniture away from the child.
   d. Observe and record behaviour immediately following the seizure.
   e. Call 911.

Critical Thinking Question

1. After resuscitation in the emergency department, following a fall down the stairs, the child has regained consciousness, is interacting with the mother, and has stable vital signs. The mother states, "Now that my child is okay I want to take him home." What is the best response of the nurse?

REFERENCES

Amit, M., & Canadian Paediatric Society (CPS), Community Paediatrics Committee. (2009). Vision screening in infants, children and youth. *Paediatrics & Child Health, 14*(4), 246–248. Reaffirmed 2018.

Brown, J., & Fishman, L. (2017). Kid care on the slopes. *Contemporary Pediatrics, 34*(1), 22–26.

Canadian League Against Epilepsy. (n.d.). *General information*. Retrieved from https://claegroup.org/General-Information

Canadian Retinoblastoma Society. (2009). National retinoblastoma strategy Canadian guidelines for care. *Canadian Journal of Ophthalmology, 44*(Suppl. 2), S1–88. https://doi.org/10.3129/i09-194.

DeGiorgio, C. M., Markovic, D., Mazumder, R., et al. (2017). Ranking the leading risk factors for sudden unexpected death in epilepsy. *Frontiers in Neurology, 8*, 1–6. https://doi.org/10.3389/fneur.2017.00473.

Epilepsy Foundation. (2018). *Ketogenic diet*. Retrieved from https://www.epilepsy.com/learn/treating-seizures-and-epilepsy/dietary-therapies/ketogenic-diet.

Farrell, C. A., & Canadian Paediatric Society (CPS), Acute Care Committee. (2013). Management of the paediatric patient with acute head trauma. *Paediatrics & Child Health, 18*(5), 253–258. Reaffirmed 2018. Retrieved from https://www.cps.ca/en/documents/position/paediatric-patient-with-acute-head-trauma.

Govindan, M., Mohney, G. B., Diehl, N. N., et al. (2005). Incidence and types of childhood exotropia: A population-based study. *Ophthalmology, 112*, 104–108.

Haddad, J., & Keesecker, S. (2016). The ear. In R. Kliegman, B. Stanton, J. St. Geme, et al. (Eds.), *Nelson textbook of pediatrics*. (20th ed.). Philadelphia: Saunders.

Hartman, M. E., & Cheifetz, I. M. (2016). Pediatric emergencies and resuscitation. In R. Kliegman, B. Stanton, J. St. Geme, et al. (Eds.), *Nelson textbook of pediatrics*. (20th ed.). Philadelphia: Saunders.

Kinsman, S., & Johnston, M. (2016). Congenital anomalies of the central nervous system. In R. Kliegman, B. Stanton, J. St. Geme, et al. (Eds.), *Nelson textbook of pediatrics*. (20th ed.). Philadelphia: Saunders.

Leis, J. A., Rutka, J. A., & Gold, W. L. (2015). Aminoglycoside -induced ototoxicity. *Canadian Medical Association Journal, 187*(1), E52. Retrieved from http://www.cmaj.ca/content/cmaj/187/1/E52.full.pdf.

Le Saux, N., Robinson, J. L., & Canadian Paediatric Society (CPS), Infection Diseases and Immunization Committee. (2016). Management of acute otitis media in children six months of age and older. *Paediatrics & Child Health, 21*(1), 39–44. Retrieved from https://www.cps.ca/en/documents/position/acute-otitis-media.

Lifesaving Society. (2017). *Canadian drowning report*. Retrieved from http://www.lifesavingsociety.com/media/264742/98cdndrowningreport_2017rev_web.pdf.

Mikati, M., & Hani, A. (2016). Seizures in childhood. In R. Kliegman, B. Stanton, J. St. Geme, et al. (Eds.), *Nelson textbook of pediatrics*. (20th ed.). Philadelphia: Saunders.

Norton, C., Feltz, S., Brocker, A., et al. (2013). Tackling long term consequences of concussion. *Nursing, 43*(1), 5053.

Olitsky, S., Hug, D., Plummer, L., et al. (2016). Disorders of the eye. In R. Kliegman, B. Stanton, J. St. Geme, et al. (Eds.), *Nelson textbook of pediatrics*. (20th ed.). Philadelphia: Saunders.

Patel, H., Feldman, M., & Canadian Paediatric Society (CPS), Community Paediatrics Committee. (2011). Universal newborn hearing screening. *Paediatrics & Child Health, 16*(5), 301–305. Reaffirmed 2018.

Public Health Agency of Canada (PHAC). (2017). *Epilepsy in Canada*. Retrieved from https://www.canada.ca/content/dam/phac-aspc/documents/services/publications/diseases-conditions/64-03-17-2021-Epilepsy-in-Canada-EN-FINAL.pdf.

Rosenfeld, R., Schwartz, S., & Pynnonen, M. (2013). Clinical practice guideline: Tympanostomy tubes in children. *Otolaryngology–Head and Neck Surgery, 149*, s1–s35.

Sams, C. (2017). Cerebral dysfunction. In S. Perry, M. Hockenberry, D. Lowdermilk, et al. (Eds.), *Maternal child nursing care in Canada*. (2nd ed.). Toronto, ON: Elsevier.

Scott, O. (2015). *Strabismus (Squint)*. Retrieved from https://patient.info/pdf/1691.pdf.

Scheffer, I. E., Berkovic, S., Capovilla, G., et al. (2017). ILAE classification of the epilepsies: Position paper of the ILAE Commission for Classification and Terminology. *Epilepsia, 58*(4), 512–521. https://doi.org/10.1111/epi.13709.

24 The Child With a Musculoskeletal Condition

http://evolve.elsevier.com/Canada/Leifer

Cheryl A. Sams

Objectives

1. Define each key term listed.
2. Discuss the musculoskeletal differences between the child and adult and how they influence orthopedic treatment and nursing care.
3. Describe age-specific changes that occur in the musculoskeletal system during growth and development.
4. Describe the management of soft tissue injuries.
5. Discuss the types of fractures commonly seen in children and their effect on growth and development.
6. Discuss the nursing care of a child in a cast.
7. Describe a neurovascular check.
8. Differentiate between Buck skin traction and Russell traction.
9. Compile a nursing care plan for the child who is immobilized by traction.
10. Describe the early signs of developmental dysplasia of the hip.
11. Identify two symptoms of Duchenne muscular dystrophy.
12. Describe the symptoms, treatment, and nursing care for the child with osteosarcoma.
13. Describe two topics applicable to home care of the child with juvenile idiopathic arthritis.
14. Describe three nursing care measures required to maintain skin integrity for an adolescent in a cast or brace for scoliosis.
15. Describe three types of child abuse.
16. Identify symptoms of abuse and neglect in children.
17. Identify two cultural or medical practices that may be misinterpreted as child abuse.

Key Terms

arthroscopy
Bryant traction
Buck skin traction
clubfoot
compartment syndrome
compound fracture
developmental dysplasia of the hip (DDH)
epiphysis (ĕ-PĬF-ă-sĭs)
gait
greenstick fracture
hematoma (hē-mă-TŌ-mă)
Milwaukee brace
muscular dystrophies
neurovascular checks
Ortolani sign
osteomyelitis
Pavlik harness
Russell traction
scoliosis
spica cast
spiral fracture

THE MUSCULOSKELETAL SYSTEM

The musculoskeletal system supports the body and provides for movement. The muscular and skeletal systems work together to enable a person to sit, stand, walk, and remain upright. In addition, muscles move air into and out of the lungs, move blood through vessels, and move food through the digestive tract. They also produce heat, which aids in numerous body chemical reactions. Bones act as levers and provide support. Red blood cells are produced in the bone marrow, and minerals such as calcium and phosphorus are also stored there.

The musculoskeletal system arises from the mesoderm in the embryo. A great portion of skeletal growth occurs between the fourth and eighth weeks of fetal life. As the limbs elongate before birth, muscle masses form in the extremities. The Ballard scoring system (see Figs. 12.2 and 12.3) is one measure of assessing neuromuscular maturity at birth. Testing various reflexes is another.

Locomotion develops gradually and in an orderly manner in the growing child. A marked deceleration of growth is always a signal for investigation.

MUSCULOSKELTAL SYSTEM: DIFFERENCES BETWEEN THE CHILD AND THE ADULT

Fig. 24.1 describes some differences between the child's and the adult's skeletal and muscular systems. Skeletal maturity and chronological age often differ. The pediatric skeletal system differs from the adult skeletal system in that bone is not completely ossified, epiphyses are present, and the periosteum is thicker

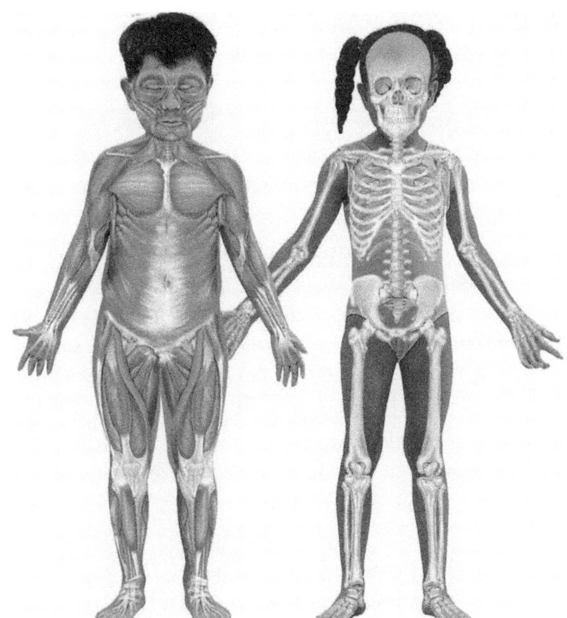

MUSCULOSKELETAL SYSTEM

- Skeletal growth is most rapid during infancy and adolescence. Assessing growth and development is an integral part of the physical examination for children.
- The bones of children are more resilient, tend to bend, and may deform before breaking.
- The blood supply to bone in children is rich; therefore healing occurs more quickly. Their periosteum is thick, and osteogenic activity is high.
- Epiphyseal plate fractures in children can disrupt the growth of bones.
- Musculoskeletal problems may be growth related.
- Rapid growth of the skeletal frame of children can cause deformities to become more severe.

Fig. 24.1 Some musculoskeletal system differences between the child and the adult. The muscular system consists of the large skeletal muscles that enable movement as well as the cardiac muscle of the heart and the smooth muscle of the internal organs. The skeletal system consists of bones and cartilage. This system helps to support and protect the body. (Art overlay courtesy Observatory Group, Cincinnati, Ohio.)

and produces callus more rapidly than in the adult. The lower mineral content of the child's bone and its greater porosity increase the bone's strength. However, rotational or angular forces can stress ligaments that insert at the epiphyseal area of the bone, and injury to the epiphysis can affect bone growth. Because of the presence of the epiphysis and hyperemia caused by the trauma, bone overgrowth is common in healing fractures of children younger than 10 years of age. At birth, the thoracic and sacral areas of the child's spine are convex curves. When the child sits and stands these curves must change to be concave, or kyphosis or lordosis will result.

OBSERVATION AND ASSESSMENT OF THE MUSCULOSKELETAL SYSTEM IN THE GROWING CHILD

To assess the musculoskeletal system of the growing child and to identify deviations, the nurse must have a basic understanding of the effect of growth, neurological development, and motor milestones at various ages. The newborn hip has limited internal rotation range of motion (ROM). The legs are maintained in a flexed position, and the lower leg has an internal rotation (internal tibial torsion) caused by the effects of uterine positioning; this can last 4 to 6 months. The general curvature of the newborn spine is a convex primary "C" curve, in the shape of the letter C. When the developing infant strengthens the neck muscles, a secondary curve of the upper spine is formed. The final lumbar curve, which becomes a double "S" lordosis curve in the lower back, forms when the child starts to creep and crawl. It is important for the young child to have maximum opportunity to creep and crawl and play on the stomach to develop proper postural alignment (see Fig. 15.1). The newborn's feet normally turn inward *(varus)* or outward *(valgus)*, but the turning-in self-corrects when the sole of the foot is stroked. The toddler's feet appear flat because of the presence of a fat pad at the arch.

Any delay in neurological development can cause a delay in the mastery of motor skills, which can result in altered skeletal growth. Assessment of the musculoskeletal system includes observation, palpation, ROM, and gait assessment in children who can walk. Children who do not walk independently by 18 months of age may have a developmental delay and should be referred to a health care provider for follow-up.

OBSERVATION OF GAIT

The **gait** is a characteristic manner of walking. The toddler who begins to walk has a wide, unstable gait. The arms do not swing with the walking motion. By 18 months of age the wide base narrows and the walk is more stable. An unusual gait before 18 months requires that the child be assessed by a health care provider. By 4 years of age the child can hop on one foot and arm swings occur with walking. By 6 years of age, the gait resembles the adult walk with equal stride lengths and associated arm swing. The trunk is centred over the legs, and movement is symmetrical. When a child favours one side, pain may be present. Toe walking after 3 years of age can indicate a muscle problem.

In most cases, excessive in-toeing, or pointing of the toe inward, will resolve by 4 years of age. These children trip and fall easily. Teaching proper sitting and body mechanics is the treatment of choice.

Participation in ballet classes and skating may enhance hip flexibility. If the problem does not resolve, a brace may be prescribed. Failure to treat can result in hip, knee, or back problems in adulthood.

Young children appear bowlegged or knock-kneed, with the knees turned inward until 5 years of age. Bowing is seldom pathological. The ligaments that support the arch are not mature before 6 years of age; therefore, the child may appear to have flat feet. If the condition interferes with walking, an orthotic appliance can be prescribed for the child to wear inside the shoes. When the flat foot is painful, a referral for follow-up examination should be made.

The role of the nurse with regard to children's gait is to reassure parents that unless there is associated pain or a problem with motor or nerve functions, many minor abnormal-appearing alignments will spontaneously resolve with activity.

OBSERVATION OF MUSCLE TONE

The nurse should assess symmetry of movement and the strength and contour of the body and extremities. Having the child push away the examiner's hand with their foot or hand can test the strength of the extremities.

NEUROLOGICAL EXAMINATION

A neurological assessment is a vital part of a comprehensive musculoskeletal examination. An assessment of reflexes, a sensory assessment, and the presence or absence of spasms should be noted (see Chapter 23 for further discussion).

DIAGNOSTIC TESTS AND TREATMENTS

Radiographic Studies

X-ray films are taken to confirm a suspected pathological condition, and the affected area is compared with the unaffected area.

Bone scans

Bone scans are helpful in identifying pathological conditions that may not clearly be seen on a routine X-ray study, such as septic arthritis or tumours.

Computed tomography

Computed tomography (CT) provides a cross-sectional picture of the bone and its relationship to other structures within the area of examination.

Magnetic resonance imaging

Magnetic resonance imaging (MRI) does not involve harmful radiation. MRIs produce detailed pictures of the brain, spinal cord, and soft tissue lesions, including a slipped femoral epiphysis.

Ultrasound

Ultrasound involves use of sound waves to produce a picture of whatever is being scanned. It is used to rule out foreign bodies in soft tissues, joint effusions, and developmental dysplasia of the hip.

Laboratory Tests and Treatments

A complete blood count (CBC) and erythrocyte sedimentation rate (ESR) may rule out septic arthritis or osteomyelitis. C-reactive protein and rheumatoid factor (RF) may help in diagnosing rheumatological disorders.

A thorough history is necessary to determine the basis for musculoskeletal concerns, which are often insidious. The nurse must determine the history of the injury; the location of pain; when symptoms started; any weakness, numbness, or loss of function in an extremity; and whether the problem is affecting the daily activities of the child.

Arthroscopy is commonly performed on adolescents with sports injuries. The health care provider is able to look inside the joint (usually the knee or shoulder) with the use of fibre-optic cameras, to determine the extent of injury. The area is inspected, foreign particles are removed, or repairs are made to the torn menisci. A bone biopsy may show a malignancy. Muscle biopsy may detect muscular dystrophy.

PEDIATRIC TRAUMA

SOFT TISSUE INJURIES

Soft tissue injuries usually accompany traumatic fractures in the child at play or the adolescent involved in sports activities and include the following:

- *Contusion*: A tearing of subcutaneous tissue resulting in hemorrhage, edema, and pain. The escape of blood into the soft tissue is referred to as a **hematoma**, or a bruise.
- *Sprain*: When the ligament is torn or stretched away from the bone at the point of trauma, there may be resulting damage to blood vessels, muscles, and nerves. Swelling, disability, and pain are major signs of a sprain.
- *Strain*: A microscopic tear to the muscle or tendon can occur over time and result in edema and pain.

Treatment of Soft Tissue Injuries

Soft tissue injuries should be treated immediately to limit damage from edema and bleeding. Functional bracing and early mobilization provide support and stability, which allow for better ROM, a quicker return to sports, and higher patient satisfaction, in comparison to immobilization. A cold pack and elastic wrap will reduce edema and bleeding and relieve pain and should be applied at *15-minute intervals* one to three times a day, in the first 36 hours after injury (McTimoney, Purcell, & Canadian Paediatric Society (CPS), Paediatric Sports and Exercise Medicine, 2007).

After a 15-minute period, ischemia can occur and impede the tissue perfusion. Nonsteroidal anti-inflammatory drugs (NSAIDs) such as ibuprofen

(Advil) can be used to manage pain and swelling. Gentle ROM exercises can be used to strength a joint. Elevating the extremity above heart level reduces edema. When an elastic bandage is used for compression, a priority nursing responsibility is to perform frequent neurovascular checks to ensure adequate tissue perfusion (see discussion below, in Nursing Care of a Child in a Cast). The child can return to normal activity when there is full range of movement and full muscle strength. For example, a sprained ankle can be tested by having the child hop on the injured leg five times and running in a zigzag pattern (About Kids Health, 2009a).

Memory Jogger

Principles of managing soft tissue injuries (PRICE) include the following:
Protection
Relative rest
Ice
Compression
Elevation

McTimoney, M., Purcell, L., & Canadian Paediatric Society (CPS), Paediatric Sports and Exercise Medicine. (2007). Ankle sprains in the paediatric athlete. *Paediatrics & Child Health*, 12(2), 133–355.

PREVENTION OF PEDIATRIC TRAUMA

While accidents are common in childhood, much can be done to prevent morbidity and mortality due to accidents. Parents are responsible for maintaining a safe environment for their children. Nurses can provide education to parents and schoolteachers about how to prevent accidental injury and maintain a safe environment.

The proper use of pedestrian safety practices, car seat restraints, bicycle helmets and other athletic protective gear, pool fences, window bars, deadbolt locks, and locks on cabinets can prevent many injuries to children. Pediatric trauma can cause permanent disability or premature death.

Nursing assessment and interventions can assist the injured child toward recovery. The nurse also has a community responsibility to support legislation that would promote safe environments for children. The Canadian Paediatric Society, the Children's Health and Safety Association, and Parachute, an organization that promotes prevention of injuries and works to save lives, are national organizations in Canada that provide many important tips and resources to help families prevent childhood injuries and traumas.

TRAUMATIC FRACTURES

Pathophysiology

A *fracture* is a break in a bone and is often caused by accidents. It is characterized by pain, tenderness on movement, and swelling. Discoloration, limited movement, and numbness may also occur. In a closed *simple fracture,* the bone is broken, but the skin over the area is not. In an *open* **compound fracture**, a wound in the skin accompanies the broken bone, and there is an added danger of infection. A **greenstick fracture** is an incomplete fracture in which one side of the bone is broken and the other is bent. This type of fracture is common in children because their bones are soft, flexible, and more likely to splinter. In a *complete fracture* the bone is entirely broken across its width. Fig. 24.2 illustrates various types of fractures. When an X-ray film shows multiple fractures at various stages of healing, child abuse should be suspected. See discussion about child abuse later in the chapter.

A fracture heals more rapidly in a child than it does in an adult. The child's periosteum is stronger and thicker, and there is less stiffness on mobilization. Injury to the cartilaginous **epiphysis**, the growth plate found at the ends of the long bones, is serious if it happens during childhood because it may interfere with longitudinal growth. A fat embolism can occur within a few hours after fractures of the long bones or multiple fractures, when fat particles escape from the site into the circulation and lodge in the lung. Although it is more common in adults than in children, the nurse must observe for signs and symptoms of fat embolism in children.

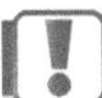
Safety Alert!

The nurse must watch for signs of a fat embolism, which is a medical emergency. Symptoms include a change in mental status, respiratory distress, tachypnea, crackles and wheezes on auscultating the lungs, rapid pulse, fever, and petechiae over the chest, neck, upper arms, or abdomen.

Fractures of the Femur in Early Childhood

The femur (thigh bone) is the largest and strongest bone of the body. It is one of the most prevalent serious breaks that occur during early childhood. Any fracture of the lower extremities in an infant who is not ambulatory suggests a nonaccidental injury or child abuse (Baldwin, Wells, & Dormans, 2016). A forceful twisting motion of the femur causes a **spiral fracture**. When the history of an injury does not correlate with X-ray findings, child abuse should be suspected, because spiral fractures can be the result of manual twisting of the extremity.

The child will usually show signs of pain and tenderness when the leg is moved and they cannot bear weight on it. X-ray films confirm the diagnosis. Skin traction occasionally may be used to reduce the fracture and keep the bones in proper alignment, and a cast may be applied.

Safety Alert!

A spiral femur fracture in a young child may indicate child abuse and must be referred to an assessment team.

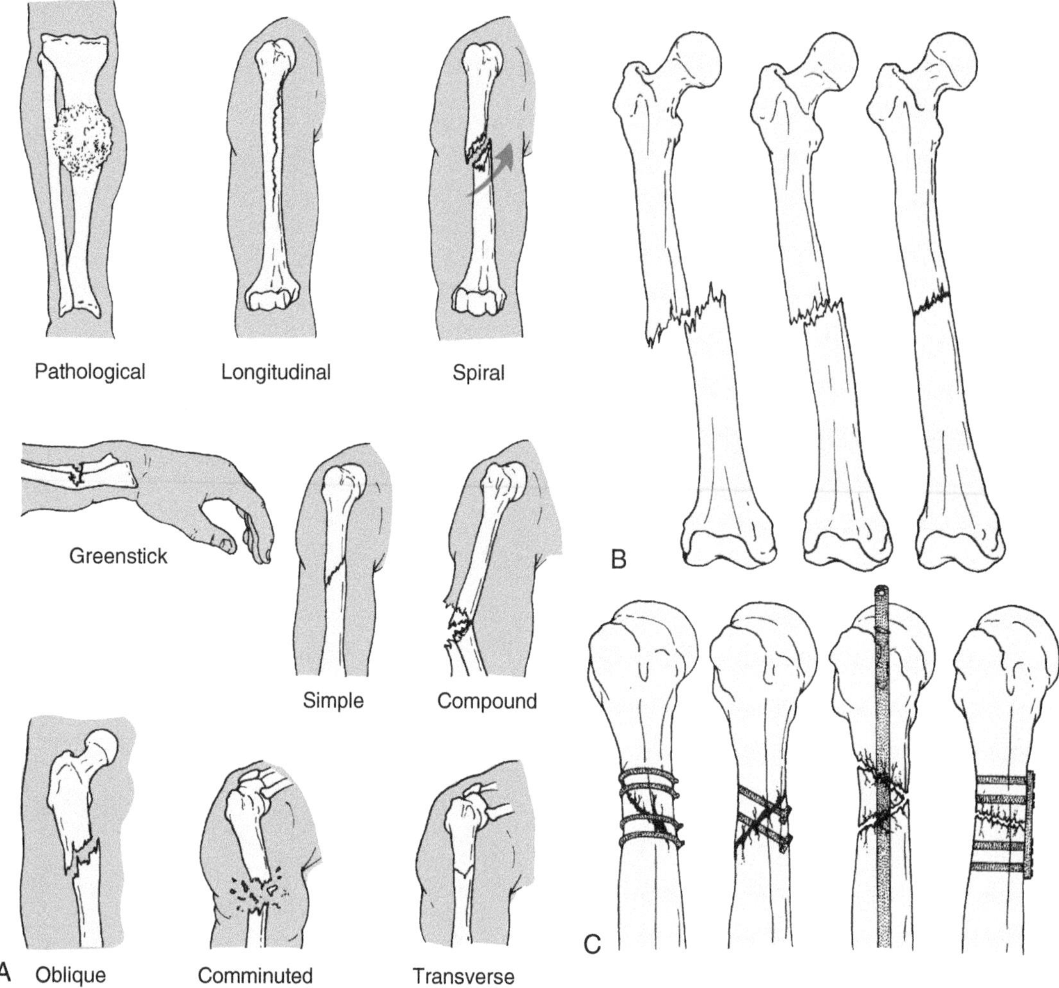

Fig. 24.2 **A,** Types of fractures. **B,** Reduction of a fractured bone. A gradual pull is exerted on the distal (lower) fragment of the bone until it is in alignment with the proximal fragment. **C,** Various methods of internal fixations, using plates, pins, nails, and screws to hold fragments of bone in place. (Redrawn from deWit, S. C. [1992]. *Keane's essentials of medical-surgical nursing* [3rd ed.]. Philadelphia: Saunders.)

Treatment of Fractures With Casts

A *cast* is a device used to immobilize a bone fracture site, usually including the joints above and below the fracture. Casts are constructed of plaster of Paris or a synthetic material such as fibreglass. Fibreglass casts are lighter than plaster casts and come in various bright colours. The fibreglass cast is water resistant if properly lined and can be washed and dried. The plaster cast will deteriorate if it becomes wet. When applied, the fibreglass cast dries within half an hour, compared to the plaster cast, which dries from the inside out and takes 24 to 48 hours to dry. The plaster cast must be carefully handled with open palms and extended fingers to prevent indents that can create pressure areas on the skin and not covered during this drying time. The plaster cast consists of crinoline, which has powdered plaster in its meshwork. It is placed in warm water before being applied over cotton wadding or a stockinette. The wet plaster of Paris hardens as it dries.

Nursing care of a child in a cast

When a cast is applied to an extremity, the toes or fingers are left exposed for observation. The nurse must assess them for neurovascular checks (capillary refill and signs of poor circulation, pallor, cyanosis, swelling, coldness, numbness, pain, or burning) (see discussion below). If circulation is impaired, the health care provider may split the cast to relieve the pressure, or the cast may need to be removed and reapplied. The nurse must also report irritation of the skin around the edges of the cast and lack of movement of the toes. Waterproof adhesive tape may be placed around the edges of the cast to prevent skin irritation.

If the cast is applied to an infant, the cast may need to be removed and reapplied, as an infant grows rapidly. Parents should be taught how to check for circulation impairments, which could be caused by a tight cast.

If surgery on tendons and bones has been performed, the nurse must also observe the cast for evidence of bleeding. If a discoloured area appears on the cast, it is circled, and the time is recorded. Further bleeding can then be estimated. If bleeding is noted, the patient's vital signs are checked and compared with preoperative readings.

Nursing responsibilities include elevating the affected extremity on a pillow and performing frequent neurovascular checks on the distal digits (Skill 24.1).

Skill 24.1 Neurovascular Checks

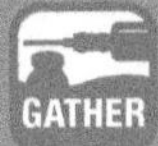

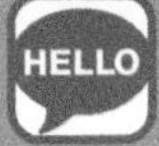

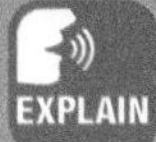

PURPOSE

To determine if tissue perfusion is adequate

STEPS

Assess each of the following:

1. *Pain:* Assess and record the location and quality of pain. Initiate pain-control strategies and medication as soon as possible. Pain at the trauma site that does not respond to medication may indicate a serious complication called compartment syndrome.
2. *Pulselessness or capillary refill of greater than 3 seconds:* Compare the quality of the pulse on the affected extremity to that on the unaffected extremity. A strong pulse indicates good blood flow necessary for healing. A compressed nail bed should return to its original colour in *less than 3 seconds.* The findings should be compared with the unaffected extremity and the results recorded frequently. Any delay in capillary refill time should be reported promptly.

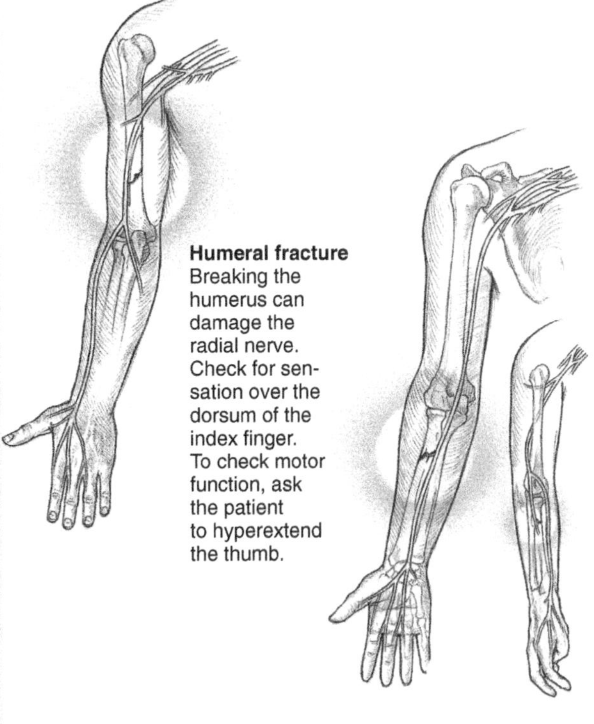

Humeral fracture
Breaking the humerus can damage the radial nerve. Check for sensation over the dorsum of the index finger. To check motor function, ask the patient to hyperextend the thumb.

Radial fracture
A break in the radius can damage the medial as well as the radial nerve. Besides checking sensory and motor function of the radial nerve, evaluate medial nerve function: Check for sensation on the palmar surface of the fingers and the thumb half of the palm. To check motor function, ask the patient to touch the thumb to the tip of the little finger.

Ulnar fracture
Breaking the ulna can damage the ulnar nerve. Check sensation on the ulnar border of the hand from the little finger to the ring finger. To check motor function, ask the patient to abduct, or spread, his or her fingers.

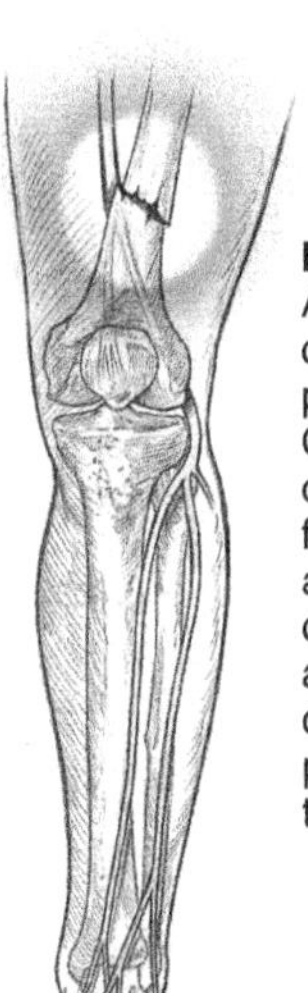

Femoral fracture
A break in the femur can damage the peroneal nerve. Check for sensation over the top of the foot between the first and second toes. To check motor function, ask the patient to dorsiflex the foot, pointing his or her toes toward the head.

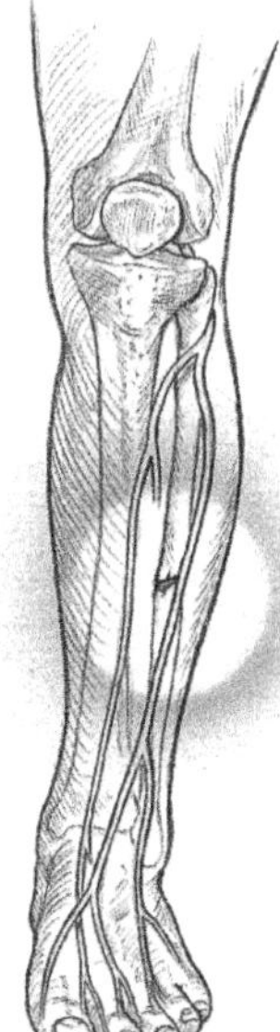

Fibular fracture
Breaking the fibula also can damage the peroneal nerve. Lack of sensation between the first and second toes on top of the foot or an inability to dorsiflex the foot is a sign of peroneal nerve damage.

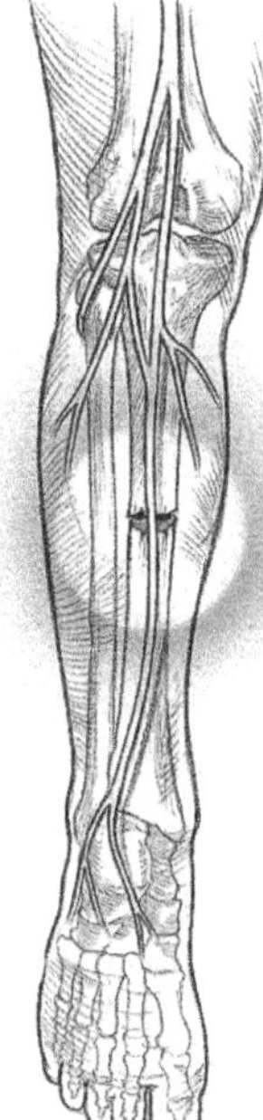

Tibial fracture
A break in the tibia can damage the tibial nerve. To check for sensory damage, ask the patient if the medial side of his foot feels warm. To evaluate motor function, ask this patient to plantarflex the foot, pointing the toes down.

Checking for nerve damage. Nerve damage can result from trauma, and the motor sensory status of the extremity should be assessed and recorded frequently. (Courtesy Bert Oppenheim.)

Skill 24.1 Neurovascular Checks—cont'd

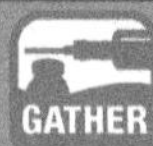

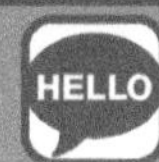

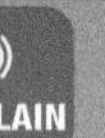

3. *Paresthesia:* Reduced sensation to touch (numbness or tingling) at a site distal to the fracture may indicate poor tissue perfusion and should be reported.
4. *Pallor or cyanosis:* Pallor at the site distal to the fracture can indicate arterial insufficiency, whereas cyanosis of the site distal to the fracture can indicate venous stasis. Cold temperature can also indicate inadequate blood flow. Adequate blood supply and vascular drainage are essential for optimal healing.
5. *Paralysis:* Arterial occlusion can cause anoxia of the muscles and reflex vasospasm, which, when unnoticed, could result in contractures and paralysis. Test the toes and fingers distal to the fracture site for movement. Because nerve injury can occur as a complication of skeletal fractures, the movement associated with specific nerve supply should also be tested.
6. *Pressure:* Assess for swelling and tenseness.

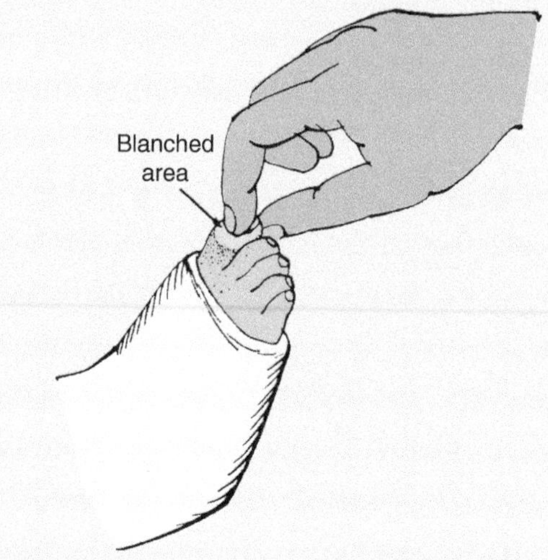

From Leifer, G. [1992]. Principles and techniques in pediatric nursing. Philadelphia: Saunders.

Before discharge, the nurse teaches the child and parents how to care for the cast and how to support the cast, to prevent the extremity from assuming a dependent position that could compromise circulation. The child is taught safe transfer from bed to wheelchair and safe crutch-walking techniques (e.g., being sure to keep the body weight on the hands and not the axillae). Parents are also taught how to check whether the cast is too loose or too tight and has compromised circulation. The parents need to be informed about when to return to the clinic or health care provider.

The child should be prepared for the experience of cast removal, because the cast cutter can appear and sound threatening. After cast removal, the skin can be expected to be dry and caked. Lotion and soothing baths are advised. Nursing care of traumatic injuries to the musculoskeletal system also includes providing emotional support regarding body image, maintenance of skin integrity, encouraging independence, and providing developmentally appropriate activities related to school progress and prevention of future injuries.

Neurovascular checks. A priority nursing responsibility in the care of a child with a fracture who has a cast or Ace bandage or who has traction in place is to perform **neurovascular checks** at regular intervals (see Skill 24.1). Any abnormalities should be reported promptly so that early intervention can prevent complications from developing.

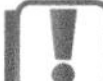

Safety Alert!

The *neurovascular check* for tissue perfusion and compartment syndrome is performed on the toes or fingers distal to an injury or cast, comparing the limbs bilaterally. This check includes the following:

- Pain and point of tenderness—moderate or severe
- Pulselessness or capillary refill is greater than 3 seconds
- Pallor or cyanosis or cold temperature
- Paresthesia—numbness or tingling, or pins-and-needles sensation distal to the injured site
- Paralysis
- Pressure and swelling

From Binder, Ball, London, et al., 2017.

Assessing for compartment syndrome. **Compartment syndrome** is a progressive loss of tissue perfusion caused by an increase in pressure resulting from edema or swelling that presses on the vessels and tissues. Circulation is compromised, and the neurovascular check is abnormal.

Compartment syndrome can be caused by a cast that is too tight and compromises circulation, or by excessive edema that causes ischemia. Often, surgical intervention (fasciotomy) is required to relieve pressure and to restore circulation. An important nursing responsibility is to provide frequent neurovascular checks on the distal fingers or toes of any injured limb to enable early intervention.

Treatment of Fractures With Traction

Most bone fractures are manually reduced or surgically pinned in place and a cast is applied. Traction is avoided whenever possible because it involves long-term bed rest and resulting complications. Traction is used when the cast cannot maintain alignment of the two bone fragments. Skeletal muscles act as a splint for the fracture. Traction aligns the injured bone by the use of weights and counter-traction. Immobilization is maintained until the bones fuse.

Traction in the younger child

Bryant traction may be used for treating fractures of the femur in children less than 2 years of age. Weights and pulleys suspend the legs vertically (Fig. 24.3). The weight of the child supplies the counter-traction.

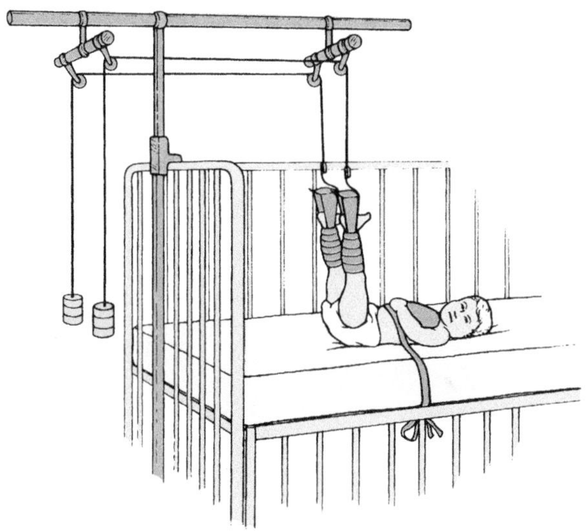

Fig. 24.3 Bryant traction is used for the young child who has a fractured femur. Note that the buttocks are slightly off the bed to facilitate counter-traction.

Traction in the older child

Buck skin traction (Buck's extension) is a type of skin traction used in fractures of the femur and in hip and knee contractures. It pulls the hip and leg into extension. The child's body supplies counter-traction; therefore, it is essential that the child not slip down in bed and that the bed not be placed in high-Fowler's position.

Russell traction is similar to Buck skin traction. In Russell traction, however, a sling is positioned under the knee, which suspends the distal thigh above the bed (Fig. 24.4). Skin traction is applied to the lower extremity. Pull is in two directions, vertically from the knee sling and longitudinally from the footplate (Fig. 24.5). This prevents posterior subluxation of the tibia on the femur, which can occur in children who are in traction.

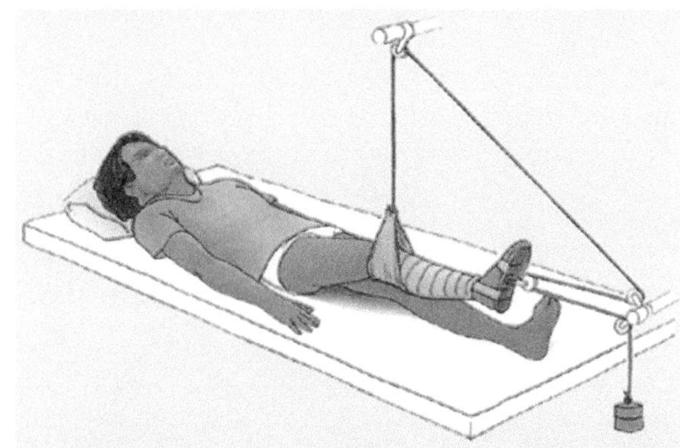

Fig. 24.4 Russell traction. A skin traction system applied to the lower extremity using a footplate and a knee sling. When there are separate weights attached to both the footplate and the knee sling, it is known as a *split Russell traction*. (From Bowden, V. R., Dickey, S. B., & Greenberg, S. C. [1998]. *Children and their families: The continuum of care.* Philadelphia: Saunders.)

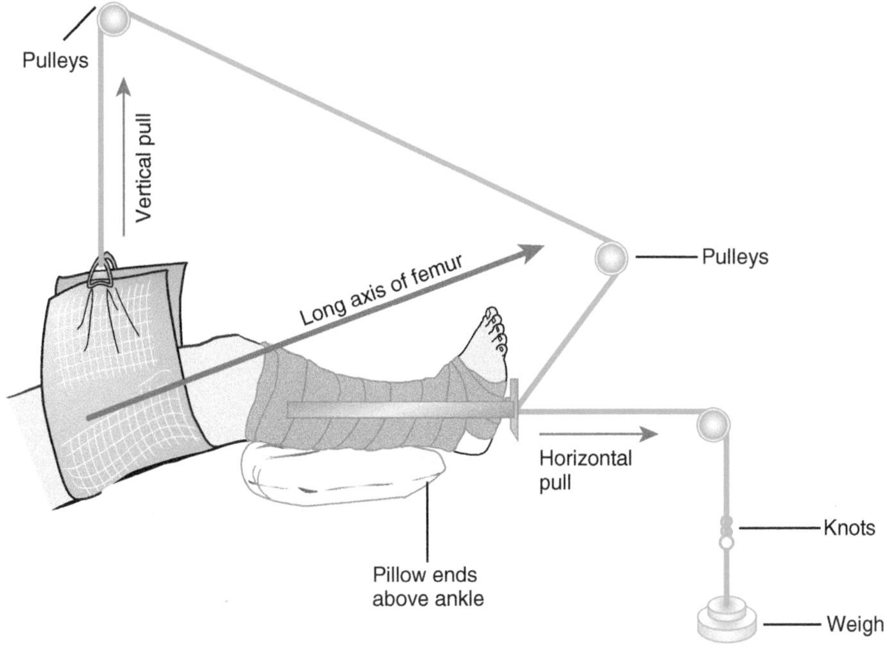

Fig. 24.5 Forces involved in traction. The placement of pulleys and the angle of the joints determine the line of pull. In this case, the combined vertical and horizontal pull results in a pull on the long axis of the femur to reduce fracture displacement.

Balanced suspension using the *Thomas splint* and *Pearson attachments* is used to treat diseases of the hip as well as fractures in older children and adolescents.

In *skeletal traction,* a Steinmann pin or Kirschner wire is inserted into the bone, and traction is applied to the pin. "Ninety-ninety" (or ninety degree–ninety degree) traction with a boot cast or sling on the lower leg may be used (Fig. 24.6). Crutchfield, or Barton, tongs may be used in the skull to provide cervical traction (Fig. 24.7). Daily observation and cleansing of the pin site is essential. Skeletal traction carries the added risk of infection from skin bacteria that may cause osteomyelitis. Health organizations have their own protocols and use either an antiseptic cleaner or normal saline to clean the pin site and the frequency of cleaning varies.

The child in traction experiences certain effects as a result of immobilization (Fig. 24.8). The nurse must focus care on preventing any of these complications.

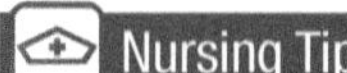 Nursing Tip

Checklist for a traction apparatus:

- Weights hanging freely
- Weights out of reach of the child
- Ropes on the pulleys
- Knots not resting against pulleys
- Bed linens not on traction ropes
- Counter-traction in place
- Apparatus does not touch foot of bed

Nursing care of a child in traction

The nurse needs to observe the traction ropes to be sure they are intact and in the wheel grooves of the pulleys and that the child's body is in good alignment. In Bryant traction, the legs should be at right angles to the body, with the buttocks raised sufficiently to clear the bed. In all types of traction, elastic bandages should be neither too loose nor too tight. Continuous traction is necessary so the weights are not removed after they

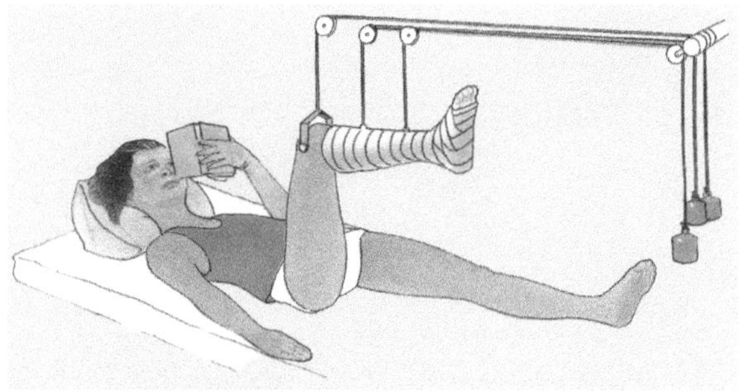

Fig. 24.6 Ninety degree–ninety degree skeletal traction. A wire pin is inserted into the distal segment of the femur. The lower leg may be placed in a boot cast or is supported by a sling. (From Bowden, V. R., Dickey, S. B., & Greenberg, S. C. [1998]. *Children and their families: The continuum of care.* Philadelphia: Saunders.)

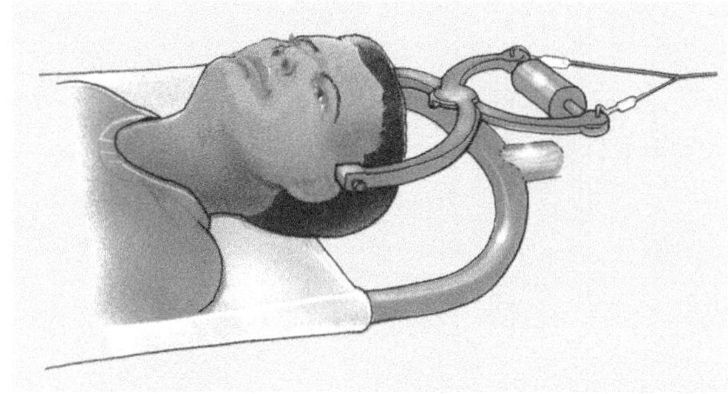

Fig. 24.7 Cervical traction. A special bed may be used to turn a patient who is in cervical traction. (From Bowden, V. R., Dickey, S. B., & Greenberg, S. C. [1998]. *Children and their families: The continuum of care.* Philadelphia: Saunders.)

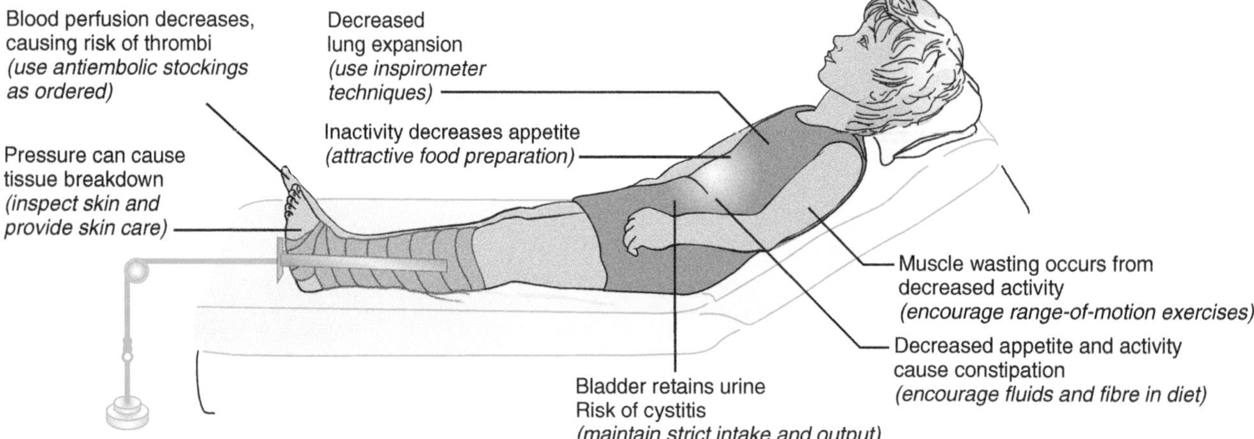
Prolonged treatment requires absence from school (request home tutor, maintain written or e-mail contact with friends)
Blood perfusion decreases, causing risk of thrombi (use antiembolic stockings as ordered)
Decreased lung expansion (use inspirometer techniques)
Inactivity decreases appetite (attractive food preparation)
Pressure can cause tissue breakdown (inspect skin and provide skin care)
Muscle wasting occurs from decreased activity (encourage range-of-motion exercises)
Decreased appetite and activity cause constipation (encourage fluids and fibre in diet)
Bladder retains urine Risk of cystitis (maintain strict intake and output)

Fig. 24.8 Overcoming the effects of immobility on a child.

are applied. The weights must hang free, and they are *not* lifted or supported when the bed is moved.

Safety Alert!

The nurse should never lift or remove weights from the traction apparatus during the delivery of patient care.

The nurse must perform frequent neurovascular checks of the toes to ensure that they are warm and that their colour is good (see Skill 24.1). Observations of conditions such as cyanosis, numbness, or irritation from attachments; tight bandages; severe pain; hypoxia or the absence of pulse rates in the extremities should be reported immediately to the health care provider. A specific and serious complication of any traction is *Volkmann's ischemia* (*iskhein,* "to hold back," and *haima,* "blood"), which occurs when the circulation is obstructed. When the legs are elevated overhead, as in Bryant traction, there is gravitational vascular drainage. Arterial occlusion can cause anoxia of the muscles and reflex vasospasm, which, when unnoticed, could result in contractures and paralysis.

The child must be provided good skin hygiene. Sheepskin padding may also be used. The sheets are pulled taut and are kept free of crumbs. Because the child in traction is unable to sit upright when eating, special precautions to prevent choking and aspiration during mealtime are priority nursing responsibilities. The child should be encouraged to drink plenty of fluids and to eat foods that are high in roughage to prevent constipation caused by a lack of exercise. Stool softeners may be necessary. A fracture bedpan is a very shallow pan that can be more easily placed under the child with a cast or traction for bowel movements, and a careful record is kept of eliminations.

Deep-breathing exercises should also be encouraged, to prevent collection of fluid in the lungs caused by the child's immobility. These exercises may be done by blowing bubbles or blowing a pinwheel.

Nursing Tip

Checklist for the patient in traction:

- Body in alignment
- Head of bed no higher than 20 degrees (for counter-traction)
- Range of motion (ROM) of unaffected parts checked at regular intervals
- Antiembolism stockings in place as ordered
- Neurovascular checks performed regularly
- Skin integrity monitored regularly
- Pain and its relief by medication documented
- Measures to prevent constipation
- Use of trapeze bar, an overhead grab bar to help a child change position
- Frequent position changes are encouraged

Diversional therapy is important because hospitalization may be lengthy. Toys may be securely suspended over the child's head so they are within easy reach. The child in a crib should be taken to the playroom in the crib, when possible, so the child can play and enjoy some socialization.

DVDs, electronic tablets, computer games, stories, and other forms of entertainment are important aspects of a total nursing care plan. Pain control is essential. Parents are encouraged to assist with care of the child as much as they are able. When prolonged hospitalization is necessary, the child's school should be contacted to provide appropriate study materials so that the child can stay up-to-date at school.

Nursing Care Plan 24.1 describes interventions for the child in traction.

CONGENITAL MALFORMATIONS

The following conditions present at birth and require specialized nursing care for the newborn.

CLUBFOOT

Pathophysiology

Clubfoot, one of the most common deformities of the skeletal system, is a congenital anomaly characterized by a foot that has been twisted inward or outward. The incidence is about 1 in 1 000 live births in North America (Winell & Davidson, 2016). Many mild forms are caused by improper position in the uterus, and these usually clear up with stretching exercises. In contrast, true clubfoot does not respond to simple exercise.

Several types are recognized. Talipes (*talus,* "heel," and *pes,* "foot") equinovarus (*equinus,* "extension," and *varus,* "bent inward") is seen in 95% of patients. The feet are turned inward, and the child walks on the toes and the outer borders of the feet. It generally involves both feet (Fig. 24.9).

Treatment and Nursing Care

The treatment of clubfoot must be started as early as possible, or the bones and muscles will continue to

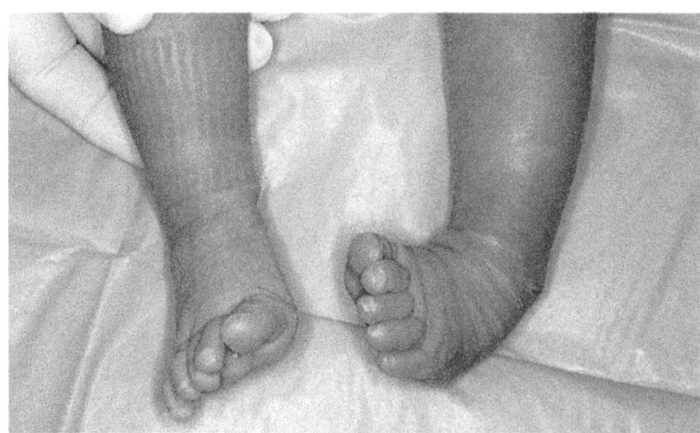

Fig. 24.9 Clubfoot. A child with a clubfoot, showing a flexed ankle, turned heel, and adducted forefoot. (From Bowden, V. R., Dickey, S. B., & Greenberg, S. C. [1998]. *Children and their families: The continuum of care*. Philadelphia: Saunders.)

Nursing Care Plan 24.1 The Child in Traction

PATIENT DATA

A 6-year-old child is admitted with a fractured femur after falling from a tree while playing. His leg is placed in Steinmann pin traction.

Selected Nursing Diagnosis Reduced physical mobility

Goals	Nursing Interventions	Rationales
Child will demonstrate knowledge and understanding of the traction equipment and treatment protocol.	Draw picture of fracture for child and explain traction apparatus.	An understanding of condition and of the type of traction used reduces anxiety and promotes assistance with treatment protocol.
	Place call light within easy reach of child.	It is frightening to be immobilized; a call light provides reassurance that help is at hand.
Child will not develop complications of immobility as evidenced by intact skin and absence of respiratory and urinary tract infections.	Change position as traction allows every 2 hours.	Position changes every 2 hours help to prevent skin breakdown.
	Encourage exercise through play by doing pull-ups on trapeze apparatus.	Exercise will help to prevent atrophy, joint contractures, and muscle weakness.
	Institute range-of-motion (ROM) exercises on unaffected extremities.	Unaffected limbs need exercise to prevent stiffness, muscle atrophy, and deformities.
	Encourage self-care.	Self-care promotes self-directed wellness.
	Encourage deep breathing with incentive spirometer or a toy.	Deep-breathing exercises help to prevent pneumonia and atelectasis.
	Observe for urinary tract infection.	Kidney filtration slows with immobilization; immobility causes minerals (e.g., calcium) to leave bones and pool in renal pelvis; stasis of urine is likely to occur, causing renal calculi.
Child will have a bowel movement on a regular basis.	Provide high-fibre diet and stool softeners as ordered.	Bulk improves stool consistency and prevents constipation. Stool softeners prevent straining during defecation.
	Provide adequate fluids; monitor intake and output.	Increased fluids are necessary to hydrate body, and they decrease the risk of urine stasis and constipation.

Selected Nursing Diagnosis Acute pain

Goals	Nursing Interventions	Rationales
Child will be comfortable as evidenced by a decrease in irritability, crying, body posturing, and anorexia. Older child verbalizes relief of pain.	Administer pain medication before activity and before pain escalates.	Child may be unable to verbalize pain. Premedication for pain allows for muscle relaxation and participation in activities.
	Allow choice in method of pain relief, if possible.	Allowing some choice, if there is one, promotes self-control.
	Encourage child to hold favourite possession.	Favourite possessions are comforting.
	Distract child with electronic tablet or computer games as age appropriate.	Distraction from a problem reduces stress and tension.
	Listen and communicate with child.	Listening to the child gives the nurse clues about the amount of pain; nonverbal cues are important in infants and toddlers.
	Use touch as a comfort measure.	Touch is particularly important in infants and toddlers but is comforting for all ages; proceed with caution if there is reason to suspect abuse.

Nursing Care Plan 24.1 The Child in Traction—cont'd

Goals	Nursing Interventions	Rationales
	Involve family in supporting child's ability to cope with pain.	Child trusts family; family members may be able to suggest favourite types of comfort for child.
	Consider cultural background in relation to pain expression.	In some cultures, showing pain is considered cowardly.
	Monitor vital signs.	A change in vital signs can indicate pain, infection, or poor tissue perfusion.
	Provide support and education to family members.	Family members who understand and participate in care can help the child to develop effective coping skills.

Selected Nursing Diagnosis Potential for tissue trauma as a result of immobility, traction, poor circulation

Goals	Nursing Interventions	Rationales
Skin will remain intact with no evidence of breakdown.	Inspect skin regularly.	Provides for early assessment of developing skin problems.
Circulation of affected extremity will be adequate as evidenced by normal capillary refill, equal and strong peripheral pulses, and sensation and motion in extremity.	Check capillary refill of nail beds in affected extremity.	Impaired tissue perfusion will result in an increased capillary refill time.
	Have child wiggle toes or fingers of affected extremity to determine sensation and motion.	Wiggling toes and fingers demonstrates extent of mobility and sensation.
	Inspect elastic bandages for wrinkles or looseness.	Excessive tightness or wrinkles in bandages can cause swelling and irritation of underlying tissue.
	Use sheepskin underneath hips and back.	Sheepskin may protect susceptible areas, such as bony prominences on sacrum.
	Monitor traction device, including ropes, pulleys, and weights.	To maintain effective traction, weights must be hanging freely, ropes must be securely on pulleys, and the traction device must be free of friction.
	Maintain body alignment.	Proper body alignment maintains a pull on the long axis of the bone.
	Inspect pin sites for redness, swelling, or discharge; provide pin care according to protocol.	Early intervention can prevent infection; pin care removes debris that can lead to infection or osteomyelitis.

Selected Nursing Diagnosis Potentail for delayed growth and development as a result of hospitalization and separation from family and friends

Goals	Nursing Interventions	Rationales
Child's developmental level will be maintained.	Allow child to choose age-appropriate games.	Allowing child to choose activities increases active participation.
	Encourage peer contact.	Children, particularly those of school age and adolescents, must remain in contact with their peers to prevent feelings of isolation.
	Involve child-life specialist or schoolteacher to provide appropriate learning activities.	Maintaining age-appropriate studies will allow the child to rejoin peers in school.

develop abnormally. Conservative treatment that consists of splinting or casting to hold the foot in the right position is performed during infancy. Passive stretching exercises may also be recommended. If these methods are not effective by age 3 months, surgery may be indicated. After surgery, the cast is changed approximately every 3 weeks to bring the foot gradually into position. When the cast is removed for the final time, exercise and use of special shoes may be indicated.

The infant with a clubfoot is under medical supervision for a long time. Parents must be instructed in developmental behaviours of the infant as well as the clinical aspects of care. Ongoing support is paramount.

The nurse is an important figure in the long-term care of the patient with clubfoot. Nurses review the normal growth and development of children in the patient's age range to anticipate problems and to educate caretakers. Children in a cast may be slow in developing certain motor abilities. Education concerning the therapy and referral for follow-up care are important nursing responsibilities.

Nursing Tip

In the long-term care of orthopedic patients, educating the parents about orthopedic devices, cast care, exercise, hygiene, and treatment goals is necessary. The nurse needs to explain the importance of frequent clinic visits, reinforce health care providers' information, and clarify directions as necessary.

DEVELOPMENTAL DYSPLASIA OF THE HIP

Pathophysiology

Developmental dysplasia of the hip (DDH) is a common orthopedic deformity. The term *hip dysplasia* is a broad description applied to various degrees of deformity: subluxation or dislocation, either partial or complete. The head of the femur is partly or completely displaced as a result of a shallow hip socket (acetabulum). Hereditary and environmental factors appear to be causal factors. Hip malformation, joint laxity, breech position, and maternal hormones may all contribute (Sankar, Horn, Wells, et al., 2016a).

DDH occurs in approximately 1 in 1 000 White children. Black, Southern Chinese, and Korean children seem to be less affected. DDH occurs in females 80% of the time (Canadian Orthopaedic Foundation, 2017). Newborn infants seldom have complete dislocation. However, the child beginning to walk exerts pressure on the hip, which can cause complete dislocation. Therefore, early detection and treatment are of particular importance so that treatment can be started before ossification occurs.

There is a high risk for DDH in cultures in which the newborn is wrapped snugly with the hips in adduction and extension. There is a lower risk for DDH in cultures in which the infant is carried straddled on the mother's waist with the infant's hips flexed and widely abducted. In Canada, Indigenous populations such as the Inuit, who tightly swaddle infants on cradle boards, have a higher rate of DDH (Canadian Orthopaedic Foundation, 2017). The infant may be at risk if it was in a breech position in utero or has a family history of a relative under 40 years of age who required a hip replacement (Krader, 2017).

Manifestations

A dislocation of the hip is commonly discovered at the periodic health examination of the infant during the first or second month of life. One of the most reliable signs is a limited abduction of the leg on the affected side. When the infant is placed on the back with knees and hips flexed, the health care provider can press the thigh of the normal hip backward until it almost touches the examining table. This can be accomplished only partially on the affected side. The knee on the side of the dislocation is lower, and the skin folds of the thigh are deeper and often asymmetrical (Fig. 24.10). When the infant is in a prone position, one buttock appears higher than the other.

A health care provider performs a *Barlow test* to detect an unstable hip in the newborn. The health care provider adducts and extends the hips while stabilizing the pelvis and may "feel" the dislocation occur as the femur leaves the acetabulum.

In infants with developmental dislocation of the hip, the health care provider can actually feel and hear the femoral head slip back into the acetabulum under gentle pressure. This is called the **Ortolani sign** or Ortolani click and is also considered diagnostic of the disorder. The child who is walking and has had no treatment displays a characteristic limp. Bilateral dislocation may occur; however, unilateral dislocation is more common. Radiographic studies confirm the diagnosis.

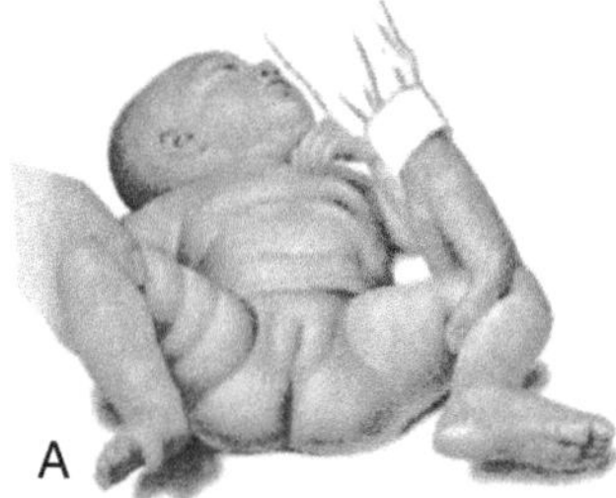

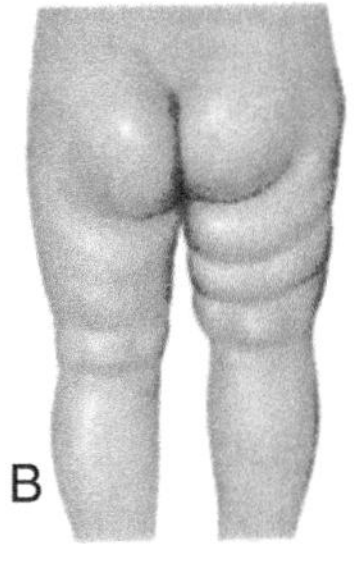

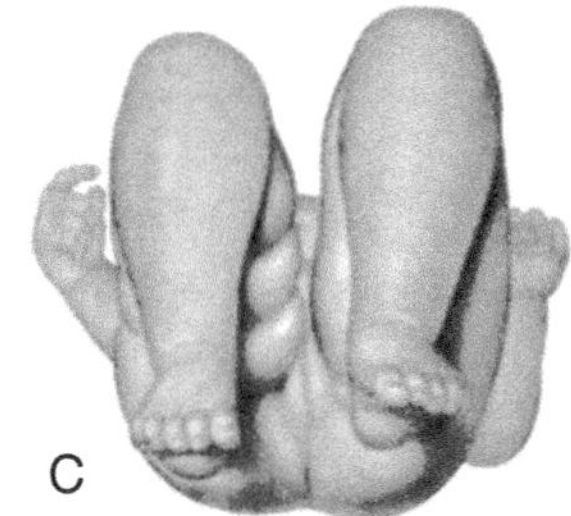

Fig. 24.10 Early signs of dislocation of the right hip. **A,** Limitation of abduction. **B,** Asymmetry of skin folds. **C,** Shortening of femur. (From Ross Laboratories. [1986]. *Clinical education aid no. 15*. Columbus, Ohio: Ross Laboratories. Reproduced with permission of Ross Laboratories.)

Safety Alert!

The Ortolani and Barlow tests for DDH should only be performed by a skilled and experienced health care provider (physician or nurse practitioner), because forcing or manipulating the affected hip can cause a permanent dislocation in the newborn.

Treatment

Treatment begins immediately on detection of the dislocation. The hips are maintained in constant flexion and abduction for 4 to 8 weeks to keep the head of the femur within the hip socket. This constant pressure enlarges and deepens the acetabulum; thus, it can correct the dislocation.

Long-term immobilization is done using a **Pavlik harness** (Fig. 24.11). Traction may be necessary if the dislocation is severe or is not detected until the child begins to walk. This pulls the head of the femur down to the correct position opposite the acetabulum and helps to overcome muscle spasm. Parents need to be taught how to care for their child without removing the harness. The harness must stay on 24 hours a day without removing it for diaper changes or tub baths. The child can have sponge baths without soaking the straps. After drying the skin, cornstarch applied under the straps helps avoid irritation. Loose clothing goes on top of the harness. The child's blanket should not be bundled or wrapped. The child needs to have the position changed alternately from stomach to back and keep the hips and knees in position while being breastfed. The skin needs to be inspected daily to ensure that there is no pressure causing redness while keeping the hips and knees in position (About Kids Health, 2009b).

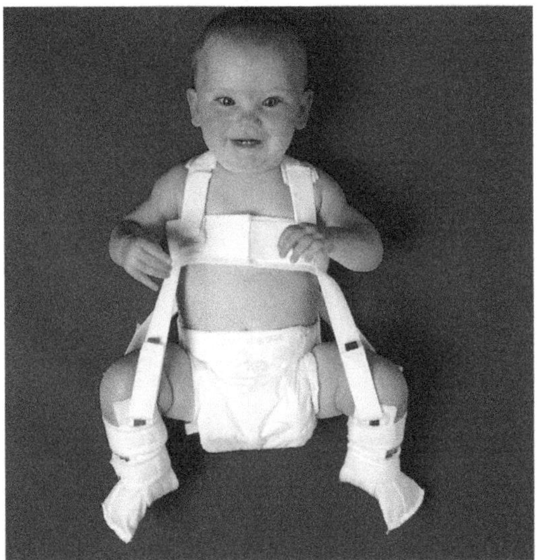

Fig. 24.11 The Pavlik harness is used with infants aged 1 to 6 months to maintain the hips in a position of flexion and abduction. (Courtesy Wheaton Brace Co., Carol Stream, Illinois.)

Casting in a froglike position is then done. This type of cast, known as a body **spica cast**, is shown in Fig. 24.12, *A*. The length of time spent in a cast varies according to the child's progress and growth and the condition of the cast; however, it is usually several months. During this time, the cast may be changed about every 6 weeks. Open reduction of the dislocation or repair of the shelf of the hipbone is performed in infants over 18 months of age who do not respond to treatment. After surgery, a hip spica cast may be applied to keep the femur in the correct position. The body hip spica cast encircles the waist and extends to the ankles or toes. Neurovascular checks need to be performed; see discussion of cast care earlier in the chapter. It is particularly important to pedal the edges of the cast to protect the diaper area of the cast. Nursing Care Plan 24.2 provides selected nursing diagnoses and interventions for the patient with a spica cast.

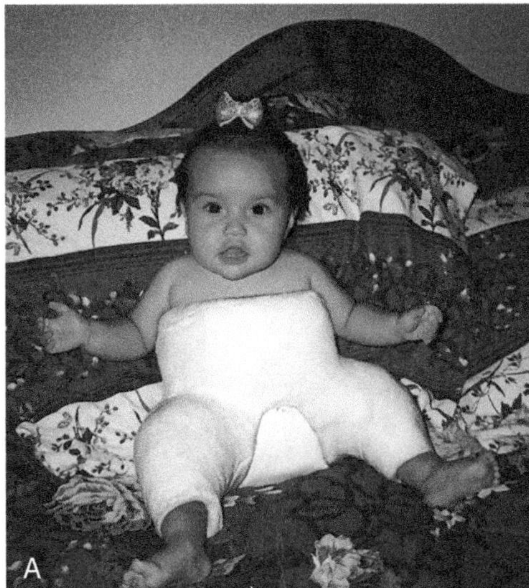

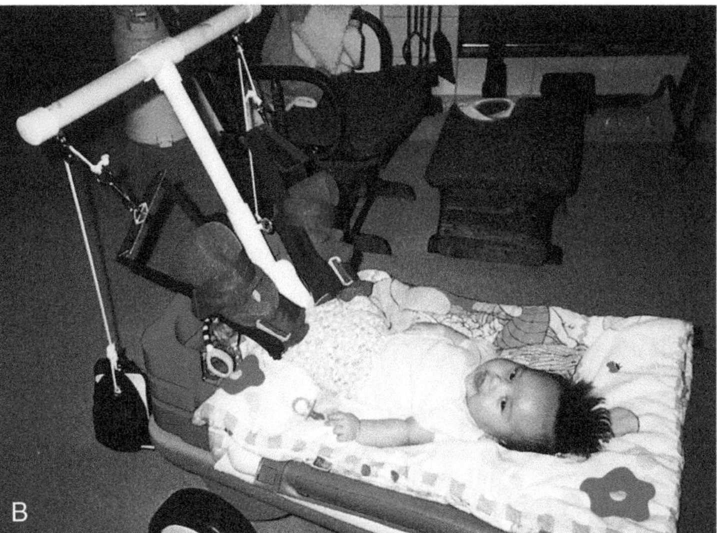

Fig. 24.12 **A,** Infant in a spica body cast. This cast maintains the legs in a froglike position and is used to treat developmental dysplasia of the hip. Note that the infant is able to move her toes freely. A diaper tucked inside prevents the cast from becoming soiled with urine or feces. **B,** Traction is sometimes necessary before surgery or casting. Home care enables the child to be in familiar surroundings that will nurture growth and development.

Nursing Care Plan 24.2 The Infant or Child With a Spica Cast

PATIENT DATA
A child returns from the cast room after having a spica cast applied. The child is scheduled for discharge after the cast is dry.

Selected Nursing Diagnosis Potential ineffective tissue perfusion as a result of cast constriction

Goals	Nursing Interventions	Rationales
Tissues and circulation will appear adequate as evidenced by pink, warm skin, appropriate capillary refill, and lack of numbness or swelling.	Observe exposed extremities and skin distal to the cast every 30 minutes for the first few hours of a new cast and every 1 to 4 hours thereafter; watch for signs of pallor, cyanosis, swelling, coldness, numbness, pain, or burning.	Circulation can be impaired, leading to ischemia. Peripheral nerves, in contrast to muscles, do not degenerate with disuse, but loss of *innervation* can take place if nerves are damaged by pressure or if the blood supply is disrupted.
	Circle any drainage on cast with date and time; monitor and record findings.	An increase in size of circle indicates further bleeding or possibly a draining infection.
	Observe nonverbal communication for signs of pain; ask older child if pain is experienced.	Unrelieved pain, especially after a few days, may indicate *compartment syndrome;* compartment syndrome appears in a group of muscles and fascia where an increase in pressure within this closed space may disrupt circulation within the space.
Parents will understand signs of inadequate circulation and explain importance of seeking immediate assistance if these signs appear.	Educate parents and patient, if old enough, in all of the above.	Education reduces stress for parents and patient.
	Provide written instructions.	Written instructions provide reinforcement and help to ensure the success of other interventions.

Selected Nursing Diagnosis Risk for injury as a result of awkwardness and weight of cast

Goals	Nursing Interventions	Rationales
Patient will remain safe and as independent as possible.	Inform child when turning as to how and when you are going to proceed (e.g., "ready, set, go").	Involving child in procedure, as age appropriate, gives them a sense of control; procedure will go more smoothly.
	Leave articles and toys within reach.	Child will not need to strain or move awkwardly to reach articles; patient will feel greater control if articles can be obtained independently.
	Provide information regarding car seats that may be adapted to accommodate a small child in a spica cast.	These children need protection in a car.

Nursing Care

The nurse must carefully assess each infant to detect signs of a hip dysplasia:

- When the infant is prone, the nurse observes the buttocks for variation in size.
- The legs of the infant should be equal in length.
- The infant should be kicking both legs, not just one leg.
- The depth and number of skin folds of the infant's upper thighs should be symmetrical.
- In the well-baby clinic, the nurse should note the posture and gait of older children and record observations.

Infants who progress well with the Pavlik harness remain at home, with regular visits to the health care provider. The parents need guidance on the care and application of the Pavlik harness. They should be encouraged to ask questions of the clinic nurse and health care provider.

The hip spica cast

Nursing care needs to be adapted for the child in a hip spica cast. Firm, plastic-covered pillows are required. These are placed beneath the curvatures of the cast for support. Older children may benefit from an overhead bar and trapeze. A fracture pan should be available at the bedside for toileting as developmentally appropriate.

The head of the patient's bed is slightly elevated so that urine or feces drain away from the body of the cast. One should not use pillows to elevate the head or shoulders of a child in a body cast, because this

Skill 24.2 Technique for Turning the Child in a Body Cast

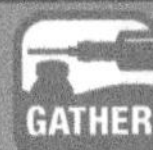

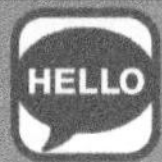

PURPOSE

To change position of child for comfort and prevention of pressure areas on skin

STEPS

Two people, one on each side of the bed, are needed to turn a child in a body cast, as follows:

1. Move the child to the edge of the bed as far as possible so that the nurse who will receive the child is farther away from them.
2. The nurse nearest to the child places one hand under the head and back and one hand under the leg part of the cast and turns the child to the midway point on the side.
3. The nurse farthest away from the child then accepts the support of the child and cast as turning is completed.

thrusts the patient's chest against the cast and causes discomfort or respiratory difficulty. Frequent changes of position are important; immobilized patients must be turned often. Infants may be held in the parent's or nurse's lap after the cast has dried. A ride on a wagon or stretcher to the playroom or around the hospital provides changes of position and scenery.

The supporting bar between the legs should not be used as a lever when turning the child (Skill 24.2). Whenever possible, the older child should be on their abdomen during mealtime to facilitate swallowing and self-feeding. When placing a child in a body cast on a fracture pan, the upper back and legs are supported with pillows so that body alignment is maintained.

Itching is often a problem for the patient in a body cast. If at all possible, a strip of gauze is placed beneath the cast before it is applied; this gauze extends through the opened area required for toilet needs. It is gently moved back and forth to relieve itching. When the strip becomes soiled, a clean one is tied to one end of the soiled gauze and pulled through the cast; this soiled portion is then removed. Other methods to relieve itch that might cause injury to the skin beneath the cast are discouraged, because any break in the skin under a cast is difficult to heal.

Toys small enough to be "hidden" inside the cast should not be given to the child. Toys that can be used when the child is in a prone position are best.

The child with this long-term condition requires help in meeting their everyday needs. Dressing and clothing may be a problem. The child cannot fit into regular furniture or much of the play equipment enjoyed by other children. Transportation can be difficult. A special wagon built up with pillows may be used (see Fig. 24.12, *B*). The child should be included in everyday family and play activities to encourage normal growth and development. A referral for home health care should be made on discharge.

DISORDERS AND DYSFUNCTION OF THE MUSCULOSKELETAL SYSTEM

OSTEOMYELITIS

Pathophysiology

Osteomyelitis is an infection of the bone that generally occurs in children younger than 1 year of age and in those between 5 and 14 years of age. Long bones contain few phagocytic cells (white blood cells [WBCs]) to fight bacteria that may enter the bone from another part of the body. The inflammation produces an exudate that collects under the marrow and cortex of the bone.

Staphylococcus aureus is the organism most often responsible for osteomyelitis in all age groups, with community-acquired methicillin-resistant *Staphylococcus aureus* (MRSA) accounting for almost 50% of the cases (Kaplan, 2016). Other causative organisms include group A streptococci and pneumococci. Osteomyelitis may be preceded by a local injury to the bone, such as an open fracture, burn, or contamination during surgery. It may also follow a furuncle, impetigo, and abscessed teeth. In newborns, a heel puncture or scalp vein monitor can be the predisposing site of infection. Infective emboli may travel to the small arteries of the bone, setting up local destruction and abscess. For this reason, a careful search for infection in other bones and soft tissues is necessary.

The vessels in the affected area are compressed, and thrombosis occurs, producing ischemia and pain. The collection of pus under the periosteum of the bone can elevate the periosteum, which can result in necrosis of that part of the bone. If the pus reaches the epiphysis of the bone in infants, infection can travel to the joint space, causing septic arthritis of that joint.

Local inflammation and increased pressure from the distended periosteum can cause pain. Older children can localize the pain and may limp. Younger children and infants will show decreased voluntary movement of that extremity. Associated muscle spasms can cause limited active ROM. The child may refuse to stand or walk. Signs of local inflammation may be present.

A detailed history may show possible sources of primary infection. Blood cultures to identify the organism may be valuable if the child has not been given antibiotics for the primary infection. A urine test for the presence of bacterial antigens and a tissue biopsy may be helpful to establish the diagnosis.

Diagnosis

In osteomyelitis there is an elevation in WBC count and ESR. X-ray examination may initially fail to reveal the infection. A microbiology culture of aspirated drainage or a bone scan may be diagnostic.

Treatment and Nursing Care

Prompt and vigorous treatment is essential to ensure a favourable prognosis. IV antibiotics are prescribed for a 4- to 6-week period. High doses of antibiotics are required; a nursing responsibility is to monitor the infant or child for toxic responses and to ensure the long-term ability to take the medication. The joint may be drained of pus arthroscopically or surgically to reduce pressure and to prevent bone necrosis. A complication should be suspected if fever lasts beyond 5 days.

The use of appropriate pain-relieving medications and gentle handling to minimize pain are essential. The child should be positioned comfortably with the limb supported by pillows or blanket rolls.

Bed rest is followed by wheelchair access, but weight-bearing should be avoided. Diversional therapy, physical therapy, and tutorial assistance for school-age children should be provided so that they can return to their classes and classmates after discharge. Close interaction with home care providers is indicated. Passive ROM and physical therapy is important. A normal ESR test is predictive of healing.

DUCHENNE MUSCULAR DYSTROPHY

Pathophysiology

The **muscular dystrophies** are a group of disorders in which progressive muscle degeneration occurs. The childhood form (Duchenne muscular dystrophy [DMD]) is the most common type. It has an incidence of about 1 in 3 600 newborns (Sarnat, 2016). DMD is a sex-linked recessive inherited disorder that occurs mainly in boys. It is very rare that females develop DMD and if they do, it is in a milder form of muscular weakness (Sarnat, 2016). Dystrophin, a protein in skeletal muscle, is absent. Becker pseudohypertrophic muscular dystrophy occurs later in childhood, progresses more slowly, and is not as common as DMD.

Manifestations

Symptoms are noted generally between 2 and 6 years of age; however, there may be a history of delayed motor development during infancy. The calf muscles in particular become hypertrophied. The term *pseudo-hypertrophic* (*pseudo,* "false," and *hypertrophy,* "enlargement") refers to this characteristic. Other signs include progressive weakness as evidenced by frequent falling, clumsiness, contractures of the ankles and hips, and *Gower sign* (a characteristic way of rising from the floor by using the hands and arms to "walk" up the body from a squatting position due to lack of thigh and hip muscle strength).

Laboratory findings show marked increases in serum creatine phosphokinase. Muscle biopsy shows a degeneration of muscle fibres and their replacement by fat and connective tissue and is considered diagnostic. A *myelogram* (a graphic record of muscle contraction as a result of electrical stimulation) shows decreases in the amplitude and duration of motor unit potentials. A serum blood polymerase chain reaction (PCR) for the gene mutation is diagnostic for this condition. The disease becomes progressively worse, and the permanent use of a wheelchair may be necessary. Death usually results from cardiac failure or respiratory tract infection. Intellectual impairment is not uncommon.

Treatment and Nursing Care

Treatment is mainly supportive to prevent contractures and to maintain quality of life. Cardiac and respiratory complications are common. A multidisciplinary team should provide psychological support, nutritional support, physiotherapy, social and financial assistance, and, when necessary, respite and hospice care. The use of prednisone has shown some promise if given early when the child is still ambulatory and has been shown to keep children ambulatory longer (Sarnat, 2016). Muscular Dystrophy Canada provides information and support for children and their families.

Compared with other children with disabilities, some children with muscular dystrophy may appear passive and withdrawn. Early on, depression may be seen because the child cannot compete with peers. Social and emotional pressures on the child and family are great.

SLIPPED CAPITAL FEMORAL EPIPHYSIS

Pathophysiology

A *slipped capital femoral epiphysis* (SCFE), also known as *coxa vara,* is the spontaneous displacement of the epiphysis of the femur. It most often occurs during rapid growth of the preadolescent and is not related to trauma. The elevated level of circulating hormones of puberty, combined with the mechanical load of excess weight on the epiphysis, results in the displacement of the head of the femur in relation to the femoral neck. Increased rates of obesity have correlated with increased rates of the occurrence of SCFE, as more than 80% of children with SCFE are obese (Sankar, Horn, Wells, et al., 2016c). The epiphysis of the femur widens, and then the femoral head and epiphysis remain in the acetabulum. The head of the femur then rotates and displaces. Symptoms include thigh pain and a limp or the inability to bear weight on the involved leg. An X-ray study confirms diagnosis.

Treatment

The child is not allowed to bear weight, and surgery is scheduled to insert a screw to stabilize the bone. Serious complications may include disturbance of circulation to the epiphysis, resulting in necrosis of the head of the femur.

Nursing Care

The general principles of caring for a child who is in a cast or traction, as discussed earlier, and of preoperative and postoperative care are used. The nurse assists in performing ROM activities, guides gradual resumption of weight-bearing with the help of crutches, and encourages referrals to maintain school studies. Education concerning management of weight is important postoperatively.

LEGG-CALVÉ-PERTHES DISEASE

Pathophysiology

Legg-Calvé-Perthes disease (LCPD) is a hip disorder. It results from temporary interruption of the blood supply to the proximal femoral epiphysis, leading to osteonecrosis and femoral head deformity. The incidence is approximately 1 in 1 200 (Sankar, Horn, Wells, et al., 2016b). The disease is seen most commonly in boys between 4 and 8 years of age. LCPD is unilateral in about 90% of cases. Healing occurs spontaneously during 2 to 4 years; however, marked distortion of the head of the femur may lead to an imperfect joint or degenerative arthritis of the hip in later life. Symptoms include thigh and knee pain, a painless limp, and limitation of motion. X-ray films and bone scans confirm the diagnosis.

Treatment

LCPD is a self-limiting disorder that heals spontaneously, but slowly, throughout the course of 4 years. The treatment involves keeping the femoral head deep in the hip socket while it heals and preventing weight-bearing. This is accomplished through the use of ambulation-abduction casts or braces that prevent subluxation (*sub*, "beneath," and *luxatio*, "dislocation") and enable the acetabulum to mould the healing head in such a way that it does not become deformed.

Nursing Care

Nursing considerations depend on the age of the patient and the type of treatment. The general principles of traction, cast, and brace care are used when immobilization of the child is necessary. Teaching and counselling are directed toward a holistic understanding of and interest in the child and family. Total immobility or partial mobility is particularly trying for children. In some cases, surgical immobilization is required.

OSTEOSARCOMA

Pathophysiology

Osteosarcoma (*osteo*, "bone," *sarx*, "flesh," and *oma*, "tumour") is a primary malignant tumour of the long bones. The two most common types of bone tumours in children are osteosarcoma and Ewing sarcoma. The mean age of onset of osteosarcoma is between 10 and 15 years of age and occurs most commonly in tall adolescents in the midst of rapid bone growth. The cause is genetic, with children having a history of retinoblastoma at highest risk. Metastasis occurs quickly because of the high vascularity of bone tissue. The lungs are the primary site of metastasis; the brain and other bone tissue are also sites of metastasis.

Manifestations

The patient experiences pain and swelling at the site. In adolescents, this is often attributed to a sports injury or "growing pains." Flexing the extremity may lessen the pain. Later, a pathological fracture may occur. Diagnosis is confirmed by X-ray. A complete physical examination, including CT and a bone scan, is performed.

Treatment and Nursing Care

Treatment of the patient with osteosarcoma consists of surgery, chemotherapy, and radiation. Radical resection or amputation may be necessary. Internal prostheses are available for most sites. Long-term survival is possible with early diagnosis and treatment. Among children aged 0 to 14 years who are diagnosed with osteosarcoma (occurring at any site in the body), 70% are expected to live for at least 5 years after their diagnosis (Canadian Cancer Society, 2019).

The nursing care is similar to that for other types of cancer. Problems with body image are particularly important to the self-conscious adolescent. If amputation is necessary, the family and patient will need much support. The nurse should anticipate anger, fear, and grief. Immediately after surgery the stump dressing must be observed frequently for signs of bleeding. Vital signs are monitored. The child is positioned as ordered by the surgeon.

Phantom limb pain may be experienced, which is the continued sensation of pain in the limb even though the limb is no longer there. It occurs because nerve tracts continue to report pain. This pain is very real, and an analgesic may be necessary. Rehabilitation measures follow surgical recovery.

EWING SARCOMA

Pathophysiology

Ewing sarcoma is a malignant growth that occurs in the marrow of the long bones. It occurs mainly in older school-age children and early adolescents. Among children aged 0 to 14 years who are diagnosed with Ewing sarcoma, 70% are expected to live for at least 5 years after their diagnosis (Canadian Cancer Society, 2019). When metastasis is present on diagnosis, the prognosis is poor. The primary sites for metastasis are the lungs and long bones.

Treatment and Nursing Care

Amputation is not generally recommended for Ewing sarcoma because the tumour is sensitive to radiation therapy and chemotherapy. The child is taught to not bear weight on the involved bone during therapy, to help prevent pathological fractures. Patients must be prepared for the effects of radiation therapy and chemotherapy. The nurse should support the family members in their efforts to cope with the diagnosis. Long-term follow-up care is important in detecting the late effects of the treatment.

JUVENILE IDIOPATHIC ARTHRITIS

Pathophysiology

Juvenile idiopathic arthritis (JIA), previously called *juvenile rheumatoid arthritis,* is the most common arthritic condition of childhood. It is a systemic autoimmune disease that involves the joints, connective tissues, and viscera, and it differs somewhat from adult rheumatoid arthritis. It is not a rare disease: 3 in every 1 000 Canadian children develop JIA. Multiple genes are involved, with an external trigger that initiates signs and symptoms such as a sports injury or bacterial or viral infection treated with antibiotics (Wu, Bryan, & Rabinovich, 2016).

Manifestations and Types

JIA has several distinct classifications (Wu et al., 2016):

1. *Oligoarthritis* involves four or fewer joints, and uveitis (inflammation of the eye) is common in about 30% of affected children.
2. *Polyarthritis* involves five or more joints, and uveitis occurs in about 10% of these children.
3. *Systemic arthritis* is characterized by fever, rash, and joint inflammation. Uveitis occurs in about 10% of these children. The *systemic* form is manifested by intermittent spiking fever above 39.5°C (103°F) persisting for more than 10 days, a nonpruritic macular rash, abdominal pain, an elevated ESR, C-reactive protein in laboratory tests, presence of antinuclear antibodies, and possibly an enlarged liver and spleen. It occurs most often in children ages 1 to 3 years and 8 to 10 years. Joint symptoms may be absent at onset, but usually arthritis develops in most patients.

Treatment

The goals of therapy are to accomplish the following:

- Reduce joint pain and swelling
- Promote mobility and preserve joint function
- Promote growth and development
- Promote independent functioning
- Help the child and family to adjust to living with a chronic illness

Medications such as NSAIDs and methotrexate may also be provided. The child should undergo frequent laboratory tests to monitor closely for adverse effects. Steroids may be administered for incapacitating arthritis, uveitis, or life-threatening complications. Immunosuppressants, such as etanercept, adalimubab, canakinumab, and tocilizumab, may be prescribed. Nursing interventions include preventing infection and close observation for serious adverse effects that can occur.

Nursing Care

The nurse functions as a member of a multidisciplinary health care team that includes the pediatrician, rheumatologist, social worker, physiotherapist, occupational therapist, psychologist, ophthalmologist, and community nurses. Physical and occupational therapy preserve joint function and mobility. Occupational therapy helps with activities of daily living. Resting in a bed with a supportive, flat mattress is helpful. Resting splints during sleep can prevent flexion contractures from developing. Moist heat and exercise are advised, and whirlpool baths and hot packs relieve pain and stiffness. Therapeutic play facilitates the ability to complete exercise regimens. Swimming can help maintain joint mobility. Sleep, rest, and general health measures are important.

Teachers can be contacted to help promote normal growth and development in school-related activities. Unnecessary restrictions should be avoided because they can lead to rebellion and difficulty following through with treatment. JIA may inhibit the child's social interactions and can interfere with development of a positive self-concept. The Arthritis Society of Canada provides services to parents and nurses involved in patient care.

This long-term disease is characterized by periods of remission and exacerbations. Nurses can serve as advocates for the child; that is, they can help alleviate stress by recognizing the impact of the disease and by openly communicating with the child, the family, and other members of the health care team. Nurses need to support the child and family as they live with this disease.

TORTICOLLIS (WRY NECK)

Pathophysiology

Torticollis (*tortus,* "twisted," and *collium,* "neck") is a condition in which neck motion is limited and the cervical spine is rotated because of shortening of the sternocleidomastoid muscle. It can be either congenital or acquired and can also be either acute or chronic. The most common type is a congenital anomaly in which the sternocleidomastoid muscle is injured during birth. It is associated with breech and forceps birth and may be seen in conjunction with other birth defects, such as congenital hip dysplasia.

Manifestations

In congenital torticollis, the symptoms are present at birth. The infant holds the head to the side of the muscle involved. The chin is tilted in the opposite direction.

There is a hard, palpable mass of dense fibrotic tissue (fibroma) within the muscle. Passive stretching, ROM exercises, and physical therapy may be indicated. Feeding and playing with the infant can encourage turning to the desired side for correction. Surgical correction is indicated if the condition persists beyond 2 years of age (O'Toole & Spiegel, 2016).

Acquired torticollis is seen in older children. It may be associated with injury, inflammation, neurological disorders, and other causes. Nursing intervention is primarily that of detection. Infants who have limited head movement require further investigation.

SCOLIOSIS

Pathophysiology

The most prevalent of the three skeletal abnormalities shown in Fig. 24.13 is scoliosis. **Scoliosis** refers to an S-shaped curvature of the spine. During adolescence, scoliosis is more common in girls. Many curvatures are not progressive and may necessitate only periodic evaluation. Untreated progressive scoliosis may lead to back pain, fatigue, disability, and heart and lung complications. Skeletal deterioration does not stop with maturity and may be aggravated by pregnancy.

There are two types of scoliosis: functional and structural. *Functional scoliosis* is usually caused by poor posture, not by spinal disease. The curve is flexible and easily correctable. Structural or fixed scoliosis is caused by changes in the shape of the vertebrae or thorax. It is usually accompanied by rotation of the spine. The hips and shoulders may appear uneven. The patient cannot correct the condition by standing in a straighter posture.

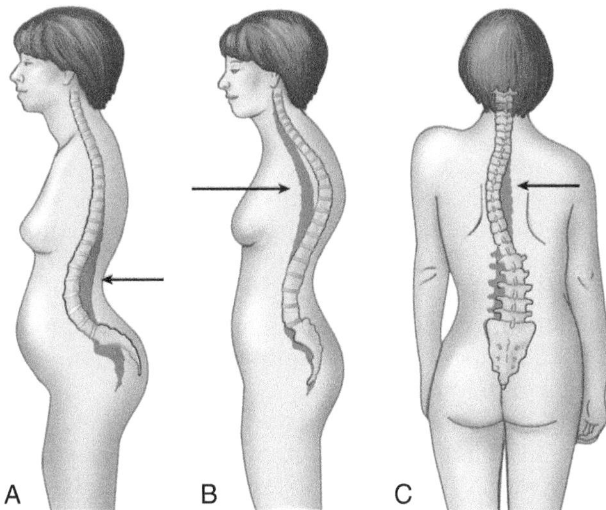

Fig. 24.13 Abnormal spinal curvatures. **A,** *Lordosis,* known as "sway back," is commonly seen during pregnancy. **B,** *Kyphosis,* known as "hunchback," is an increased roundness in the thoracic curve commonly found in older persons. **C,** *Scoliosis,* an abnormal side-to-side curvature of the spine, is commonly found in adolescents. (From Patton, K. T., & Thibodeau, G. A. [2015]. *Anatomy & physiology* [9th ed.]. St. Louis: Mosby.)

Idiopathic scoliosis is a curve of at least 10 degrees noted on an anterior-posterior spinal X-ray. The specific cause is unknown, but genetic, hormonal, anatomical, and functional factors are thought to play a role. Eighty percent of idiopathic scoliosis affects children 11 years of age and older.

Signs and Symptoms

Symptoms develop slowly and are not painful, so detection usually occurs during an assessment, which reveals shoulders that are different heights, a one-sided rib bump, and a prominent scapula. This asymmetry is seen from the back when the child leans forward. Definitive diagnosis is made by a spinal X-ray study while the child is in an upright position.

Treatment

There is evidence that asymptomatic individuals have a mild clinical course and that interventions such as braces and exercise may not improve back pain or quality of life. Potential harms include unnecessary medical evaluations and psychological adverse effects, especially related to wearing corrective braces. Therefore, routine screening is not recommended unless the child has symptoms or it is found incidentally (Greig, Constantin, LeBlanc, et al., 2016). In scoliosis, one shoulder is noted to be higher than the other, a scapula may be prominent, the arm-to-body spaces may be unequal, or a hip may protrude; one arm may appear longer than the other when the person bends forward. Referrals are made as indicated for those who may require further assessment and treatment.

If treatment is required, it is aimed at correcting the curvature and preventing more severe scoliosis. Curves up to 20 degrees do not necessitate treatment but are carefully followed with exercise to increase muscle tone and posture. Curves between 20 and 40 degrees may require the use of a **Milwaukee brace** (Fig. 24.14). This apparatus exerts pressure on the chin,

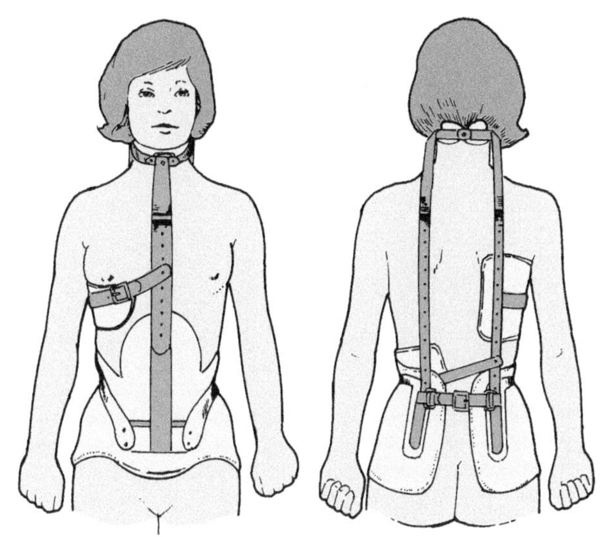

Fig. 24.14 The Milwaukee brace.

pelvis, and convex (arched) side of the spine. It is worn approximately 16 to 23 hours a day and is worn *over* a cotton T-shirt without seams to protect the skin. The brace should be worn as tightly as possible. It is important for the child to bathe daily and apply rubbing alcohol with the hands to all parts of the skin that the brace covers. The skin needs to be closely observed for reddened areas where the brace is tight. The brace can be washed with soap and water (Cincinnati Children's, 2018).

An underarm modification of the brace (the Boston brace) is proving effective for patients with low curvatures. It is less cumbersome and is more acceptable to the self-conscious young person. Transcutaneous electrical muscle stimulation (TENS) and exercise have also proven effective in the treatment of scoliosis (Mistovich & Spiegel, 2016).

Severe scoliosis beyond a curvature of 45 degrees necessitates surgery to fuse the bones and stop progression of the deformity. A Harrington rod, Dwyer instrument, or Luque wires may be inserted for immobilization during the time required for the fusion to become solid. Halo traction may be used when there is associated weakness or paralysis of the neck and trunk muscles (Fig. 24.15); this traction is also used in treating cervical fractures and fusions. An anterior-posterior plastic shell or orthotic may be worn for several months until the spine is stable. Helping the teen cope with a body brace and maintain a positive self-image is an important and challenging aspect of care.

Vertebral expandable prosthetic titanium rib (VEPTR) surgery expands the thoracic space and is indicated in patients with severe spinal curves that restrict lung function. This treatment allows for the patient's development of maximum height, before spinal fusion is necessary. The use of "growing rods" is another approach to treatment, in which expandable rods are placed subcutaneously and lengthened as the child grows until skeletal maturity occurs (Mistovich & Spiegel, 2016).

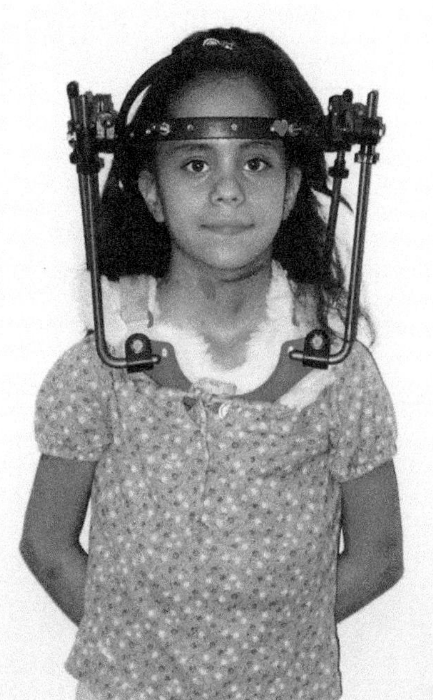

Fig. 24.15 Halo traction. This halo jacket and apparatus is used for cervical fractures and spinal disorders. (Courtesy Pat Spier, RN-C.)

 Nursing Tip

Nurses should teach patients that insertion of a Harrington rod or other metal device may delay the patient at an airport or other security scanner because the metal could activate the alarm.

Nursing Care

For adolescents undergoing spinal fusion, routine preoperative nursing care is necessary. Much postoperative nursing care is directly related to decreasing the physical results of immobilization (see Fig. 24.8). The body systems become sluggish because of inactivity. This is evidenced in the gastrointestinal tract by anorexia, irregularity, and constipation. Allowing the adolescent to select foods with the aid of the dietitian is helpful in improving appetite. Increasing fluid intake reduces constipation. The adolescent and parents need to be introduced to the multidisciplinary health care team. Postoperative exercise, physical therapy, and promotion of adolescent school and developmental tasks are essential aspects of nursing care.

SPORTS INJURIES

Many adolescents participate in athletic activities. The CPS recommends that a complete physical examination be given every 1 to 2 years for all children ages 6 to 17 years (Greig et al., 2016). The research regarding sports-specific examination prior to participating in athletics is not conclusive that it will prevent health-related conditions (O'Brien, 2017), so this type of examination is not generally recommended.

Prevention

Several factors help to prevent sports injuries. Some of these are adequate warm-up and cool-down periods; year-round conditioning; careful selection of activity according to physical maturity, size, and skill required; proper supervision by adults; safe, well-fitting protective equipment; and avoidance of participation when in pain or injured.

It is important that health care providers include safety topics in their discussions with children and their parents (Greig et al., 2016). For example, the use of safety helmets is strongly recommended by the CPS and is mandated in some provinces and territories for sports such as cycling, snowboarding, skiing, snowmobiling, skateboarding, using all-terrain vehicles, and skating. Trampolines can also be the site of significant injuries. Skiing and snowboarding combined are the second leading cause of sport- and recreation-related injury hospitalizations in the winter

(18%) and spring months (10%) in Ontario, surpassed only by snowmobile injuries. There is increasing concern regarding the frequency and severity of hockey-related injuries, particularly concussions. Concussions are discussed in more detail in Chapter 23. Body-checking is identified as the major action associated with youth hockey injuries, including concussions. The CPS recommends that body-checking not be allowed until players are 13 to 14 years of age to decrease the risks of injury and concussion, as well as eliminating body-checking from non-elite youth ice hockey (Houghton, Emery, CPS Healthy Active Living Committee, 2016).

Proper diet and fluid intake are also necessary. In addition, sun safety is an important factor in preventing dehydration and injury to skin.

A few of the more common sports-related injuries are listed in Table 24.1. The nurse has a major role in educating and directing parents and children to sources of accurate information to ensure that the physical, emotional, and maturational levels of the adolescent are appropriate for the activity (see Health Promotion box). Parents are encouraged to inquire about the capabilities of coaches or supervising personnel and the availability of emergency services before the beginning of a competition.

Table 24.1 Common Sports Injuries

TYPE	DESCRIPTION
Concussion	Any blow to the head followed by alterations in mental functioning should be treated as a possible concussion; observe carefully for sequelae (See Chapter 23 for further discussion).
"Stingers" or "burners"	A common neck injury when a player hits another in the head in such sports as football or soccer; caused by brachial plexus trauma; feels like an electrical jolt; usually mild and disappears suddenly. Restrict sports activity until symptoms disappear; reassess protective gear.
Injured knee	Usually a result of stress on the knee ligaments; potentially serious; should be evaluated by an experienced trainer or health care provider. It may necessitate arthroscopic surgery.
Sprain or strained ankle	May injure growth plate. X-ray films are important in adolescents.
Muscle cramps	Caused by injury, alterations in blood flow, or electrolyte deficiencies. It is important to warm up before activity and ensure fluid intake is adequate.
Shin splints	Pain and discomfort in lower leg caused by repeated running on a hard surface such as concrete. Avoid such activity; use well-fitting shoes; decrease inflammation by rest.

Health Promotion

Selected Recreational Activities and Their Risks

ACTIVITY	RISK
Gymnastics	Common problems associated with children engaging in competitive gymnastics are delayed menstruation and eating disorders. Trauma and overuse injuries of the large joints and spine are common. Injury prevention includes muscle-strengthening exercises, flexibility exercises, and use of wrist braces. Nutritional planning and education are essential.
Ballet	Common problems associated with ballet include delayed menarche and development of eating disorders. There is a high risk for stress fractures, strains, shin splints, and spinal deviations. Injury prevention includes skilled coaching, and nutrition planning and education.
Wrestling	Placement in a wrestling match is based on weight. A bingeing-and-purging behaviour is commonly found in athletes participating in wrestling. Concussions, neck strains, and spinal injuries are common. Skin dermatitis and infection occur from contact with floor mats. Skilled coaching and nutrition education and planning are important.
Football	Improvements in techniques, protective equipment, and game exercises have decreased serious injuries in children participating on football teams.
Hockey	Injuries can occur from both collisions with other athletes and collisions with pucks or sticks. Proper protective equipment and sporting rules help decrease the seriousness of injuries.
Basketball, volleyball	These are jumping sports that involve injury risk to ankles, knees, and fingers. Ankle sprain, tendonitis, stress fractures, and blisters are common complications of these sports.
Running	Running involves repeated, poorly absorbed foot impact. Muscle fatigue, environmental temperature, and running surface contribute to development of injuries. Engaging in proper exercises before running, using good impact-absorbing shoes, cross-training, and adequate rest are essential. Shin splints involve pain over the anterior tibia and result from tearing the collagenous fibres that connect muscle to bone. Shoe orthotics, running on a soft surface, cross-training, and rest are the priorities in managing shin splints.
Skiing, snowboarding	Injuries are usually related to falls. Better equipment, the use of helmets, controlled slope conditions, and separation of skiers by skill level all contribute to a decreased rate of injury.
Cheerleading	This activity involves acrobatics, pyramid climbing, and tossing. Falls can result in injuries such as sprains, fractures, dislocations, and head injuries. Safety instruction is important, and a certified coach should be present.

VIOLENCE

Violence has become a problem that affects children of all social classes across the nation. Family violence includes intimate partner violence and child abuse, neglect, and maltreatment. In homes where intimate partner violence or child abuse occurs, children learn the behaviours they may practice when they become adults, and the abuse cycle continues. Parents who are abusive are not usually psychotic or criminal. They may have a knowledge deficit about child care needs and child growth and development. Abusive parents are often without a support system and are perhaps alone, angry, or in crisis, or have unrealistic expectations.

Community violence can be seen in some neighbourhoods where gang activity is present, and even non–gang-related adolescents arm themselves with guns and knives for protection.

Preschoolers who are repeatedly allowed to watch violent programs on television or play aggressive computer games may be learning antisocial coping skills that they will use as they grow and mature. Parents should control the time spent watching television and the content of programs watched, so that television exposure results in the acquisition of knowledge, skills, and information that will motivate learning (CPS, 2017).

CHILD ABUSE

In Canada, *child abuse* is defined as harm or risk of harm to a child who is under the care of a trusted individual or who is dependent on that individual. These individuals include a parent, sibling, teacher, caregiver, guardian, or other relatives. Harm may occur by the individual acting directly (acts of commission) or through the person's neglect to provide an element of care that is necessary to ensure healthy child growth and development (acts of omission) (Health Canada, 2012). The abuse and maltreatment have long-term consequences for the child and the family.

There are five types of child maltreatment. Table 24.2 contains descriptions of the different types of child maltreatment along with the statistics for each type of abuse.

Child abuse continues to be a very serious situation in Canada, and around the world. The rates of child abuse are difficult to estimate and are often underreported. As well, the provinces and territories collect the information in different ways, which can make comparisons across Canada hard to evaluate. Statistics Canada has reported that there are 267 child victims of family violence for every 100 000 Canadians under 18 years of age (Sinha & Statistics Canada, 2015). Statistics Canada's self-reported data from child victims indicate that the number of child victims has been on the decline, to a rate of 13% since 1940 (Hango & Statistics Canada, 2017). Canadian Indigenous children have been identified as a major at-risk group and have four times the maltreatment rate for non-Indigenous children (Public Health Agency of Canada [PHAC], 2010).

 **Health Promotion**

Factors That May Contribute to or Trigger Child Abuse

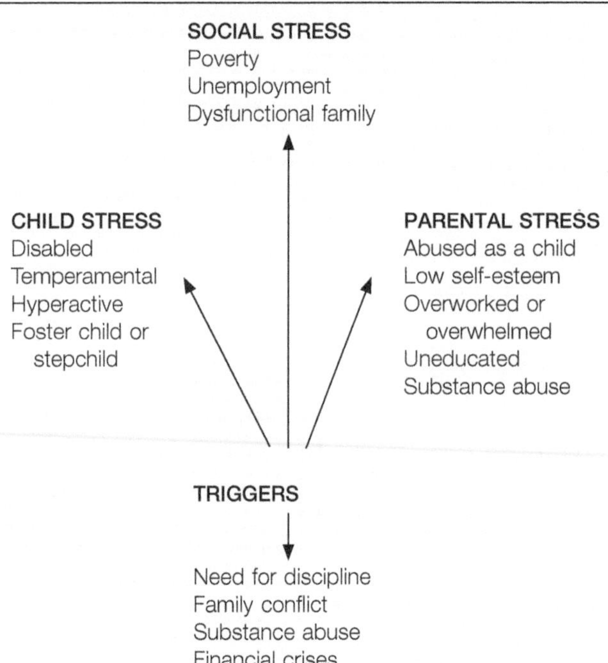

Checking for nerve damage. Nerve damage can result from trauma, and the motor sensory status of the extremity should be assessed and recorded frequently. (Courtesy Bert Oppenheim.)

Note: Abusive parents usually love their children but respond to stress and triggers that provoke abusive behaviour.

Legal and Ethical Considerations

Nurses and other health care providers are often the individuals who identify potential or actual abuse. They play an important role with the child and family to ensure the child's safety and in helping the child and family cope with the situation. In Canada, everyone has a legal duty to report suspected child abuse. This citizen reporting responsibility is built into the legislation of the individual provinces and territories. The legislation and process for notifying authorities varies slightly between individual provinces and territories. It is essential that nurses learn the legal and ethical responsibilities that govern their practice province or territory. Most provinces and territories have penalties for failure to report suspected child abuse. Referrals usually are made to the local child protective services, and a caseworker is assigned.

All persons who report suspected abuse or neglect are given immunity from criminal prosecution and civil liability if the report is made in good faith. Many professionals, such as health care providers, nurses, and social workers, are mandated to report child abuse. Please see Additional Learning Resources at the end of the chapter for the Government of Canada's guide on how to address child maltreatment.

Nursing Care and Interventions

Nursing interventions for high-risk children are of utmost importance (Box 24.1). One approach currently taken is to identify high-risk infants and parents during

Table 24.2 **Types of Maltreatment and Child Abuse**

CATEGORY (% REPORTED)	DEFINITION	SOME EXAMPLES
Physical abuse (assault) (20%)	The application of unreasonable force by an adult or youth to any part of a child's body	Harsh physical discipline, forceful shaking, pushing, choking, stabbing, and the excessive use of restraints
Sexual abuse (3%)	Involvement of a child, by an adult or youth, in an act of sexual gratification, or exposure of a child to sexual contact, activity, or behaviour	Penetration, attempted penetration, oral sex, fondling, sex talk, voyeurism, and sexual exploitation
Neglect (34%)	Failure by a parent or caregiver to provide the physical or psychological necessities of life to a child	Failure to supervise, leading to physical harm or to sexual harm; permitting criminal behaviour; physical neglect; medical neglect; failure to provide psychological treatment; abandonment; and educational neglect
Emotional harm (9%)	Adult behaviour that harms a child psychologically, emotionally, or spiritually	Hostile or unreasonable and abusive treatment, frequent or extreme verbal abuse (that may include threatening and demeaning or insulting behaviours)
Exposure to family violence (34%)	Circumstances that allow a child to be aware of violence occurring between a caregiver and their partner or between other family members	Allowing a child to see, hear, or otherwise be exposed to signs of the violence

Data from Public Health Agency of Canada. (2018). *Family violence: How big is the problem in Canada?* Retrieved from https://www.canada.ca/en/public-health/services/health-promotion/stop-family-violence/problem-canada.html.

Box 24.1 **Nursing Interventions for Abused and Neglected Children and Adolescents**

TEACH CHILD ANXIETY-REDUCING TECHNIQUES

- Relaxation skills
- How to relax to music
- Visual imagery
- How to use exercise to reduce anxiety
- To talk to safe, appropriate people about feelings
- To choose, build, and maintain positive support systems
- To ensure personal safety
- To set boundaries
- To establish a safe, supportive relationship
- To clarify expectations and rules
- Self-soothing techniques

ASSIST CHILD IN MANAGING THEIR FEELINGS

- Identify feelings
- Express feelings appropriately
- Modulate and control feelings
- Identify events that elicit strong positive and negative feelings
- Express feelings verbally instead of physically
- Normalize feelings resulting from abuse
- Share feelings appropriately with peer group
- Find commonality and support within group for feelings resulting from abuse

TEACH CHILD ASSERTIVENESS SKILLS

- Identify differences between assertiveness, passivity, and aggression
- Practice assertiveness skills
- Identify boundaries
- Understand when someone violates boundaries
- Practice responses when someone violates boundaries

ASSIST CHILD IN DEVELOPING PROBLEM-SOLVING SKILLS

- Provide simple problem-solving model
- Increase awareness of child's control and decision making
- Teach child to generate a list of possible solutions to problem situations
- Help child look at consequences of each solution
- Help child make the best choice
- Help child give positive and gentle negative feedback to self
- Coach problem solving with actual situations as much as possible
- Teach about good touch and bad touch
- Teach refusal skills
- Teach age-appropriate sexual expression
- Teach the effects of substance abuse

ASSIST CHILD IN VALUE BUILDING AND CLARIFICATION

- Define values
- Identify role of values
- Assist child in identifying and verbalizing values
- Help link child's values to child's actions
- Assist child in development of values
- Help child practice value-based decision-making

ASSIST CHILD IN ENHANCING THEIR COPING MECHANISMS

- Teach child to practice positive self-talk
- Help child set realistic expectations for self
- Assist child in learning to nurture self
- Teach child to practice relaxation
- Teach child to practice assertiveness and appropriate expression of feelings
- Assist child in learning to accept defeat and failure
- Help child identify and build skills and hobbies
- Encourage child to identify and focus on strengths
- Help child set and accomplish goals
- Assist child in developing organizational skills

Data from Santrock, J. (2011). *Child development* (13th ed.). Philadelphia: McGraw-Hill; DiMarco, M., & Melnyk, B. (2009). The mental health needs of children and adolescents. *Archives of Psychiatric Nursing, 23*, 334–336; Storch, E., & Elder, J. (2009). Introduction to special series on child and adolescent mental health. *Pediatric Nursing, 24*, 1–2.

the prenatal and perinatal periods. Public health departments provide closer follow-up of mothers and newborns who are assessed to be at risk.

Nurses in obstetrical units and clinics have the opportunity to observe parents and their abilities to cope. The history of the parent(s), desirability of the pregnancy, number of children already in the family, financial and personal stability of the family, types of support systems, and other factors may have a bearing on parenting knowledge and skills. Pertinent observations include a description of parent–newborn interaction. Both verbal and nonverbal communications are important, as is the level of body and eye contact. Lack of interest, indifference, or negative comments about the sex, looks, or temperament of the infant could be significant.

A collaborative team approach is necessary. This may include services such as family planning, protective services, day care centres, homemakers, parenting classes, self-help groups, family counselling, child advocates, and a continued effort to reduce the incidence of preterm birth. Other related areas include financial assistance, employment services, transportation, emotional support and encouragement, and long-term follow-up care.

Individual nurses can help to detect child abuse by maintaining a vigilant approach in their work settings. Record keeping should be *factual* and *objective.* The pediatric nurse should make a point of reviewing old records of their patients, which may show repeated hospitalizations, X-ray films of multiple fractures, persistent feeding problems, a history of failure to thrive, and a history of chronic absenteeism from school. Neglect or delay in seeking medical attention for a child or failure to obtain immunization and well-child care can be significant findings. Children who seem overly upset about being discharged must be brought to the attention of the health care provider.

The abused child should be approached quietly and preparation for any treatment carefully explained in advance. The number of caretakers should be kept to a minimum. The child may be able to express some hostility and fear through play or drawing. It is not unusual for abused children to be unresponsive or openly hostile or to show affection indiscriminately. Direct questioning is kept to a minimum. Praise is used when appropriate. Activities that promote physical and sensory development are encouraged. The nurse should avoid speaking to the child about the parents in a negative manner. Other professionals need to be consulted about setting limits for poor behaviour.

There can be two victims in cases of child abuse: the child *and* the abuser. Because of personal problems, the abuser often leads an isolated life. Some have themselves been battered or neglected as children. Many have unrealistic expectations about the child's intelligence and capabilities. There may be a role reversal in which the child becomes the comforter. Although removing the child from the home is one answer, many authorities believe this can be more detrimental in the long run.

Being open to parents during this type of crisis is difficult but essential if the nurse wishes to be part of the solution rather than part of the problem. When placement in a foster home is necessary, parents experience grief, loss, and remorse. The child also mourns the loss of the family, even though there has been abuse. The nurse should be aware of the child's needs and facilitate the expression of feelings of loss.

! Safety Alert!

Bruises and hematomas heal in various stages, indicated according to colour:

- 1 to 2 days: swollen, tender
- 2 to 5 days: red or purple
- 5 to 7 days: green
- 7 to 10 days: yellow
- 10 to 14 days: brown
- 14 to 28 days: clear

It is important to ask yourself, "Does the bruise match the caregiver's explanation of what happened and when? Are there multiple bruises in different stages of healing?"

Cultural and Medical Issues

Multiple factors should be considered when evaluating the child who has been abused. It is essential that the nurse gather a detailed history and accurate data on children who have been injured. For example, some children may have bruising from physical activities such as sports.

A careful and sensitive history is essential. The nurse should be aware that what appears to be a cigarette burn could be a single lesion of impetigo. Mongolian spots can be mistaken for bruises. A severe diaper rash caused by a fungal infection can look like a scald burn. In some cases, loving parents can injure infants when shaking them to wake or feed them. They are not aware of the danger of shaken baby syndrome.

Some cultural practices can be interpreted as physical abuse if the nurse is not aware of traditional healing practices. For example, "coining" of the body by some cultures to allay disease can cause welts on the body (see Chapter 21). Burning small areas of the skin to treat enuresis is practiced by some Asian cultures. Forced kneeling may be a type of discipline technique. Some Yemenite Jews treat infections by placing garlic preparations on the wrists, which can result in blisters.

The nurse should document all signs of abuse and interaction as well as verbal comments between the child and parents (Fig. 24.16). Child protective services should oversee any investigation that is warranted. Providing support to the parents and child, including an opportunity to talk in privacy, and planning for follow-up care are basic nursing responsibilities. Parent education concerning growth and development is valuable.

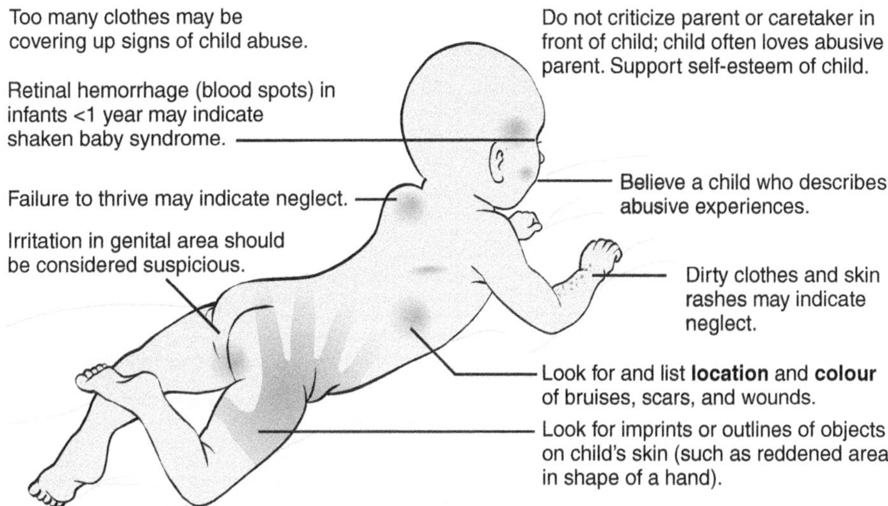
Too many clothes may be covering up signs of child abuse.
Retinal hemorrhage (blood spots) in infants <1 year may indicate shaken baby syndrome.
Failure to thrive may indicate neglect.
Irritation in genital area should be considered suspicious.
Do not criticize parent or caretaker in front of child; child often loves abusive parent. Support self-esteem of child.
Believe a child who describes abusive experiences.
Dirty clothes and skin rashes may indicate neglect.
Look for and list **location** and **colour** of bruises, scars, and wounds.
Look for imprints or outlines of objects on child's skin (such as reddened area in shape of a hand).
Divide the body into four planes: front, back, right side, and left side.
Injuries occurring in more than 1 plane should be considered suspicious.

Fig. 24.16 Assessing for child abuse. The nurse should be alert for inconsistent statements about injuries, bruises at various stages of healing, delay in seeking care, and a history that is not compatible with injury or development.

Get Ready for the Certification Examination!

Key Points

- The age, neurological development, and motor milestones achieved will influence the nursing assessment of the musculoskeletal system in a growing child.
- The normal gait of a toddler is wide and unstable. By 6 years of age, the gait resembles an adult walk.
- Injury to the epiphyseal plate at the ends of long bones is serious during childhood because it may interfere with longitudinal growth.
- In an open compound fracture, a wound in the skin accompanies the broken bone, and there is added danger of infection.
- Any delay in neurological development can cause a delay in mastery of motor skills, which can result in altered skeletal growth.
- Children who do not walk by 18 months of age should be referred for follow-up care.
- Protection and relative rest, ice, compression, and elevation are the principles of managing soft tissue injuries.
- Pain over a muscle area that does not respond to medication may indicate a complication known as compartment syndrome.
- A neurovascular check includes colour, warmth, capillary refill time, movement, pulse, sensation, swelling, and pain.
- Frequent neurovascular checks should be performed on the distal digits of a patient with a cast to determine adequate tissue perfusion.
- Immobility causes a deceleration of body metabolism along with many other issues.
- Tutorial assistance should be provided to school-age children who are hospitalized or immobilized for long periods of time.
- Nursing care includes providing emotional support regarding body image, maintenance of skin integrity, encouraging independence, and providing developmentally appropriate activities related to school progress and prevention of future injuries.
- A complication of any traction is an arterial occlusion termed Volkmann's ischemia.
- Legg-Calvé-Perthes disease affects the blood supply to the head of the femur.
- Clubfoot is a congenital malformation that may require casting or physiotherapy.
- A positive Barlow test and Ortolani sign are indicative of developmental dysplasia of the hip.
- The body spica cast encircles the waist and extends to the ankles or toes. It is used to treat developmental dysplasia of the hip.
- Juvenile idiopathic arthritis is the most common arthritic condition of childhood.
- Juvenile idiopathic arthritis can inhibit social interaction and the development of a positive self-image.
- Treatment of scoliosis may include bracing, exercise, and surgery (spinal fusion) although asymptomatic children may not require treatment.
- Adolescents who participate in sports are subject to injuries such as concussions and ligament injuries. Activities must be selected carefully according to physical maturity, size, and skill required.
- A spiral fracture of the femur or humerus may be a sign of child abuse.
- Child abuse may be physical, emotional, or sexual; it may involve neglect or exposure to family violence.

Additional Learning Resources

evolve Go to your Evolve website (http://evolve.elsevier.com/Canada/Leifer) for the following learning resources:

- Answer Key for Critical Thinking Questions
- Answer Key for Textbook Review Questions
- Audio Glossary
- Interactive Review Questions
- Skills Performance Checklists
- Video clips and more!

Online Resources

- Arthritis Society, *Stop Childhood Arthritis:* https://www.arthritis.ca/campaigns/stop-childhood-arthritis
- Canadian Centre for Child Protection, *Resources:* https://www.protectchildren.ca/en/resources-research/#research
- Canadian Orthopaedic Foundation, *Parents' Guide to Clubfoot and Its Treatment Using the Ponseti Method:* http://whenithurtstomove.org/wp-content/uploads/Clubfoot-Booklet_2015-EN.pdf
- Children's Health and Safety Association, *Children's Health and Safety Information:* https://www.safekid.org/en/
- Government of Canada, *Child Maltreatment: A "What to Do" Guide for Professionals Who Work With Children:* https://www.canada.ca/en/public-health/services/health-promotion/stop-family-violence/prevention-resource-centre/children/child-maltreatment-what-guide-professionals-who-work-children.html
- Muscular Dystrophy Canada: http://www.muscle.ca/
- Parachute: http://www.parachutecanada.org/

Review Questions

1. Which type of fracture in a young child may be indicative of child abuse?
   a. Greenstick fracture of the tibia
   b. Spiral fracture of the femur
   c. Pathological fracture of the fibula
   d. Aligned fracture of the wrist
2. A teenager who had a cast applied after a tibia fracture states that his pain medication is not working and his pain is still a 9 or 10. The nurse notices some edema of the toes and a capillary refill of 6 seconds. Which of the following would be the priority nursing action?
   a. Call the health care provider immediately.
   b. Check if there is an order for a stronger pain medication.
   c. Try nonpharmacological techniques of pain relief.
   d. Explain to the teen that a new fracture is expected to be painful the first day.
3. A neurovascular check for tissue perfusion includes which observations? *(Select all that apply.)*
   a. Pulse
   b. Colour
   c. Capillary refill
   d. Movement and sensation
   e. Equal pupil size of eyes
4. Which condition involves an abnormal S-shaped curvature of the spine seen in school-age children?
   a. Sclerosis
   b. Sciatica
   c. Scabies
   d. Scoliosis
5. A nurse assessing a yellow bruise knows that the injury is approximately how many days old?
   a. 2
   b. 5 to 7
   c. 7 to 10
   d. 10 to 14
6. A nurse would teach which information to the parents of a preschool child who has had an above-the-knee cast applied? *(Select all that apply.)*
   a. Use fingertips to lift the cast until it is fully dry.
   b. Keep small toys out of the child's reach.
   c. Place a heating pad on the toes if they feel cold.
   d. Elevate the leg on pillows.
   e. Contact the health care provider if the child states a feeling of numbness.

Critical Thinking Questions

1. The nurse enters the room of a child who is in skeletal traction for a fractured femur. He is sitting in a high-Fowler's position watching television and eating snacks. What nursing observations relating to the traction would the nurse make, and what interventions are necessary?
2. A mother brings her 2-year-old child to the clinic stating that the spica cast has a strong, unpleasant odour. The child has a temperature of 37.8°C (100°F). He appears to be in no acute distress and is playing with a small toy car in one hand and has a half-eaten cracker in the other hand. What nursing intervention is indicated?

REFERENCES

About Kids Health. (2009a). *Ankle sprains*. Retrieved from https://www.aboutkidshealth.ca/anklesprain.

About Kids Health. (2009b). *Pavlik harness orthosis*. Retrieved from https://www.aboutkidshealth.ca/Article?contentid=971&language=English.

Baldwin, K. D., Wells, L., & Dormans, J. P. (2016). Common fractures. In R. M. Kliegman, B. F. Stanton, J. W. St. Geme, et al. (Eds.), *Nelson textbook of pediatrics* (20th ed.). Philadelphia: Saunders.

Binder, R. C. M., Ball, J. W., London, M. C., et al. (2017). *Clinical skills manual for maternity and pediatric nursing* (5th ed.). Toronto, ON: Pearson.

Canadian Cancer Society. (2019). *What is childhood bone cancer?* Retrieved from http://www.cancer.ca/en/cancer-information/cancer-type/bone-childhood/childhood-bone-cancer/?region=on.

Canadian Orthopaedic Foundation. (2017). *Hip dysplasia*. Retrieved from https://whenithurtstomove.org/about-orthopaedics/joint-anatomy/hip/hip-dysplasia.

Canadian Paediatric Society (CPS). (2017). Position statement: Screen time and young children: Promoting health and development in a digital world. *Paediatrics & Child Health, 22*(8), 461–468. Retrieved from https://www.cps.ca/en/documents/position/screen-time-and-young-children.

Cincinnati Children's. (2018). *Milwaukee brace*. Retrieved from https://www.cincinnatichildrens.org/health/m/milwaukee.

Greig, A. A., Constantin, E., LeBlanc, C. M., et al. (2016). An update to the Greig Health Record: Executive summary. *Paediatrics & Child Health, 21*(5), 265–268. Retrieved from https://www.cps.ca/en/documents/position/greig-executive-summary.

Hango, D., & Statistics Canada. (2017). *Childhood physical abuse: Differences by birth cohort*. Retrieved by https://www.statcan.gc.ca/pub/75-006-x/2017001/article/54869-eng.htm.

Health Canada. (2012). *Child maltreatment in Canada*. Retrieved from https://www.canada.ca/en/public-health/services/health-promotion/stop-family-violence/prevention-resource-centre/children/child-maltreatment-canada.html.

Houghton, K. M., Emery, C. A., & Canadian Paediatric Society (CPS), Healthy Active Living Committee. (2016). Bodychecking in youth ice hockey. *Paediatrics & Child Health, 17*(9), 509. Retrieved from https://www.cps.ca/en/documents/position/bodychecking-ice-hockey.

Kaplan, S. (2016). Osteomyelitis. In R. M. Kliegman, B. F. Stanton, J. W. St. Geme, et al. (Eds.), *Nelson textbook of pediatrics* (20th ed.). Philadelphia: Saunders.

Krader, G. C. (2017). Developmental dysplasia of the hip. *Contemporary Pediatrics, 34*(6), 31–37.

McTimoney, M., Purcell, L., & Canadian Paediatric Society (CPS), Paediatric Sports and Exercise Medicine. (2007). Ankle sprains in the paediatric athlete. *Paediatrics & Child Health, 12*(2), 133–355. Retrieved from https://www.cps.ca/en/documents/position/ankle-sprains-athlete.

Mistovich, R. J., & Spiegel, D. A. (2016). Congenital scoliosis. In R. M. Kliegman, B. F. Stanton, J. W. St. Geme, et al. (Eds.), *Nelson textbook of pediatrics* (20th ed.). Philadelphia: Saunders.

O'Brien, K. (2017). *Screening programs are unlikely to prevent sudden cardiac arrest among competitive athletes, new study suggests.* Updated 2017. Toronto: St. Michaels' Hospital. Retrieved from http://stmichaelshospital.com/media/detail.php?source=hospital_news/2017/1115.

O'Toole, P., & Spiegel, D. (2016). Torticollis. In R. M. Kliegman, B. F. Stanton, J. W. St. Geme, et al. (Eds.), *Nelson textbook of pediatrics* (20th ed.). Philadelphia: Saunders.

Public Health Agency of Canada (PHAC). (2010). *Canadian incidence study of reported child abuse and neglect 2008: Major findings*. Retrieved from http://cwrp.ca/sites/default/files/publications/en/CIS-2008-rprt-eng.pdf.

Sankar, W., Horn, D., Wells, L., et al. (2016a). Developmental dysplasia of the hip. In R. M. Kliegman, B. F. Stanton, J. W. St. Geme, et al. (Eds.), *Nelson textbook of pediatrics* (20th ed.). Philadelphia: Saunders.

Sankar, W., Horn, D., Wells, L., et al. (2016b). Legg-Calvé-Perthes disease. In R. M. Kliegman, B. F. Stanton, J. W. St. Geme, et al. (Eds.), *Nelson textbook of pediatrics* (20th ed.). Philadelphia: Saunders.

Sankar, W., Horn, D., Wells, L., et al. (2016c). Slipped capital femoral epiphysis. In R. M. Kliegman, B. F. Stanton, J. W. St. Geme, et al. (Eds.), *Nelson textbook of pediatrics* (20th ed.). Philadelphia: Saunders.

Sarnat, H. B. (2016). Muscular dystrophies. In R. M. Kliegman, B. F. Stanton, J. W. St. Geme, et al. (Eds.), *Nelson textbook of pediatrics* (20th ed.). Philadelphia: Saunders.

Sinha, M., & Statistics Canada. (2015). *Section 4: Family violence against children and youth*. Retrieved from https://www.statcan.gc.ca/pub/85-002-x/2013001/article/11805/11805-4-eng.htm.

Winell, J. J., & Davidson, R. S. (2016). Talipes equinovarus (clubfoot). In R. M. Kliegman, B. F. Stanton, J. W. St. Geme, et al. (Eds.), *Nelson textbook of pediatrics* (20th ed.). Philadelphia: Saunders.

Wu, E., Bryan, A., & Rabinovich, E. (2016). Juvenile idiopathic arthritis. In R. M. Kliegman, B. F. Stanton, J. W. St. Geme, et al. (Eds.), *Nelson textbook of pediatrics* (20th ed.). Philadelphia: Saunders.

25 The Child With a Respiratory Condition

http://evolve.elsevier.com/Canada/Leifer

Cheryl A. Sams

Objectives

1. Define each key term listed.
2. Distinguish the differences between the respiratory tract of the infant and that of the adult.
3. Review the signs and symptoms of respiratory distress in infants and children.
4. Describe how sinusitis in children is different from that in adults.
5. Discuss the nursing care of a child with common respiratory conditions.
6. Recognize the precautions involved in the care of a child diagnosed with epiglottitis.
7. Discuss the nursing care of a child with a pneumothorax.
8. Describe smoke inhalation injury as it relates to delivery of nursing care.
9. Discuss the postoperative care of a child who has had a tonsillectomy.
10. Describe the characteristic manifestations of allergic rhinitis.
11. Assess the control of environmental exposure to allergens in the home of a child with asthma.
12. Discuss the role of sports and physical exercise for the asthmatic child.
13. List at least five goals of asthma therapy.
14. Provide four nursing goals in the care of a child with cystic fibrosis.
15. Review the prevention of bronchopulmonary dysplasia.
16. Discuss the prevention of sudden infant death syndrome (SIDS).

Key Terms

alveoli (ăl-VĒ-ō-lī)
atelectasis (ă-tĕ-LĔK-tă-sĭs)
carbon dioxide narcosis
clubbing of the fingers
coryza (kō-RĪ-ză)
diffusion
dysphagia (dĭs-FĀ-jhă)
meconium ileus
orthopnea (ŏr-thŏp-NĒ-ă)
perfusion
pursed-lip breathing
reactive airway disease (RAD)
spirometry
stridor (STRĪ-dŏr)
surfactant (sŭr-FĂK-tănt)
tachycardia tachypnea (tăk-ĭp-NĒ-ă)
ventilation

THE RESPIRATORY SYSTEM

DEVELOPMENT OF THE RESPIRATORY TRACT

Pulmonary structures differentiate in an orderly fashion during fetal life. This makes it possible to determine at what point a particular defect may have occurred. The trachea and the esophagus originate as one hollow tube; gradually, by 4 weeks of gestation, a septum forms to completely separate them. If the septum fails to form completely, a tracheoesophageal fistula occurs (see Chapter 28). By the seventh week of fetal life the diaphragm forms and separates the chest from the abdominal cavity. If the diaphragm fails to close completely, a diaphragmatic hernia allows the abdominal contents (intestines, spleen, and stomach) to enter the chest cavity and prevents the lungs from expanding fully. Alveoli and capillaries, which are necessary for gas exchange in the human body, are formed between 24 and 28 weeks of gestation.

At the twenty-fourth week, the formed alveolar cells begin to produce surfactant. **Surfactant** is composed of lecithin and sphingomyelin and prevents the alveoli from collapsing during respirations after birth. A premature birth is accompanied by problems with respiratory gas exchange. During fetal life, the lungs are filled with a fluid that has a low surface tension and viscosity; this is rapidly absorbed after birth. Spontaneous respiratory movements occur in the fetus, although gas exchange occurs via placental circulation. When surfactant is present in the lungs, the respiratory movements force some of the surfactant into the amniotic fluid. At about 35 weeks of gestation, the lecithin component is twice that of the sphingomyelin component. The analysis of the lecithin/sphingomyelin ratio (L/S ratio) by amniocentesis (see Table 5.1) is one method of determining fetal maturity and the ability of the fetus to survive outside the uterus.

The differences between the respiratory tracts of the growing infant and the adult are shown in Table 25.1 and Fig. 25.1.

NORMAL RESPIRATION

The process of normal respiration involves ventilation, diffusion, and perfusion. **Ventilation** is the process of inspiration and expiration, **diffusion** is the movement of oxygen and carbon dioxide between the alveoli and the red blood cells, and **perfusion** is the distribution of the oxygen to the body tissues.

In ventilation, the process of breathing air into and out of the lungs, the ribs and diaphragm allow for inspiration of air. Air enters the body through the nares, or nostrils. The mucous membranes and cilia that line the respiratory tract warm, moisten, and filter the air as it passes to the pharynx. The pharynx contains the tonsils, which assist in infection control. The larynx at the upper end of the trachea contains the epiglottis, the glottis, and the vocal cords, which prevent food and fluids from entering the trachea and allow voice sounds. The trachea is encircled by smooth muscle and cartilage to maintain patency and carries the air to the bronchi and then to the smaller bronchioles. The bronchioles continue to divide and lead to small, thin air sacs (alveoli) that are kept open on inspiration by the air contained in them. During expiration, when the air sacs collapse, surfactant prevents the walls from sticking together, allowing for reinflation. The volume of air inhaled with each breath is related to body size.

Ventilation is affected by several elements and their interaction with one another:

- *Intercostal muscles, diaphragm, ribs:* These allow chest expansion and contraction. Expansion of the chest lowers pressure in the chest cavity, and air flows from the higher pressure of the atmosphere into the lower pressure of the chest cavity. The opposite occurs during expiration.
- *Brain:* The vagus nerve and the respiratory centres in the medulla of the brain regulate rhythmic

Table 25.1 Differences in the Respiratory Tracts of the Growing Infant and the Adult

DIFFERENCE	SIGNIFICANCE
The infant relies primarily on the abdominal muscles and the diaphragm for breathing. The intercostal muscles only stabilize the chest wall.	Assessment of respiration is best accomplished by monitoring the rise and fall of the abdomen along with auscultating the chest, until 3 years of age, when thoracic breathing begins. Adult types of breathing patterns are typically developed by 7 years of age. Substernal retraction is a sign of respiratory distress in infants.
In infants, the diaphragm is attached higher than in the adult and is stretched longer, limiting its ability to contract forcefully.	Abdominal distention from feeding or gas can interfere with movement of the diaphragm.
The infant depends on the accessory muscles for respiratory efforts.	Muscle fatigue can result in respiratory arrest.
Infants are nose breathers and do not breathe through the mouth unless crying.	Swelling of the nasal mucosa will interfere with sucking and will cause irritability.
In infants, the tissue below the vocal cords is not firm, and portions of the larynx are very narrow.	Any edema or swelling can cause respiratory obstruction.
In infants, the cartilage that maintains the patency of the airway is soft, not firm.	Vagal nerve stimulation or muscle constriction can cause collapse of the airway and respiratory obstruction.
The larynx and trachea are higher in the chest in infancy and descend slowly as the child grows.	Positioning the infant or child for airway clearance and resuscitation is different than for adults. Excess flexion or extension of the neck can cause respiratory obstruction.
Alveoli in the lung divide and thin as the child grows and develops, resulting in increased surface area for gas exchange. The number of alveoli present at puberty is nine times that found in the infant.	Less surface area in the alveoli is available for gas exchange, which predisposes infants and young children to respiratory distress.
Infants and young children have a small airway diameter.	Edema or muscle spasm can rapidly cause respiratory obstruction.
Newborns and infants produce less respiratory mucus (which serves as a cleansing agent).	Infants and children are more susceptible to respiratory infections.
Infants have a smaller amount of developed smooth muscle lining the airway than do older children and adults.	Bronchospasm may not occur in infants, and therefore wheezing may not be a presenting sign of a narrowed airway.
In infants, the respiratory rate is higher and the breathing pattern is irregular.	Meaningful assessment of respiration must be related to the age of the child. Irregular respirations with short periods of apnea is a normal pattern for a young infant but abnormal for an adult.

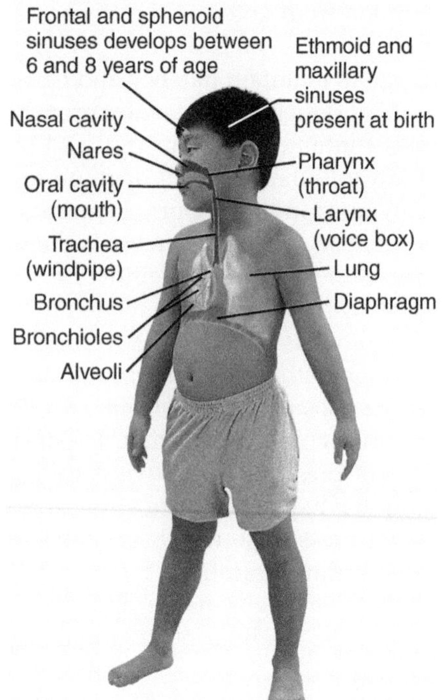

RESPIRATORY SYSTEM

- Respiratory rates are higher in children.
- Diaphragmatic abdominal breathing is common in infants.
- Oxygen consumption is high in children in proportion to body size; metabolic rate is higher than in adults.
- Airway diameter is smaller in children, which increases the potential for obstruction.
- Mucous membranes of airways are highly vascular and are susceptible to trauma, edema, and spasm.
- Surfactant is lacking in preterm infants, which contributes to respiratory distress syndrome.
- Accessory muscles of respiration are not as strong in children, particularly in infants.
- Chest wall retractions are common in infants with respiratory problems because the chest wall is supple.

Fig. 25.1 Respiratory tract in children. (Art overlay courtesy Observatory Group, Cincinnati, Ohio.)

respiratory movements. Signals sent to the respiratory centre will increase or decrease respiratory rates.

- *Chemoreceptors:* These sensors respond to changes in the oxygen (O_2) saturation of the blood by sending a signal to the pons in the brainstem, which is stimulated to increase respirations when the oxygen saturation is low.

Gas exchange occurs in the alveoli through diffusion to the bloodstream. Once oxygen is in the bloodstream, it needs to be delivered to the body tissues through the process of perfusion. Blood circulates to the capillary beds of tissue and oxygen is removed at this point.

Note that a high carbon dioxide (CO_2) level in the blood and a low oxygen saturation stimulate the brain to increase the respiratory rate. In chronic lung disease, however, the receptors become tolerant to the high carbon dioxide and low oxygen concentrations in the blood. Administration of supplemental oxygen increases the oxygen saturation level and may result in a decreased respiratory effort (**carbon dioxide narcosis**), leading to respiratory failure.

Procedures that may be performed on the child with a respiratory condition include throat and nasopharyngeal cultures, bronchoscopy, lung biopsy, arterial blood gas (Pao_2, $Paco_2$) and pH analysis, pulse oximetry, and various pulmonary function tests (PFTs). Chest X-ray films, computed tomography (CT), radioisotope scanning, bronchography, and angiography may prove useful, depending on symptoms. The inspection, percussion, and auscultation procedures performed by the nurse are important in data collection.

DISORDERS OF THE RESPIRATORY SYSTEM

Nasopharyngitis

Pathophysiology

A cold, also known as acute **coryza**, is the most common infection of the respiratory tract. It can be caused by different viruses, including the rhinoviruses, respiratory syncytial virus (RSV), adenoviruses, influenzas, and parainfluenza, which are spread from one child to another by sneezing, coughing, or direct contact. The age, state of nutrition, and general health of the child contribute to the susceptibility level.

The viruses are spread by contact with contaminated fingers that touch the conjunctiva of the eyes or the mucous membranes of the mouth. Routine hand hygiene practices, especially before rubbing the nose or sucking the fingers, can help prevent the spread of the common cold.

The common cold differs from allergic rhinitis in that a child who has allergic rhinitis has no fever, no purulent nasal discharge, and no reddened mucous membranes. Sneezing, watery eyes, and itching of the skin are the primary manifestations of *allergic rhinitis.* The infection is self-limiting and usually lasts from 4 days up to 10 days, if there are complications. Young children have immature immune systems and are more susceptible to catching viral illnesses. Children under 2 years of age can get as many as 8 to 10 colds yearly. Viruses are spread easily in close, indoor spaces, such as day care centres and schools, by direct and indirect contact (Canadian Paediatric Society [CPS], 2016).

Manifestations

The symptoms of a cold in an infant or small child are different from those in an adult. Children's air passages are smaller and more easily obstructed. The virus causes inflammation and edema of the membranes of the upper respiratory tract, which damage cilia and prevent the drainage of mucus. Fever as high as 40°C (104°F) is not uncommon in children younger than 3 years of age. Nasal discharge, irritability, sore throat, cough, and general discomfort are present, and there may be vomiting and diarrhea. The diagnosis is complicated by the fact that many infectious diseases resemble the common cold during their onset. Complications of a cold include bronchitis, bronchiolitis, pneumonitis, and ear infections.

Treatment and nursing care

There is no cure for the common cold. Treatment should begin early, when a cold is suspected. The following treatment is designed to relieve symptoms:

- *Rest:* Fatigue should be prevented; activities that limit activity are encouraged. The nurse should consider the age and developmental level of the child and the activity level involved in their play when designing appropriate activities and guiding parents in the home care of their child.
- *Clear airways:* Congested nasal passages cause discomfort and may impede breastfeeding or sucking from a bottle. Because fluid consumption is essential to prevent fever and dehydration, the airways must be cleared before feeding and before bedtime to provide a restful sleep. The nurse can teach the parents that instilling a few drops of saline solution into the nose and then suctioning with a bulb syringe (see Skill 11.3) is the best way to clear the nostrils. The bulb syringe should be cleaned frequently with warm, soapy water, rinsed well, and hung downward to dry, in order to prevent infection. Medicated nose drops can be irritating to the mucosa of a young child's nasal passages. Use of nose drops with an oily base should be avoided because they are readily aspirated and can cause respiratory problems. Rebound congestion can be avoided by limiting the use of medicated nose drops to no more than 3 days. Use of over-the-counter combination cold remedies should be avoided; if used, the label should be checked for safe dosage. Parents can elevate the child's head of the bed to promote drainage.
- *Adequate fluid intake:* Anorexia is common in children with nasopharyngitis. Intake of fluids should be encouraged to prevent dehydration. Cool, bland liquids are usually tolerated well in a child who has a sore throat.
- *Prevention of fever:* Ibuprofen (Motrin or Advil) or acetaminophen (Tylenol) can be administered when a high fever accompanies a cold.
- *Skin care:* A petroleum-based ointment can be applied to the nares and upper lip to prevent skin irritation from a nasal discharge.
- *Immunizations*: Immunizations do not prevent colds, but they will help prevent some of the complications, such as bacterial infections of the ears or lungs. Influenza (flu) vaccine protects against the flu but not against other respiratory viruses.

Follow-up with a health care provider is required when the child:

- Is breathing rapidly or seems to be working hard to breathe or has blue lips.
- Is coughing, leading to choking or vomiting.
- Has one or both eyes stuck shut with dried yellow pus upon wakening.
- Is much sleepier than usual, doesn't want to feed or play, or is very fussy and cannot be comforted, or has thick or coloured (yellow, green) discharge from the nose for more than 10 to 14 days.
- Has signs of a middle ear infection (ear pain, drainage from the ear) (CPS, 2016).

Children under 3 months old should see a health care provider in the following situations:

- Trouble breathing
- Not eating or is vomiting
- Fever (temperature of 38.5°C [101.3°F] or higher)

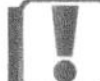

Safety Alert!

Parents should be cautioned to check the label of any medication for appropriate dosages and to use the measuring devices that are supplied with the medication.

Moist air soothes an inflamed nose and throat. An electric cold-air humidifier is safe and convenient. It must be cleaned and disinfected daily.

The older child is taught the proper way to remove nasal secretions from the nose. The mouth is opened slightly, and secretions are gently blown out through both nostrils at the same time. This method prevents the infection from being forced into the eustachian tubes. Antibiotics are not effective against the common cold because it is viral in origin.

Otitis media is an inflammation of the middle ear. The middle ear is connected to the throat by the eustachian tube, which provides drainage of middle ear secretions into the nasopharynx and equalizes pressure between the middle ear and the outside atmosphere. When the lining of the eustachian tube becomes infected as a complication of nasopharyngitis, otitis media often develops, usually following an upper respiratory infection. Infants are more prone to middle ear infections because their eustachian tubes are shorter, straighter, and wider than those of older children or adults. For a detailed discussion of otitis media, see Chapter 23.

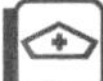

Nursing Tip

Children and parents can be taught the following techniques to prevent the spread of infection:

- Wash their hands frequently and use hand sanitizers, particularly after coughing and sneezing
- Not to touch eyes, nose, or mouth when coughing
- Cough and sneeze into their sleeves, or a tissue, rather than their hands
- Dispose of used tissues immediately
- Keep household surfaces and toys clean
- No sharing of food, dishes, and utensils

Acute Pharyngitis

Pathophysiology

Acute pharyngitis is an inflammation of the structures in the throat. This infection is common among children between 5 and 10 years of age. In approximately 80% of cases the causative organism is a virus. Group A beta-hemolytic streptococcus (strep throat) is the most common bacterial cause for sore throat, although it is uncommon in children under 3 years of age.

Manifestations, treatment, and nursing care

Symptoms include fever, malaise, **dysphagia** (*dys,* "difficult," and *phagia,* "swallowing"), and anorexia. It is difficult to distinguish viral from bacterial types by symptoms only. Conjunctivitis, rhinitis, cough, and hoarseness with a gradual onset and persisting no longer than 5 days are characteristic of viral pharyngitis. In a child over 3 years of age, streptococcal pharyngitis characteristically includes high fever (40°C [104°F]) and difficulty swallowing, and it may last longer than 1 week. Strep throat is determined by throat culture.

When the culture is positive, antimicrobial therapy such as penicillin is administered orally for 10 days. It is important that the nurse carefully explain to parents the need for the child to finish all the medication. Clindamycin or erythromycin may be prescribed if the child is allergic to penicillin. Acetaminophen or ibuprofen may be taken to relieve soreness of the throat. If the child is old enough to gargle, a solution of warm water and salt may be used.

Prompt treatment of strep throat is important to prevent serious complications such as rheumatic fever, glomerulonephritis, peritonsillar abscess, otitis media, mastoiditis, meningitis, osteomyelitis, or pneumonia. The persistence of a positive streptococcal culture after careful follow-up and therapy may indicate that the child is a group A beta-hemolytic streptococcus carrier. However, it may also mean that the child did not complete the 10-day course of medication or that a medication-resistant organism has evolved. The child with strep throat is no longer infectious to others after medication therapy has begun and fever has decreased.

Sinusitis

The maxillary and ethmoid sinuses are most often involved in childhood sinusitis. An acute sinusitis is suspected when an upper respiratory infection lasts longer than 10 days, with a daytime cough. The proximity of this sinus to the tooth roots often results in tooth pain when the sinus is infected. Halitosis is often present. Untreated sinusitis can lead to periorbital cellulitis, because the infection spreads from the ethmoid sinus to the subperiosteal space around the eye. Treatment typically involves a 10- to 14-day course of antibiotic therapy.

Croup Syndromes

Pathophysiology

Croup is a general term applied to a number of conditions whose chief symptom is a "barking" (croupy) cough and varying degrees of inspiratory **stridor** (a harsh, high-pitched sound). When the larynx is involved, the clinical picture becomes more intense because of possible alterations in respiratory status, such as airway obstruction, acute respiratory failure, and hypoxia (Fig. 25.2). Acute viral spasmodic laryngitis is the milder form of the syndrome. Acute laryngotracheobronchitis is the most common serious form; it is also referred to as *subglottic croup.*

The area below the glottis is firm cartilage and therefore cannot expand outward when edema occurs, as other regions of the respiratory tract can. For that reason, subglottic edema that occurs with epiglottitis or bacterial tracheitis results in acute respiratory obstruction (Roosevelt, 2016). Croup can be benign or acute.

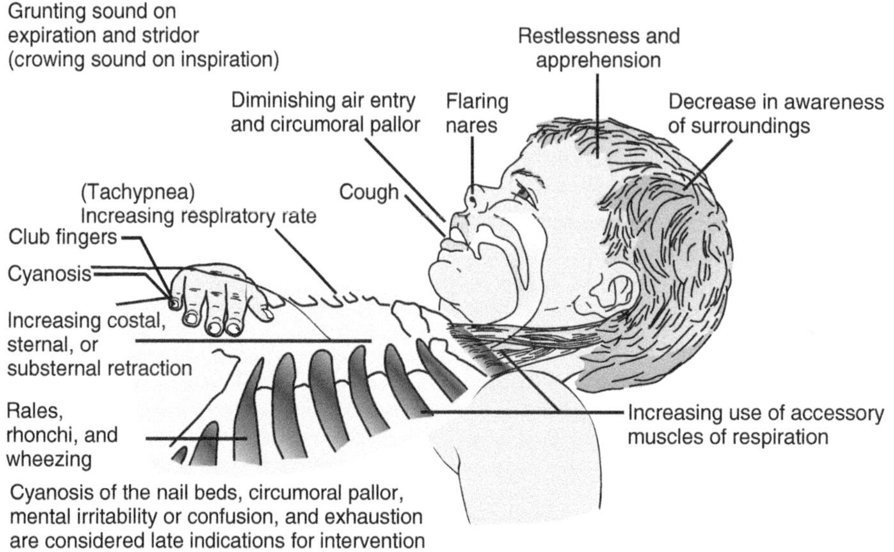

Fig. 25.2 Signs of respiratory distress in infants and children.

Benign croup is frightening but rarely life-threatening. Acute croup can develop into a respiratory emergency.

Benign crouplike conditions

Congenital laryngeal stridor (laryngomalacia). Some infants are born with a weakness of the airway walls and a floppy epiglottis that causes a stridor on inspiration. There may be inspiratory retractions. The symptoms lessen when the infant is placed prone or propped in the side-lying position. Respiratory infection and crying may cause the symptoms to become frightening to the parents. The condition usually clears spontaneously as the child grows and the muscles strengthen. The nurse should provide reassurance and suggest slow, small feedings for the infant.

Spasmodic laryngitis (spasmodic croup). Spasmodic croup usually occurs in children between 1 and 3 years of age and can be caused by a virus, allergy, or psychological trigger. Very often, gastroesophageal reflux (GER) will trigger an attack. Spasmodic croup has a sudden onset, usually at night, and is characterized by a barking, brassy cough and respiratory distress. The child appears anxious, and the parents often become frightened. The attack lasts a few hours, and by morning the child appears normal and is in no distress. Increasing humidity and providing fluids are helpful treatment measures.

Acute croup

Laryngotracheobronchitis. The viral condition laryngotracheobronchitis is manifested by edema, destruction of respiratory cilia, and exudate, resulting in respiratory obstruction. A mild upper respiratory infection usually precedes the development of a characteristic barking or brassy cough. Stridor develops, and classic symptoms of respiratory distress follow (see Fig. 25.2). The infant prefers to be held upright or sit up in bed (orthopnea). Crying and agitation worsen the symptoms. Hypoxia can develop and can be accompanied by tachycardia and diminished breath sounds.

Treatment and nursing care. When the child is treated at home, parents are often instructed to take their child outside if it is cold. Breathing the cool air may relieve some of the symptoms. It is also important to encourage oral fluids.

If symptoms of respiratory distress continue, the child needs to be hospitalized. In the past, humidified, cool mist was used to try to reduce laryngospasm, but there is no evidence that it is effective (Ortiz-Alvarez & CPS Acute Care Committee, 2017). Intravenous (IV) fluids may be prescribed to prevent dehydration and to decrease the risk of vomiting and aspiration that can occur after a coughing episode. Antipyretics help to reduce a fever and manage discomfort. Organization of care is essential to enable the child to have long periods of rest. The child is placed on a cardiorespiratory monitor, and vital signs are observed closely. Oxygen is provided to reduce hypoxia (see Chapter 20). Oxygen saturation is monitored, and saturation levels are maintained above 90% (see Skill 12.1 for pulse oximeter sensor application).

Opiates are contraindicated because they depress respiration. Sedatives are also contraindicated because increased restlessness is a primary sign of increased respiratory obstruction, and sedatives can mask the signs of restlessness. Corticosteroids are prescribed for children with croup; the symptoms usually improve in 2 to 3 hours after a single dose of dexamethasone (Ortiz-Alvarez & CPS Acute Care Committee, 2017). Corticosteroids reduce the edema caused by inflammation and are used to prevent further destruction of ciliated epithelium in children hospitalized with croup. Nebulized epinephrine may be used to relieve the symptoms of respiratory obstruction (Fig. 25.3).

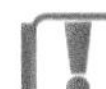 **Safety Alert!**

Respiratory illness is always potentially more serious in children than in adults.

Epiglottitis

Pathophysiology

Epiglottitis is a swelling of the tissues above the vocal cords, that is, *supraglottic swelling*. This results in narrowing of the airway inlet, with the possibility of total obstruction. It is caused by parainfluenza A and B, adenovirus, RSV, and *H. influenzae* type B. It most often occurs in children 3 to 6 years of age. It can occur in any season. The course is rapid and progressive. Blood gases fluctuate and there is leukocytosis. **Epiglottitis is a life-threatening medical emergency.**

Manifestations

The onset of epiglottitis is abrupt, and the child presents with classic symptoms. The child insists on sitting up,

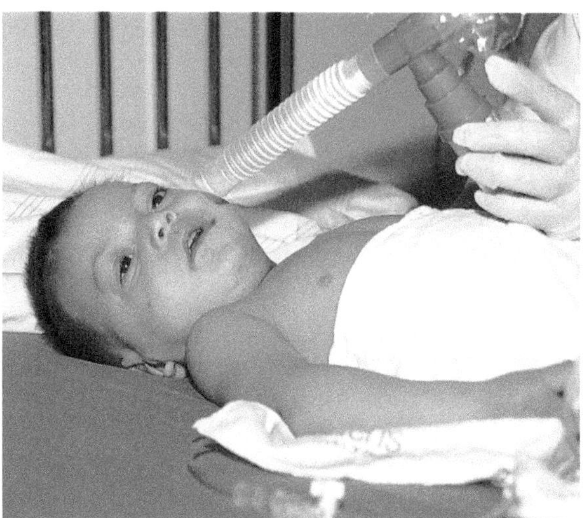

Fig. 25.3 A child receiving aerosol therapy (medicated nebulizer treatments). (From McKinney, E. S., James, S. R., Murray, S. S., Nelson, K., & Ashwill, J. W. [2017]. *Maternal-child nursing* [5th ed.]. Philadelphia: Saunders.)

leans forward with the mouth open, and drools saliva because of the difficulty in swallowing. The child appears wide-eyed, anxious, and restless, and they may emit a froglike croaking sound on inspiration. A cough is absent. Inspection of the throat shows an enlarged, reddened edematous epiglottis, much like a "beefy-red thumb." However, the examining tongue blade may trigger a laryngospasm and result in sudden respiratory arrest.

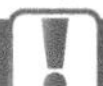

Safety Alert!

It is a primary nursing responsibility to be sure there is a tracheotomy set at the bedside before any examination of the throat is attempted in a child with suspected epiglottitis.

Treatment

The treatment of choice is immediate tracheotomy or endotracheal intubation and oxygen to prevent hypoxia, brain damage, and sudden death caused by respiratory arrest. Parenteral antibiotic therapy usually results in a dramatic improvement within a few days.

Prevention

The Government of Canada (2018) recommends that *H. influenzae* type B conjugate vaccines be administered beginning at 2 months of age as part of a regular immunization program for all children. This type of program has decreased the incidence of acute epiglottitis in children.

Bronchitis

Pathophysiology

A study of the respiratory system shows that the air tubes leading to the lungs resemble an upside-down tree. The trachea is the main trunk, with the bronchi, bronchioles, and alveoli being the branches. These passages proceed from large to small and are lined with a continuous membrane. If there is an infection of the bronchial tree, it is seldom confined to one area but more often involves other structures.

Acute bronchitis is an infection of the bronchi. It seldom occurs as a primary infection but is usually secondary to a cold or other communicable disease. It is caused by a variety of organisms. Poor nutrition, allergy, and chronic infection of the respiratory tract may precipitate this condition. Most patients are younger than 4 years of age.

Manifestations

The gradual onset of an unproductive "hacking" cough is preceded by an upper respiratory infection or cold. The cough may become productive with purulent sputum. Children less than 7 years of age cannot voluntarily cough and usually swallow their sputum.

Treatment

The use of cough suppressants before bedtime may be helpful in promoting restful sleep. Antihistamines, expectorants, and antibiotics are usually not helpful. Most children recover uneventfully with symptomatic care at home.

Bronchiolitis

Pathophysiology

Acute bronchiolitis is a viral infection of the small airways (bronchioles) in the lower respiratory tract. It is the most common cause for admission to hospital in the first year of life. It occurs in infants and children 6 months to 2 years of age, with peak incidence at 6 months of age. The small diameters of the bronchioles in the infant are susceptible to obstruction when inflammation results in edema and excess mucus. The obstruction often leads to atelectasis. The gas exchange in the lungs becomes impaired, and hypoxia can occur.

Manifestations

An upper respiratory infection or cold with a mild fever and serous (clear) nasal discharge is followed by the development of a wheezing cough and signs of respiratory distress. The increase in respiratory rate interferes with successful feeding, and the child becomes irritable and dehydrated. RSV is the causative organism in 50% of cases in infants. An apneic episode is usually the cause of hospitalization. Infants who have bronchiolitis may develop a hyperreactive airway or asthma later in life.

Treatment and nursing care

The treatment of an infant with bronchiolitis is symptomatic and similar to that of the child with croup. A semi-Fowler's position with a slightly hyperextended neck facilitates respirations. Oral feedings are often supplemented by IV fluids. Intake and output are recorded. The CPS recommends that when a child is not improving, nebulized epinephrine may be administered and frequent nasal suctioning may be helpful. High-flow nasal cannula oxygen may also be started (Friedman, Rider, Walton, et al., 2014/2018). Frequent assessment of vital signs and monitoring of oxygen saturation levels are essential.

Influenza

The influenza virus causes a respiratory infection that is responsible for many hospitalizations and deaths of children, especially those with underlying medical conditions such as asthma, cystic fibrosis, sickle cell anemia, Kawasaki disease, and any disorder that compromises respiratory function. The virus is spread via droplets, with coughing, sneezing, and contaminated surfaces being the methods of transmission. It is considered a seasonal virus, occurring between October and March in the northern hemisphere and between April and September in the southern hemisphere. The incubation period is 1 to 4 days and is considered contagious beginning 1 day before and throughout the duration of the infection. Every year, three to four influenza subtypes circulate with influenza A and B viruses.

Vaccines are manufactured each year, guided by predictions of the dominating type. The CPS highly recommends annual vaccinations during the flu season for infants aged 6 months through adulthood (Moore & CPS Infectious Diseases and Immunization Committee, 2018). Two types of influenza vaccines are available in Canada: inactivated influenza vaccines (IIV) for intramuscular (IM) injection and an intranasal, live attenuated influenza vaccine (LAIV) (Moore CPS Infectious Diseases and Immunization Committee, 2018). LAIV, because it is a live vaccine, is contraindicated in individuals with an immune-compromising condition or severe asthma, children who are on chronic acetylsalicylic acid, because of the association with Reye's syndrome during influenza season, and children under 2 years of age (Moore & CPS Infectious Diseases and Immunization Committee, 2018).

Signs and symptoms are similar to those of other viral infections, and complications of pneumonia and bacterial infections can lead to serious illness in both children and adults. It can be difficult to differentiate symptoms of the common cold from those of influenza. Influenza symptoms include a sudden fever with chills and shakes and muscle aches; common cold symptoms include a mild fever without the muscle aching.

Treatment

Influenza A or B can be diagnosed by means of a nasal swab or a nasopharyngeal wash. Office-based testing strips are effective in accurately diagnosing influenza A or B and RSV within 10 minutes (Allen & CPS Infectious Diseases and Immunization Committee, 2013/2018).

Treatment should be started within 48 hours of the first signs and symptoms. In Canada, medications that can be used to help treat symptoms of influenza A and B include oseltamivir (Tamiflu), which is given orally for patients as young as newborn, and inhaled or IV zanamivir (Relenza) for patients over 7 years of age. For severely ill patients, zanamivir administered intravenously is preferred to inhaled medication (Allen & CPS Infectious Diseases and Immunization Committee, 2013/2018). These neuraminidase inhibitors prevent the release of influenza A or B viruses from infected cells.

Respiratory Syncytial Virus

RSV is responsible for 50% of cases of bronchiolitis in infants and young children and is the most common cause of viral pneumonia. RSV is the single most important respiratory pathogen in infancy. RSV occurs worldwide and causes annual epidemics during the winter months. Most children who are infected with RSV develop it before their second birthday, and reinfection is common, especially in children attending day care centres. Infants between 2 and 7 months of age can become seriously ill with this condition because their airways are so small and prone to obstruction by the thick mucus produced. In developed countries, 1 to 3% of all infants are hospitalized with RSV infection (Robinson, Le Saux, & CPS Infectious Diseases and Immunization Committee, 2015/2018). Researchers in the Canadian north have identified that Inuit children are at risk for RSV for the following reasons: maternal smoking during pregnancy, residing in rural communities, being of full Inuit lineage, and overcrowding (Banerji, Greenberg, White, et al., 2009). Older children and adults do not get as seriously ill and continue to go to work or school, becoming carriers and spreading the infection. A low-grade fever, cough, and rhinorrhea (running nose) are the initial symptoms that gradually progress to respiratory distress. Chest X-rays are usually normal.

Transmission

RSV is spread by direct contact with respiratory secretions, usually by contaminated hands to the mucous membranes (eyes, mouth, nose). RSV survives for more than 6 hours on countertops, tissues, and soap bars. RSV is not spread via the airborne route. The incubation period is approximately 2 to 8 days. Reinfection is common, as infection does not result in immunity (Robinson et al., 2015/2018). Good hand hygiene, encouraging breastfeeding, and avoidance of passive tobacco smoke are the main aspects of prevention.

Health care–acquired infection can be a major problem, because caregivers may be carrying the organism. For this reason, an infant diagnosed with RSV infection is placed on transmission-based *contact isolation* precautions to prevent the spread of RSV to other sick children.

Diagnosis

An examination of naso- or nasopharyngeal secretions for RSV using direct rapid immunofluorescent antibody staining (DFA) or enzyme-linked immunosorbent assay (ELISA) techniques for antigen detection can be performed while the child waits so that the diagnosis is established before the child is admitted to the pediatric unit. The specimen is placed on ice and sent immediately to the laboratory. A chest X-ray will usually show hyperinflation.

Prevention

Prevention of RSV is available via a monoclonal antibody, palivizumab (Synagis), given in monthly IM injections. This medication is started at the onset of RSV season and is terminated at the end of the season (the season usually lasts from November through March). The CPS practice guidelines state that candidates for preventive therapy include infants with bronchopulmonary dysplasia, severe immunodeficiencies, or significant congenital heart disease and those on continuous mechanical respiratory support (Robinson et al., 2015/2018).

The powder form of palivizumab should be administered within 6 hours of reconstitution because it is preservative free. The provinces and territories have their own policies to manage palivizumab distribution and administration. RSV immunoglobulin may be used for high-risk infants, such as preterm newborns with bronchopulmonary dysplasia.

Treatment and nursing care

The care of infants with RSV infection should be assigned to personnel who are not caring for other patients that may be at high risk for adverse response to RSV. Infection prevention and control techniques are used to prevent the spread of infection to others on the unit. Additional contact precautions need to be carried out to prevent fomite spread. Frequent hand hygiene is essential. Liquid soap dispensers should be available at the sink, because the organism survives for a long time on a dry bar of soap.

Support of the infant and family

It is important for the nurse to have effective communication skills to provide support for parents of the infant who is seriously ill. The parents should be familiarized with respiratory equipment and encouraged to participate in the care and feeding of the infant. Adults who have RSV can shed the virus for 1 week after the infection, and precautions should be taken if that adult is caring for the infant.

Symptomatic care

Addressing ineffective breathing is the nursing priority for an infant hospitalized with RSV infection. Reporting **tachypnea** (increased respiration) and **tachycardia** (increased heart rate) is essential, because these vital sign changes may indicate hypoxemia. It is also important to auscultate breath sounds and to report wheezing, rales, or rhonchi. A child who has been wheezing and suddenly has a "quiet chest" on auscultation may be at risk for respiratory arrest. The higher pitched the wheeze, the more constricted the airway. Signs of respiratory distress should be assessed and reported.

Oxygen saturation levels are monitored, and oxygen is administered at levels needed to maintain a minimum of 90 to 95% saturation. Suctioning of mucus may be necessary to maintain a patent airway.

Monitoring of IV fluids and recording intake and output are essential to prevent dehydration. Urine output should be a minimum of 1 to 2 mL/kg/hr for infants and children. Clear-liquid electrolyte formulas may be prescribed for infants at risk of dehydration. The child should be weighed daily to detect early signs of dehydration.

Inhaled bronchodilators or steroids are not helpful in relation to RSV infections.

Complications

Infants who have a small airway size and are severely ill and hospitalized with RSV infection may be at risk for wheezing and **reactive airway disease (RAD)** later in life. Asthma is difficult to diagnose in young children, and it is not clear whether early, severe RSV wheezing disease causes some cases of asthma or whether patients who will develop asthma first present with symptoms when provoked by RSV infection during infancy. However, results from a recent long-term follow-up study of infants who received palivizumab prophylaxis suggested that prevention of severe RSV infection reduces the incidence of RAD later in life (Crowe, 2016).

Pneumonia

Pathophysiology

Pneumonia or *pneumonitis* is an inflammation of the lungs in which the **alveoli** (air sacs) become filled with exudate and surfactant may be reduced. The affected portion of the lung does not receive enough air. Breathing is shallow. As a result, the bloodstream does not have sufficient oxygen.

Pneumonia may occur as the initial or primary disease, or it may complicate another illness, in which case it is termed *secondary pneumonia*. There are many types of pneumonia. Classification may be by causative organism (i.e., bacterial or viral) or by the part of the respiratory system involved (i.e., lobar or bronchial). Group B streptococcus is the most common cause of pneumonia in newborns, whereas *Chlamydia* is a common cause of pneumonia in infants 3 weeks to 3 months of age. The incidence of *H. influenzae* type B infection has been decreasing with current immunization programs. RSV, rhinovirus, adenovirus, and pneumococcus are other organisms that are responsible for pneumonia in infants and children. Immunocompromised children may develop pneumonia caused by a Gram-negative organism or a fungus such as *Pneumocystis jiroveci* (formerly known as *Pneumocystis carinii*).

> **Nursing Tip**
>
> The pneumococcal conjugate 13-valent (Pneu-C-13) vaccine is recommended for children beginning at 2 months of age, using a three- or four-dose schedule (depending on province or territory). The 23-valent pneumococcal vaccine (Pneu-P-23) provides protection for children older than 2 years who have chronic disease or are immunosuppressed.

Toddlers often aspirate small foreign bodies such as peanuts or popcorn and develop *aspiration pneumonia* as a result; therefore, such foods are to be discouraged for this age group.

Lipoid pneumonia occurs when the infant inhales an oil-based substance into the airways. It is less common today because children are seldom given cod liver oil or castor oil routinely as they were in the past. Nose drops with an oil base must not be used for children because the oil can be aspirated and can cause lipoid pneumonia. A child who drinks kerosene may also develop a type of pneumonia.

Hypostatic pneumonia may occur in patients who have poor circulation in their lungs and remain in one position too long. The child recovering from anaesthesia must be turned frequently to stimulate circulation through the lungs. Early ambulation also accomplishes this.

Manifestations

The symptoms of pneumonia vary with the patient's age and the causative organism. They may develop suddenly or may be preceded by an upper respiratory tract infection. The cough is dry at first, but it gradually becomes productive. Fever rises as high as 39.5° to 40°C (103° to 104°F) and may fluctuate widely during a 24-hour period. The respiratory rate may increase *(tachypnea)*. Respirations are shallow as the child attempts to reduce the amount of chest pain. The chest pain may be caused by a pleural irritation or a musculoskeletal irritation from frequent coughing. Sternal retractions may be seen when the accessory muscles of respiration are used. The nostrils may flare. The child is listless, has a poor appetite, and tends to lie on the affected side.

X-rays confirm the diagnosis and determine whether there are complications such as atelectasis. A differential white blood cell (WBC) count is routinely performed. Blood specimens show a marked increase in the number of WBCs (16 to 40 × 10^9/L). Culture specimens may be obtained from the nose, the throat, or sputum.

Treatment

Treatment depends on the causative organism. Antipyretics are given to reduce fever. Oxygen is administered for dyspnea or cyanosis. When this treatment is begun early, the child is less restless and does not require as many sedatives or medications to relieve pain. Because medication therapy has become so effective, many uncomplicated cases can be treated at home. Fluid intake should be increased, particularly clear fluids and "flattened" soft drinks. Pediazole (a combination of erythromycin ethylsuccinate and sulfisoxazole acetyl) may be prescribed for infants younger than 6 months of age, but amoxicillin is the medication of choice for children up to 5 years of age.

Rest, fluids, and a cough suppressant before bedtime are the basics of home care. Parent education concerning the need to complete all medication prescribed is essential. Tobacco use in the environment should be avoided, and the need for *H. influenzae* type B (Hib) immunizations should be stressed. The proper use and disposal of tissues, coughing or sneezing into the sleeve, and the modelling of proper hand hygiene techniques are preventive measures the nurse should teach the family.

Nursing care

Nursing care for the hospitalized child for all types of pneumonia is basically the same. The age of the patient determines the nurse's approach and the type of equipment used. The infant receives oxygen in an isolette or via oxygen hood, whereas the older child requires nebulized low-flow oxygen via a mask or nasal cannula. Rest is an important part of the treatment. The nurse must organize care so that the child is not disturbed unnecessarily. Planned, quiet activities for the child are recommended.

The nurse needs to check vital signs at regular intervals. When a child is flushed with fever, heavy clothing and blankets should be removed. The nurse should encourage the child to take fluids, flavoured popsicles, or small sips of water frequently. If vomiting persists, parenteral fluids are given.

Pneumothorax

Pathophysiology

A *pneumothorax* is a collection of air in the pleural space which creates a pressure that collapses part of a lung. The most common form is a spontaneous pneumothorax, which is an accumulation of air in the pleural space without an apparent reason. It is caused by the following conditions: rupture of the small blebs on the visceral pleural space, trauma, tuberculosis, and chronic obstructive pulmonary disease (COPD), such as cystic fibrosis. It occurs mostly in adolescents who are tall and thin but can also occur in young children with no apparent precipitating cause. A pneumothorax may be closed or open when there is an unsealed opening in the chest wall, and it may be accompanied by a hemothorax when blood collects.

Manifestations

The child with a pneumothorax may have sudden or gradual onset of symptoms. Chest pain may be present, as well as signs of respiratory distress such as paleness or cyanosis, tachypnea, nasal flaring, in-drawing, and grunting. There may be asymmetrical chest wall movements with decreased or absent sounds or hyperresonance on the affected side, as well as tachycardia.

A chest X-ray reveals air in the pleural space. Arterial blood gases show hypoxemia and respiratory alkalosis. Electrocardiogram (ECG) changes may be present.

Treatment

Treatment depends on the cause and severity of the pneumothorax. In mild cases, re-expansion can be achieved using a conservative approach, with bed rest, oxygen therapy, and close monitoring of the child's vital signs.

In more severe cases, needle aspiration of the pleural space with a large-bore needle may be required. Alternatively, insertion of a chest tube between the ribs into the leaking air space can be performed. The tube is connected to a wall suction with a disposable chest drainage mechanism such as a pleurovac. The drainage system will draw out the leaking air and fluid to keep the lung re-expanded until the lung heals and stops the air leak. A pleurovac closed drainage system is often used at a pressure of 20 mm Hg suction (see Fig. 26.6). It is composed of three chambers next to one another with water pressure and a one-way valve to prevent air and fluid from flowing backward into the chest cavity.

Nursing care

The nurse needs to assess the child's respiratory status frequently along with pulse oximetry. The chest tube should be taped well with an occlusive dressing and is not routinely changed. Assessment of tube patency and fluid drainage is important. The chest tube should not be clamped or the pleurovac be disconnected from the wall suction or the suction turned off, because fluid or air may recollect.

Safety Alert!

A pair of hemostats should be at the bedside in case of dislocation of the chest tube. If dislocated, the tube should be clamped off.

Smoke Inhalation Injury and Carbon Monoxide Poisoning

Smoke inhalation injury may cause carbon monoxide poisoning. Poisonous substances inhaled from burning material may also cause pathological disturbance. There are three stages of inhalation injury:

1. Pulmonary insufficiency in the first 6 hours
2. Pulmonary edema from 6 to 72 hours
3. Bronchopneumonia after 72 hours, which may cause *atelectasis* (areas of collapse in the lung)

When the child is injured by fire and burns are evident around the face or mouth, heat injury to the upper airway should be suspected. Burned materials can be carried deep into the respiratory tract in the form of insoluble gases and may cause chemical injury. Smoke from burning synthetic materials and plastic are especially toxic to the airways. Severe exposure to these chemicals can inhibit secretion of surfactant and cause a hyaline membrane to form, resulting in acute respiratory distress syndrome (ARDS). Carbon monoxide is not toxic to the lungs, but, by combining with hemoglobin to form carboxyhemoglobin (COHb), it prevents oxygen from binding to hemoglobin and thus inhibits cellular respiration.

Safety Alert!

Pulse oximetry readings are of little value in carbon monoxide poisoning because pulse oximetry does not detect COHb and readings may appear normal.

Treatment of carbon monoxide poisoning is often symptomatic and includes oxygen administration, careful monitoring of intake and output, and frequent assessments of arterial blood gas reports. In severe carbon monoxide poisoning hyperbaric oxygenation (see Chapter 21) may be the treatment of choice.

Safety Alert!

Respiratory arrest can occur suddenly in children who have smoke inhalation injuries. An intubation tray should be readily available.

Health Promotion

Parents should be encouraged to have working smoke and carbon monoxide detectors in their homes and to test them at least twice a year.

Tonsillitis and Adenoiditis

Pathophysiology

The tonsils and adenoids, located in the pharynx (throat), are made of lymph tissue and are part of the body's defense mechanism against infection. The symptoms of tonsillitis include difficulty in swallowing and breathing. Enlarged adenoids block the nasal passage, resulting in mouth breathing. Other symptoms are similar to those of nasopharyngitis. Nursing care involves providing salt water gargles; throat lozenges (if age appropriate); a cool, liquid diet; and acetaminophen or ibuprofen to promote comfort. Antibiotics are not usually prescribed unless a throat culture is positive for the streptococcal organism.

Treatment

The removal of the tonsils and adenoids, referred to as a "T&A," is not routinely recommended for children. It is thought that the condition may correct itself if surgery is postponed, because the tissues become smaller as the child grows. A *tonsillectomy* (removal of the palatine tonsils) is indicated only if persistent airway obstruction, repeated infections, or difficulty in breathing occurs. The surgery is not performed during an acute infectious episode because inflamed tissue responds poorly to surgery.

Age-appropriate explanations should be provided to children to prepare them for the surgery. Wording should be carefully selected, because young children may associate being "put to sleep" for the operation with their sick pet being "put to sleep" and never heard from again (see Chapter 19). The presence of loose teeth should be reported to the anaesthesiologist because there may be a danger of aspiration during the surgical procedure. Identification bands are applied, and routine preoperative care is initiated and documented.

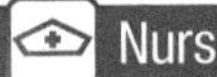

Nursing Tip

Frequent swallowing while the child is sleeping is an early sign of bleeding after a tonsillectomy.

Postoperative care

To facilitate drainage immediately after surgery, the child is placed partly on the side and partly on the abdomen, with the knee of the uppermost leg flexed to hold the position. The child is watched carefully for evidence of bleeding, such as an increase in pulse rate and respirations, restlessness, *frequent swallowing* (which may be from blood trickling down the back of the child's throat), or vomiting of bright red blood. An ice collar may be applied for comfort. The child's face and hands are wiped with a warm washcloth, and the hospital gown and linen are changed whenever necessary. Small amounts of clear liquids are given as tolerated. Red- or brown-coloured juices are avoided because they make it difficult to evaluate the content of emesis and the presence of blood. A popsicle may appeal to the child. If these are well tolerated, progression to a soft diet is begun. The child is kept quiet for the remainder of the day. A small child may nestle on a parent's lap.

Coughing, clearing the throat, and blowing the nose should be avoided to decrease the risk of precipitating bleeding at the operative site. Appropriate pain relief is important and will help to minimize crying, which may further irritate the throat. Hemorrhage is the most common postoperative complication.

Same-day surgery is the usual setting for a tonsillectomy, with the child returning home after a few hours. Postoperative antibiotic treatments are not usually prescribed (Wetmore, 2016). The nurse should not assume that because the surgery is minor it does not involve certain risks.

Written instructions are given to the parents when the child is discharged. The child should be kept quiet for a few days and should receive nourishing fluids and soft foods. After this, the child may continue to take a nap or to have a rest period so that they have sufficient convalescent time. Acetaminophen or ibuprofen may be administered to reduce throat discomfort. Gargling and highly seasoned food should be avoided during the first postoperative week. Parents need to know signs of tonsillar hemorrhage that can occur up to 14 days postsurgery.

Nursing Tip

After a tonsillectomy, milk and milk products may coat the throat and cause the child to "clear" the throat, further irritating the operative site.

Allergic Rhinitis

Allergic rhinitis is an inflammation of the nasal mucosa caused by an allergic response. It often occurs during specific seasons and is referred to as *hay fever.* While allergic rhinitis is not a life-threatening condition and does not necessitate hospitalization, it occurs in 10% of children and accounts for many school absences.

Pathophysiology

The mast cells in the nasal mucosa respond to an antigen by releasing mediators such as histamine, which cause edema and increased mucous secretion. A generalized parasympathetic response can follow. The child may have a genetic predisposition to develop the allergy, and exposure to the allergen triggers the response.

Manifestations

The characteristic signs of allergic rhinitis include nasal congestion, a clear, watery nasal discharge, sneezing, and itching of the eyes and are often called the "allergic salute" (Fig. 25.4).

Diagnosis

Laboratory tests of the mucous membranes of the nose show the presence of eosinophils, and skin sensitization testing may be positive for specific allergens. The history shows seasonal occurrence, family history of allergy or asthma, typical appearance, and absence of fever or purulent drainage.

Treatment and nursing care

Symptomatic treatment revolves around the use of nonsedating antihistamine medications and decongestants to reduce edema of the nasal mucous membranes

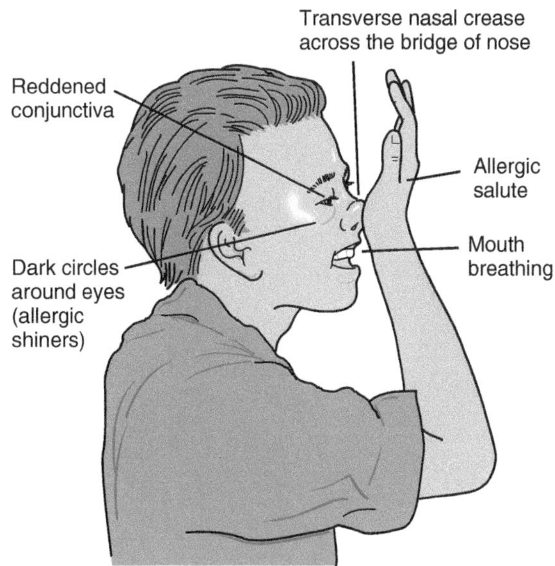

Fig. 25.4 The allergic salute. Signs of allergic rhinitis include a typical rubbing of the nose in response to nasal discharge *(allergic salute)*, darkened circles under the eyes *(allergic shiners)* caused by an obstruction of lymphatic and vein flow, and a *transverse crease* across the bridge of the nose resulting from the allergic salutes.

without creating sedation. Topical medications should not be used because of a "rebound effect" that occurs with long-term use. Prophylactic therapy with cromolyn inhalants or glucocorticoid nasal sprays may be prescribed if antihistamines are not effective, but this type of medication requires daily administration and collaboration between parent and child. Immunotherapy for identified allergens may be prescribed. Carbinoxamine maleate is a liquid sustained-release histamine H1 receptor blocker indicated for the relief of allergic rhinitis in children older than 2 years of age. It may be mildly sedating and is prescribed on an every 12-hour dosage schedule. Leukotriene antagonist medications have also been effective in the treatment of allergic rhinitis (Milgrom & Sicherer, 2016).

The main goals of nursing care are to help the parent identify the difference between an allergy and a cold and to provide a referral for medical care and support during the long-term allergy testing and immunotherapy process. Teaching the family about controlling environmental exposure to allergens is very important. Dust control, prevention of contact with animal dander, the use of air conditioners and high-efficiency particulate air (HEPA) filters in the home, and the planning of vacation locales that do not present pollen challenges are some of the important topics to discuss with the family.

Asthma

Pathophysiology

Asthma is a syndrome caused by increased responsiveness of the tracheobronchial tree to various stimuli that results in reversible, *paroxysmal* (intermittent) constriction of the airways. Asthma can be manifested by one of four main components:

- Bronchospasm
- Edema and mucus
- Inflammation
- Airway reactivity

The medication prescribed by the health care provider is individualized to treat the asthmatic component that the child is manifesting. For example, inhaled corticosteroids may be prescribed for children with RAD, whereas an inhaled bronchodilator is the treatment of choice for bronchospasm. A child with asthma can develop one or more of the components of the asthma syndrome.

Asthma may have a genetic or allergic origin with many environmental risk factors included. Asthma is the leading cause of school absenteeism, emergency department visits, and hospitalization. In Canada, children with asthma have 275 000 emergency visits each year. The asthma rate in developed countries has quadrupled over the past 20 years (Canadian Institutes of Health Research [CIHR], 2016). Although asthma may occur at any age, about 80% of children who have asthma have their first symptoms before 5 years of age.

Factors that may lead to the development of asthma include the following (Government of Canada, 2015):

- Family history of allergy and allergic disorders (including hay fever, asthma, and eczema)
- High exposure to airborne allergens (pets, house dust mites, cockroaches, mould) in the first years of life in susceptible children
- Exposure to tobacco smoke, including during pregnancy
- Frequent respiratory infections early in life
- Low birth weight and respiratory distress syndrome (RDS)

Asthma is a recurrent and reversible obstruction of the airways in which bronchospasm, mucosal edema, and secretion of and plugging by mucus contribute to significant narrowing of the airways and subsequently impaired gas exchange (Fig. 25.5). Both large and small airways may be involved.

The onset of asthma may be triggered by house dust, animal dander, wool, feathers, pollen, mould, passive smoking, strong odours (as from wet paint, wood stoves, or fireplaces), and certain foods. Vigorous physical activity (especially in cold weather) and rapid changes in temperature and humidity may precipitate an attack. Viral infections may also be

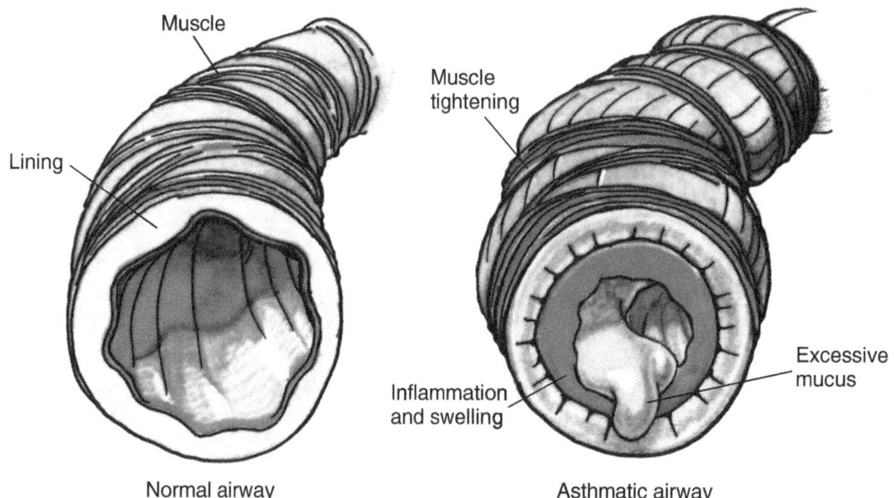

Fig. 25.5 An asthmatic airway compared to a normal airway. (From Bowden, V. R., Dickey, S. B., & Greenberg, S. C. [1998]. *Children and their families: The continuum of care.* Philadelphia: Saunders.)

responsible. Emotional upsets, which affect smooth muscle and vasomotor tone (*vas*, "vessel," and *motor*, "mover"), are closely intertwined with the condition. Environmental factors such as smoking combined with a genetic disposition may trigger the onset of asthma. Medications, such as aspirin, nonsteroidal anti-inflammatory drugs (NSAIDs), antibiotics, and beta blockers, can be triggers, as well as foods such as sulphite preservatives, nuts, milk, or dairy products. Whatever the precipitating cause, the response of the airways is similar. As the attack worsens, arterial blood gases change. $Paco_2$ rises and the blood pH falls, increasing respiratory acidosis and producing a strain on the heart.

Diagnosis

A history, physical examination, and response to bronchodilator therapy are the first diagnostic tools. An elevated level of eosinophils in the blood is typical. Eosinophils in the sputum are also diagnostic. Allergy skin testing and a radioallergosorbent test (RAST) are measures that can identify a sensitivity to allergens. Exercise testing and PFTs help to diagnose asthma and assess the progress of the syndrome. Medications tailored to the individual symptoms are usually prescribed.

Asthma is rarely diagnosed in infancy; the increased susceptibility of infants to respiratory obstruction and dyspnea in response to many different illnesses has many causes:

- Decreased smooth muscle of an infant's airway
- Presence of increased mucous glands in the bronchi
- Normally narrow lumen of the normal airway
- Lack of muscle elasticity in the airway
- Fatigue-prone and overworked diaphragmatic muscle on which infant respiration depends

The symptom of wheezing in infancy can be caused by GER, cystic fibrosis, or the chronic aspiration often seen in developmentally delayed infants, or it may be a manifestation of a milk or food allergy.

Manifestations

The symptoms of asthma may begin slowly or abruptly. The CPS classifies asthma into mild, moderate, or severe categories (Ortiz-Alverez, Mikrogianakis, & CPS Acute Care Committee, 2012/2017). Obstruction is most severe during expiration because the airways become smaller during this phase of respiration. The trapped air in the lung causes hyperinflation and results in an increase in the effort needed for breathing. This increased work of breathing can eventually put a strain on the heart. The hypoxia and resulting acidosis can then cause general pulmonary vasoconstriction that damages alveoli, decreases surfactant, and causes a chronic respiratory problem.

In acute episodes the patient coughs, wheezes, and has difficulty breathing, particularly during expiration. The child may state that their chin, neck, or chest itches. Signs of air hunger, such as flaring of the nostrils, and the use of the accessory muscles of respiration (chest and abdominal muscles) may be evident. Orthopnea appears. The child is restless, perspires, and sometimes has symptoms of abdominal pain; participation in activities decreases. Pulse and respirations are increased, and rales (abnormal respiratory sounds) may be heard in the chest. Inflammation of the nose and sinuses may accompany asthma.

Asthma attacks often happen during the night and are frightening for both the child and the parents. Chronic asthma is manifested by discoloration beneath the eyes (allergic shiners), slight eyelid eczema, and mouth breathing.

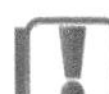 **Safety Alert!**

Shortness of breath accompanied by restricted breath sounds and a rising respiratory rate may indicate imminent respiratory failure and should be reported promptly to the health care provider.

Treatment and long-term management

The management of childhood asthma involves assessing; monitoring; education; environmental control; medication, and reduction of exacerbations while maintaining normal growth and development and childhood lifestyles. Asthma Canada provides guidelines and an asthma action plan to help children and their families manage their asthma (Fig. 25.6). The plan is modified with the health care provider and is based on frequency and severity of symptoms and results of peak flow monitoring and sets out how the child should adjust the medication depending on how controlled the asthma is. The plan is divided into different zones. Green zone is when the child is free of asthma symptoms. Yellow zone is when the child has asthma symptoms. Red is when the child is in danger with an asthmatic attack and needs help.

The main goals of asthma therapy include the following (Fig. 25.7):

- Maintain a near-normal pulmonary function.
- Maintain a near-normal activity level.
- Prevent chronic signs and symptoms.
- Prevent exacerbations that necessitate hospital treatment.
- Prevent adverse responses to medication.
- Promote self-care and monitoring consistent with developmental level.

Medications

There are two types of medications used for outpatient treatment of asthma: controllers (or preventers), which are taken to reduce inflammation in the airways and are taken daily, and relievers ("rescue") to help alleviate symptoms quickly (Table 25.2). An asthma specialist is usually responsible for the follow-up care of the child with asthma.

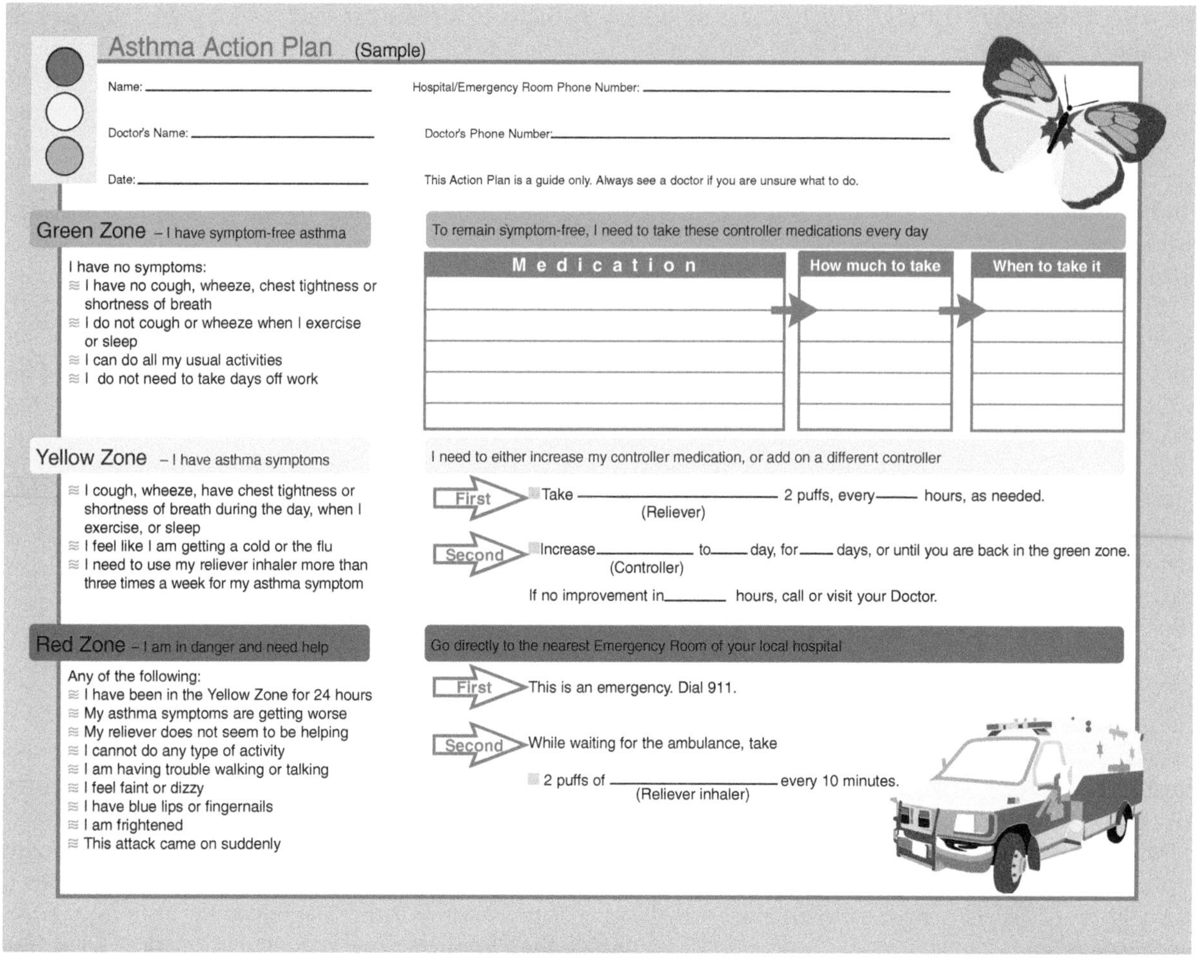

Asthma Action Plan (Sample)

Name: ____________ Hospital/Emergency Room Phone Number: ____________

Doctor's Name: ____________ Doctor's Phone Number: ____________

Date: ____________ This Action Plan is a guide only. Always see a doctor if you are unsure what to do.

Green Zone – I have symptom-free asthma

I have no symptoms:
- I have no cough, wheeze, chest tightness or shortness of breath
- I do not cough or wheeze when I exercise or sleep
- I can do all my usual activities
- I do not need to take days off work

To remain symptom-free, I need to take these controller medications every day

Medication	How much to take	When to take it

Yellow Zone – I have asthma symptoms

- I cough, wheeze, have chest tightness or shortness of breath during the day, when I exercise, or sleep
- I feel like I am getting a cold or the flu
- I need to use my reliever inhaler more than three times a week for my asthma symptom

I need to either increase my controller medication, or add on a different controller

First: Take ____________ (Reliever) 2 puffs, every ____ hours, as needed.

Second: Increase ____________ (Controller) to ____ day, for ____ days, or until you are back in the green zone.

If no improvement in ____ hours, call or visit your Doctor.

Red Zone – I am in danger and need help

Any of the following:
- I have been in the Yellow Zone for 24 hours
- My asthma symptoms are getting worse
- My reliever does not seem to be helping
- I cannot do any type of activity
- I am having trouble walking or talking
- I feel faint or dizzy
- I have blue lips or fingernails
- I am frightened
- This attack came on suddenly

Go directly to the nearest Emergency Room of your local hospital

First: This is an emergency. Dial 911.

Second: While waiting for the ambulance, take 2 puffs of ____________ (Reliever inhaler) every 10 minutes.

Fig. 25.6 A sample of the Asthma Canada Action Plan. An Asthma Action Plan is an individualized series of steps a child can take to manage asthma when it gets out of control. (From Asthma Canada. [n.d.]. *Asthma action plan.* Retrieved from https://asthma.ca/wp-content/uploads/2017/08/AsthmaActionPlan_ENG.pdf.)

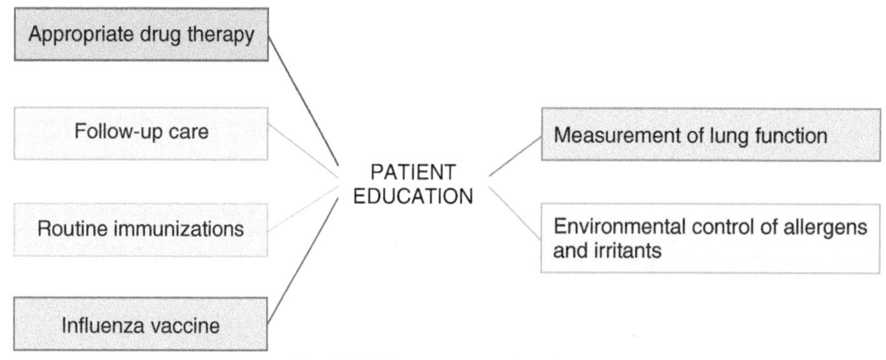

Fig. 25.7 Management of asthma.

The nurse should teach the family how to use the inhalation devises and the precautions concerning frequency of dosages. The nurse should also instruct the family in medication–medication interactions (Table 25.3).

Slow inhalation of an inhaled medication enables the medication to reach the lower airway. Rapid inhalation causes some of the dose to be lost by being deposited on the sides of the pharynx. The respiratory therapist in the hospital may administer nebulized inhalation therapy, and home care units are also available.

Nursing care

The parents and child are taught about the importance of environmental control, such as avoiding pet dander, mould, smoking, stuffed toys, and dust. Humidity in living areas of the house should be controlled to between 25 and 50%, because excess humidity (above

Table 25.2 **Selected Medications Commonly Used to Treat Asthma**

MEDICATION	ACTIONS	NURSING CONSIDERATIONS
Rescue Medications		
Short-Acting Beta$_2$ Agonists (SABA)		
Salbutamol (nebulizer or metered-dose inhaler [MDI])	Bronchodilator acts in 5–10 minutes	Child should hold breath 5–10 seconds after inhaling or use spacer. Child should rinse mouth after administration. Observe for tachycardia, headache, and nervousness.
Inhaled Steroids		
Beclomethasone (MDI or nebulizer)	Anti-inflammatory; reduces mucus in airway	Administer with spacer. Clean inhaler between uses. Child should rinse mouth after dose. Observe for gastrointestinal distress such as stomach upset, nausea, and vomiting.
Combination corticosteroid (budesonide) and long-acting bronchodilator	Used for rescue when symptoms get worse but also taken as a controller to reduce symptoms over time	
Oral Corticosteroids		
Prednisone; prednisolone (oral)	Decreases signs of inflammation Enhances bronchodilation	Give with food to reduce gastric irritation. Administer in early morning when normal hormones peak. Prolonged therapy and high doses may cause immunosuppression.
Anticholinergic		
Ipratropium (Atrovent) (MDI or nebulizer)	Bronchodilation and decreases mucus within 30–90 minutes	Child should rinse mouth to relieve bitter taste. Observe for dry mouth, tachycardia.
Daily Medications (Controllers)		
Long-Acting Beta$_2$ Agonists (LABA)		
Salmeterol; formoterol (dry powder inhaler)	Keeps airways open and muscles relaxed. They help to prevent asthma episodes (attacks).	Long-acting bronchodilators work slowly, over a 12-hour period; not used during acute episodes. Take 30–60 minutes before exercise. Observe for tachycardia, tremor.
Mast Call Inhibitors		
Cromolyn sodium Nedocromil sodium (MDI or nebulizer)	Anti-inflammatory; inhibit response to allergens and exercise-induced asthma	Do not use during acute episode. Must use several times a day on a regular basis to prevent attacks. Observe for nasal congestion; throat irritation.
Leukotriene Receptor Agonists (LTRA)		
Montelukast or zafirlukast (oral)	Anti-inflammatory; provides protection against bronchoconstriction	Administer in evening. Mix granules in applesauce or ice cream (not liquids) or chew tablet. Administer between meals. Do not give with theophylline or warfarin unless advised by health care provider.
Methylxanthines		
Theophylline (oral)	Bronchodilator that works directly on airway muscles—not commonly used in treatment of asthma	It is taken in the evening if shortness of breath disturbs sleep, or regularly if asthma is severe. Do not crush or chew tablet. Monitor blood levels. Watch for dysrhythmia and tremors.
Immunotherapy		
Omalizumab	An antibody that blocks allergic reactions	Used for child older than 12 years. Injections given every 2 weeks, based on immunoglobulin E (IgE) levels. Given subcutaneously. Child should be observed for 30 minutes after injection for anaphylaxis. Observe for neuropsychiatric adverse effects such as aggressive behaviour, suicidal ideation.

Table 25.2 Selected Medications Commonly Used to Treat Asthma—cont'd

MEDICATION	ACTIONS	NURSING CONSIDERATIONS
Mepolizumab	A monoclonal anti-IL-5 antibody approved by Health Canada for children over 12 years of age with severe recurrent asthmatic exacerbation due to eosinophilic airway inflammation	Given intravenously or subcutaneously to lower eosinophil levels. Given every 4 weeks. Observe for herpes zoster virus infections and allergic responses.

Data from Asthma Canada. (2015). *Asthma medications*. Retrieved from https://www.lung.ca/lung-health/lung-disease/asthma/medications; Liu, A. H., Covar, R. A., Spahn, J. D., & Sicherer, S. H. (2016). Childhood asthma. In R. Kliegman, B. Stanton, J. St. Geme, et al. (Eds.), *Nelson textbook of pediatrics* (20th ed.). Philadelphia: Saunders; Wilson, B. A., & Shannon, M. (2017). *Nurses drug guide, 2017*. Toronto, ON: Pearson.

Table 25.3 Asthma Medication Interactions

ASTHMA MEDICATION	INTERACTING SUBSTANCE	EFFECT
Ephedrine	Antihypertensive medications	Decrease antihypertensive effects
	Antidepressants—monoamine oxidase inhibitors (MAOIs) such as phenelzine, tranylcypromine	Can cause a rise in blood pressure
	Antacids	Increase serum level of ephedrine
	Ammonium chloride expectorants	Reduce effectiveness of ephedrine
	Steroids	Lessen steroid effectiveness
Epinephrine	Antidepressants—tricyclics (e.g., imipramine, amitriptyline and MAOIs)	Can cause tachycardia, high blood pressure, and cardiac dysrhythmia
	Beta-adrenergic blockers, such as propranolol	Can cause high blood pressure
	Digitalis	Can cause cardiac dysrhythmia
Theophylline	Allopurinol (Zyloprim)	Can cause tachycardia and allopurinol toxicity
	Antibiotics (specifically erythromycin)	Can cause theophylline toxicity
	Antibacterials (ciprofloxacin)	May increase theophylline levels significantly
	Rifampin	Decreases effectiveness of theophylline
	Cimetidine (Tagamet)	Can cause theophylline toxicity
	Phenytoin (Dilantin)	Can decrease effect of both medications
	Phenobarbital	Decreases effect of theophylline
	Ephedrine	Can cause dysrhythmia and nervousness
	Beta-adrenergic blockers, such as propranolol	Decrease effect of theophylline
	Oral contraceptives	Can increase theophylline blood levels
	High-fat foods	Increase absorption of theophylline

50%) promotes mould growth. Dust collectors such as carpets, upholstery, or drapes should not be in the bedroom of an asthmatic child. Mattress covers, foam rubber pillows, and cotton blankets are preferred. Wool, down, and feather-stuffed items should be avoided. Upholstery, drapes, and carpets can be sprayed every 3 months with benzyl benzoate to kill dust mites, followed by cleaning and vacuuming. The use of HEPA air-filtering devices in the bedroom and HEPA filters in the vacuum is advisable. Identifying triggers of asthma for each child is helpful in controlling symptoms.

Children can be taught to monitor their own lung function with the use of a peak flow meter at home (Skill 25.1). Involvement in self-care aids in the ability to follow through with required care and results in better control of asthmatic symptoms.

The parents and teachers should not exclude the child from physical activity in school for fear of triggering an asthmatic attack. In children with exercise induced asthma, pretreatment with a short acting beta-agonist before scheduled physical education or activity may prevent the asthma attack. Swimming is best tolerated, probably because of the high humidity in the air inhaled, and the exhaling of air underwater is similar to "pursed-lip" exhaling. Sports such as baseball, short sprints, and gymnastics are well tolerated, because the activity is intense but short. Individuals with asthma are less able to tolerate prolonged intense activity such as jogging, lap running, race running, or basketball. Pre-exercise puffs of a prescribed inhaler and a warm-up before vigorous exercise can enable the child to participate more fully in age-appropriate school physical exercise. Many Olympic athletes have successfully managed their asthma symptoms. The promotion of normal growth and development is a basic goal in asthma care, and participation with peers is important.

Skill 25.1 Using the Peak Flow Meter

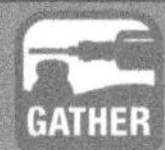

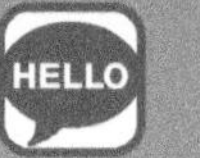

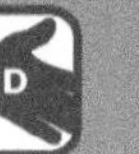

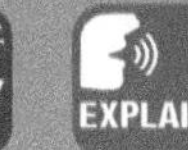

WASH

PURPOSE

To monitor lung function

STEPS

1. Be sure the arrow points to 0 or is at the bottom of the numbered scale.
2. Instruct the child to close their mouth over the mouthpiece.
3. Instruct the child to take a deep breath and blow as hard as possible into the peak flow meter.
4. Observe and record the score or measurement on the peak flow meter.
5. Repeat three times and report the highest of the three readings.
6. Compare the score with previous scores and correlate with the plan of care.
7. Document for future reference.

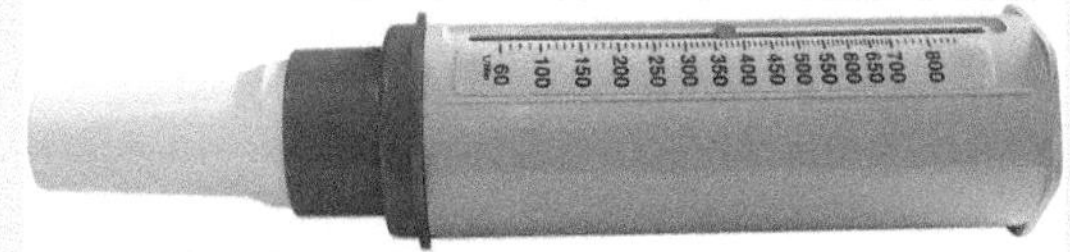

Using the peak flow meter. Assessments should be done daily at home. The reading in the morning should be within 20% of the evening reading. (Source: iStock.com/MarkUK97)

More severe asthma attacks often require hospitalization. The nurse should limit conversation with the child during the emergency period to questions that can be answered "yes" or "no." The nurse should also organize tasks so that the child obtains sufficient rest. Oxygen reduces hypoxia and improves the patient's colour. Nasal prongs, a hood, or a facial mask can be used to administer the oxygen.

If the child is in respiratory distress on admission, oxygen is administered per the health care provider's protocol, and the child is positioned comfortably. One method is to place a pillow on the overbed table and have the child extend the arms over it, elbows bent. This is a comfortable position and allows maximum use of the accessory muscles of breathing. Lung sounds are assessed for rhonchi, wheezing, or rales. Arterial blood gases and vital signs are monitored. The child is evaluated for clinical improvement (quieter, slower respirations, relaxed facial expressions, cessation of retractions).

! Medication Alert!

Oxygen is a medication, and administration should be correlated with monitoring of oxygen saturation levels. Too little oxygen can result in hypoxia; too much oxygen can result in lung damage.

Nursing Tip

A child may become nervous and restless after receiving short-acting $beta_2$ agonist (SABA) medication. It is important to keep the child as calm and quiet as possible.

Diet. Oral fluids are encouraged because they help to liquefy secretions and are needed to compensate for fluid loss from dyspnea and diaphoresis. Carbonated beverages, such as ginger ale and colas, should be avoided when the child is wheezing. Beverages are served at room temperature because cold liquids can trigger reflex bronchospasm. Milk products are avoided because they tend to increase the production of mucus. Intake and output should be recorded. The patient is observed for cracked lips, the absence of tears, poor skin turgor, and a decrease in urine output, all of which signal dehydration.

A well-balanced diet and adequate fluids are necessary for general health. Ample time should be allowed for meals because respiratory distress may interfere with eating. Eating antioxidant foods may be helpful in lowering asthma symptoms, but basically a diet that maintains normal weight is essential, as obesity is related to the development of asthma.

Self-care. The child should be taught self-care. The importance of exercise to strengthen vulnerable lungs is emphasized. *Pursed-lip breathing* (blowing out as if blowing a kiss) and biofeedback are also helpful. The child is taught to observe "personal triggers" that are forewarnings of an attack and how to use the peak flow meter. Other aspects of care include how to administer metered-dose inhalers (MDIs) and understanding medications and their possible adverse effects. Specific information about how often and when to use inhalers is paramount.

Smartphone applications offer free information and reminders to take medications to increase ability to adhere to the medication regimen. Please see Additional Resources at the end of the chapter for online information.

The child should be encouraged to discuss daily school routines. The health care provider needs to be seen regularly to evaluate progress and to readjust medications as needed. The nurse reviews the signs of respiratory infection with the child and where, when, and whom to call for help. Early attention to symptoms may prevent escalation of the disease.

Nursing Tip

The principles of asthma treatment are as follows:
- Daily monitoring
- Symptom diary
- Treatment plan with active participation of the child
- Identification and avoidance of triggers

Nursing Tip

The goal of treatment is to maintain long-term asthma control, using the least amount of medication to avoid adverse events, and to maintain a normal developmental lifestyle with no more than one acute episode a year.

Spirometry. Spirometry measures air flow and volume during a forced exhalation at a maximal effort into a spirometer. Spirometry provides an objective measure of pulmonary functions in children over 6 years of age who are developmentally able to participate in testing. It should be used at 6-month intervals to assess progress. Spirometry reveals underlying inflammation that may not be clinically evident. This test should take place in a clinic during follow-up care (Nierengarten 2016).

Routine monitoring of airway obstruction should be part of comprehensive asthma management. A 6-year-old can self-test with adult supervision. Assessment with a peak flow meter that measures the rate at which air is expelled from the lungs is useful, and a diary of peak flow readings (PFRs) should be brought to the health care provider at each follow-up visit to monitor for changes in lung function. The nurse should be alert to the fact that some older children and adolescents may have difficulty adhering to the guidelines for PFR and may cause false results by manipulating the unit.

Metered-dose inhalers (MDIs). An MDI consists of a pump consisting of a mouthpiece and an actuator (or holder) into which a medicine canister is inserted. Asthma Canada (2019) recommends that spacers always be used with MDIs, rather than just the MDI alone, as the medicine often ends up in the mouth, throat, stomach, and lungs. With a spacer on the inhaler, more medication is delivered to the lungs without the systemic adverse effects (Fig. 25.8). The use of a spacer slows the movement of the medicine, allowing more time to inhale the medicine. Spacers with masks are available for infants and young children.

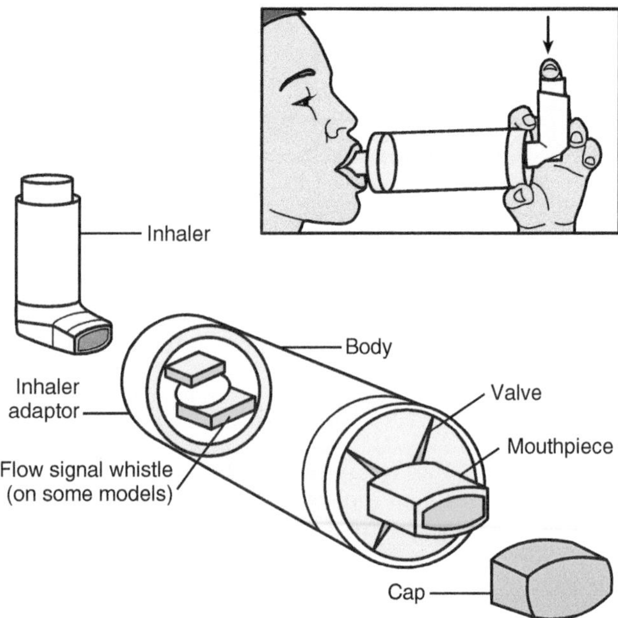

Fig. 25.8 A spacer is recommended to be used with an inhaler. This allows for more medication to be delivered to the child. (From Asthma Canada. [2018]. *Spacers*. Retrieved from https://www.asthma.ca/spacers.)

Practice to acquaint the child with the treatment and to reduce stress of using it is helpful, because crying reduces delivery of medication to the lungs (Skill 25.2). Parents should be taught to use distractions such as books, music, or toys to minimize crying.

Dry powder inhalers are popular because more medications are coming in powder form and often the dose administered does not need to be coordinated with inhalation and a spacer cannot be used. The powder inhalation technique is different; the child needs to have a tight seal around the mouth and inhale rapidly and deeply. The child should be taught to rinse the mouth after steroid inhalation to prevent the development of candidiasis. Activators should be cleaned regularly.

Most near-empty inhaler canisters will float in a bowl of water. Some canisters have an alert system to notify the user of remaining doses available in the canister. Knowing the canister content level enables the child to request a refill and avoid missing medication doses. A nebulizer machine can be used in the home when inhalers are not appropriate for the individual child.

The nurse should help the child see connections between triggers, medicines, and signs of respiratory distress. For example, did the peak flow drop after contact with a cat or rabbit? Does the peak flow always change with a cold? Any time there is a change in peak flow, the child should know to look for a cause that triggered it.

During every clinic visit, the nurse should have the child demonstrate the use of the inhaler or spacer and reinforce the principles involved.

Skill 25.2 Using a Metered-Dose Inhaler (MDI) and Spacer (AeroChamber)

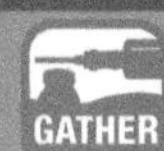

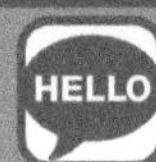

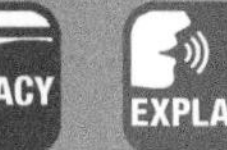

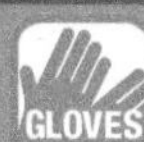

GLOVES

PURPOSE

To promote home self-care

STEPS

Metered-Dose Inhaler With an AeroChamber

1. Attach the AeroChamber to the upright MDI and shake vigorously (see Fig. 25.8).
2. Apply the mask to the face tightly for a good seal or insert mouthpiece with lips around it tightly.
3. Take slow, regular breaths if the child is old enough to understand instructions.
4. Depress the inhaler firmly to release the medication.
5. Hold AeroChamber in place for six breaths and then administer a second puff.
6. Wait 1 minute between puffs as bronchodilator is being administered.
7. Remove from face or mouth.

Medication Alert!

Medicated inhalers should be used as prescribed. Overuse can be dangerous.

Status Asthmaticus

Status asthmaticus is continued severe respiratory distress that is not responsive to medications, including epinephrine and aminophylline. **This is a medical emergency.** The child requires immediate admission to the critical care unit. Oxygen is administered via nasal cannula or hood. Vital signs and the flow of IV medications are carefully monitored.

Following the prescribed medical regimen, promptly seeking medical care when indicated, minimizing exposure to known allergens, wearing a medical identification bracelet, and having a written plan for crisis management can minimize the life-threatening occurrence of status asthmaticus.

Cystic Fibrosis

Pathophysiology

Cystic fibrosis (CF) is a major worldwide cause of serious chronic lung disease in children. CF is the most common fatal genetic disease that affects children and young adults in Canada. Currently, there is no cure. It occurs in approximately 1 in every 3 600 children born in Canada. There are more than 4 100 Canadians presently attending specialized CF clinics (Cystic Fibrosis Canada, 2019a). With advances in research, the estimated median survival age for Canadians with CF is now 53.5 years, which is among the highest in the world. In North America, CF mostly affects Whites but also includes individuals from mixed African-White, Mexican-White, and Indian-White ancestries (Li, Sun, Corey, et al., 2011). It is an inherited recessive trait, with both parents carrying a gene for the disease. Newborn screening for CF is performed in all provinces except for Quebec and some areas of Nunavut. Research has shown that newborn screening and early treatment lead to better long-term health in people with CF in the first 5 years of life compared to those diagnosed later (Mak, Sykes, Stephenson, et al., 2016). A sweat chloride test is considered diagnostic.

The basic defect in CF is an exocrine gland dysfunction that includes (1) increased viscosity (thickness) of mucous gland secretions and (2) a loss of electrolytes in sweat because of an abnormal chloride movement. CF is considered a multisystem disease that affects each of the following systems, because of the thick, viscid secretions:

- Respiratory system (lung involvement)
- Digestive system (pancreatic involvement)
- Skin (sweat glands)
- Reproductive system

See further discussion below regarding the impact on each of these systems.

Manifestations

The manifestations of CF are illustrated in Fig. 25.9.

Lung involvement. The small and large air passages of the lungs become clogged with mucus. There is widespread obstruction of the bronchioles. It is difficult for the child to breathe; expiration is especially difficult. More and more air becomes trapped in the lungs *(obstructive emphysema),* and small areas of collapse (**atelectasis**) may occur. Eventually, the chest assumes a barrel shape, with increased diameter across the front and back. The thick secretions in the lungs and response of tissues to infections cause hypoxia that can result in heart failure. The right ventricle of the heart, which supplies the lungs, may become strained and enlarged. **Clubbing of the fingers** and toes (see Fig. 26.4), a compensatory response indicating a chronic lack of oxygen, may be present. *Staphylococcus* and *Pseudomonas* infections can easily occur in the lungs, which provide a suitable medium for the organism's growth. This causes more thickening of the abnormal secretions, irritates and damages lung tissues, and further increases lung obstruction.

Emphysema, wheezes, and respiratory distress are common. The child is irritable and tires easily. There

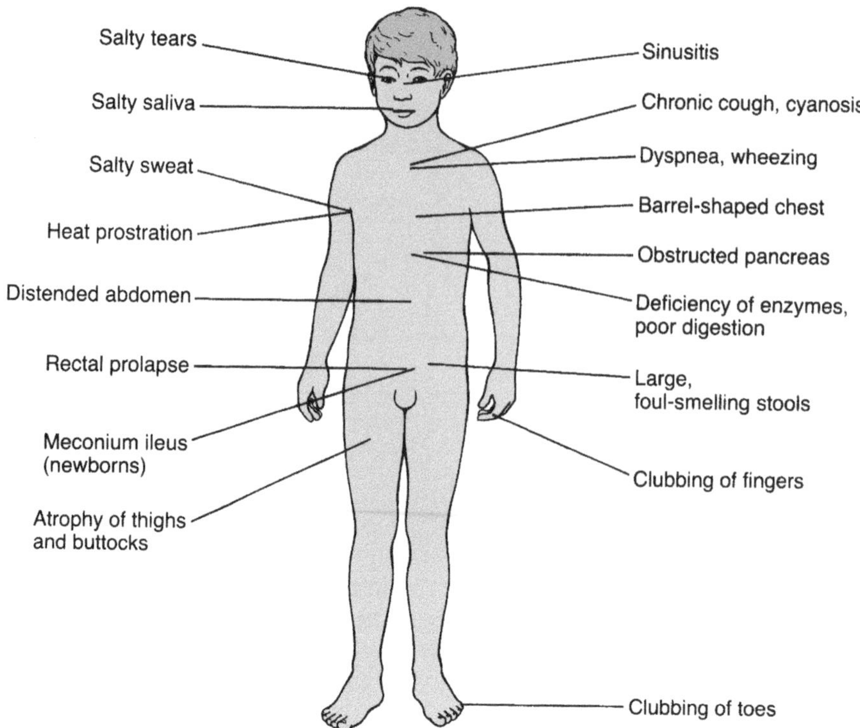

Fig. 25.9 Manifestations of cystic fibrosis.

is a gradual change in physical appearance. Evidence of obstructive emphysema, atelectasis, and fibrosis of lung tissue may also be present. The prognosis for survival depends on the extent of lung damage. However, this is only part of the picture, because CF also affects the pancreas and sweat glands.

Pancreatic involvement. The pancreas lies behind the stomach. Some of its cells secrete pancreatic enzymes that drain from the pancreatic duct into the duodenum in the same area in which bile enters. Changes occurring in the pancreas result from obstruction by thickened secretions that block the flow of pancreatic digestive enzymes. As a result, foodstuffs, particularly fats and proteins, are not properly digested and used by the body.

The stools in infants may be loose and light in colour. Because of impaired digestion and food absorption, the feces of the child become large, frothy, and foul smelling. The child does not gain weight despite a good appetite and may look undernourished. The abdomen becomes distended, and the buttocks and thighs *atrophy* (waste away) as fat disappears from the main deposit sites.

Thick, impacted feces can cause rectal prolapse. Pancreatic, liver, and biliary obstruction occur. A condition known as **meconium ileus** exists when the intestine of the newborn becomes obstructed with abnormally thick meconium while in utero. This condition is caused by the absence of pancreatic enzymes that normally digest proteins in the meconium. The abnormal, putty-like stool sticks to the walls of the intestine, causing blockage. The presenting symptoms develop within hours after birth. The absence of stools and the presence of vomiting and of abdominal distention can indicate intestinal obstruction. X-ray films confirm the diagnosis.

Sweat glands. The sweat, tears, and saliva of the patient with CF become abnormally salty because of an increase in sodium chloride levels. Up to about 20 years of age, more than 60 mmol/L of sodium chloride in sweat is diagnostic of CF. Levels of 40 to 60 mmol/L are highly suggestive, especially in children less than 3 months of age. The analysis of sweat is a major aid in diagnosing the condition. Because these children lose large amounts of salt through perspiration, they must be watched for heat prostration. Liberal amounts of salt should be included with food, and extra fluids and salt should be provided during hot weather.

Reproductive system. Sexual development may be delayed in these patients. Males are generally sterile, but sexual function is unimpaired. Adolescent girls may experience secondary amenorrhea during exacerbations. Infertility problems are common in CF due to the thick secretions that decrease sperm motility in males, and the thick cervical mucus can inhibit sperm from reaching the fallopian tubes in females.

Complications

CF is often responsible for rectal prolapse in infants and children, partly because of poor muscle tone in the rectal area and because of the excessive leanness of the buttocks of the patient.

As the disease progresses, the liver may become hard, nodular, and enlarged. *Cor pulmonale* (*cor*, "heart," and *pulmon*, "lung"), which is heart strain caused by improper lung function, is often a cause of death. There is a deficiency of vitamin A because the child is unable to absorb fats from which this vitamin is obtained.The incidence of diabetes mellitus (CF-related diabetes) is greater in children with CF than in the general population. It may be caused by the changes in the pancreas and decreased blood supply over time.

Treatment and nursing care

Respiratory relief. Patients with CF often require oxygen therapy, which is discussed in Chapter 20. Inhalation therapy to deliver medication as well as to pediatric hydrate the lower respiratory tract is prescribed, and intermittent aerosol therapy is administered to promote the removal of secretions. Antimicrobials may be administered as a preventive measure against respiratory infection. Nursing Care Plan 25.1 summarizes interventions for the patient with CF.

Nursing Care Plan 25.1 The Pediatric Patient With Cystic Fibrosis

PATIENT DATA

A 5-year-old child diagnosed with cystic fibrosis is admitted to the pediatric unit. The child has loose, foul-smelling stools, a persistent cough with some nasal flaring, and chest retractions.

Selected Nursing Diagnosis Difficulty breathing as a result of thick mucus in respiratory tract due to cystic fibrosis as evidenced by thick mucus production, unproductive or minimal cough, and adventitious breath sounds (wheezes, crackles, dyspnea, tachypnea, cyanosis)

Goals	Nursing Interventions	Rationales
Child will have a patent airway as demonstrated by effective cough, thin respiratory secretions, age-appropriate respiratory rate and effort, and O_2 saturation >92% on room air.	Observe respiratory status (rate, depth, effort, breath sounds, O_2 saturation, and skin colour) *at least* every 4 hours.	Allows for early detection of and intervention for changes in child's respiratory status.
	Administer humidified O_2 as ordered by health care provider; monitor O_2 saturation frequently.	Humidification helps to thin and loosen secretions. In chronic obstructive respiratory diseases, the respiratory centre in the brain becomes tolerant of low O_2 saturation in the blood. Administering high concentrations of O_2 to a child with chronic lung disease can lead to carbon dioxide narcosis.
	Administer bronchodilators and expectorants as ordered by health care provider.	These medications help the thinning, loosening, and expectoration of respiratory mucus.
	Encourage age-appropriate oral intake of fluids.	Helps to decrease the viscosity (thickness) of secretions.
	Perform chest physiotherapy (CPT) and postural drainage (PD) every 4 hours or as needed. Perform CPT/PD 1 hour before or 2 hours after meals.	CPT and PD help to mobilize secretions and to increase oxygenation. Performing 1 hour before or 2 hours after meals lessens the risk of vomiting and aspiration.
	Teach the child how to do coughing and deep-breathing exercises. Use play therapy whenever possible. For example, using an inspirometer, "blow up" the fingers of a clean glove.	Children younger than age 7 years cannot voluntarily produce an effective cough. Coughing and deep-breathing exercises help expand the lungs and mobilize secretions.
	Teach parents and caregivers *not* to give over-the-counter (OTC) medications, especially cough suppressants, to the child with cystic fibrosis.	Cough-suppressant medication inhibits the cough reflex, leading to secretions being retained and the possibility of respiratory infection.

Selected Nursing Diagnosis Potential for inadequate nutrition due to a decrease in the availability of pancreatic enzymes; poor intestinal absorption of nutritional intake; anorexia secondary to cystic fibrosis as evidenced by decreased oral intake, weight loss or failure to thrive, diarrhea, steatorrhea, or constipation

Goals	Nursing Interventions	Rationales
Child will be able to ingest age-appropriate nutrition and maintain weight or gain height and weight according to the normal growth and development charts. Stools will be of normal colour, consistency, and amount for age.	Determine child's normal feeding patterns, dietary likes and dislikes, and activity level.	Knowing the child's preferences and activity level will aid in the plan of care for feeding the child.

Continued

Nursing Care Plan 25.1 The Pediatric Patient With Cystic Fibrosis—cont'd

Goals	Nursing Interventions	Rationales
	Administer pancreatic replacement enzymes and fat-soluble vitamin supplements as directed by the health care provider before meals and snacks.	Digestive and nutritional therapy consists of replacement of pancreatic enzymes and dietary adjustments. Administering supplemental fat-soluble vitamins is necessary because of the inability of the body to absorb fats.
	Teach the child (and parents) *not* to chew the capsules or "beads" but to swallow the medication whole; if using powder form, to sprinkle over a nonfat, nonprotein food, such as applesauce. Do not mix enzymes with hot (heated) foods, high-starch, or high-acid–containing foods. Wipe any powder from oral mucosa or lips.	Pancreatic enzymes are inactivated by heat, and acids are known to degrade the enzymes. Wipe the excess powder off mucosa to prevent excoriation or breakdown of mucosal membranes.
	Note colour, consistency, amount, and frequency of stools. Notify the health care provider of any changes (e.g., diarrhea, constipation, or steatorrhea).	Pancreatic enzymes are known to cause constipation if taken in high doses, or they can cause steatorrhea from malabsorption of fats and proteins or because of low intake of the enzymes.

Selected Nursing Diagnosis Potential for family stress due to chronicity of disease, need for outside support, the risk of life-threatening complications as evidenced by frequent health care provider office visits or hospitalizations, a diminished focus on other siblings in the home, and the need for therapeutic interventions and adherence to home care routines

Goals	Nursing Interventions	Rationales
Family members will verbalize their feelings about the impact cystic fibrosis has on them; will be able to comply with the therapeutic treatment plan; and will use available resources within their community to assist in the care and treatment of their child.	Determine the educational level and amount of knowledge each family member has on cystic fibrosis *before* planning any family interventions or teaching sessions.	Educational level will help to determine the type of teaching methods to be used (i.e., written, visual, hands-on, auditory). Having this information in advance helps the nurse to map out the plan of care and teaching. It also prevents the repetition of the same information and guides the nurse as to the amount of teaching and information required or needed by the family.
	Determine the level of impact that the disease has had on the family.	Guides the nurse in selecting appropriate referrals to community or sup port agencies needed by the family.
	Teach or review with the family the skills required in the daily care of the child with cystic fibrosis—for example, assessing respiratory rate and status, CPT and PD methods, monitoring stools, caring for skin, and medication administration.	Return demonstration enables the nurse to evaluate the ability of the family to provide effective home care.

It is important to sterilize airway clearance equipment by taking all pieces apart and washing them with soapy water, rinsing with sterile water, sterilizing with hot or cold techniques, and storing them in a closed plastic bag to avoid growth of infective material. Refer to Additional Learning Resources at the end of this chapter for the cleaning technique recommended by Cystic Fibrosis Canada.

An inhaler that acts as a mucous clearance device can be used in the home care of these children. Bronchodilators are used to increase the width of the bronchi, allowing free passage of air into the lungs. Recombinant human deoxyribonuclease dornase alfa, in a single daily aerosol dose, is effective in decreasing thickness of secretions, thereby improving pulmonary function.

There are many airway clearance techniques that can be individualized for each person with CF, including the following:

- Active cycle of breathing technique, which comprises a cycle of breathing control, chest expansion exercises, and the forced expiratory technique or huffing to expel thick mucus
- Autogenic drainage technique, in which the airflow is used while breathing out to move mucus from the small to larger airways, where it can be cleared
- Positive expiratory pressure, in which individuals breathe through a face mask or mouthpiece attached to a resistor, which causes pressure to keep the airways open, allowing mucus to be cleared
- Oscillating positive expiratory pressure involves breathing repeatedly through a device, which causes pressure and vibrations in the airways to help loosen and move mucus out (Cystic Fibrosis Canada, 2019b).

Postural drainage and chest-clapping therapy are also of value (Fig. 25.10). The physiotherapist or respiratory therapist performs these procedures during hospitalization. When postural drainage and chest clapping are done properly, the secretions in the chest are moved up and out. This technique should be explained to the parents, so they can continue the procedure when the child returns home. These procedures are done after nebulization and at least 2 hours after eating. General aerobic exercise is beneficial for the patient, as well as weight training (Egan, Green, & Voynow, 2016). Play activities such as somersaults and headstands within the child's endurance limits are therapeutic.

Breathing exercises may also be recommended for the older child. **Pursed-lip breathing** is one technique that is simple and effective. The patient is instructed to inhale through the nose, then to exhale through the mouth with the lips pursed as if whistling. Exhalation should be at least twice as long as inhalation. (For example, if it takes 3 seconds to breathe in, 6 seconds are taken to allow all the air to escape.) The child is taught not to force the air out but to let it escape naturally.

Prevention of respiratory infections is essential. The child must be kept away from patients and personnel who may have infections. The period of hospitalization is kept brief, if possible, to avoid cross-infection. The necessary immunizations against childhood diseases should be given to this child (see Chapter 32).

Lung transplants have been performed in patients with CF with good success. In 2016, 45 individuals with CF received transplants; their median age was 31.2 years.

Nursing Tip

Chest physiotherapy should be performed *between* meals.

Diet. The maintenance of adequate nutrition is essential. The diet should be high in tolerated fat, protein, and calories. The administration of insulin has been shown to maintain an adequate nutritional status in some children. Supplemental enzymes are provided with the food to aid in digestion, and fat-soluble vitamins and iron may be prescribed. The child's weight should be monitored and intake and output recorded. Infants can breastfeed with added enzyme intake. Formula-fed infants do best with a higher calorie-per-gram formula. Parenteral alimentation (total parenteral nutrition [TPN]) may be indicated in some cases. Weekly growth hormone therapy can improve nutritional outcomes (Egan et al., 2016).

An oral pancreatic preparation, such as pancrelipase (Viokase), is given to the child with each meal and snack to replace the pancreatic enzymes that the child's body cannot produce. This medication is considered specific for the disease because it helps the child digest and absorb food, thus improving the condition of the stools. If the child is ill and not eating, the medication is withheld. When meals are erratic, such as during vacations, medication is given when the largest amount of food will be consumed. High doses have been associated with the development of gastrointestinal strictures, thus the child should be monitored. Vitamins A, D, E, and K, iron, and zinc supplements are also prescribed. In 2012, a medication, ivacaftor (Kalydeco), was approved by Health Canada for children 6 years and older who have a specific genetic mutation (CFTR) identified (Cystic Fibrosis Canada, 2019a). The medication is given orally with a fat-containing food such as eggs, butter, cheese, whole milk, or yogurt. The medication should not be administered with antibiotics such as rifampin, seizure medications such as phenobarbital or phenytoin, or herbal supplements such as St. John's wort, as they may decrease effectiveness of the medication. Grapefruit juice should be avoided. Liver enzymes should be monitored.

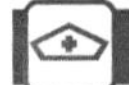
Nursing Tip

Pancreatic enzyme powder should be given with applesauce or other nonstarch, nonfat, nonprotein food.

General hygiene. The nurse must pay special attention to the skin of the child with CF. The diaper area is cleansed after each bowel movement. An ointment to protect the skin is advisable because the character of the stool subjects the diaper area to irritation. The buttocks should be exposed to air when a rash occurs. Because the child has little fat and muscle, their position must be changed frequently, especially if the child is weak and cannot get out of bed. Frequent changes of position also prevent the development of pneumonia.

The child should wear light clothing to avoid becoming overheated; it should be loose to allow freedom of movement. Good oral hygiene is necessary because the teeth may be in poor condition from dietary deficiencies. Mouth care is given after postural drainage because foul mucus may be raised, leaving an unpleasant taste in the patient's mouth.

Long-term care. The goals of care include minimizing pulmonary complications, ensuring adequate nutrition, promoting growth and development, and assisting the family in adjusting to the long-term care required at home. This care can be taxing financially, physically, and emotionally. The parents must distribute their time and energy within the family yet give careful attention to their sick child or, sometimes, chil-

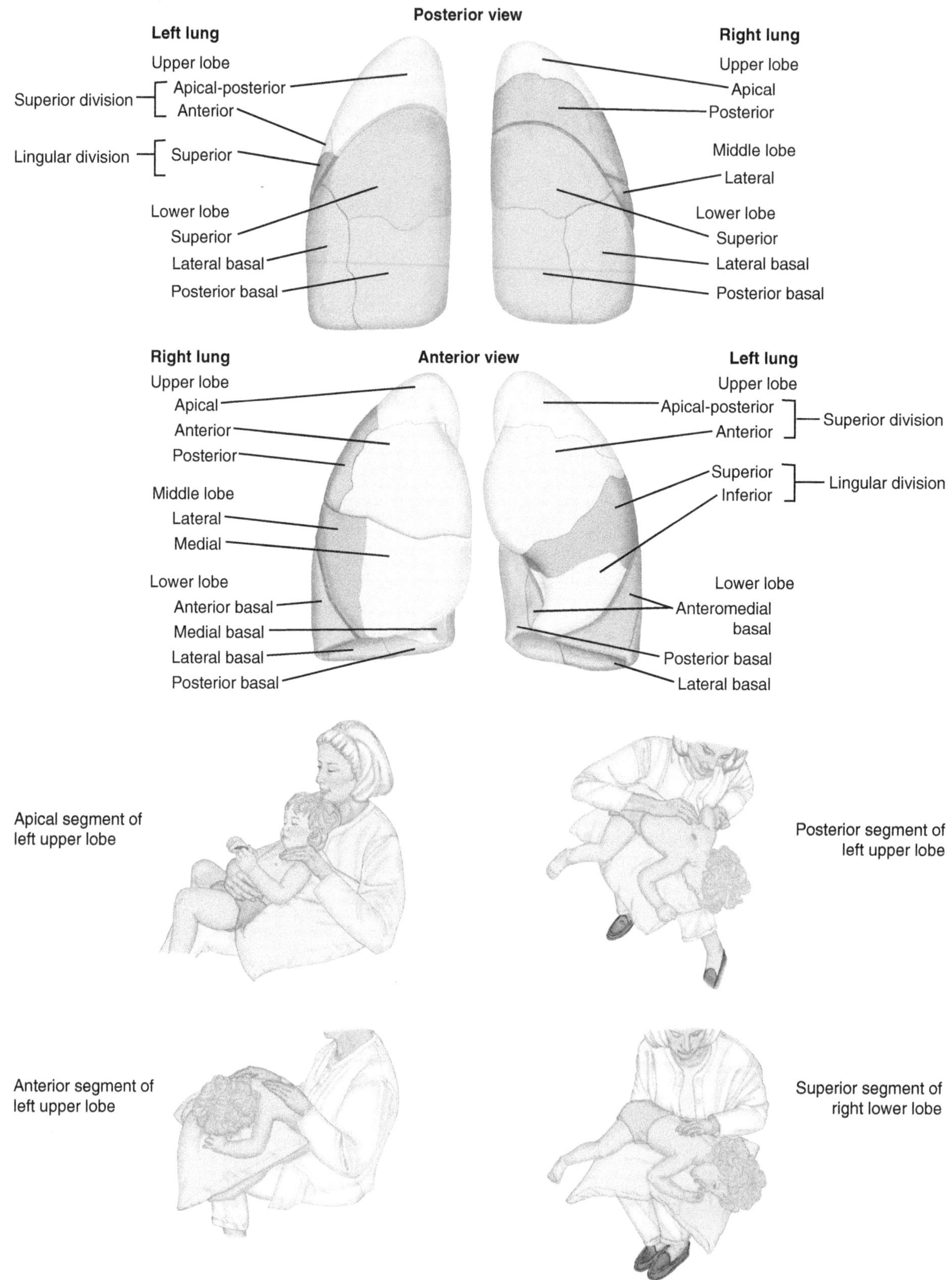

Fig. 25.10 Postural drainage. The positions for postural drainage are correlated with the segment being drained. (From McKinney, E. S., James, S. R., Murray, S. S., Nelson, K., & Ashwill, J. W. [2017]. *Maternal-child nursing* [5th ed.]. Philadelphia: Saunders.)

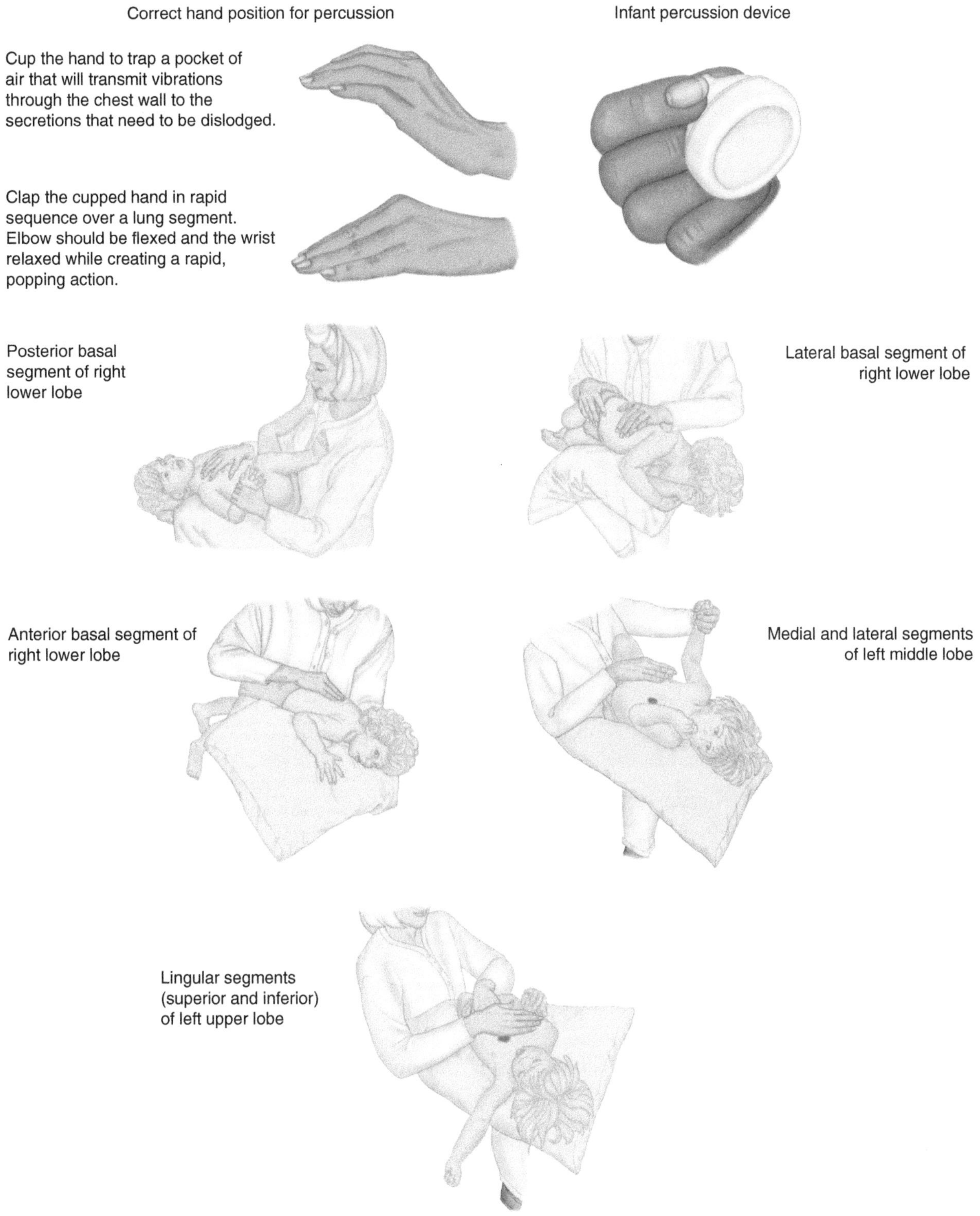

Correct hand position for percussion

Cup the hand to trap a pocket of air that will transmit vibrations through the chest wall to the secretions that need to be dislodged.

Clap the cupped hand in rapid sequence over a lung segment. Elbow should be flexed and the wrist relaxed while creating a rapid, popping action.

Infant percussion device

Posterior basal segment of right lower lobe

Lateral basal segment of right lower lobe

Anterior basal segment of right lower lobe

Medial and lateral segments of left middle lobe

Lingular segments (superior and inferior) of left upper lobe

Fig. 25.10, Cont'd

dren. Coping techniques must be developed and used.

Parents need explicit instructions regarding diet, medication, postural drainage, prevention of infection, rest, and continued medical supervision. Many families require the assistance of a social worker to secure funds for equipment and medications. Genetic counselling is also advised.

Emotional support. The child who is chronically ill can find it hard to accept restricted activity. The amount and types of diversion required vary in CF because the disease affects children of all ages and varies in severity.

Children generally benefit from simple, straightforward answers to questions about their illnesses. An uncomplicated diagram might be helpful. They should know why they must take medications with each meal, use the nebulizer, and have postural drainage. They should see and handle the unfamiliar equipment necessary for care.

The young child usually finds it more difficult to be separated from parents during hospitalization. Even when the prognosis is grave, a child's courage is sustained if parents are there. Rooming-in is encouraged whenever possible. Close contact by mail, telephone, text, or email with friends, school, church, and clubs is important for the school-age child. It is helpful for patients to develop an activity that they enjoy, such as music or art, as this can increase feelings of worth and provide outlets for the frustration of living with the disease. Consideration must be given to ways of fostering love, acceptance, trust, fair play, security, freedom of choice, creativity, and maintenance of self-identity.

Bronchopulmonary Dysplasia

Pathophysiology

Bronchopulmonary dysplasia (BPD) is a fibrosis, or thickening, of the alveolar walls and the bronchiolar epithelium. It occurs in premature infants (less than 32 weeks) who have abnormal or arrested lung development and who receive ventilation and oxygen for more than 28 days to survive (Lestrud, 2016). Swelling of the tissues causes edema, and the respiratory cilia are paralyzed by the high oxygen concentrations and lose their ability to clear mucus from the airways. Respiratory obstruction, mucous plugs, and atelectasis follow.

Prevention

Respiratory distress in the newborn is the major reason that oxygen and ventilators are used for prolonged periods. The main cause of respiratory distress in the newborn is prematurity. The goal of treatment for respiratory distress in the newborn should be to administer only the amount of oxygen required to prevent hypoxia, at the minimum necessary ventilator pressures, so as to prevent tissue trauma. The use of antenatal steroids to hasten lung development during preterm labour and the administration of surfactant within 15 minutes after birth in a very premature infant may prevent respiratory distress that would necessitate oxygen and prolonged ventilation treatment.

Symptoms

Symptoms of chronic respiratory distress include the following:

- Wheezing
- Retractions
- Cyanosis on exertion
- Use of accessory respiratory muscles
- Clubbing of the fingers (see Fig. 26.4)
- Failure to thrive
- Irritability caused by hypoxia

Treatment

After BPD has developed, the goal of therapy is to reduce inflammation of the airway and to wean the infant from the mechanical ventilator. The infant may become oxygen dependent and develop reactive airway bronchoconstriction. Noninvasive ventilation techniques such as positive pressure ventilation (PPV) with nasal continuous positive airway pressure (CPAP) has been found to decrease the risk of barotrauma and oxygen toxicity. Right-sided heart failure may also develop. Fluid restriction, bronchodilators, and diuretics may be prescribed. A tracheostomy may also be needed. Nasogastric tube feedings may be required to conserve energy while maintaining adequate nutrition. Infants with BPD often develop respiratory stridor and retractions with even minor respiratory infections, which result in repeated hospitalizations.

Ongoing home care is required, and respiratory problems persist through adulthood. Maintaining optimum growth and development is a challenge. Education and support of the family for a technology-dependent child at home are essential, as is a multidisciplinary health care team approach.

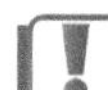
Safety Alert!

When oxygen is used in the home, the family should be taught safety precautions to prevent fire and injury.

Sudden Infant Death Syndrome

Sudden infant death syndrome (SIDS) is clinically defined as the sudden, unexpected death of an apparently healthy infant younger than 1 year of age, for which a routine autopsy fails to identify the cause. It is also referred to as "crib death" or sudden unexplained infant death (SUID). It is the leading cause of postneonatal deaths between 1 and 12 months. The peak incidence is between 2 and 4 months of age. The clinical features of the disease remain constant:

- Death occurs during sleep.
- The infant does not cry or make other sounds of distress.

The risk for SIDS is 6.6 times higher when children sleep on their stomach than on their back. Other risk factors for SIDS include intrauterine exposure to environmental tobacco use, and the use of alcohol or illicit substances by the mother. The use of soft mattresses, pillows, and comforters in the crib and an overheated environment are also risk factors for SIDS. The practice of bed sharing with the infant and parent is a significant risk factor for SIDS. Breastfeeding may help protect the infant from SIDS, and the use of pacifiers reduces the risk. Male infants are more at risk for SIDS. Premature or preterm infants may have a reduced arousal response that contributes to the development of SIDS. A newborn that has experienced an apparent life-threatening event (ALTE), which is sudden apnea, cyanosis, hypotonia, and gasping, also presents a significant risk factor for SIDS. Infants should have some time in the prone position (tummy time) when awake and should be observed.

The occurrence of SIDS in Canada has decreased significantly since the 1992 initiation of the "Safe Sleep" campaign, which urges parents to place their babies on their back for sleep. The decline in rates of SIDS may be partly a result of changes in parental behaviour, such as placing infants on their back to sleep and decreasing maternal smoking during pregnancy (Government of Canada, CPS, Canadian Foundation for the Study of Infant Deaths, et al., 2018). SIDS rates are roughly three times higher than the national rate among Indigenous populations (Asuri, Ryan, & Arbour, 2011). The higher rate may be due to a number of factors, including poverty, poor living conditions, overcrowding, lack of access to prenatal care, and smoking during pregnancy (Sheppard, Shapiro, Bushnik, et al., 2017).

Prevention

Infants should be placed in a supine position on a firm mattress with no extra bedding, pillows, or bumper pads surrounding the infant. The crib should meet Canadian regulations. Nurses need to be role models in health care facilities for the "Safe Sleep" campaign by placing infants on their back for sleep.

The use of a pacifier may be protective although recommendations are to use a pacifier after breastfeeding has been well established (Ponti & CPS Community Paediatrics Committee, 2003/2018). For high-risk infants, home apnea monitors have been used to warn parents of an impending problem and enable them to try to resuscitate the infant manually, but the effectiveness as a SIDS prevention has not been established. All parents are recommended to have training in cardiopulmonary resuscitation (CPR). Infants who share a room with a parent or caregiver have a lower risk of SIDs, but sharing the bed is discouraged (CPS, Canadian Foundation for Study of Infant Deaths, Canadian Institute for Child Health, et al., 2011).

When infants are in car seats, care should be taken to avoid flexion of the infant's head so that the chin rests on the chest, as this can cause oxygen desaturation and hypoxia. Car seats should not be used as a prolonged sleeping arrangement (CPS et al., 2011). When an infant is placed in a "sling carrier," care should be taken that the infant's face is above the fabric and the nose and mouth are unobstructed.

Safety Alert!

The Canadian Paediatric Society recommends that all healthy infants be placed on their backs for sleep to help prevent the occurrence of SIDS.

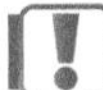

Safety Alert!

Infants should not remain in car seats for a prolonged period of time because when the infant's chin rests on the chest, hypoxia can occur.

Nursing care

When an infant succumbs to SIDS, in talking with the grieving parents, the nurse must convey some important facts: that the infant died of a disease entity called sudden infant death syndrome, that currently the disease cannot be predicted or prevented, and that they are *not* responsible for the child's death. The parents need time to say good-bye to their child. They should be encouraged to hold and rock the infant, shed tears, and assist in burial preparations. This process is conducive to the resolution of grief.

Parents can experience much guilt and are catapulted into a totally unexpected bereavement that creates the need for numerous explanations to relatives and friends. Often needless blame has been placed on one parent by the other or by relatives. There have been crib deaths for which parents have been mistakenly charged with child abuse. The family babysitter and health care provider may also be targets of attack. Emergency department personnel must be especially sensitive and supportive during this crisis.

Get Ready for the Certification Examination!

Key Points

- Routine hand hygiene can prevent the spread of the common cold.
- Quiet play may be more restful than confinement to bed for toddlers and young children.
- Use of nose drops with an oil base should be avoided.
- The maxillary and ethmoid sinuses are most often involved in childhood sinusitis.
- Periorbital cellulitis is a complication of childhood sinusitis.
- Laryngomalacia and acute spasmodic laryngitis are benign forms of croup.
- Laryngotracheobronchitis and epiglottitis are acute types of croup.
- A tongue blade examination of the throat can cause sudden respiratory arrest in a child with epiglottitis.
- Pneumothorax symptoms are sudden or gradual onset of symptoms with asymmetrical chest movements.
- Pulse oximetry readings are of little value in carbon monoxide poisoning.
- An intubation tray should be readily available at the bedside for infants with carbon monoxide poisoning.
- Frequent swallowing while the child is sleeping is an early sign of bleeding immediately after a tonsillectomy.

- Coughing, clearing the throat, and blowing the nose should be avoided in the immediate postoperative period after a tonsillectomy.
- Symptoms of asthma can be prevented when children and families are taught appropriate environmental control and how to avoid triggers.
- Swimming and sports activities that involve intermittent activity are well tolerated by asthmatic children.
- Cystic fibrosis is a multisystem disease characterized by an increased viscosity of mucous gland secretions.
- Bulky, frothy, foul-smelling stools are characteristic of cystic fibrosis.
- An infant should be positioned for sleep on the back, on a firm mattress without pillows or blankets. A car seat should not be used as a prolonged sleeping arrangement for infants.

Additional Learning Resources

evolve Go to your Evolve website (http://evolve.elsevier.com/Canada/Leifer) for the following learning resources:

- Answer Key for Critical Thinking Questions
- Answer Key for Textbook Review Questions
- Audio Glossary
- Interactive Review Questions
- Skills Performance Checklists
- Video clips and more!

Online Resources

- Asthma Canada, *Guidelines for the Diagnosis and Management of Asthma:* https://www.asthma.ca/get-help/asthma-3/control/asthma-action-plan
- Centers for Disease Control and Prevention, *Respiratory Syncytial Virus Infection (RSV):* https://www.cdc.gov/rsv
- Cystic Fibrosis Canada, *Clinical Care Guidelines:* https://www.cff.org/Care/Clinical-Care-Guidelines/

Review Questions

1. Which is a priority nursing diagnosis in a child admitted with acute asthma?
   a. Risk for infection
   b. Imbalanced nutrition
   c. Ineffective breathing pattern
   d. Disturbed body image
2. Which sign or symptom observed in a sleeping 2-year-old child immediately after a tonsillectomy necessitates reporting and follow-up care?
   a. A pulse of 110 beats/min
   b. A blood pressure of 96/64 mm Hg
   c. Nausea
   d. Frequent swallowing
3. The nurse is reinforcing teaching concerning the use of a cromolyn sodium inhaler for a 10-year-old with asthma. What should the nurse emphasize?
   a. You should use the inhaler whenever you feel some difficulty in breathing.
   b. You should use the inhaler between meals.
   c. You should use the inhaler regularly every day even if you are symptom free.
   d. You can discontinue using the inhaler when you are feeling stronger.
4. A health care provider is preparing to examine the throat of a child diagnosed with acute epiglottitis. What is the nursing priority?
   a. Have a tracheotomy set at the bedside.
   b. Immobilize the child's head.
   c. Restrain the child's arms.
   d. Have oxygen available.
5. An infant is admitted with a diagnosis of respiratory syncytial virus (RSV) infection. Which type of isolation would the nurse prepare for the child?
   a. Routine precautions
   b. Droplet precautions
   c. Contact precautions
   d. Airborne infection isolation precautions
6. Which of the following foods would be appropriate to offer a child following a tonsillectomy? *(Select all that apply.)*
   a. Low-fat milk
   b. Orange juice
   c. Clear carbonated soft drink
   d. Vanilla flavoured popsicle
   e. Yellow gelatin

Critical Thinking Question

1. The father of a child diagnosed with cystic fibrosis visits his child in the hospital. He states that he thinks the hospital food does not agree with his child because he notices the child has a loose stool with a very bad odour. None of his other children have that type of stool. He brought some loperamide pills from the drugstore to give to the child. What is the best response of the nurse?

REFERENCES

Allen, U. D., & Canadian Paediatric Society (CPS), Infectious Diseases and Immunization Committee. (2013). The use of antiviral drugs for influenza: Guidance for practitioners, 2012/2013; Paediatric summary. *Paediatrics & Child Health, 18*(3), 155–158. Reaffirmed 2018. Retrieved from https://www.ncbi.nlm.nih.gov/pmc/articles/PMC3680290/.

Asthma Canada. (2019). *Delivery devices: Home delivery devices*. Retrieved from https://www.asthma.ca/get-help/asthma-3/treatment/how-to-use/.

Asuri, S., Ryan, A. C., & Arbour, L. (2011). *Report 1—Sleep practices among Inuit infants and the prevention of SIDS*. Retrieved from https://www.itk.ca/wp-content/uploads/2016/07/2011-Report-Sleep-Practices-among-Inuit-Infants-and-the-Prevention-of-SIDS.pdf.

Banerji, A., Greenberg, D., White, L., et al. (2009). Risk factors and viruses associated with hospitalization due to lower respiratory tract infections in Canadian Inuit children. A case control study. *Pediatric Infectious Disease Journal, 28*(8), 102 697–701. https://doi.org/10.1097/INF.0b013e31819f1f89.

Canadian Institutes of Health Research (CIHR). (2016). *Could asthma start with your gut? How our gut bugs can influence our health*. Retrieved from http://www.cihr-irsc.gc.ca/e/49726.html.

Canadian Paediatric Society (CPS). (2016). *Colds in children*. Retrieved from https://www.caringforkids.cps.ca/handouts/colds_in_children.

Canadian Paediatric Society (CPS), Canadian Foundation for Study of Infant Deaths, Canadian Institute for Child Health., et al. (2011). *Joint statement on safe sleep: Preventing sudden infant deaths in Canada*. Ottawa: PHAC. Retrieved from http://www.phac-aspc.gc.ca/hp-ps/dca-dea/stages-etapes/childhood-enfance_0-2/sids/pdf/jsss-ecss2011-eng.pdf.

Crowe, J. (2016). Respiratory syncytial virus. In R. Kliegman, B. Stanton, J. St. Geme, et al. (Eds.), *Nelson textbook of pediatrics* (20th ed.). Philadelphia: Saunders.

Cystic Fibrosis Canada. (2019a). *What is cystic fibrosis?* Retrieved from http://www.cysticfibrosis.ca/about-cf/what-is-cystic-fibrosis.

Cystic Fibrosis Canada. (2019b). *Introduction to treatment options*. Retrieved from http://www.cysticfibrosis.ca/about-cf/living-with-cystic-fibrosis/introduction-to-treatment-options.

Egan, M., Green, D., & Voynow, J. (2016). Cystic fibrosis. In R. Kliegman, B. Stanton, J. St. Geme, et al. (Eds.), *Nelson textbook of pediatrics* (20th ed.). Philadelphia: Saunders.

Friedman, J. N., Rieder, M. J., Walton, J. M., et al. (2014). *Canadian Pediatric Society Position statement: Bronchiolitis: Recommendations for diagnosis, monitoring and management of children one to 24 months of age*. Reaffirmed 2018. Retrieved from https://www.cps.ca/en/documents/position/bronchiolitis.

Government of Canada. (2015). *Asthma*. Retrieved from https://www.canada.ca/en/public-health/services/chronic-diseases/chronic-respiratory-diseases/asthma.html.

Government of Canada. (2018). *Canadian immunization guide: Part 1—Key immunization information*. Retrieved from https://www.canada.ca/en/public-health/services/canadian-immunization-guide.html.

Government of Canada, Canadian Paediatric Society (CPS), the Canadian Foundation for the Study of Infant Deaths., et al. (2018). *Joint statement on safe sleep: Preventing sudden infant deaths in Canada*. Retrieved from https://www.canada.ca/en/public-health/services/health-promotion/childhood-adolescence/stages-childhood/infancy-birth-two-years/safe-sleep/joint-statement-on-safe-sleep.html.

Lestrud, S. (2016). Bronchopulmonary dysplasia. In R. Kliegman, B. Stanton, J. St. Geme, et al. (Eds.), *Nelson textbook of pediatrics* (20th ed.). Philadelphia: Saunders.

Li, W., Sun, L., Corey, M., et al. (2011). Understanding the population structure of North American patients with cystic fibrosis. *Clinical Genetics, 79*(2), 136–146. https://doi.org/10.1111/j.1399-0004.2010.01502.x.

Mak, D. Y. F., Sykes, J., Stephenson, A. L., et al. (2016). The benefits of newborn screening for cystic fibrosis: The Canadian experience. *Journal of Cystic Fibrosis, 15*(3), 302–308. https://doi.org/10.1016/j.jcf.2016.04.001.

Milgrom, H., & Sicherer, S. (2016). Allergic rhinitis. In R. Kliegman, B. Stanton, J. St. Geme, et al. (Eds.), *Nelson textbook of pediatrics* (20th ed.). Philadelphia: Saunders.

Moore, D. L., & Canadian Paediatric Society (CPS), Infectious Diseases and Immunization Committee. (2018). Vaccine recommendations for children and youth for the 2017/2018 influenza season. *Paediatrics & Child Health, 23*(1), e10–e13. Retrieved from https://academic.oup.com/pch/article/23/1/e10/4860355.

Nierengarten, M. (2016). Spirometry established asthma control in kids. *Contemporary Pediatrics, 33*(3), 20–24.

Ortiz-Alvarez, O., & Canadian Paediatric Society (CPS), Acute Care Committee. (2017). Acute management of croup in the emergency department. *Paediatrics & Child Health, 22*(3), 166–169.

Ortiz-Alvarez, O., Mikrogianakis, A., & Canadian Paediatric Society (CPS), Acute Care Committee. (2012). Managing the paediatric patient with an acute asthma exacerbation. *Paediatrics & Child Health, 17*(5), 251–255. Reaffirmed 2017.

Ponti, M., & Canadian Paediatrics Society (CPS), Community Paediatrics Committee. (2003). Recommendations for the use of pacifiers. *Paediatrics & Child Health, 8*(8), 515–519. Reaffirmed 2018. Retrieved from https://www.cps.ca/en/documents/position/pacifiers.

Robinson, J. L., Le Saux, N., & Canadian Paediatric Society (CPS), Infectious Diseases and Immunization Committee. (2015). Preventing hospitalizations for respiratory syncytial virus infection. *Paediatrics & Child Health, 20*(6), 321–326. Reaffirmed 2018. Retrieved from https://www.cps.ca/en/-documents/position/preventing-hospitalizations-for-rsv-infections.

Roosevelt, G. E. (2016). Acute inflammatory upper airway obstruction (croup, epiglottitis, laryngitis, and bacterial tracheitis). In R. Kliegman, B. Stanton, J. St. Geme, et al. (Eds.), *Nelson textbook of pediatrics* (20th ed.). Philadelphia: Saunders.

Sheppard, A. J., Shapiro, G. D., Bushnik, T., et al. (2017). *Birth outcomes among First Nations, Inuit and Métis populations*. Retrieved from https://www150.statcan.gc.ca/n1/pub/82-003-x/2017011/article/54886-eng.htm.

Wetmore, R. (2016). Tonsils and adenoids. In R. Kliegman, B. Stanton, J. St. Geme, et al. (Eds.), *Nelson textbook of pediatrics* (20th ed.). Philadelphia: Saunders.

26 The Child With a Cardiovascular Condition

http://evolve.elsevier.com/Canada/Leifer

Keri-Ann Berga

Objectives

1. Define each key term listed.
2. Distinguish the differences between the cardiovascular system of the infant and that of the adult.
3. List the general signs and symptoms of congenital heart disease.
4. Describe screening techniques used for early identification of critical congenital heart disease.
5. Differentiate between atrial septal defect, ventricular septal defect, patent ductus arteriosus, coarctation of the aorta, and tetralogy of Fallot.
6. Discuss six nursing goals relevant to the child with heart failure.
7. List the symptoms of rheumatic fever.
8. Discuss the prevention of rheumatic fever.
9. Discuss hypertension in childhood.
10. Differentiate between primary and secondary hypertension.
11. Identify factors that can prevent hypertension.
12. Describe heart-healthy guidelines for children.
13. Recognize the manifestation of Kawasaki disease and the related nursing care.

Key Terms

acquired heart disease
carditis (kăhr-DĪ-tĭs)
chorea (kŏ-RĒ-ă)
congenital heart disease (CHD)
critical congenital heart disease (CCHD)
DASH diet
hemodynamics (hē-mō-dī-NĂM-ĭks)
hypothermia (hī-pō-THŬR-mē-ă)
Jones criteria
polyarthritis
polycythemia (pŏl-ē-sī-THĒ-mē-ă)
pulse pressure
rheumatic fever (RF)
shunt
stenosis
stroke volume
tachycardia
tachypnea
"tet" spells
thoracotomy (thŏ-ră-KŎT-ō-mē)

THE CARDIOVASCULAR SYSTEM

The cardiovascular system consists of the heart, the blood, and the blood vessels. The heart is a muscular organ with four chambers, with the primary purpose of pumping blood throughout the body. The cardiovascular system develops between the third and the eighth weeks of gestation. It is the first system to function in intrauterine life. There are various critical developmental moments that need to occur during this time.

Following the anatomical development of the heart in utero, there are various physiological changes that must occur at birth for normal transition from fetal to newborn life. Establishing respirations is critical to the newborn's transition, as lungs become the organ of gas exchange after separation from maternal uteroplacental circulation. Over 90% of newborns make the transition from intrauterine life to extrauterine life without difficulty, requiring little to no assistance. Health care providers who care for newborns immediately after birth should have knowledge about newborn transition and should have skills in newborn resuscitation (Weiner & Zaichkin, 2016). See Fig. 3.7 for changes that occur in cardiovascular circulation at birth.

Because of anatomical and physiological immaturity, the cardiovascular system of the child differs from that of the adult. Fig. 26.1 summarizes some of these differences.

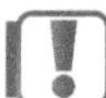

Safety Alert!

Pulse, respiration, blood pressure, and hematological values vary with the age of the child. Nurses need to be aware of what is appropriate for each age group.

SIGNS REALTED TO SUSPECTED CARDIAC PATHOLOGY

Although signs and symptoms of specific congenital heart diseases relate to the specific pathology involved, several signs and symptoms are common to most infants with congenital cardiac problems. When the nurse assesses the child, the following observations should be reported:

- Failure to thrive or poor weight gain
- Cyanosis, pallor

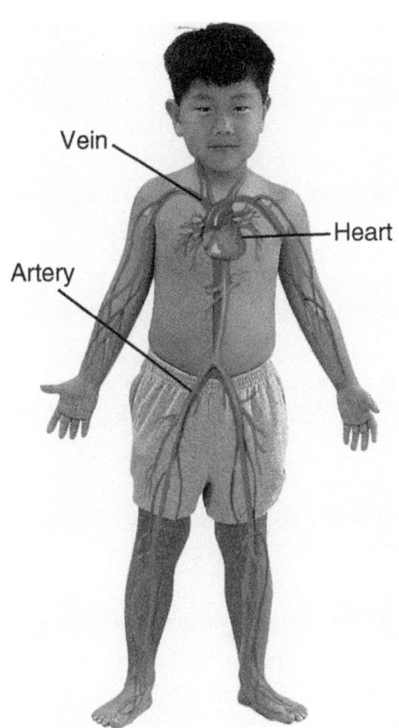

Vein
Heart
Artery
CARDIOVASCULAR SYSTEM
• Pulse, respiration, blood pressure, and hematological values vary with the age of the child.
• Chest walls are thin in infants and young children because of the relative lack of subcutaneous and muscle tissue compared with older children. "Innocent" murmurs can be heard in structurally normal hearts.
• The newborn's circulation differs from fetal circulation; if adaptations do not take place, congenital heart problems may arise.
• Capillary function is immature in newborns. It takes several weeks for the small capillaries to expand and contract in response to external temperatures.
• The heart rate is higher in newborns and infants than in adults.
• Children have limited ability to increase stroke volume in response to decreased cardiac output.
• Most heart conditions in children result from defects in embryonic structure.

Fig. 26.1 Summary of some cardiovascular system differences between the child and the adult. The cardiovascular system consists of the heart, blood, and blood vessels. As the heart beats, blood, oxygen, and nutrients are transported to all the tissues of the body, and waste products are removed. (Art overlay courtesy Observatory Group, Cincinnati, Ohio.)

- Visually observed pulsations in the neck veins
- Tachypnea, dyspnea
- Irregular pulse rate
- Clubbing of fingers
- Fatigue during feeding or activity
- Excessive perspiration, especially over forehead

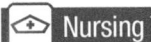

Bradycardia may be a sign that cardiovascular arrest is imminent in children with hypoxia.

CONGENITAL HEART DISEASE

When cardiovascular development is incomplete, heart defects or malformations may occur. Only about 10 to 15% of the etiologies of congenital heart disease (CHD) are known (Butler, Carvan, & Johnson, 2016). In about 8% of children with a CHD there is a clear genetic cause, and many cases are associated with chromosomal abnormalities. Children with other syndromes (e.g., Marfan, Williams, and DiGeorge syndromes) account for about 3% of children with CHD. Environmental factors account for about 2% of CHD, with fetal exposure to teratogens such as antiepileptic medications, warfarin, or alcohol or exposure to viral infections (e.g., rubella or cytomegalovirus) causing alteration in fetal development. In the remaining 85% there is no clear cause; it is thought to be multifactorial in nature, with inheritance, predisposition, and environmental triggers being responsible (Blackburn, 2013). Fetal echocardiography may detect intrauterine cardiac malformations in high-risk cases.

Critical congenital heart disease (CCHD) accounts for about 25% of all CHD that is diagnosed in Canada. CCHD can be any potentially life-threatening, duct-dependent defect by which infants will die or that will require surgical repair or intervention within the first 28 days of life to optimize health outcomes (Amsbaugh, Scott, & Foss, 2015; Wong, Fournier, Fruitman, et al., 2017).

Acquired heart disease occurs *after* birth, as a result of a defect or illness.

Pathophysiology

CHDs are not a problem for the fetus because the fetal–maternal circulation compensates for all fetal oxygen needs. At birth, however, the infant's circulatory system must take over and provide for the child's own oxygen needs. Any heart defect or patent (open) fetal pathways in the cardiovascular system after birth produce signs and symptoms that indicate an anatomical heart defect. CHD occurs in approximately 8 to 12 of 1 000 births, and 50% of these infants show signs and symptoms before the first year of life (Narvey, Wong, & Fournier, 2017; Wong et al., 2017). Some defects, such as mitral valve prolapse, may not manifest until later in life.

Of the congenital anomalies, heart defects are the principal cause of death during the first year of life. Therefore, nurses must stress the need for good prenatal care, advocate for access to care, and encourage parents to ensure regular checkups at well-baby clinics. Many heart murmurs have been detected early in infancy at periodic checkups.

Diagnosis

The appearance of clinical symptoms and the results of diagnostic tests aid in the diagnosis of CHD (Table 26.1). Early diagnosis of CCHD continues to be important for early intervention and treatment and optimal health outcomes. Pulse oximetry screening is safe, noninvasive, easy to perform, and proven to enhance detection

Table 26.1 Diagnostic Tests Used in Congenital Heart Disease

TEST	DEFINITION	VALUE
Angiocardiography (selective)	Serial X-ray films of the heart and great vessels after injection of an opaque substance; a radiopaque catheter is moved into the heart chambers, and contrast medium is injected in specific areas	Abnormal communications in the heart can be observed; the course of the blood through the heart and great vessels can be traced.
Aortography	X-ray films of the aorta after injection of an opaque material	Useful in showing patent ductus arteriosus.
Radionuclide angiocardiography	Noninvasive nuclear procedure that permits visualization of the course of blood through the heart	May be used as a precardiac catheterization screening study; provides assessment of congenital and acquired cardiovascular lesions and monitors the effects of therapy. Intravenous (IV) access is necessary to permit injection of the radionuclide.
Cardiac catheterization	A radiopaque catheter is passed through the femoral artery directly into the heart and large vessels	Shows blood pressure within the heart; health care provider can examine the heart closely with the tip of the catheter to detect abnormalities. Blood samples can be obtained to determine oxygen content.
Chest X-ray film	A radiographic image of a body structure	Provides a permanent record; shows abnormalities in the shape and position of heart.
Cineangiocardiography	Motion pictures of images recorded by fluoroscopy	Useful recording and monitoring device.
Echocardiography	The use of ultrasound to produce an image of sound waves of the heart; transducer is placed directly on chest; sounds are analyzed	Noninvasive procedure; localizes murmurs. It determines if heart is structurally normal.
Electrocardiogram	Tracing of heart action by electrocardiography	Detects variations in heart action and shows the condition of the heart muscle. It may also be used as a monitoring device during cardiac catheterization.
Magnetic resonance imaging (three-dimensional [3-D] imaging)	Noninvasive imaging technique that uses low-energy radio waves in combination with a magnetic field to generate signals that produce tomographic images	Useful in diagnosing coarctation of the aorta.

of CCHDs that have a hypoxemia component, such as hypoplastic left heart syndrome (HLHS), pulmonary atresia with intact septum, tricuspid atresia, total anomalous pulmonary venous connection (TAPVC), tetralogy of Fallot (TOF), transposition of the great arteries (TGA), and truncus arteriosus (Amsbaugh et al., 2015; Narvey et al., 2017; Wong et al., 2017). These are often referred to as *cyanotic heart diseases.*

Newborn screening recommendations

The Canadian Paediatric Society (CPS) recommends that pulse oximetry screening (POS) be initiated in all term and late preterm infants (gestational age 34 weeks up to full-term infants). Box 26.1 lists the conditions that can be detected using pulse oximetry in infants. POS can be performed any time after birth; however, the CPS recommends that it be completed between 24 and 36 hours of life in all asymptomatic newborns. If it is not possible to screen an infant during this time, it is still best to screen prior to 24 hours than to not screen at all.

Box 26.1 Heart Lesions Detectable Using Pulse Oximetry Screening

MOST CONSISTENTLT CYANOTIC

- Hypoplastic left heart syndrome
- Pulmonary atresia with intact ventricular septum
- Total anomalous pulmonary venous return
- Tetralogy of Fallot
- Transposition of the great arteries
- Tricuspid atresia
- Truncus arteriosus

MAY BE CYANOTIC

- Coarctation of the aorta
- Double outlet right ventricle
- Ebstein anomaly
- Interrupted aortic arch
- Defects with single ventricle physiology

Adapted from Narvey, M., Wong, K., Fournier, A., & Canadian Paediatric Society, Fetus and Newborn Committee. (2017). Pulse oximetry screening in newborns to enhance detection of critical congenital heart disease. *Paediatrics & Child Health, 22*(8), 494–498. Retrieved from https://www.cps.ca/en/documents/position/pulse-oximetry-screening

Oxygen saturations should be checked in the right hand and either foot of all newborns, and any differences in oxygen saturations should be assessed (Narvey et al., 2017). General screening can be completed in about 5 minutes. Refer to Fig. 26.2 for the screening algorithm that should be followed.

Newborns with failed screening results require thorough assessment by the most responsible health care provider. An assessment that includes four limb blood pressures, an electrocardiogram (ECG), and a chest X-ray may be helpful. If not already initiated, a pediatrician should be consulted, and when the most likely cause for a failed screening result appears to have a cardiac origin or remains unclear, a consult with pediatric cardiology followed by an echocardiogram is required to rule out CCHD.

Since many centres in Canada require transport to a tertiary centre, it is important that nurses help minimize false-positive test results by completing this screening assessment carefully and within the recommended time period, if possible.

Treatment

The treatment of most cardiac defects is surgical. A **thoracotomy** (chest incision) is performed, and the use of a cardiopulmonary bypass machine and hypothermia during the procedure minimizes blood loss and enhances patient recovery. **Hypothermia** (*hypo,* "under," and *thermal,* "heat") reduces the temperature of body tissues, resulting in a decreased need for oxygen. The cardiopulmonary bypass machine provides oxygenation of the body tissues while the surgeon stops the heart to perform surgery. Heart transplants may be the treatment of choice in cases such as a three-chambered heart. Interventional cardiac catheterization can correct some heart defects without open heart surgery.

Classification

Heart defects can be divided into two categories: cyanotic and acyanotic. A more accurate classification is based on the effect of the defect on blood circulation. The study of blood circulation is termed **hemodynamics** (*hemo,* "blood," and *dynamics,* "power"). Blood always flows from an area of high pressure to an area of low pressure and takes the path of least resistance. Physiologically, defects can be organized into (1) lesions that increase pulmonary blood flow, (2) lesions that restrict blood flow, and (3) lesions that decrease pulmonary blood flow. There are also lesions that result in mixed oxygenated and nonoxygenated blood. A **shunt** refers to the flow of blood through an abnormal opening

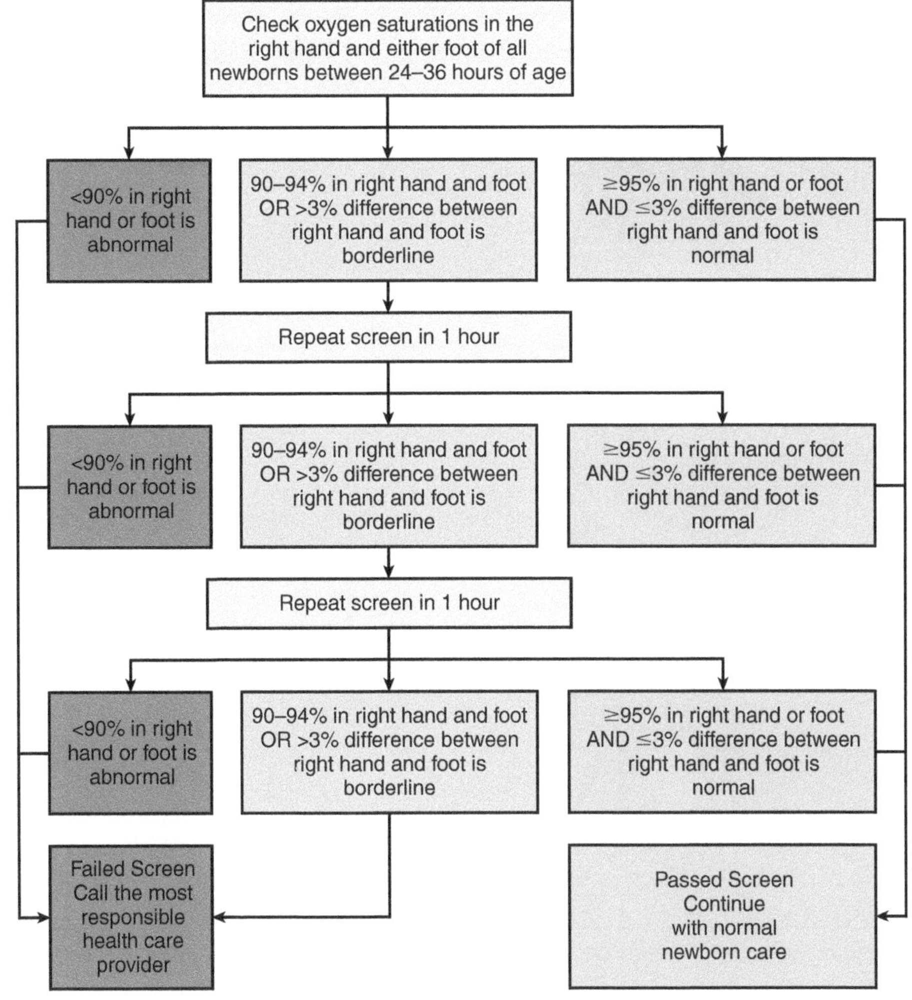

Fig. 26.2 Pulse oximetry screening algorithm. (From Narvey, M., Wong, K., Fournier, A., & Canadian Paediatric Society Fetus and Newborn Committee. [2017]. Pulse oximetry screening in newborns to enhance detection of critical congenital heart disease *Paediatrics & Child Health, 22*[8], 494–498. Retrieved from https://www.cps.ca/en/documents/position/pulse-oximetry-screening)

between two vessels of the heart. Fig. 26.3 compares the normal heart and the heart with various congenital defects.

Defects that increase pulmonary blood flow

Heart defects that cause the blood to return to the right ventricle and recirculate through the lungs before exiting the left ventricle through the aorta are known as defects that increase pulmonary blood flow. For example, the defect in the atrial septum in the fetus allows blood to flow from the right atrium through the defect into the left atrium, providing a bypass of the lungs. After birth, the pressure is higher in the left atrium; if the atrial opening persists, the blood flows back into the right atrium *(left-to-right shunt)* and then recirculates to the lungs, causing increased pulmonary flow. Some defects that increase pulmonary flow are atrial septal defect, ventricular septal defect, and patent ductus arteriosus (see Fig. 26.3). In heart defects that result in increased pulmonary flow because of a left-to-right shunt, the oxygenated blood recirculates to the lungs, and cyanosis is rare.

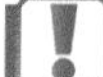

Safety Alert!

In congenital heart disease, cyanosis is *not always* a clinical sign.

Atrial septal defect. Atrial septal defect (ASD) involves an abnormal opening between the right and left atria. Blood that already contains oxygen is forced from the left atrium back to the right atrium. Most patients do not have symptoms. The defect may be recognized when a murmur is heard during a routine health examination. Cardiac catheterization, ECG, and echocardiography may be performed to help confirm the diagnosis. Spontaneous closure sometimes occurs.

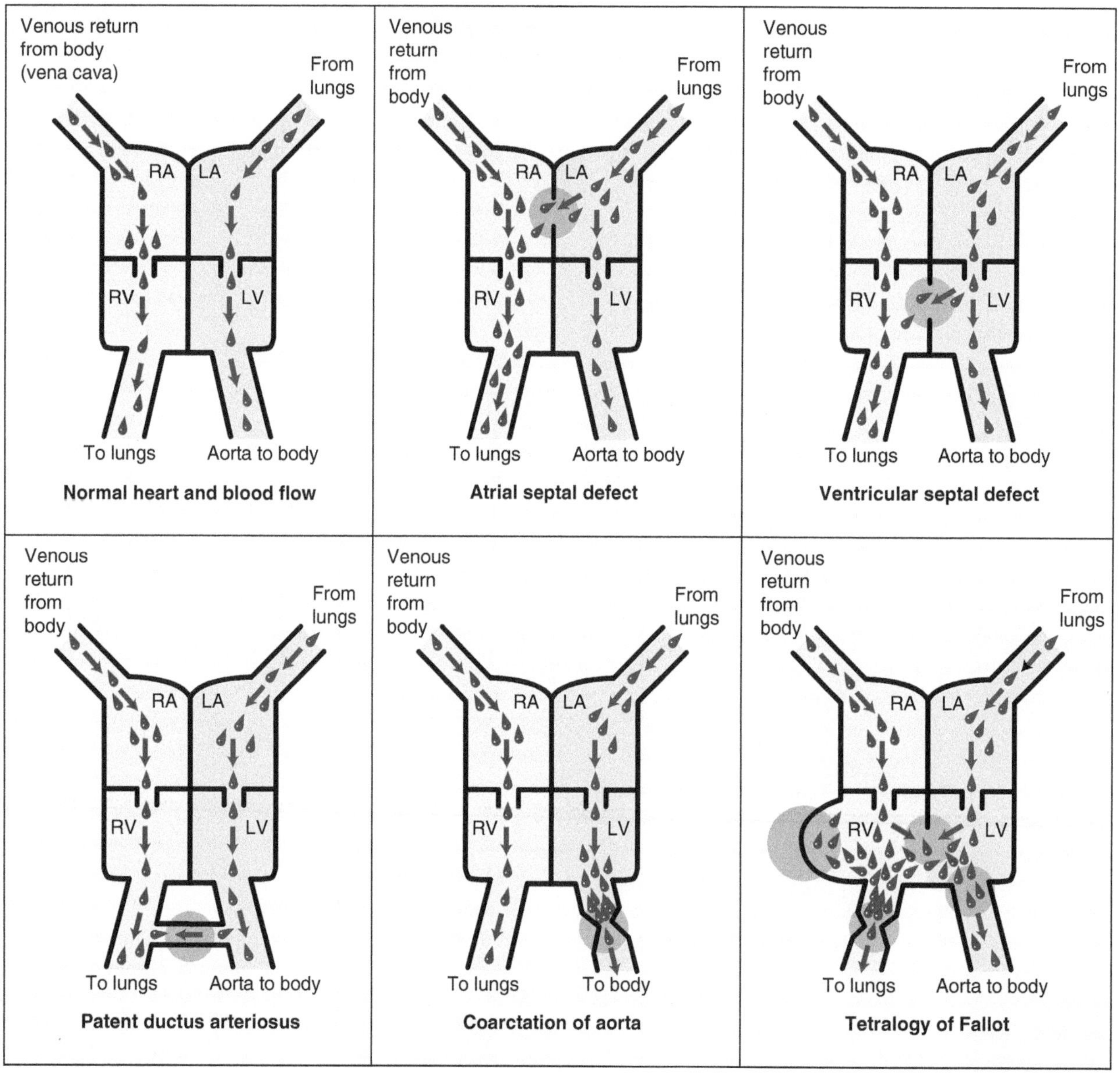

Fig. 26.3 The normal heart and various congenital heart defects. *LA*, Left atrium; *LV*, left ventricle; *RA*, right atrium; *RV*, right ventricle.

The surgical repair involves application of a surgical Dacron patch or repair with open cardiac surgery or robotic surgery using a portion of the pericardium to secure a patch. Nonsurgical closure during cardiac catheterization can sometimes be accomplished. Continued cardiology follow-up is necessary. Low-dose aspirin therapy is usually prescribed for 6 months after repair. Untreated children are at risk for stroke. Children usually recover well from ASD repairs.

Ventricular septal defect. Ventricular septal defect (VSD) is the most common heart anomaly, in which there is an opening between the right and left ventricles of the heart. Increased pressure within the left ventricle forces blood back into the right ventricle (left-to-right shunt). A loud, harsh murmur combined with a systolic thrill is characteristic of this defect. The condition may be mild or severe. It is often associated with other defects. Many children with small defects may experience spontaneous closure during the first year of life as a result of growth.

Early surgical intervention has a low risk for most infants, and the prognosis is excellent. Normal growth and development are usually achieved within 1 or 2 years after surgery.

Open heart surgery is performed under hypothermia. With the use of the heart–lung bypass machine the condition can be corrected in a fairly dry or bloodless field. The hole is ligated (closed) with sutures or a synthetic patch.

Patent ductus arteriosus. The circulation of the fetus differs from that of the newborn in that most of the fetal blood bypasses the lungs. The ductus arteriosus is the passageway (shunt) through which the blood crosses from the pulmonary artery to the aorta and avoids the deflated lungs. This vessel closes shortly after birth; when it does not close, blood continues to pass from the aorta, where the pressure is higher, into the pulmonary artery. This causes oxygenated blood to recycle through the lungs, overburdening the pulmonary circulation and making the heart pump harder.

The symptoms of patent ductus arteriosus (PDA) may go unnoticed during infancy. As the child grows, dyspnea is experienced, the radial pulse becomes full and bounding on exertion, and there is an unusually wide range between systolic and diastolic blood pressures. This is referred to as the **pulse pressure**. A characteristic machinery type of murmur may be heard. A two-dimensional echocardiogram is useful in visualizing and determining blood flow across the PDA.

PDA is one of the more common cardiac anomalies. It occurs twice as frequently in girls as in boys. Premature infants with hypoxia often respond to intravenous (IV) indomethacin or IV ibuprofen drug therapy that results in closure of the PDA. The ductus may be ligated via the visually assisted thoracoscopic surgery (VATS) technique. Nonsurgical options include the insertion of coils to occlude the PDA, which is done in a cardiac catheterization lab. Prostaglandin E_1 may be administered to maintain patency of the ductus arteriosus until surgery can be performed when an anomaly such as hypoplastic heart is diagnosed in the newborn. The prognosis is excellent.

Defects that restrict ventricular blood flow

Some congenital cardiac defects can restrict blood flow from the ventricles because of a **stenosis** (narrowing) of a vessel.

Coarctation of the aorta. The word *coarctation* means "a tightening." In coarctation of the aorta, there is a constriction or narrowing of the aortic arch or of the descending aorta (i.e., the blood meets an obstruction) (see Fig. 26.3). Hemodynamics consist of increased pressure proximal to the defect and decreased pressure distally. The characteristic symptoms are a marked difference in the blood pressure and pulses of the upper and lower extremities. The patient may not develop symptoms until late in childhood. Some children may state they have leg pain after exercise. X-ray examination may show cardiac enlargement and "notching" of the ribs, caused by vessels developed as collateral circulation. Two-dimensional echocardiography can aid in the diagnosis. If the condition is untreated, hypertension, heart failure (HF), and infective endocarditis may develop. Treatment depends on the type and severity of the defect. Infants who have associated HF are treated medically until the optimal time for surgery.

Percutaneous balloon angioplasty is the treatment of choice for older children, and stents can be inserted to maintain patency. The surgeon resects the narrowed portion of the aorta and joins its ends. The joining is called an *anastomosis*. As in PDA, closed heart surgery is performed because the structures are outside the heart. The prognosis is good if there are no other defects and the child's physical condition is favourable at the time of surgery. If restenosis occurs after surgery for coarctation, a balloon angioplasty can relieve the obstruction.

The nurse should observe the child after coarctation surgery for the development of hypertension and abdominal pain associated with nausea and vomiting, leukocytosis, and gastrointestinal bleeding or obstruction. Antihypertensive medications, steroids, and nasogastric tube decompression are the priority treatments for these postsurgical complications.

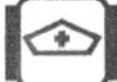 **Nursing Tip**

The systolic blood pressure is normally 10–15 mm Hg higher in the legs than the arms. Systolic blood pressure that is lower in the legs than in the arms should be reported, as this could be a sign of coarctation of the aorta.

 **Safety Alert!**

A significant difference in the blood pressure between the upper extremities and the lower extremities is a characteristic sign of coarctation of the aorta.

Defects that decrease pulmonary blood flow

A decrease in pulmonary blood flow occurs when a congenital heart anomaly allows blood that has not passed through the lungs *(unoxygenated blood)* to enter the aorta and the general circulation. Cyanosis caused by the presence of unoxygenated blood in the circulation is a characteristic feature of this type of congenital heart anomaly.

Tetralogy of Fallot. *Tetra* means "four." In *tetralogy of Fallot* there are four defects:

1. Stenosis or narrowing of the pulmonary artery, which decreases the blood flow to the lungs
2. Hypertrophy of the right ventricle, which enlarges because it must work harder to pump blood through the narrow pulmonary artery
3. Dextroposition (*dextro,* "right," and *position*) of the aorta, in which the aorta is displaced to the right and blood from both ventricles enters it
4. VSD (see Fig. 26.3)

When venous blood enters the aorta, the child displays symptoms of cardiac problems. Cyanosis increases with age, and clubbing of the fingers and toes is seen (Fig. 26.4).

The child rests in a "squatting" position to breathe more easily. This position alters systemic venous return. Feeding problems, growth restriction, frequent respiratory infections, and severe dyspnea on exertion are prevalent. The red blood cells (RBCs) of the body increase, causing **polycythemia** (*poly,* "many," *cyt,* "cells," and *hema,* "blood") to compensate for the lack of oxygen.

Narrowing of the pulmonary artery causes HF as a result of the increased muscular force necessary to propel blood through the narrowed orifice. When unoxygenated blood enters the general circulation, *hypoxia* occurs and may be manifested by cyanosis.

The increased oxygen consumption and decreased energy and ability to eat result in failure to thrive.

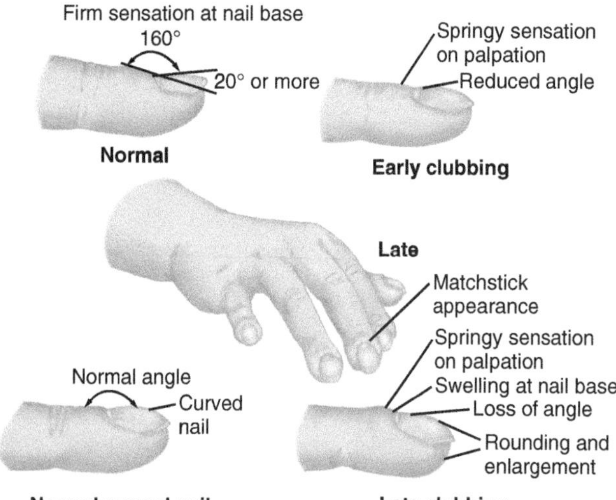

Fig. 26.4 Clubbing of the fingernails may indicate chronic hypoxemia. (From James, S. R., Nelson, K., & Ashwill, A. [2012]. *Nursing care of children: Principles and practices* [4th ed.]. Philadelphia: Saunders.)

Multiple hospitalizations, cyanotic skin, and limited energy can impede growth and development both physically and socially.

Paroxysmal hypercyanotic episodes, or **"tet" spells**, occur during the first 2 years of life. Spontaneous cyanosis, respiratory distress, weakness, and syncope occur. They can last a few minutes to a few hours and are followed by lethargy and sleep. Parents and day care personnel must be instructed to place the child in a knee–chest position when a tet spell occurs (Fig. 26.5). Often the child will pause and voluntarily squat in position until the attack abates. Recovery from the tet spell is usually rapid.

Diagnosis of TOF is confirmed by a chest X-ray study that shows a typical boot-shaped heart. An ECG, three-dimensional echocardiography, and cardiac catheterization aid in confirming the diagnosis.

Complications such as cerebral thrombosis caused by polycythemia (thickened blood as a result of increased RBCs) are a problem, especially if dehydration occurs. Iron deficiency anemia develops because of decreased appetite and increased energy required to suck or eat. Bacterial endocarditis can occur but can be prevented with prophylactic antibiotic therapy.

Treatment is designed to increase pulmonary blood flow to relieve hypoxia. A Blalock-Taussig (B-T) surgical procedure (temporary shunt) can be performed successfully on newborns or premature infants. Open heart surgery allows for total correction of all defects and is usually performed, with excellent results, at 4 months to 2 years of age. The nurse should be observant for signs of HF and an irregular heartbeat postoperatively.

Nursing Tip

There are four defects in tetralogy of Fallot:

1. Pulmonary artery stenosis
2. Hypertrophy of the right ventricle
3. Dextroposition of aorta
4. Ventricular septal defect

Defects that cause mixed pathology

Hypoplastic left heart syndrome. In hypoplastic left heart syndrome there is an underdevelopment of the left side of the heart, usually resulting in an absent or nonfunctional left ventricle and hypoplasia of the ascending aorta. This condition can be diagnosed before birth and the infant placed immediately on a transplant list so that surgery can be performed soon after birth. The initial survival of the infant depends on a patent foramen ovale and ductus arteriosus to provide a pathway for oxygenated blood to the general body system. Prostaglandin E_1 is administered to maintain patency of the ductus arteriosus. Other serious congenital anomalies may be present, and the infant should be carefully assessed.

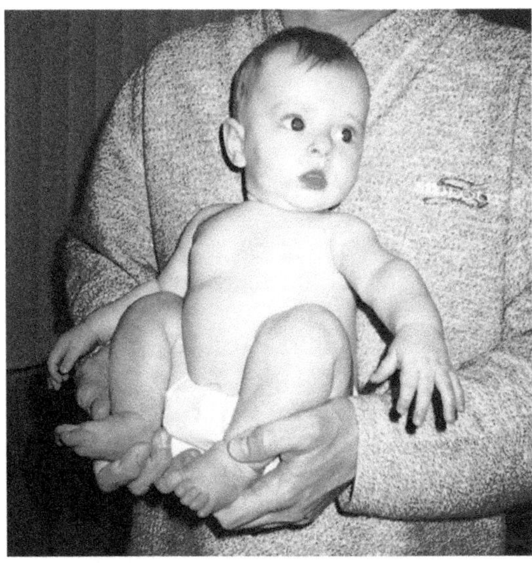
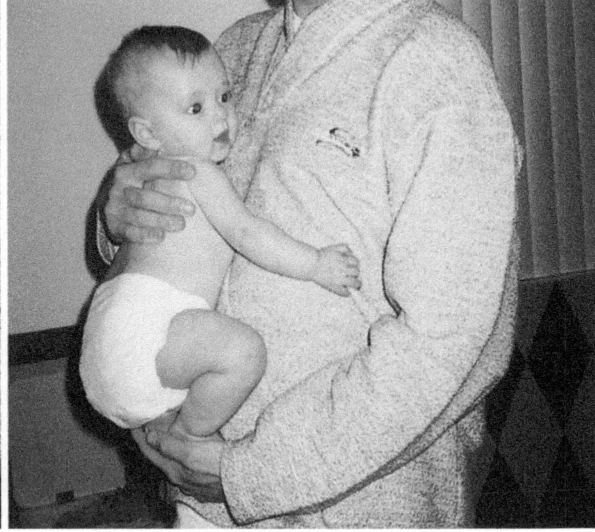

Fig. 26.5 Tet position. Infants and children with tetralogy of Fallot can have paroxysmal hypercyanosis or "tet" spells. Placing the child in the tet position (a knee–chest position) will relieve these symptoms. Older children will spontaneously squat when a tet spell occurs.

Symptoms include a greyish-blue colour of the skin and mucous membranes and signs of HF, including dyspnea, weak pulses, and a cardiac murmur. Survival beyond the first few months of life without intervention is rare. A three-stage surgical procedure can be life-saving if a heart is not available for transplant. With the advent of successful heart transplants, however, the prognosis for these infants is much brighter, and emphasis is placed on maintaining life and hope until an appropriate heart is available for transplant. After a transplant, immunosuppressive therapy to prevent organ rejection is required.

General Treatment and Nursing Care of Children With Congenital Heart Disease

Recent technological advances have enabled therapeutic catheterization procedures for valvuloplasty, angioplasty, and other corrections of pediatric heart pathologies as alternatives to open heart surgery. After the procedure, the nursing care involves monitoring vital signs, observing for thrombosis formation, assessing peripheral (i.e., femoral and pedal) pulses, and performing neurovascular checks of each limb. This neurovascular assessment is often referred to as the "6 P's," which includes assessing for any **p**ain, **p**allor, **p**ulselessness, **p**aresthesia, **p**ressure, and **p**aralysis, which may indicate severe occlusion or peripheral vascular insufficiencies (see Skill 24.1). In most cases, hospitalization after cardiac catheterization is limited to 2 or 3 days.

Emotional support of the family and education concerning what to do and expect during and after therapy is a nursing responsibility. Parents must be guided to understand that the child should not be overprotected or restricted from normal activities related to optimum growth and development. Fear and anxiety can be transferred from the parents to the child. Education concerning general health, hygiene, dental care, balanced diet, and routine immunizations should be emphasized. Immunizations after cardiac transplantation must be placed on hold.

Immunizations are also not recommended immediately before cardiac transplant, because immune-suppressants are used to prevent rejection of the transplanted heart, and the child's ability to manufacture antibodies in response to routine immunizations will be impaired.

Dental health care in children with heart disease is important to prevent bacteremia, which can cause bacterial endocarditis. Antibiotics are usually required before dental care.

Competitive sports may need to be avoided for children with congenital heart disease, because the pressure for a team win can interfere with the child's need to stop activity if specific symptoms arise. Some children benefit from being transported to school so that energy can be consumed *during* school activities rather than by walking to and from school.

Nutritional guidance is aimed at preventing anemia and promoting optimal growth and development. Parents should be instructed in the techniques of preventing dehydration in children with polycythemia. Care must be taken during the hot summer months to ensure the child's fluid requirements are met by replacing fluid lost from sweating. Vacations to high altitudes or very cold environments may cause adverse responses in a child who is already hypoxic or who has cardiac problems.

Cardiac surgery—if needed to repair a defect that causes HF—is generally performed at a pediatric centre where the necessary equipment is available. Chest tubes may be used postoperatively to remove secretions and air from the pleural cavity and to allow re-expansion of the lungs. These are attached to underwater-seal drainage systems or to a commercially manufactured disposable system such as Pleur-evac (Fig. 26.6). Units for infants and older children are available. This system must be *airtight* to prevent collapse of the lung. Drainage systems **are always kept below the level of the chest** to prevent the backflow of secretions. This is especially important during transportation. **Two padded Kelly clamps must be available at all times** for emergency clamping of tubes. These are applied to the tubes as close as possible to the child's chest if a break in the system occurs.

Cardiac transplants are a treatment option when other treatments fail. Infection and rejection of the new tissue are the most common causes of death post-transplant.

Postoperative cardiac care usually takes place in a critical care unit, where high-technology monitoring minimizes complications. The practical nurse will have contact with the child who is returning for postoperative checkups or is on a home care program after discharge. Providing routine supportive care, encouraging appropriate medical follow-up, and designing activities that promote optimal growth and development are primary goals of care.

> **Medication Alert!**
>
> Complementary and alternative health modalities (CAHM) therapy with ginkgo, ginseng, and St. John's wort may interact with medications used for congenital heart disease and should not be used (Holcomb, 2009).

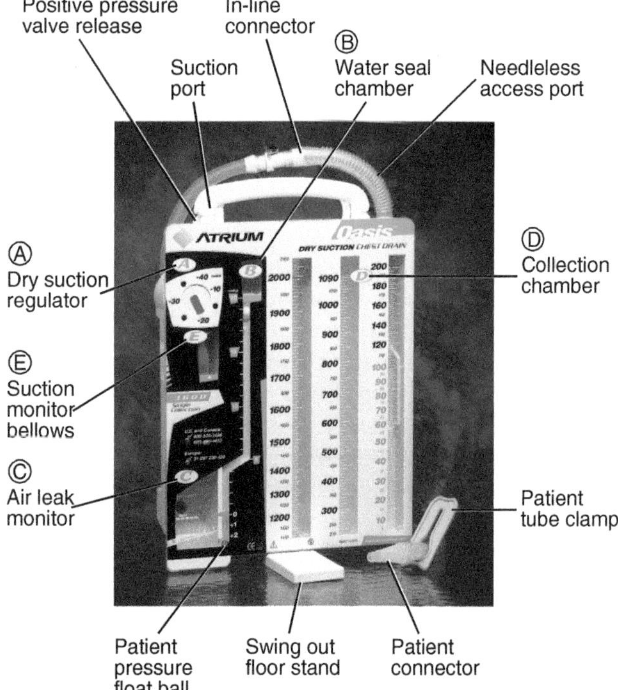

Fig. 26.6 Chest tube with underwater seal drainage system. (Courtesy Atrium Medical Corp. From Potter, P. A., & Perry, A. G. [2016]. *Fundamentals of nursing* [9th ed., p. 998]. St. Louis: Elsevier.)

ACQUIRED HEART DISEASES

Acquired heart disease is a cardiac condition that occurs *after* birth. It may be a complication of a congenital heart disease or a response to respiratory infection, sepsis, hypertension, or severe anemia.

Heart Failure

Heart failure is defined as cardiac output inadequate to meet the metabolic needs of the body.

Manifestations

Manifestations of HF depend on the side of the heart affected. The *right side* of the heart moves unoxygenated blood to the pulmonary circulation. A failure results in the backup of blood in the systemic venous system. The *left side* of the heart moves oxygenated blood from the pulmonary circulation to the systemic circulation. A failure results in backup into the lung. When the body tries to compensate for the problems, peripheral vasoconstriction occurs and results in cold or blue hands and feet, tachycardia, and tachypnea. Although HF may start as a right- or left-sided failure, eventually *both* sides become involved.

Signs and symptoms may differ somewhat and are more subtle in infants. Some of these signs are cyanosis, pallor, rapid respiration, rapid pulse, feeding difficulties, fatigue, a weak cry, excessive perspiration (especially on the forehead), failure to gain weight, edema, and frequent respiratory infections.

> **Safety Alert!**
>
> Early signs of heart failure in infants that should be reported include the following:
> - Tachycardia at rest
> - Fatigue during feeding
> - Sweating around scalp and forehead
> - Dyspnea
> - Sudden weight gain

Cyanosis. When observing the patient's colour, the nurse should note whether the cyanosis is general or localized. If it is localized, the exact location is recorded in the nurse's notes—for example, hands, feet, lips, or around the mouth. Is the cyanosis deep or light? Is it constant or transient? Sometimes colour improves during crying, and sometimes it gets worse; this is significant to note during the health history, as an improvement in cyanosis during crying may indicate another structural anomaly, such as choanal atresia, and if it worsens, it may indicate a cyanotic congenital heart defect. If overt cyanosis is not apparent in the infant with dark-coloured skin, the palms of the hands and bottoms of the feet are observed. Clubbing of the fingers and toes (see Fig. 26.4) may be evident as a result of blood pooling in the capillaries of the extremities in children with chronic hypoxia. The skin may be very pale or mottled. Sweating, particularly of the head, may be seen.

Rapid respiration. Rapid respiration is called ***tachypnea***. A rate of more than 60 breaths/min in a newborn at rest indicates distress. The amount of *dyspnea*, or shortness of breath, varies. In more acute cases, dyspnea is accompanied by flaring of the nostrils, mouth breathing, grunting, and sternal retractions. The infant has more trouble breathing when flat in bed than when held upright. Air hunger is evidenced if the child is irritable and restless. The cry is weak and hoarse. (Refer to Appendix A for normal vital signs.)

Rapid pulse. A rapid pulse is termed tachycardia. An increase in pulse rate is one of the first signs of HF. The heart is pumping harder in an effort to increase its output and to provide sufficient oxygen to all the tissues of the body. Cardiac output can be increased by one of two mechanisms: tachycardia or increased stroke volume. Stroke volume is the amount of blood ejected during one contraction. Because infants and small children have a limited ability to increase stroke volume, their heart rate must increase to meet the demand.

Feeding difficulties. These infants tire easily when feeding and may stop sucking after a small amount. When placed in the crib, they cry and appear hungry. They may choke and gag during feedings; sucking is difficult because of their inability to breathe.

Poor weight gain. The child fails to gain weight. A sudden increase in weight may indicate edema and the beginning of HF.

Edema. Blood flow to the kidneys is decreased, and the glomerular filtration rate slows. This causes both fluid and sodium to be retained. The nurse should watch for puffiness about the eyes and, occasionally, in the legs, feet, and abdomen. Urine output may decrease.

Frequent respiratory tract infections. Resistance is very low. Slight infections can be highly dangerous because the heart and lungs are already compromised. Immunizations are reviewed and updated as needed. The nurse should prevent exposure to other children who have upper respiratory tract infections and other illnesses.

Treatment and nursing care

The initial treatment is focused on correcting the cause of HF. The nursing goals significant to the care of children with HF are the following:

- Reduce the work of the heart
- Improve respirations
- Maintain proper nutrition
- Prevent infection
- Reduce the anxiety of the patient
- Support and instruct the parents

The nurse must organize care so that the infant is not unnecessarily disturbed. A complete bath and linen change for an infant with a serious heart defect may not be a priority. The infant is fed early if crying and late if asleep. The health care provider will order the position in which the infant is to be placed. In some cases, the knee–chest position facilitates breathing; in other cases, the Fowler position may be helpful. Feedings are small and frequent. A soft nipple with holes large enough to prevent the infant from tiring should be provided. Often, formulas with increased caloric density are used, owing to increased metabolic demand. In some cases, nasogastric tube feedings are advantageous because they are less tiring for the child. Oxygen is administered to relieve dyspnea. As breathing becomes easier, the infant should begin to relax. A soft voice and gentle care are soothing. Whenever possible, the infant should be held and comforted during feedings.

Digitoxin (Digitaline) and digoxin (Lanoxin) are common oral digitalis preparations that are sometimes used. These medications slow and strengthen the heartbeat. The nurse needs to count the patient's *pulse for 1 full minute* before administering them. A resting apical pulse is most accurate. As a rule, if the pulse rate of an infant or child is below 100 beats/min, the medication is withheld and the health care provider is notified. In older children, the pulse rate should be more than 70 beats/min. Because the pulse rate varies with the age of the child, the health care provider needs to specify in the written medication order at what heart rate the nurse should withhold the medication. It is important to refer to the health care agency's policy and procedure for specific information and recommendations for administration of this medication. The health care provider should be notified when the medication is withheld.

The health care provider should be contacted if the patient vomits. Digitalis administration is not repeated until the health care provider confirms that it is safe to do so. Tachycardia and irregularities in the rhythm of the pulse are significant and should be reported. Symptoms of toxicity include nausea, vomiting, anorexia, irregularity in rate and rhythm of the pulse, and a sudden change in pulse. If the infant is discharged while still receiving medication, the parents need to be taught how to take the pulse and what signs to be alert for when administering the medication.

A group of medications called *angiotensin-converting enzyme inhibitors (ACE-I)* can be prescribed as first-line treatment. Captopril, enalapril, and lisinopril are examples of these medications. The nurse should observe for signs of hypotension, cough, renal dysfunction, and hyperkalemia. Serum potassium should be carefully monitored.

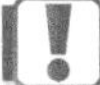
Medication Alert!

Two nurses must check dosage of medications such as digoxin. A single dose larger than 0.05 mg, or 50 mcg, should be reconfirmed with the health care provider.

Diuretics such as furosemide (Lasix) or chlorothiazide (Diuril) are useful in reducing edema. Careful monitoring of serum electrolyte levels prevents electrolyte imbalance, particularly potassium depletion. Parents of older patients should be taught to recognize foods high in potassium, such as bananas, oranges, milk, potatoes, and prune juice. Diapers should be weighed to determine urine output. Daily weighing of the infant also helps the health care provider to determine the effectiveness of the diuresis. Spironolactone (Aldactone) is another diuretic that may be prescribed and does not require potassium supplementation.

IV medications such as nitroprusside must be administered in the critical care unit as the blood pressure must be constantly monitored. Beta-adrenergic agonists such as dopamine, dobutamine, and isoproterenol are also used in the critical care unit setting. Refer to Table 26.2 to review commonly administered cardiovascular medications.

Table 26.2 Commonly Administered Cardiac Medications

CARDIAC MEDICATION CLASSIFICATION	ACTION	COMMENTS	NURSING CARE CONSIDERATIONS
Diuretics	Furosemide (Lasix)—Blocks reabsorption of sodium and water in proximal renal tubule and interferes with reabsorption of sodium and may be used in heart failure	Diuretic medications reduce the kidneys' reabsorption of sodium and water, thus lowering circulating fluid volume and lowering blood pressure. This may also be the medication type of choice in severe heart failure. They cause excretion of chloride and potassium (hypokalemia may precipitate digitalis toxicity).	Begin to record output as soon as a diuretic medication is given. Observe for dehydration caused by profound diuresis. Observe for adverse effects (nausea and vomiting, diarrhea, ototoxicity, hypokalemia, dermatitis, postural hypotension). Encourage foods high in potassium or give potassium supplements. Monitor chloride and acid–base balance with long-term therapy. Observe for signs of digoxin toxicity.
	Chlorothiazide (Diuril)—Acts directly on distal tubules to decrease sodium, water, potassium, chloride, and bicarbonate absorption and may be used in heart failure	This medication is used less frequently. It causes hypokalemia, acidosis from large doses.	Observe for adverse effects (nausea, weakness, dizziness, paresthesia, muscle cramps, skin eruptions, hypokalemia, acidosis). Encourage foods high in potassium or give potassium supplements, or both.
	Spironolactone (Aldactone)—Blocks action of aldosterone, which promotes retention of sodium and excretion of potassium and may be used in heart failure	Weak diuretic. Has potassium-sparing effect; frequently used with thiazides, furosemide. It is poorly absorbed from the gastrointestinal tract. It takes several days to achieve maximum actions.	Observe for adverse effects (skin rash, drowsiness, ataxia, hyperkalemia). Do not administer potassium supplements.
Inotropic agent	Digitalis glycoside (digoxin)—Improves contractility of the heart and may be used in heart failure. Other inotropes may be administered in a critical care setting.	In children, digoxin is used almost exclusively, because of its more rapid onset of action and decreased risk of toxicity as a result of its relatively short half-life of 1½ days compared with other digitalis preparations. It is available as an elixir (50 mcg/mL) for oral administration.	Because digoxin has a very narrow margin of safety, the dosage must be calculated exactly. Premature infants are more sensitive to digoxin and require smaller dosages because their impaired renal excretion causes the medication to accumulate in the blood faster than in full-term infants and children. Observe for signs of toxicity, especially bradycardia and vomiting. Refer to your health care agency's policy and procedure for administration of this medication.

Continued

Table 26.2 Commonly Administered Cardiac Medications—cont'd

CARDIAC MEDICATION CLASSIFICATION	ACTION	COMMENTS	NURSING CARE CONSIDERATIONS
Angiotensin-converting enzyme (ACE) inhibitors	ACE inhibitors reduce the afterload on the heart, making it easier for the heart to pump and may be used in heart failure. Common ACE inhibitor antihypertensives: Lisinopril Fosinopril Enalapril Captopril	ACE inhibitors hinder the normal function of the renin-angiotensin system in the kidney so that instead of vasoconstriction, vasodilation occurs. Vasodilation results in decreased pulmonary and systemic vascular resistance, decreased blood pressure, a reduction in afterload, and decreased right atrial and left atrial pressures. Renal blood flow is then improved, which enhances diuresis.	Monitor blood pressure and pulse. Take 1 hour prior to meals to increase absorption. Monitor laboratory results prior to and after initiation—serum potassium, creatinine, complete blood count. Contraindicated in pregnancy. Adverse effects may include a cough and, rarely, angioedema (captopril). Advise to avoid rapid position changes (may initially cause dizziness). Patient should stay well hydrated.
Calcium channel blockers	Calcium channel blockers reduce systemic vascular resistance through relaxation of arterial smooth muscle. Common calcium channel blockers: Amlodipine (Norvasc) Nifedipine (Adalat)	Calcium channel blockers may be used to treat hypertension because of their main mechanism of relaxing smooth muscle by blocking calcium entry. The result of this mechanism is systemic vasodilation.	May increase heart rate. Do not crush nifedipine (extended release). Adverse effects may include constipation, peripheral edema. Use with caution with other antihypertensives as hypotension may result.

Adapted from Bernstein, D. (2016). Heart failure. In R. M. Kliegman, B. F. Stanton, J. St. Geme, et al. (Eds.), *Nelson textbook of pediatrics* (20th ed.). Philadelphia: Saunders; Hogarth, A. (2017). Cardiovascular dysfunction. In S. Perry, M. Hockenberry, D. Lowdermilk et al. (Eds.). *Maternal child nursing care in Canada* (2nd ed.). Toronto, ON: Elsevier; Hockenberry, M. J., & Wilson, D. (2015). *Wong's essentials of pediatric nursing* (10th ed.). St. Louis, MO: Mosby/Elsevier.

Arrhythmia is a serious complication of patients with heart pathology; the use of an implantable cardioverter-defibrillator can be life-saving (Bernstein, 2016a).

Safety Alert!

Before administering a digoxin medication, the resting apical pulse should be counted for 1-full minute.

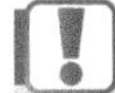

Safety Alert!

ACE Inhibitors

Because ACE inhibitors also block the action of aldosterone, the addition of potassium supplements or spironolactone to the medications regimen of patients taking diuretics and an ACE inhibitor may cause hyperkalemia.

An accurate record of intake and output is essential. Signs of dehydration such as thirst, fever, decreased skin turgor, apathy, sunken eyes or fontanelle, dry skin, dry tongue, dry mucous membranes, and decreased urination should be brought to the immediate attention of the health care provider. Pneumonia can occur rapidly. Fever, irritability, and an increase in respiratory distress may indicate this condition. The child's position should be changed regularly to help prevent hypostatic pneumonia.

The nurse working in a cardiac unit assesses the child frequently for complications of cardiac and respiratory failure and should be competent in cardiopulmonary resuscitation (CPR) techniques and the necessary modifications required for pediatric patients (Pediatric Advanced Life Support [PALS] certification).

The parents of the child need support and understanding throughout the long period of the child's illness. Because the heart is the body's major vital organ, this type of diagnosis causes much apprehension. The health care provider must reassure the parents without minimizing the danger involved.

The patterns formed during infancy can build the framework of a healthy personality for the patient. Children who have heart conditions and who are well integrated into family life have a decided advantage over children who are made to think they are invalids. Routine naps and early bedtimes provide adequate rest for most children.

As children grow, they usually set their own limits on the amount of activity they can handle. Prompt treatment of infections is important. A suitable diet with adequate fluids is necessary. Eating iron-rich foods is encouraged. Dental care should be regular. All-day attendance in school may be too tiring for the child; therefore, special arrangements may be necessary. The child needs careful evaluation before any type of minor surgery is performed.

Detailed discharge planning and coordination of community services can be of value to the family.

Rheumatic Fever

Pathophysiology

Rheumatic fever (RF) is a systemic disease involving the joints, heart, central nervous system (CNS), skin, and subcutaneous tissues. It belongs to a group of disorders known as *collagen diseases.* Their common feature is the destruction of connective tissue. RF is particularly detrimental to the heart, causing scarring of the mitral valves. Its peak incidence is between 5 and 15 years of age. RF is common worldwide in lower-income groups and where overcrowded conditions exist. It is more prevalent during winter and spring, and carrier rates among school-age children are believed to be higher during these seasons. RF is an autoimmune disease that occurs as a complication of untreated group A beta-hemolytic streptococcus infection of the throat.

Rheumatic heart disease was largely eliminated from Canada over the course of the twentieth century; however, the disease still remains a lethal problem in Canada and beyond, particularly for people living in geographic areas that have impoverished living conditions related to housing, lacking clean water and inadequate access to health care services, and having a long-standing history of culture loss, racism, and stigmatization (Canadian Institutes of Health Research [CIHR], 2018; Greenwood & de Leeuw, 2012). For example, for Indigenous people living in the area around Sioux Lookout in Ontario, the likelihood of contracting RF is 75 times greater than for the non-Indigenous Canadian population (Gordon, Kirlew, Schreiber, et al., 2015). Similarly, in Manitoba, Indigenous children are at a higher risk of contracting RF than non-Indigenous children (Schantz, Buffo, Soni, et al., 2013). This discrepancy has highlighted the need for more aggressive diagnosis and treatment of streptococcal pharyngitis and reiterates the importance of assessment of social and structural determinants of health, as well as providing and advocating for accessible health care.

Manifestations

Symptoms of RF range from mild to severe and may not occur until 1 to 6 weeks after a strep throat infection (Fig. 26.7). The classic symptoms are *migratory poly arthritis* (wandering joint pains), skin eruptions, chorea (a nervous disorder), and inflammation of the heart. Subcutaneous nodules may appear beneath the skin but are less common in children. Abdominal pain, often mistaken for appendicitis, sometimes occurs. Fever varies from slight to very high. Pallor, fatigue, anorexia, and unexplained nosebleeds may be seen. An elevated antistreptolysin O (ASO) titre is a standard diagnostic test for RF.

RF tends to recur, and each attack carries the threat of further damage to the heart. The recurrences are most frequent during the first 5 years after the initial attack, and they decline rapidly thereafter.

Migratory polyarthritis. The **polyarthritis** (*poly,* "many," *arthr,* "joint," and *itis,* "inflammation of") seen in RF is distinctive in that it does not result in permanent deformity to the joint. It involves mainly the larger joints: knees, elbows, ankles, wrists, and shoulders. The joints become painful and tender and are difficult to move. The symptoms last for a few days, disappear without treatment, and frequently return in another joint. This pattern may continue for a few weeks. The symptoms tend to be more severe in older children. The joint may be visibly swollen and inflamed. On diagnosis, salicylates are administered to relieve the pain.

Skin eruptions. *Erythema marginatum,* the rash seen in RF, consists of small, red circles with red-coloured margins, a pale centre, and wavy lines appearing on the trunk and abdomen. They appear and disappear rapidly and are significant in diagnosing the disease.

Sydenham chorea. **Chorea**, or "Saint Vitus dance," is a disorder of the CNS characterized by involuntary, purposeless movements of the muscles. It may occur as an acute rheumatic involvement of the brain. Sydenham chorea is primarily seen in prepubertal girls.

Attacks of chorea, which begin slowly, may be preceded by increased tension and behavioural problems. The child becomes "clumsy," may stumble and spill things,

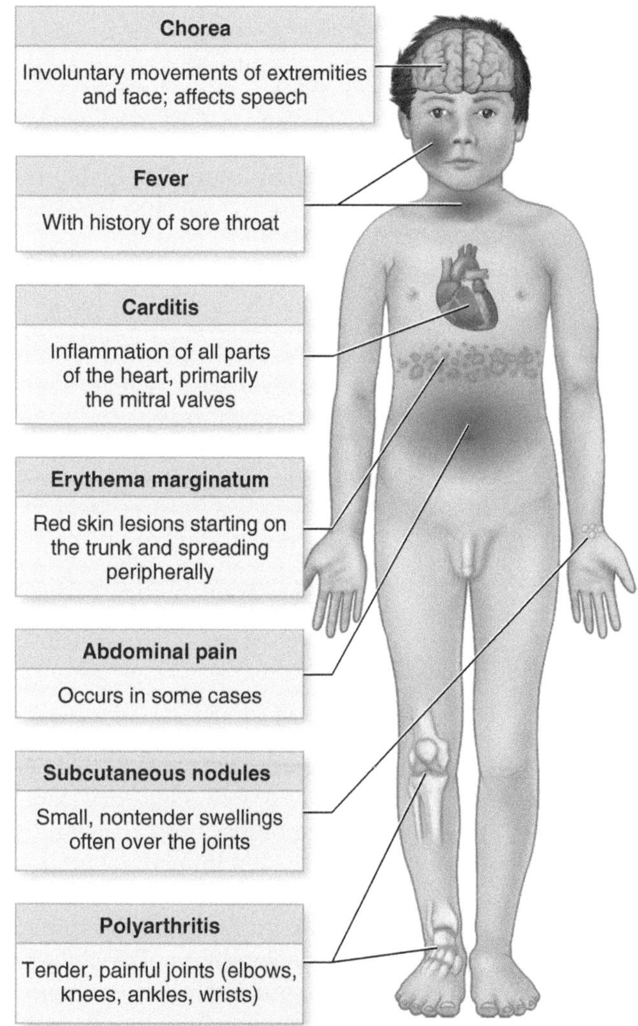

Fig. 26.7 Manifestations of rheumatic fever. (From Silvestri, L. A. [2017]. *Saunders Canadian comprehensive review for the NCLEX-RN® examination* [1st ed., p. 485]. St. Louis: Mosby.)

and may have difficulty buttoning clothes and writing. When the facial muscles are involved, grimaces occur. The child may laugh and cry inappropriately. In severe cases, the patient may become completely incapacitated, and deterioration in speech may be noticeable.

Treatment of Sydenham chorea is directed toward the relief of symptoms. The condition usually disappears spontaneously within weeks to months. Medication may also be required. The presence of Sydenham chorea alone can support the diagnosis of RF.

Rheumatic carditis. **Carditis**, an inflammation of the heart, is a manifestation of RF that can be fatal. It occurs more often in the young child. The tissues that cover the heart and the heart valves are affected. The heart muscle (myocardium) may be involved, as may the pericardium and the endocardium. The *mitral valve,* which is located between the left atrium and the left ventricle, is often involved. When this valve becomes narrowed, the condition is called *mitral stenosis.* Myocardial lesions called *Aschoff's bodies* are also characteristic of the disease. The burden on the heart is great, because it must pump harder to circulate the blood. As a result, it may become enlarged. Symptoms of poor circulation and HF may appear.

The child has an irregular, low-grade fever, is pale and listless, and has a poor appetite. Moderate anemia and weight loss are apparent. The child may experience dyspnea on exertion. The pulse and respiration rates are out of proportion to the body temperature. A soft murmur may be detected over the apex of the heart.

Diagnosis

The diagnosis of RF is difficult to make; for this reason, the **Jones criteria** have been developed and used and modified throughout the years (Box 26.2). The presence of two major criteria or one major and two minor criteria, supported by evidence of recent streptococcal infection, indicates a high probability of RF. A careful physical examination is performed, and a complete history of the patient is obtained. Certain blood tests are helpful. The erythrocyte sedimentation rate (ESR) is elevated. Abnormal proteins, such as C-reactive protein, may also be evident in the blood serum. Leukocytosis may occur but is not regularly present. Antibodies against the streptococci (measured by ASO titre) may also be detected. Additional studies may include chest X-rays, throat culture, and pulmonary function tests. The ECG, a graphic record of the electrical changes caused by the beating of the heart, is very useful. Changes in conductivity, particularly a prolonged P-R interval (indicating a first-degree heart block), may reflect carditis. These tests are repeated throughout the course of the disease so that the health care provider may determine when the active stage has subsided. Refer to Appendix B for further details of normal laboratory value ranges.

Box 26.2 Modified Jones Criteria

A positive diagnosis of rheumatic fever cannot be made without the presence of two major criteria, or one major and two minor criteria, plus a history of streptococcal infection.

MAJOR CRITERIA

- Carditis
- Polyarthritis
- Erythema marginatum
- Chorea
- Subcutaneous nodules

MINOR CRITERIA

- Fever
- Arthralgia
- Previous history of rheumatic heart disease
- Elevated erythrocyte sedimentation rate
- Leukocytosis
- Abnormal electrocardiogram (altered P-R interval)
- Positive test for C-reactive protein

Nursing Tip

A useful mnemonic for remembering the Jones criteria is:

MAJOR CRITERIA	MINOR CRITERIA
Joint (arthritis)	**P**-R interval
Obvious carditis	**E**SR elevated
Nodules subcutaneous	**A**rthralgia
Erythema marginatum	**C**RP elevated
Sydenham's chorea	**E**levated temperature (fever)

Treatment and nursing care

Treatment is aimed at preventing permanent damage to the heart. Treatment involves antibacterial therapy, physical and mental rest, relief of pain and fever, and management of HF, should it occur. Initial antibacterial therapy is directed toward eliminating the streptococcal infection. Penicillin is the medication of choice (given for a 10-day period) unless the patient is sensitive to it, in which case erythromycin is substituted.

Elimination of infection through medication is followed by long-term *chemoprophylaxis* (prevention of disease by medications). Anti-inflammatory medications are used to decrease fever and pain. Aspirin is the medication of choice for joint disease without evidence of carditis. The use of steroids is reserved for severe cardiac symptoms or when aspirin does not relieve cardiac pain. Concerns during therapy include aspirin toxicity and the effects of aspirin on blood clotting. Mild signs of Cushing disease, such as moon face, acne, and hirsutism (increased hairiness), should be anticipated with the use of steroids. Phenobarbital is effective in managing chorea. Padded side rails are used to protect the patient who experiences spasms. If HF occurs, symptomatic treatment is provided.

Bed rest during the initial attack is recommended until the ESR returns to normal levels. The amount of work the heart must do should be limited by resting the entire body. In this way, the circulation of the heart is slower, and the heart does not need to work as fast or as hard as when a child is active. The nurse should teach parents and children about the need for rest and the types of play activity appropriate during home care.

Table 26.3 Procedures in Which Infective Endocarditis Prophylaxis Is Recommended

DENTAL PROCEDURES	RESPIRATORY TRACT PROCEDURES	GASTROINTESTINAL TRACT PROCEDURES	GENITOURINARY TRACT PROCEDURES	SKIN PROCEDURES
All dental procedures that involve the manipulation of gingival tissue, the periapical region of teeth, or the perforation of the oral mucosa	Invasive procedures of the respiratory tract that involves incision or biopsy of the respiratory mucosa, such as tonsillectomy and adenoidectomy and bronchoscopy involving an incision of the respiratory tract mucosa	*High-risk patients only:* Gastrointestinal (GI) or genitourinary (GU) tract infection, or for those who receive antibiotic therapy to prevent wound infection or sepsis associated with a GI or GU tract procedure	*High-risk patients only:* Elective cystoscopy or other urinary tract manipulation and those who have an enterococcal urinary tract infection or colonization, antibiotic therapy to eradicate enterococci from the urine before the procedure may be considered	*For procedures on infected skin, skin structure, or musculoskeletal tissue only:* The antibiotic regimen should include coverage against staphylococci and group A streptococci

Adapted from Allen, U. D., & Canadian Paediatric Society, Infectious Diseases and Immunization Committee. (2010). Infective endocarditis: Updated guidelines. *Pediatrics & Child Health, 15*(4), 205–208. (Reaffirmed in 2018). Heart Association. (2018). *Infective (bacterial) endocarditis wallet card*. Retrieved from http://www.heart.org/idc/groups/heart-public/@wcm/@hcm/documents/downloadable/ucm_307644.pdf.

Nursing activities should be organized to ensure as few interruptions as possible to prevent tiring the patient. A bed cradle can be used to prevent pressure on painful extremities. Care includes special attention to the skin, especially over bony prominences; back care; good oral hygiene; and small, frequent feedings of nourishing foods. Maintaining healthy teeth and preventing cavities is of special importance. The patient with RF is particularly susceptible to *subacute bacterial endocarditis,* which can occur as a complication of dental or other procedures likely to cause bleeding or infection. Prophylactic antibiotic treatment is required before any dental procedure.

Nutrition consists of small servings that are increased as the child's appetite improves. A record of fluid intake and output is kept, because overhydration may tax the heart.

All efforts should be made to provide emotional support for the child and family. The child may also need assistance from the school to continue school studies.

Prevention

Prevention of infection and prompt treatment of group A beta-hemolytic streptococcal infections can prevent the occurrence of RF. All throat infections should be cultured. After a diagnosis of strep throat is established, the nurse should stress the need to complete antibiotic therapy even if symptoms disappear and the child "feels better." Close medical supervision and follow-up care are essential. The prognosis is favourable.

Infective (Bacterial) Endocarditis

Infective endocarditis (IE) previously referred to as bacterial endocarditis (BE). IE is an infection of the valves and inner lining of the heart, which can potentially damage or destroy the heart valves, with high morbidity and mortality for affected patients (Bernstein, 2016b; Chow, Ateah, Scott, et al., 2013). It is most commonly seen in children with congenital heart defects or prosthetic valves. Endocarditis can also occur without any known risk factors, commonly affecting the mitral or aortic valve. The incidence of IE appears to have increased in the pediatric population, most likely because of improved survival among children at risk for IE (those with congenital heart defects and hospitalized infants) (Allen & CPS Infectious Diseases and Immunization Committee, 2010/2018).

The most common causative agents are *Streptococcus viridans* and *Staphylococcus aureus*. The presentation of IE varies among individuals. Signs and symptoms may include fever, malaise, a new murmur, and the findings of vegetations (caused by turbulent blood flow and subsequent damage of the endothelium) on echocardiography (Bernstein, 2016b). Positive blood cultures are present in most patients; however, endocarditis can also be present despite negative blood cultures, especially if antibiotics have already been given.

Complete antibiotic or antifungal treatment of the causative organism is necessary, and treatment may last up to 4 to 7 weeks. Prevention of IE in a susceptible child is vital and involves antibiotic prophylaxis. Children susceptible to IE include those with the following conditions (Allen & CPS Infectious Diseases and Immunization Committee, 2010/2018):

- Prosthetic cardiac valves
- Previous IE
- Unrepaired cyanotic CHD
- Completely repaired congenital heart defect with prosthetic material or device, during the first 6 months after the procedure
- Repaired CHD with residual defects at the site or adjacent to the site of a prosthetic patch or prosthetic device
- Cardiac transplant recipients with cardiac valvulopathy
- Rheumatic heart disease if prosthetic valves or prosthetic material was used in valve repair

Table 26.3 lists procedures in which IE prophylaxis is recommended.

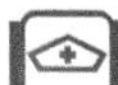

Nursing Tip

The nurse should teach parents about the need for prophylactic antibiotic therapy before any procedure included in Table 26.3 is done.

Systemic Hypertension

Pathophysiology

Hypertension, or high blood pressure, is being seen more often during childhood and adolescence. Blood pressure is a product of peripheral vascular resistance and cardiac output. An increase in cardiac output or peripheral resistance results in an increase in blood pressure. Systemic blood pressure increases with age and is correlated with age, sex, and height throughout childhood and adolescence. (See Appendix A for blood pressure measurements in children.) An abnormal blood pressure reading should be measured and confirmed by auscultation on three different occasions before a diagnosis is made (Flynn, Kaelber, Baker-Smith, et al., 2017). *Hypertension* is defined as the consistent elevation of blood pressure beyond values considered to be the upper limits of normal. The two major categories are essential hypertension (no identifiable cause) and secondary hypertension (subsequent to an identifiable cause). Hypertension in children and adolescents is defined as having a systolic or diastolic blood pressure that consistently falls at or over the ninety-fifth percentile. This group is further delineated as follows:

Stage 1 is defined by blood pressure between the ninety-fifth and ninety-ninth percentiles plus 5 mm Hg.

Stage 2 is defined by blood pressure greater than the ninety-ninth percentile plus 5 mm Hg (Dionne, Harris, Benoit, et al., 2017).

Hypertension is referred to as *secondary* when a disease process can explain the increased pressure. Renal, congenital, vascular, and endocrine disorders represent the majority of illnesses that account for secondary hypertension. Primary, or *essential* hypertension implies that no known underlying disease is present. Nevertheless, heredity, obesity, stress, and a poor diet and exercise pattern can contribute to any type of hypertension. (See Chapter 20 for skills and techniques in obtaining blood pressure in children.)

There is increasing evidence that essential hypertension, though not generally seen until adolescence or adulthood, may have its roots in childhood and, perhaps, during fetal development. Prevention is thus significant in reducing the incidence of stroke or myocardial infarction as a person ages. The assessment of blood pressure levels should be part of every physical examination during childhood for children over 3 years of age.

Hypertension is more prevalent in children whose parents have high blood pressure. High blood pressure in children is usually discovered during a routine physical examination. Measuring blood pressure in young children requires careful attention to cuff size. Refer to Chapter 20 on how to assess blood pressure in children.

Nursing Tip

Using the proper-size blood pressure cuff is essential to obtaining an accurate blood pressure in children. The bladder length of the cuff should be 80–100% of the circumference of the arm, and the width should be at least 40% (Dionne et al., 2017).

Treatment and nursing care

It is a nursing responsibility to refer any child who has a blood pressure measurement at or above the ninetieth percentile to the primary health care provider for follow-up care. The initial treatment and nursing care involve lifestyle management that includes nutritional counselling, weight reduction, and an age-appropriate program of aerobic exercise. Adolescents should be counselled on the adverse effects of medications, alcohol, and tobacco on blood pressure. There is evidence that the ingestion of caffeine and the use of over-the-counter medications such as non-steroidal anti-inflammatory drugs (NSAIDs), some herbal and nutritional supplements, and hormonal contraceptives may be associated with the development of hypertension in children and adolescents (Dionne et al., 2017; Flynn et al., 2017).

The **D**ietary **A**pproach to **S**top **H**ypertension, or **DASH diet**, is prescribed as initial lifestyle management. The DASH diet is basically a plant-based diet that is high in fruits and vegetables, low-fat milk products, grains, fish, poultry, and lean red meat; low sodium and some sugar and sweets are allowed (Dionne et al., 2017). Sedentary activities should be limited to 2 hours per day, and at least 30 to 60 minutes of active daily exercise is recommended for children. The initial nonpharmacological treatment goal is to reduce blood pressure to below the ninetieth percentile, maintain a normal body mass index (BMI), avoid excess sodium intake, consume a DASH diet, and participate in regular physical activity. The parents and child should be educated in lifestyle changes to ensure active involvement in the child's care.

Stage 2 hypertension includes the above management along with the addition of prescribed antihypertensive medication. This could include an ACE inhibitor such as captopril (Capoten), a long-acting calcium channel blocker such as felodipine (Plendil), an angiotensin receptor blocker (ARB) such as candesartan (Atacand), or a thiazide diuretic.

Children and adolescents with hypertension may participate in competitive sports once hypertensive target organ effects and cardiovascular risk have been assessed (Flynn et al., 2017). Medication therapy may not be effective in adolescents, who often have difficulty taking medication for long-term regimens. The nurse should support the adolescent and parents by providing encouragement of diet, medication, and exercise prescriptions.

Prevention

The main focus of a hypertensive prevention program is patient education. Community health fairs should offer opportunities for blood pressure screening. Blood pressure measurement should be assessed regularly for children older than 3 years old. Risk factors such as obesity, elevated serum cholesterol levels, sedentary lifestyle, and drug, alcohol, or tobacco use and intake of salty foods should be discussed.

Health Promotion

Nonpharmacological Methods for Preventing and Treating High Blood Pressure

- Aerobic exercise for 60 minutes at least three to five times per week
- Reduction of sedentary activities, such as surfing on the computer, watching television, and playing video games
- Weight reduction; maintaining a normal body mass index (BMI)
- Dietary management with the DASH diet
- Avoiding excess salty foods
- Adequate intake of potassium and calcium
- Avoidance of smoking and being in the presence of others smoking

Dyslipidemia

Pathophysiology

Dyslipidemia refers to any abnormality in the lipid levels of the body and includes high cholesterol, triglycerides, or fat phospholipids. *Hyperlipidemia,* the most common dyslipidemia, refers to excessive lipids (fat and fatlike substances) in the blood. Lipoproteins contain lipids and proteins and include the following:

- *Low-density lipoproteins (LDL),* which contain low amounts of triglycerides, a high level of cholesterol, and some protein. LDL carries cholesterol to the cells, which aids in cellular metabolism and steroid production.
- *High-density lipoproteins (HDL)* contain low amounts of triglycerides, little cholesterol, and high levels of protein. HDL carries cholesterol to the liver for excretion.

Diagnosis

In Canada, the Canadian Cardiovascular Society (CCS) does not currently recommend universal screening for hypercholesterolemia. The CCS suggests targeted screening in children and adolescents with such cardiovascular risk factors as a positive family history of dyslipidemia or cardiovascular disease, obesity, smoking, hypertension, or type 2 diabetes (Genest, Hegele, Bergeron, et al., 2014). Screening the plasma lipid profile (Table 26.4) in children with a positive family history and with poor lifestyle or cardiovascular risk factors might help motivate the adoption of preventive strategies (Genest et al., 2014).

Treatment and nursing care

Most children with high triglycerides are obese. Therefore, reduction of calories, increase in fibre in the diet, and regular exercise should be stressed in their education. An active prevention program for all children and adolescents

Health Promotion

Heart-Healthy Guidelines for Children in Canada

PHYSICAL ACTIVITY

- Children of all ages benefit from physical activity. The type and amount of activity they need change as they grow. For healthy growth and development, infants and preschoolers should be active several times during the day.
- Children and teens should accumulate 60 minutes of moderate- to vigorous-intensity physical activity daily. They should engage in vigorous-intensity activities at least 3 days per week.
- Children should also do activities that strengthen their muscles and bones at least 3 days per week.
- Children should reduce time spent sitting daily (screen time, driving in cars).
- Parents should be good role models related to physical activity and screen time.

ACTIVITY RECOMMENDATIONS BASED ON AGE

Infants (Less Than 1 Year)

- Being physically active several times in a variety of ways, particularly through interactive floor-based play—more is better. For those not yet mobile, this includes at least 30 minutes of tummy time spread throughout the day while awake.

Toddlers (1–2 Years)

- At least 180 minutes spent in a variety of physical activities at any intensity, including energetic play, spread throughout the day—more is better.

Preschoolers (3–4 Years)

- At least 180 minutes spent in a variety of physical activities spread throughout the day, of which at least 60 minutes is energetic play—more is better.

Children and Youth (5–17 Years)

- Moderate to vigorous physical activity—an accumulation of at least 60 minutes per day of moderate to vigorous physical activity involving a variety of aerobic activities. Vigorous physical activities and muscle and bone strengthening activities should be incorporated at least 3 days per week.

Data from Canadian Society for Exercise Physiology. (2018). *Canadian 24-hour movement guidelines for children and youth*. Retrieved from http://www.csepguidelines.ca; Heart and Stroke. (2018). *Heart healthy activity*. Retrieved from http://www.heartandstroke.ca/get-healthy/healthy-kids/heart-healthy-activity.

Table 26.4 Average Lipid Profile Levels in Childhood

	TOTAL CHOLESTEROL MMOL/L (MG/DL)	TRIGLYCERIDES MMOL/L (MG/DL)	LDL MMOL/L (MG/DL)	HDL MMOL/L (MG/DL)
Newborn	1.758 (68)	0.395 (35)	0.749 (29)	0.905 (35)
1–9 years	4.0–4.27 (155–165)	0.621–0.734 (55–65)	2.405–2.586 (93–100)	1.371–1.448 (53–56)
10–14 years	4.14 (160)	0.699–0.8123 (62–72)	2.508 (97)	1.345–1.422 (52–55)
15–19 years	3.88–4.14 (150–160)	0.824–0.881 (73–78)	2.431–2.483 (94–96)	1.189–1.345 (46–52)

is essential. Lifelong healthy eating habits should be nurtured early and practiced by the entire family. Children less than 2 years of age should not have a fat-restricted diet because calories and fats are necessary for CNS growth and development. The Heart and Stroke Foundation of Canada recommendations for heart-healthy guidelines are presented in the Health Promotion box.

Nursing Tip

Developing rapport and motivational interviewing in the clinic or during hospitalization provide excellent opportunities for the nurse to review heart-healthy information. Reviews of family history, lifestyle, and eating patterns are suitable interventions, even in the absence of high risks.

Kawasaki Disease

Kawasaki disease (KD) (mucocutaneous lymph node syndrome) occurs worldwide and is the leading cause of acquired cardiovascular disease in most developed countries (Son & Newberger, 2016). It usually affects children less than 5 years of age. Studies have shown that no known microbe is associated with KD, although it may be a response to a mild asymptomatic viral infection in children with a genetic predisposition (Son, & Newberger, 2016). KD is not spread from person to person. Clinical signs and symptoms make the diagnosis; specific laboratory findings are not diagnostic.

KD causes inflammation of the vessels in the cardiovascular system. The inflammation weakens the walls of the vessels and often results in an *aneurysm* (an abnormal dilation of the wall of a blood vessel). Aneurysms can cause thrombi (blood clots) to form, resulting in serious complications. Approximately 40% of untreated children develop aneurysms of the coronary vessels, which can be life-threatening. For this reason, it is essential that a diagnosis of KD be made as early as possible.

Manifestations

The onset is abrupt with a sustained fever, sometimes above 40°C (104°F), that does not respond to antipyretics or antibiotics. The fever lasts for more than 5 days. Conjunctivitis without discharge, fissured lips, a "strawberry tongue" (enlarged reddened papilla on the tongue), inflamed mouth and pharyngeal membranes, and enlarged nontender lymph nodes are seen. An erythematous skin rash develops, with swollen hands and desquamation (peeling) of the palms and soles (Fig. 26.8). The child can be very irritable and may develop signs of cardiac problems. Abnormalities in an echocardiogram can be detected by the tenth day. Laboratory results may show an elevated C-reactive protein, ESR, and white blood count.

Treatment and nursing care

Intravenous immune globulin (IVIG) administered early in the illness can prevent the development of coronary artery pathology. Salicylate therapy (aspirin) is prescribed for its antithrombus properties. If the child does not respond to IVIG therapy and aspirin, a second dose of IVIG may be prescribed or cyclosporine may be added to the treatment. Prednisolone may be used, but its effectiveness has not been proven (Son & Newberger, 2016).

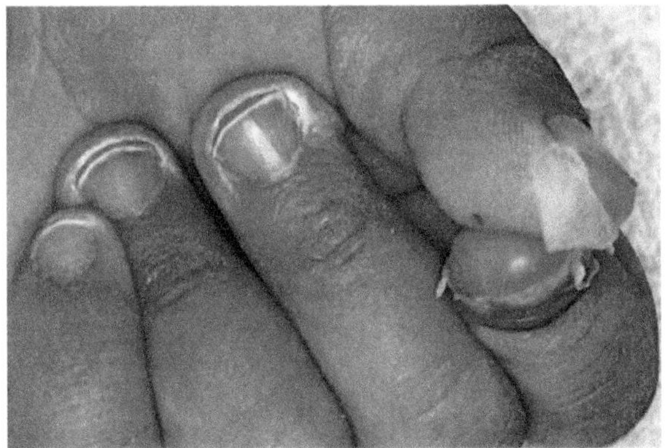

Fig. 26.8 Peeling of the fingertips. The appearance of fingertip or toe tip peeling is characteristic of the subacute phase of Kawasaki disease. (From Zitelli, B. J., McIntire, S., & Nowalk, A. [2018]. *Zitelli and Davis' atlas of pediatric physical diagnosis* [7th ed.]. Philadelphia: Elsevier.)

Nursing care is symptomatic and supportive. Parent teaching should be reinforced concerning the need to postpone active routine immunizations for 11 months after the administration of IG, which is an immunosuppressant.

Long-term, low-dose aspirin therapy may be prescribed to prevent clot formation. It may be difficult for the child to adhere to a long-term regimen in which medication must be taken when the child feels "well." The nurse should reinforce parent teaching concerning the recognition of cardiac problems and updating their CPR skills.

FOLLOW-UP CARE FOR CHILDREN WITH ACQUIRED AND CONGENITAL HEART DISEASE

Children with acquired and congenital heart disease may be at greater risk for neurodevelopmental delays related to changes in oxygenation and blood flow affecting brain development and functioning. For children with complex CHD, neurodevelopmental disabilities are common, affecting approximately half of the survivors as they mature (Wernovsky & Licht, 2016). Since there have been great advances in early diagnosis, operative techniques, and critical care, infants and children with CHD are more likely to live longer into adulthood (Larson & Doyle, 2018). For this reason, longitudinal follow-up with cardiologists, pediatricians, and primary care providers is key to long-term health and the early identification of cardiac or other health-related problems. Children may also be referred to child development specialists as required.

Some Canadian children's hospitals offer satellite and outreach clinics for patients and families living in rural or remote areas to enhance access and to save families from travelling far distances for care (Children's Hospital of Eastern Ontario [CHEO], 2018). There are also a variety of specialized summer camps offered for pediatric cardiology patients, which provide children who have CHD with the opportunity to be active, have fun, experience camp life, and connect with other children, all while in a safe environment (Alberta Health Services, 2018; CHEO, 2018).

The nurse plays an essential role in providing health teaching information to families at discharge regarding the importance of follow-up care, available community resources, and what the family can expect at their upcoming appointments.

Get Ready for the Certification Examination!

Key Points

- Signs and symptoms of congenital heart abnormalities in infants include dyspnea, difficulty with feedings, choking spells, recurrent respiratory infections, cyanosis, poor weight gain, clubbing of the fingers and toes, and heart murmurs.
- Congenital heart disease may be caused by genetic factors, maternal factors such as drug use or illness, or environmental factors. Acquired heart disease occurs after birth as a response to a defect or illness.
- Congenital heart defects that result in a recirculation of blood to the lungs do not usually produce cyanosis as a clinical sign.
- A congenital heart defect can cause an increase in pulmonary blood flow, a decrease in pulmonary blood flow, or an obstruction of blood flow.
- Blood pressure in the legs is normally 10–20% higher than the brachial artery blood pressure. A lack of difference in the blood pressure between the arm and leg may be a sign of coarctation of the aorta in the infant.
- The defects in tetralogy of Fallot include pulmonary artery stenosis, hypertrophy of the right ventricle, dextroposition of the aorta, and a ventricular septal defect.
- Hypercyanotic "tet" spells are relieved by placing the child in a knee–chest position.
- Signs of heart failure in infants include tachycardia, at-rest fatigue during feedings, and perspiration around the forehead.
- The nursing goals significant to the care of children with heart failure are to (1) reduce the work of the heart, (2) improve respiration, (3) maintain proper nutrition, (4) prevent infection, (5) reduce anxiety of the parent, and (6) support growth and development.
- Two nurses must check the dose of digoxin before administration. A dose exceeding 0.05 mg should be reconfirmed with the health care provider.
- Chest tube drainage systems must always be kept below the level of the chest.
- The major Jones criteria diagnostic of rheumatic fever include polyarthritis, erythema marginatum, Sydenham chorea, and rheumatic carditis.
- It is essential to use the correct size blood pressure cuff when assessing the blood pressure of infants and children.
- The DASH diet; daily aerobic activity; and maintenance of a normal BMI are the cornerstones of lifestyle modifications that can control hypertension.
- Hypertension is classified as stage 1 hypertension or stage 2 hypertension.
- Young infants should *not* have a fat-restricted diet because fat is needed for central nervous system growth and development.

Additional Learning Resources

evolve Go to your Evolve website (http://evolve.elsevier.com/Canada/Leifer) for the following learning resources:

- Answer Key for Critical Thinking Questions
- Answer Key for Textbook Review Questions
- Audio Glossary
- Interactive Review Questions
- Skills Performance Checklists
- Video clips and more!

Online Resource

- Heart and Stroke Foundation of Canada: http://www.heartandstroke.ca

Review Questions

1. When administering digoxin to an infant, the medication should be withheld and the health care provider notified in which of the following situations? *(Select all that apply.)*
   a. Pulse rate is below 60 beats/min.
   b. Infant is dyspneic.
   c. Pulse rate is below 100 beats/min.
   d. Respiratory rate is above 40 breaths/min.
2. An infant with tetralogy of Fallot is experiencing a tet spell involving cyanosis and dyspnea. In which position should the infant be placed?
   a. Fowler
   b. Knee-chest
   c. Trendelenburg
   d. Prone
3. Which can best prevent rheumatic fever?
   a. Keeping children with fever home
   b. Sending children with sore throats home from school
   c. Having sore throats cultured as soon as possible
   d. Treating all colds with antibiotics

4. Which of the following conditions would a nurse assess for in a child admitted with possible Kawasaki disease?
   a. Cardiac dysrhythmia
   b. Decreased urine output
   c. Peeling skin on fingers
   d. Decreased level of consciousness
5. A child who has had heart surgery returns to the pediatric unit with a chest tube attached to an underwater seal drainage system in place. What is a priority nursing responsibility when caring for a child with chest tubes?
   a. Empty the chest tube drainage each shift.
   b. Clamp the chest tubes when turning the patient.
   c. Place the drainage system on the bed when moving the bed.
   d. Keep the drainage system below the chest level at all times.
6. The nurse is recording the vital signs of an infant admitted with signs of respiratory distress. Which observations should be reported to the health care provider? *(Select all that apply.)*
   a. Blood pressure is higher in the legs than in the arms
   b. Blood pressure is lower in the legs than in the arms
   c. Cyanosis of the lips
   d. Respiratory rate of 35 breaths per minute

Critical Thinking Questions

1. A child who was diagnosed with Kawasaki disease is discharged home with directions to take a low-dose aspirin tablet once a day. The parent states that she heard that aspirin is contraindicated for use in children and asks if she can substitute acetaminophen instead. What is the best response by the nurse?
2. A parent states that her 4-month-old infant is scheduled for heart transplant surgery in the next few weeks. She states that the infant is now due for her second immunization series and asks if the child will be better protected if she has the immunizations now before she has the surgery. What is the best response by the nurse?

REFERENCES

Alberta Health Services. (2018). *Hearts in right place at special summer camp*. Retrieved from https://www.albertahealthservices.ca/news/Page14598.aspx.

Allen, U. D., & Canadian Paediatric Society (CPS), Infectious Diseases and Immunization Committee. (2010). Infective endocarditis: Updated guidelines. *Paediatrics and Child Health, 15*(4), 205–208. Reaffirmed 2018.

Amsbaugh, S., Scott, S. D., & Foss, K. (2015). Pulse oximetry screening for critical congenital heart disease: Bringing evidence into practice. *Journal of Pediatric Nursing, 30*(4), 591–597.

Bernstein, D. (2016a). Heart failure. In R. M. Kliegman, B. F. Stanton, J. W. St. Geme, et al. (Eds.), *Nelson textbook of pediatrics* (20th ed.). Philadelphia: Saunders.

Bernstein, D. (2016b). Infective endocarditis. In R. M. Kliegman, B. F. Stanton, J. W. St. Geme, et al. (Eds.), *Nelson textbook of pediatrics* (20th ed.). Philadelphia: Saunders.

Blackburn, S. (2013). *Maternal, fetal, & neonatal physiology: A clinical perspective*. Maryland Heights, MO: Elsevier Saunders.

Butler, M. R., Carvan, M. J., & Johnson, T. S. (2016). Understanding genetics and pediatric cardiac health. *Journal of Pediatric Nursing, 31*, 3–10.

Children's Hospital of Eastern Ontario (CHEO). (2018). *Cardiology*. Retrieved from http://www.cheo.on.ca/en/aboutcardiology.

Chow, J., Ateah, C., Scott, S., et al. (2013). *Canadian maternity and pediatric nursing*. Philadelphia, PA: Wolters Kluwer/ Lippincott Williams & Wilkins.

Canadian Institutes of Health Research (CIHR). (2018). *Pathways to health equity for Aboriginal peoples: Overview*. Retrieved from http://www.cihr-irsc.gc.ca/e/47003.html.

Dionne, J. M., Harris, K. C., Benoit, G., et al. (2017). Hypertension. Canada's 2017 guidelines for the diagnosis, assessment, prevention, and treatment of pediatric hypertension. *Canadian Journal of Cardiology, 33*(5), 577–585.

Flynn, T., Kaelber, D., Baker-Smith, C., et al. (2017). Clinical practice guideline for screening and management of high blood pressure in children and adolescents. *Pediatrics, 140*(3), 1–74. Retrieved from http://pediatrics.aappublications.org/content/pediatrics/140/3/e20171904.full.pdf.

Genest, G., Hegele, R. A., Bergeron, J., et al. (2014). Canadian Cardiovascular Society position statement on familial hypercholesterolemia. *Canadian Journal of Cardiology, 30*(12), 1471–1481.

Gordon, J., Kirlew, M., Schreiber, Y., et al. (2015). Acute rheumatic fever in First Nations communities in northwestern Ontario: Social determinants of health "bite the heart." *Canadian Family Physician, 61*, 881–886.

Greenwood, M. L., & de Leeuw, S. N. (2012). Social determinants of health and the future well-being of Aboriginal children in Canada. *Paediatrics and Child Health, 17*(7), 381–384.

Holcomb, S. (2009). Common herb–drug interactions: What you should know. *Nurse Practitioner, 34*(5), 25–29.

Larson, J. A., & Doyle, E. A. (2018). Transitional care for young adults with congenital heart disease: A case study. *Journal of Pediatric Health Care, 32*(2), 195–200.

Narvey, N., Wong, K. K., & Fournier, A. (2017). Pulse oximetry screening in newborns to enhance detection of critical congenital heart disease. *Paediatrics and Child Health, 8*(27), 494–498.

Schantz, D. I., Buffo, I., Soni, R., et al. (2013). The changing incidence of acute rheumatic fever in the province of Manitoba. *Canadian Journal of Cardiology, 29*(10), S90.

Son, M., & Newburger, J. (2016). Kawasaki disease. In R. M. Kliegman, B. F. Stanton, J. W. St. Geme, et al. (Eds.), *Nelson textbook of pediatrics* (20th ed.). Philadelphia: Saunders.

Weiner, G. M., & Zaichkin, J. (2016). *Textbook of neonatal resuscitation. American Academy of Pediatrics*. Retrieved from http://reader.aappublications.org/textbook-of-neonatal-resuscitation-nrp-7th-ed/2.

Wernovsky, G., & Licht, D. J. (2016). Neurodevelopmental outcomes in children with congenital heart disease—What can we impact? *Pediatric Critical Care Medicine, 17*(1), S232–S242.

Wong, K. K., Fournier, A., Fruitman, D. S., et al. (2017). Canadian Cardiovascular Society/Canadian Pediatric Cardiology Association position statement on pulse oximetry screening in newborns to enhance detection of critical congenital heart disease. *Canadian Journal of Cardiology, 33*(2), 199–208.

The Child With a Condition of the Blood, Blood-Forming Organs, or Lymphatic System

27

Andrea Logan

http://evolve.elsevier.com/Canada/Leifer

Objectives

1. Define each key term listed.
2. Summarize the components of blood.
3. Describe two laboratory procedures commonly performed on children with blood disorders.
4. List the symptoms, prevention, and treatment of iron-deficiency anemia.
5. Review the effects of severe anemia on the heart.
6. Recommend four food sources of iron for a child with iron-deficiency anemia.
7. Discuss the pathophysiology and the signs and symptoms of sickle cell disease.
8. Describe four types of sickle cell crises.
9. Devise a nursing care plan for a child with sickle cell disease.
10. Recognize the effects on the bone marrow of increased red blood cell production caused by thalassemia.
11. Describe the pathophysiology and the signs and symptoms of hemophilia A and hemophilia B.
12. Identify the nursing interventions necessary to prevent hemarthrosis in a child with hemophilia.
13. Compare and contrast four manifestations of bleeding into the skin.
14. Recognize normal blood values of infants and children.
15. Plan the nursing care of a child with leukemia.
16. Review the nursing care of a child receiving a blood transfusion.

Key Terms

alopecia (ăl-ō-PĒ-shă)
anemia
Christmas disease
ecchymosis (ĕk-ĭ-MŌ-sĭs)
erythropoietin (ĕ-rĭth-rō-POI-ă-tĭn)
hemarthrosis (hē-măhr-THRŌ-sĭs)
hematoma (hē-mă-TŌ-mă)
hematopoiesis (hē-mă-tō-poi-Ē-sĭs)
hemosiderosis (hē-mō-sĭd-ŭr-Ō-sĭs)
lymphadenopathy (lĭm-făd-ĕn-ŎP-ă-thē)
oncologists
petechiae (pĕ-TĒ-kē-ă)
purpura (PŬR-pyŭ-ră)
sickle cell crises
splenomegaly (splĕ-nō-MĔG-ă-lē)

HEMATOLOGICAL SYSTEM

The blood and blood-forming organs make up the hematological system. Blood is vital to all body functions. *Blood dyscrasias* or disorders occur when blood components fail to form correctly or when blood values exceed or fail to meet normal standards (refer to Appendix B).

Plasma and blood cells are formed at about the second week of gestation, primarily in the yolk sac. Later, blood forms in the spleen, liver, thymus, lymph system, and bone marrow. In the fetus, blood is formed primarily in the liver until the last trimester of pregnancy. During childhood, the red blood cells (RBCs) are formed in the marrow of the long bones (such as the tibia and femur); by adolescence, **hematopoiesis** (blood formation) takes place in the marrow of the ribs, sternum, vertebrae, pelvis, skull, clavicle, and scapulae. The rate of RBC production is regulated by **erythropoietin**. The liver of the fetus produces this substance, but at birth the kidneys take over erythropoietin production. The blood volume of a newborn is approximately 85 mL/kg weight. The newborn has a high hemoglobin and RBC count at birth because of the high erythropoietin level, placental shift of blood to the vascular system at birth, and low extracellular fluid volume. A high white blood cell (WBC) level is evident at birth but decreases by 1 week to a stable level. The vitamin K level is low in the newborn and is required for the development of several blood clotting factors, therefore vitamin K is usually administered within the first 6 hours after birth.

The lymphatic system includes lymphocytes, lymphatic vessels, lymph nodes, the spleen, the tonsils, the adenoids, and the thymus gland. The lymphatic system drains regions of the body to lymph nodes, where infectious organisms are destroyed and antibody production is stimulated. Lymph nodes are not palpable in the newborn, but the cervical, auxiliary, and inguinal nodes may be palpable by childhood. Lymphadenopathy is an enlargement of lymph nodes that is indicative of infection or disease. Fig. 27.1 summarizes some of the differences between the child's and the adult's lymphatic systems.

Fig. 27.2 depicts the main types of blood cells in the circulating blood. Circulating blood consists of two portions: plasma and formed elements. The formed elements are erythrocytes (RBCs), leukocytes (WBCs), and thrombocytes (platelets). Erythrocytes primarily transport oxygen and carbon dioxide to and from the lungs and tissues. Leukocytes act as the body's defense against infections. Thrombocytes, along with portions of blood plasma, are involved with blood coagulation. In the young child, every available space in the bone marrow is involved with blood formation.

Lymphocytes, unlike other WBCs, are produced in the lymphoid tissues of the body. They travel in the circulation but are more commonly found in the lymph tissue. They are released into the body to fight infection and to provide immunity. Their numbers greatly increase in chronic inflammatory conditions. The spleen is the largest organ of the lymphatic system. One of the main functions of the spleen is to bring blood into contact with lymphocytes. Aside from trauma and rupture, the most commonly seen pathological condition of the spleen is enlargement. This is termed splenomegaly. The spleen enlarges during infections, congenital and acquired hemolytic anemias, and liver malfunction.

Bone marrow aspiration is a procedure helpful in determining disorders of the blood. Numerous types of blood counts are used as well. Many are specific to a particular disease. The skin is sometimes an indicator of certain conditions of the blood. Petechiae (pinpoint hemorrhagic spots) and purpura (large petechiae) can be seen, and these conditions should alert the nurse to the possibility of blood dyscrasias. The liver and spleen should be assessed by palpation and percussion to determine whether they are enlarged.

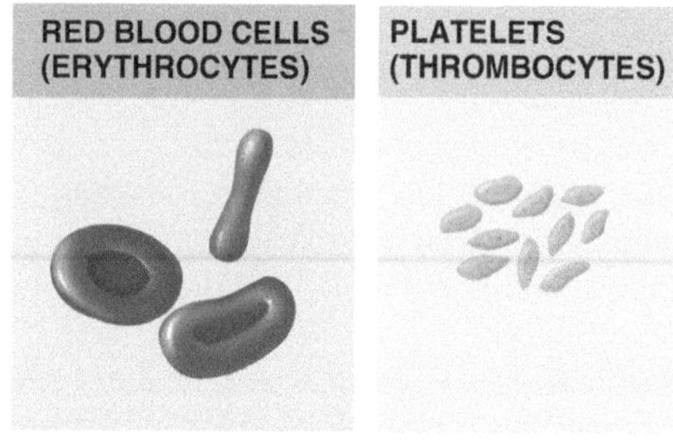

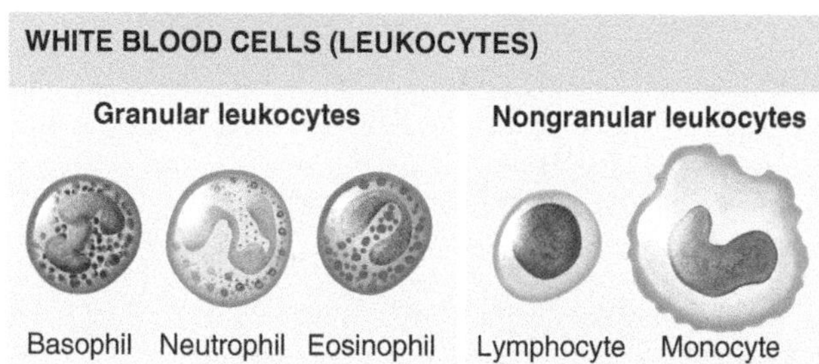

Fig. 27.2 The formed elements of the blood. Red blood cells (RBCs; erythrocytes), white blood cells (WBCs; leukocytes), and platelets (thrombocytes) constitute the formed elements of the blood. (From Patton, K. T., & Thibodeau, G. A. [2016]. *Anatomy and physiology* [9th ed.]. St. Louis: Mosby.)

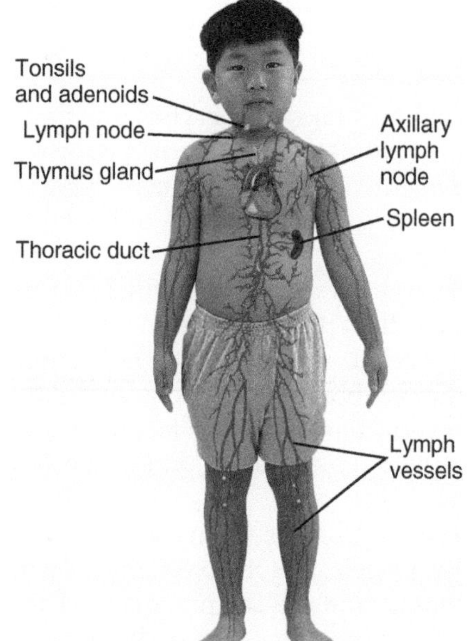

LYMPHATIC SYSTEM

- The increased size of tonsils and adenoids is normal in preschool and school-age children and is one of the body's defense mechanisms.
- The thymus gland is important in the development of the immune response in newborns.
- Preterm and term infants are at greater risk for viral and bacterial infections because of immature T-cell activity.

Fig. 27.1 Summary of lymphatic system differences between the child and the adult. The lymphatic system is a subsystem of the circulatory system. It returns excess tissue fluid to the blood and defends the body against disease. (Art overlay courtesy Observatory Group, Cincinnati, Ohio.)

ANEMIAS

Anemia can result from many different underlying causes. A reduction in the amount of circulating hemoglobin reduces the oxygen-carrying ability of the blood. A hemoglobin level below 80 g/L results in an increased cardiac output and a shunting of blood from the periphery of the body to the vital organs. Pallor, weakness, tachypnea, shortness of breath, and heart failure can result.

IRON-DEFICIENCY ANEMIA

Pathophysiology

Iron deficiency is a common nutritional deficiency in children, with low rates in Canada, although there are certain Indigenous populations in which rates are higher (Abdullah, Zlotkin, Parkin, et al., 2011). The increased prevalence of iron-deficiency anemia (IDA) in these populations may be related to a high consumption of evaporated milk and cow's milk after 6 months of age, prolonged exclusive breastfeeding, and high rates of *Helicobacter pylori* infection. Other high-risk groups include children from families of low socioeconomic status, children of Chinese background, infants of low birth weight, and children who consume whole cow's milk before 12 months of age (Abdullah et al., 2011).

This form of anemia is caused by insufficient amounts of iron in the body. The incidence is highest during infancy and adolescence—two rapid growth periods. **Anemia** (*an*, "without," and *emia*, "blood") is a condition in which there is a reduction in the amount and size of the RBCs, in the amount of hemoglobin, or both. IDA may be caused by severe hemorrhage, the child's inability to absorb the iron received, excessive growth requirements, drinking large quantities of milk per day (greater than 500 mL), or an inadequate diet (Parkin, DeGroot, Maguire, et al., 2016). Feeding whole cow's milk to young infants can precipitate gastrointestinal bleeding, which can also result in anemia.

Prevention of IDA begins with good prenatal care to ensure that the mother has a suitable intake of iron during pregnancy. During the first few months after birth, the newborn relies on iron that was stored in their body during fetal life. Preterm infants may be deprived of a sufficient supply because iron is obtained late in the prenatal period. In addition, the iron stores of low-birth-weight infants and infants from multiple births are relatively small.

The highest incidence of IDA occurs from the ninth to the twenty-fourth months. During this rapid growth period, the infant outgrows the limited iron reserve that was in the body; in addition, foods high in iron may not have been introduced. Feeding problems or inadequate access to healthy food also contribute to this deficiency. Infants who are fed larger quantities of breastmilk or formula receive very little iron. Iron-rich foods should be introduced as the first food at 6 months of age (see Chapter 14). Examples of appropriate food include eggs, meat, leafy green vegetables, iron-fortified cereal, dried fruits (apricots, peaches, prunes, raisins), dry beans, crushed nuts, and whole-grain bread. Iron-fortified cereals eaten out of the box provide a nutritious snack. Unfortunately, the body does not absorb all the iron found in a food source. The bioavailability of iron in vegetables is less than that in meat.

Manifestations

The symptoms of IDA are pallor, irritability, anorexia, fatigue or a decrease in activity, and, in more serious cases, shortness of breath. Blood tests for anemia may include RBC and reticulocyte count, hemoglobin and hematocrit levels, and determination of morphological cell changes and iron concentration. The stool may be tested for occult blood. A dietary history is also obtained. Occasionally, a slight heart murmur is heard. The spleen may be enlarged.

Untreated IDA progresses slowly, and in severe cases the heart muscle becomes too weak to function. If this happens, heart failure follows. Children with longstanding anemia may have impaired normal growth and development, including effects on mental development and functioning. Screening procedures may be suggested between 6 and 12 months for at-risk children (Abdullah et al., 2011).

Treatment

IDA responds well to treatment. Elemental iron is administered orally two or three times daily between meals. Vitamin C aids in the absorption of iron; therefore, providing juice when administering iron is suggested. Liquid preparations of elemental iron are taken through a straw to prevent temporary discoloration of the teeth. (Some iron preparations without this disadvantage are available.) The toddler needs solid foods that are rich sources of iron, such as meat and green vegetables.

Nursing Tip

Oral iron supplements should not be ingested with milk or milk products because milk interferes with iron absorption. Iron supplements should be administered 1 hour before or 2 hours after milk or milk product ingestion.

Parent Education

Parents need explicit instructions regarding proper foods for the infant. The nurse should stress the importance of breastfeeding exclusively for the first 6 months, and up to 2 years or longer with appropriate solid foods to support nutritional and immunological needs as well as healthy growth and development (Critch & Canadian Paediatric Society (CPS) Nutrition and Gastroenterology Committee, 2014/2017). Nurses can address three potentially modifiable feeding practices that are associated with IDA: (1) cow's milk consumption greater than 500 mL/day; (2) daytime bottle use beyond 12 months of age; and (3) bottle use in bed (Parkin et al., 2016). Solid food intake should be reviewed and specific iron-enriched nutrients suggested. The nurse needs to take into consideration financial, ethnic, and family preferences when developing teaching plans. Behaviour concerns at mealtime may also have to be addressed.

The stools of infants who are taking oral iron supplements are tarry green. An absence of this finding may indicate the child is not receiving an adequate amount of the medication. To increase absorption, these preparations should be given between meals, when digestive acid concentration is highest. It is important to emphasize that both dietary changes and supplemental iron therapy are necessary to eradicate IDA. Good dietary practices must be lifelong to maintain good health. Periodic evaluation of the child's blood status is recommended.

Safety Alert!

Prevent iron poisoning in children by keeping preparations well out of reach. Educate parents about this hazard.

SICKLE CELL DISEASE

Pathophysiology

Sickle cell disease is an inherited defect in the formation of hemoglobin. Canadians of South American, Indian, Mediterranean, Middle Eastern, African, Turkish, and Caribbean heritage are affected by sickle cell disease (Sickle Cell Disease Association of Canada [SCDAC], n.d.). It is believed that the gene for sickle cell disease developed in these populations as protection against malaria. While the rates vary according to province, approximately 1 in 2 500 babies will be born with sickle cell disease in Canada (SCDAC, n.d.). Sickling (clumping) caused by decreased blood oxygen levels may be triggered by dehydration, infection, physical or emotional stress, or exposure to cold or very hot temperatures. Laboratory examination of the affected child's blood shows that the RBC has changed its shape to resemble that of a sickle blade, from which the name of the disorder is derived (Fig. 27.3).

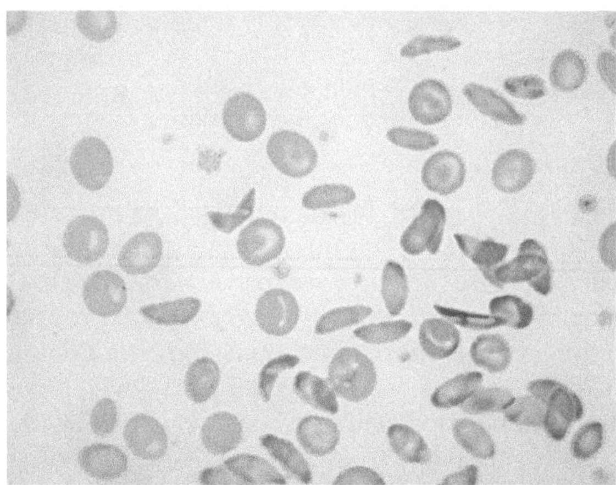

Fig. 27.3 Scanning electron micrograph of erythrocytes. Note that the normal red blood cell is round. The sickle-shaped cell can clump as it flows through the circulation, causing a vaso-occlusive sickle cell crisis. (From Zitelli, B. J., et al. [2018]. *Zitelli and Davis' atlas of pediatric physical diagnosis* [7th ed.]. Philadelphia: Saunders.)

Sickle cells contain an abnormal form of hemoglobin termed *hemoglobin S* (the sickling type). The membranes of these cells are fragile and easily destroyed. Their crescent shape makes it difficult for them to pass through the capillaries, causing a pileup of cells in the small vessels. This clumping may lead to a thrombosis (clot) and cause an obstruction. *Infarcts,* or areas of dead tissue, may result when the tissue is denied proper blood supply. These generally develop in the spleen but may also be seen in other areas of the body, such as the brain, heart, lungs, gastrointestinal tract, kidneys, joints, and bones. The patient feels acute pain in the affected area.

There are two types of sickle cell disease: an asymptomatic version (sickle cell trait) and much more severe forms that can necessitate intermittent hospitalization (sickle cell anemia).

Sickle cell trait

In this form of the disease, the blood of the patient contains a mixture of normal (hemoglobin A) and sickle (hemoglobin S) hemoglobins. This form is the more common type. The proportions of hemoglobin S are low because the disease is inherited from only one parent. The health care provider can distinguish sickle cell trait from the more severe disease by means of electrophoresis, a study of the patient's RBCs and hemoglobin. Sickling is more rapid and extreme with sickle cell disease. In sickle cell trait, the hemoglobin and RBC counts are normal.

Sickle cell trait does not develop into sickle cell disease. Although there is no need to treat the patient with sickle cell trait, the patient is a carrier, and genetic counselling is important.

Sickle cell anemia

This severe form of sickle cell disease results when the abnormality is inherited from both parents (Fig. 27.4). Each offspring has a one in four chance of inheriting the disease (which is not the same as one in four children inheriting it). In general, the clinical symptoms do not appear until the last part of the first year of life, which is directly related to fetal hemoglobin levels from birth. There may be an unusual swelling of the fingers and toes. The specific symptoms of sickle cell disease are caused by the abnormal sickle cell shape that causes clumping and obstruction in the vessels and ischemia to the organs or areas affected.

Chronic anemia occurs. Depending on the form of the disease, the hemoglobin level can range from 70 to 90 g/L or, on occasion, lower. The child is pale, tires easily, and has little appetite. These manifestations of anemia are complicated by characteristic episodes called **sickle cell crises**, which are painful and can be fatal. Specific types of crises have been identified. They differ in their pathological causes and manifestations and may necessitate somewhat different treatments

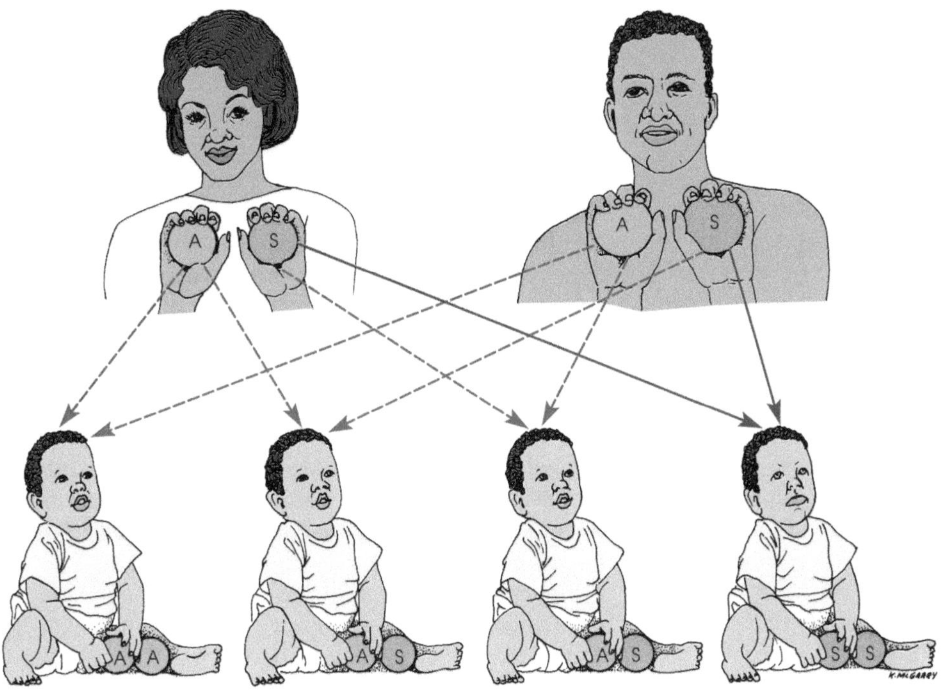

Fig. 27.4 Transmission of sickle cell disease from parents to children. Parents who are carriers of the sickle cell trait do not show symptoms of the disease because hemoglobin A (the normal form of hemoglobin) in their red blood cells protects them from hemoglobin S (the sickling form). When two carriers become parents, however, the possibilities are as follows: One child in four will inherit all normal hemoglobin and thus be free of the disease (AA); two children in four will inherit both hemoglobin A and hemoglobin S and thus become carriers (AS) of the trait (similar to their parents); and one child in four will inherit all sickling hemoglobin and thus be affected by sickle cell disease (SS).

Table 27.1 Types of Sickle Cell Crises

TYPE	COMMENT
Vaso-occlusive (painful crises)	Most common type; there is an obstruction of blood flow by cells, infarctions, and some degree of vasospasm. Dactylitis, painful joints and extremities, abdominal pain (infarction or bleeding within liver, spleen, abdominal lymph node), central nervous system strokes, pulmonary disease, or priapism may be present. Morphine is commonly prescribed with intravenous hydration.
Splenic sequestration	Large amounts of blood pool in the liver and spleen. Spleen becomes massive. Abdominal pain occurs. Circulatory collapse and shock can be present. Children between 8 months and 5 years of age are particularly susceptible. Death may occur within hours of appearance of symptoms. Minor episodes may resolve spontaneously. Splenectomy may be indicated for children who have one or more severe crises.
Aplastic crises	Bone marrow stops producing red blood cells (RBCs); a number of infections may precipitate this (usually viral, e.g., parvovirus). Decreased reticulocyte count may be present. Child may be transfused with fresh packed RBCs if severe anemia occurs.
Hyperhemolytic	Rapid rate of hemolysis is superimposed on an already severe process; rare condition. Functional hyposplenism and overwhelming infection occur. Progressive fibrosis of spleen reduces its function; patient becomes more susceptible to infection.

Data from Jackson-Allen, P., Vessey, J., & Schapiro, N. (2010). *Primary care of the child with a chronic condition* (5th ed.). Philadelphia: Mosby; DeBaun, M., Frei-Jones, M., & Vichinsky, E. (2016). Hemoglobinopathies. In R. Kliegman, B. Stanton, J. St. Geme, et al. (Eds.), *Nelson textbook of pediatrics* (20th ed.). Philadelphia: Saunders.

(Table 27.1). Unfortunately, in some cases the sickle cell crisis is the first obvious manifestation of the condition. The patient appears acutely ill. The symptoms depend on the location of the sickling, and there could be severe abdominal pain, muscle spasms, leg pain, painful swollen joints, and hypoxia. Fever, vomiting, hematuria, convulsions, stiff neck, coma, or paralysis can result, depending on the organs involved. Children with sickle cell disease have a risk for stroke as a complication of a vaso-occlusive sickle cell crisis. The sickle cell crises recur periodically throughout childhood; however, they tend to decrease with age and proper management.

Patients should be kept in good health between episodes. Immunizations of these children are particularly important and should be kept up to date. They include those for *Haemophilus influenzae*, meningitis, hepatitis A, and hepatitis B, as well as the pneumococcal and yearly influenza vaccine. Patients should refrain from becoming overly tired. They also should avoid situations such as flying in an unpressurized airplane or exercising at a high altitude, because oxygen concentrations in their blood are already reduced. Extra stress and exposure to cold may lower resistance, causing additional problems. Overheating, which can lead to dehydration, is also to be avoided. Oral intake of iron is of no value in reducing symptoms.

Nursing Tip

During sickle cell crises, anticipate the child's need for tissue oxygenation, hydration, rest, protection from infection, pain control, blood transfusion, and emotional support for this life-threatening illness.

Diagnosis

Sickle cell disease can be detected before birth by chorionic villi sampling (CVS) and amniocentesis (Vacca & Blank, 2017). (See Chapter 4 for further discussion on prenatal testing). Early diagnosis by screening of all newborns in Canada allows for early detection before symptoms occur (see Newborn Screening, in Chapter 11). The newborn screen is conducted from a heel stick at birth. Hemoglobin electrophoresis ("fingerprinting") is used when the newborn screen result is positive. This procedure separates and records the various peptide patterns of the blood. It distinguishes between patients with the trait and those with the disease.

Treatment and Nursing Care

When the infant or child is hospitalized during a crisis, the treatment is supportive and symptomatic. The patient is confined to bed. Analgesics are provided to relieve pain. Children in severe pain may need an intravenous (IV) infusion containing an opioid, such as morphine. A patient-controlled analgesia (PCA) pump enables older children to maintain control of their pain and participate in care. Every effort is made to combat dehydration and acidosis. Small blood transfusions may be administered to increase the hemoglobin count, but the results are only temporary, and the patient and family should be aware of the risks of donor blood transfusion. Packed RBCs are often given with the goal of keeping the abnormal RBCs at the level of 30% of total hemoglobin (Vacca & Blank, 2017). An accurate record of intake and output should be kept. The patient's body position needs to be changed frequently but gently.

Oral hydroxyurea with once-daily dosing is the only approved drug treatment for sickle cell disease in Canada. This medication increases circulating fetal hemoglobin in the blood, decreases the adhesiveness of the RBCs, and increases the size of the RBCs, which results in increased blood flow. As the medication is metabolized, nitric oxide is released, which causes vasodilation. Hydroxyurea therapy reduces the occurrence of vaso-occlusion and associated pain, as well as the need for transfusions and hospitalizations (Vacca & Blank, 2017).

A complete blood count (CBC) is done monthly and monitored for neutropenia, which may increase the risk for infection. Maintaining adequate hydration is important, as dehydration can increase sickling. When bed rest is necessary, venous thrombosis prophylaxis should be initiated to prevent development of blood clots and ischemic strokes. Hematopoietic stem cell transplantation (HSCT) may provide a cure in the near future, but is still being investigated.

Sickle cell disease may take a wide variety of courses. As always, the individual patient's progress is followed. Sometimes it is difficult to distinguish between abdominal pain caused by a sickle cell crisis and abdominal pain caused by appendicitis. The nurse must remember that pain experienced by a child with sickle cell disease may also be caused by an unrelated condition.

Prevention of infection and prevention of dehydration are very important goals in the care of a child with sickle cell disease. Infants and children with sickle cell disease often have functional asplenia and impaired immune function, and bacteremia (sepsis) is a leading cause of death in this group. Oral penicillin prophylaxis before any invasive treatment, including dental care, is advised.

Hemosiderosis (the deposit of iron into organs and tissues in the body) is a complication of this type of hemolytic disease. The medication deferoxamine mesylate (Desferal) binds with iron and allows its excretion via the kidney. An oral form is also available. An exchange transfusion may reduce the number of circulating sickle cells and prevent complications such as thrombus formation and stroke.

The main goals of nursing care are to observe for sickling, dehydration, hypoxia, and infection, which can cause a sickle cell crisis. Erythropoietin can increase the production of normal hemoglobin and reduce complications.

Surgery

The use of splenectomy in children with sickle cell disease has been conservative. A recurrence of acute splenic sequestration becomes less likely after 5 years of age. Routine splenectomy is not recommended because the spleen generally atrophies on its own because of fibrotic changes that take place in patients with sickle cell disease. HSCT can cure sickle cell disease, but this therapy is currently available only to those with a human leukocyte antigen (HLA)–compatible sibling and has limited availability in Canada (Field, Vichinsky, & DeBaun, 2018).

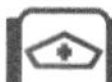

Nursing Tip

It is essential to teach parents the signs and symptoms of dehydration, hypoxia, and infection to prevent the occurrence of sickle cell crisis. Encouraging regular follow-ups with the sickle cell health care team is also of importance in preventing complications.

> **! Safety Alert!**
>
> Cold compresses should not be used to relieve pain in a child with sickle cell anemia, because cold promotes sickling and ischemia, and ischemic tissues have reduced sensation. Therefore, damage can occur.

THALASSEMIA

Pathophysiology

The *thalassemias* are a group of hereditary blood disorders in which the patient's body cannot produce sufficient adult hemoglobin. The RBCs are abnormal in size and shape and are rapidly destroyed. This abnormality results in chronic anemia. The body attempts to compensate by producing large amounts of fetal hemoglobin. Thalassemias are caused by a deficiency in the normal synthesis of hemoglobin polypeptide chains. They are categorized according to the Greek letters designating the polypeptide chain affected, but α- and β-thalassemia are the most common forms.

The thalassemia that involves impaired production of beta chains is known as *β-thalassemia*. This variety consists of two forms: thalassemia minor and thalassemia major. Thalassemia major is also called *Cooley's anemia*. Thalassemia occurs mainly in persons of Mediterranean origin and of African, Middle Eastern, and Asian descent. The term is derived from the Greek *thalassa*, which means "sea." Thalassemia can also occur from spontaneous mutations.

Thalassemia minor

Thalassemia minor, which is also termed *β-thalassemia trait*, occurs when the child inherits a thalassemia gene from only one parent *(heterozygous inheritance)*. It is associated with mild anemia. These patients are often misdiagnosed as having an IDA. Symptoms are minimal. The patient is pale, and the spleen may be enlarged. The patient may lead a normal life, with the illness going undetected. This condition is of genetic importance, particularly if both parents are carriers of the trait.

Thalassemia major (Cooley's anemia)

When two thalassemia genes are inherited *(homozygous inheritance)*, the child is born with a more serious form of the disease. A progressive, severe anemia becomes evident around 6 months of life, however, newborn screening (available in select provinces for hemoglobinopathies) assists in earlier detection and treatment.

The child may be pale and irritable, has poor growth and development, and has a poor appetite and difficulty sleeping. Jaundice, which at first is mild, progresses to a muddy bronze colour resulting from *hemosiderosis*, a deposit of iron (released by blood cell destruction) into the tissues. Abdominal distention occurs, which causes pressure on the organs of the chest. Cardiac failure caused by the profound anemia is a constant threat. The liver and spleen enlarge as defective RBCs are destroyed and a compensatory mechanism occurs known as *extramedullary hematopoiesis*. Bone marrow space also enlarges to compensate for an increased production of blood cells. *Hematopoietic (hema*, "blood," and *poiesis*, "to make") defects and a massive expansion of the bone marrow in the face and skull result in changes in the facial contour that give the child a characteristic appearance (Fig. 27.5). The teeth protrude because of an overgrowth of the upper jawbone; the bone becomes thin and is subject to pathological fracture.

Diagnosis is aided by a family history of thalassemia, radiographic bone growth studies, and blood tests. Hemoglobin electrophoresis is helpful in diagnosing the type, but genetic testing is more helpful in determining the severity of the various thalassemias. Prenatal screening and diagnosis are available, and genetic counselling is advised.

Treatment and Nursing Care

The goals of care for children with thalassemia are to (1) maintain hemoglobin levels at 90 g/L to prevent overgrowth of bone marrow and resultant deformities and (2) provide for growth and development and normal physical activity. Some patients require splenectomy, but that increases the risk for blood clots and infection.

The mainstay of treatment for thalassemia major is frequent (every 3 to 4 weeks) blood transfusions to maintain the hemoglobin level above 95 to 105 g/L. As a result of repeated blood transfusions, excessive deposits of iron may be stored in the tissues. This is termed *hemochromatosis* and is seen especially in the spleen, liver, heart, pancreas, and pituitary glands. Deferasirox (Exjade or Jadenu) is a chelating medication that is given orally once a day. It can be toxic to the kidneys. Other chelating medications include

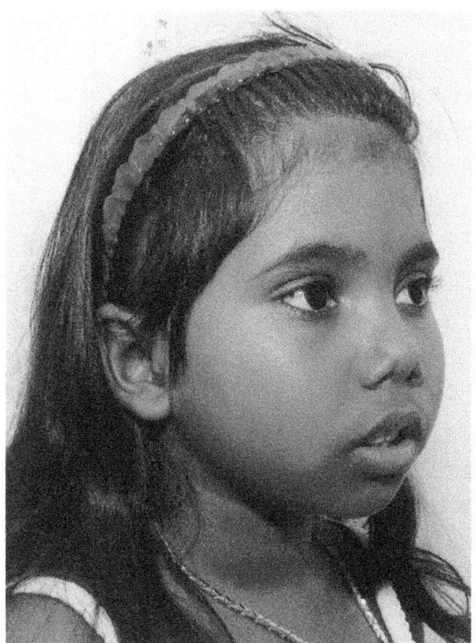

Fig. 27.5 Appearance of child with thalassemia. Note the overgrowth of the upper jawbone (maxillary hyperplasia). (From Hockenberry, M. J., & Wilson, D. [2015]. *Wong's nursing care of infants and children* [10th ed.]. St. Louis: Mosby.)

deferoxamine mesylate (Desferal), given intravenously or subcutaneously. This medication causes red discoloration of the urine. Blurred vision or ringing in the ears should be reported. These chelating drugs can be given in combination to more efficiently excrete excess iron in the body and prevent hemosiderosis (DeBaun, Frei-Jones, & Vichinsky, 2016). An antimetabolite, hydroxyurea, increases normal hemoglobin production, which is used successfully in sickle cell anemia and is sometimes used in thalassemia with varied affect.

Nursing care involves observation of the patient during a blood transfusion. Whenever possible, to provide security and trust, the same nurse cares for the patient during transfusions, blood tests, and other unpleasant procedures. Children are taught to regulate their activities according to their own tolerance.

The emotional health of the child and parents calls for special consideration by the nurse. Every attempt must be made to ease the strain of this prolonged illness. Home care arrangements can be provided through community agencies. The family can be referred to support groups for support and education. Older children need special support to accept changes in their body image caused by the disease. Suggestions applicable to the care of the chronically ill child are discussed in Chapter 22. For the most part, these children go on to live normal and healthy lives while maintaining monthly transfusion regimes and adherence to their chelation medication regimens.

BLEEDING DISORDERS

HEMOPHILIA

Pathophysiology

Hemophilia is one of the oldest hereditary diseases known to humanity. In this disorder, the blood does not clot normally, and even the slightest injury can cause severe bleeding. This congenital disorder is confined almost exclusively to males but is transmitted by symptom-free females.

Hemophilia is inherited as a sex-linked recessive trait. It is termed *sex-linked* because the defective gene is located on the X, or female, chromosome. Different combinations of genes account for the fact that some children inherit the disease, some become carriers, and others neither inherit nor carry the trait. New mutations do occur, and the reason for this is unclear. Fetal blood sampling detects hemophilia. Some carrier women can also be identified.

There are several types of hemophilia. More than 10 identified factors in blood are involved in the clotting mechanism. A deficiency in any one of the factors will interfere with normal blood clotting. The two most common types of hemophilia are *hemophilia B*, or **Christmas disease** (a factor IX deficiency), and *hemophilia A* (a deficiency in factor VIII). This discussion is limited to classic hemophilia, or hemophilia A, which accounts for approximately 85% of cases (Scott, 2016).

Hemophilia A is caused by a deficiency of coagulation factor VIII, or antihemophilic globulin (AHG). The severity of the disease depends on the level of factor VIII in the plasma of the patient's blood. Some patients' lives are endangered by minor injury, whereas a child with a mild case of hemophilia might just bruise a little more easily than the normal person. The degree of severity tends to remain constant within a given family. The aim of therapy is to increase the level of factor VIII high enough to ensure clotting. It is possible to determine the level of factor VIII in the blood by means of a test called *partial thromboplastin time (PTT)*, which can help to diagnose and assess the child's condition.

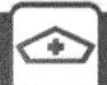 **Nursing Tip**

A classic symptom of hemophilia is bleeding into the joints (hemarthrosis).

Manifestations

Hemophilia can be diagnosed at birth because maternal factor VIII cannot cross the placenta and be transferred to the fetus. However, it is usually not apparent in the newborn unless abnormal bleeding occurs at the umbilical cord or after circumcision. As the child grows older and becomes more subject to injury, the slightest bruise or cut can induce extensive bleeding. Normal blood clots in about 3 to 6 minutes. In a patient with severe hemophilia, however, the time required for clotting may be 1 hour or longer.

Anemia, leukocytosis, and a moderate increase in the number of platelets may be seen in the hemorrhaging child. There may also be signs of shock. Spontaneous hematuria is seen. Death can result from excessive bleeding anywhere in the body, but particularly when hemorrhage into the brain or neck occurs. Severe headache, vomiting, and disorientation may reflect cranial bleeding. Bleeding into the neck can cause airway obstruction. Bleeding into the ears and eyes can affect hearing and vision. Bleeding into the spinal column can lead to paralysis.

The circumstances leading to diagnosis may be the inability of a parent to stop a child's bleeding from a cut around the mouth or gums. A deciduous tooth loss may precipitate problems in a child who has a bleeding disorder. Hematomas may develop after immunizations. An injured knee, elbow, or ankle presents particular problems. Hemorrhage into the joint cavity, or **hemarthrosis** (*hema*, "blood," *arthron*, "joint," and *osis*, "condition of"), is considered a classic symptom of hemophilia. The effusion (*ex*, "out," and *fundere*, "to pour") into the joint is very painful because of the pressure buildup. Repeated hemorrhages may cause permanent deformities that could incapacitate the child. This deformity is sometimes referred to as an *ankylosis* (*ankyle*, "stiff joint," and *osis*, "condition of").

Treatment and Nursing Care

In a newborn with a family history of hemophilia, heel sticks and intramuscular injections are not delayed to prevent bleeding and tissue injury, but the nurse should use the smallest gauge needle and apply pressure for 10 minutes afterward. Circumcision is delayed or avoided in this patient population.

The principal therapy for hemophilia is to prevent bleeding by replacing the missing factor (Traore, Chan, Webert, et al., 2014). The development of recombinant antihemophilic factor, a synthetic product, has eliminated the need for repeated blood transfusions and its theoretical accompanying dangers (such as human immunodeficiency virus [HIV] and hepatitis infection). Diagnosed infants may receive prophylactic factor replacements to prevent hemarthrosis. The prophylactic dose depends on the type and severity of hemophilia as well as the product type. Desmopressin acetate (DDAVP) is usually administered subcutaneously or intravenously, intranasal is an option but the absorption rate is less effective than the other routes. DDAVP can be given before a procedure or activity or it can be used to treat bleeds. It increases factor VIII in the blood, which leads to decreased bleeding and may be the treatment of choice for mild cases of hemophilia. Tranexamic acid is an antifibrinolytic agent that can be used for mucocutaneous bleeds with the exception of urological bleeds. An example would be to control bleeding that might occur because of dental care.

The use of aspirin and nonsteroidal anti-inflammatory drugs (NSAIDs) that affect platelets should be avoided. Prophylactic therapy and education concerning the prevention of injuries that can cause bleeding enable the hemophiliac child to live a normal life. Because young children often fall while playing, padding their play outfits can protect the joints of knees, hips, and elbows. Appropriate sports activities should be selected to prevent undue injury and the risk of bleeding into joints. When bleeding does occur, the traditional approach to care includes **p**rotection, **r**est, **i**ce, **c**ompression, and **e**levation (PRICE). There is some controversy about using ice; ice probably decreases the pain but it may cause vasoconstriction of vessels, thus the important factors to decrease bleeding may not get to the injury as quickly. A medical alert identification band should be worn at all times.

A factor VIII concentrate (Kovaltry) used to treat hemophilia A disease and factor IX concentrate to treat hemophilia B (Rixubis) are currently approved to control and prevent bleeding in hemophilia (Scott, 2016). Gene therapy offers hope in the near future.

Home care programs supervised by a comprehensive health care team are the treatment support of choice. These greatly reduce the cost of treatment and decrease the risk of psychological trauma. Using a multidisciplinary approach to care assists families in developing healthy coping strategies to manage a child who has a chronic illness.

It is difficult for parents not to be overly protective. The struggle to protect these children and still foster independence and a sense of autonomy may seem monumental to parents, especially those who work away from home. Allowing children to participate in decision making about their care and focusing on their strengths are helpful. See Chapter 22 for further discussion of caring for children with a chronic illness.

Parent groups and professional counselling may provide support to enable children and parents to develop a healthy attitude toward the child's medical condition.

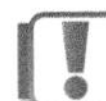
Safety Alert!

Drugs that contain salicylates and NSAIDs are contraindicated for use in children with hemophilia.

PLATELET DISORDERS

The reduction or destruction of platelets in the body interferes with the clotting mechanism. Skin lesions that are common to these disorders include petechiae, a bluish, nonblanching, pinpoint-sized lesion; purpura, groups of adjoining petechiae; **ecchymosis**, an isolated bluish lesion larger than a petechia; and **hematoma**, a raised ecchymosis.

Immune Thrombocytopenia

Pathophysiology

Immune thrombocytopenia (ITP) (formerly called *idiopathic thrombocytopenic purpura*) is an autoimmune platelet disorder that occurs in childhood. It is the most common of the *purpuras*, which is a group of disorders affecting the numbers of platelets or their function. The cause is unknown, but it is thought to be an autoimmune system reaction preceded by a viral infection. Platelets become coated with antiplatelet antibody, are "perceived" as foreign material, and are eventually destroyed by the spleen. ITP occurs in all age groups, with the main incidence between 1 and 4 years of age (Scott, 2016).

Manifestations

The classic symptoms of ITP are slowed blood clotting and easy bruising, which result in *petechiae* (pinpoint hemorrhagic spots beneath the skin) and *purpura* (hemorrhage into the skin). Approximately 30% of patients also have nosebleeds. There may have been a recent history of a viral respiratory infection. The interval between exposure and onset is about 2 to 4 weeks. The platelet count can be below 20×10^9 /L (normal range is between 150×10^9 /L and 400×10^9 /L). Anemia may be present if bleeding has occurred, but other blood components are normal. A bone marrow aspiration to rule out leukemia may be indicated if abnormal WBCs are present in a routine blood test.

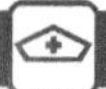
Nursing Tip

The bruises of immune thrombocytopenia (ITP) must be distinguished from those of child abuse.

Treatment and nursing care

When platelet counts are low, the greatest danger is spontaneous intracranial bleeding. Neurological assessments are therefore a priority of care. Treatment is not indicated in most cases of ITP. Spontaneous remission occurs in about 3 to 6 months. A few children progress to chronic ITP. Medications that interfere with platelet function should be avoided to prevent bleeding. These include aspirin and NSAIDs. Activity is limited during the acute stage to prevent bruises from falls and trauma. Nursing considerations for the more acutely ill child focus on observing the patient for signs of bleeding. The child should use soft toothbrushes for oral hygiene to minimize tissue trauma.

Platelet infusion is usually not provided because the disease process destroys them. Corticosteroids such as prednisone may be prescribed as a first-line of treatment. IV gamma globulin (IVIG) may be used as a second-line of therapy to elevate platelet counts. In some patients, infusion with anti-D antibody may be an effective treatment for Rh-positive patients who still have a spleen and are nonanemic.

Complications of ITP include bleeding from the gastrointestinal tract, hemarthrosis, and intracranial hemorrhage. Mortality in childhood ITP is less than 1%. It is important for children to receive recommended immunizations against the viral diseases of childhood to prevent this complication from occurring.

Safety Alert!

After administration of anti-D antibody, the child should be observed for 1 hour for fever, chills, headache, or alteration in vital signs.

HENOCH-SCHÖNLEIN PURPURA (HSP)

HSP is a vasculitis that occurs in 14 to 20/100 000 children per year between 3 and 10 years of age (Ardoin & Fells, 2016). It is an autoimmune illness that involves inflammation of the blood vessels with multi-organ involvement and signs and symptoms of petechiae and palpable (raised) purpura and ecchymosis, mostly in the lower extremities. Abdominal pain, gastrointestinal bleeding, and hematuria may occur. Risk factors can be respiratory illness, use of NSAIDs, or food allergies (Misha, 2017). There is no thrombocytopenia in this condition.

Most cases are mild and respond to general supportive care, with adequate hydration, nutrition, and pain control. Steroids may be prescribed to assist with severe joint and abdominal pain, but they do not prevent renal involvement (Guo & Lam, 2016). Monthly urinalysis tests should be performed for at least 6 months to monitor renal involvement.

DISORDERS OF WHITE BLOOD CELLS

LEUKEMIA

Leukemia refers to a group of malignant diseases of the bone marrow and lymphatic system. There are many types and classifications, each with its own therapy and prognosis. Acute lymphoblastic leukemia (ALL) is the most common type of leukemia diagnosed in young children, and it occurs more often in boys than girls. The classification of ALL depends on the characteristics of the malignant cells in the bone marrow. The classification is important to the design of the individual treatment and prognosis (Friehling, Ritchey, Tubergen, et al., 2016). Acute myelogenous leukemia (AML) is less common and usually occurs more often in girls than boys. Rare types of childhood leukemias can also develop, including chronic lymphoblastic leukemia (CLL) and chronic myelogenous leukemia (CML) (Canadian Cancer Society, 2019). The discussion in this text refers to ALL, the most common type of childhood leukemia.

Survival rates for children diagnosed with leukemia have greatly improved. However, close monitoring of late adverse effects of leukemia therapy is essential, and long-term follow-up care should be monitored.

Pathophysiology

Leukemia (*leuko,* "white," and *emia,* "blood") is a malignant disease of the blood-forming organs of the body that results in an uncontrolled growth of immature WBCs. The immature cells are termed *blasts,* or *stem cells.* This term comes from the Greek *blastos,* meaning "germ" or "formative cell." Leukemia is the most common form of childhood cancer. It was considered fatal in the past, but the prognosis has improved greatly with modern treatments and medication.

The leukemias involve a disruption of bone marrow function caused by the overproduction of immature WBCs in the marrow. Although the WBC count can be very high, the cells are immature and do not function as healthy WBCs to fight infection; increased susceptibility to infection results. The WBCs take over the centres that are designed to form RBCs, and anemia results. When the WBCs infiltrate and take over the marrow centres that form platelets, the reduced platelet counts cause bleeding tendencies. The invasion of the bone marrow causes weakening of the bone, and pathological fractures can occur.

Leukemia cells can infiltrate the spleen, liver, and lymph glands, resulting in fibrosis and diminished function. The cancerous cells invade the central nervous system and other organs, draining these organs of their nutrients and finally causing metabolic starvation of the body.

Manifestations

The most common symptoms during the initial phase of leukemia are low-grade fever; repeated infections; pallor; bruising tendency; leg, bone and joint pain; lethargy; abdominal pain; and enlargement of lymph nodes. These symptoms may develop gradually or may be sudden in onset. As the disease progresses, the liver and spleen become enlarged. The skin may have an unusual lemon-yellow colour. Petechiae and purpura may be early objective symptoms. Anorexia, vomiting, and weight loss are not as common at diagnosis but can also occur. The kidneys and testicles may enlarge, and the patient may develop hematuria, anemia, and thrombocytopenia.

Because the WBCs are not functioning normally, bacteria easily invade the body. Ulcerations develop around the mucous membranes of the mouth and anal regions and have a tendency to bleed (Fig. 27.6).

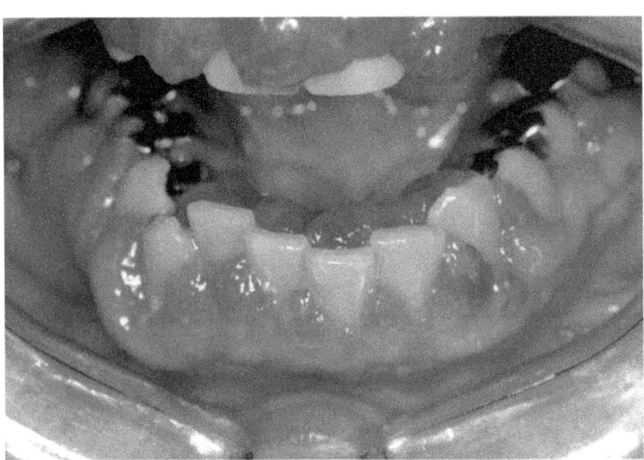

Fig. 27.6 The mouth lesions of leukemia. (From Regezi, J. A., Sciubba, J. J., & Jordan, R. C. K. [2017]. *Oral pathology: Clinical pathologic correlations* [7th ed.]. St. Louis: Saunders.)

Anemia becomes severe despite transfusions. The child may die as a direct result of the disease or from secondary infection. The symptoms are similar regardless of the type of WBC affected, but they vary widely with each patient depending on the parts of the body involved.

Diagnosis

The diagnosis of leukemia is based on the history and symptoms of the patient and the results of extensive blood tests that demonstrate the presence of leukemic blast cells in the blood, bone marrow, or other tissues. Because many WBCs and RBCs are formed in the bone marrow, a bone marrow aspiration is commonly performed. A piece of bone marrow is aspirated from the sternum or, more often in children, from the iliac crest. A special needle is used to obtain the sample, and the marrow is studied in the laboratory (Fig. 27.7). X-ray films of the long bones show changes. After the diagnosis has been confirmed, a spinal tap determines central nervous system involvement. Kidney and liver function studies are also performed because normal functioning of these organs is absolutely necessary for chemotherapy to be safely used in treating the disease.

Treatment and Nursing Care

Long-term care is provided on an outpatient basis whenever possible. The treatment of a child with cancer involves the interdisciplinary health care team (pediatrician, pathologist, oncologist, nurse, nurse practitioner, radiotherapist, nutritionist, psychologist, and school personnel). Pediatric **oncologists** (health care providers who specialize in the treatment of tumours) are challenged with the treatment of cancer in children because radiation, surgery, and chemotherapy often have adverse effects on growth and development.

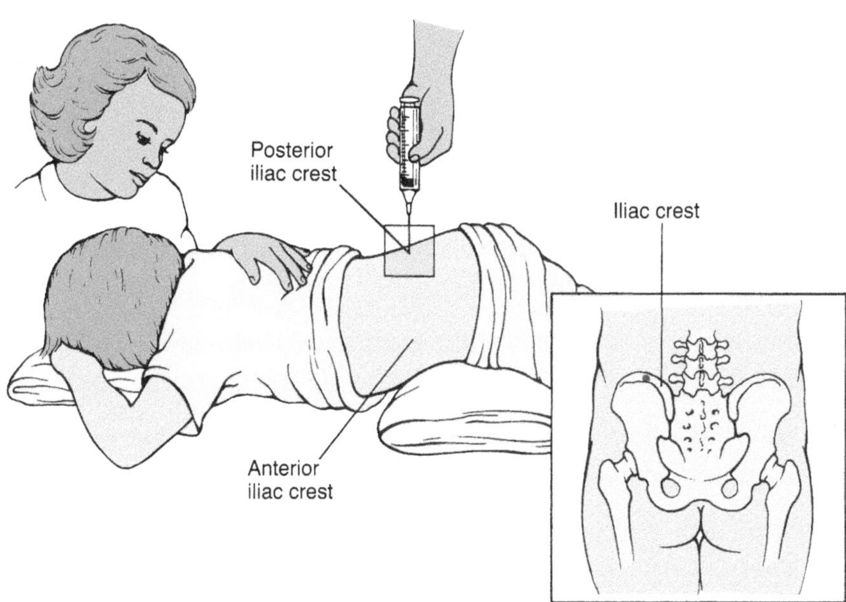

Fig. 27.7 Bone marrow aspiration. Because many white blood cells and red blood cells are formed in the bone marrow, a bone marrow aspiration can determine the type and quantity of cells present and help to rule out or to confirm a serious disease.

Most children with cancer are treated in large medical centres to maximize the availability of high technology and newer treatment methods. Chemotherapy is performed in specialized units with specially trained and certified personnel.

Although multi-agent chemotherapy may be effective in reducing leukemic cells, the adverse and long-term effects of treatments must be addressed. In chemotherapy, bone marrow suppression makes it essential for the family to be taught about infection prevention. Neutropenia may require protective isolation precautions. Adequate hydration should be emphasized to minimize kidney damage. Active routine immunizations must be delayed while the child is receiving immunosuppressive medications, because the body will not be able to manufacture antigens as expected. Parents should report any exposure to infections such as chicken pox so that immunoglobulin can be administered. Chicken pox can be life-threatening to a child who is immunosuppressed.

Nausea and vomiting are common complications of chemotherapy and result in decreased appetite, weight loss, and generalized weakness. Presenting the child's favourite foods in an attractive manner may help stimulate the appetite. Total parenteral nutrition (TPN) may be indicated to support nutritional needs. An intake and output record is maintained, and meticulous oral hygiene must be provided.

Because hair loss (**alopecia**) is an adverse effect of chemotherapy, the child can be offered a hat or a wig to help preserve a positive body image. School tutoring and counselling should be continuous in the hospital setting and in the home during home care to provide optimal growth and development. The nurse should refer parents to available support groups. The Ronald McDonald house and hospice programs can help parents and families cope with this illness.

Nursing Tip

Four priority challenges in the care of children with leukemia are (1) the complications of anemia from decreased red blood cell (RBC) production, (2) infection from neutropenia, (3) bleeding from decreased platelets, and (4) fractures resulting from the involvement of the bone marrow.

Radiation and chemotherapy target specific cells. Box 27.1 discusses different types of chemotherapy.

The list of medications for treatment of ALL is growing. A combination of medications are used to induce remissions. The therapeutic effects of some medications are of short duration, therefore, it is necessary to use additional medications that help to maintain the remissions. The steroid prednisone has the adverse effects of masking the symptoms of infection, increasing fluid retention, inducing personality changes, and causing the child's face to take on a moon-shaped appearance. Methotrexate and mercaptopurine are useful in maintaining remissions because they act against chemicals vital to the life of the WBC. These powerful medications produce adverse effects of varying degrees, such as nausea, diarrhea, rash, alopecia, fever, anuria, anemia, and bone marrow depression. Peripheral neuropathy may be signalled by severe constipation caused by decreased nerve sensations to the bowel. The nurse should consult a pharmacology text for information about the particular medications used for the patient, to anticipate potential problems.

A bone marrow transplant may be useful. An *autologous* transplant uses the child's own bone marrow that has been purged of malignant cells. An *allogeneic* bone marrow transplant is taken from a donor who matches the child. Transplanted marrow rejection is a risk. When the child is hospitalized, protective environmental precautions and additional precautions may prevent health care–associated infections.

Box 27.1 Different Phases of Chemotherapy

- **Induction chemotherapy:** The goal of induction chemotherapy for childhood acute lymphoblastic leukemia (ALL) is to bring about remission by killing all the leukemia cells, or blasts, in the blood, bone marrow, and cerebrospinal fluid (CSF).
- **Consolidation chemotherapy:** The goal of consolidation therapy is to kill any leukemia cells, or blasts, that are still in the blood or bone marrow once complete remission has been reached. It helps prevent recurrence in distant sites, such as the central nervous system (CNS) or testicles.
- **Interim maintenance chemotherapy:** An interim maintenance phase usually follows consolidation chemotherapy. This phase is similar to a standard maintenance cycle. It allows the bone marrow to recover while maintaining remission.
- **Delayed intensification chemotherapy:** In the delayed intensification, or reinduction, phase more intense chemotherapy is given before maintenance chemotherapy starts. It helps to prevent leukemia from recurring.
- **Maintenance chemotherapy:** Once the other treatment phases lower the number of leukemia cells, or blasts, maintenance chemotherapy begins. During this final phase, chemotherapy is given at a low level of intensity (lower doses given less frequently) over a longer period of time, to maintain remission.
- **Central nervous system therapy:** CNS therapy is given during all phases of treatment for childhood ALL. It helps prevent any leukemia cells, or blasts, from spreading to the CNS and kills any leukemia cells in the CNS.

Source: Canadian Cancer Society. (2018). *Treatments for childhood ALL*. Retrieved from http://www.cancer.ca/en/cancer-information/cancer-type/leukemia-childhood/treatment/acute-lymphocytic-leukemia-all/?region=on.

HSCT has been used successfully in children with ALL who do not respond to chemotherapy. After transplant, prevention of infection is the challenge for the health care team. HSCT is a risky procedure because the immune system of the child must first be destroyed before the transplant procedure starts. However, approximately 90% of children with leukemia are cured (Tubergen, Bleyer, Ritchkey, et al., 2016).

Children's anxiety often centres on their symptoms. They fear that the treatments necessary to correct their problems may be painful, as indeed some are, such as venipunctures, bone marrow aspirations, and blood transfusions. Their trust in others is in a precarious balance. Nurses must inform the child of what they are about to do and why it is necessary. The explanation is given in terms the child will understand.

The child may ask the nurse the inevitable question, "Am I going to die?" One suggestion is to reply with a question, such as "Why do you ask that? Do you feel sick today?" This may encourage the child to verbalize feelings. The nurse who encourages patients to discuss their concerns will find opportunities to clear up misconceptions and to decrease children's feelings of isolation.

The patient is assessed frequently for signs of infection. Particular attention is paid to potential sites of infection, such as the patient's mucous membranes and puncture breaks in the skin from laboratory or therapeutic procedures. Pierced ears or other pierced body parts are observed for inflammation. Vital signs are observed for subtle variances, because steroid therapy may mask these indicators. The patient should be turned often and observed for skin breakdown, particularly in the perianal area. Nutritious meals and supplemental feedings that are high in protein and calories should be offered. Parents and children need to be taught what they should look for and report.

Thrombocytopenic bleeding is a common complication of leukemia. The nurse needs to observe the patient's skin for petechiae and ecchymosis. Nosebleeds are common and are treated by the application of cold and pressure.

The mouth is inspected daily for ulcerations and bleeding from the gums. It may be rinsed with a prescribed solution. Commercial mouthwashes should be used with caution because they may alter normal flora and may cause fungal overgrowth. A water pick is helpful in massaging and toughening the gums.

If the child is comatose, mouth care supplies are kept at the bedside. A soft tooth sponge is helpful. The nurse may also clean food particles from the child's teeth with a piece of gauze wrapped around a gloved finger. Lip balm should be applied to dry, cracked lips.

For further discussion of caring for the child who is dying, see Chapter 22.

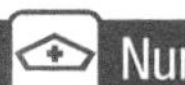 **Nursing Tip**

Bleeding from the nose or mouth may be evidenced by a soiled pillowcase or sheet.

HODGKIN LYMPHOMA

Pathophysiology

Hodgkin lymphoma (HL) is a malignancy of the reticuloendothelial and lymphatic systems. It primarily involves the lymph nodes. It may metastasize to the spleen, liver, bone marrow, lungs, or other parts of the body. The presence of giant multinucleated cells called *Reed-Sternberg cells* is diagnostic of the disease. HL is rarely seen before 5 years of age, with the incidence increasing during adolescence and early adulthood. It is more common in boys than in girls. It may have a genetic origin or may be linked to a viral infection such as Epstein-Barr virus (EBV) (Hochberg, Giulino-Roth, & Cairo, 2016).

Manifestations

The presenting symptom of HL is generally a painless lump along the neck, above the clavicle. Characteristically, there are few other manifestations. In general, the patient or parents first note the swelling. In more advanced cases, there may be unexplained low-grade fever, chronic cough (if compression of the trachea), anorexia, unexplained weight loss, night sweats, general malaise, rash, and itching. Diagnosis is confirmed by excisional biopsy of the node. The stages of HL are defined in Table 27.2.

Treatment

Well-established treatment regimens are now being used to treat this illness. Both radiation therapy and chemotherapy are used in accordance with the clinical stage of the disease and will be decided on by the oncologist. Therapy needs to be monitored. Long-term prognosis is excellent, but long-term effects of therapy have to be monitored. Stem cell transplant may be a treatment option for children with primary progressive (also called resistant) or recurrent childhood classic HL.

Nursing Care

Nursing care is mainly directed toward symptomatic relief of the adverse effects of radiation therapy and chemotherapy. Education of the patient and family is paramount because most patients are cared for in the home. The nurse should explain the many diagnostic tests to be performed and prepare the child for the typical procedures and their aftereffects. After a lymphangiogram, for example, the skin and urine may take on a bluish colour.

Table 27.2 Criteria for Staging Hodgkin Lymphoma

STAGE	CRITERIA
I	Restricted to single site or localized in a group of lymph nodes; asymptomatic
II	Involves two or more lymph nodes in area or on same side of diaphragm
III	Involves lymph node regions on both sides of diaphragm; involves adjacent organ or spleen
IV	Is diffuse disease; least favourable prognosis

Children and parents should be prepared to handle the impact on self-image. The school should be contacted to implement a schedule that will promote growth and development while preventing overfatigue. A common adverse effect of irradiation is malaise. The adolescent tires easily, may be irritable, and have a loss of appetite. The skin in the treated area may be sensitive and must be protected against exposure to sunlight and irritation. After treatment, a sun-blocking agent containing para-aminobenzoic acid (PABA) should be used to prevent burning. The attending health care provider may prescribe an ointment to relieve itching. Nothing should be applied to the treatment area without the recommendation of the health care provider. There may be diarrhea after abdominal irradiation. The patient needs to be reassured that they do *not* become radioactive during or after therapy.

Emotional support of the adolescent is age appropriate. Nurses must be particularly prepared for periods of anger, which may be directed at them. Suitable outlets, such as the use of a punching bag, allow for the safe direction of anger; routine use helps to prevent a buildup of tension. The patient generally regulates their own activity. The health care provider advises the patient if special precautions are necessary.

The appearance of secondary sexual characteristics and menstruation may be delayed in pubescent patients. Sterility is often an adverse effect of treatment and can be a source of anxiety. Adolescents may be interested in sperm banking before immunosuppressive therapy is initiated. The nurse needs to respect the patient's concerns and can be most effective by listening empathically.

Care of a child receiving a transfusion

Platelets and packed RBCs may be given to a child. Hemolytic reactions caused by mismatched blood are rare. Nevertheless, the nurse should positively identify donor and recipient blood types and groups on labels and the patient's chart together with another licensed professional. Blood is infused through a blood filter to exclude impurities. Medications are *never* added to blood. Blood is administered *slowly*. The IV site is frequently checked for infiltration. The patient is observed for *signs of transfusion reaction,* which include *chills, itching, rash, fever, headache,* and *pain* in the back. If such a reaction or reactions occur, the tubing should be clamped off immediately, the line kept open with normal saline solution, and the health care team notified. Every health care facility has policies and procedures specific to blood transfusions, and it is the nurse's responsibility to know and follow these guidelines.

Transfusions with piggyback setups are common. A stopcock connects blood, normal saline, or other suitable IV solutions. When a blood transfusion must be stopped, tube patency can be maintained by opening the saline line. Necessary emergency medications can thus be administered and the site preserved for future infusions. Often a second IV site will be started to prevent having to stop a transfusion.

Circulatory overload is always a danger with children. An infusion pump is routinely used to regulate blood flow. Dyspnea, precordial pain, crackles, cyanosis, dry cough, and distended neck veins are indicative of circulatory overload. Apprehension can also be a warning signal of air emboli or electrolyte disturbance. The nurse must maintain a high level of alertness for such signs, particularly in children whose conditions warrant repeated transfusions. If a reaction occurs, the blood bag and tubing are saved and returned to the blood bank.

Most transfusion reactions occur within the first 10 minutes of administration; nevertheless, the patient must be carefully monitored throughout this treatment. Diphenhydramine (Benadryl) may be ordered for allergic reactions. Oxygen may be necessary to relieve dyspnea and cyanosis. To prevent cardiac dysrhythmias, a blood warmer must warm blood transfusions that are administered through central lines.

Baseline data (temperature, pulse, respiration, and blood pressure) are established before transfusion, and the nurse needs to monitor for changes. Suitable diversions can minimize the child's boredom during transfusion; often the parents can assist with this.

Nursing Tip

If a blood transfusion reaction occurs, stop the infusion, keep the vein open with normal saline solution, and notify the health care team immediately. Take the patient's vital signs, stay at the bedside, and observe the patient closely.

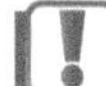

Safety Alert!

Medications are never added to blood transfusions, and the drip rate should be slow.

Get Ready for the Certification Examination!

Key Points

- Circulating blood consists of two portions: plasma and formed elements.
- Bone marrow aspiration is one procedure that is helpful in determining disorders of the blood.
- A nutritional deficiency disorder in some children in Canada is iron-deficiency anemia.
- Sickle cell disease is an inherited defect in the formation of hemoglobin. The cells become crescent shaped and clump together.
- Massive expansion of the bone marrow in thalassemia causes changes in the contour of the child's skull and face.
- Hemophilia A results from a deficiency in coagulation factor VIII, and hemophilia B (Christmas disease) involves a deficiency in factor IX.
- Hemarthrosis (bleeding into the joints) is a characteristic sign of hemophilia A.
- Hemosiderosis (deposits of iron in the organs and tissues) is a complication of multiple transfusions in hemolytic blood disorders.
- Petechiae are bluish pinpoint lesions on the skin. Purpuras are groups of adjoining petechiae, ecchymosis is an isolated bluish lesion larger than a petechiae, and a hematoma is a raised ecchymosis.
- Leukemia is the most common form of childhood cancer.
- Four priority challenges in the care of a child with leukemia are anemia, bleeding, infection, and fractures.
- Diagnostic procedures for patients with blood disorders are often invasive or painful. The nurse needs to prepare and support the patient and family during these procedures.
- Maintenance of schooling, adequate hydration and nutrition, prevention of infection, promotion of a positive self-image, and meticulous oral hygiene are essential components of nursing care for a child with leukemia.
- Reed-Sternberg cells are diagnostic for Hodgkin lymphoma.
- Signs of transfusion reactions include chills, itching rash, fever, and headache.

Additional Learning Resources

evolve Go to your Evolve website (http://evolve.elsevier.com/Canada/Leifer) for the following learning resources:

- Answer Key for Critical Thinking Questions
- Answer Key for Textbook Review Questions
- Audio Glossary
- Interactive Review Questions
- Skills Performance Checklists
- Video clips and more!

Online Resources

- Canadian Cancer Society: http://www.cancer.ca/en/?region=on
- Canadian Hemophilia Society: https://www.hemophilia.ca/
- Sickle Cell Disease Association of Canada: https://www.sicklecelldisease.ca/

Review Questions

1. When the patient experiences apprehension and urticaria while receiving a blood transfusion, what is the priority intervention by the nurse?
   a. Slow the transfusion and take the patient's vital signs.
   b. Observe the child for further transfusion reactions.
   c. Stop the transfusion, allow normal saline solution to run slowly, and notify the health care team immediately.
   d. Stop what they are doing and obtain the patient's history.
2. A child who is in a vaso-occlusive crisis caused by sickle cell anemia is experiencing acute pain. Which medication would the nurse most likely administer?
   a. Morphine
   b. Demerol
   c. NSAID
   d. Tylenol
3. Which principle should the nurse teach the parent concerning administering liquid iron preparations to the child with iron-deficiency anemia?
   a. Allow the preparation to mix with saliva and bathe the teeth before swallowing.
   b. Warm the medication before administering.
   c. Administer between meals.
   d. Administer in the bottle of formula.
4. With which of the following is thalassemia major (Cooley's anemia) primarily treated?
   a. A diet high in iron
   b. Multiple blood transfusions
   c. Bed rest until the sedimentation rate is normal
   d. Oxygen therapy
5. What is a characteristic manifestation of Hodgkin lymphoma?
   a. Petechiae
   b. Erythematous rash
   c. Enlarged lymph nodes
   d. Pallor
6. Which orders written for a child admitted with a diagnosis of sickle cell anemia should the nurse question? *(Select all that apply.).*
   a. Restrict fluids
   b. Provide a high-calorie, high-protein diet.
   c. Administer meperidine (Demerol) 25 mg IM for pain q6h
   d. Administer oxygen at 2 litres via nasal cannula prn.

REFERENCES

Abdullah, K., Zlotkin, S., Parkin, P., et al. (2011). *Iron-deficiency anemia in children*. Retrieved from: https://www.cpsp.cps.ca/uploads/publications/RA-iron-deficiency-anemia.pdf.

Ardoin, S., & Fells, E. (2016). Henoch-Schönlein purpura. In R. Kliegman, B. Stanton, J. St. Geme, et al. (Eds.), *Nelson textbook of pediatrics* (20th ed.). Philadelphia: Saunders.

Canadian Cancer Society. (2019). *What is childhood leukemia?* Retrieved from: https://www.cancer.ca/en/cancer-information/cancer-type/leukemia-childhood/childhood-leukemia/?region=on#.

Critch, J. N., & Canadian Paediatric Society (CPS), Nutrition and Gastroenterology Committee. (2014). Nutrition for healthy term infants, six to 24 months: An overview. *Paediatrics & Child Health, 19*(10), 547–549. Reaffirmed 2017.

DeBaun, M., Frei-Jones, M., & Vichinsky, E. (2016). Thalassemia syndromes. In R. Kliegman, B. Stanton, J. St. Geme, et al. (Eds.), *Nelson textbook of pediatrics* (20th ed.). Philadelphia: Saunders.

Field, J., Vichinsky, E., & DeBaun, M. (2018). Overview of the management and prognosis of sickle cell disease. *UpToDate*. Retrieved from: https://www.uptodate.com/contents/overview-of-the-management-and-prognosis-of-sickle-cell-disease.

Friehling, E., Ritchey, K., Tubergen, D., et al. (2016). Acute lymphoblastic leukemia. In R. Kliegman, B. Stanton, J. St. Geme, et al. (Eds.), *Nelson textbook of pediatrics* (20th ed.). Philadelphia: Saunders.

Guo, D., & Lam, J. M. (2016). Henoch-Schonlein purpura. *Canadian Medical Association Journal, 188*(15), E939.

Hochberg, J., Giulino-Roth, L., & Cairo, M. (2016). Hodgkin's lymphoma. In R. Kliegman, B. Stanton, J. St. Geme, et al. (Eds.), *Nelson textbook of pediatrics* (20th ed.). Philadelphia: Saunders.

Misha, B. (2017). Henoch-Schönlein purpura. *Consultant, 57*(3), 184–186.

Parkin, P. C., DeGroot, J., Maguire, J. L., et al. (2016). Severe iron-deficiency anaemia and feeding practices in young children. *Public Health Nutrition, 19*(4), 716–722. https://doi.org/10.1017/S1368980015001639.

Scott, J. P. (2016). Idiopathic (autoimmune) thrombocytopenic purpura. In R. Kliegman, B. Stanton, J. St. Geme, et al. (Eds.), *Nelson textbook of pediatrics* (20th ed.). Philadelphia: Saunders.

Sickle Cell Disease Association of Canada (SCDAC). (n.d.). *Advocacy and awareness*. Retrieved from: http://www.sicklecelldisease.ca/advocacy_awareness.php

Traore, A. N., Chan, A., Webert, K., et al. (2014). First analysis of 10-year trends in national factor concentrates usage in haemophilia: Data from CHARMS, the Canadian Hemophilia Assessment and Resource Management System. *Haemophilia, 20*(4), e251–e259. https://doi.org/10.1111/hae.12477.

Tubergen, D., Bleyer, A., Ritchkey, K., et al. (2016). Leukemias. In R. Kliegman, B. Stanton, J. St. Geme, et al. (Eds.), *Nelson textbook of pediatrics* (20th ed.). Philadelphia: Saunders.

Vacca, V., & Blank, L. (2017). Sickle cell disease: Where are we now? *Nursing, 47*(4), 26–34.

The Child With a Gastrointestinal Condition

28

Lisa Keenan-Lindsay

http://evolve.elsevier.com/Canada/Leifer

Objectives

1. Define each key term listed.
2. Discuss three common gastrointestinal anomalies in infants.
3. Describe the postoperative nursing care of an infant with hypertrophic pyloric stenosis.
4. Discuss the dietary management of celiac disease.
5. Describe the symptoms, treatment, and nursing care of a child with Hirschsprung disease.
6. Describe the treatment and nursing care of a child with intussusception.
7. Interpret the nursing management of an infant with gastroesophageal reflux.
8. Outline the nursing care of a child with esophageal atresia and tracheoesophageal fistula.
9. Differentiate between cleft lip and cleft palate.
10. Explain why infants and young children become dehydrated more easily than adults.
11. Differentiate between three types of dehydration.
12. Understand how nutritional deficiencies influence growth and development.
13. Review the prevention of the spread of thrush in infants and children.
14. Trace the route of the pinworm cycle and describe how reinfection takes place.
15. Prepare a teaching plan for the prevention of poisoning in children.
16. List two measures to reduce the effect of acetaminophen poisoning in children.
17. Indicate the primary source of lead poisoning.

Key Terms

anasarca (ăn-ă-SĂHR-kă)
anthelmintics (ănt-hĕl-MĬN-tĭkz)
cheiloplasty (KĪ-lō-plăs-tē)
cleft lip
cleft palate
colitis
colonoscopy
currant jelly stools
encopresis (ĕn-kō-PRĒ-sĭs)
endoscopy
enterocolitis (ĕn-tĕr-ō-kō-LĪ-tĭs)
esophageal atresia (EA)
failure to thrive (FTT)
gastroenteritis
herniorrhaphy (hŭr-nē-ŎR-ă-fē)
Hirschsprung disease
homeostasis (hō-mē-ō-STĀ-sĭs)
hypertonic (hī-pŭr-TŎN-ĭk)
hypertrophic pyloric stenosis
hypotonic (hī-pō-TŎN-ĭk)
imperforate anus
incarcerated hernia
inguinal hernia
intussusception
isotonic (ī-sō-TŎN-ĭk)
kwashiorkor
Meckel's diverticulum
parenteral fluids (pă-RĔN-tŭr-ăl)
pica
plumbism
polyhydramnios (pŏl-ē-hī-DRĂM-nē-ōs)
projectile vomiting
pruritus
rebound tenderness
reflux
sigmoidoscopy
tracheoesophageal fistula (TEF)

THE GASTROINTESTINAL TRACT

The gastrointestinal (GI) tract transports and metabolizes nutrients necessary for the life of cells in the body. It extends from the mouth to the anus. Nutrients are broken down into absorbable products by enzymes from various digestive organs. The primitive digestive tube is formed by the yolk sac and is divided into the foregut, the midgut, and the hindgut. The foregut evolves into the pharynx, the lower respiratory tract, the esophagus, the stomach, the duodenum, and the beginning of the common bile duct. The midgut elongates in the fifth fetal week to form the primary intestinal loop. The remainder of the large colon is derived from the primitive hindgut. The liver, pancreas, and biliary tree evolve from the foregut. The anal membrane ruptures at 8 weeks of gestation, forming the anal canal and anal opening.

The anatomy of the digestive tract, with some of the differences between that of the child and that of the adult, is depicted in Fig. 28.1. As the child grows, the GI capacity increases. A newborn infant has the stomach capacity of 10 to 20 mL; a 1-month-old infant has

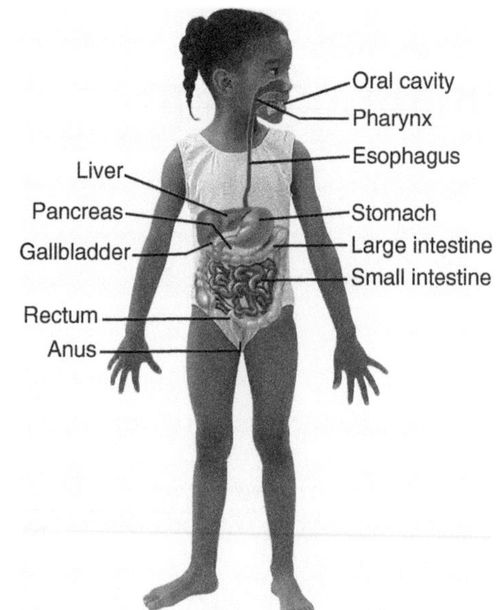

GASTROINTESTINAL SYSTEM

- At birth the resistance of the newborn's intestinal tract to bacterial and viral infection is incompletely developed.
- As children grow, they have higher nutritional, metabolic, and energy needs.
- Children with nausea and vomiting dehydrate more quickly than do adults with those symptoms.
- The infant's stomach is small and empties rapidly.
- Newborns produce little saliva until 3 months of age.
- Swallowing is a reflex for the first 3 months.
- Hepatic efficiency in the newborn is immature, sometimes causing jaundice.
- The infant's fat absorption is poor because of a decreased pool of bile acid.

Fig. 28.1 Some of the gastrointestinal system differences between the child and adult. The digestive system consists of the digestive tract and the glands that secrete digestive juices into the digestive tract. This system mechanically and chemically breaks down food and eliminates wastes. (Art overlay courtesy Observatory Group, Cincinnati, Ohio.)

the stomach capacity of 90 to 150 mL; a 1-year-old infant has the stomach capacity of 210 to 360 mL; and a 2-year-old has a stomach capacity of approximately 500 mL. The adult stomach has a capacity of 2000 to 3000 mL. Many enzymes necessary for digestion are deficient until 4 to 6 months of age.

Understanding the physiology of the pediatric digestive tract is the basis for developing a plan for introducing new foods during the first year and avoiding problems that can occur with overfeeding.

DIAGNOSTIC AND IMAGING TESTS OF THE GASTROINTESTINAL TRACT

A number of procedures are available to determine GI disorders. Laboratory work, such as a complete blood count (CBC) with differential, will show anemia, infections, and some chronic illnesses. An elevated erythrocyte sedimentation rate (ESR) is indicative of inflammation. A comprehensive chemical panel will show electrolyte and chemical imbalances. Often-used X-ray studies include GI series, barium enema, and flat plates of the abdomen.

Endoscopy

There are four types of endoscopy typically used in pediatrics that allow for the direct visualization of the GI tract. Preparation for the tests includes a clear liquid diet and bowel preparation the day before.

Capsule endoscopy

Capsule endoscopy requires the child to swallow a capsule that contains a camera that takes pictures as it passes through the entire GI tract, propelled by natural peristalsis. A wireless device is worn on the outside of the body that records these pictures. The device is returned to the health care provider for analysis. The capsule is removed through the normal defecation process within 72 hours.

Gastroscopy, sigmoidoscopy, and colonoscopy

A more invasive form of endoscopy allows direct visualization of the GI tract through the insertion of a flexible lighted tube that has a camera at its tip and is inserted through the mouth (upper GI) or the rectum (sigmoidoscopy or colonoscopy, respectively). The health care provider looks through the scope or on a computer monitor to visualize the GI tract. It is also valuable for obtaining biopsies, removing foreign objects, and cauterizing bleeding vessels.

Nursing care

Nursing responsibilities include assisting with the diet and bowel cleansing the day before and documenting the passage of the capsule, if noted, and returning the electronic recording device to the appropriate health care provider or department. Nurses also assist in the performance of these diagnostic tests.

Laboratory Tests and Diagnostic Imaging

Stool cultures and rectal biopsy are also important diagnostic tools. Ultrasonography is a noninvasive procedure useful in visualizing intestinal organs and masses, particularly of the liver and pancreas. Some liver function blood tests include alanine aminotransferase (ALT), aspartate aminotransferase (AST), prothrombin time (PT), and partial thromboplastin time (PTT). Liver biopsy may also be indicated. Overall malabsorption tests, such as the 72-hour fecal fat test and the Schilling test (which can determine the absorption capacity of the lower ileum), are also useful.

Breath Tests

A hydrogen breath test is used to diagnose abnormal bacterial growth in the intestines or carbohydrate malabsorption, and a urea breath test measures the amount of carbon dioxide present in exhaled air. Depending on the test, the child may be given a liquid or a capsule to swallow. Certain gases are measured either in the exhaled air into a "balloon" or via a blood draw. For more detailed information concerning preparation for various tests, refer to a laboratory diagnostics textbook.

Signs and Symptoms of Gastrointestinal Disorders

Symptoms of GI disorders may be manifested by systemic signs, such as failure to thrive (FTT— failure to develop according to established growth parameters such as height, weight, and head circumference) or jaundice. **Pruritus** (itching) in the absence of allergy may indicate liver dysfunction. Local manifestations of a GI disorder include pain, vomiting, diarrhea, constipation, rectal bleeding, and hematemesis.

Developmental delays in children should be investigated to determine whether they are related to the GI system. Skin problems in these patients may be related to pruritus from liver disease, irritation from frequent bowel movements, or other disorders. Pain and discomfort may occur during acute episodes; however, they may also result from medication adverse effects, or they may be referred pain. General nursing interventions focus on providing adequate nutrition and freedom from infection, which can result from malnutrition or depressed immune function.

DISORDERS AND DYSFUNCTION OF THE GASTROINTESTINAL TRACT

OBSTRUCTIVE DISORDERS

Hypertrophic Pyloric Stenosis (HPS)

Pathophysiology

Hypertrophic pyloric stenosis (narrowing) is an obstruction at the lower end of the stomach (pylorus) caused by an overgrowth (hypertrophy) of the circular muscles of the pylorus or by spasms of the sphincter. This condition is commonly classified as a congenital anomaly; however, it is not present at birth and the symptoms do not appear until the infant is 2 to 5 weeks old. HPS is the most common condition of the digestive tract in infancy that requires surgery (Fig. 28.2). Its incidence is higher in boys than in girls, and there is a genetic predisposition. It is more common in full-term than in preterm infants and is seen less frequently in Black and Asian infants than in White infants (Hunter & Liacouras, 2016). The cause has not been established. HPS is associated with many conditions.

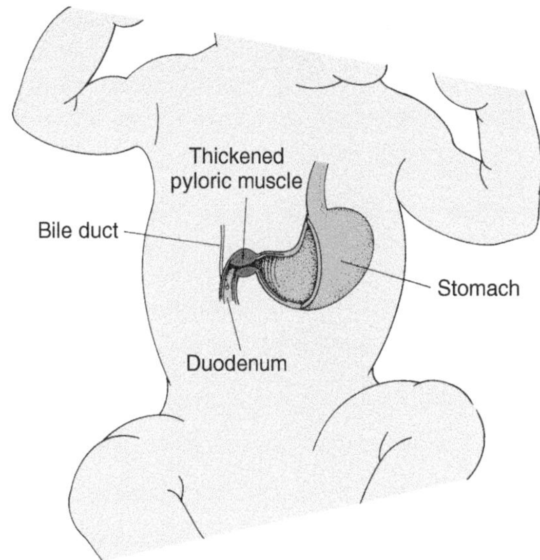

Fig. 28.2 Pyloric stenosis. Hypertrophy or thickening of the pyloric sphincter blocks passage of the stomach contents, causing the infant to regurgitate forcefully. Serious electrolyte imbalances ultimately occur, and surgery is necessary to correct the condition. (From Betz, C., Hunsburger, M., & Wright, S. [1994]. *Family-centered nursing care of children* [2nd ed.]. Philadelphia: Saunders.)

Manifestations

Vomiting is a common symptom of this disorder. The force progresses until most of the food is ejected a considerable distance from the mouth. This is termed **projectile vomiting**, and it occurs immediately after feeding. The vomitus contains mucus and ingested milk. The infant is constantly hungry and will eat again immediately after vomiting. Dehydration as evidenced by a sunken fontanelle, decreased skin turgor, and decreased urination, as well as malnutrition, can develop. An olive-shaped mass may be felt in the right upper quadrant of the abdomen. Ultrasonography is commonly used for diagnostic purposes because it is noninvasive and accurate. If ultrasound scanning fails to demonstrate a hypertrophied pylorus, upper GI radiography should be done to rule out other causes of vomiting. In severe cases, the outline of the distended stomach and peristaltic waves are visible during feeding.

Treatment

The surgery performed for HPS is a pyloromyotomy (*pylorus*, "lower orifice of the stomach," *myo*, "muscle," and *tomy*, "incision of"), known as the *Fredet-Ramstedt procedure*. It involves cutting into the hypertrophied muscle but not through the mucous membrane of the bowel. Therefore, the infant will not need nasogastric decompression postoperatively and will be able to resume oral feedings 3 to 6 hours after surgery.

Nursing care

The dehydrated infant is given intravenous (IV) fluids preoperatively to restore fluid and electrolyte balance. If this is not done, shock may occur during surgery. The infant is burped *before* as well as *during* feedings to remove any gas accumulated in the stomach. The feeding is done slowly, and the infant should be handled gently and as little as possible. Charting of the feeding includes time, type, and amount offered; the amount taken and retained; and the type and amount of vomiting. The nurse should also note whether the infant appeared hungry after the feeding or if vomiting occurred again.

The nurse needs to obtain and record a baseline weight and weigh the infant at about the same time each morning. Other factors to be charted include the type and number of stools and the colour of urine and frequency of voiding (intake and output). The infant's position is changed frequently because they may be weak and vulnerable to pneumonia. All procedures designed to protect from infection must be strictly performed.

The care of the infant after surgery includes a careful observation of vital signs and the administration of IV fluids. The wound site is inspected frequently (see Chapter 20 for postoperative care). The health care provider prescribes oral feedings of small amounts of clear liquid that gradually increases to breastmilk or formula, as tolerated. Overfeeding should be avoided, and the nurse needs to review feeding techniques with parents (Clinical Pathway 28.1). The diaper is placed low over the abdomen to prevent contamination of the wound site.

Clinical Pathway 28.1 An Interdisciplinary Plan of Care for the Infant With Pyloric Stenosis

Nursing Diagnosis	Day: Admission	Day: Postop 1	Day: Postop 2
PATIENT AND FAMILY INTERMEDIATE OUTCOMES			
Dehydration as a result of persistent vomiting	Child shows improved fluid and electrolyte balance.	Child demonstrates normal fluid and electrolyte balance, as evidenced by normal urine output (1 mL/kg/hr), moist mucous membranes, good skin turgor, and laboratory values within normal limits.	→
Nutritional deficits as a result persistent vomiting	Child stops vomiting.	Child ingests and retains small amounts of breastmilk or formula.	Child ingests and retains sufficient nutrients to meet dietary needs.
Acute pain as a result incision, muscle cutting, and manipulation during surgery		Child has signs of pain recognized and interventions are promptly implemented. Child experiences minimal levels of pain.	→
Education needs due to treatments, surgery, postoperative care	Parents verbalize understanding of treatments and surgery.	Parents verbalize understanding of postoperative pain management, feeding, and incision care.	Parents verbalize understanding of home care and follow-up needs.
CARE INTERVENTION CATEGORIES			
Laboratory values	CBC, electrolytes Repeat electrolytes prn to monitor Cl and CO_2 values.		
Medications and IVs	IV fluids: maintenance and replacement Provide acetaminophen or morphine prn for pain.	Saline- or heparin-lock IV when tolerating PO fluids.	Discontinue IV if tolerating PO fluids.
Nutrition	NPO	Administer 10 mL oral electrolyte solution after recovery from anaesthesia; start pyloric refeeding protocol (increasing feeding volumes from clear fluids to breastmilk or diluted formula to full-strength formula); repeat previous step if emesis x1, notify surgeon if emesis x2.	Provide breastmilk or full-strength formula at normal feeding volumes.

Clinical Pathway 28.1 An Interdisciplinary Plan of Care for the Infant With Pyloric Stenosis—cont'd

Nursing Diagnosis	Day: Admission	Day: Postop 1	Day: Postop 2
Pain management	Provide acetaminophen or morphine (see "Medications and IVs" earlier in this table). Flex knees; position to avoid stretching abdominal muscles. Burp frequently to avoid abdominal distention.	→	→
Radiology	Ultrasound of abdomen and barium study as needed to confirm diagnosis		
Teaching and discharge planning	Teach parents about preoperative care routines. Teach parents about surgical routines; review postoperative care.	Teach parents methods of pain assessment and management; reintroduce feedings; provide incision care. Assess supplies that will be needed at home (medications, dressings) and ability of parents to obtain them.	Evaluate parent's ability to manage pain, feeding, and caring for incision; review techniques prn. Discharge child when full oral feedings are tolerated.
Vital signs and baseline parameters	Vital signs with blood pressure on admission and q4h	→	→
	Daily weight	→	→
	Urine specific gravity each shift	→	→
	Intake and output	→	→

CBC, Complete blood count; *Cl*, chloride; CO_2, carbon dioxide; *IV*, intravenous route; *NG*, nasogastric; *NPO*, nothing by mouth; *PO*, by mouth; prn, as needed.
Modified from Bowden, V. R., Dickey, S. B., & Greenberg, C. S. (1998). *Children and their families: The continuum of care*. Philadelphia: Saunders.

Imperforate Anus

Pathophysiology

Anorectal malformations occur in about 1 of every 5 000 live births (Blackburn, 2013). The lower GI tract and the anus arise from two different tissues. Early in fetal life the two tissues meet and join; the tissue separating them then perforates, allowing for a passageway between the lower GI tract and the anus. When this perforation does not occur, the lower end of the GI tract and the anus end in blind pouches. This is called **imperforate anus**. There are several types of imperforate anus, ranging from a stenosis to complete separation or failure of the anus to form.

Manifestations

A routine part of the newborn assessment is determining the patency of the anus. Failure to pass meconium in the first 24 hours must be reported.

Treatment and nursing care

Diagnosis may be confirmed by abdominal ultrasonography. After a diagnosis of imperforate anus is established, the infant is given nothing by mouth (NPO) and is prepared for surgery. The initial surgical procedure may be a colostomy. Subsequent surgery can re-establish the patency of the anal canal and possibly protect the ability for continence. If the child has anal stenosis the treatment is usually manual dilation of the anus.

Intussusception

Pathophysiology

Intussusception (*intus*, "within," and *suscipere*, "to receive") is a slipping of one part of the intestine into another part just below it (Fig. 28.3). It is often seen at the ileocecal valve, where the small intestine opens into the ascending colon. The mesentery, a double fan–shaped fold of peritoneum that covers most of the intestine and is filled with blood vessels and nerves, is also pulled along and edema occurs. At first this telescoping of the bowel causes intestinal obstruction, but strangulation takes place as peristalsis forces the structures more tightly. This portion may burst, causing peritonitis.

Intussusception generally occurs most often in boys from 3 months to 2 years of age and who are otherwise healthy. Its frequency decreases after 3 years of age. Occasionally, the condition corrects itself without

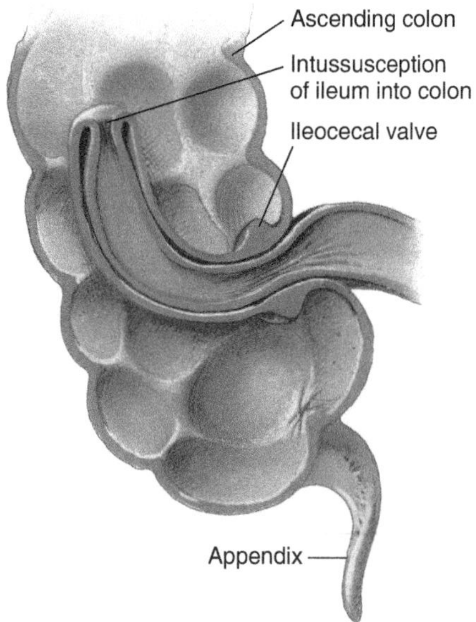

Fig. 28.3 Intussusception. The most common type begins at or near the ileocecal valve, with this part of the intestines (bowel) pushing into the cecum and on to the colon. At first the obstruction is partial, but complete obstruction occurs as the bowel becomes inflamed and edematous. (From McKinney, E. S., et al. [2005]. *Nursing care of children: Principles and practice* [2nd ed.]. Philadelphia: Saunders.)

treatment. This is termed a *spontaneous reduction*. However, because the condition puts the child's life in danger, the health care provider does not waste time waiting for correction to occur. The prognosis is good when the patient is treated within 24 hours.

Manifestations

In typical cases, the onset is sudden. The infant feels severe paroxysmal pain in the abdomen, as evidenced by loud cries, straining efforts, and kicking and drawing of the legs toward the abdomen. At first there is comfort between pains, but the intervals shorten and the condition becomes worse. The child vomits. The stomach contents are green or greenish yellow (this results from bile stain), and the contents are described as bilious. Bowel movements diminish, and little flatus is passed. Movements of blood and mucus that contain no feces are common about 12 hours after the onset of the obstruction; these are termed **currant jelly stools**. An abdominal mass may be palpable. Rectal bleeding may occur.

Treatment and nursing care

Intussusception is an emergency, and because of the severity of symptoms, most parents contact a health care provider promptly. An ultrasound may indicate the mass. A pneumoenema (air enema) with or without water-soluble contrast or ultrasound-guided hydrostatic (saline) enema is used to reduce the defect; the advantage of the latter is that no ionizing radiation is needed. The recurrence rate after this procedure is approximately 10% (Kennedy & Liacouras, 2016).

If surgery is required, a bowel resection is performed and the affected area is removed. The cut end of the ileum is joined to the cut end of the colon; this procedure is called an *anastomosis*. Routine preoperative and postoperative care is discussed in Chapter 20.

Meckel's Diverticulum

Pathophysiology

During fetal life, the intestine is attached to the yolk sac by the vitelline duct. A small, blind pouch may form if this duct fails to disappear completely. This condition is termed **Meckel's diverticulum**. It usually occurs near the ileocecal valve, and it may be connected to the umbilicus by a cord. A fistula may also form. This sac is subject to inflammation, much like the appendix. This disorder is the most common congenital malformation of the GI tract.

Manifestations

Symptoms may occur at any age but appear most often before 2 years of age. Painless bleeding from the rectum is the most common sign. Bright red or dark red blood is more usual than tarry stools. Abdominal pain may or may not be present. An ultrasound, computed tomography (CT) scan, mesenteric angiography, or radionucleotide scintigraphy is used for diagnosis. X-ray films are not helpful, because the pouch is so small that it may not appear on the screen.

Treatment and nursing care

The diverticulum is removed by surgery. Nursing care is the same as for the patient undergoing exploration of the abdomen. Because this condition appears suddenly and bleeding causes parental anxiety, emotional support is of particular importance.

STRUCTURAL DEFECTS

Esophageal Atresia (EA)/Tracheoesophageal Fistula (TEF)

Pathophysiology

Esophageal atresia and **tracheoesophageal fistula** are caused by a failure of the tissues of the GI tract to separate properly from the respiratory tract early in prenatal life. They may occur individually or in combination with each other. EA with or without a TEF is the most common type of esophageal malformation. There are five types of EA/TEF (Fig. 28.4):

1. The upper esophagus and the lower esophagus (leading from the stomach) end in a blind pouch—esophageal atresia (see Fig. 28.4, *A*).
2. The upper esophagus ends in a blind pouch; the lower esophagus (leading from the stomach) connects to the trachea (see Fig. 28.4, *C*).
3. The upper esophagus is attached to the trachea; the lower esophagus (leading from the stomach) is also attached to the trachea (see Fig. 28.4, *D, E*).

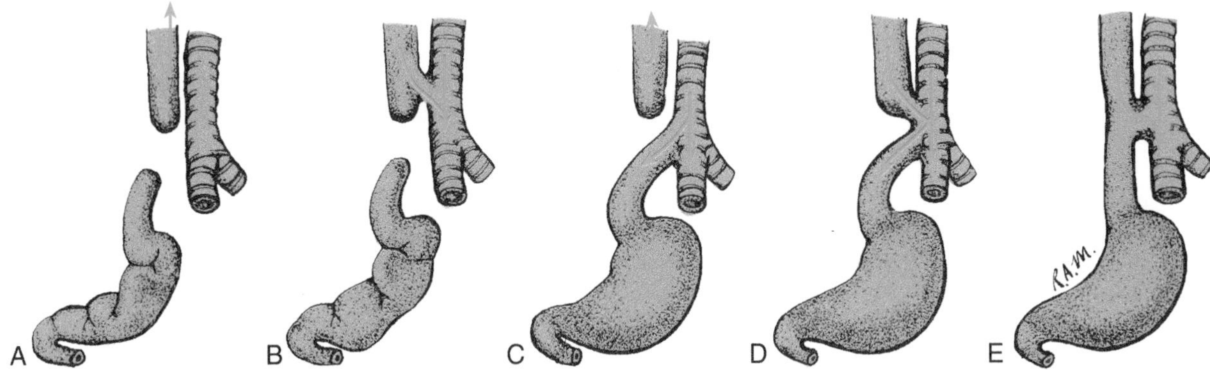

Fig. 28.4 The five most common types of esophageal atresia and tracheosesophageal fistula. **A,** Esophageal atresia (blind pouch at each end). **B,** Fistula from upper esophageal segment to trachea. **C,** Esophageal pouch and distal segment is connected to the trachea. **D,** Fistula to upper and lower segment of esophagus from the trachea. **E,** Normal esophagus and trachea connected by a fistula.

4. The upper esophagus connects to the trachea; the lower esophagus (leading from the stomach) ends in a blind pouch (see Fig. 28.4, *B*).

The diagnosis of this condition is based on clinical manifestations and is confirmed by X-ray study. TEF occurs in approximately 1.7 of 10 000 live births (Khan & Orenstein, 2016a).

Manifestations

The earliest sign of EA/TEF occurs prenatally, when the mother develops polyhydramnios. When the upper esophagus ends in a blind pouch, the fetus cannot swallow the amniotic fluid, resulting in an accumulation of fluid in the amniotic sac (polyhydramnios). After birth, the infant will vomit and choke when the first feeding is introduced. Because the upper end of the esophagus ends in a blind pouch in an EA (see Fig. 28.4, *A*), the newborn cannot swallow accumulated secretions and will appear to be drooling. Although drooling after age 3 months is related to teething, drooling in a newborn is pathological and is related to atresia. If the upper esophagus enters the trachea (TEF), the first feeding will enter the trachea and result in coughing, choking, cyanosis, and apnea. If the lower end of the esophagus (from the stomach) enters the trachea, air will enter the stomach each time the infant breathes, causing abdominal distention.

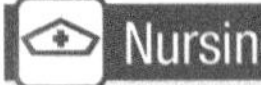 **Nursing Tip**

Drooling in the newborn is pathological because the salivary glands do not develop for several months.

Treatment and nursing care

The nursing goals involve preventing pneumonia, choking, and apnea in the newborn. Assessment of every newborn during the first feeding is essential. If symptoms are noted, the infant is placed NPO, suctioned to clear the airway, and positioned to drain mucus from the nose and throat. Surgical repair is essential for survival.

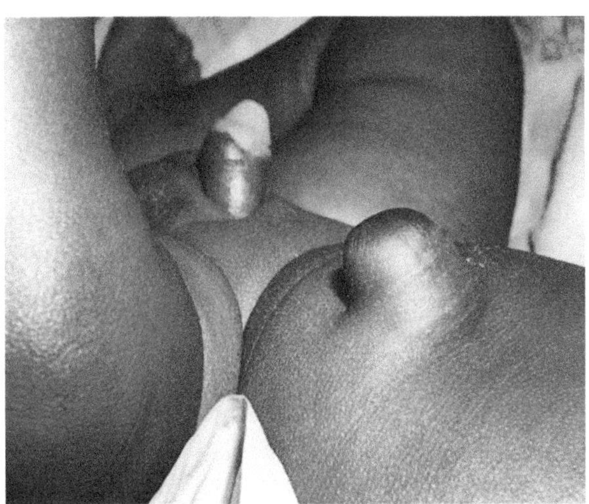

Fig. 28.5 An umbilical hernia in an infant boy.

Hernia

Pathophysiology

An inguinal hernia is a protrusion of part of the abdominal contents through the inguinal canal in the groin. It is more common in boys than in girls. It is also commonly seen in preterm infants. An *umbilical* hernia is a protrusion of a portion of intestine through the umbilical ring (an opening in the muscular area of the abdomen through which the umbilical vessels pass; Fig. 28.5). This type of hernia appears as a soft swelling covered by skin, which protrudes when the infant cries or strains. Hernias may be present at birth (congenital) or may be acquired, and they can vary in size. A hernia is called *reducible* if it can be put back into place by gentle pressure; if this cannot be done, it is called an *irreducible* or an incarcerated hernia. Incarceration (constriction) occurs more often in infants less than 10 months of age. Hernias may be bilateral.

Manifestations

The infant with a hernia may be relatively free of symptoms. Irritability, fretfulness, and constipation are sometimes evident. The diagnosis is made when physical examination shows a mass in the area that reappears from time to time, particularly when the child cries or strains. A *strangulated* hernia occurs when the intestine becomes caught in the passage and the blood supply is diminished. This happens more often during the first 6 months of life. Vomiting and severe abdominal pain are present. Emergency surgery is necessary if strangulation occurs, and in some cases a bowel resection is performed.

Treatment and nursing care

Hernias are successfully repaired by the surgical operation called a **herniorrhaphy**. This is a relatively simple procedure and is well tolerated by the child. Most children are scheduled for procedures in same-day surgery units. The benefits of this method are both economic and psychological. Parents bring the fasting child to the hospital about 1 hour before surgery. Parents remain with the child during the entire time except during the actual procedure. They are encouraged to assist in routine postoperative care.

Sometimes a waterproof collodion dressing, which looks like clear nail polish, is applied, but often no dressing is applied to the wound. Postoperative care is directed toward keeping the wound clean. Diapers are left open for this purpose. Wet diapers are changed frequently.

Cleft Lip

Pathophysiology

Cleft lip and cleft palate are common congenital anomalies and occur in about 1 in 600 births (Government of Canada, 2013). A **cleft lip** is characterized by a fissure or opening in the upper lip. It is a result of the failure of the maxillary and median nasal processes to unite during embryonic development, usually between the seventh and eighth weeks of gestation. In many cases, it seems to be caused by autosomal dominant hereditary predisposition, but occasionally it can be caused by environmental influences during the stage of oral development. This condition appears more frequently in boys than in girls, and there is a high incidence in certain ethnic groups, including the Indigenous population. It may occur on one or both sides of the lip. The extent of the defect may vary from slight to severe. Sometimes it is accompanied by a cleft palate—a fissure in the midline of the roof of the mouth (Fig. 28.6).

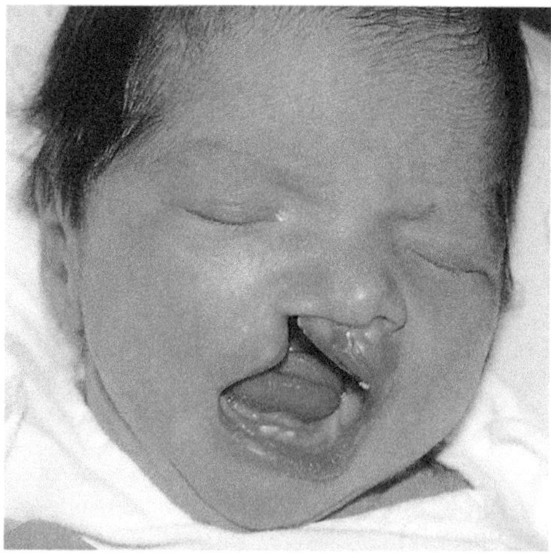

Fig. 28.6 An infant with a unilateral cleft lip and palate. (Courtesy Dr. A. E. Chudley, Section of Genetics and Metabolism, Department of Pediatrics and Child Health, Children's Hospital and University of Manitoba, Winnipeg, Manitoba, Canada. From Moore, K. L., Persaud, T. V. N., & Torchia, M. G. [2016]. *The developing human: Clinically oriented embryology* [10th ed.]. Philadelphia: Saunders.)

Treatment and nursing care

The initial treatment for cleft lip is a surgical repair known as **cheiloplasty**. The cleft lip is repaired at approximately 3 months of age or when weight gain is established and the infant is free of infection (Tinanoff, 2016). Surgery improves the infant's sucking ability and also changes the infant's appearance.

Routine preoperative care is performed. Any signs of oral, respiratory, or systemic infection are noted and reported. The surgeon may order elbow immobilizers to prevent the infant from scratching the lip and to acquaint the infant with them because they may be necessary postoperatively. A syringe with a rubber tip, a long nipple with a large hole attached to a squeeze bottle, or a soft sippy cup may be used to feed the infant breastmilk or formula before surgery to allow them to get used to these methods, because some health care providers may want the infant to avoid sucking motions to keep from applying tension on the suture line.

Postoperative nursing care

Postoperative nursing goals for the infant undergoing a cheiloplasty include the following:

- Preventing the infant from crying, which could cause tension on the suture line. Depending on the health care provider, sucking may also be prevented for the first 7 to 10 days.
- Resuming feeding when tolerated. Feeding in an upright position in a car seat may be helpful.
- Careful positioning on the back or side to prevent injury to the operative site.
- Preventing infection and scarring by gentle cleansing of the suture line to prevent crusts from forming.
- Preventing injury to the operative site by using elbow immobilizers. A Logan bow (a device used to immobilize the upper lip) may be applied for a short time postoperatively.
- Providing for the infant's emotional needs by cuddling and other forms of affection. This is of particular importance because the infant cannot obtain the usual satisfactions from sucking.
- Providing appropriate pain relief and sedation, which may be required for active infants.

Feeding

The infant may be breastfed immediately after surgery with good lactation support for the mother. Some centres may advocate feedings by dropper until the wound is completely healed (7 to 10 days). Care should be taken to avoid touching the suture line when inserting the medicine dropper. Placing a small amount of breastmilk or formula into the infant's mouth and allowing time for swallowing will prevent aspiration. Offering small amounts of sterile water will cleanse the mouth after feeding. The incision is gently cleaned with saline solution, and an ointment may be applied to the skin as prescribed. Holding the infant during feedings, burping frequently, and placing the infant in an infant seat after feeding or on the right side propped with a rolled blanket may enhance digestion. The mother who has breastfed her infant preoperatively and has been assisted with feedings during hospitalization will feel more confident after discharge. The immediate improvement as a result of surgery can be encouraging to the parents, particularly if the child must have further surgery for cleft palate repair.

Cleft Palate

Pathophysiology

A **cleft palate** is a failure of the hard palate to fuse at the midline during the seventh to twelfth weeks of gestation. This separation forms a passageway between the nasopharynx and the nose, which not only complicates feeding but also easily leads to infections of the respiratory tract and middle ear that can result in hearing loss. It is generally responsible for speech difficulties that occur in later life. The cleft may not be readily apparent at birth, and for this reason careful examination of the oral cavity and upper palate at birth is essential. Feeding is a problem because the cleft prevents negative pressure from being formed within the mouth, which is necessary for successful sucking.

Treatment and nursing care

The goals of therapy are union of the cleft, improved feeding, improved speech, improved dental development, and the nurturing of a positive self-image. Some surgeons prefer to operate before 1 year of age, so that speech patterns are minimally affected and tooth buds are protected (Tinanoff, 2016). If surgery has been deferred, a dental speech appliance may be used to facilitate communication. This appliance must be changed periodically as the child grows.

Treatment of the child with a cleft lip and palate requires multidisciplinary teamwork with a surgeon, pediatrician, pediatric dentist, orthodontist, nurse, psychologist, speech therapist, and social worker. The emotional problems that sometimes occur with this condition may require more extensive attention than does the repair itself. A child born with a facial deformity may encounter many problems. Feedings are difficult and may require special nipples. As the child grows, irregular tooth eruptions, drooling, delayed speech, and the need for intermittent hospitalization and frequent clinic appointments can be difficult to manage for some families.

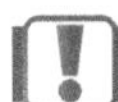
Safety Alert!

Suctioning the mouth should be avoided in infants who have a cleft palate repair.

Psychosocial adjustment of the family

A parent's first reaction to a disfigured newborn may be one of shock, disappointment, and guilt. Some parents may wish to hide the child from relatives and friends. The developing child may sense the parents' feelings and acquire a negative self-image. The patient and family need understanding, a concrete basis for hope, and practical advice. Family stress often occurs because of the multiple surgeries that may be required throughout childhood.

Follow-up care and home care

In large cities, special cleft palate clinics may be available in which several specialists can work together in convenient consultation. The parents should be instructed about the resources available in the province in which they live. AboutFace is a resource for families with a child with facial differences.

Postoperative treatment and nursing care

Nutrition. Fluids are taken by a cup, through a gravity feeder, or by breastfeeding. Breastfeeding may begin within the first day after surgery without complication to the wound (Reilly, Reid, Skeat, et al., 2013). The diet is progressive, at first consisting of clear fluids and then full fluids. By the time of discharge, a soft diet can generally be taken. Hot foods and liquids are avoided to prevent injury to the operative site. The patient must not suck on a straw. When feeding with a spoon, the nurse should place the spoon into the side of the mouth. The spoon must not touch the roof of the mouth. The nurse needs to teach parents to keep objects such as the child's thumb, tongue blades, toast, cookies, forks, and pacifiers out of the mouth. Elbow immobilizers may be used to keep the child from placing their fingers or objects in the mouth.

The older infant or child may be discharged on a blenderized or soft diet, and parents are instructed to continue the diet until the surgeon directs them otherwise. Parents should be cautioned against allowing the child to eat hard items (e.g., toast, hard cookies, and potato chips) that can damage the repaired palate (Hogarth, 2017).

Oral hygiene. The mouth must be kept clean at all times. Feedings are followed by a little water. The surgeon may prescribe a mild antiseptic mouthwash.

Speech. Children who have undergone extensive repairs or have associated deafness may require support from a speech/language therapist. The therapist evaluates the child and assists the parents in specific activities that facilitate speech development. It is helpful for the child that people speak slowly and distinctly to the child.

Diversion. Crying is to be prevented as much as possible in the immediate postoperative period. Play should be quiet. The nurse can provide distractions by reading, drawing, or colouring with the child.

Complications. Ear infections and dental decay may accompany cleft palate. Parents should be instructed to take the child to the health care provider at the first sign of earache. Regular visits to the dentist should be scheduled. Throughout the long-term care, a stable goal in the care of this infant is to promote optimal growth and development and to establish positive self-esteem.

MALABSORPTION SYNDROMES

Celiac Disease

Pathophysiology

Celiac disease is also known as *gluten-induced enteropathy, gluten-induced sensitivity,* or *sprue* and is the leading malabsorption problem in children; the incidence has been shown to be 1 in 266, as a result of improved screening tests (McCabe, Toughill, Parkhill, et al., 2012). It is an autoimmune genetic illness that affects the small intestine because of gluten intolerance and resolves with removal of gluten from the diet.

Gluten is a complex of water-insoluble proteins (gliadin and glutenin) found in wheat, barley, and rye. A gluten-free diet is an essential treatment for celiac disease to prevent the development of other autoimmune diseases, including GI cancer in later life. Children with an allergy to wheat or with a gluten sensitivity may also benefit from a gluten-free diet, under close supervision of a dietitian to ensure adequate vitamin, mineral, and fibre intake. Since hidden glutens are often found in many prepared foods, candy, ice cream, and food starch, it is important for the parents and child to be taught how to read packaging labels.

Manifestations

Symptoms are not evident until 6 months to 2 years of age, when foods containing gluten are introduced to the infant. Repeated exposure to gluten damages the villi in the mucous membranes of the intestine, resulting in malabsorption of food and vitamins. The infant presents with growth failure and diarrhea. Stools are large, bulky, foul-smelling, and frothy because of undigested contents. The infant is irritable. Diagnosis is confirmed by serum immunoglobulin A (IgA) antigliadin antibody, anti-tissue transglutaminase (tTg), and an increased fecal fat content. The characteristic profile of a child with a malabsorption syndrome is abdominal distention with atrophy of the buttocks (Fig. 28.7).

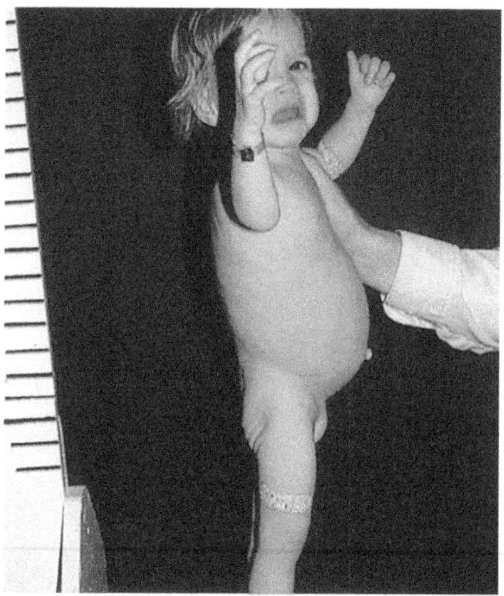

Fig. 28.7 A child with celiac disease. Note that the classic profile of a child with a malabsorption syndrome is an enlarged abdomen with atrophy of the buttocks. (From Zitelli, B. J., McIntire, S., & Nowalk, A. [2018]. *Zitelli and Davis' atlas of pediatric physical diagnosis* [7th ed.]. Philadelphia: Saunders.)

Celiac disease is classified into four types:

1. *Classic celiac disease* involves atrophy of the villi of the small intestine and is characterized by malabsorption, diarrhea, abdominal pain, and weight loss.
2. *Atypical celiac disease* involves the duodenum and includes mild GI symptoms such as reflux and bloating. Malabsorption is manifested by anemia, fatigue, and peripheral nerve problems. Osteoporosis, short stature, and infertility are also signs of atypical celiac disease.
3. *Silent celiac disease* is diagnosed when the atrophy of the intestinal villi is discovered by endoscopy or biopsy that may be done for other reasons, or by a positive blood test.
4. *Latent celiac disease* may not have atrophy of the intestinal villi but may manifest a wheat sensitivity by a recurring rash. These patients are at risk of developing celiac disease in the future.

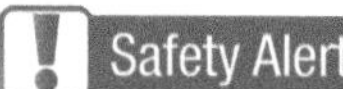

Safety Alert!

A bulky, frothy stool may indicate malabsorption.

Treatment and nursing care

The treatment for celiac disease involves a lifelong diet restricted in wheat, rye, and barley. Often, oats are avoided because they are routinely contaminated with wheat during the growing and processing (Branski, Troncone, & Fasano, 2016). In order for a food to be considered gluten free, it has to have less than 20 parts per million of gluten in the food (Government of Canada, 2017).

Nurses must teach the family the importance of dietary adherence, because tiny amounts of gluten can cause damage to the villi of the intestines. Maintaining a gluten-free diet is a challenge, because gluten is often expressed on labels as a "malt," and it is in emulsifiers, stabilizers, meat substitutes, and thickening agents in many processed foods, soups, and candy. A dietitian can aid in identifying foods that are gluten free. Long-term bowel pathology can occur if dietary adherence is not lifelong.

See Additional Learning Resources at the end of the chapter for more information.

DISORDERS OF MOTILITY

Hirschsprung Disease (HD)

Pathophysiology

Hirschsprung disease, or congenital aganglionic megacolon, occurs when there is an absence of ganglionic innervation to the muscle of a segment of the bowel. This usually happens in the lower portion of the sigmoid colon. Because of the absence of nerve cells, there is a lack of normal peristalsis. This results in chronic constipation. Ribbonlike stools are seen as a result of feces passing through the narrow segment. The portion of the bowel nearest to the obstruction dilates, causing abdominal distention (Fig. 28.8). It is seen more often in boys than girls, and it has familial tendencies. The incidence is approximately 1 in 5 000 live births (Fiorino & Liacouras, 2016). There is a higher incidence in children with Down syndrome.

Manifestations

In the newborn, failure to pass meconium stools within 24 to 48 hours may be a symptom of HD. In the infant, constipation, ribbonlike stools, abdominal distention, anorexia, vomiting, and failure to thrive may be evident. Often the parent brings the young child to the clinic after trying several over-the-counter laxatives to treat the constipation without success. If the child

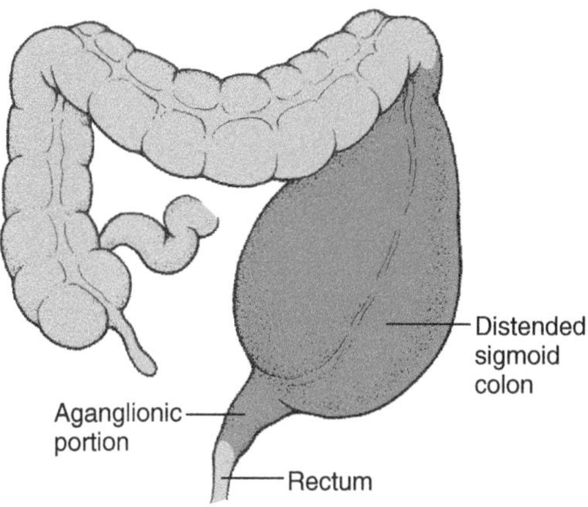

Fig. 28.8 Hirschsprung disease (megacolon). There is no ganglionic nerve innervation or peristalsis in the narrowed section. The adjacent bowel becomes enlarged, causing distention of the abdomen. (From Bowden, V. R., Dickey, S. B., & Greenberg, S. C. [1998]. *Children and their families: The continuum of care.* Philadelphia: Saunders.)

is untreated, other signs of intestinal obstruction and shock might be seen.

Treatment and nursing care

HD is treated by surgery. The impaired part of the colon is removed, and an anastomosis of the intestine is performed. In newborns, a temporary colostomy may be necessary, and more extensive repair may follow at about 12 to 18 months of age. Closure of the colostomy follows in a few months. Parents and the child need to learn care of the ostomy if this is required.

Nursing care is age dependent. In the newborn, detection is a high priority. As the child grows older, careful attention to a history of constipation and diarrhea is important. Signs of undernutrition, abdominal distention, and poor feedings are suspect.

Postoperative care of children is discussed in Chapter 20. Constipation and fecal incontinence may be chronic problems in a few patients after surgical correction for HD; this can significantly impact quality of life for some children.

Diarrhea

Pathophysiology

Diarrhea in the infant cannot be defined in the same way as diarrhea in the adult. The number of stools per day is not often significant in the infant. Diarrhea in infancy is a sudden increase in stools from the infant's normal pattern, with a fluid consistency and a colour that is green or contains mucus or blood. *Acute sudden diarrhea* is most often caused by an inflammation, an infection, or as a response to a medication, food, or poisoning. *Chronic diarrhea* lasts for more than 2 weeks and may be indicative of a malabsorption problem, long-term inflammatory disease, or allergic responses. *Infectious diarrhea* is caused by viral, bacterial, or parasitic infection and is also known as *gastroenteritis* (see discussion below). The priority problem in diarrhea is dehydration and acid–base imbalance.

The most common noninfectious causes of diarrhea involve food intolerance, overfeeding, improper formula preparation, or ingestion of high amounts of sorbitol (a substance found in sweetened "sugar-free" products). Sometimes parents need help in interpreting food labels to avoid foods to which their child may be allergic. Table 28.1 lists some terms that often need clarification for parents of a child who is food intolerant.

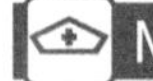

Nursing Tip

Green, watery stools may indicate diarrhea in infants.

Manifestations

The symptoms of diarrhea may be mild or extremely severe. The stools are watery and are expelled with force (explosive stools). They may be yellowish green.

The infant becomes listless, refuses to eat, and loses weight. The temperature may be elevated, and the infant may vomit. Dehydration is evidenced by sunken eyes and fontanelle and by dry skin, tongue, and mucous membranes. Urine output is decreased. In severe cases, the excessive loss of bicarbonate from the GI tract results in acidosis.

Treatment and nursing care

Treatment of diarrhea is focused on identifying and eradicating the cause. The main goals of care include assessing fluid and electrolyte imbalance, rehydration,

Table 28.1 Clarifying Food Labels

INGREDIENT LISTED	MAY CONTAIN
Binder	Egg
Bulking agent	Soy
Casein	Cow's milk (often in canned tuna)
Coagulant	Egg
Emulsifier	Egg
Protein extender	Soy

and reintroduction of an adequate diet. Nursing responsibilities include teaching caregivers proper and age-appropriate diet and feeding techniques. Oral rehydrating solutions (ORS) are recommended as first-line therapy for dehydration from diarrhea as they promote reabsorption of sodium and water (Leung, Prince, and Canadian Paediatric Society (CPS), Nutrition and Gastroenterology Committee, 2006/2016). ORS are given in small, frequent feedings. After being rehydrated, the child should be given an age-appropriate diet (Leung et al., 2006/2016). Breastfeeding is encouraged.

Mild diarrhea in older children may be treated at home under a health care provider's direction.

Gastroenteritis

Pathophysiology

Gastroenteritis is infectious diarrhea and involves an inflammation of the stomach and the intestines; **colitis** involves an inflammation of the colon; **enterocolitis** involves an inflammation of the colon and the small intestine. *Rotavirus* is the most common cause of gastroenteritis among children and can be severe in young children. It is often spreads in day care centres. Other causes of infectious diarrhea include Norwalk virus and *E. coli,* which are food-borne pathogens; *Salmonella,* from contaminated food or pet contact (especially turtles); and *Shigella.*

C. difficile, a spore-forming, anaerobic Gram-positive bacillus, is the most common cause of diarrhea associated with antimicrobial therapy and so is considered a health care–associated condition. Symptoms may include abdominal pain, fever, and bloody diarrhea. *C. difficile* is a reportable disease, which allows rates to be tracked (Public Health Agency of Canada, 2013).

Giardia lamblia is an intestinal protozoan that causes diarrhea and is more common in toddlers. It is spread by contaminated water, unsanitary conditions, and fecal contamination by animals.

Treatment and nursing care

C. difficile diarrhea may be treated with nitazoxanide, an anti-infective medication. The use of probiotics during broad-spectrum antibiotic treatment may prevent the development of diarrhea caused by *rotavirus* and *C. difficile* infection (Marchand & CPS Nutrition and Gastroenterology Committee, 2012/2019).

The nursing care of gastroenteritis includes maintaining intake and output records and providing skin care and frequent diaper changes to prevent excoriation from the frequent stools. Parents should be taught about the importance of good hand hygiene, proper food handling, and principles of cleanliness and infection prevention. The infant should be weighed daily, observed for dehydration or overhydration, and kept warm. Contact precautions should be used to prevent the spread of infection. Nursing Care Plan 28.1 provides nursing interventions for care of a child with gastroenteritis.

Nursing Tip

To prevent foodborne diarrhea, parents should be taught to keep perishable foods refrigerated, avoid thawing frozen food at room temperature for more than 2 hours, cook meat thoroughly, and wash hands, utensils, and work areas with soap and water.

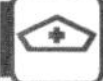

Nursing Tip

Hand hygiene with soap and water rather than an alcohol-based hand sanitizer is recommended when caring for patients with *C. difficile* diarrhea. The environment should be cleaned with a bleach disinfectant by staff.

Vomiting

Pathophysiology

Vomiting, a common symptom during infancy and childhood, results from sudden contractions of the diaphragm and the muscles of the stomach. It must be evaluated in relation to the child's overall health status. Persistent vomiting requires investigation because it results in dehydration and electrolyte imbalance. The continuous loss of hydrochloric acid and sodium chloride from the stomach can cause alkalosis.

Nursing Care Plan 28.1 The Child With Gastroenteritis

PATIENT DATA

An 11-month-old infant is admitted with a history of diarrhea for several days and vomiting related to food ingestion. A diaper rash is evident, and skin tissue turgor is poor.

Selected Nursing Diagnosis Dehydration as a result of diarrhea and/or vomiting, as seen by weight loss, output greater than intake, emesis, liquid stools, decreased urine output, abdominal distention/rebound tenderness, excoriation of perianal mucosa, hypotension, increased pulse rate, change in skin turgor, lethargy, irritability

Goals	Nursing Interventions	Rationales
Infant's or child's weight will be within 5% of normal baseline. Bowel movements will be reduced in number within 24 hours of nursing intervention. Urine output will be above 1 mL/kg/hr. Infant or child will be free from fluid and electrolyte imbalance.	Weigh infant or child daily. Monitor vital signs (e.g., temperature, pulse rate, respirations, blood pressure, and skin turgor). Record intake and output accurately, including ice chips, intravenous (IV) fluids, gelatins, or other food products that become watery at room temperature. Observe and monitor IV fluid administration. Notify health care provider of decreased number of stools, ability to drink liquids without emesis; increased urine output, and improvement in vital signs and skin turgor. Obtain fresh stool specimen, if ordered, and send to laboratory for analysis. After child is rehydrated, resume a normal diet for age.	Daily *accurate* weights are necessary to ascertain the amount of fluids lost through liquid stools and vomiting. Helps determine if the infant or child is responding appropriately to medical and nursing interventions. Accurate recording of intake and output is necessary to determine the amount of fluid replacement required. Fluid depletion occurs very rapidly in infants and small children because they have different proportions of both body water and fat than an adult. IV fluids may be needed to prevent dehydration, electrolyte imbalance, shock, and death. Prevents overhydration of infant or child. A fresh sample is required to determine if there are any ova (eggs) or parasites in the stool that could be the cause of the gastroenteritis. Rehydration fluids help to decrease the mobility of the colon and decrease the risk of water toxicity.

Selected Nursing Diagnosis Skin breakdown as a result of frequency of stools, as seen by excoriation of skin and tissue in perianal area, erythema, pain with each stooling; burning or pain in perianal area

Goals	Nursing Interventions	Rationales
Infant or child will show improvement or resolution of erythema and exhibit tissue that is intact and free from secondary infection.	Change diapers or underwear as soon as a stooling occurs; cleanse perianal area with warm water using a soft cloth free of any alcohol. Leave buttocks exposed to air whenever possible (usually *after* the diarrhea slows down or stops). Apply soothing ointment to affected area (*after* thorough cleansing) sparingly. If medicated powders are prescribed or used, teach the parent to put powder in the hand and then apply on the infant's or child's buttocks and to keep powder container away from the infant or child.	Liquid stools generally contain high amounts of acids. The longer the stool is in contact with the infant's or child's skin, the greater the risk of excoriated tissue. Alcohol can be very painful on impaired tissue. Air helps to keep the skin dry and free from any irritation such as from diapers or underwear rubbing on the skin. The ointment is a protective barrier on the infant's or child's skin. If the ointment is placed on uncleansed skin, the infant or child is at increased risk of excoriation. If powder is "sprayed" onto the buttocks, the infant or child is at risk of inhaling the powder.

Selected Nursing Diagnosis Potential need for parental education related to diarrhea in infants and children if there is lack of previous experience

Continued

Nursing Care Plan 28.1 The Child With Gastroenteritis (Diarrhea and Vomiting)—cont'd

Goals	Nursing Interventions	Rationales
Parents will verbalize understanding of the dietary needs, potential complications, and method of treatment for gastroenteritis or diarrhea.	Instruct parents on proper methods of making, reconstituting, and storing formulas, oral fluid replacements, and foods.	Ensure that parents understand that improper handling or storing of food products can increase the risk of further gastroenteritis.
	Teach and reinforce proper hand hygiene techniques, especially after handling soiled diapers and clothing and before preparing and/or eating a meal.	Hand hygiene is the first line of defense in preventing the spread of infection.
	Explain that dehydration occurs rapidly in infants and small children. Thus parents need to seek help from their health care provider early on to prevent potential hospitalization and further complications.	Early detection and interventions prevent more severe complications from the dehydration that occurs with gastroenteritis.
	Teach parents that some over-the-counter remedies for vomiting and diarrhea can be harmful to infants and small children.	Absorbents such as kaolin and pectin may alter the consistency and appearance of stools, decreasing the frequency of evacuation; however, they may mask actual fluid loss.

CRITICAL THINKING QUESTION

1. An 11-month-old infant is brought to the clinic. The mother states that he has watery diarrhea, and the nurse notices that his eyes are sunken and that his skin turgor is only fair. The mother tells the nurse she wants to give an antidiarrheal medicine that she has at home and asks how much to give. What is the best response of the nurse?

In this condition, the acid–base balance of the body becomes disturbed because of a loss of chlorides and potassium.

Manifestations

The child may vomit from various causes, including toxic ingestions, food intolerances and allergies, mechanical obstruction of the GI tract, metabolic disorders, and psychogenic problems. Other causes of vomiting are systemic illness such as increased intracranial pressure or infection. Complications that occur from vomiting include dehydration, electrolyte disturbances, malnutrition, and aspiration. In aspiration, vomitus is drawn into the air passages on inspiration, causing immediate death in extreme cases. Health professionals and laypersons should become familiar with life-saving procedures such as cardiopulmonary resuscitation (CPR) for use in such emergencies.

Treatment and nursing care

The key to treatment is addressing the cause of the vomiting and preventing complications that can occur. To prevent vomiting, the nurse or caregiver must carefully feed and burp the infant. Treatments are avoided immediately after feedings. An infant with vomiting should be handled as little as possible after feedings and may need to be placed on the right side following feeding to prevent aspiration. When an older child begins to vomit, the head is turned to one side, and an emesis basin and tissues are provided.

Factors to be charted include amount, colour (e.g., bloody, bile-stained), and consistency of vomitus, and force, time, and frequency of vomiting and whether or not it was preceded by nausea or feedings. IV fluids may be given. Sips of water are provided according to the child's tolerance and condition and gradually increased when the vomiting stops. The child's intake and output need to be carefully recorded so that the health care provider can compare the urine output with the total fluid intake.

Antiemetics may be required; these include ondansetron (Zofran), trimethobenzamide (Tigan), metoclopramide (Reglan), and promethazine (Phenergan). They may be prescribed when vomiting is persistent.

Gastroesophageal Reflux

Pathophysiology

Gastroesophageal reflux (GER) results when the lower esophageal sphincter is relaxed or not competent, which allows stomach contents to be easily regurgitated into the esophagus.

Many infants have this condition to a small degree, with symptoms peaking at 4 months and resolving at around 12 months of age, when the child stands upright and eats more solid foods. Gastroesophageal reflux disease (GERD) implies there is tissue damage or symptoms resulting from GER and may include growth failure, bleeding, or dysphagia.

Manifestations

In the infant, symptoms include vomiting, weight loss, and failure to thrive. The vomiting occurs within the first and second weeks of life. The infant is fussy and hungry. Respiratory problems can occur when vomiting stimulates the closure of the epiglottis and the infant presents with apnea. Aspiration of vomitus can also occur.

Treatment and nursing care

A careful history is taken with a focus on when the vomiting started, type of feeding, type of vomiting, feeding techniques, and the infant's eating in general. Tests used to determine the presence of GER include scintigraphy, which involves the infant drinking a radioactively labelled formula, and following the path of the fluid with imaging studies to determine the presence of reflux or poor swallowing coordination. One of the most definitive diagnostic tests is 24-hour esophageal pH monitoring, which helps to determine the acuity of the disease and the course of treatment to prevent esophagitis.

Therapy depends on the severity of symptoms. Most parents need only reassurance and education about feeding the infant. Teaching should include careful burping, avoiding overfeeding (which distends the stomach), and proper positioning. GER is less common in children who are breastfed. Breastfeeding can usually continue with the infant put in an upright position for 2 hours after feeding.

Parents are instructed to burp the infant frequently. Formula feedings can be thickened with rice cereal (5 to 15 mL per 30 mL of formula) or a commercial thickening additive. Adding rice cereal to the formula increases the caloric density from 20 to 27 calories per 30 mL. However, there may be an association between thickened formula and the development of necrotizing enterocolitis in preterm infants (Khan & Orenstein, 2016b).

After being fed, the infant should be placed in an upright position or propped on the left side. The body is inclined about 30 degrees, and the infant may be held in place by a Fowler's sling (Fig. 28.9). Sitting upright in an infant seat or swing is not recommended because it increases intra-abdominal pressure. The upright prone position has been recommended for the infant with GER when awake and monitored. The supine (back) sleep position is recommended for all healthy infants.

Medications that relax the pyloric sphincter and promote stomach emptying may be used. A proton pump inhibitor (PPI) such as omeprazole (Prilosec) and chronic antacid therapy should be avoided (Khan & Orenstein, 2016b). The medication should be administered before meals. Adverse effects such as drowsiness or restlessness can occur.

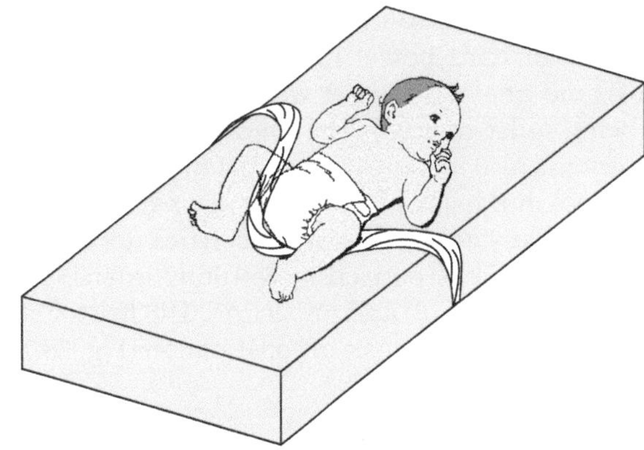

Fig. 28.9 Fowler's sling. Fowler's sling is used to maintain Fowler's position and to prevent the infant from sliding down to the foot of the bed. The bed is in Fowler's position; the rolled blanket is tucked under the mattress on each side at armpit level; when the infant is in the side-lying position or prone, the legs straddle the sling to maintain positioning.

 **Nursing Tip**

Infants with GER should be placed upright at a 30-degree angle when observed but should be placed supine for sleep.

Constipation

Pathophysiology

Constipation is defecation that is difficult or infrequent, with the passage of hard, dry fecal material. There may be associated symptoms, such as abdominal discomfort or blood-streaked stools.

Manifestations

The frequency of bowel movements varies widely in children. There may be periods of diarrhea or encopresis (constipation with fecal soiling). Constipation may be a symptom of other disorders, particularly obstructive conditions. Diet, culture, and social, psychological, and familial patterns may also influence its occurrence. The daily use of laxatives and enemas should be discouraged. Many children use the bathroom every day, but they may be hurried and have an incomplete bowel movement. Some children are embarrassed or even afraid to use school or public bathrooms.

Constipation is defined variably, but involves infrequent, difficult, painful or incomplete evacuation of hard stools (Rowan-Legg & CPS Community Paediatrics Committee, 2011/2018). The term *functional constipation* describes all children in whom constipation does not have an organic etiology. Functional constipation is commonly the result of withholding of feces in a child who wants to avoid painful defecation (Rowan-Legg & CPS Community Paediatrics Committee, 2011/2018).

Functional constipation is diagnosed according to the ROME IV criteria. For children under 4 years of age, this includes less than two defecations per week, a history of hard bowel movements, large-diameter stools, and one episode per week of incontinence (after being toilet trained). For children over 4 years of age, criteria also include evidence of the child trying to hold stool in (Hyams, Di Lorenzo, Saaps, et al., 2016). Continued distention lessens the reflex to evacuate stool and weakens peristalsis, resulting in encopresis (an overflow of stool) and impaction. The Bristol Stool chart aids in the diagnosis of constipation (Fig. 28.10).

Treatment and nursing care

The goal of treatment is to produce soft, painless stools and to prevent reaccumulation of feces. Education, behavioural modification, daily maintenance stool softeners, and dietary modification are all important components of therapy (Rowan-Legg & CPS Community Paediatrics Committee, 2011/2018).

Evaluation begins with a thorough history of dietary and bowel habits. The frequency, colour, and consistency of the stool are noted. The nurse should inquire about any medication the child may be taking. The parents should be asked to define what they mean by constipation. Parent teaching on how to prevent constipation is important.

Fecal disimpaction may be necessary at the outset of treatment and may be achieved by either oral or rectal medication (Rowan-Legg & CPS Community Paediatrics Committee, 2011/2018).

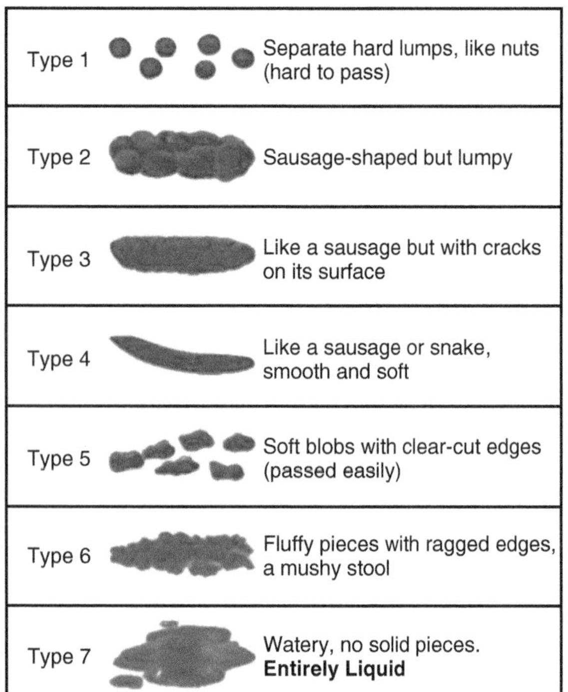

Bristol Stool Chart
Type 1
Separate hard lumps, like nuts (hard to pass)
Type 2
Sausage-shaped but lumpy
Type 3
Like a sausage but with cracks on its surface
Type 4
Like a sausage or snake, smooth and soft
Type 5
Soft blobs with clear-cut edges (passed easily)
Type 6
Fluffy pieces with ragged edges, a mushy stool
Type 7
Watery, no solid pieces. Entirely Liquid

Fig. 28.10 The Bristol Stool chart shows normal and abnormal stools. (Courtesy Elder, J. [2016]. Enuresis and voiding dysfunction. In R. Kliegman, B. Stanton, J. St. Geme, et al. [Eds.], *Nelson textbook of pediatrics* [20th ed.]. Philadelphia: Saunders.)

Dietary modification includes adding more roughage to the diet. Foods high in fibre include whole-grain breads and cereals, raw vegetables and fruits, bran, and popcorn for older children. Some infants respond to intake of formula with a high iron content by developing constipation. Changing to a low-iron formula may be helpful. Increasing fluid intake is also important.

The child should be encouraged to try to move the bowels at the same time each day to establish a routine. The child should not be hurried. Increased exercise may help sedentary children with constipation. The use of stool softeners, fluids, diet, and behaviour modification can prevent a chronic functional constipation problem from occurring. Polyethylene glycol is a safe, effective and well-tolerated long-term treatment for constipation (Rowan-Legg & CPS Community Paediatrics Committee, 2011/2018).

FLUID AND ELECTROLYTE IMBALANCE

Principles of Fluid Balance in Children

Infants and small children have different proportions of body water and body fat from those of adults (Fig. 28.11), and the water needs and water losses of the infant (per unit of body weight) are greater. In children less than 2 years of age, surface area is particularly important in fluid and electrolyte balance because more water is lost through the skin than through the kidneys. The surface area of the infant is two to three times greater than that of the adult in proportion to body volume or body weight. Metabolic rate and heat production are also two to three times greater in infants per kilogram of body weight. This causes more waste products to be produced, which must be diluted to be excreted. It also stimulates respiration, which causes increased evaporation through the lungs. Compared with adults, a greater percentage of body water in children less than 2 years of age is contained in the extracellular compartment.

Fluid turnover is rapid, and dehydration occurs more quickly in infants than in adults. The infant cannot survive as long as the adult in the presence of continued water depletion. A sick infant does not adapt as rapidly to shifts in intake and output because the kidneys lack maturity; they are less able to concentrate urine and require more water than an adult's kidneys to excrete a given amount of solute. Disturbances of the GI tract often lead to vomiting and diarrhea. Electrolyte balance depends on fluid balance and cardiovascular, renal, adrenal, pituitary, parathyroid, and pulmonary regulatory mechanisms. Many of these mechanisms are maturing in the developing child and are unable to react at full capacity under the stress of illness, such as diarrhea and vomiting. Signs of dehydration in a child may not be evident until the fluid loss reaches 4%, and severe dehydration may not be evident until the fluid loss reaches 10% (Table 28.2).

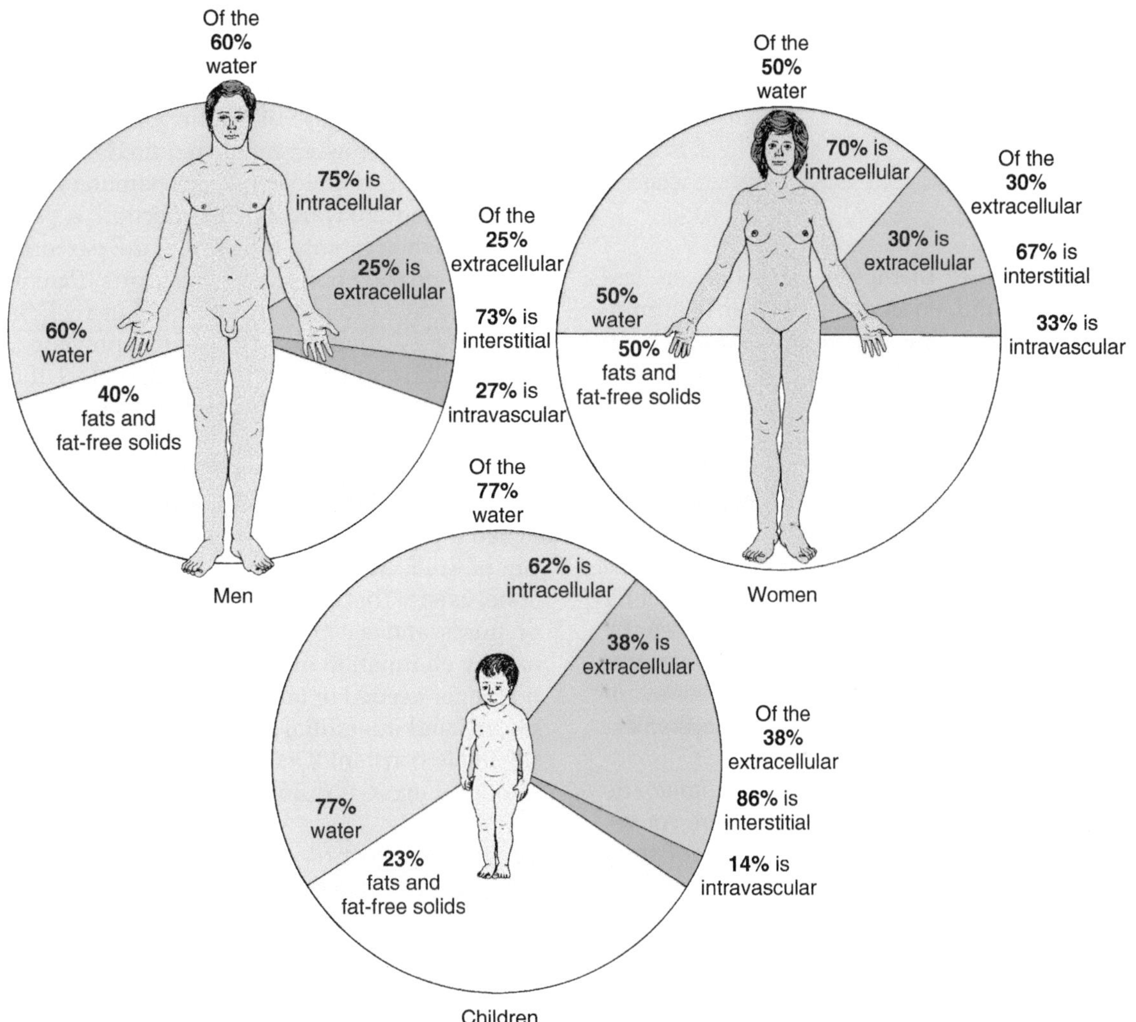

Fig. 28.11 Relationship of body water and body solids to the body weight in the adult man and woman and in the child.

Table 28.2 Signs of Isotonic, Hypertonic, and Hypotonic Dehydration

	SIGNS OF DEHYDRATION		
AREA OF ASSESSMENT	**ISOTONIC**	**HYPERTONIC**	**HYPOTONIC**
Weight loss	*Mild dehydration:* Up to 5% weight loss *Moderate dehydration:* 5 to 10% weight loss *Severe dehydration:* More than 10% weight loss		
Behaviour	Irritable and lethargic	Irritable when disturbed; lethargic	Lethargic to delirious; coma
Skin turgor	Decreased elasticity	Firm turgor; "foam rubber" feel	Very poor turgor; clammy
Mucous membranes	Dry	Parched	Clammy
Eyeballs and fontanelle	Sunken and soft	Sunken	Sunken and soft
Tearing and salivation	Absent or decreased	Absent or decreased	Absent or decreased
Thirst	Present	Marked	Present
Urine	Decreased output; serum globulin (SG) elevated	Normal to decreased output; SG elevated or decreased	Decreased output; SG elevated
Body temperature	Subnormal to elevated	Elevated	Subnormal
Respirations	Rapid	Rapid	Rapid
Blood pressure	Normal to low	Normal to low	Very low
Pulse	Rapid	Rapid	Rapid
Blood chemistry	BUN increased Na decreased K normal or increased Cl decreased pH usually decreased	BUN increased Na decreased K decreased Cl low during correction Ca decreased	BUN increased Na decreased K varies or increased Cl decreased

BUN, Blood urea nitrogen; *Ca,* calcium; *Cl,* chloride; *K,* potassium; *Na,* sodium.
Data from Bender, B., Skoe, C., & Ozuah, P. (2005). Oral rehydration therapy. *Contemporary Pediatrics*, *22*(4), 72–76; Greenbaum, L. A. (2016). Deficit therapy. In R. M. Kliegman, B. F. Stanton, J. W. St. Geme, et al. (Eds.), *Nelson textbook of pediatrics* (20th ed.). Philadelphia: Saunders.

Safety Alert!

An accurate intake and output record must be kept for all children with vomiting or diarrhea.

Oral fluids

ORS are preferred to IV therapy because they are less traumatic for the child, cheaper, and easier to administer. They can also be administered in a variety of settings, including the home (Leung, Prince, & CPS Nutrition and Gastroenterology Committee, 2006/2016). Nurses must use their ingenuity to coax sick children to take enough fluids, because they may refuse food and water and do not understand the importance of such intake for recovery. Toddlers and infants are not capable of drinking by themselves. The nurse must find time to offer them fluids and be patient and gently persistent in this effort. Liquids are offered frequently and in small amounts. Brightly coloured containers and drinking straws may help. ORS options are available in varied flavours and in frozen forms that are more acceptable to the young child.

Premixed ORS, rather than powdered or homemade ones, should be used. ORS powders are more convenient to store, less expensive, and have a longer shelf life than ORS fluids, but they must be mixed precisely to avoid changes in glucose and electrolyte concentrations (Leung et al., 2006/2016). Carbonated drinks and sweetened fruit juices are discouraged because of their high carbohydrate content, very low electrolyte content, and high osmolarity. Plain water should not be offered to children with acute gastroenteritis to avoid hyponatremia and hypoglycemia (Leung et al., 2006/2016).

Oral rehydration fluids are usually given as 1 millilitre of ORS for every gram of output. Replacement fluid needs are usually estimated as 10 mL/kg for each stool and 2 mL/kg for each emesis. Children without dehydration should continue to be fed an age-appropriate diet. Children with dehydration should be fed an age-appropriate diet as soon as they have been rehydrated (Leung et al., 2006/2016).

The nurse needs to keep an accurate record of the patient's intake and output. General hygiene and principles of preventing diarrhea should be discussed with the parents.

Parenteral fluids

Parenteral fluids (*para,* "beside or apart from," and *enteron,* "intestine") are fluids given by some route other than the digestive tract. They are necessary when vomiting or loss of consciousness accompanies sickness or when the GI system requires rest. Parenteral fluids are needed in severe cases of vomiting and diarrhea in which the loss of water and electrolytes will lead to death if untreated. They also provide a means for the safe and effective administration of prescribed parenteral medications. Solutions given parenterally must be sterile to prevent a general or local infection. The nurse must be aware of the importance of parenteral therapy and the assessments required.

The infant or child receiving parenteral fluids continues to require warmth and affection. A pacifier may be used when infants are NPO, if the parents agree, in order to provide non-nutritive sucking. Parents should be encouraged to pick up and hold or rock their child receiving IV therapy. Arm boards prevent the child from pulling out the IV line and protect the tubing. Parenteral therapy is discussed in Chapter 20.

Dehydration

Pathophysiology

When a person is in good health, the intake and output of fluids are balanced and **homeostasis** (a uniform state) exists. This is accomplished by appropriate shifts of fluids and electrolytes across cellular membranes and by elimination of products of metabolism that are no longer needed or are in excess. The volume of blood plasma and interstitial and intracellular fluids remains relatively constant. Dehydration occurs whenever fluid output exceeds fluid intake, regardless of the cause.

Manifestations

Disorders of fluids and electrolytes—sodium (Na^+), potassium (K^+), calcium (Ca^{++}), and magnesium (Mg^{++})—are more complex in growing children. A newborn's total weight consists of approximately 77% water, compared with 60% in adults (Fig. 28.11). This varies with the amount of fat. In addition, the daily turnover of water in infants is equal to almost 24% of total body water, compared with about 6% in adults. An infant's body surface in comparison to weight is three times that of the older child; therefore, the infant is subject to greater evaporation of water from the skin. The younger the patient, the higher the metabolic rate and the more unstable the heat-regulating mechanisms. Elevations in temperature also increase the rate of water loss. Rapid respirations speed up this process; when diarrhea is present, additional fluid is lost in the stools.

Immaturity of the kidneys impairs the infant's ability to conserve water. The average urine output in infants and children is listed in Table 28.3. The average urine output in children is 1 to 2 mL/kg/hr, and the output for older children is a minimum of 30 mL/hr. An important nursing responsibility is to document the intake and output of hospitalized infants and children.

Preterm and newborn infants are also more susceptible to dehydration from variations in room temperature and humidity. When this is coupled with higher fluid losses, life-threatening deficits can ensue within a few hours (Table 28.4).

Problems of fluid and electrolyte disturbance require evaluation of the type and severity of dehydration, clinical observation of the patient, and chemical analysis of the blood. The types of dehydration are classified according to the level of serum sodium, which depends on the relative losses of water and electrolytes. These types are usually termed **isotonic** (the person has lost equal amounts of fluids and electrolytes), **hypotonic** (the person has lost more electrolytes than fluid), and **hypertonic** (more fluids are lost than electrolytes) (see Table 28.2). These classifications are important, because each form of dehydration is associated with different relative losses from intracellular fluid (ICF) and extracellular fluid (ECF) compartments, and each requires certain modifications in treatment.

! Safety Alert!

Life-threatening deficits can occur within a few hours of dehydration and fluid loss. Close assessment and reporting of signs and symptoms of dehydration are essential.

Treatment and nursing care

Maintenance fluid therapy replaces normal water and electrolyte losses, and *deficit therapy* restores preexisting body fluid and electrolyte deficiencies. The composition of IV fluids and the amount and rate of flow are important in preventing complications.

There are two methods for calculating pediatric maintenance fluid rates. It is the responsibility of the health care provider to order daily fluid requirement, but the nurse should double check the order for accuracy (The Hospital for Sick Kids [SickKids], n.d.).

- Formula method: (100 mL for each of the first 10 kg) + (50 mL for each kg 11–20) + (20 mL for each additional kg) / 24 hour
- 4 / 2 / 1 Method: (4 mL/kg for the first 10 kg) + (2 mL/kg for kg 11–20) + (1 mL/kg for every kg above 20) = hourly rate

Shock (hypovolemia) is the greatest threat to life in isotonic dehydration. The electrolyte content of oral fluids is particularly significant in the care of infants and small children who have disorders of fluid balance and are receiving infusions. Commercially prepared electrolyte solutions, or ORS, are available. Children with hypotonic dehydration (excess water with sodium electrolyte depletion) are at risk for water intoxication. This can also occur if tap water enemas are given to small children.

Potassium is lost in almost all degrees of dehydration. Replacement potassium is administered only after normal urinary excretion is confirmed.

Documentation must include accurate assessment of intake and output, vital signs, daily weight, skin and fontanelles, mucous membranes, and level of consciousness.

Nursing Tip

Intake and output records include information concerning oral and parenteral intake, suction, wound drainage, vomiting, urine and stool, and sweating. All of this must be documented accurately.

Nursing Tip

One way of determining fluid loss in infants is to weigh a wet diaper and then weigh a dry diaper of the same type and size and to mark the weight on the outside of the dry diaper. Subtract the weight of the dry diaper from the weight of the wet diaper, and record results on the intake and output record. Include both urine and liquid stools (1 g = 1 mL of output).

Table 28.3 Average Daily Excretion of Urine (Approximate)

AGE	MILLILITRES (ML)	FLUID OUNCES
Days 1 and 2	30–60	1–2
Days 3–10	100–300	3–10
Day 10–2 months	250–450	9–15
2 months–1 year	400–500	14–17
1–3 years	500–600	17–20
3–5 years	600–700	20–24
5–8 years	650–1000	22–34
8–14 years	800–1400	27–47

Table 28.4 Estimation of Dehydration

	DEGREE		
CLINICAL SIGN	**MILD**	**MODERATE**	**SEVERE**
Weight loss (%)	5	10	15
Behaviour	Normal	Irritable	Hyperirritable to lethargic
Thirst	Slight	Moderate	Intense
Mucous membranes	May be normal	Dry	Parched
Tears	Present	Decreased	Absent
Anterior fontanelle	Flat	+/–	Sunken
Skin turgor	Normal	+/–	Decreased
Urinary output	Normal	Decreased	Minimal

Data from Greenbaum, L. A. (2016). Deficit therapy. In R. M. Kliegman, B. F. Stanton, J. W. St. Geme, et al. (Eds.), *Nelson textbook of pediatrics* (20th ed.). Philadelphia: Saunders.

Safety Alert!

The nurse must document that at least one void has occurred before IV potassium is administered.

Electrolyte Imbalance

The nurse must be able to assess the electrolyte needs of the child. When fluid snacks or nourishment are ordered, the selection of fluid can influence the treatment given for dehydration. For example, if the child has a hypertonic type of dehydration (which means there is excess sodium) and the nurse offers the child tomato juice, the high sodium content of tomato juice will negatively affect the child's prescribed treatment. If the child has hypotonic dehydration (which means the child has deficient electrolytes) and the nurse offers plain water, this will also have a negative impact on the child's care. Therefore, it is a nursing responsibility to correlate laboratory findings of the individual child with fluids and foods offered to the child.

Overhydration

Pathophysiology

Overhydration results when the body receives more fluid than it can excrete. This can occur in patients with normal kidneys who receive IV fluids too rapidly. It also can occur in a patient receiving acceptable rates of fluid, especially when the patient's illness is related to disorders of fluid mechanism.

Manifestations

Edema is the presence of excess fluid in the interstitial (*interstitium,* "a thing standing between") spaces. Interstitial fluid is similar to plasma, but it contains little protein. In healthy persons, it responds well to shifts in fluid balance. Any factor causing sodium retention can cause edema. The flow of blood out of the interstitial compartments also depends on adequate circulation of blood and lymph. Low protein levels can also disturb osmotic cellular pressure, causing edema. This is seen in patients with nephrosis, in which large amounts of albumin are lost.

Trauma to or infections of the head can cause cerebral edema, which can be life-threatening. **Anasarca** (*ana,* "throughout," and *sarx,* "flesh") is a severe generalized edema.

Treatment and nursing care

Edema in infants may first be seen about the eyes and in the presacral, occipital, or genital areas. In pitting edema, the nurse notices an impression in the skin that lasts for several seconds after exerting gentle pressure with the finger.

Early detection and management of edema are essential. Taking an accurate weight daily is indispensable, as is close attention to body weight changes. Vital signs, physical appearance, and changes in urine character or output are noted.

Infants receiving IV therapy have their IV and oral intakes recorded. If the oral intake falls below prescribed rates, the IV rate is increased. If the oral intake exceeds prescribed levels, the IV rate is decreased or the IV is converted to a heparin or saline lock to maintain patency and prevent overhydration.

NUTRITIONAL DEFICIENCIES

Because infancy is a period of rapid growth, poor nutrition is particularly dangerous at this time. Severe vitamin deficiencies are rare in North America although occasionally do occur. Fig. 28.12, *A*, shows a child with general, moderate malnutrition. Severe malnutrition is a concern in many developing countries. Sometimes the infant's body is unable to use food even though the diet is adequate. An example of this is celiac disease, in which the intestines are unable to handle fats and starches. Severe malnutrition may also be seen in failure to thrive.

Failure to Thrive

Pathophysiology

Failure to thrive (FTT) describes infants and children who, without an obvious cause, fail to gain and often lose weight. FTT be classified according to

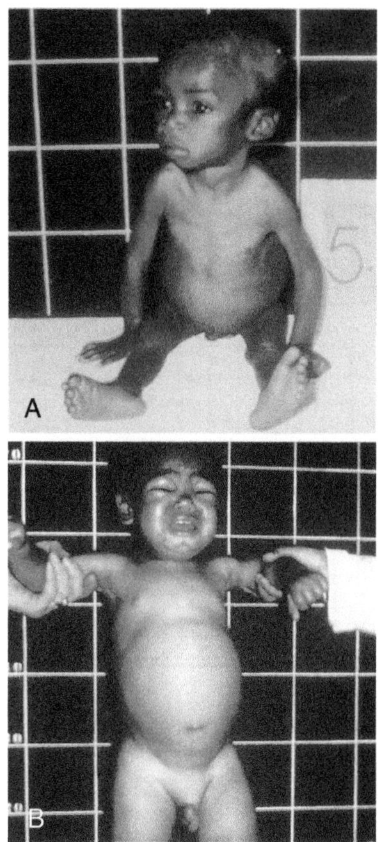

Fig. 28.12 **A,** Failure to thrive is a general nutritional-calorie deficiency. Note the profound wasting found in malnutrition or starvation. **B,** Kwashiorkor, caused by a protein deficiency. The infant has generalized edema with a white streak in the hair. (From Zitelli, B. J., McIntire, S., & Nowalk, A. [2018]. *Zitelli and Davis' atlas of pediatric physical diagnosis* [7th ed.]. Philadelphia: Saunders.)

pathophysiology in the following categories: (1) inadequate caloric intake—due to incorrect formula preparation, neglect, food fads, excessive juice consumption, poverty, behavioural problems affecting eating, or central nervous system problems affecting intake; (2) inadequate absorption—as in cystic fibrosis, celiac disease, vitamin or mineral deficiencies, biliary atresia, or hepatic disease; (3) increased metabolism—hyperthyroidism, congenital heart defects, or chronic immunodeficiency; and (4) defective utilization—as in genetic anomalies such as trisomy 21 or 18, congenital infection, or metabolic storage diseases (Cole & Lanham, 2011).

Infants who fail to thrive are often admitted to the hospital for evaluation with presenting symptoms of weight loss or failure to gain, irritability, and disturbances of food intake such as anorexia or pica (abnormal consumption of nonfood materials). Vomiting, diarrhea, and general neuromuscular spasticity sometimes accompany the condition. These children fall below the fifth percentile in weight and height on standard growth charts. Their development may be delayed. The child has a complete workup to identify reasons for FTT, and the cause is treated.

Manifestations

In some cases of FTT there may be a disturbance in the caregiver–child relationship. The situation is complex and may be associated with relationship discord, economic pressures, lack of parental knowledge, and low stress tolerance. Alcohol and drug use can be present. Infants may suffer from the inability to establish a sense of trust in their caregivers. Their coping abilities are affected by a lack of nurturing. Obvious neglect and physical abuse may be present.

Prevention of this type of FTT consists chiefly of social measures such as parenting classes, family planning, and early recognition of and support for families at risk. All children should receive routine health assessments. The pregnancy history may show circumstances that contribute to a lack of bonding, such as an unplanned pregnancy. Planning interventions that will enhance parent–infant interaction is an important nursing responsibility.

Treatment and nursing care

Treatment involves a multidisciplinary approach in accordance with the circumstances; that is, the health care provider, the nurse, the social worker, the family agency, and the counsellor may all participate. If the child requires hospitalization, one nurse per shift is selected to increase nurturing and interaction with the infant and parent.

It is vital to provide support to the caregiver. Listening and helping the caregiver to understand their feelings and frustrations, and helping them to explore their choices, can facilitate parental attachment. The nurse needs to encourage the caregiver to assist with the daily care of the child. The child's uniqueness and responses to the parent are stressed. The nurse should point out developmental patterns and provide anticipatory guidance in this area. Community resources are important to provide to support families when they are at home.

The prognosis of this condition is uncertain. Because later cognitive and motor function is affected by malnourishment in infancy, many of these children may be below normal in intellectual development, have poorer language development and less developed reading skills, attain lower social maturity, and have a higher incidence of behavioural disturbances (Breen-Reid, 2017).

Kwashiorkor

Kwashiorkor is a protein deficiency that is very rare in Canada. In kwashiorkor, there is a severe deficiency of protein in the diet despite the fact that the number of calories consumed may be nearly adequate. It belongs to a class of disorders termed *protein-energy malnutrition* (see Fig. 28.12, *B*). The child fails to grow normally. The muscles become weak and wasted. There is edema of the abdomen that may become generalized. Diarrhea, skin infections, irritability, anorexia, and vomiting may be present. The hair becomes thin and dry. Because protein is the basis of melanin, which is a substance that provides colour to hair, melanin becomes deficient. This is the reason that the earliest sign of this protein malnutrition is a white streak in the hair of the child (depigmentation). The child looks apathetic and weak with a protuberant abdomen and a reddish-brown scaling of the skin.

Rickets

Pathophysiology

Rickets is a disease of infancy and childhood caused by deficient amounts of vitamin D. Vitamin D and exposure to sunshine are necessary for the proper absorption and metabolism of calcium and phosphorus, which are needed for the normal growth of bones.

Vitamin D–deficiency rickets continues to be a concern in Canada, especially among Indigenous peoples. The Canadian Paediatric Society (CPS) (Godel & CPS First Nations, Inuit and Métis Health Committee, 2007/2017) has identified the following risk factors in children:

- Children exclusively breastfed by mothers with an inadequate intake of vitamin D or mothers who had vitamin D deficiency during pregnancy
- Children with dark skin pigmentation
- Diets that are low in sources of vitamin D and calcium
- Children who live in northern communities (They have less exposure to sunlight due to lack of sunlight hours and covering the skin during sunlight hours to prevent black fly, mosquito, or other bites.)

- Children who live in polluted urban sites
- Children who cover the skin for religious purposes

Manifestations

The classic symptoms of rickets are bowlegs; knock-knees; beading of the ribs, called the *rachitic rosary;* and improper formation of the teeth.

Treatment and nursing care

The nurse should guide parents in the need for a well-balanced diet, exercise, and exposure to outdoor sunlight. All breastfed infants should receive 400 IU of vitamin D daily and this amount should be increased in children who live in northern communities (Health Canada, 2019).

Scurvy

Scurvy is a disease caused by insufficient fruits and vegetables that contain vitamin C in the diet; it is very rare in Canada. The symptoms of scurvy include joint pains, bleeding gums, loose teeth, and lack of energy. Good sources of vitamin C are citrus fruits and raw, leafy vegetables. Vitamin C is easily destroyed by heat and exposure to air. Small amounts of water should be used for cooking vegetables to prevent vitamin C from being destroyed, because it is also water-soluble. The vitamin is not stored in the body, and daily intake from food sources is required.

INFLAMMATORY DISORDERS

Appendicitis

The most common reason for emergency abdominal surgery in childhood is appendicitis. The challenge in diagnosing appendicitis is that rupture or perforation of the appendix can occur with serious complications within 36 hours after the onset of abdominal pain. A delay in diagnosis often occurs because the younger child is unable to localize or express the symptoms experienced. Therefore, the incidence of ruptured appendix is high in young children and after 12 days of symptoms.

Pathophysiology and manifestations

The appendix is a small appendage arising from the cecum; it is located on the right side of the abdomen. The lumen may become obstructed with fecal matter, with lymphoid tissue after a viral illness, or with parasites. There is stasis, increased swelling, edema, and growth of organisms. The initial pain perceived is usually periumbilical and increases within a 4-hour period. When the inflammation spreads to the peritoneum, the pain localizes in the right lower quadrant (RLQ) of the abdomen. The appendix may become gangrenous or rupture, causing peritonitis and septicemia. Vomiting may occur after periumbilical pain starts, whereas in children with gastroenteritis, vomiting precedes abdominal pain. Infrequent mucus diarrhea may occur because of intestinal irritation caused by developing peritonitis. Frequent watery stools are associated with gastroenteritis. Fever is not a reliable sign of appendicitis in children.

On examination, the most intense pain will be at McBurney point, located midway between the anterior superior iliac crest and the umbilicus. Other diagnostic signs include the following:

- Guarding: There is a tightening of the abdominal muscles or rigidity of the abdomen on palpation.
- **Rebound tenderness**: Pressing the RLQ with rapid release of pressure causes severe pain.
- Pain on lifting the thigh while in the supine position is caused by muscle irritation.
- Pain in the RLQ when palpated and pain on rectal examination often occur.

Laboratory tests may be undertaken to confirm the diagnosis and to rule out other possible diagnoses. A urinalysis will rule out a urinary tract infection. C-reactive protein levels will be increased after 12 hours if any infection is present. An ultrasound will show a thickened appendix and a soft tissue mass in the RLQ, and it is used to rule out an ovarian cyst in females who may exhibit similar clinical signs. A CT scan with rectal contrast (CTRC) administered via the rectum may be used to confirm the enlarged appendix. A culture of the stool may be performed to rule out gastroenteritis. A laboratory evaluation of the white blood cell (WBC) count will show an increased WBC count with neutrophils increased 75%, but this may not be helpful in diagnosing an unperforated appendix.

Signs of ruptured appendix and peritonitis include sudden relief of acute pain, rigid guarding of the abdomen, abdominal distention, tachycardia, chills, and irritability.

Treatment and nursing care

Observing the behaviour of the child in relation to their developmental level and using pain scales can help assess the pain level. A warmed stethoscope should be used when auscultating the abdomen of a child; it is less frightening than the approaching fingers of the hand. The child and family need to be prepared for the diagnostic tests and the possibility of surgery. They should be informed of the reason for NPO status until the need for surgery is determined.

Nonoperative care, including IV antibiotic therapy and percutaneous drainage of fluid, is successful in 80% of patients; however, readmission with intra-abdominal abscesses after this procedure continues to be a problem. Therefore, the nonoperative approach remains controversial (Aiken & Oldham, 2016). The nurse should explain to the child and parents what to expect in this care and discuss coping mechanisms.

Postoperative care is similar to that for any abdominal surgery. IV therapy is gradually replaced with fluids and food. A drain may be present at the wound site if perforation has occurred, and a frequent change of dressings may be necessary. Pain management, prevention of infection, and early ambulation are the primary goals.

INFECTIONS

Thrush (Oral Candidiasis)

Pathophysiology

Thrush is an infection of the mucous membranes of the mouth that is caused by the fungus *Candida.* This organism is normally present in the mother's vagina and is nonpathogenic. However, the altered conditions in the vagina produced by pregnancy may lead to the development of candidiasis vaginitis. The mucous membranes of the infant's mouth may become infected by direct contact with this infection during birth or by contact with the caregiver's or nurse's contaminated hands. Cross-infection of other newborns may result. The infection can also be passed from the mother's nipples to the infant's mouth.

Manifestations

White patches that resemble milk curds appear on the tongue, inner lips, gums, and oral mucosa. They are painless but cannot be wiped away. Anorexia may be present. The systemic symptoms are mild if the infection remains in the mouth; however, it can pass along the mucous membranes into the GI tract, causing inflammation of the esophagus and the stomach. Pneumonitis may also develop. *Epstein's pearls,* which are small, white, epithelial cysts that appear along both sides of the midline of the hard palate, are sometimes mistaken for thrush. These are harmless and gradually disappear.

Treatment and nursing care

A thrush infection responds well to the local application of an antifungal suspension such as nystatin (Mycostatin). The mouth is swabbed three or four times a day between feedings with a sterile applicator moistened with the prescribed solution. With proper care, the condition disappears within a few days after its onset. In some cases, a single dose of fluconazole is the treatment for recurrent cases in combination with nystatin (Ericson, Smith, & Benjamin, 2016).

Newborns suspected of having thrush are cared for using routine precautions. Individual feeding equipment is necessary, and the equipment should be sterile. Disposable bottles, disposable nipples, and pacifiers, are preferred for use.

Candida infection of the diaper area presents as a bright red, sharply demarcated diaper rash. Nystatin cream is often prescribed.

> **Nursing Tip**
>
> In the home, parents are taught to drop nystatin or other medication slowly into the side of the infant's mouth. Medication must remain in contact with "patches" as long as possible. Instruct parents to watch for dehydration (e.g., decrease in number of wet diapers) that can result from the infant's refusal to take fluids because of mouth discomfort.

Enterobiasis (Pinworms)

Pathophysiology

Of the several varieties of worms that affect humans, the most common is the pinworm, *Enterobius vermicularis* (*enteron,* "intestine," *bios,* "life," and *vermis,* "wormlike"). It is seen more often in toddlers but it can develop in older children and adults. The pinworm looks like a white thread about 0.8 cm long. It lives in the lower intestine but comes out of the anus to lay its eggs, generally during the night. These eggs become infective a few hours after they have been deposited. This type of parasite spreads from one person to another, particularly where large groups of children are in close contact with one another. The route of entry is the mouth; the child becomes infected by ingesting the eggs. Reinfection takes place by way of contact from the rectum to the fingers to the mouth or by way of the rectum to the clothing to the fingers to the mouth.

Manifestations

The parent may notice that the child scratches the anal area and may state they have significant itching. There may be associated irritability and restlessness. Weight loss, poor appetite, and fretfulness during the night can develop. The rectal area may become irritated from scratching. A special pinworm diagnostic tape or paddle, or a tongue blade covered with cellophane tape, sticky side out, may be placed against the anal region to obtain pinworm eggs (the "Scotch tape test"). This is done early in the morning, before the child has a bowel movement, bathes, or scratches the anal area with the fingers. The tape is put on a glass slide and examined under a microscope. The eggs are typical of pinworms.

Treatment and nursing care

Several effective **anthelmintics** (*anti,* "against," and *helminth,* "worms") are available. Mebendazole (Vermox) is a single-dose, chewable tablet and is the medication of choice for children older than 2 years of age. Pyrantel pamoate (Combantrin) also controls the infestation. Pyrvinium pamoate (Vanquin) suspension, a one-dose treatment, is an alternative medication; nurses should advise parents that pyrvinium pamoate stains and turns the stools red.

The main nursing responsibility is the education of the patient and family concerning the prevention of worm infestation through general hygiene, food handling, and environmental controls. The child must be taught to wash the hands thoroughly after bowel movements. The child's fingernails are kept short. A soothing ointment is applied to the rectal area. The patient should wear clean underwear that fits snugly to prevent scratching the anus with the fingers.

All symptomatic members of the family should be treated for this condition to prevent reinfection. Pregnant women should not take mebendazole and should consult a health care provider before taking any alternative medication. The toilet seats in the home should be scrubbed daily. Cloth diapers and bed linens need to be washed in hot water.

POISONING

For Canadians of all ages, poisoning is the fifth leading cause of injury deaths, hospitalizations, and emergency room visits. Researchers estimate that half of all poison exposures occur among children younger than 6 years of age (Parachute, n.d.). The use of child-resistant medication packaging and limited doses per container contributes to the decline in poisoning among young children.

Poison Control Centres

The telephone number of the provincial poison control centre is listed in the telephone directory and online and should be posted near the phone in all homes and added to cellular phone contacts. The Canadian Association of Poison Control Centres has all the provincial centres listed. These centres can identify the antidote or treatment needed for specific poisons.

Parents are advised to call the poison control centre first to determine the next steps. Sometimes treatment can be started at home. If the child needs be taken to the hospital, the container of the substance ingested should be brought to the hospital. Table 28.5 indicates how to assess the type of toxic substance ingested according to the odour of the vomitus.

 **Safety Alert!**

The provincial poison control centre phone number should be listed on cell phones and kept in prominent places in the home or business of all caregivers.

Principles of Care

Prevention of poisoning is best accomplished through a multifaceted approach combining education, enforcement, and environmental modifications (Parachute, n.d.). Effective poison prevention emphasizes the following key aspects:

- Poison prevention education for families
- The safe storage of potentially poisonous substances
- Limiting the quantity of potentially harmful over-the-counter medications that can be purchased in a single package
- Mandatory carbon monoxide alarms in all residences
- The establishment and coordination of data surveillance and collection

Goals in the primary management of poisoning are the following:

- Remove access to the poison.
- Prevent further absorption.
- Call the poison control centre.
- Provide supportive care—seek medical help.

If poisoning does occur, nursing care involves assessment, parent and patient support, and monitoring of the patient. Treatment of poisoning includes prevention of absorption, enhancement of excretion of the poison from the body, maintenance of fluid and electrolyte balance, and cardiopulmonary stabilization.

Table 28.5 Detecting Poison by Specific Odour of Breath or Vomitus

ODOUR OF VOMITUS	POSSIBLE CONTENT
Sweet	Chloroform, acetone
Bitter almond	Cyanide
Pear	Chloral hydrate
Garlic	Organophosphate (chemical fertilizer), arsenic
Shoe polish	Nitrobenzene
Violet	Turpentine
Rotten egg	Natural gas leak

Note: The nurse should report and document the specific odour of breath or vomitus, which can be helpful in determining the specific poison contained in the substance ingested.

Data modified from Baddock, N. R. (2000). Detection of poisoning by substances other than drugs: A neglected art. *Annals of Clinical Biochemistry, 37*, 146–157.

Gastrointestinal decontamination (GID)

GID is used if necessary, depending on the type of poison ingested. GID is used to remove the ingested poison, by adsorbing the toxin with activated charcoal, performing gastric lavage, or increasing bowel motility (catharsis) (Hogarth, 2017). Some poisons have specific antidotes that would be administered.

Activated charcoal. Activated charcoal provides a large absorptive area that combines with many toxins in the stomach to prevent absorption and facilitate excretion from the body. It is a powder that is mixed with water or saline to make a slurry syrup, flavoured with chocolate or a diet soft drink to make it more palatable. Many children vomit after receiving a dose, thus it is not used after ingestion of a caustic substance. An assessment of a clear protective airway before administration is essential. Activated charcoal may be administered via nasogastric tube if the patient is unconscious. Activated charcoal is best administered within 30 to 60 minutes of ingestion in order for it to be effective.

Gastric lavage. Gastric lavage involves placing a tube into the stomach, aspirating the contents, and flushing the stomach with a fluid such as normal saline. Gastric lavage is rarely effective more than 1 hour after the ingestion. The procedure can cause bradycardia due to a vagal response and delay administration of specific antidotes. It is no longer recommended as a routine treatment for poisoning, as it is associated with serious complications, though may be recommended in certain situations.

Whole bowel irrigation. Whole bowel irrigation involves instilling (usually by nasal gastric tube) large volumes of a polyethylene glycol electrolyte solution (Go-LYTELY) to flush the entire GI tract. It is most effective with slowly absorbed toxins and toxins that do not respond to activated charcoal. Nursing responsibilities include maintaining an open airway, ensuring bowel sounds are present before administering, observing for abdominal distention and excretion of stool, and monitoring the fluid and electrolyte balance.

Other methods of excreting toxins. Enhanced elimination of toxins can be used if a toxin is already absorbed in the body and may prevent organ damage. Techniques include the following:

Alkalization of the urine involves IV administration of bicarbonates that trap the toxin in the renal tubules and enhance excretion. Monitoring for adverse effects such as altered fluid and electrolytes is essential.

Hemodialysis requires the use of a machine and dialyzer (referred to as an "artificial kidney") to remove fluid and waste products from the blood and to correct electrolyte imbalances.

Peritoneal dialysis (*peritoneum* and *dialysis*, "passing of a solute through a membrane") is a therapeutic measure in which the solution is infused into the abdominal cavity and then drained after a set number of hours. This therapy uses the principles of osmosis and diffusion through the semipermeable peritoneal membrane, with the purpose of removing toxic substances from the blood.

Intralipid emulsion treatment infusing a 20% intralipid substance, similar to that used in total parenteral nutrition (TPN), can be used in combination with fat-soluble medications and has shown promise in the treatment of overdose of specific medications.

Poisonous Plants

Many common plants used in home landscapes can be poisonous to the young child exploring in the backyard.

Health Promotion

Common Household Plants That Are Poisonous

PLANTS	CAUSE SYMPTOMS SIMILAR TO
Azalea Buttercup Marigold	Aconite poisoning
Lantana Jimsonweed	Atropine poisoning
Sweet pea Black mountain laurel	Curare poisoning
Apricot pits Peach pits Elderberry	Cyanide poisoning
Camellia seeds Foxglove Oleander	Symptoms similar to digitalis poisoning
Goldenrod Nightshade Poinsettia	Nitrate poisoning
Laurel Water hemlock	Resin poisoning
Camellia Marigold Tulips Violets	Salicylate poisoning

Note: These plants should not be used to landscape the backyard of homes with young children, who may place the leaves or flowers in their mouth.

Medications

Medications prescribed for family members and left within the reach of children are often the cause of accidental poisoning. Many over-the-counter medications are considered harmless by parents but can be deadly to toddlers, even in small doses (Table 28.6). Even a small amount of an oral hypoglycemic medication can lower blood sugar in a small child and can result in a coma. Herbal remedies can also be poisonous to small children. Common antidotes for specific poisonings are listed in Box 28.1.

The nurse must realize the danger of medication poisoning and must constantly practice and teach

Table 28.6 Selected Over-the-Counter Medications That Can Be Deadly to Young Children

GENERIC NAME	TRADE NAME	TOXICITY
Benzocaine	Orajel	Methemoglobinemia Seizures
Camphor	Vicks VapoRub	Central nervous system (CNS) depression Seizures
Diphenoxylate	Lomotil	CNS depression
Methyl salicylate	Oil of wintergreen Icy–Hot balm Arthritis ointments	Cardiovascular collapse
Tetrahydrozoline hydrochloride	Visine eye drops; Murine	Tachycardia; seizures

Data modified from http://www.healthsafety.com/articles/toxic-medicine.

Box 28.1 Common Antidotes to Specific Poisons

POISON	ANTIDOTE
Acetaminophen	Mucomyst (*N*-acetylcysteine)
Opioids	Naloxone (Narcan)
Salicylates, tricyclic antidepressants, and benzodiazepines	Sodium bicarbonate
Lead, arsenic, and inorganic mercury	BAL (Dimercaprol) Calcium disodium Dimercaptosuccinic acid
Iron	Deferoxamine
Ethylene glycol Methanol	Fomepizole
Calcium channel blocker	Insulin and calcium salts
Beta blockers	Glucagon and insulin
Heparin	Protamine sulfate

Note: Early intervention with antidotes is important in managing the poisoning in a child. Responses to the antidote administered must be clearly observed and documented.

Data adapted from California Poison Control System. (2017). *Antidotes*. Retrieved from https://calpoison.org/topics/antidotes; and Vera, M. (2012). *Common drugs and their antidotes.* Retrieved from https://nurseslabs.com/list-of-common-drugs-their-antidotes-that-nurses-should-know/.

safety measures to prevent tragedies. Treatment rooms, utility rooms, and medication storage areas should be scrutinized to ensure that nothing harmful is within the reach of ambulatory children.

Acetaminophen poisoning

Acetaminophen (Tylenol) has now replaced aspirin as the most commonly ingested medication that causes toxicity. This is because it is so widely used and because aspirin, which has been associated with Reye syndrome, is no longer recommended for fever in children with flulike symptoms. Acetaminophen is also found as an ingredient in multidrug medications, which, if taken with concentrated acetaminophen, can result in an overdose. Because acetaminophen is metabolized in the liver, overdose results in hepatic destruction. With early treatment, most children recover without complications.

Treatment and nursing care. Manifestations of acetaminophen overdose are often nonspecific. A history and laboratory findings often lead to the diagnosis. Nursing responsibilities for patients with acute poisoning are shown in Table 28.7.

Medical intervention is necessary if the single ingested dose exceeds 200 mg/kg in children and greater than 7.5 to 10 g in adolescents (Kostic, 2016). Treatment should be started within 24 hours of ingestion. Blood levels usually peak 4 to 6 hours after ingestion and, depending on the serum acetaminophen level, *N*-acetylcysteine (Mucomyst) may be prescribed. This medicine has a bad smell and taste, and the patient needs coaxing and support to assist with administration. The medicine may be mixed with a soft drink or juice. Treatment within 8 hours of ingestion can reduce the risk of liver damage, but a delay of more than 24 hours may increase the risk of liver damage. Levels of liver enzymes (ALT and AST) usually peak within 96 hours and are monitored along with prothrombin times.

Prevention of overdose is of utmost importance. Even in uncomplicated cases, the child is subjected to unpleasant, stressful procedures. A history of accidental or intentional ingestion will guide the path of follow-up care.

Nonsteroidal anti-inflammatory drug (NSAID) poisoning

Anti-inflammatory medications such as ibuprofen (Motrin or Advil) inhibit prostaglandin synthesis. Overdose symptoms can include GI irritation, reduced kidney function, and platelet dysfunction. Ingestion of over 400 mg/kg can cause altered mental status and metabolic acidosis. Initial manifestations include nausea, vomiting, and abdominal pain. Supportive care, including use of antiemetics and medications that reduce stomach acids as indicated, is the primary therapy for NSAID toxicity. Decontamination with activated charcoal should be considered if a patient presents within 1 to 2 hour of a potentially toxic ingestion (Kostic, 2016).

Salicylate poisoning

Aspirin (acetylsalicylic acid) poisoning is seen less often than in the past because of safety packaging and the increased use of acetaminophen. Nevertheless, aspirin is often used in many homes as it is present in many muscle and sports creams such as oil of wintergreen (methyl salicylate) that can be swallowed by the curious child. It is sometimes used as a home remedy for arthritic pain. Even a dose as small as 5 mL can cause a child's death.

Salicylate acts rapidly but is excreted slowly. Ingestion of 150 mg/kg of body weight causes symptoms. Although most cases of aspirin poisoning are emergencies, a child may unknowingly be poisoned by the cumulative effect of aspirin. The use of several aspirin-containing products at once, such as over-the-counter cold remedies combined with aspirin, can be hazardous. Time-release aspirin is especially dangerous because the symptoms of poisoning are delayed. Therefore, it is wise to read labels carefully and to administer aspirin sparingly. It is even better to use it only under a health care provider's direction. Nausea, vomiting,

Table 28.7 Anticipated Care for Poisoning

SYMPTOMS	INTERVENTION
Absorption	Assist with initial treatment and gastrointestinal decontamination
Central nervous system: restlessness, agitation, seizures, coma	Seizure precautions, document LOC and response
Respiratory: airway obstruction, hypoventilation, hypoxia	Cardiopulmonary resuscitation, oxygen saturation monitoring, oxygen therapy, keep artificial airway handy
Cardiovascular: difficulties with electrolytes, blood urea nitrogen, creatinine, glucose	Monitor vital signs and laboratory results
Gastrointestinal: difficulty swallowing, abdominal pain	NPO status; monitor bowel sounds and diarrhea
Kidney problems	Monitor intake and output; monitor IV lines
Hypothermia or hyperthermia	Cooling blanket, monitor body temperature
Child: physical response or psychological trauma Parents: guilt, anger, family dysfunction	Crisis intervention Counselling, teaching, referral

IV, Intravenous; *LOC*, level of consciousness; *NPO*, nothing by mouth.

ringing in the ears (tinnitus), and tachycardia (rapid heartbeat) are all symptoms of overdose; seeking medical intervention as soon as possible is essential.

Treatment and nursing care. Vitamin K may be administered to control bleeding.

Lead Poisoning

Pathophysiology

Lead poisoning (**plumbism**) results when a child repeatedly ingests or absorbs substances containing lead. Canadians are exposed to low levels of lead through food, drinking water, air, dust, soil, and products. Although blood lead levels (BLLs) have declined by over 70% in Canada since 1978–1979, lead is still widely detected in the Canadian population (Health Canada, 2009). Canada has eliminated the use of lead in gasoline and household paint and banned the use of solder to seal food and beverage cans. Lead-based paint may still be present in older homes. For infants and children, ingestion of nonfood items containing lead (such as dust, lead-based paint, soil, and products), along with food and drinking water, are the greatest sources of exposure to lead in the environment (Health Canada, 2009). Lead poisoning is most common in children between 18 months and 3 years of age.

To lessen lead exposure, parents should be taught to do the following (Government of Canada, 2016):

- Always let tap water run until it is cold before using it for drinking, cooking, and especially for making baby formula. This is very important after water has been sitting in the pipes for long periods of time, like first thing in the morning.
- Don't use water from the hot water tap for cooking or drinking. Use cold water instead.
- Clean the house regularly to remove dust and particles that may contain lead. This is especially important for surfaces that young children might touch often.
- Do not keep food or drinks in lead crystal containers for any length of time. Do not serve pregnant women or children drinks in crystal glasses. Babies should never drink from lead crystal.
- Do not use glazed glass or ceramic dishes bought outside of Canada for serving food or drinks. They may contain higher levels of lead than are allowed in Canada.
- Remove any horizontal PVC (plastic) mini-blinds made in Asia or Mexico from the home if children in the home are 6 years of age or younger.
- Discourage children from putting things into their mouths unless they are intended to be mouthed (like food and pacifiers).
- If working in a smelter, refinery, or any other industry where you may be exposed to high levels of lead, shower and change clothing before going home. Have BLL checked regularly.
- Never burn waste oil, coloured newsprint, battery casings, or wood covered with lead paint in or near the home, because lead fumes may be released. Dispose of them through municipal hazardous waste program.
- If lead solder is used in a hobby (like making stained glass windows), use a good-quality breathing mask, keep surfaces clean, and keep children and pregnant women out of the area. Perform hand hygiene after handling lead solder.
- Avoid eating wild animals that have been shot with lead bullets. Use nonlead bullets and shots when hunting for food.

Lead is a neurotoxin and can have a lasting effect on the nervous system, especially the brain. Increased lead levels, even 5 mcg/dL, can cause cognitive and behavioural problems. Health Canada provides information to reduce exposure to lead.

Manifestations

The symptoms occur gradually and range from mild to severe. The lead settles in the soft tissues and bones and is excreted in the urine. In the beginning, signs such as weakness, weight loss, anorexia, pallor, irritability, vomiting, abdominal pain, and constipation may be seen. In later stages, signs of anemia and nervous system involvement, such as muscular incoordination, neuritis, convulsions, and encephalitis, are seen. Being exposed to lead during pregnancy can lead to problems in the newborn.

Treatment and nursing care

Blood and urine tests are performed to determine the amount of lead in the system. Lead is especially toxic to the synthesis of heme in the blood; heme is necessary for hemoglobin formation and for the functioning of renal tubules. BLL is the primary screening test. X-ray films of the bones may show further deposits of lead. The child's history may reveal *pica,* a condition in which the child has a distorted appetite and eats a variety of things that most persons consider unpalatable, such as sand, grass, wool, glass, plaster, coal, animal droppings, and paint from furniture.

Treatment is aimed at reducing the concentration of lead in the tissues and blood. Chelating agents combine with lead in the blood to safely excrete them from the body. Chelation treatment is administered if lead levels exceed 45 mcg/dL. Adequate hydration is essential when receiving chelation therapy. Medications used can include the following:

- Calcium disodium edetate (CaNa2EDTA or calcium EDTA) and succimer (Chemet, meso-2,3 dimercaptosuccinic acid [DMSA])
- British anti-Lewisite (BAL, dimercaprol, dimercaptopropanol) is used in conjunction with EDTA; contraindicated if peanut allergy or glucose 6-phosphate dehydrogenase (G6PD) deficiency

- D-penicillamine (Cuprimine) given orally, contraindicated in penicillin allergy and renal insufficiency, requires monitoring of renal function and blood counts

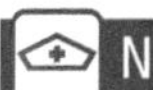 **Nursing Tip**

Treatment for lead poisoning prevents further harm but does not reverse any harm already done.

The prognosis depends on the extent of poisoning. All children with elevated lead blood levels must be followed to evaluate developmental and intellectual milestone achievement. Prevention of this condition is of foremost importance. Health Canada (2009) recommends lead-level screening in areas where there are unusual sources of lead exposure, such as a historic or ongoing problem of soil contamination from a smelter or where higher blood lead levels have been observed.

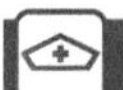 **Nursing Tip**

Documentation of adequate urine output is essential during chelation therapy.

FOREIGN BODY INGESTION

Approximately 80% of all foreign body ingestion occurs in children between 6 months and 3 years of age. Most foreign bodies ingested pass through the GI tract, but others require surgical removal. The high level of curiosity of the young child and the tendency to place objects in the mouth increase the susceptibility to accidental ingestion of a nonfood object. Unless the object is sharp or large, passage through the GI tract may be possible and can take up to 4 to 6 days. The child is cared for at home, and the nurse should emphasize the importance of cutting and examining each stool until the object is passed successfully.

The nurse should caution parents not to use laxatives and to maintain a normal diet to prevent the intestinal spasms that may precipitate an obstruction. Parents should be instructed to notify the health care provider if abdominal pain or vomiting occurs. Follow-up care and teaching concerning safety in the environment and the prevention of ingesting or inhaling foreign bodies are priority nursing responsibilities.

Get Ready for the Certification Examination!

Key Points

- Pyloric stenosis is caused by hypertrophy of the pyloric muscles and is manifested by projectile vomiting.
- Nursing care for the child with pyloric stenosis involves frequent assessment, careful feeding, positioning on the right side after feedings, and education and support of the parents.
- The first stool of the newborn should be documented to record the patency of the anus.
- The newborn should be closely observed for signs of tracheoesophageal fistula (TEF), which include coughing, choking, cyanosis, and apnea during feedings.
- Drooling in the newborn may be a sign of an obstructed esophagus or TEF.
- Currant jelly stools characterize intussusception.
- Postoperative nursing care of the infant with a cleft lip includes preventing the infant from crying, which could impair healing of the suture line.
- Large, bulky, frothy stools are characteristic of malabsorption syndromes.
- Celiac disease is caused by a genetic sensitivity to gluten in the diet.
- Hirschsprung disease occurs when there is an absence of ganglionic innervation of the muscle of a bowel segment.
- The treatment of gastroesophageal reflux includes thickened feedings, burping, and maintaining Fowler position.
- A diarrheal stool in an infant is manifested by a watery consistency and a greenish colour with the possible presence of mucus or blood. Frequency of bowel movements, by itself, is not an indication of diarrhea in infants.
- *C. difficile* is a health care–associated diarrhea that may occur with antimicrobial therapy.
- Hand hygiene with soap and water rather than an alcohol-based hand sanitizer is recommended when caring for patients with *C. difficile* diarrhea. Contact precautions are recommended, and the environment should be cleaned with a bleach disinfectant by housekeeping staff.
- Teaching parents basic hygienic practices, hand hygiene, and proper animal handling can prevent outbreaks of gastroenteritis.
- The functions of the gastrointestinal tract have a great influence on the fluid and electrolyte balance in infants and children.
- The higher daily exchange of water that occurs in infants leaves them less volume reserve when they are dehydrated.
- Oral rehydrating solutions are commercially prepared electrolyte solutions.
- Isotonic dehydration is the loss of equal amounts of water and electrolytes. Hypertonic dehydration is the loss of more water than electrolytes. Hypotonic dehydration is the loss of more electrolytes than water.
- Infants who receive nourishment by the IV route should be picked up and held and allowed to suck on a pacifier, if agreed to by the parents.
- An intake and output record includes accurate documentation of information concerning oral and parenteral intake and suction, wound drainage, sweating, vomiting, urine, and stool output.

- Kwashiorkor is a protein deficiency characterized by a depigmented (white) streak of hair.
- Disposable nipples, pacifiers, and bottles should be used for infants with thrush.
- Pinworm is diagnosed by a "Scotch tape test." Preventing the child from scratching the anal area is an essential part of breaking the cycle of worm reinfestation.
- The nurse should teach parents not to store poisonous substances in food containers.
- Prevention of accidental poisoning should be part of every plan for teaching parents.
- Lead poisoning (plumbism) can cause neurological damage.

Additional Learning Resources

evolve Go to your Evolve website (http://evolve.elsevier.com/Canada/Leifer) for the following learning resources:

- Answer Key for Critical Thinking Questions
- Answer Key for Textbook Review Questions
- Audio Glossary
- Fluids & Electrolytes tutorial
- Interactive Review Questions
- Skills Performance Checklists
- Video clips and more!

Online Resources

- AboutFace—A resource for people with facial differences: https://www.aboutface.ca/
- Canadian Association of Poison Control Centres: http://www.capcc.ca/en
- Canadian Celiac Association: http://www.celiac.ca
- Health Canada, *What Is Lead?:* https://www.canada.ca/en/health-canada/services/environmental-workplace-health/environmental-contaminants/lead.html

Review Questions

1. What does the pathological disturbance of pyloric stenosis result from?
   a. Edema of the pyloric muscle
   b. Ischemia of the pyloric muscle
   c. Hypertrophy of the pyloric muscle
   d. Neoplastic obstruction
2. Which menu selections are best for a child diagnosed with celiac disease?
   a. Pizza and chocolate cake
   b. Spaghetti and blueberry muffin
   c. Chicken sandwich on whole-wheat bread
   d. Corn tortilla and fresh fruit
3. A nurse is monitoring a 2-year-old child for signs of dehydration. Which of the following techniques of monitoring body temperature is appropriate? *(Select all that apply.)*
   a. Axillary
   b. Rectal
   c. Tympanic
   d. Temporal artery
   e. Stroking the forehead
4. How are pinworms diagnosed?
   a. Seeing the worm in the stool
   b. A blood antigen level
   c. A "Scotch tape test" in the early morning
   d. A stool laboratory examination obtained at the hour of sleep
5. A nurse would teach which priority topic to parents of a child who ingested a foreign body?
   a. Encouraging the use of mild laxatives every night
   b. Slicing each stool passed to observe for the foreign body
   c. Encouraging a daily enema until the foreign body is passed
   d. Keeping the child NPO until the foreign body is passed
6. A nurse would include which of the following when providing postoperative care to an infant who has had a cheiloplasty? *(Select all that apply.)*
   a. Feed formula using a soft nipple.
   b. Apply elbow immobilizers.
   c. Provide pain relief measures.
   d. Position infant on its abdomen.

REFERENCES

Aiken, J., & Oldham, K. (2016). Acute appendicitis. In R. M. Kliegman, B. F. Stanton, J. W. St. Geme, et al. (Eds.), *Nelson textbook of pediatrics* (20th ed.). Philadelphia: Saunders.

Blackburn, S. (2013). *Maternal, fetal, and neonatal physiology: A clinical perspective* (4th ed.). St. Louis: Saunders.

Branski, D., Troncone, R., & Fasano, A. (2016). Celiac disease. In R. M. Kliegman, B. F. Stanton, J. W. St. Geme, et al. (Eds.), *Nelson textbook of pediatrics* (20th ed.). Philadelphia: Saunders.

Breen-Reid, K. M. (2017). The infant and family. In S. Perry, M. Hockenberry, D. Lowdermilk, et al. (Eds.), *Maternal child nursing care in Canada* (2nd ed.). Toronto, ON: Elsevier.

Cole, S. Z., & Lanham, J. S. (2011). Failure to thrive: An update. *American Family Physician, 83*(7), 829–834.

Ericson, J., Smith, P. B., & Benjamin, D. (2016). Infections in immunocompetent children and adolescents. In R. M. Kliegman, B. F. Stanton, J. W. St. Geme, et al. (Eds.), *Nelson textbook of pediatrics* (20th ed.). Philadelphia: Saunders.

Fiorino, K., & Liacouras, C. (2016). Congenital aganglionic megacolon (Hirschsprung disease). In R. M. Kliegman, B. F. Stanton, J. W. St. Geme, et al. (Eds.), *Nelson textbook of pediatrics* (20th ed.). Philadelphia: Saunders.

Godel, J. C., & Canadian Paediatric Society (CPS), First Nations, Inuit and Métis Health Committee. (2007). Vitamin D supplementation: Recommendations for Canadian mothers and infants. *Paediatrics & Child Health, 12*(7), 583–589. Reaffirmed 2017. Retrieved from: http://www.cps.ca/documents/position/vitamin-d.

Government of Canada. (2013). *Congenital anomalies in Canada 2013—A perinatal health report*. Retrieved from: http://publications.gc.ca/site/eng/443924/publication.html.

Government of Canada. (2016). *Reduce your exposure to lead*. Retrieved from: https://www.canada.ca/en/health-canada/services/home-garden-safety/reduce-your-exposure-lead.html.

Government of Canada. (2017). *Canadian Food Inspection Agency (CFIA): Compliance and enforcement of gluten-free claims*. Retrieved from: http://www.inspection.gc.ca/food/labelling/food-labelling-for-industry/allergens-and-gluten/gluten-free-claims/eng/1340194596012/1340194681961.

Health Canada. (2009). *Lead information package—Some commonly asked questions about lead and human health*. Retrieved from: https://www.canada.ca/en/health-canada/services/environmental-workplace-health/environmental-contaminants/lead/lead-information-package-some-commonly-asked-questions-about-lead-human-health.html#a51.

Health Canada. (2019). *Vitamin D and calcium: Updated dietary reference intakes*. Retrieved from: http://www.hc-sc.gc.ca/fn-an/nutrition/vitamin/vita-d-eng.php#a15.

Hogarth, A. (2017). Gastrointestinal dysfunction. In S. Perry, M. Hockenberry, D. Lowdermilk, et al. (Eds.), *Maternal child nursing care in Canada* (2nd ed.). Toronto, ON: Elsevier.

Hunter, A. K., & Liacouras, C. A. (2016). Hypertrophic pyloric stenosis. In R. M. Kliegman, B. F. Stanton, J. W. St. Geme, et al. (Eds.), *Nelson textbook of pediatrics* (20th ed.). Philadelphia: Saunders.

Hyams, J. S., Di Lorenzo, C., Saps, M., et al. (2016). Childhood functional gastrointestinal disorders: Child/adolescent. *Gastroenterology, 150*, 1456–1468.

Kennedy, M., & Liacouras, C. A. (2016). Intussusception. In R. M. Kliegman, B. F. Stanton, J. W. St. Geme, et al. (Eds.), *Nelson textbook of pediatrics* (20th ed.). Philadelphia: Saunders.

Khan, S., & Orenstein, S. R. (2016a). Esophageal atresia and tracheoesophageal fistula. In R. M. Kliegman, B. F. Stanton, J. W. St. Geme, et al. (Eds.), *Nelson textbook of pediatrics* (20th ed.). Philadelphia: Saunders.

Khan, S., & Orensetin, S. R. (2016b). Gastroesophageal reflux disease. In R. M. Kliegman, B. F. Stanton, J. W. St. Geme, et al. (Eds.), *Nelson textbook of pediatrics* (20th ed.). Philadelphia: Saunders.

Kostic, M. (2016). Poisoning. In R. M. Kliegman, B. F. Stanton, J. W. St. Geme, et al. (Eds.), *Nelson textbook of pediatrics* (20th ed.). Philadelphia: Saunders.

Leung, A., Prince, T., & Canadian Paediatric Society (CPS), Nutrition and Gastroenterology Committee. (2006). Oral rehydration therapy and early refeeding in the management of childhood gastroenteritis. *Journal of Paediatric and Child Health, 11*(8), 529. Reaffirmed 2016.

Marchand, V., & Canadian Paediatric Society (CPS), Nutrition and Gastroenterology Committee. (2012). Using probiotics in the paediatric population. *Paediatrics & Child Health, 17*(10), 575. Reaffirmed 2019. Retrieved from: http://www.cps.ca/en/documents/position/probiotics-in-the-paediatric-population.

McCabe, M. A., Toughill, E. H., Parkhill, A. M., et al. (2012). Celiac disease: A medical puzzle. *American Journal of Nursing, 112*(19), 34–44.

Parachute (n.d.). *Poison prevention*. Retrieved from: http://www.parachutecanada.org/policy/item/261

Public Health Agency of Canada. (2013). *The Chief Public Officer's report on the state of public health in Canada 2013—Healthcare-associated infections—Due diligence*. Retrieved from: https://www.canada.ca/en/public-health/corporate/publications/chief-public-health-officer-reports-state-public-health-canada/chief-public-health-officer-report-on-state-public-health-canada-2013-infectious-disease-never-ending-threat/healthcare-associated-infections-due-diligence.html.

Reilly, S., Reid, J., Skeat, J., et al. (2013). ABM clinical protocol #18: Guidelines for breastfeeding infants with cleft lip, cleft palate, or cleft lip and palate. *Breastfeeding Medicine, 8*(4), 349–353. https://doi.org/10.1089/bfm.2013.9988.

Rowan-Legg, A., & Canadian Paediatric Society (CPS), Community Paediatrics Committee. (2011). Managing functional constipation in children. *Paediatrics & Child Health, 6*(10), 661–665. Reaffirmed 2018. Retrieved from: http://www.cps.ca/en/documents/position/functional-constipation.

The Hospital for Sick Children (SickKids). (n.d.). *Calculating maintenance fluid rates*. Retrieved from: http://www.sickkids.ca/Nursing/Education-and-learning/Nursing-Student-Orientation/module-two-clinical-care/paediatric-iv-therapy/Calculating-Maintenance-Fluid-Rates/index.html

Tinanoff, N. (2016). Cleft lip and palate. In R. M. Kliegman, B. F. Stanton, J. W. St. Geme, et al. (Eds.), *Nelson textbook of pediatrics* (20th ed.). Philadelphia: Saunders.

The Child With a Genitourinary Condition

29

Andrea Logan

http://evolve.elsevier.com/Canada/Leifer

Objectives

1. Define each key term listed.
2. Name the functional unit of the kidney.
3. Recognize normal urine output for pediatric patients of various ages.
4. Describe four urological diagnostic procedures.
5. Recognize urinary tract anomalies in infants.
6. Discuss the cause and prevention of urinary tract infections in children.
7. Discuss the skin care pertinent to the child with nephrosis.
8. Explain any alterations in diet applicable to the child with nephrosis.
9. Differentiate between nephrosis and acute glomerulonephritis.
10. Outline the nursing care for a child who is diagnosed with having Wilms tumour.
11. Discuss the impact of undescended testes on fertility.
12. Discuss the impact of genitourinary surgery on the growth and development of children at various ages.

Key Terms

chordee (KŎR-dē)
cryptorchidism (krĭp-TŎR-kĭ-dĭz-ŭm)
cystometrogram (sĭs-tō-MĔT-rō-grăm)
dysuria (dĭs-YŪ-rē-ă)
enuresis (ĕn-yū-RĒ-sĭs)
epispadias (ĕp-ĭ-SPĀ-dē-ŭs)
frequency
glomeruli (glō-MĔR-yū-lī)
hydrocele (HĪ-drō-sēl)
hydronephrosis (hī-drō-nĕ-FRŌ-sĭs)
hyperkalemia (hī-pŭr-kă-LĒ-mē-ă)
hypoalbuminemia (hī-pō-ăl-byū-mĭn-Ē-mē-ă)
hypospadias (hī-pō-SPĀ-dē-ŭs)
micturition (mĭk-tū-RĬSH-ŭn)
nephron (NĔF-rŏn)
nocturia (nŏk-TŪ-rē-ă)
oliguria (ŏl-ĭ-GŪ-rē-ă)
orchiopexy (ŏr-kē-ō-PĔK-sē)
paraphimosis (păr-ă-fī-MŌ-sĭs)
phimosis (fī-MŌ-sĭs)
polyuria (pŏl-ē-YŪ-rē-ă)
pyelonephritis (pī-ĕ-lō-nĕ-FRĪ-tĭs)
testicular torsion (tĕs-TĬK-yū-lăr TŎR-shŭn)
ureteritis (yū-rē-tŭr-Ī-tĭs)
urethritis (yū-rĕ-THRĪ-tĭs)
urgency
vesicoureteral reflux (vĕs-ĭ-kō-yū-RĒ-tŭr-ăl RĒ-flŭks)
Wilms tumour

DEVELOPMENT OF THE URINARY TRACT

Soon after implantation, the embryonic mass differentiates into three distinct layers of cells: the *ectoderm, mesoderm,* and *endoderm.* The urinary and reproductive organs originate from the mesoderm. At approximately the third month of gestation the fetal kidney begins to secrete urine. The amount gradually increases as the fetus matures and comprises a portion of the amniotic fluid volume. An absence or small amount of amniotic fluid (oligohydramnios) may indicate genitourinary difficulties.

The urinary system consists of two kidneys, two ureters, the urinary bladder, and the urethra. Fig. 29.1 depicts these structures and illustrates how they differ in the developing child and in the adult. The function of the kidneys is to rid the body of waste products and to maintain body fluid homeostasis (Fig. 29.2). The kidneys also produce substances that stimulate red blood cell formation in the bone marrow (e.g., erythropoietin-stimulating factor [ESF]), as well as renin, which regulates blood pressure. Microscopically, the functional unit of the kidneys is the **nephron**. Each kidney contains more than one million nephrons. Although the newborn's kidneys are immature, they function quite effectively. Nevertheless, the functional limitations must be considered carefully when the newborn is premature or ill. This applies especially to the administration of medications, breastmilk or formula, and parenteral fluids. The expected urine output for children is approximately 1 to 2 mL/kg/hr. For older children 30 mL/hr is the minimum normal output. This volume may vary slightly depending on the child's condition.

The bladder capacity increases from 50 mL at birth to approximately 700 mL in adulthood.

There is an unexplained relationship between low-set ears in the newborn and urinary tract anomalies.

URINARY SYSTEM

- Fluid is of greater importance to the body chemistry of infants and small children, because it constitutes a larger fraction of their total body weight.
- Glomerular filtration and absorption are relatively low until 1 to 2 years of age. Infants are more prone to fluid volume excess and dehydration.
- Kidneys are more susceptible to trauma in children, because they usually do not have as much fat padding.
- Kidney function is immature until after 2 years of age.

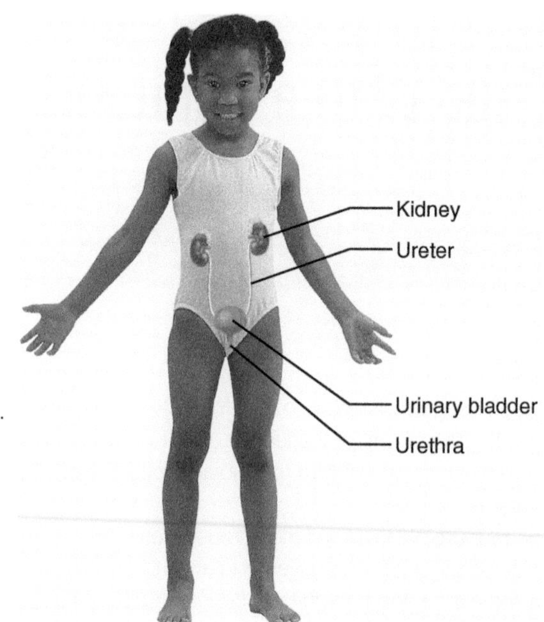

Fig. 29.1 Summary of some urinary system differences between the child and the adult. The urinary system is the main excretory system. The kidneys remove wastes and excess materials from the blood and produce urine. This system helps to regulate blood chemistry. (Art overlay courtesy Observatory Group, Cincinnati, Ohio.)

System	Organ	Excretion
Urinary	Kidney	Nitrogen compounds Toxins Water Electrolytes
Integumentary	Skin—sweat glands	Nitrogen compounds Water Electrolytes
Respiratory	Lung	Carbon dioxide Water
Digestive	Intestine	Digestive wastes Bile pigments Salts of heavy metals

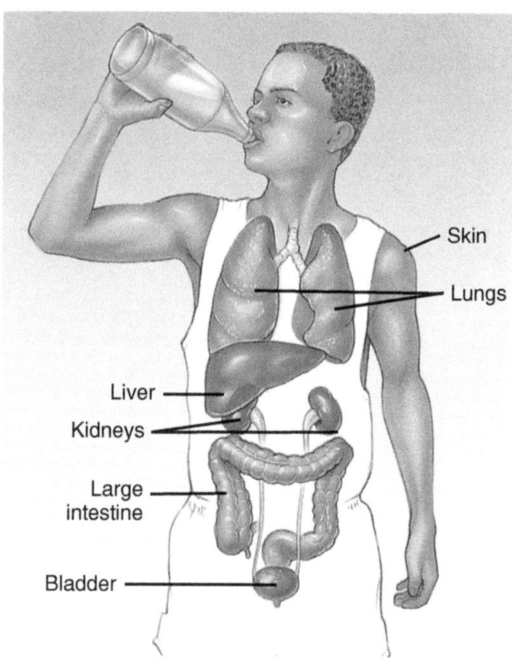

Fig. 29.2 The urinary system's chief function is to regulate the volume and composition of body fluids and to excrete unwanted materials, but it is not the only system in the body that is able to excrete unneeded substances. The table in this figure compares the excretory functions of several systems. Although all of these systems contribute to the body's effort to remove wastes, only the urinary system can finely adjust the water and electrolyte balance to the degree required for normal homeostasis of body fluids. (From Thibodeau, G. A., & Patton, K. T. [2016]. *Anatomy & physiology* [9th ed.]. St. Louis: Mosby.)

Because the kidney and the ear develop at about the same time in fetal life, an abnormality of the ear can be a signal that an abnormality of the urinary tract may also be present. Therefore, low-set ears may be a "red flag" to indicate that further assessment would be warranted. When assessing the newborn, an imaginary line should be drawn between the outer canthus of the eye and the ear. The line should cross the tip of the auricle. If the tip of the auricle falls below this line, the assessment should be recorded and reported (see Fig. 11.9).

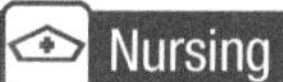

Nursing Tip

Most newborns urinate within the first 24 hours of life. Documenting and reporting the presence or absence of urination is very important to future care.

DEVELOPMENT OF THE REPRODUCTIVE SYSTEMS

The reproductive system provides for continuance of the species. Members of each gender are equipped with gonads (which provide reproductive cells) and a set of accessory organs. The gonads (ovaries in the female and testes in the male) produce sex cells and hormones that affect the reproductive organs and other body systems. Fig. 29.3 shows the female and male reproductive systems and lists some of the differences in these systems between children and adults.

Sex is genetically determined at the time of fertilization. The presence of a Y chromosome is essential for the development of the testes and their hormones. Sex differentiation in the embryo occurs early. The organs specific to the male or female child develop. Before this, the embryo has neither male nor female characteristics. The development of the ovaries occurs later than that of the testes. By the twelfth week the external genitalia of the fetus are often recognizably male or female.

Several tests are helpful in diagnosing conditions of the reproductive tract. These include a Papanicolaou (Pap) smear, serological blood tests, cultures, ultrasound procedures, pregnancy tests, and routine blood and urine tests.

Menstrual disorders and premenstrual syndrome are discussed in Chapter 2. Sexually transmitted infections are discussed in Chapters 2 and 32.

ASSESSMENT OF URINARY TRACT FUNCTION

Urological diagnostic procedures include urinalysis, ultrasonography, intravenous (IV) pyelogram, and computed tomography (CT) scan of the kidneys. Renal biopsy is used to diagnose the extent of kidney disease. A *uroflow* is an assessment procedure used to determine the rate of urine flow. The child voids into a receptacle, and a uroflowmeter graphs the volume and pressure. This is useful in diagnosing stricture or scarring. Cytoscopy is useful for investigating congenital abnormalities or acquired lesions in the bladder and lower urinary tract. Radiographic examination of the bladder and urethra before and during micturition (voiding) is called *voiding cystourethrography.* The cystometrogram and the urethral pressure profile are used to assess bladder capacity and function. Both tests require catheterization and infusion of sterile water. Common laboratory tests used in the assessment of urinary tract function are reviewed in Table 29.1.

Terms commonly used to describe urinary dysfunction include the following:

- Dysuria: difficulty in urination
- Frequency: abnormal number of voids in a short period
- Urgency: strong urges to void, often despite inability to do so
- Nocturia: awakening during the night to void
- Enuresis: uncontrolled voiding after bladder control has been established
- Polyuria: increased urine output (>3 mL/kg/hr)
- Oliguria: decreased urine output (<1 mL/kg/hr)

URINARY TRACT DYSFUNCTION

Phimosis

Pathophysiology

Phimosis is defined as a scarring and thickening of the foreskin that prevents retraction back over the glans (Fig. 29.4). Phimosis may occur secondary to recurrent

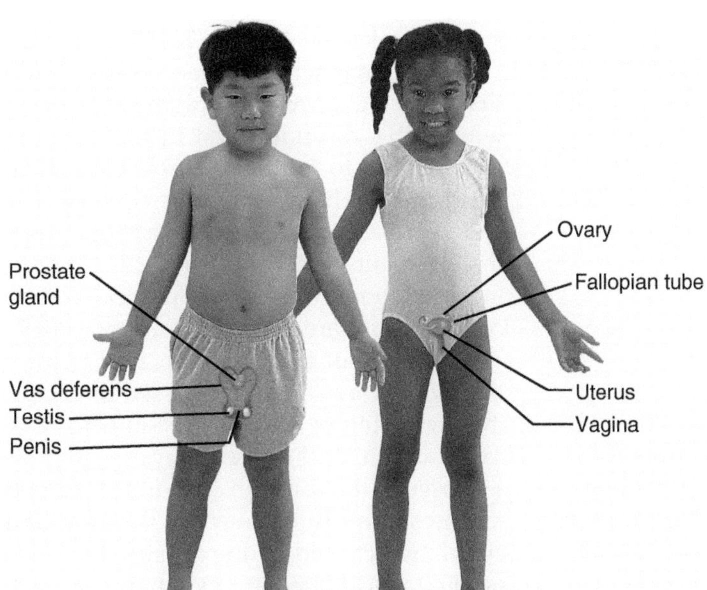

REPRODUCTIVE SYSTEM

- The genitals in preterm females may appear swollen. The labia minora may protrude beyond the labia majora.
- The testicles may appear large at birth in proportion to the size of the infant. They may fail to move into the scrotum, causing a condition termed *undescended testes.*
- The foreskin may be tight at birth, causing phimosis.
- The sex organs do not mature until the onset of puberty.
- Secondary sex characteristics occur with the onset of puberty.

Fig. 29.3 Summary of some reproductive system differences between the child and the adult male and female. Each reproductive system consists of gonads and associated structures. The reproductive system maintains sexual characteristics and provides for perpetuation of the species. (Art overlay courtesy Observatory Group, Cincinnati, Ohio.)

Table 29.1 **Common Laboratory Tests for Urinary Tract Function**

TEST	NORMAL LEVELS*	SIGNIFICANCE OF DEVIATION
Blood		
Blood urea nitrogen (BUN)	<1 year: 2.9–10.0 mmol/L 1 year: 1.8–5.4 mmol/L ≥2 years: 2.9–7.1 mmol/L	High BUN level indicates renal disease, dehydration, need for steroid therapy
Uric acid	Female: 120–360 mmol/L Male <14 years: 120–360 mmol/L Male ≥14 years: 180–420 mmol/L	Renal disease
Creatinine	≤6 days: 19–99 mcmol/L 7–60 days: 10–56 mcmol/L 2 month–5 years: <36 mcmol/L 6–9 years: <53 mcmol/L 10–3 years: <79 mcmol/L ≥14 years: <98 mcmol/L	Severe renal disease
Urine (ideally first morning void)		
Blood	Negative or "trace nonhemolyzed"	Trauma, infection, stones
Casts	Negative/Occasional (breakdown of types of casts beyond this chapter)	Glomerular disease, pyelonephritis
Leukocyte esterase	Negative	Infection
Nitrites	Negative	Negative result does not rule out infection
Ketones	Negative or trace	Stress; diabetes mellitus; metabolic disorders
Glucose	Negative	Diabetes mellitus
Protein	≤ Trace	Glomerular kidney disease
pH	5–9	Potassium deficiency, electrolyte imbalance
Specific gravity	1.010–1.025	Dehydration Overhydration, renal disease, pituitary malfunction

HPF, High-powered field.
White blood cells (WBCs): >2/HPF may signify infection or inflammation. Red blood cells (RBCs): >5/HPF is abnormal.
*Values for different age groups are indicated only when relevant.
From Dipchand, A. I., Friedman, J. N., Gupta, S., Bismilla, Z., & Lam, C. (2010). *The Hospital for Sick Children handbook of pediatrics* (11th ed.). Toronto, ON: Elsevier.

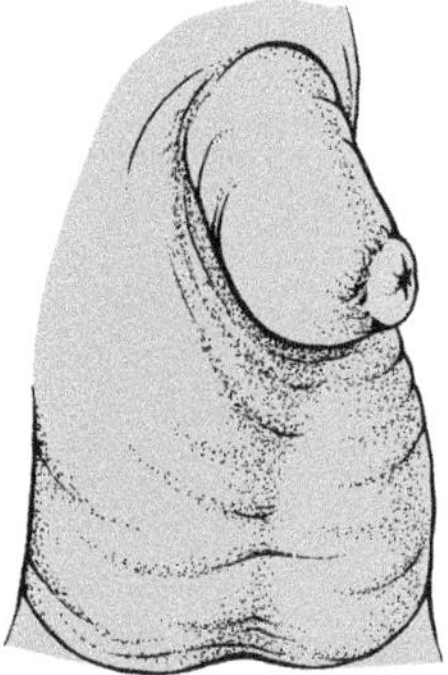

Fig. 29.4 Phimosis. The foreskin is advanced and fixed; it cannot be retracted over the glans.

infections, inflammation, or lichen sclerosis. Phimosis needs to be differentiated from the normal nonretractile foreskin (Sorokan, Finlay, Jefferies, et al., 2015/2018). This is normal in newborns and usually disappears by 3 years of age. In some children, this narrowing may obstruct the stream of urine, causing dribbling, irritation, or ballooning of the foreskin while urinating. Topical steroids or circumcision can correct the condition.

Treatment and nursing care

First-line treatment for phimosis is the use of topical steroids to the foreskin, which works in up to 80% of cases, avoiding circumcision. The use of topical steroids leads to thinning of the tissue and releases adhesions (Sorokan et al., 2015/2018).

When circumcision is necessary, careful explanations and reassurance should be provided to the child who is able to understand them. The nurse needs to be sensitive to the child's embarrassment and fear. Postoperatively, the penis is covered with a petroleum gauze. Circumcision is painful, thus proper pain management must be considered. Complications can include minor bleeding and local infection; severe complications are rare (Sorokan et al., 2015/2018).

Cleansing of the uncircumcised penis and retraction of the foreskin are discussed in Chapter 11. Forcible retraction of a tight foreskin is to be avoided because it can lead to paraphimosis (Fig. 29.5). When this occurs, the foreskin cannot be returned to its normal position. There may be swelling and impaired circulation caused by the constriction. This condition necessitates immediate evaluation by a health care provider.

Hypospadias and Epispadias

Pathophysiology

Hypospadias is a congenital defect in which the urinary meatus is located not at the end of the penis but on the

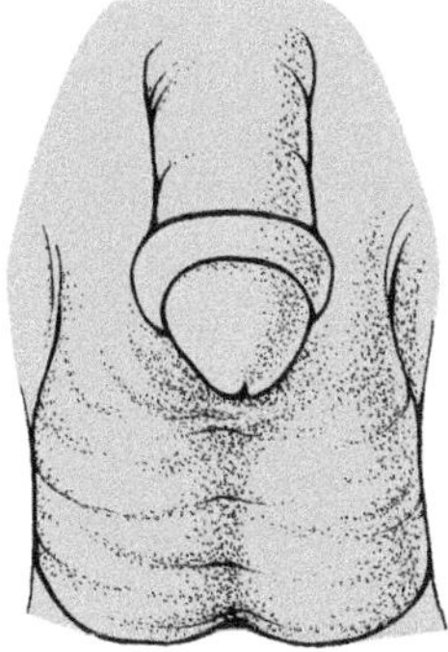

Fig. 29.5 Paraphimosis. The foreskin is retracted and fixed; it cannot be returned to its original position. Constriction impedes circulation.

lower shaft. In mild cases, it lies just below the tip of the penis, but it may be found at the midshaft or near the penile–scrotal junction (Fig. 29.6, *B*). With **epispadias**, the opening of the urinary meatus is on the upper surface of the penis (Fig. 29.6, *A*). Unlike epispadias, hypospadias is fairly common, occurring in 1 out of 200 newborn boys (Keays & Dave, 2017). Hypospadias may be accompanied by **chordee**, a downward curvature of the penis caused by a fibrotic band of tissue (Fig. 29.6, *C*).

Treatment and nursing care

The nurse may discover hypospadias or epispadias during the newborn assessment; however, mild cases may not be noticed immediately. In mild cases, surgery may not be required for either condition unless the location and extent of the defect are such that the child will not be able to stand to void or the defect would cause psychological problems or difficulties in future sexual relations.

Treatment consists of surgical repair and is usually performed between 6 and 18 months of age, before a child can stand to urinate. Most techniques can be performed during same-day surgery. Circumcision at birth is to be avoided in these children, because the foreskin may be useful in the repair.

Postoperatively, the infant may be double diapered, with the inner diaper collecting stool and the outer diaper collecting urine to protect the operative site. The parents should be instructed to avoid holding the infant straddled on their hip to avoid pressure on the operative site. Pain should be treated with the appropriate medication.

Exstrophy of the Bladder

Pathophysiology

In exstrophy of the bladder, the lower portion of the abdominal wall and the anterior wall of the bladder are missing. As a result, the bladder lies open and exposed on the abdomen. Exstrophy is caused by a failure of the midline to close during embryonic development. Other congenital anomalies may also be present. This anomaly occurs in 1 out of 35 000 to 40 000 live births and is twice as common in boys as in girls (Elder, 2016a).

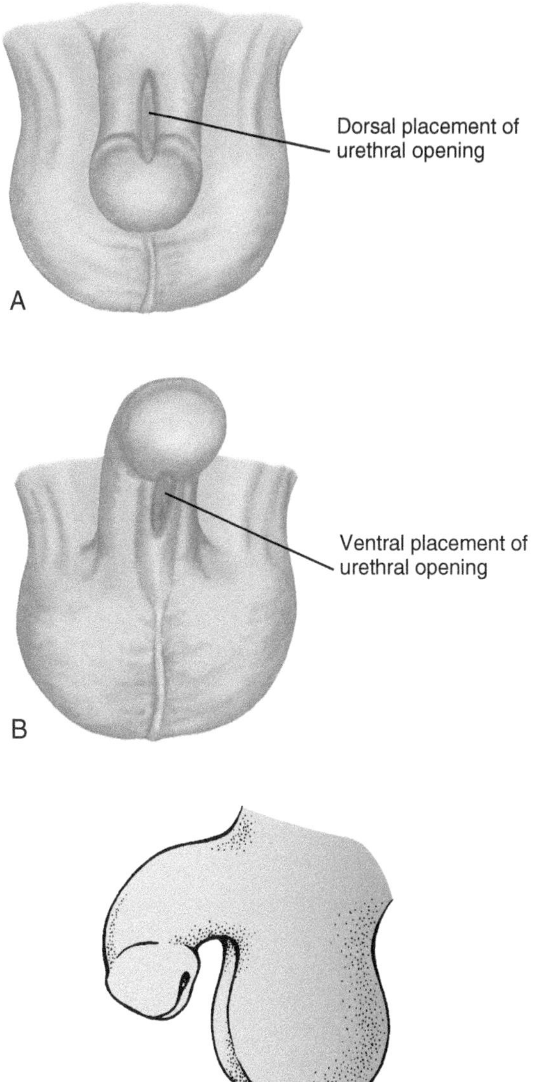

Fig. 29.6 **A,** Epispadias. **B,** Hypospadias. **C,** Chordee. (From James, S. R., Nelson, K. A., Murray, S. S., & Ashwill, J. W. [2013]. *Nursing care of children: Principles and practice* [4th ed.]. St. Louis: Saunders.)

Manifestations

This disorder is noticeable by fetal ultrasound. The defect may range from a small cutaneous fistula in the abdominal wall to complete exstrophy (the turning inside out of an organ). Urine leaks continually from the bladder. The skin around the bladder becomes excoriated.

Treatment and nursing care

The bladder is covered with a plastic shield or appropriate dressing to protect its mucosa but still to allow for urinary drainage. This also protects the bladder from irritation by bedclothes or diapers. Ointment is applied to protect the skin. Diapers are generally placed under rather than around the infant. The infant is positioned on their back or side so that urine drains freely. Antibiotics are given to prevent infection.

Ideally, surgical closure is performed during the first 48 hours of life. Parents may require psychological support and guidance in caring for the infant. Support and health teaching are a necessity as the infant will require continued follow-up visits, diagnostic screening, and interventions to support potential long-term effects and to prevent long-term complications such as continence and libido-related issues (Alsowayan, Capolicchio, Jednak, et al., 2016).

Obstructive Uropathy

Pathophysiology

Many conditions, such as calculi (stones), tumours, strictures, and scarring, may cause an obstruction of the normal flow of urine. These conditions may be congenital or acquired, and blockage may be either partial or complete. One or both kidneys may be affected. The pathological changes depend on the nature and location of the problem. **Hydronephrosis** (*hydro,* "water," and *nephro,* "kidney") is the distention of the renal pelvis as a result of an obstruction. The pelvis of the kidney becomes enlarged, and cysts form. This may eventually damage renal nephrons, resulting in deterioration of the kidneys. *Polycystic kidney* refers to a condition in which large, fluid-filled cysts form in place of healthy kidney tissue in the fetus. This is inherited as an autosomal recessive trait.

Kidney damage can result in an inability of the kidney to concentrate urine, resulting in metabolic acidosis. Urine that is not excreted promptly can promote the growth of organisms that cause urinary tract infection.

Treatment and nursing care

Urinary diversion is necessary in certain conditions and may be accomplished through several procedures (Table 29.2). This type of surgery can be a source of great apprehension for parents. The physical care of the child with a urinary stoma (artificially created opening or passage) presents hygiene and skin concerns. Frequent trips to the health care provider may add to the strain of everyday life.

Stress from the urinary diversion is age related. The toddler may be unable to attain toilet independence. The school-age child may feel different from others and may have a distorted body image. The adolescent may have lowered self-esteem and be concerned about sexuality. Parents with affected newborns may grieve the loss of a perfect child and experience concerns about the length and quality of the infant's life.

The nurse needs to anticipate the impact of this type of diagnosis and incorporate suitable psychological interventions into daily care. Providing emotional support and teaching parents how to prevent infection are priorities of care.

Assessing for a distended bladder. To assess for a distended bladder, the nurse gently palpates below the umbilicus, moving toward the symphysis pubis. The normal bladder is not palpable because it lies behind the symphysis pubis.

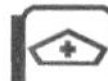 **Nursing Tip**

The bladder capacity of a child can be approximated by the following formula:

Age in years × 30 mL + 60 mL = Millilitres of bladder volume or capacity.

Acute Urinary Tract Infection

Pathophysiology

In the newborn period, uncircumcised boys have a slightly higher incidence of urinary tract infections (UTIs), although the risk of UTI declines rapidly in males after the first few months of life to an incidence of 1 in 1 000 by 1 year of age (Sorokan et al., 2015/2018). It is important to teach parents proper care of the circumcised and uncircumcised penis and the principles of perineal care (see Chapter 11).

Table 29.2 Surgical Procedures Used in Urinary Diversion

PROCEDURE	DEFINITION
Ureterostomy	Ureters are surgically diverted to an opening (stoma) on outside abdominal wall. This allows urine to drain into a collection device.
Ileal or colon conduit (artificial channel)	Conduit diverts urine at the ureter, bypassing the bladder and urethra; ureters are removed from the bladder and attached to the ileum or colon, which then acts as bladder; there is no voluntary control of voiding. Patient has a stoma, which is larger and not as prone to stenosis as a ureterostomy; child wears an ileostomy appliance. **Note:** Urine from conduit may appear cloudy from secretions of bowel conduit; this is not a sign of urinary tract infection.
Nephrostomy	Tube passes through flank into pelvis of kidney; this allows urine to be drained from the pelvis (bypassing ureter, bladder, and urethra; drains into ostomy bag).
Suprapubic tube placement	A suprapubic tube is placed above the symphysis pubis into the bladder to provide urinary drainage.
Vesicostomy	A surgical opening is made into the bladder between the umbilicus and pubis; the bladder wall is brought to surface of abdomen.

Several factors account for the preponderance of UTIs in girls. In girls, the incidence of UTIs is highest in the infant/toddler years and with toilet learning. The short urethra in girls and the urinary meatus being close to the rectum increase the risk for contamination by fecal bacteria. The wearing of close-fitting nylon underwear, the use of bubble baths, the retention of urine, and vaginitis also contribute to development of UTIs. Sexual abuse should be considered in young girls with repeated infections. Of all infections, 75 to 90% are caused by *Escherichia coli*, followed by *Klebsiella* sp. and *Proteus* sp. (Elder, 2016c). The following terms are used to describe the location and nature of urinary tract disturbances:

- **Urethritis**: infection of the urethra
- *Cystitis:* inflammation of the bladder
- *Bacteriuria:* bacteria in the urine
- **Pyelonephritis**: infection of the kidney and the renal pelvis
- **Ureteritis**: infection of the ureters
- **Vesicoureteral reflux**: backward flow of urine into the ureters

Certain chemical and physical factors are important to note in relation to UTIs. Normal urine is acidic. Alkaline urine favours the growth of pathogens. Urine that remains in the bladder for a prolonged period of time serves as an excellent medium for bacterial growth.

Vesicoureteral reflux. *Vesicoureteral reflux (VUR)* refers to the abnormal retrograde flow of urine from the bladder to the ureters during a void (see Fig. 29.7). After the void, urine flows back into the bladder, where urinary stasis occurs that allows growth of bacteria, leading to UTI. The bacteria have access to the kidneys during subsequent reflux; pyelonephritis and renal scarring can result.

Manifestations and diagnosis

The signs and symptoms of UTI are age dependent. The infant may be admitted with only a high fever or accompanying vomiting and chills. A urine specimen for culture is obtained before antibiotics are administered. Specimens must be processed promptly or refrigerated to prevent contamination. Urine specimens should not be collected from the diaper because the chemicals and gels contained in the diaper fabric may alter the results of some tests. Urine specimens in infants must be obtained via urinary catheterization to obtain the most accurate results.

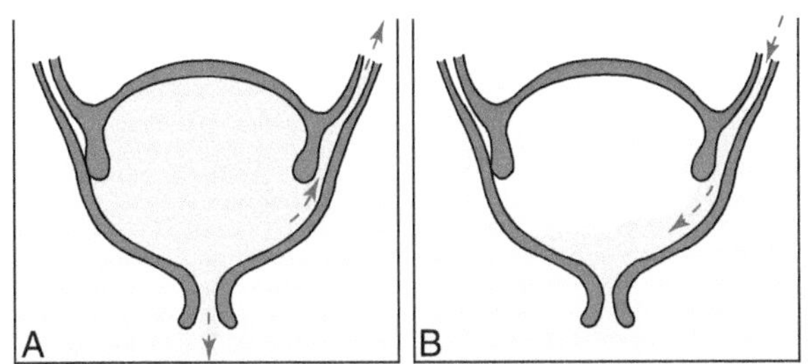

Fig. 29.7 Vesicoureteral reflux. **A,** Congenital abnormalities of the junction between the bladder and the ureters can force urine to flow backward into the ureters during voiding. **B,** After voiding, residual urine from the ureter remains in the bladder.

Obtaining urine samples from children who are not toilet independent requires urethral catheterization or, less often, suprapubic aspiration (SPA). In children who are toilet-independent, a midstream urine specimen is obtained after cleansing the urethral meatus. A renal/bladder ultrasound (RBUS) is recommended, and a voiding cystourethrogram (VCUG) may be ordered if the ultrasound is abnormal, showing indications of selected renal abnormalities or obstruction or high-grade VUR (Robinson, Finlay, Lang, et al., 2014/2017).

Treatment and nursing care

Infants with UTIs who are less than 2 to 3 months of age, toxic-looking children, or children who have complicated UTIs are hospitalized, observed, and treated with IV antibiotics (Robinson et al., 2014/2017). Most infants and children are now treated as outpatients with oral antibiotics, assuming they are likely to receive and tolerate every dose (Robinson et al., 2014/2017). If infants are sent home on oral antibiotics, close follow-up and health teaching are required. Children under 2 years of age should have a RBUS after their first febrile UTI to identify significant renal abnormalities or severe VUR (Robinson et al., 2014/2017). Infants with low-grade VUR usually outgrow this spontaneously, but they are monitored regularly as outpatients. Severe VUR can require an endoscopic procedure to prevent retrograde flow of urine. Open surgical interventions are reserved mostly for significant anatomical defects.

Acute cystitis is treated promptly to prevent development of pyelonephritis and kidney damage. Until the specific organism causing the infection is identified, broad-spectrum antibiotics are initially prescribed. Prophylactic medication is no longer routine but may be prescribed in certain circumstances with a nephrology consultation for infants under 1 year of age or if the infant has repeated UTIs to prevent kidney scarring (Wu, Huang, Fu, et al., 2016).

Methods of preventing UTIs need to be taught to caregivers and to the patient, if age appropriate. The nurse should stress the need for proper amounts of fluid intake to maintain sterility and flushing of the bladder, and encourage regular voiding regimes throughout the day. Nursing Care Plan 29.1 presents the nursing considerations appropriate for these patients. The prognosis is excellent with prompt treatment. Monitoring vital signs, including blood pressure, and providing anticipatory guidance help to decrease the stress of the children and parents.

Nursing Care Plan 29.1 The Child With a Urinary Tract Infection

Patient Data

A school-age girl is brought to the clinic stating she feels burning on urination. Her mother states the child fears going to the bathroom because "it will hurt."

Selected Nursing Diagnosis Abnormal urinary elimination as a result of dysuria

Goals	Nursing Interventions	Rationales
Child will state no symptoms of frequency, urgency, or pain on urination. Child will not strain or fret before voiding.	Administer antibiotics as prescribed.	Antibiotics are chosen according to urine culture and sensitivity and local susceptibility patterns; phenazopyridine may be given to decrease dysuria.
Child will verbalize reasons for frequent bladder emptying.	Encourage complete bladder emptying; explain necessity for this, as age appropriate.	Retained urine in the bladder is very susceptible to the growth of organisms.
	Remind child to void frequently	Under normal conditions the bladder flushes away organisms by regularly ridding itself of urine; this prevents organisms from accumulating and invading nearby structures. The convalescent bladder is less resistant to invasion than is a healthy bladder.
	Encourage fluids.	Child may be febrile; increasing fluids decreases the concentration of solutes and alleviates urinary stasis.
	Keep accurate intake and output records.	This is essential to determine the progress of treatment, because the kidneys and bladder play an important part in fluid balance.
	Teach child how to collect urine specimens, if age appropriate. Asking the female child to sit backward on the toilet seat enables the labia to spread and may prevent contamination (Robinson et al., 2014/2017)	Education ensures that the specimen will be correctly obtained without contamination.
	Provide privacy.	Children must be given the same courtesy as adults because they are sensitive and embarrassed by body exposure and body functions.

Selected Nursing Diagnosis Possible need for education regarding hygiene measures useful in prevention of urinary tract infection (UTI)

Goals	Nursing Interventions	Rationales
Girl will demonstrate on doll how to wipe herself after voiding. Child will verbalize methods to accomplish this.	Instruct girl of importance of wiping self from front to back.	Good perineal hygiene prevents fecal contamination of urethra.
	Emphasize need to avoid bubble baths.	The oils in these products are known to irritate the urethra.
	Encourage the use of showers.	These hygienic measures are helpful in preventing infection.
	Explain the need for cotton underwear.	Cotton underwear is more absorbent.
	Suggest juices (e.g., apple, cranberry) to maintain acidity of urine. Diet of meats, cheese, prunes, cranberries, plums, and whole grains is also beneficial (acid ash–producing foods).	Acidifying urine decreases the rate of bacterial multiplication.

Nursing Care Plan 29.1 The Child With a Urinary Tract Infection—cont'd

Goals	Nursing Interventions	Rationales
	Recommend frequent pad change for menstruating girls and proper genital cleansing during period.	Old, pooled blood fosters the growth of organisms; proper cleansing helps to prevent irritation.

Selected Nursing Diagnosis Need for parental support and education as a result of child requiring follow-up care

Goals	Nursing Interventions	Rationales
Parents will verbalize necessity for continued supervision and medication.	Teach parents to administer medication as prescribed and to continue for the time recommended by the health care provider.	Typical course of antibiotic treatment is 7–10 days; emphasize the need to complete prescribed dosage.
	Suggest that patient avoid using hot tubs or whirlpool baths.	May be potential sources of infection.
	Remind parents of necessity of adequate hydration for child.	Children dehydrate very quickly.
	Teach parents that any unexplained fever should be assessed for recurrence of a UTI	Unexplained fever could be due to a recurrent UTI and needs to be assessed and treated (Robinson et al., 2014/2017).

CRITICAL THINKING QUESTION

1. A mother comes to the clinic with her 5-year-old child who has a urinary tract infection for the second time in 3 months. The nurse notices that the child is wearing spandex sports shorts and is carrying a doll. She is holding a bottled water container that is filled with fruit punch. What teaching interventions could the nurse initiate?

Nursing Tip

Interventions to prevent urinary tract infection (UTI) include the following:

- Cleanse perineum with each diaper change.
- Wipe perineum from front to back.
- Avoid bubble baths.
- Have child urinate immediately after a bath.
- Encourage child to empty bladder frequently throughout the day—have a voiding routine.
- Treat constipation with a diet rich in fibre and good level of hydration; if required, the use of polyethylene glycol is recommended.
- Wear cotton underwear.
- Wear loose-fitting pants.
- Offer child adequate fluid intake (diuresis increases antibacterial properties of the renal medulla).

Nephrotic Syndrome

Pathophysiology

Nephrotic syndrome refers to a number of different types of kidney conditions that are distinguished by the presence of marked amounts of protein in the urine, high cholesterol, edema, and hypoalbuminemia. *Minimal change nephrotic syndrome (MCNS),* found in approximately 85% of cases, responds well to steroid therapy.

MCNS is more common in boys than in girls and is seen most often in children 3 to 9 years of age (Andolino & Reid-Adam, 2015). The specific cause is unknown, but it often occurs following a recent viral infection. The prognosis is good in steroid-responsive patients. Most children experience periods of relapse until the disease resolves itself. There is an 80% favourable prognosis over the long term.

Manifestations

The characteristic symptoms of MCNS are proteinuria and edema. This occurs slowly; the child does not appear to be sick. It is first noticed around the eyes and ankles and later becomes generalized. The gravity-dependent edema shifts with the position of the child, especially during sleep. The child gains weight because of the accumulation of fluid. The abdomen may become distended (ascites). The child can become pale, irritable, and listless and has a poor appetite. Blood pressure is usually normal.

Urine examination shows massive albumin (protein) and some results can display a few microscopic red blood cells. Gross hematuria is uncommon and should be investigated for other diagnoses. The **glomeruli**, the working units of the kidneys that filter the blood, become damaged and allow albumin and blood cells to enter the urine. The level of protein in the blood falls; this is termed **hypoalbuminemia** (*hypo,* "below," *albumin,* and *emia,* "blood"). Diagnosis of nephrotic syndrome includes a triad of hypoalbuminemia, hypercholesterolemia, and proteinuria.

Treatment

The goals of treatment include minimizing edema, preventing infection, reducing the loss of protein in the urine, and preventing toxicity from the medication prescribed.

Control of edema. The child with nephrosis is given medications designed to reduce proteinuria and, consequently, edema. Steroid therapy is currently used for this purpose. High-dose oral prednisone (60 mg/m^2/day) is initially given. The dosage is reduced for maintenance therapy, slowly tapering down the dose, which continues for 1 to 2 months. Because steroids mask signs of infection, the patient must be watched closely for more subtle symptoms of illness. Children are prone to infection due to suppression of the immune system. Other adverse effects include weight gain, increased appetite, behaviour changes, excess hair growth, and hypertension.

The nurse needs to watch for temperature variations and changes in behaviour. Suspicion of infection should be promptly reported because septicemia is life-threatening. Prompt antimicrobial therapy is begun when an acute bacterial infection is recognized. Diuretics are given in severe cases or worsening edema that impairs ambulation, along with fluid restrictions for a short period of time. Frequent follow-ups are required. Immunosuppressive therapy, for example, cyclophosphamide, mycophenolate mofetil, and tacrolimus, may be used for some steroid-resistant children (Andolino & Reid-Adam, 2015; Pais & Avner, 2016).

! Safety Alert!

When steroids are administered, the immune system is depressed. Care should be taken to limit exposure to infections.

Diet. An attractively served, well-balanced diet is desirable. Parents are instructed to offer a low-salt diet while the child is receiving prednisone therapy to prevent edema and hypertension. Fluids are not usually restricted except when massive edema is present. A normal protein intake is recommended. Obesity should be avoided in children who receive long-term steroids.

Nursing care

The nursing care of the child with MCNS has added importance because the disease necessitates long-term therapy and the child has increased susceptibility to infection. The child may be periodically hospitalized and become a familiar personality to hospital personnel.

The nurse can provide supportive care to the parents and child throughout the course of this disease. The child is treated at home whenever possible and is brought to the hospital for outpatient follow-up and special therapy only. Parents are instructed to keep a daily record of the child's first morning urinary protein levels and the child's medications. Signs of infection, abnormal weight gain, and increased protein in the urine must be reported promptly. Good skin care is especially important during periods of marked edema. After the acute stage of the illness subsides, the child is allowed to participate in normal childhood activities.

Monitoring intake and output. The child's intake and output must be strictly charted. Parents should be taught to inform the nurse of how much fluid has been taken. The importance of keeping proper fluid balance sheets (i.e., intake and output records) for patients with diseases of the kidneys cannot be overemphasized.

To measure an infant patient's urine output, diapers are weighed before their application and after removal (1 g = 1 mL). A careful check of the number of voids is of particular value. The character, odour, and colour of the urine are also important to note. If a 24-hour urine collection is ordered, *every* voided specimen within that time must be saved, or the test will not be valid. The specimens are collected in a large bottle or container that is correctly labelled. Some tests require special care or that certain preservatives be added to the container; these instructions should be clarified before the procedure begins.

Nursing Tip

Remember to measure and record urine specimens sent to the laboratory.

Weight and protection from infection. The patient is weighed two or three times weekly to determine changes in the degree of edema. The child is weighed on the same scale each time and at about the same time of day. Abdominal girth (circumference) should also be measured daily.

Nurses need to make every effort to protect the child from exposure to upper respiratory tract infections. Children with nephrotic syndrome are given pneumococcal vaccinations along with a yearly influenza vaccine to prevent infection. Vaccinations with live vaccines are contraindicated in children receiving steroid therapy because they are immunosuppressed and unable to respond to the vaccination; they must wait 3 months post-treatment to receive these vaccines. Household contacts may be vaccinated with live vaccines, but the child with nephrotic syndrome should avoid exposure for 3 to 6 weeks to respiratory or gastrointestinal secretions of those vaccinated (Pais & Avner, 2016).

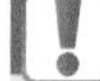

Safety Alert!

Children receiving steroid therapy should not receive live virus vaccines and should avoid for 3 to 6 weeks contact with respiratory or gastrointestinal secretions of household contacts who have recently been vaccinated with live virus vaccines.

The vital signs of a patient with nephrotic syndrome need to be taken regularly. Ordinarily, there is no temperature elevation unless an infection is present. Blood pressure usually remains normal. Nurses must provide parental guidance and support. The child with nephrosis is kept under close medical supervision throughout an extended period. Home care is preferred, with parents being taught monitoring skills and close outpatient follow-up.

Acute Glomerulonephritis

Pathophysiology

Acute glomerulonephritis (AGN) is an allergic reaction (antigen-antibody) to a group A beta-hemolytic streptococcal infection. It may appear after the patient has had a strep infection, scarlet fever, or skin infections. The body's immune mechanisms appear to be important in its development. Antibodies produced to fight the invading organisms also react against the glomerular tissue. Glomerulonephritis is a common form of nephritis in children, and it occurs most often in children aged 5 to 12 years of age, although the rates of AGN have decreased in industrialized countries, probably because of improved hygiene (Pan & Avner, 2016). Both kidneys are usually affected.

Within the bulb of each nephron lies a cluster of capillaries called the *glomerulus.* It is these structures that are affected, as the name implies. They become inflamed and sometimes blocked, permitting red blood cells and protein (which are normally retained) to enter the urine. The kidneys become pale and slightly enlarged. Table 29.3 compares nephrosis with AGN.

The prognosis for AGN is excellent. The acute phase of the disease may last 6 to 8 weeks. Patients with protracted cases may show urinary changes for as long as 1 year, but they experience complete recovery. The possibility of complications involving severe prolonged hypertension can lead to intracranial bleeding and necessitates careful monitoring and care of each patient.

Manifestations

From 1 to 3 weeks after a streptococcal infection has occurred, the parent may notice that the child has periorbital edema when awakening in the morning and that the child's urine is smoky brown or bloody. This can be frightening to the parent and child, and most parents immediately seek medical advice. Urine output may be decreased *(oliguria).* The urine specific gravity is high, and albumin, red and white blood cells, and casts may be found on examination. The blood urea nitrogen (BUN) level is elevated, as are the serum creatinine level and the sedimentation rate. The serum complement level (C3) is usually reduced. **Hyperkalemia** (excessive potassium in the blood) may produce cardiac toxicity. Hypertension may occur. An antistreptolysin (ASO) titre, if positive, evidences a recent streptococcal infection.

Treatment and nursing care

Although children may feel well, activity should be limited until gross hematuria subsides. The urine needs to be examined regularly. Every effort should be made to prevent children from becoming overly tired, chilled, or exposed to infection. Because renal function is impaired, there is a danger of accumulating nitrogenous wastes and sodium in the body. Dietary sodium and fluid restrictions are based on the hypertension and edema present. Foods high in potassium, such as bananas, are restricted during periods of oliguria.

Prevention of infection and fatigue, maintenance of accurate intake and output records, and frequent monitoring of vital signs are essential. Monitoring of responses to diuretics or antihypertensives that may be prescribed is also important.

Although glomerulonephritis is generally benign, it can be a source of anguish for the parents and child. If the patient is treated at home, the parents must plan quiet activities to keep the child occupied. They must understand the importance of continued medical supervision, because follow-up urine and blood tests are necessary to assess progress toward recovery. All children with hypertension should be monitored for

Table 29.3 Comparison Between Nephrosis and Acute Glomerulonephritis

	NEPHROSIS	ACUTE GLOMERULONEPHRITIS
Cause	Unknown, may be thymus T-cell dysfunction	Response to infection with group A beta-hemolytic streptococci
Edema	Massive edema Anasarca: whole-body edema Ascites: fluid in abdominal cavity	Periorbital edema (puffiness of eyes)
Blood pressure	Usually normal	Usually moderately elevated
Urine tests	Proteinuria Trace of blood	Trace of protein Hematuria (resolves within 1 month, but urinary symptoms may persist for 1 year)
Pallor	Degree of pallor is greater than expected in relation to degree of anemia (appearance resulting from edematous tissue)	Pallor related to anemia

Note: The signs and symptoms of nephrosis and acute glomerulonephritis are similar. Careful analysis and comparisons show significant differences. Either condition can lead to renal failure and its consequences.

signs of increased intracranial pressure. Most children recover completely with no sequelae.

Wilms Tumour

Pathophysiology

Wilms tumour, or *nephroblastoma* (*nephro*, "kidney," *blasto*, "bud," and *oma*, "tumour"), is one of the most common malignant renal tumours of early life. It is thought to have a genetic basis.

About two-thirds of these growths are discovered before the child is 3 years of age. As with some other malignancies, there are few or no symptoms during the early stages of growth. A mass in the abdomen is generally discovered by a parent or by the health care provider during a routine checkup. Radiographic examinations of the kidneys (most importantly, IV pyelograms) show a growth and verify that the remaining kidney is normal. The tumour compresses kidney tissue and is usually encapsulated. Renal damage may cause hypertension. Wilms tumor seldom affects both kidneys.

Treatment and nursing care

Treatment of patients with Wilms tumour usually consists of a combination of surgery, radiation therapy, and chemotherapy. The kidney and tumour are removed as soon as possible after the diagnosis has been confirmed. In some cases, preoperative chemotherapy may be done to shrink the tumour (Daw, Huff, & Anderson, 2016). Meticulous surgical technique avoids rupture of the capsule around the kidney.

General nursing measures for the comfort of the patient need to be implemented. One important consideration pertaining to this condition is the avoidance of all unnecessary handling of the abdomen, because rupture of the capsule can cause the tumour to spread. The health care provider should explain this to the parents, and in the hospital a sign should be placed on the bed or crib: "Do not palpate abdomen." Chemotherapy and, depending on staging, radiation therapy after surgery are usually completed at a specialized cancer centre. Postoperatively, contact sports should be avoided to prevent damage to the remaining kidney.

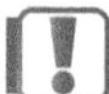

Safety Alert!

Abdominal palpation as part of the assessment of a child with Wilms tumour is omitted.

Hydrocele

Pathophysiology

A **hydrocele** (*hydro*, "water," and *cele*, "tumour") is an excessive amount of fluid in the sac that surrounds the testicle, and it causes the scrotum to swell (Fig. 29.8). When the testes descend into the scrotum in utero, the *processus vaginalis* (a fold of tissue) precedes them. This tissue ordinarily fuses, separating the peritoneal cavity from the scrotum. When this fusion does not take place, however, peritoneal fluid may enter the inguinal canal. Its appearance in the newborn is not uncommon, and in many cases the condition corrects itself by 1 year of age.

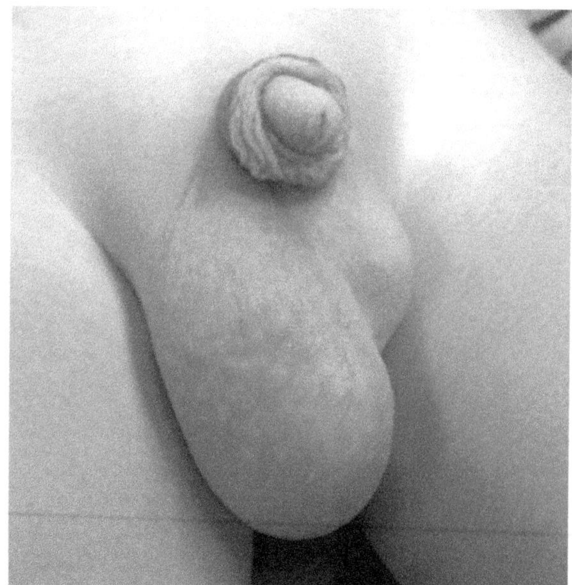

Fig. 29.8 Hydrocele A newborn with a large right hydrocele. (From Kleigman, R. M., Stanton, B.F., St. Geme, J.W. et al. (Eds.). et al. [2016]. *Nelson textbook of pediatrics* [20th ed.]. Philadelphia: Elsevier.)

Treatment

A chronic hydrocele that persists beyond 1 to 2 years is corrected by surgery (Elder, 2016b). Routine postoperative nursing care is provided. This is outlined in Chapter 20. Same-day surgery may be arranged.

Cryptorchidism (Undescended Testis)

Pathophysiology

The testes are the male sex glands. These two oval bodies begin their development in the embryo within the abdominal cavity, just below the kidneys. Their function is to produce spermatozoa (male sex cells) and male hormones, particularly testosterone. Toward the end of the seventh fetal month, the testes begin to descend along a pathway into the scrotum. If this descent does not take place normally, the testes may remain in the abdomen or the inguinal canal. This condition is common in approximately 30% of low-birth-weight infants (Elder, 2016b). When one or both testes fail to lower into the scrotum, the condition is termed **cryptorchidism** (*kryptos*, "hidden," and *orchi*, "testis"). The unilateral form is more common.

Because the testes are warmer in the abdomen than in the scrotum, the sperm cells begin to deteriorate. If both testes are affected, sterility results. Inguinal hernia often accompanies this condition. Acute scrotal pain may indicate a **testicular torsion** (twisting), which necessitates immediate surgery to preserve testicular function.

Treatment and nursing care

Usually, a testis or the testes spontaneously descend within 3 to 6 months of life, but if not, an operation called an **orchidopexy** (*orchio,* "testicle," and *pexy,* "fixation") may be performed by 6 to 18 months of age (Braga, Lorenzo, & Romao, 2017).

Although an orchidopexy improves the condition, the fertility rate among these patients may be reduced. Hormonal therapy is not usually effective in causing the testis to descend and is not recommended as first-line therapy (Braga et al., 2017). When the child returns from surgery, care is taken to prevent contamination of the suture line, and scrotal support is maintained.

Home Care Considerations

Monitoring of the urine output and prevention of infection should be taught to parents. Self-image support may be needed.

The psychological approach of the nurse to the patient and his family is important because of the embarrassment they may feel. People may ask the child why he is undergoing surgery when there is no visible evidence of trauma. This problem is often compounded by the fact that the older child may have been told not to discuss his condition; in addition, his understanding of his problem and just what is going to happen in surgery may be vague. Therefore, the nurse caring for the child should know what he has been told and how he feels about his operation, to give emotional support. Terminology needs to be clarified. The nurse can assure the child that his penis will not be involved in the surgery.

The parents, too, may have anxieties that they cannot verbalize. A thoughtful, sensitive nurse who tries to anticipate related feelings and fears can promote the child's adjustment.

IMPACT OF URINARY OR GENITAL SURGERY ON GROWTH AND DEVELOPMENT

Surgery of the urinary or genital tract can affect a child's growth and development. Preschoolers may perceive the treatment as punishment. Separation anxiety during hospitalization can peak, and preventive strategies to address such anxiety should be explained to the parents. The body image of the child must be assertively maintained whenever surgery is delayed beyond infancy.

Between 3 and 6 years of age, the child becomes curious about sexual differences. Surgical interventions during this stage of development necessitate guidance and preparation to minimize the negative impact on growth and development.

During home care, tub baths may be contraindicated, dressings to "private parts" of the body must be inspected daily, and restrictions on play activities that involve straddle toys (e.g., tricycles, rocking horses) are necessary.

Adolescents may be concerned about the effects of surgery on their appearance and sexual abilities.

Get Ready for the Certification Examination!

Key Points

- The functional unit of the kidney is the nephron.
- The minimum urine output for young children it is 1–2 mL/kg/hr and a minimum of 30 mL/hr for adolescents.
- Children with hypospadias are born with the urethral opening on the undersurface of the penis.
- Bladder exstrophy is a serious congenital defect in which the bladder lies exposed on the lower portion of the abdominal wall. Surgical correction of this defect is life-saving.
- Obstruction of the urinary tract may lead to hydronephrosis, a distention of the kidney pelvis. This is a serious condition because it could eventually lead to kidney failure if left untreated.
- To prevent fecal contamination of the urinary tract, girls are taught to wipe the perineal area from front to back after urination.
- Normally, urine flows from the ureters into the bladder, and almost no flow re-enters the ureters.
- Repeated urinary tract infections or improper position of the ureters or sphincters in the bladder at birth may result in the reflux of urine into the ureters.
- Ascites is an abnormal collection of fluid in the peritoneal cavity. It is seen in advanced cases of nephrosis and in other conditions.
- The accurate charting of intake and output for patients with kidney problems is absolutely essential to their treatment and recovery. This includes ostomy and urinary drainage.
- Accurate blood pressure measurements will detect hypertension, a condition often associated with kidney problems.
- Routine abdominal palpation is omitted for a child diagnosed with Wilms tumour.
- A hydrocele is an excessive amount of fluid in the sac that surrounds the testicle. This causes the scrotum to swell.
- Undescended testes *(cryptorchidism)* refers to a condition in which the testes do not lower into the scrotum during the fetal period but remain in the abdomen or the inguinal canal after birth.
- Early treatment of cryptorchidism is necessary to preserve testicular function.

Additional Learning Resources

evolve Go to your Evolve website (http://evolve.elsevier.com/Canada/Leifer) for the following learning resources:

- Answer Key for Critical Thinking Questions
- Answer Key for Textbook Review Questions

- Audio Glossary
- Fluids & Electrolytes tutorial
- Interactive Review Questions
- Skills Performance Checklists
- Video clips and more!

Online Resources

- About Kids Health, *Hypospadias Repair: Taking Care of Your Child at Home After the Operation:* https://www.aboutkidshealth.ca/Article?contentid=1215&language=English
- The Kidney Foundation of Canada: https://www.kidney.ca/

Review Questions

1. The nurse understands that genitourinary surgery affects growth and development. When caring for a 4-year-old child postoperatively, a priority nursing responsibility would include which of the following?
   a. Strategies to preserve the child's body image
   b. Assurances that appearance and sexual function will not be affected
   c. Providing age-appropriate toys such as tricycles
   d. Preventing embarrassment by limiting visitation of family and friends
2. The administration of prednisone to children with nephrosis creates which problem?
   a. Intolerance to foods
   b. Increased risk of infection
   c. Increased periorbital edema
   d. Weight loss
3. What is a priority nursing responsibility in the care of a child with Wilms tumour?
   a. Maintain accurate intake and output records.
   b. Omit abdominal palpation during daily assessments.
   c. Maintain strict bed rest.
   d. Assess neurological function.
4. A nurse is caring for a child diagnosed with nephrosis. Symptoms that are characteristic of nephrosis include which of the following? *(Select all that apply.)*
   a. Massive proteinuria
   b. Edema
   c. A positive antistreptolysin titer
   d. Bacteriuria
5. A 2½-year-old child is being discharged after a hypospadias repair. Which of the following should the nurse teach the parents postoperatively? *(Select all that apply.)*
   a. Leave the diaper off until the site is healed.
   b. Restrict fluids to reduce output for 1 week.
   c. Continue with toilet learning.
   d. Avoid holding the infant straddling on the hip.
   e. Avoid tricycle riding as a play activity.

REFERENCES

Alsowayan, O., Capolicchio, J. P., Jednak, R., et al. (2016). Long-term functional outcomes after bladder exstrophy repair: A single, low-volume centre experience. *Canadian Urology Association Journal*, *10*(3-4), E94–E98.

Andolino, T. P., & Reid-Adam, J. (2015). Nephrotic syndrome. *Pediatrics in Review*, *36*(3), 117–126.

Braga, L. H., Lorenzo, A. J., & Romao, L. P. (2017). Canadian Urological Association–Pediatric Urologists of Canada (CUA-PUC) guideline for the diagnosis, management, and follow-up of cryptorchidism. *Canadian Urological Association Journal*, *11*(7), E251–E260.

Daw, N. C., Huff, V., & Anderson, P. M. (2016). Wilms tumor. In R. M. Kliegman, B. F. Stanton, J. W. St. Geme, et al. (Eds.), *Nelson textbook of pediatrics* (20th ed.). Philadelphia: Saunders.

Elder, J. (2016a). Anomalies of the bladder. In R. M. Kliegman, B. F. Stanton, J. W. St. Geme, et al. (Eds.), *Nelson textbook of pediatrics* (20th ed.). Philadelphia: Saunders.

Elder, J. (2016b). Disorders and anomalies of the scrotal contents. In R. M. Kliegman, B. F. Stanton, J. W. St. Geme, et al. (Eds.), *Nelson textbook of pediatrics* (20th ed.). Philadelphia: Saunders.

Elder, J. (2016c). Urinary tract infections. In R. M. Kliegman, B. F. Stanton, J. W. St. Geme, et al. (Eds.), *Nelson textbook of pediatrics* (20th ed.). Philadelphia: Saunders.

Keays, M. A., & Dave, S. (2017). Current hypospadias management: Diagnosis, surgical management, and long-term patient-centred outcomes. *Canadian Urological Association Journal*, *11*(Suppl. 1-2), S48–S53.

Pais, P., & Avner, E. (2016). Nephrotic syndrome. In R. M. Kliegman, B. F. Stanton, J. W. St. Geme, et al. (Eds.), *Nelson textbook of pediatrics* (20th ed.). Philadelphia: Saunders.

Pan, C. G., & Avner, E. (2016). Acute poststreptococcal glomerulonephritis. In R. M. Kliegman, B. F. Stanton, J. W. St. Geme, et al. (Eds.), *Nelson textbook of pediatrics* (20th ed.). Philadelphia: Saunders.

Robinson, J. L., Finlay, J. C., Lang, M. E., et al. (2014). Urinary tract infection in infants and children: Diagnosis and management. *Paediatrics & Child Health*, *19*(6), 315–319. Reaffirmed 2017.

Sorokan, S. T., Finlay, J. C., Jefferies, A. L., et al. (2015). Newborn male circumcision. *Paediatrics & Child Health*, *20*(6), 311–315. Reaffirmed 2018.

Wu, T. H., Huang, F. L., Fu, L. S., et al. (2016). Treatment of recurrent complicated urinary tract infections in children with vesicoureteral reflux. *Journal Microbiology, Immunology, & Infection*, *49*(5), 717–722.

The Child With a Skin Condition

30

Cheryl A. Sams

http://evolve.elsevier.com/Canada/Leifer

Objectives

1. Define each key term listed.
2. Describe the differences between the skin of the infant and that of the adult.
3. Identify common congenital skin lesions and infections.
4. Outline the nursing care of various microbial infections of the skin.
5. Describe two topical agents used to treat acne.
6. Summarize the nursing care for a child who has infantile eczema and state the rationale for each nursing measure.
7. Identify the principles of topical therapy.
8. Differentiate between the various types of topical medication.
9. Discuss the prevention and care of pediculosis, scabies, and bedbugs.
10. Differentiate among first-, second-, and third-degree burns—the anatomical structures involved, the appearance, the level of sensation, and the first aid required.
11. Describe how the response of the child with burns differs from that of the adult.
12. Describe the emergency treatment of three types of burns.
13. List five objectives of the nurse who is caring for the burned child.
14. Discuss the prevention and treatment of sunburn and frostbite.

Key Terms

alopecia (ăl-ō-PĒ-shă)
autograft (ĂW-tō-grăft)
chilblain (CHĬL-blān)
comedo (KŎM-ĕ-dō)
crust
Curling ulcer (KŬR-lĭngz ŬL-sŭr)
debridement (dĕ-BRĒD-mnt)
dermabrasion (dŭrm-ă-BRĀ-zhŭn)
ecchymosis (ĕk-ĭ-MŌ-sĭs)
emollient (ĕ-MŎL-ē-ŭnt)
eschar (ĔS-kăhr)
exanthem (ĕg-ZĂN-thŭm)
frostbite
heterograft (HĔT-ŭr-ō-grăft)
hives
homografts (HŌ-mō-grăfts)
ileus (ĬL-ē-ŭs)
isograft (Ī-sō-grăft)
lanugo
macule (MĂK-yūl)
methicillin-resistant *Staphylococcus aureus* (MRSA) (mĕth-ĭ-SĬL-ĭn rē-zĭs-tĕnt stăf-ĭ-lō-KŎK-ŭs ĂW-rē-ŭs)
milia
mongolian spot
nevi
papule (PĂP-yūl)
pediculosis (pĕ-dĭk-yū-LŌ-sĭs)
pruritus (prū-RĪ-tŭs)
pustule (PŬS-tyūl)
sebum
stye
total body surface area (TBSA)
vernix caseosa
vesicle (VĔS-ĭ-kŭl)
wheal (WĒL)
xenografts (ZĒ-nō-grăfts)

SKIN DEVELOPMENT AND FUNCTIONS

The main function of the skin is protection. It acts as the body's first line of defense against disease. It prevents the passage of harmful physical and chemical agents and prevents the loss of water and electrolytes. It also has the capacity to regenerate and repair itself. The skin and the structures derived from it, such as hair and fingernails, are known as the integumentary system. Fig. 30.1 depicts these structures and how they differ in the developing child and in the adult.

Four basic skin sensations—pain, temperature, touch, and pressure—are felt by the skin in conjunction with the nervous system. The skin also secretes sebum, which helps to protect and maintain its texture. The outer surface of the skin is acidic, with a pH of 4.5 to 6.5, to protect the skin from pathological bacteria that thrive in an alkaline environment.

The skin is composed of two layers: the epidermis (derived from the ectoderm) and the dermis (derived from the mesoderm). Vernix caseosa is a cheeselike substance that covers the fetus until birth. This protects the fetal skin from maceration as the fetus floats in the amniotic fluid. The fetal skin is at first so transparent that blood vessels are clearly visible. Downy lanugo

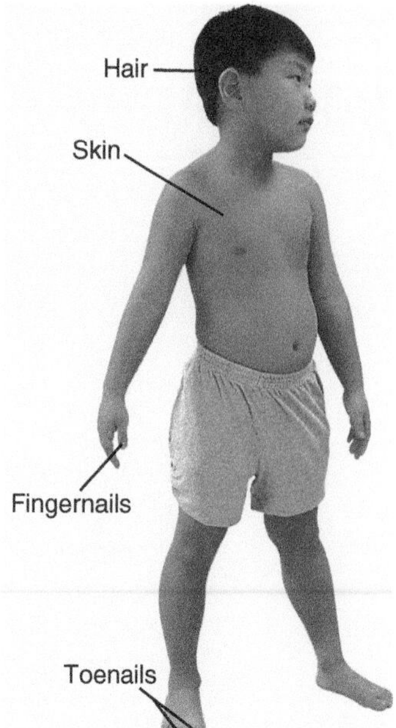

INTEGUMENTARY SYSTEM

- The thin epidermis in infants blisters easily, absorption is dramatically greater, and infections occur more readily.
- Sebaceous glands do not begin producing sebum until about 8 to 10 years of age. Without lubrication, the skin is more dry and chaps more easily.
- Skin infections are more likely to produce systemic symptoms.
- Preterm and term newborns have less subcutaneous fat; therefore they are more sensitive to heat and cold.
- At birth the skin is alkaline, increasing susceptibility to infection.
- The ability to perspire through the skin matures by 3 years of age, and axillary perspiration begins near puberty. Therefore thermoregulation may be a problem in children.

Fig. 30.1 Summary of some differences between the child and the adult in the integumentary system. The integumentary system consists of the skin and the structures derived from it. This system protects the body, helps to regulate body temperature, and receives stimuli such as pressure, pain, and temperature. (Art overlay courtesy Observatory Group, Cincinnati, Ohio.)

hair begins to develop at about 13 to 16 weeks, especially on the head. At 21 to 24 weeks the skin is reddish and wrinkled, with little subcutaneous fat. Adipose tissue forms during later weeks. At birth, the subcutaneous glands are well developed, and the skin is pink and smooth and has a polished look. It is thinner than the skin of an adult.

Maintaining skin integrity is not only important for physical health but also for self-esteem and therefore has both a psychological and a physiological component. This is particularly evident in patients with facial disfigurement.

SKIN DISORDERS AND VARIATIONS

Certain skin conditions in children may be associated with age, as in the case of milia, which is normal to be seen in infants and acne in adolescents. A skin condition may be a manifestation of a systemic disease, such as chickenpox. Some lesions, such as strawberry nevi and mongolian spots, are congenital. Other skin lesions, such as those seen in rubella and fifth disease, are self-limited and do not necessitate treatment.

There are great individual differences in skin texture, colour, pH, and moisture. Skin colour is an important diagnostic criterion in cases of liver disease, heart conditions, child abuse, and for overall assessment. Complete blood counts and serum electrolyte levels are helpful in diagnosing skin conditions. Skin tests are used in diagnosing allergies. Skin scrapings are used for microscopic examination. The *Wood's light* is an instrument used to diagnose certain skin conditions. It reflects a particular colour according to the organism present.

Hair condition is important to observe. Hair is inspected for colour, texture, quality, distribution, and elasticity. Hair may become dry and brittle and may lack luster owing to inadequate nutrition. Hair may begin to fall out or even change colour during illness or the ingestion of certain medications.

The nurse should describe the lesions with regard to size, colour, configuration (e.g., butterfly rash), presence of pain or itching, distribution (e.g., arms, legs, behind ears), and whether the rash is general or local. Hives, a general rash that appears abruptly, is often an allergic or medication reaction. The condition of the skin around the lesions is also significant, as is the skin turgor. Managing itching is a key component in preventing secondary infection that can result from scratching. Dressings and ointments are applied as prescribed. Preventing infections is a consideration in the case of open wounds. Treatment of physiological jaundice is covered in Chapter 12. Skin disorders related to communicable diseases are discussed in Chapter 32.

Many childhood infectious diseases, such as measles, German measles, and chickenpox, involve the presence of an exanthem (a skin rash). Box 30.1 identifies terms used to describe some conditions of the skin that the nurse may witness. Some rashes begin as one lesion and evolve into others. For example, the sequence of chickenpox rash is macule to papule, to vesicle, and then to crust. A stye is an infection of the sebaceous gland of the eyelash (Fig. 30.2). The nurse should document any birthmarks or skin lesions on admission. Skin conditions may be acute or chronic.

CONGENITAL LESIONS

Strawberry Nevus

Strawberry nevus (Fig. 30.3) is a common hemangioma (consisting of dilated capillaries in the dermal space) that may not become apparent until a few weeks after birth. Although it is harmless and usually disappears without treatment, it can be disturbing to parents,

Box 30.1 Terms Used to Describe Skin Conditions

Macule: Flat rash (freckles)

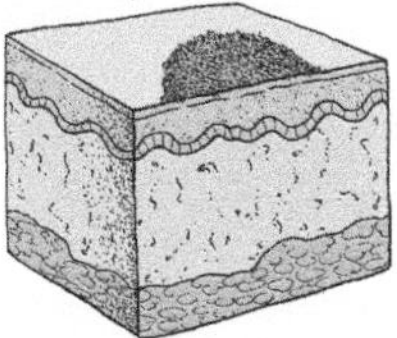

Vesicle: Elevated, fluid-filled blister (cold sore, chickenpox)

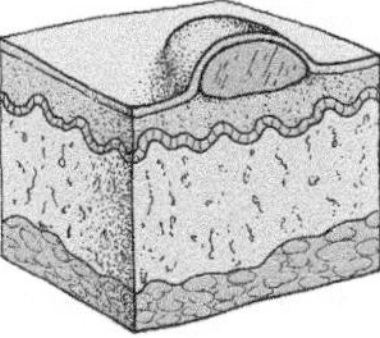

Crust: Scab

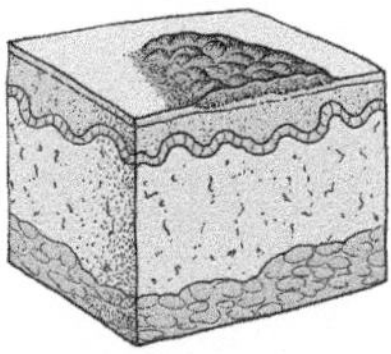

Papule: Elevated area (pimple)

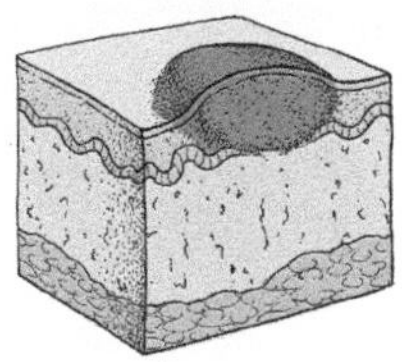

Pustule: Elevated, pus filled (impetigo, acne)

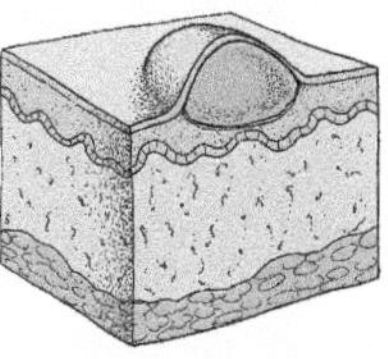

Wheal: Raised red, irregular (mosquito bite, allergic reactions)

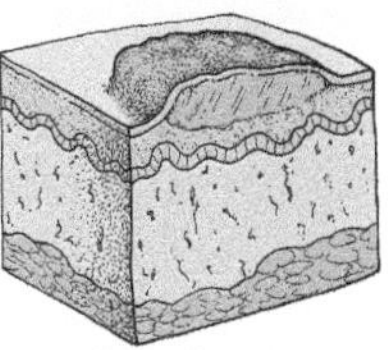

Ecchymosis: Black and blue-purple mark (bruise)

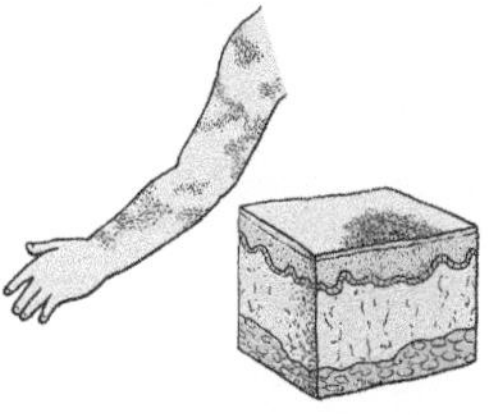

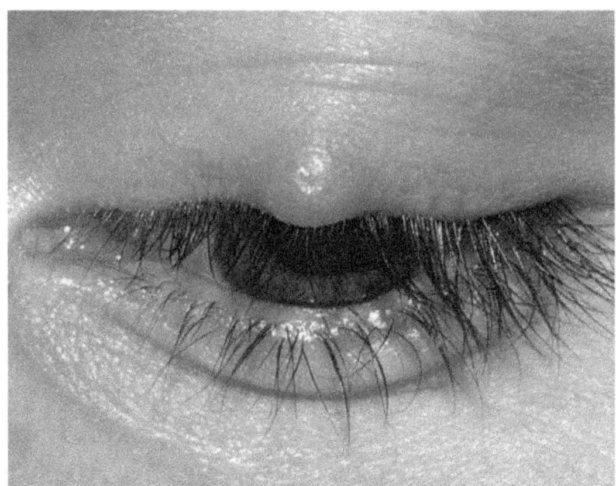

Fig. 30.2 A stye, or hordeolum, is an inflammation of the sebaceous gland of the eyelid that is commonly seen in infants and children. (From Zitelli, B. J., et al. [2018]. *Zitelli and Davis' atlas of pediatric physical diagnosis* [7th ed.]. St. Louis: Elsevier.)

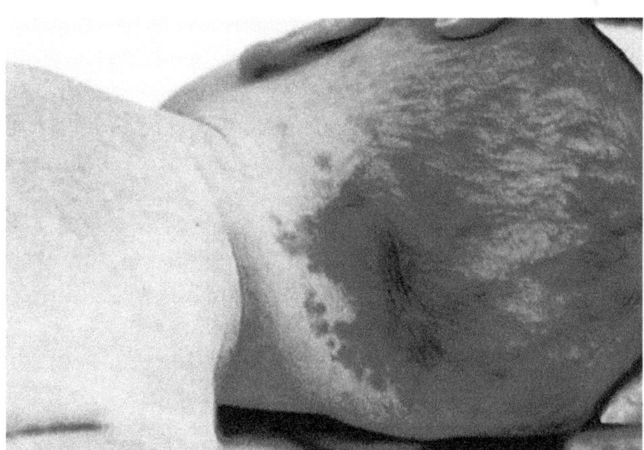

Fig. 30.3 Strawberry nevus. It usually fades within the first 1 to 2 years of life. (From Swartz, M. H. [2014]. *Textbook of physical diagnosis: History and examination* [7th ed.]. Philadelphia: Saunders.)

especially when it appears on the head or face. At first it is flat, but it gradually it becomes raised. The lesion is bright red, elevated, and sharply demarcated. The lesions gradually blanch, with 60% disappearing spontaneously by 5 years of age and 90% disappearing by 9 years of age.

Laser treatment or excision may be considered if the area becomes ulcerated. After laser surgery, the skin may appear black for 7 to 10 days. Salicylates should be avoided, and sun exposure should be minimized. The nurse needs to offer support and reassurance to parents and provide information.

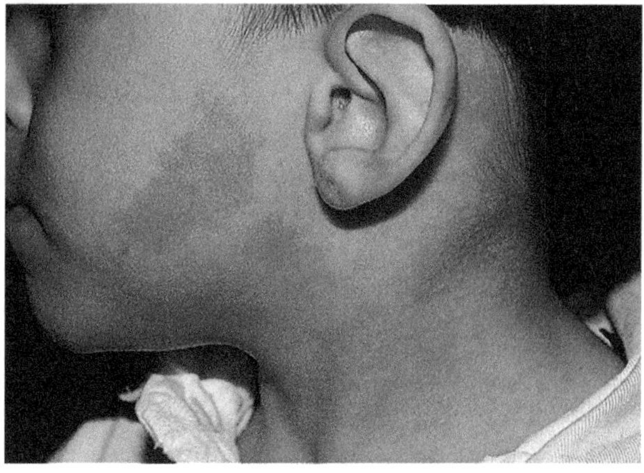

Fig. 30.4 Port-wine stain. (From Weston, W. L., Lane, A. T., & Morelli, J. G. [2007]. *Color textbook of pediatric dermatology* [4th ed.]. St. Louis: Mosby.)

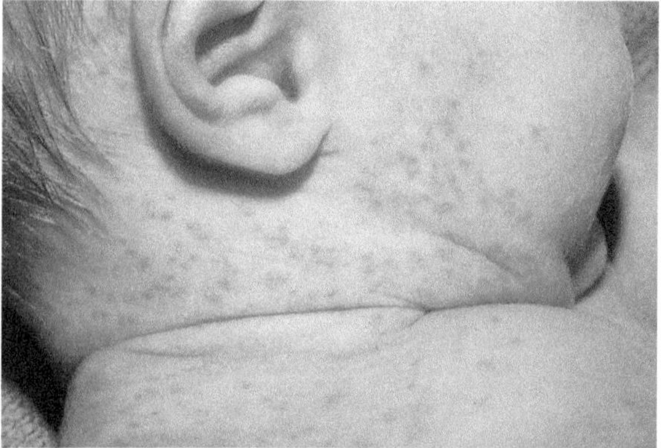

Fig. 30.5 Miliaria. Note the many tiny pustular lesions in the folds of the neck. (From Zitelli, B. J., et al. [2018]. *Zitelli and Davis' atlas of pediatric physical diagnosis* [7th ed.]. St. Louis: Elsevier.)

Port-Wine Nevus

Port-wine nevi (Fig. 30.4) are present at birth and are caused by dilated dermal capillaries. The lesions are flat, sharply demarcated, and purple to pink in colour. The lesion darkens as the child grows older. If the area is small, cosmetics may disguise the lesion. If the area is large, laser surgery may be considered.

SKIN MANIFESTATIONS OF ILLNESS

- *Café-au-lait macules* occur in 10 to 20% of people and are light brown, oval patches on the skin. Multiple café-au-lait macules are associated with neurofibromatosis (a chromosomal abnormality) and tuberous sclerosis.
- *Hypopigmented macules* are whitish oval- or leaf-shaped macules. Multiple hypopigmented macules are associated with tuberous sclerosis.
- *Butterfly rash* over the nose and cheeks can be associated with photosensitivity and may be associated with systemic lupus erythematosus (SLE).
- *Scaling skin eruption* around the mouth in a horseshoe-shaped distribution around the chin and cheeks, or as a perianal rash and involving papules and scales, is associated with zinc deficiency in infants. It also is associated with diarrhea and failure to thrive.
- *Vascular birthmarks* such as hemangioma resemble a bruise that changes in appearance through the years. Hemangiomas around the chin may be associated with airway problems, and those appearing around the lumbar region may be associated with spinal problems. Some hemangiomas can be treated with topical timolol maleate, which is a beta blocker and used as an alternative to oral propranolol (Püttgen, Lucky, Adams, et al., 2016).

SKIN CONDITIONS

Miliaria

Miliaria (prickly heat) refers to a rash caused by excess body heat and moisture (Fig. 30.5). There is retention of sweat in the sweat glands, which have become blocked or inflamed. Rupture or leakage into the skin causes the inflamed response. It appears suddenly as tiny, pinhead-sized, reddened papules with occasional clear vesicles. It may be accompanied by pruritus (itching). It is seen in infants during hot weather or in newborns who sleep in rooms that are too warm. It often occurs in the diaper area or in the folds of the skin where moisture accumulates. Plastic enclosures on diapers hold in body warmth that results in a rash. This harmless condition may be reversed by removing extra clothing, bathing, skin care, and frequent diaper changes.

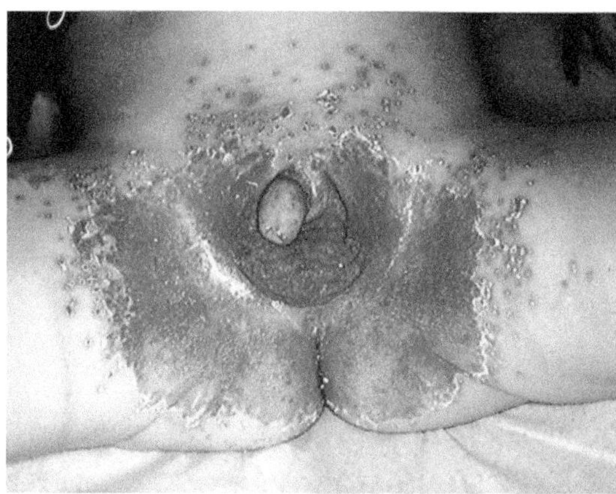

Fig. 30.6 Intertrigo. Red, moist patches have sharply demarcated borders and some loose scales, usually in the genital area and extending along the inguinal and gluteal folds. Urine, feces, heat, and moisture aggravate this lesion. (From Hurwitz, S. [2016]. *Clinical pediatric dermatology: A textbook of skin disorders of childhood and adolescence* [5th ed.]. St. Louis: Elsevier.)

Intertrigo

Intertrigo (*in*, "into," and *terere*, "to rub") is the medical term for chafing. It is a dermatitis that occurs in the folds of the skin (Fig. 30.6). The patches are red and moist and are usually located along the neck and in the inguinal and gluteal folds. Urine, feces, heat, and moisture aggravate this condition. Obese children are more prone to intertrigo. Prevention consists of keeping the affected areas clean and *dry*. The child should have diapers removed and the area exposed to air and light as much as possible. Maceration of the skin can lead to secondary infections. Intertrigo is often accompanied by a *Candida* (yeast) infection. Protection of the diaper area with zinc oxide cream or an unscented barrier cream such as petroleum jelly and removal of the cream with mineral oil rather than water may prevent *Candida* infection of the skin folds.

Seborrheic Dermatitis

Pathophysiology

Seborrheic dermatitis is an inflammation of the skin that involves the sebaceous glands (Fig. 30.7). Thick, yellow, oily, adherent, crustlike scales on the scalp and the forehead characterize this condition. The skin beneath the patches may be red (erythematous). Less often it may involve the eyelids, the external ear, and the inguinal area. Secondary bacterial and yeast infections may occur. It is seen in newborns, in infants, and at puberty. In newborns, it is commonly known as "cradle cap." It is seen in infants with sensitive skin, even when the head and hair are washed frequently. Seborrhea resembles eczema, but it usually does not itch and there is a negative family history. In adolescents, it is more localized and is usually confined to the scalp.

Treatment

Treatment consists of shampooing with a nonmedicated shampoo on a regular basis, but not too often or the scalp will dry out. Applying baby oil or olive oil to the head the evening before and shampooing in the morning may soften scales in newborns. The scalp is rinsed well. A soft brush is helpful in removing loose particles from the hair. If the infant has dry, scaling, thickened skin over the forehead, on the cheeks, and behind the ears, an unscented moisturizer can be used two to three times a day on the skin. A mild hydrocortisone cream (0.5%) is safe and usually effective (Canadian Paediatric Society [CPS], 2017). A dandruff-control shampoo containing selenium or an azole are useful and can be used for adolescents. The response to therapy is usually rapid.

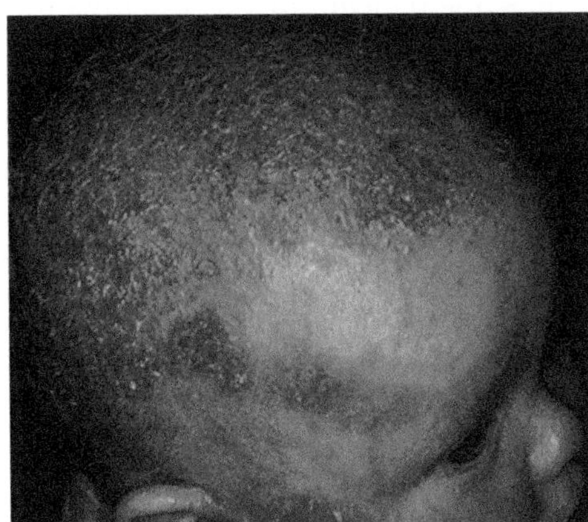

Fig. 30.7 Seborrheic dermatitis (cradle cap). Thick, yellow, greasy adherent scales appear on the scalp and forehead. There is no itching (pruritus). (From Hurwitz, S. [2016]. *Clinical pediatric dermatology: A textbook of skin disorders of childhood and adolescence* [5th ed.]. St. Louis: Elsevier.)

Diaper Dermatitis

Pathophysiology

Diaper dermatitis (diaper rash) is a commonly seen condition that results from prolonged contact of the skin to a mixture of urine and feces. The urine increases the pH of the skin, resulting in increased sensitivity to fecal enzymes. If the skin remains moist inside the soiled diaper, the skin may become more likely to develop a *Candida albicans* infection. The rash of simple diaper dermatitis may appear as an erythema (redness); however, a beefy red rash in the diaper area may be indicative of a *Candida* (thrush) infection and necessitates prompt treatment (Fig. 30.8). Disposable diapers contain a super-absorbent gel material that helps maintain normal skin pH, so their use can reduce the occurrence of diaper dermatitis.

Treatment and nursing care

It is easier to prevent diaper rash than to cure it. Prevention is accomplished by frequent diaper changes to limit the skin's exposure to moisture. The diaper is periodically removed to expose the skin to light and air. With each diaper change, the perineal area is gently and thoroughly cleansed (preferably with warm water) and gently dried. After bowel movements, the area is cleansed with mild soap and water. The skin folds are thoroughly washed, rinsed, and dried. A cloth, or unscented, non–alcohol-containing wipe may be used to remove feces from the skin.

Some common over-the-counter ointments for prevention of diaper dermatitis include ointments with

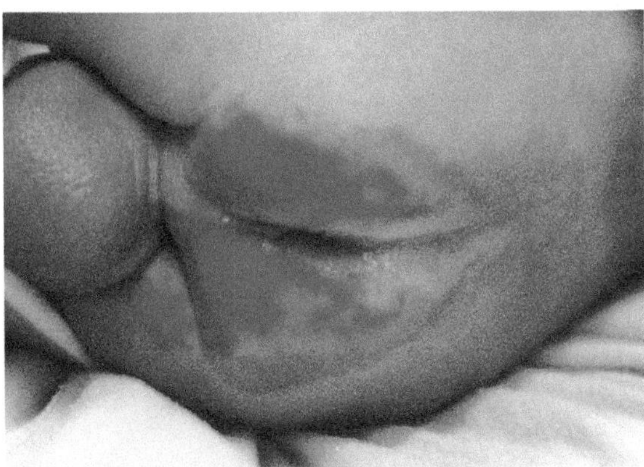

Fig. 30.8 Diaper rash (diaper dermatitis). A red, moist maculopapular rash with poorly defined borders appears in the diaper area. Rash is caused by *Candidia*. The infant may have a history of infrequent diaper changes or the use of snug rubber or plastic pants. The inflammation results from ammonia, heat, and moisture. (From Bowden, V. R., Dickey, S. B., & Greenberg, S. C. [1998]. *Children and their families: The continuum of care*. Philadelphia: Saunders.)

the active ingredients of vitamins A and D and lanolin, and other products containing zinc oxide. A thick layer of zinc oxide should be applied for an erythematous rash; an antifungal cream (Nystatin) may be added if there is evidence of candida. Aggressive scrubbing of the skin should be avoided (Bortolussi, Martin, & CPS Infectious Diseases and Immunization Committee, 2007/2018). Mineral oil can aid in removing sticky ointments. The use of corticosteroid ointments in an occluded diaper area should be avoided because skin absorption can cause systemic complications.

Acne Vulgaris

Pathophysiology

Acne is an inflammation of the sebaceous glands and hair follicles in the skin (Fig. 30.9). Because of hormonal influence, the sebaceous glands enlarge at puberty and secrete increased amounts of a fatty substance called **sebum**. Genetic factors and stress are also thought to play a part in acne's etiology. The course of acne may be brief or prolonged (lasting 10 years or longer). Preadolescent and premenstrual acne in girls is not uncommon. The principal lesions include comedones, papules, and nodulocystic growths.

A **comedo** (plural, *comedones*) is a plug of keratin, sebum, or bacteria. Keratin is a protein substance and is the main constituent of epidermis and hair. There are two types of comedones: open and closed. In the open comedo, or *blackhead,* the surface is darkened by melanin. Closed comedones, or *whiteheads,* are responsible for the inflammatory process of acne. With continued buildup, the walls of the follicle rupture, releasing their irritating contents into the surrounding skin. A pustule may appear when this develops near the exterior. This process occurs no matter how carefully the teenager washes, because surface bacteria are not involved in the pathogenesis. Acne is usually seen on the chin, the cheeks, and the forehead. It can also develop on the chest, the upper back, and the shoulders. It is often more severe in winter.

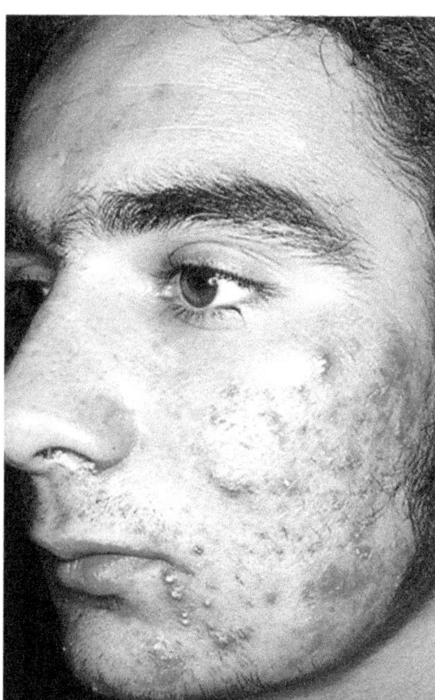

Fig. 30.9 Acne; it is the most common skin problem of adolescence. An increase in sebaceous gland activity creates increased oiliness. Open comedones (blackheads) and closed comedones (whiteheads) are common. Severe acne includes papules and nodules. The lesions can appear on the face, chest, back, and shoulders. (From Hurwitz, S. [2016]. *Clinical pediatric dermatology: A textbook of skin disorders of childhood and adolescence* [5th ed.]. St. Louis: Elsevier.)

Medication-induced acne can occur in children taking long-term steroids, phenobarbital, phenytoin, lithium, vitamin B_{12}, or medications containing iodides or bromides.

Treatment

The basic treatment of acne has changed considerably during the past few years. It is no longer thought that certain foods trigger the condition; therefore, the restriction of chocolate, peanuts, and cola drinks is unwarranted. A regular, well-balanced diet is encouraged. General hygienic measures of cleanliness, rest, and the avoidance of emotional stress may help to prevent exacerbations.

Routine skin cleansing with any mild soap or astringent cleanser is helpful. Excessive cleansing of the skin can irritate and dry the tissues. Surface bacteria do not cause acne. Squeezing pimples ruptures intact lesions and causes local inflammation and possible infection.

Medications prescribed include retinoids, such as tretinoin (Retin-A) or adapalene, which reduce peeling of follicular epithelium and help to clear existing lesions. Retinoids are available over the counter as gels, creams, and liquids and increase sun sensitivity. Benzoyl peroxide gel is antimicrobial and highly successful as a treatment. Topical clindamycin antibiotic may be prescribed for inflammatory acne.

Isotretinoin (Accutane) is given to patients with severe pustulocystic acne who have been unable to benefit from other types of treatment. It has many adverse effects; thus, the patient must be carefully monitored. It is not prescribed during pregnancy or to those at risk for pregnancy because it causes serious birth defects if it is taken when a female becomes pregnant or if she is breastfeeding. Health Canada (2016) has instituted a pregnancy prevention program that requires patients' written consent, two negative pregnancy tests before starting treatment, monthly tests during treatment and 1 month after stopping, as well as the use of two reliable methods of birth control through this period. Despite this program, pregnancies can still occur among young women taking isotretinoin. Nurses play an important role in educating young women and young men about safer sex and the risk of fetal deformities that is associated with use of isotretinoin.

Systemic antibiotics, such as tetracycline, may be prescribed for inflammatory acne. Planing of the skin to minimize scarring (**dermabrasion**) is done selectively, because it is not always successful. Estrogen-containing oral contraceptives (OCs) are also effective, because sebum production is controlled by androgens, and these OCs reduce androgen levels.

Acne may be distressing to the adolescent, particularly when the face is extensively involved. Sometimes even a minimal problem is seen as emotionally disastrous when it happens before an important event. The self-conscious young person feels different and embarrassed. The nurse who is attuned to the feelings of individuals can provide support. Although the adolescent is educated to assume responsibility for the regimen, including the parents in the education may help to prevent conflict surrounding the regimen.

Nursing Tip

Topical benzoyl peroxide and Retin-A neutralize each other when applied together.

Nursing Tip

Sun exposure can darken acne lesions in adolescents with dark skin colour, thus use of SPF sun protection is important to help prevent this.

Herpes Simplex Type I

Pathophysiology

Herpes simplex type I, a viral infection, is commonly known as a cold sore or fever blister. It may begin with a feeling of tingling, itching, or burning on the lip. Vesicles and crusts form (Fig. 30.10). Spontaneous healing occurs in about 8 to 10 days. Communicability is highest early in the formation and is spread by direct contact. Recurrence is common, because the virus lies dormant in the body until it is activated by stress, sun exposure, menstruation, fever, and other causes. Patients must become familiar with their own personal triggers. Herpes can be serious in newborns and in patients who are immunocompromised.

Genital herpes caused by the herpes virus type II and spread by sexual contact is discussed in Chapter 2 and Table 2.1.

Treatment and nursing care

Topical acyclovir or oral famciclovir or valacyclovir may reduce viral shedding and hasten healing. Topical ointments should always be applied with gloved hands. Contact precautions should be followed. Patients should be taught the importance of not picking at lesions, because this may cause spreading to other sites. They should not share lipstick and should avoid kissing while lesions are active. Sensitivity to the self-conscious adolescent who has a cold sore is important.

Infantile Eczema (Atopic Dermatitis)

Pathophysiology

Infantile eczema, or atopic dermatitis, is an inflammation of genetically hypersensitive skin (Fig. 30.11). The pathophysiology is characterized by local vasodilation in affected areas. This progresses to *spongiosis*, or the breakdown of dermal cells and the formation of intradermal vesicles. Chronic scratching produces weeping and results in lichenification, or coarsening, of the skin folds. It seems to follow a definite familial history of allergies and asthma.

Symptoms are triggered, but not caused by, substances that enter the body via the digestive tract (food), by inhalation (dust, pollen), by direct contact (wool, soap, strong sunlight), or by injections (insect bites, vaccines). Some children develop the triad of atopic dermatitis, asthma, and hay fever. The major features of atopic dermatitis is eczema, pruritus (itching), and a relapsing course with a positive family history of elevated immunoglobulin E (IgE). Laboratory studies may show an increase in IgE and eosinophil levels.

Manifestations

Although infantile eczema can occur at any age, it is more common during the first 2 years of the infant's

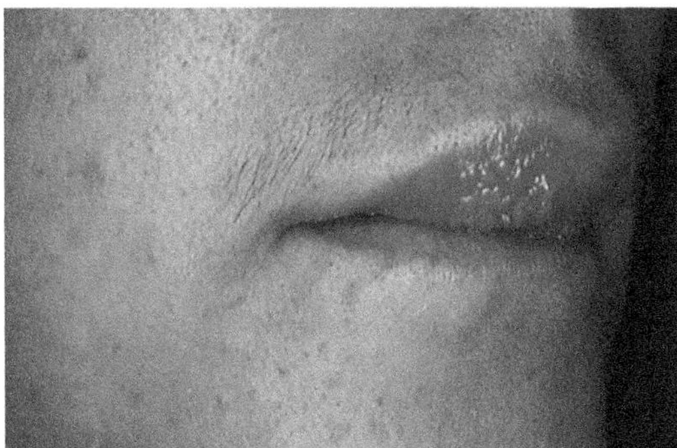

Fig. 30.10 Herpes simplex (cold sores). These begin with tingling skin and sensitivity, and they erupt with tight vesicles, then pustules, and then a crust. Lesions commonly appear on the upper lip. (From Hurwitz, S. [2016]. *Clinical pediatric dermatology: A textbook of skin disorders of childhood and adolescence* [5th ed.]. St. Louis: Elsevier.)

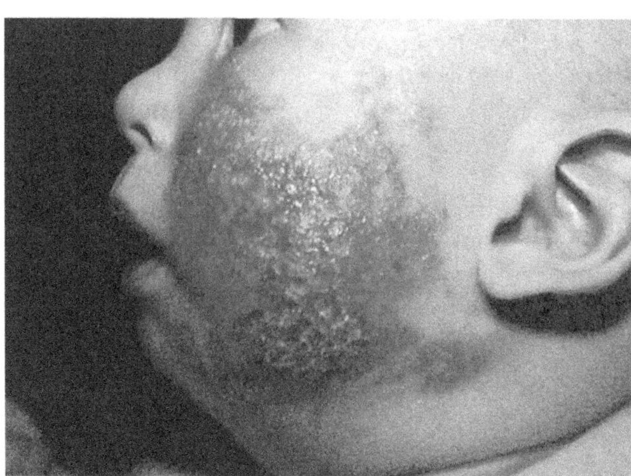

Fig. 30.11 Infantile atopic dermatitis with oozing and crusting of lesions. (From Hurwitz, S. [2016]. *Clinical pediatric dermatology: A textbook of skin disorders of childhood and adolescence* [5th ed.]. St. Louis: Elsevier.)

life. The pruritic lesions form vesicles that weep and develop a dry crust. They are more severe on the face but may occur on the entire body, particularly in the skin folds. Eczema is worse in the winter than in the summer and has periods of temporary remission.

The infant will scratch the affected area because the itching is constant, and the child can become irritable and unable to sleep. Bacterial or viral agents easily infect the lesions. Infants and children with eczema should not be exposed to adults with cold sores because the children may develop a systemic reaction with high fever and multiple vesicles on the eczematous skin. Eczema may flare up after immunization.

Food allergies

Often, a food allergy is thought to be the cause or trigger of atopic dermatitis in infants and children. The eczema caused by the sensitivity results in an impaired skin barrier and increase in sensitization (Canadian Dermatology Association, 2019a). Guidelines have been developed for prevention of food allergies that include peanuts and eggs by providing early exposure to infants at various risk levels to atopic allergy. The guidelines recommend the following:

- Do not restrict maternal diet during pregnancy or lactation.
- Breastfeed exclusively for the first 6 months of life.
- Choose a hydrolyzed cow's milk-based formula, if necessary.
- Do not delay the introduction of any specific solid food beyond 6 months of age. Later introduction of peanuts, fish, or eggs does not prevent, and may even increase, the risk of developing a food allergy.
- Regular ingestion of newly introduced foods (e.g., several times per week and with a soft, mashed consistency to prevent choking) is important to maintain tolerance.

More research is needed in order to more accurately prevent food allergies (Chan, Cummings, CPS Community Paediatrics Committee, Allergy Section, 2013/2016).

Treatment and nursing care

Treatment of the child with infantile eczema is aimed at relieving pruritus (itching), hydrating and lubricating the skin, relieving inflammation, and preventing infection. Efforts should be made to identify triggers of recurrent relapses. An emollient bath is sometimes prescribed for its soothing effect on the skin. Oatmeal and a mixture of cornstarch and baking soda are examples of emollients prescribed. The infant's hair is washed with a soap substitute rather than a shampoo. A bath oil may be used as the lesions begin to heal. This prevents the skin from becoming too dry. For correct use, bath oils should be added after the patient has soaked for a while and the skin is hydrated. In this way, moisture is sealed rather than excluded, as it is when oil is added before the patient gets into the tub. It is important to protect children from slipping on the oily tub surface.

Whenever possible, patients are treated at home because of the danger of infection in the hospital. When soap is used, a mild, nonperfumed soap is used. Glycerin-based lubricants are preferred over lanolin, which may be an irritant to an infant who is allergic to wool. White petroleum costs less and is effective. In 2017, a nonsteroidal PDE-4 inhibitor, crisaborole (Eucrisa), received Health Canada approval for the long-term treatment of mild to moderate atopic dermatitis in children over 2 years of age, which may reduce the need for steroidal creams.

Corticosteroids may be administered systemically or locally but must be monitored for adverse effects such as skin atrophy and systemic effects such as adrenal suppression. Systemic corticosteroids are not routinely used, as their use can be followed by a flare-up of atopic dermatitis when the dose is tapered or discontinued. Antibiotics may be needed if infection is present.

Medication to help relieve itching is ordered for the patient. A child who is uncomfortable and unable to sleep because of itching may be given an antihistamine. Nonsteroidal topical ointments such as pimecrolimus or tacrolimus are used for children over 2 years of age when steroids are not used or effective, but long-term use should be avoided. The types of topical medications are listed in Table 30.1.

Cyclosporine medications are immunosuppressive and increase the risk for infection. Antimetabolites such as mycophenolate mofetil or methotrexate can be prescribed in severe cases of atopic dermatitis. These medications cause immunosuppression, increase the risk for infection, and may cause bone marrow suppression.

Phototherapy may be prescribed, but long-term use may cause adverse effects. Allergen immunotherapy, prebiotics, probiotics, Chinese herbal medication, and vitamin D are all investigational approaches that require further research. Avoiding irritants and identifying environmental food triggers to inflammation for the individual child are essential for the management of atopic dermatitis.

The nurse plays a vital role in the treatment of patients with eczema. The nurse should assess the family's ability to cope with the care of the child at home. Techniques of home bathing or application of soaks combined with quiet playtime can enhance family coping. Control of itching is essential. Ointments are applied with a gloved hand to minimize contact with the skin. The fingernails of the child should be kept short, and cotton gloves or socks can be used to prevent scratching. Appropriate dress is advised, as is using cotton fabric and avoiding wool and stuffed animals because of their allergy potential. Clothes should

Table 30.1 **Types of Topical Medications**

TYPE	DEFINITION
Cream	A water-based emulsion of oil in water that is nongreasy for use on weeping lesions
Ointment	An oil-based emulsion of water in oil that is clear and greasy; used on dry skin; does not rub off easily
Lotion	A suspension of powder in water that should be shaken well before using; may cause drying of skin; often used on scalp lesions
Aerosol spray	Suspension of medication in an alcohol base; alcohol evaporates, leaving medication on the skin; effective for hairy areas
Gel	A clear, semisolid emulsion; liquefies when applied to skin
Bath oils	Bath oils are not used in pediatrics because they lubricate the sides of the tub, causing falls and injuries; the value of the treatment must be weighed against the risks involved; colloidal oatmeal baths may be soothing.

be laundered using mild soaps, avoiding products that contain fragrances or harsh chemicals.

Parents should be taught the principles of general hygiene to prevent secondary infection of the open skin lesions. A plan for identifying possible food sensitivities should be explained to parents. When a food allergen triggers eczema, stopping the food results in a clearing of the skin.

Parent teaching concerning topical therapy. Skin lesions can be pruritic (itchy), scaling, weeping, or crusted. Most skin lesions cause psychological stress, which should be addressed for both the parents and the child with the skin lesion. Prevention of secondary infection is essential, and the nurse should help the parent to identify the signs of inflammation or infection. When topical medication is applied, the lesions may change in form or colour as they heal. Parents should be advised of changes to expect and when to seek follow-up advice. The nurse should teach parents the principles and techniques of applying topical medication:

- Absorption is best when an ointment is applied after a warm bath.
- Medication should be applied by stroking in the direction of hair growth. (Circular or rubbing motions can inflame hair follicles.)
- Follow instructions on how much ointment to apply (e.g., pea-sized bead).
- The use of elbow immobilizers can prevent an infant from scratching while allowing freedom of movement.
- Do not use topical steroids when a viral infection is present.

Nursing Tip

Parents should be taught that the "kiss to make it better" can introduce organisms into a wound that can cause infection.

Staphylococcal Infection

Pathophysiology

The genus of bacteria called *Staphylococcus* comprises common bacteria that are found in dust and on the skin. Under normal conditions, they do not present a problem to the healthy body's defenses. In preterm infants and newborns, whose general resistance is low, skin infections may occur if the number of organisms increases. An abscess may form, and infection may enter the bloodstream. This condition is called *septicemia.* Pneumonia, osteomyelitis, or meningitis may result. Primary infection of the newborn may develop in the umbilicus or circumcision wound. It may occur while the newborn is in the hospital or after discharge. This infection spreads readily from one infant to another. Small pustules on the newborn must be reported immediately.

Treatment and nursing care

Antibiotics effective against the appropriate strain of *Staphylococcus* are administered. Ointments may be locally applied. In past years, the staphylococci that invaded the body developed resistance to the medications in current use. **Methicillin-resistant *Staphylococcus aureus* (MRSA)** infections are resistant to certain antibiotics and are treated under strict contact isolation precautions. The use of disposable individual equipment for patients and aseptic techniques can decrease health care–associated spread of infection.

Community-associated MRSA infections have become more common across the pediatric population. Those at risk include Indigenous children, athletes, and day care attendees, although many infected children have no risk factors (Robinson, Salvadori, & CPS Infectious Diseases and Immunization Committee, 2011/2017). Strategies are needed to decrease overcrowding and supply potable water in affected Indigenous communities in order to reduce rates of illness and infection. MRSA infection can also lead to serious morbidity and mortality (Irvine & CPS First Nations, Inuit and Métis Health Committee, 2012/2017).

Scalded skin syndrome is caused by *S. aureus.* The lesions begin with a mild erythema with sandpaper texture; vesicles appear and rupture, and peeling occurs, exposing a bright red surface. The skin looks as though it had been scalded, and child abuse is often suspected. Intravenous (IV) antibiotics, strict isolation, and prevention of secondary infection are priorities. Maintaining warmth and fluid–electrolyte balance are also important in the plan of care. Healing usually takes place without scarring.

Impetigo

Pathophysiology

Impetigo is an infectious disease of the skin caused by staphylococci or by group A beta-hemolytic streptococci. It results when the organism comes in contact with a break in the skin, such as an insect bite or laceration. The bullous form seen primarily in infants is usually staphylococcal, whereas nonbullous types, more commonly seen in children and young adults, can harbour either organism. The newborn is susceptible to this infection because resistance to skin bacteria is low. Impetigo tends to spread from one area of skin to another and is contagious.

Manifestations

The first symptoms of a bullous lesion are red papules (Fig. 30.12). These eventually become small vesicles or pustules surrounded by a reddened area. When the blister breaks, the surface beneath is raw and weeping. The lesions may occur anywhere, but are most often found around the nose and mouth and in moist areas of the body, such as the creases of the neck, the axilla, and the groin. In older children a crust may form, and scratching may cause further infection. Nephritis may occur as a complication of group A beta-hemolytic streptococcal infections.

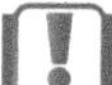 **Safety Alert!**

If a child has recurrent impetigo, the caregiver may be a nasal carrier of *S. aureus*.

Treatment and nursing care

Systemic antibiotics are administered either orally or parenterally. Parents are instructed to wash the lesions three or four times daily to remove crusts. Ointments such as mupirocin (Bactroban) may be prescribed for topical application. Prevention of the disease by treating small cuts promptly is important. The prognosis with proper treatment is good. Nursing care consists primarily of preventing this disease.

Education of parents includes reminding them of the necessity for prompt attention to minor cuts and bites. Impetigo is easily spread from person to person by direct contact with the lesions or indirectly by touching items (clothing, towels, sheets, or toys) that have been used by individuals with this skin disease. Indirect transmission is less frequent than direct person-to-person transmission. Lesions should be covered when out in public until no longer infectious.

If the diagnosis is made when the newborn is still in the hospital, the infant is isolated to prevent other newborns from becoming infected.

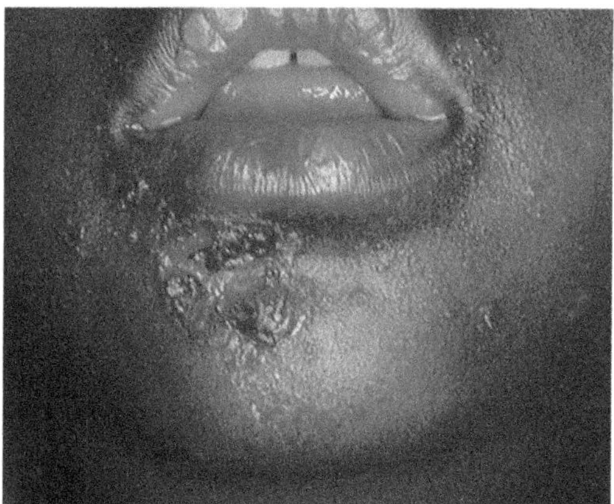

Fig. 30.12 Impetigo. This consists of moist, thin-roofed vesicles with an erythematous base. The vesicles rupture to form a thick, honey-coloured crust. It is a contagious bacterial infection of the skin that is most common in infants and children. (From Hurwitz, S. [2016]. *Clinical pediatric dermatology: A textbook of skin disorders of childhood and adolescence* [5th ed.]. St. Louis: Elsevier.)

Fungal Infections

Pathophysiology

Fungal infections are caused by several closely related fungi that have a preference for invading the stratum corneum, the hair, and the nails. Fungi are larger than bacteria. Some fungi may be transmitted from person to person and others from animal to person.

The common name for this infection is *ringworm.* Some specific fungal infections are named by combining the word *tinea,* which comes from the Latin "worm," and the Latin word denoting the part of the body involved.

Tinea capitis

Tinea capitis ("ringworm of the scalp") is seen in school-age children. Patches of **alopecia** (hair loss) characterize this condition. The hair loses pigment and may break off. The papules become pustules, which progress to red scales. There are areas of circular balding.

Diagnosis is made by history and appearance. Some strains of tinea capitis glow green under a Wood's light.

This condition is treated with griseofulvin, which is administered by mouth. It is given with or after meals to avoid gastrointestinal irritation and increase absorption. Suspensions should be well shaken. Parents are instructed to continue therapy as long as ordered and that they should not miss a dose. Exposure to the sun is to be avoided. Treatment may be necessary for 8 to 12 weeks. Children may go to school but are warned not to exchange hats, combs, or other personal items. Selenium sulfide shampoos are also used, which may eliminate the spores. This infection can be stubborn and may take several weeks to clear. Topical steroids are not used.

Tinea corporis

Tinea corporis ("ringworm of the skin") is evident as an oval scaly, inflamed ring with a clear centre. It is seen on the face, neck, arms, and hands (Fig. 30.13).

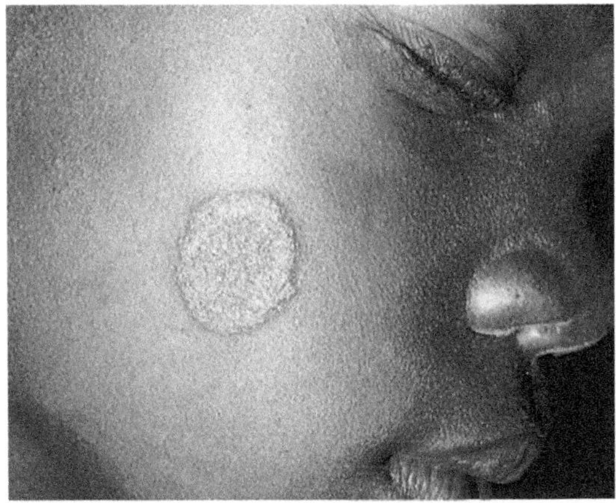

Fig. 30.13 Tinea corporis (ringworm of the body). Scales, hyperpigmented in Whites and depigmented in dark-skinned children, appear on the face, chest, abdomen, or arms, forming multiple circular lesions with clear centres. (From Hurwitz, S. [2016]. *Clinical pediatric dermatology: A textbook of skin disorders of childhood and adolescence* [5th ed.]. St. Louis: Elsevier.)

Infected pets can transmit it. Treatment consists of local application of an antifungal preparation such as clotrimazole (Canesten) for 2 to 4 weeks.

Tinea pedis

Tinea pedis refers to "athlete's foot." Lesions are located between the toes, on the instep, and on the soles. There is accompanying pruritus. It occurs more often in preadolescents and adolescents. Direct microscopic scrapings of the lesions provide the diagnosis.

Treatment consists of topical therapy with an antibacterial or antifungal preparation such as fluconazole, itraconazole, and terbinafine. Burow's solution soaks help heal vesicular or macerated lesions.

Because this condition is aggravated by heat and moisture, the feet must be carefully dried, especially between the toes. Clean cotton socks should be worn. Shoes need to be well ventilated. Plastic shoes that retain heat and moisture are to be avoided. Recurrences are common.

Tinea cruris

Tinea cruris ("thigh") affects the groin area and is commonly referred to as "jock itch." It occurs on the inner aspects of the thighs and scrotum. The initial lesion is small, raised, and scaly. It spreads, and tiny vesicles occur at the margins of the rash. Local application of the antifungal clotrimazole may be effective. General hygiene should be stressed.

Pediculosis

The infestation of humans by lice is termed **pediculosis**. There are three types: pediculosis capitis (head lice), pediculosis corporis (body lice), and pediculosis pubis (crabs or pubic lice). The various types usually remain in the part of the body designated by their name. They are transmitted from person to person or by contact with contaminated articles. Their survival depends on

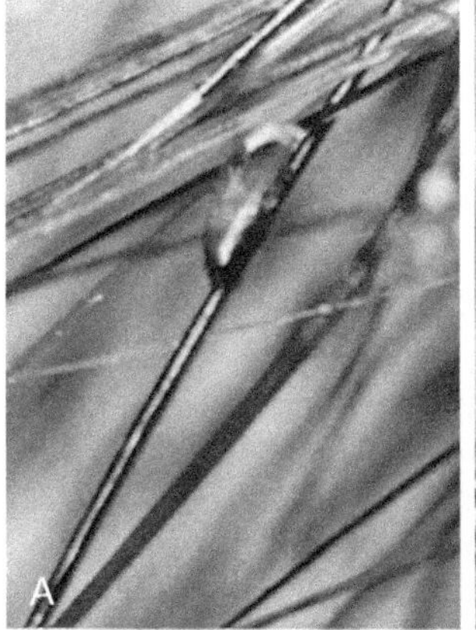

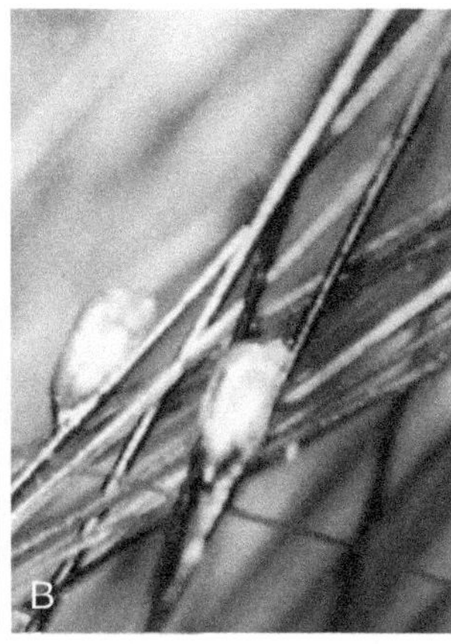

Fig. 30.14 **A,** Empty nit case. **B,** Viable nits. (Courtesy Dr. Michael Sherlock. In Zitelli, B. J., et al. [2018]. *Zitelli and Davis' atlas of pediatric physical diagnosis* [7th ed.]. St. Louis: Elsevier.)

the blood they extract from the infected person. Severe itching in the affected area is the main symptom. In all cases, treatment is aimed at ridding the patient of the parasite, treating the excoriated skin, and preventing the infestation of others. The most common form seen in children is head lice (Fig. 30.14).

Pediculosis capitis

Pathophysiology. Pediculosis capitis, commonly known as *head lice,* affects the scalp and hair. The louse lays eggs (nits) that attach to the hair and hatch within 3 or 4 days. Head lice are more common in girls than in boys because of hair length and the tendency to share combs and hair ornaments. The parasite may be acquired from hats, combs, or hairbrushes. It is easily transferred from one child to another and is seen most often in the school-age child and in preschool children who attend day care centres.

Manifestations. Children with pediculosis capitis suffer from severe itching of the scalp. They scratch their heads frequently and thus often cause further irritation. The hair becomes matted. Pustules and excoriations may be seen about the face. Nurses admitting patients to pediatric units should be on the alert for head lice. In particular, the nurse should inspect the hairline at the back of the neck and about the ears. Crusts, pediculi, nits, and dirt may cause matting of the hair and a foul odour.

Treatment and nursing care. Treatment is directed toward killing the lice, getting rid of the nits, and managing any infections of the face and scalp. Family members and playmates of the child should be examined and treated as necessary. Pediculicide shampoos may be prescribed. Pyrethrins and permethrins are insecticides that have low toxicity to humans. Isopropyl myristate/ST-cyclomethicone solution is a noninsecticidal treatment. Benzyl alcohol may be prescribed. Retreatment may be necessary in 1 week to 10 days. It has been reported that lindane (Kwell) has neurotoxic effects and thus is no longer used for infants and young children (Cummings, Finlay, McDonald, et al., 2018).

If the eyebrows and eyelashes are involved, a thick coating of petroleum jelly may be applied, followed by removal of the remaining nits. Nits on the head are removed by combing wet hair with a fine-toothed comb dipped in a 1:1 solution of white vinegar and water. The hair is then washed. In some cases, recovery is hastened by cutting the hair. Contact precautions should be followed.

Children should be cautioned against swapping caps, headscarves, and combs. Parents are taught the importance of inspecting the child's head regularly. Excluding children with nits or live lice from school or child care has no rational medical basis and is not recommended (Cummings et al., 2018). The families of children in the same classroom or child care group should be alerted to the presence of a case of head lice. Information on diagnosis and management of head lice from a credible source should be shared, along with clear messages that head lice are neither a disease risk nor a sign of lack of cleanliness (Cummings et al., 2018).

Scabies

Pathophysiology

Scabies is a parasitic infection caused by the itch mite, *Sarcoptes scabiei*. It is seen worldwide. The adult female mite, who burrows under the skin and lays eggs, causes scabies. The mite has a round body and four pairs of legs and is visible by microscopic examination. A characteristic burrow is sometimes seen under the skin, particularly between the fingers. Burrows contain the eggs and feces of the mite. Itching is intense, especially at night. A vesiculopustular lesion can occur in children.

Scabies may occur anywhere on the body but is seldom seen on the face. It thrives in moist body folds, but in young children the lesions may appear on the head, the palms, and the soles of the feet. It is spread by close personal contact, including sexual relations. It is rarely transmitted by fomites because the isolated mite dies within 2 to 3 days.

It can affect individuals at any socioeconomic level, but at a higher risk are individuals who live in overcrowded conditions or in poverty. Indigenous people are disproportionately affected because of the overcrowding and poverty that exist in many of their communities (Banerji & CPS First Nations, Inuit, and Métis Health Committee, 2015/2018).

Treatment and nursing care

Treatment consists of the application of permethrin. It can be used for children older than 2 months of age. Parents are instructed to follow the directions carefully. All family members, babysitters, and close associates require treatment. Contact isolation precautions are followed. An oral antiparasitic agent, ivermectin, has been approved for use in children weighing more than 15 kg in cases where the response to other methods is deficient. Oral ivermectin is effective but it is not available in Canada except through Health Canada's Special Access Program (Banerji & CPS First Nations, Inuit, and Métis Health Committee, 2015/2018).

Linen and clothes should be washed and dried in high heat. Stuffed toys and nonwashable items should be stored in bags for 1 week before reuse.

Hair Thinning–Traction Alopecia

Hair-style trends, such as tight braiding, tight pony tails, multiple pony tails, use of extensions, and hair twisting, contribute to "traction alopecia," which is a thinning caused by chronic pulling or twisting of the hair. When gels, pomades, or oils are also used to slick the hair back, hair follicles can be blocked and local inflammation occurs, resulting in scarring and hair loss. Acne that occurs along the forehead is seen as an early sign of this process. Recommended hair care products include those that are silicone or water based rather than oil based, which can block pores (Hilton, 2016).

Bedbugs

Pathophysiology

Bedbugs (*Cimex lectularius* and *Cimex hemipterus*, family *Cimicidae*) cause a parasitic infestation in humans around the world. Since the 1990s, the bedbug populations have been increasing on an annual basis because of an increase in global travel, trading of goods, and the rising number of insecticide-resistant bedbugs (Lai, Ho, Glick, et al., 2016). The increase in the number of bedbugs has caused a significant socioeconomic problem in public health. No causal relationship has been found between bedbugs and infectious disease transmission in humans (Lai et al., 2016).

Bedbugs are tiny, wingless brown insects up to 10 mm long with an oval, broad, flat body and a short, broad head. They are unable to jump or fly. They bite the skin and feed on the blood of sleeping humans, which deepens their colour to a blood red. The eggs are almost microscopic with a sticky coating and can be easily transferred on objects such as suitcases. The eggs hatch in 6 to 17 days and feed as soon as food is accessible. Bedbugs can survive without feeding for up to a year and a half or longer and can also live for a year or more in an environmental temperature of 21 to 28°C.

Bites can appear up to 14 days after being bitten and can occur anywhere on the body but are commonly found on the face, neck, arms, legs, and chest. Skin reactions vary from none to small itchy welts and rarely lead to severe allergic reactions.

Treatment and nursing care

It is important for nurses to encourage the child and family not to scratch the bites and keep the skin clean in order to avoid infection. Antiseptic creams or lotions, in addition to antihistamines, may be helpful.

A key treatment strategy is to remove the bedbugs from the environment. Methods include vacuuming and then steam cleaning, heating, freezing, washing, and discarding items. The Government of Canada (2015) strongly recommends hiring a licensed professional pest control operator and using registered bedbug control products to safely manage potential toxins.

INJURIES

Burns

Pathophysiology

Burns often occur during childhood. They are the leading cause of accidental death in the home for children between 1 and 4 years of age. Sometimes burns are a result of child abuse and neglect. The two times of day during which burns are most likely to occur are the early morning hours before parents awaken and after school. There are several types of burns:

- *Thermal:* caused by fire or a scalding vapor or liquid
- *Chemical:* caused by a corrosive powder or liquid
- *Electrical:* caused by electrical current passing through the body
- *Radiation:* caused by X-rays or radioactive substances

Burns can involve the skin or mucous membranes. When a child is burned by fire near the face, the flames may be inhaled, causing a burn of the mucous membrane lining the airway. Assessing for resulting edema and respiratory distress is a priority. When a bottle or food is heated in the microwave oven, "hot spots" occur that can cause burns to the mucous membranes lining the mouth.

The differences in responses of children from those of adults to a burn are as follows:

- The child's skin is thinner than that of the adult, leading to a more serious depth of burn with lower temperatures and shorter exposure than with adults.
- The large body surface area (BSA) of the child results in greater fluid, electrolyte, and heat loss.
- Immature response systems in young children can cause shock and heart failure.
- The increased basal metabolic rate (BMR) of a child results in increased protein and calorie needs.
- Less muscle and fat in the body results in protein and caloric deficiencies when oral intake is limited.
- The skin is more elastic in children, causing pulling on the scarring areas and resulting in formation of a larger scar; children may have to wear compression garments for up to 2 years. Many children are left with disfigurement, permanent disability, and emotional struggles.
- The immature immune system predisposes the child to developing infections that complicate burn treatment.
- The prolonged immobilization and treatment required for burns adversely affect growth and development.

Classification

The severity of a burn depends on the area, extent, and depth of involvement. The size of the burn is calculated as a percentage of **total body surface area (TBSA)**. Age-related charts are used for children because their body proportions differ from those of adults (Fig. 30.15). A useful rapid estimation of the BSA involved in an

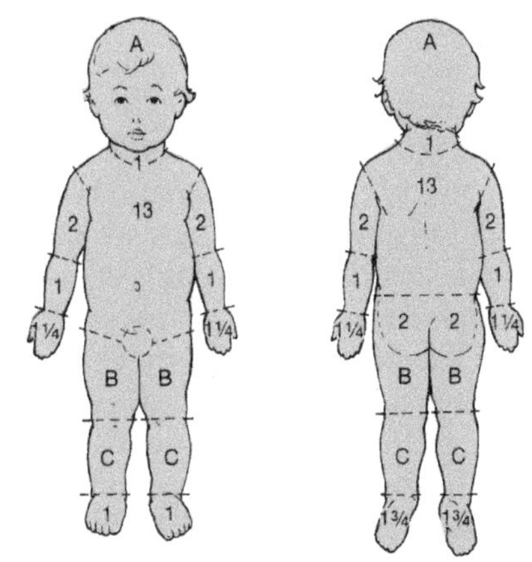

RELATIVE PERCENTAGES OF AREAS AFFECTED BY GROWTH

A

AREA	BIRTH	AGE 1 YR	AGE 5 YR
A = ½ of head	9½	8½	6½
B = ½ of one thigh	2¾	3¼	4
C = ½ of one leg	2½	2½	2¾

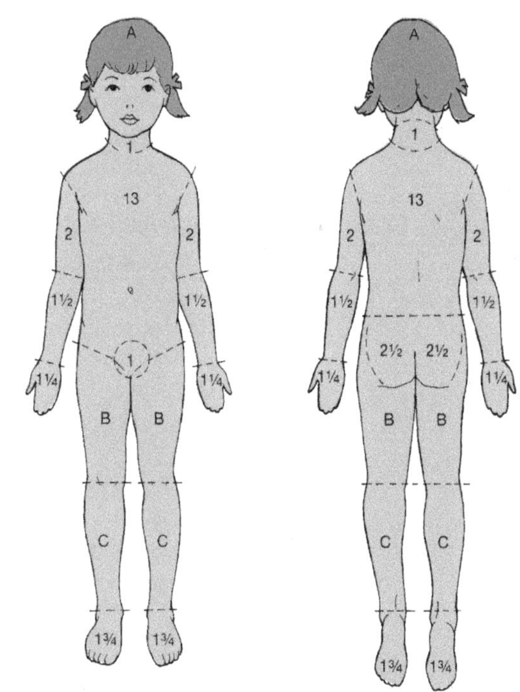

RELATIVE PERCENTAGES OF AREAS AFFECTED BY GROWTH

B

AREA	AGE 10 YR	AGE 15 YR	ADULT
A = ½ of head	5½	4½	3½
B = ½ of one thigh	4½	4½	4¾
C = ½ of one leg	3	3¼	3½

Fig. 30.15 Body surface area (BSA) charts. These charts are used to determine the developmentally related percentage of BSA burned. The percentage of BSA involved is the basis for determining the fluid and nutritional needs of the burned child. In children younger than 3 years of age, the "rule of nines" assigns the infant's head as 18% of total BSA (TBSA) and the lower extremities as 14% TBSA, with 9% assigned to each arm and 1¼% to the hands or palms. These charts are also referred to as the *Lund and Browder chart*. (From Hockenberry, M. J., & Wilson, D. [2015]. *Wong's nursing care of infants and children* [10th ed.], Figure 24-5. St. Louis: Elsevier.)

infant or child with a burn is the "rule of palm," which is the measurement of the area between the crease of the skin at the wrist to the crease at the beginning of the fingers in the palm of the hand. It is estimated to be 1% of the child's BSA.

The terms *partial thickness* and *full thickness* describe the extent of destruction of the skin. In partial-thickness burns, only some of the skin layers are damaged. Full-thickness burns are deeper and more extensive and may necessitate skin grafting. The classification of and first aid treatment for burns are summarized in Table 30.2. The volume of IV fluids needed for treatment is calculated from the estimated extent and depth of the burn. One can survive a rather extensive superficial burn, whereas a deep burn involving a smaller surface area can threaten the patient's life. Table 30.3 outlines children's responses to burn injuries.

Burns can also be complicated by fractures, soft tissue injury, or pre-existing conditions such as diabetes, obesity, epilepsy, and heart or renal disease. The "6 Cs" of burn care include clothing, cooling, cleaning, chemoprophylaxis, covering, and comforting or pain relief (Herndon & Jones, 2007). Burn treatment can be administered in an outpatient clinic, in a general hospital, or at a specialized burn centre.

Treatment

Care of electrical burns. When electricity is the cause of the injury, the child should be assessed for entry and exit lesions that may appear as a small erythematous area. The locations of the entry and exit wounds indicate the path of electricity through the body (Fig. 30.16). Muscle damage can occur, and if the electrical current passes through the heart, cardiac muscle damage can result. Deep muscle damage can cause renal impairment from myoglobinuria. The child should be observed closely for responses with electrocardiography (ECG) monitors, the recording of vital signs, and assessment of cardiac enzymes before discharge.

Nursing Tip

Electrical burns of the mouth are common in small children, who put everything into their mouths. Biting into electrical cords is not unusual. Such wounds are usually deep and leave an entrance and an exit burn. They are subject to bleeding for several weeks.

Emergency care. Community education programs emphasize the response to a child with a burn injury and should include the following instructions:

- *Stop the burning process.* Stop, drop, and roll is the sequence of care. Rolling the child in a blanket smother's the flames. A caustic powder should be brushed off before water is used to wash the area; this prevents spreading the caustic substance and enlarging the area of contact. Electricity should be turned off before touching a child who has been electrocuted.

Table 30.2 Classification and First Aid Treatment of Burns

DEGREE	ANATOMY AND DEPTH	APPEARANCE AND SENSATION	FIRST AID TREATMENT
Superficial (first)	Epidermis only	Skin red but blanches easily on pressure and refills quickly; painful, indicating tissue viability	Immerse in cool water or normal saline to halt burning process; apply an antimicrobial ointment.
Partial thickness (second)	Epidermis and much of dermis; partial thickness	Blistered, moist, pink, or red; painful, indicating tissue viability	If area is small, treat as if for first-degree burn and apply antimicrobial ointment; otherwise treat as if for deep dermal burn.
Deep dermal (deep partial thickness)	Extends deep into dermis; partial thickness but can become full thickness with infection, trauma, or poor blood supply	Mottled; red, tan, or dull white; blisters; painful, indicating tissue viability	Immerse in cool water or normal saline to halt burning process; cover with sterile dressing or clean cloth to prevent contamination and decrease pain from contact with air; avoid breaking blisters; seek medical attention immediately.
Full thickness (third)	Subdermal; involves entire skin and all its structures; full thickness	Tough, leathery, dry; does not blanch or refill; dull brown, tan, black, or pearly white; painless to touch, indicating death of tissue	Halt the burning process by immersing in cool water or normal saline or rolling in a blanket or rug. Wrap in a clean sheet or other sterile dressing; provide blanket for warmth. Have victim lie down; *do not* apply ointment or any other substance to burned area. Take patient to nearest emergency treatment centre immediately. Skin grafting may be needed.
Fourth	All skin and nerve endings are destroyed; includes muscle and bone destruction	Blood vessels and bone may be visible. Necrosis occurs.	

Table 30.3 Response to Burn Injury in Children*

RESPONSE	EFFECT
Capillary permeability increases, and hypovolemia occurs.	There is a loss of plasma, proteins, and fluids; shock occurs.
Blood flow to vital organs increases, and blood flow to periphery of body and nonvital organs decreases.	Peristalsis ceases (ileus). Curling ulcer can form in stomach.
Body metabolism increases to maintain heat.	Increased basal metabolic rate (BMR) can strain the heart by causing increased cardiac output.
Damage to red blood cells and hemolysis results in anemia.	Anemia causes increased cardiac output to maintain perfusion.
Open wounds of burn can predispose to infection. Dead tissue provides a medium for bacterial growth.	Immature immune system can be overwhelmed, and sepsis can result.
Waste products accumulate in the blood because of anemia and slow perfusion of nonvital organs.	Renal failure, cardiac failure, and pulmonary edema can complicate toxicity from burn injury.

*Thermal injuries produce both local and systemic effects.

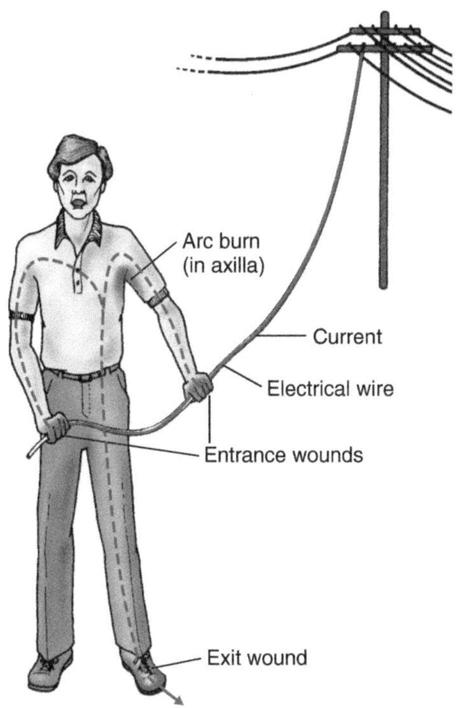

Fig. 30.16 Mechanism of electrical injury. The electrical current enters the body and travels through the heart before exiting the body. All patients with electrical injuries should have their cardiac enzymes monitored to determine if heart damage has occurred. (From Ignatavicius, D. D., & Workman, M. L. [2016]. *Medical-surgical nursing: Patient-centered collaborative care* [8th ed.]. St. Louis: Saunders.)

- *Evaluate the injury.* Check the "ABCs" (**a**irway, **b**reathing, **c**irculation) of the victim. Cardiopulmonary resuscitation (CAB—compressions-airway-breathing) is initiated as appropriate. Minor burns can be treated at home or as an outpatient; a health care provider should assess major burns.
- *Cover the burn.* The burned area should be covered with a clean cloth to minimize contact with air, reduce pain, minimize hypothermia, and prevent contamination of the wound. Burned clothing and jewellery should be removed, because metal retains heat and continues the burn injury.
- *Transport to a hospital.* Do not give any fluids by mouth, because peristalsis may have diminished in response to the burn injury. If available, IV fluids and oxygen should be administered, and the child comforted and reassured.

Safety Alert!

The child should be taught to stop, drop, and roll if the clothes become ignited.

Care of minor thermal burns. Minor burns are treated at home and followed with clinic visits until healing is complete. The wound is cleansed and an antimicrobial ointment applied with a loose dressing. Blisters are not disturbed unless a chemical burn occurred. Dressings are changed as prescribed, and the parent is advised to report any sign of infection. The status of tetanus immunization is reviewed and updated as needed. Pain relief is administered as needed.

The wound of a minor burn is usually completely healed within 20 days. Evaluation of scarring and effect on range of motion (ROM) will determine future follow-up needs. Sun exposure will increase discoloration of new skin formed in the healing process.

Care of major burns. The health care provider, nurse, respiratory therapist, and other specialists in the emergency department or, in some instances, the operating room handle the immediate treatment of shock in cases of severe burns. Priorities include establishing an airway in patients with facial burns or smoke inhalation, instituting IV lines, and assessing burn wounds and other, perhaps initially unrecognized, injuries. At times, some of these procedures are performed simultaneously.

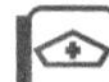
Nursing Tip

A severe burn can cause a loss of function in two of the most important properties of the skin: the ability to protect against infection and the ability to prevent loss of body fluid.

Cyanosis, singed nasal hairs, charred lips, and stridor are indications that flames may have been inhaled.

An endotracheal tube is inserted to maintain an adequate airway, although this is not required for all patients. This permits the delivery of humidified air with oxygen, easy removal of secretions from respiratory passages, and use of a pressure ventilator if needed. Sedation is administered with caution to prevent further respiratory inhibition.

If **eschar** (*eschara,* "scab") from burns on the trunk inhibits respirations, an incision called an *escharotomy* is made to prevent the restriction of chest movement. Blood gas levels, including level of carbon monoxide, are ascertained. The child is placed on sterile sheets. Attendants wear a facemask, sterile gown, and gloves.

IV infusions are begun to prevent intravascular dehydration and electrolyte imbalance. Ringer's lactate solution is often used initially. Albumin or plasma may be used when capillary permeability is restored (within 24 to 48 hours).

Laboratory studies include hematocrit and sodium chloride, potassium, carbon dioxide, blood urea nitrogen, creatinine, and serum protein levels. Blood typing and cross matching are performed. Fluid therapy requires close monitoring throughout hospitalization. To determine urine volume and characteristics, a urinary catheter is inserted and an accurate intake and output record is maintained.

The loss of fluid causes renal vasoconstriction, leading to depressed glomerular filtration and oliguria. Acute renal failure can develop without adequate therapy. Urine output is observed hourly. It varies considerably but, on average, 20 to 30 mL/hr for patients older than 2 years of age is considered adequate during the resuscitative stage. The patient's weight is recorded and used as baseline data for determining adequacy of ongoing treatment.

A nasogastric tube is inserted and is attached to low wall suction. This empties the stomach and prevents complications such as gastric dilation, vomiting, and paralytic **ileus** (intestinal muscle paralysis). The patient has nothing by mouth for the first 24 hours. Sporadic bleeding as a result of a **Curling ulcer** (stress ulcer) is not uncommon in patients with severe burns; the administration of IV antacids such as cimetidine can help to reduce its incidence. Pain control and close monitoring are essential.

Wound care. The goals of wound care include the removal of necrotic tissue to allow healing to take place, maintenance of moist conditions and adequate circulation, conservation of body heat and fluids, prevention of infection, and minimization of scar formation. The loss of skin increases the threat of infection, and fluid loss caused by evaporation can be significant. The immune system is depressed. Strict asepsis is maintained, and the wound site is treated in accordance with the health care provider's instructions. A tetanus immunization history is obtained, and tetanus prophylaxis is administered as required. Low doses of antibiotics may be prescribed to prevent streptococcal infection.

Immediate care of the wound itself includes cleansing and **debridement** (removal of dried crusts) of necrotic tissue. Cleaning a burn wound can be painful, and pain-relief measures are a priority. The wound is cleansed by tub baths or, in many cases, whirlpool baths are used to soften necrotic areas and debride the wound. The black eschar of necrotic tissue can be debrided via a whirlpool bath. Yellow eschar is not removed.

Dressings may be applied. Aquacel AG and Acticoat are silver-based antimicrobial dressings that provide a long-acting and sustained pain-relief and bacteriocidal effect, and the dressing can remain in place for several days. A partial-thickness burn is treated with antibacterial agents such as silver sulfadiazine, mafenide acetate, or bacitracin after initial assessment and cleaning. Box 30.2 lists some topical agents used in treating burn patients.

A semi-open method of burn dressing may be used, although exposure methods may be useful on accessible areas such as the face. The wound is covered by a few layers of sterile gauze that has been saturated with antibacterial ointment or cream. The gauze may be held in place by elastic netting (Fig. 30.17). When the wound is being dressed, *keep all burned surfaces separated and not touching to avoid tissue damage.* A sterile blanket may be used to prevent chilling.

Surgical debridement is done, when needed, to cleanse the wound and prepare the new granulation tissue for grafting. All infection must be cleared before skin grafting can be performed. A biological dressing or a synthetic dressing may be used to prevent fluid loss and to promote healing. The burn area is closed and resurfaced by grafting.

Box 30.2 Topical Agents Used to Treat Burn Patients

SILVER SULFADIAZINE CREAM 1%

Cream is effective against Gram-negative and Gram-positive bacteria and yeast *(Candida albicans).*
Do not use if patient is allergic to sulpha drugs.
Cream does not sting; it softens eschar.
Do not waste; cream is expensive.
Gently remove old cream before reapplying.

MAFENIDE ACETATE 10%

Agent is effective against Gram-positive and Gram-negative organisms; penetrates eschar.
Agent is painful because it draws water out of the tissues; pain may last 15 to 30 minutes or longer.
Remain with the child after application for comfort and diversion.
Do not apply to the face.
There is a potential for metabolic acidosis.

BACITRACIN

Agent is painless and is applied twice daily.
Agent is a low-cost prophylactic antibiotic.

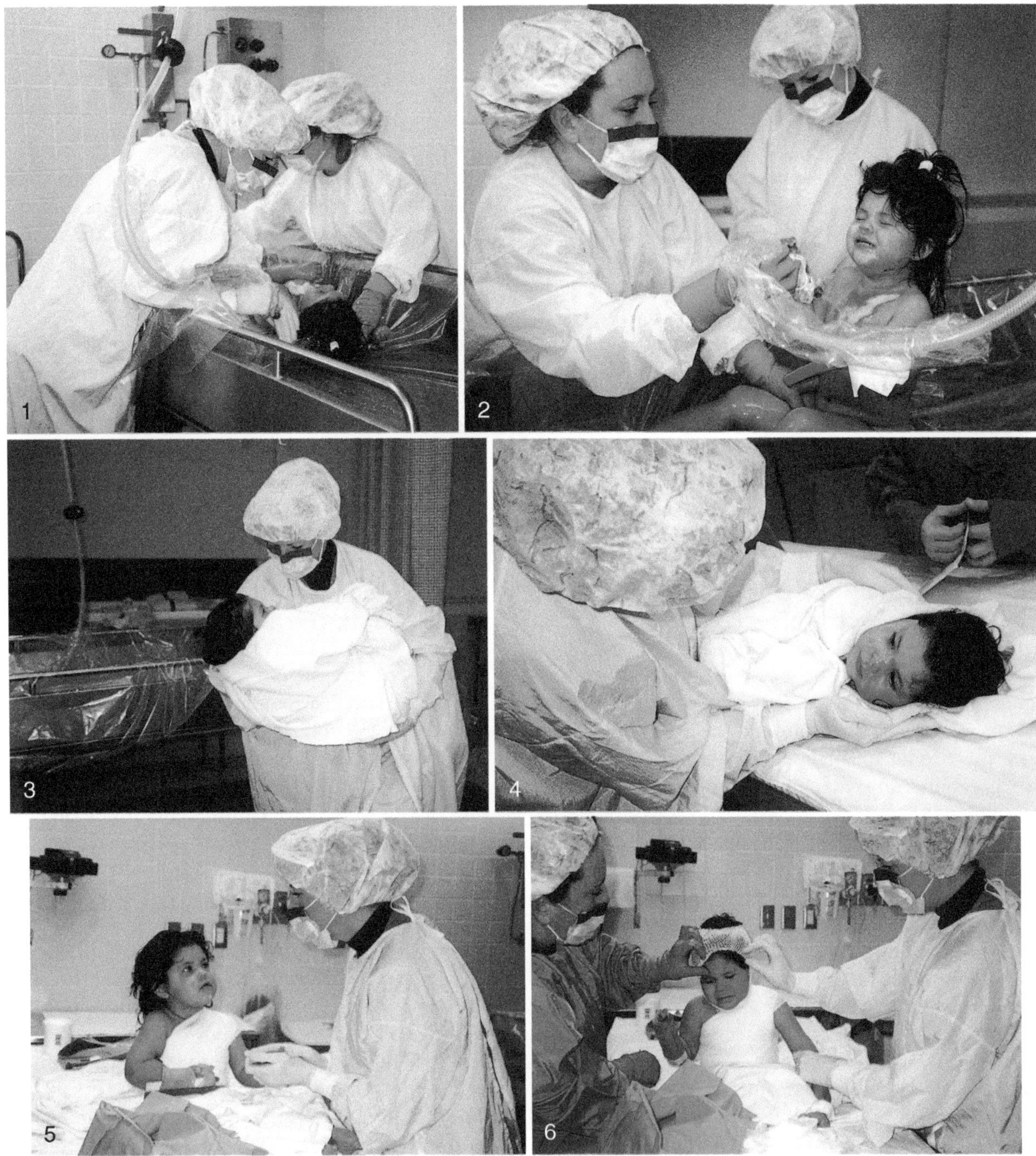

Fig. 30.17 This child is having her burn dressings changed and is undergoing whirlpool bath debridement. She is gently dried with sterile towels, and a pressure dressing is reapplied. (Photos courtesy Pat Spier, RN-C.)

Skin grafts. Temporary grafts are used during the acute stage of recovery. They protect the wound from infection and reduce fluid loss but are eventually rejected by the body. Temporary grafts include **homografts** (usually tissue from disease-free cadavers) and **heterografts** (tissues obtained from different species). Heterografts are also referred to as **xenografts** (*xeno,* "foreign," and *graft,* "slice of skin").

Many grafts are derived from pigskin, which is available commercially either fresh or frozen; these biological dressings are often used in children and are called *porcine xenografts*. They are particularly useful in partial-thickness or deep dermal burns and have greatly improved burn management. Deep dermal wounds may be preceded by tangential *(merely touching)* excision, which is a surgical technique of removing burned eschar with a dermatome. Thin layers are shaved down to the live tissues, and temporary porcine grafts are applied.

There are two types of permanent grafts: autografts and isografts. An **autograft** (*auto,* "self") is healthy tissue obtained from another part of the patient's body. An **isograft** (*iso,* "equal") is obtained from the patient's identical twin or genotype. Permanent grafts are performed during the rehabilitative stage of the patient's illness to improve appearance and function. The site from which the tissue is removed is called the *donor area*.

Advances in grafting techniques have improved the overall prognosis in burn patients and have helped to minimize scarring. A split-thickness skin graft can be prepared with the use of a dermatome. For extensive burns, it is sometimes difficult to find enough intact skin for use. Special methods such as the Tanner mesh graft may be used. In this method, a strip of split-thickness skin is run through a special cutting machine that makes multiple slits; this expands the skin to provide more coverage, which in some cases is as much as nine times the original area of the skin. The graft is sutured in place to maintain tension.

The "postage stamp" graft consists of small pieces of donor skin placed on the granulation tissue. Spaces between grafts allow for drainage and healing. Full-cover grafts are sheets of skin placed intact over the wound. These are cosmetically more effective than patch and mesh grafts but are not always available. The donor site is covered with xenograft or fine mesh gauze; it heals in about 2 weeks.

Newly grafted areas are covered with sterile dressings. Every effort is made to prevent bleeding and infection. The areas surrounding the wound are observed for edema and impaired circulation. Hyperbaric oxygen therapy can enhance the healing of grafts (see Chapter 21).

Biological dressings. Biological dressings can be applied to a noninfected burn wound within 6 hours of the injury and will peel off as the wound heals. Dressing changes are not necessary. The dressings are made from newborn foreskin fibroblast cells combined in a nylon mesh that is sterile and frozen for storage. After thawing, they cannot be refrozen. The dressings contain human or pigskin products, and hypersensitivity should be considered before use.

Vacuum-assisted wound closure is negative pressure applied to a wound after the wound is packed and sealed. Fluid from the wound exits via a suction tube into a canister. The vacuum draws out fluid, increases blood perfusion to the tissues, and decreases bacterial contamination and scarring while enhancing healing.

Posthealing care. After basic healing has occurred, a nonperfumed moisturizer cream or cocoa butter may be recommended to maintain skin moisture. Ointments containing lanolin are not advised. Sun block should be used to prevent hyperpigmentation of the newly healed skin. It may take 2 years for complete healing to occur.

Systemic antihistamines such as diphenhydramine (Benadryl) or hydroxyzine (Atarax) may be prescribed to control itching. Bicarbonate of soda baths are soothing.

 **Nursing Tip**

Disorientation, fever, and diminished bowel sounds may be early signs of sepsis.

Nursing care of the burned child

Children who have suffered extensive burns and survive the early dangers of their injuries face a long period of hospitalization and require specialized care. The various aspects of nursing care differ with the age of the patient, the area of the burn, and the type of treatment used.

Protective (reverse) isolation is instituted. All instruments that come in contact with the wound must be sterile. Ointments are applied with a sterile gloved hand or sterile tongue depressor. Care must be taken to prevent injury to granulation tissue. Analgesics are administered *before* painful procedures are performed.

The nurse must report immediately any signs of infection: elevations of temperature, pulse, and respiration; restlessness and confusion; pain; purulent drainage; and an odour emanating from the wound dressing. A careful description of the wound in the nurse's notes facilitates daily comparison and determination of progress.

The nurse must remain alert for signs of fluid overload, in particular, behavioural changes and altered sensorium. Although initially restricted to prevent nausea and vomiting, oral fluids are necessary during the convalescent stages to prevent kidney damage and to maintain body fluid requirements. The nurse needs to use ingenuity to persuade the child to take sufficient amounts of fluids. An accurate record of intake and output of fluids is kept.

The demands on the metabolism as it copes with this trauma are increased, and more calories are spent as water evaporates from the wound site. Frequent feedings of foods high in calories, protein, and iron are therefore necessary. A high-protein diet—a normal diet with added amounts of meat, milk, eggs, fish, or poultry—is usually prescribed. Iron therapy may be initiated if anemia begins to develop. High-energy meal replacement drinks are nourishing between-meal drinks for burn patients with such needs. Small amounts are offered frequently. Vitamins A, B, and C and zinc sulphate are given to hasten healing and to stimulate the appetite. Gavage feedings may be necessary. Accurate daily records of foods consumed, calorie count, and the patient's weight will help to determine their nutritional status.

The nurse needs to bear in mind that other, unaffected parts of the body need exercise and proper positioning to prevent painful contractures. The child's position should be changed every 2 to 4 hours unless contraindicated. A footboard is used to prevent foot drop. Support should be provided by means of pillows, sandbags, and rolled towels as necessary.

The physiotherapist attends to the child regularly for exercise and to keep the joints limber and healthy. The child should begin to ambulate as soon as possible. Self-help activities and mobility need to be encouraged. Pressure splints or elasticized garments help to reduce scar tissue and are sometimes worn for months after discharge.

The importance of burn prevention cannot be overemphasized. Nurses also need to be able detect burns resulting from accidents and those from child abuse. For instance, Fig. 30.18 shows the difference in appearance of a scald burn wound from an accidental spill and a scald wound that was inflicted (child abuse). Nurses have important roles in health education and prevention of burns and scalds. Table 30.4 outlines family safety tips for preventing burns.

Emotional support. A burn injury can be taxing to the child and parents. It may require long periods of hospitalization and frequent readmissions. The accident itself may be terrifying for the child but can be made even worse if caused by disobedience. Nurses need to encourage these children to express their feelings. The long-term patient requires diversions of various types. School tutors should be requested, and contact must be maintained with peers through cards, email, or social media.

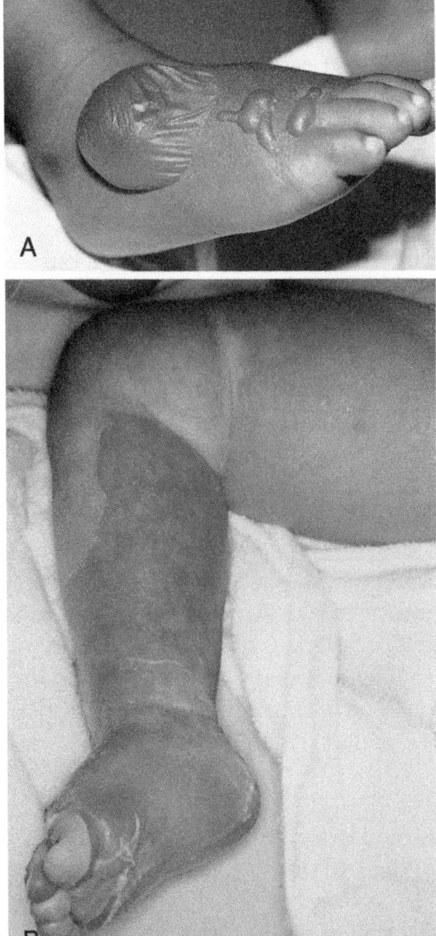

Fig. 30.18 Scald burns. **A,** An accidental scald burn. Note the droplet pattern indicating a splash. **B,** Nonaccidental scald burn. An inflicted scald reveals severe extensive second-degree burns on the entire leg. (From Zitelli, B. J., et al. [2018]. *Zitelli and Davis' atlas of pediatric physical diagnosis* [7th ed.]. St. Louis: Elsevier.)

Nurses must give constant support to the parents, who may feel guilty if the child was injured in an accident. Nurses can indicate through their manner of communication that they do not blame the parents for what has happened.

Preparation for discharge begins early and involves the multidisciplinary health care team, which may include the health care provider, nurse, public health nurse, schoolteacher, physiotherapist, psychologist, and child-life specialist. Instructions are provided regarding wound care, diet, exercise, and rest. Return appointments are made, and referral agencies are contacted. Methods to improve the physical appearance of the patient are also discussed.

Nursing Tip

In cases of car, house, or airplane fires, patients may face additional crises, such as the loss of relatives, pets, and possessions.

Sunburn

Sunburn is a common skin injury caused by overexposure to the sun, especially at midday. Sunburn can be a minor epidermal burn or a more serious partial-thickness burn with blistering. It can also include fever, nausea, and headache. Small infants have less melanin to protect their skin and need to be physically protected from excessive sun exposure. In addition, certain medications render the skin more sensitive to the sun, such as acne medications, nonsteroidal anti-inflammatory drugs (NSAIDs), and birth control pills. Melanoma is a common form of cancer that occurs as a result of frequent sun exposure without protection, thus it is important to avoid sunburn in children.

The exposure of ultraviolet (UV) radiation from indoor tanning beds before the age of 35 causes premature aging and significantly increases the risk of skin cancer, including melanoma, the deadliest form of skin cancer. In Canada, children and youth under 18 years of age are banned from commercial indoor tanning facilities, only in a few provinces (Taddeo, Stanwick, & CPS Adolescent Health Committee, 2012/2018). The CPS recommends that children and youth under the age of 18 years be prohibited by law from using commercial indoor tanning facilities, as this would be a significant cancer prevention strategy (Taddeo et al., 2012/2018).

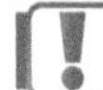
Safety Alert!

Contact the child's health care provider at once if an infant under the age of 1 year gets a severe sunburn. It is a medical emergency.

Table 30.4 Prevention of Pediatric Burns and Scald Injuries

SOURCE OF INJURY	SAFETY TIPS
Gas fireplaces	Use safety gates and barriers around the fireplace to keep children away from the glass and metal pieces of the fireplace. The glass can heat up to over 200°C in about 6 minutes. Always supervise to ensure young children cannot access the fireplace.
Smoke alarms and carbon monoxide detectors	Change the batteries yearly when the clocks change and discard the detectors after 10 years of use. Smoke alarms are a proven way to prevent injuries and death from fires. Install both alarms on every level and in every sleeping area. Vacuum the detectors occasionally.
Lighters and matches	Make sure to use child-resistant lighters and keep them out of sight and reach.
Hot liquids and scalds	Keep children away from hot liquids. Scalds are the types of burn injuries that most often send children to hospital. Scalds are burns from hot water or liquids. Young children under the age of 5 suffer 83% of all scald injuries requiring hospital admission. Use a travel coffee mug with a lid to avoid spillage onto children. Keep the child safely out of the way when you are cooking. Cook on the back burners and turn the pot handles away from the front. Keep cords from the hot water kettle and other appliances out of reach.
Hot tap water	Check water temperature at home after running the hot water tap for 2 minutes. If a lot of hot water was used recently, wait 2 hours before testing. If the water is higher than 49°C (120°F), lower water temperature. A third-degree burn (characterized by blistering, intense pain, and permanent tissue damage) will occur in children in only 5 seconds when water temperature is 60°C (140°F). At 55°C (130°F), a third-degree burn will occur in 15 seconds, while the time to produce a third-degree burn extends to at least 5 minutes when water temperature is 49°C (120°F). The temperature should not be below 50°C as it may increase the risk of Legionnaires' disease, a form of pneumonia, due to bacterial growth in the tank. That disease is caused by *Legionella* bacteria, which live in water.
Safe bath time	Always check the temperature of the water before bathing the child. Make sure to test the water with your elbow or forearm in the water. Ideally, it should feel warm, not hot. Mix the water to get rid of hot spots. Hot water guards that prevent scalding can be installed in the taps.

From Parachute. (2015). *Scalds and burns*. Retrieved from http://www.parachutecanada.org/injury-topics/topic/C18.

Goals of treatment include stopping sun exposure, treating inflammation, and rehydrating the skin. Immersion in a tepid water bath (36.7°C [98°F]) for 15 to 20 minutes is the initial treatment. A bland oil-in-water moisturizing lotion can be applied. Cool compresses, aloe vera, and calamine lotion are recommended (Dickey & Chiu, 2016).

Education is key in preventing sunburn. Covering the skin with clothing, wearing a hat, and using sunscreen liberally are recommended. Two types of products are available.

Sunscreens

Physical sunscreens that contain a cream, such as zinc oxide, magnesium dioxide, or titanium dioxide, block UV light and are usually referred to as *sunblocks*. Most sunburns are caused by UVB rays (Dickey & Chiu, 2016).

Chemical sunscreens that contain para-aminobenzoic acid (PABA), avobenzone, and ecamsule absorb UVB and UVA wavelengths and are usually labelled "Broad Spectrum Protection." Minimum SPF protection should be 30 (Canadian Dermatology Association, 2019b). (SPF is the minimal time of sunlight required to produce a mild sunburn compared to no sunscreen use.) If the individual normally burns in sun exposure after 10 minutes, the use of SPF 15 sun screen will allow 10 × 15, or 150, minutes of sun exposure before burning occurs. SPF refers to UVB rays only (Dickey & Chiu, 2016).

Sunscreen should be worn when outdoors, even when the sun is not shining brightly, and reapplied every 2 hours after swimming. Sunscreen is not recommended for infants under 6 months old, who can rub it in their eyes and mouth, so they should be covered with hats, sun-protective clothing, and sunshades (CPS, 2016).

Sunglasses

Many sunglasses block UV rays, and some block both UVA and UVB rays, known as "UV400 protection." The wrap-around style of frame provides the best protection for the eyes against the UV rays linked to cataracts and macular degeneration.

Frostbite

In exposure to extreme cold, warmth is lost in the periphery of the body before the core temperature drops, and the extremities can suffer considerable damage before the onset of potentially fatal hypothermia. **Frostbite** is the result of the freezing of a body part. Frostbitten extremities appear pale and hard and are without sensation. **Chilblain** is a cold injury with erythema and the formation of vesicles and ulcerative lesions that occur as a result of vasoconstriction.

In extreme cases of exposure to freezing temperatures, the head and the torso should be warmed before the extremities to ensure survival with minimal consequences. Sensitive skin should be handled gently. Massage is contraindicated. The extremity can be placed in the axilla or placed in warm (not hot) water. Dry clothing should be applied and muscle activity encouraged. Blankets or sleeping bags are initially used to start rewarming. Warm, moist oxygen; warming blankets; and warming baths of 37.8 to 42.2°C (100 to 108°F) are used.

A deep purple flush appears with the return of sensation, which is accompanied by extreme pain. Pain relief and monitoring of vital signs are essential. Blistering and ulcers can occur and are treated with whirlpool soaks. Skin damage is similar to that incurred with burns. Frostbite can result in *necrosis* (death) of tissue and may necessitate amputation of the extremity.

Education to prevent cold injury is essential for people living in or visiting cold climates. Public health nurses play a vital role in educating parents and children about avoiding cold-related injury. Adequate layered clothing, including hats and gloves (wool over cotton), should be worn.

Get Ready for the Certification Examination!

Key Points

- The skin is the body's first line of defense against disease.
- Certain skin conditions are symptoms of systemic disease.
- A strawberry nevus is an example of a hemangioma.
- Common skin problems in infants are diaper dermatitis, seborrheic dermatitis, and atopic dermatitis (eczema).
- Pediculosis is the term for lice. Lice may occur on the head, body, or pubic area.
- Tinea pedis, or athlete's foot, is prevented by drying the feet well, particularly between the toes, and wearing well-ventilated footwear.
- Atopic dermatitis involves itching and eczema of the skin. New guidelines to prevent food allergies that can cause atopic dermatitis have been developed.
- Absorption of a topical hydrating medication is best when applied after a warm bath.
- A severe burn can cause a loss of function in two of the most important properties of the skin: the ability to protect against infection and the ability to prevent the loss of body fluid.
- Types of burns include thermal, electrical, chemical, and radiation.
- Electrical burns carry the risk of thrombosis and tissue damage in other parts of the body.
- The severity of a burn depends on the area, extent, and depth of involvement.
- Preventing infection is an important nursing intervention for patients with burns or any skin lesion.
- A sunburn can be a minor epidural burn or a partial-thickness burn with blisters.
- Topical chemical sunscreens partially absorb the sun's UV rays and have ratings to evaluate the effectiveness of blocking these rays. Physical sun blocks are creams that block the UV rays.
- Repeated sunburns for cosmetic reasons and use of tanning booths are associated with the development of skin cancer.
- Frostbite can cause tissue damage similar to that with burns.

Additional Learning Resources

evolve Go to your Evolve website (http://evolve.elsevier.com/Canada/Leifer) for the following learning resources:

- Answer Key for Critical Thinking Questions
- Answer Key for Textbook Review Questions
- Audio Glossary
- Fluids & Electrolytes tutorial
- Interactive Review Questions
- Skills Performance Checklists
- Video clips and more!

Online Resources

- Canadian Dermatology Association: https://dermatology.ca/
- Government of Canada, *Stop Bedbugs! Start by Checking Your Room:* https://www.canada.ca/en/health-canada/services/consumer-product-safety/reports-publications/pesticides-pest-management/fact-sheets-other-resources/stop-bedbugs-start-checking-your-room.html
- Shriners Hospital, *Be Burn Aware:* https://www.shrinershospitalsforchildren.org/shc/beburnaware

Review Questions

1. Why is pain relief important for the burn patient?
   a. It prevents discomfort.
   b. The child must be kept from crying.
   c. Parents become upset.
   d. Pain contributes to shock.
2. Which are the principles of care in the treatment of infantile eczema?
   a. Hydrate skin, prevent infection, relieve itching.
   b. Keep skin dry, clean with mild soap.
   c. Use elbow immobilizers to prevent scratching, increase fluid intake.

d. Dress warmly, bathe often with clear water, administer antibiotics.

3. When caring for a child newly admitted with a major burn injury, the priority nursing responsibilities include which of the following interventions? *(Select all that apply.)*
   a. Prevent infection.
   b. Maintain accurate intake and output.
   c. Provide daily baths for cleanliness
   d. Provide a high-carbohydrate diet.
4. What is contained in an emollient bath often prescribed for children with eczema?
   a. Bath oil
   b. Glycerin soap
   c. Oatmeal
   d. Salt or saline solution
5. When instructing parents who plan to take their 5-month-old infant sunbathing at the beach, what is most important for a nurse to emphasize?
   a. Use a sunscreen with an SPF greater than 30 over exposed areas of the infant's skin.
   b. Reapply sunscreen after playing in the water.
   c. Use sunglasses to protect eyes.
   d. Use light clothes and a hat to protect against sun exposure.
6. A child is admitted with a burn injury that involves the forehead, ears, cheeks, and chests. Which of the following are essential nursing responsibilities? *(Select all that apply.)*
   a. Weigh the child.
   b. Provide oxygen and assess respirations.
   c. Apply dry, sterile dressings to burned areas.
   d. Remove eschar from burned areas.

REFERENCES

Banerji, A., & Canadian Paediatric Society (CPS), First Nations, Inuit, and Métis Health Committee. (2015). Scabies. *Paediatrics & Child Health, 20*(7), 395–398. Reaffirmed 2018. Retrieved from: https://www.cps.ca/en/documents/position/scabies.

Bortolussi, R., Martin, S., & Canadian Paediatric Society (CPS), Infectious Diseases and Immunization Committee. (2007). Antifungal agents for common outpatient paediatric infections. *Paediatrics & Child Health, 12*(10), 875–878. Reaffirmed 2018. Retrieved from: https://www.cps.ca/en/documents/position/antifungal-agents-common-infections.

Canadian Dermatology Association. (2019a). *Eczema*. Retrieved from: https://dermatology.ca/public-patients/skin/eczema/.

Canadian Dermatology Association. (2019b). *Sun safety for every day*. Retrieved from: https://dermatology.ca/public-patients/sun-protection/sun-safety-every-day/.

Canadian Paediatric Society (CPS). (2016). *Sun safety*. Retrieved from: https://www.caringforkids.cps.ca/handouts/sun_safety.

Canadian Paediatric Society (CPS). (2017). *Your baby's skin*. Retrieved from: https://www.caringforkids.cps.ca/handouts/your-babys-skin.

Chan, E. S., Cummings, C., & Canadian Paediatric Society (CPS), Community Paediatrics Committee, Allergy Section. (2013). Dietary exposures and allergy prevention in high-risk infants. *Paediatrics & Child Health, 18*(10), 545–549. Reaffirmed 2016. Retrieved from: https://www.cps.ca/en/documents/position/dietary-exposures-and-allergy-prevention-in-high-risk-infants.

Cummings, C., Finlay, J. C., MacDonald, N. E., et al. (2018). Head lice infestations: A clinical update. *Paediatrics & Child Health, 23*(1), e18–e24. Retrieved from: https://www.cps.ca/en/documents/position/head-lice.

Dickey, B., & Chiu, Y. (2016). Photosensitivity. In R. Kliegman, B. Stanton, J. St. Geme, et al. (Eds.), *Nelson textbook of pediatrics* (20th ed.). Philadelphia: Saunders.

Government of Canada. (2015). *Bedbugs—What are they?* Retrieved from: https://www.canada.ca/en/health-canada/services/pest-control-tips/bedbugs-what-are-they.html?_ga=2.165746174.1173238371.1537726332-1369007158.1523290776.

Health Canada. (2016). *Health Canada reinforces the importance of preventing pregnancy while taking the acne drug isotretinoin to avoid birth defects*. Retrieved from: http://www.healthycanadians.gc.ca/recall-alert-rappel-avis/hc-sc/2016/60096a-eng.php?_ga=2.23114234.1395626806.1526743881-1369007158.1523290776.

Herndon, D., & Jones, J. (Eds.). (2007). *Total burn care* (3rd ed.). St. Louis: Saunders.

Hilton, L. (2016). Common pediatric disorders in skin of color. *Contemporary Pediatrics, 33*(20), 30–33.

Irvine, J., & Canadian Paediatric Society (CPS), First Nations, Inuit and Métis Health Committee. (2012). Community-associated methicillin-resistant *Staphylococcus aureus* in Indigenous communities in Canada. *Paediatrics & Child Health, 17*(7), 385–386. Reaffirmed 2017. Retrieved from: https://www.cps.ca/en/documents/position/community-associated-MRSA-in-Indigenous-communities.

Lai, O., Ho, D., Glick, S., et al. (2016). Bed bugs and possible transmission of human pathogens: Systematic review. *Archives of Dermatological Research, 308*(8), 531–538. https://doi.org/10.1007/s00403-016-1661-8.

Püttgen, K., Lucky, A., Adams, D., et al. (2016). Topical timolol maleate treatment of infantile hemangiomas. *Pediatrics, 138*(3), e20160355. https://doi.org/10.1542/peds.2016-0355.

Robinson, J. L., Salvadori, M. I., & Canadian Paediatric Society (CPS), Infectious Diseases and Immunization Committee. (2011). Management of community-associated methicillin-resistant *Staphylococcus aureus* skin abscesses in children. *Paediatrics & Child Health, 16*(2), 115–116. Reaffirmed 2017. Retrieved from: https://www.cps.ca/en/documents/position-/methicillin-resistant-Staphylococcus-aureus-skin-abscesses.

Taddeo, D., Stanwick, R., & Canadian Paediatric Society (CPS), Adolescent Health Committee. (2012). Banning children and youth under the age of 18 years from commercial tanning facilities. *Paediatrics & Child Health, 17*(2), 89. Reaffirmed 2018. Retrieved from: https://www.cps.ca/en/documents/position/tanning-facilities.

The Child With a Metabolic Condition

31

Martha Cope

http://evolve.elsevier.com/Canada/Leifer

Objectives

1. Define each key term listed.
2. Relate why growth parameters are of importance to patients with a family history of endocrine disease.
3. List the symptoms of hypothyroidism in infants.
4. Discuss the dietary adjustment required for a child with diabetes insipidus.
5. Differentiate between type 1 and type 2 diabetes mellitus.
6. List three precipitating events that might cause diabetic ketoacidosis.
7. Compare the signs and symptoms of hyperglycemia and hypoglycemia.
8. Outline the educational needs of the parents and the child with diabetes mellitus in the following areas: nutrition and meal planning, exercise, blood tests, glucose monitoring, administration of insulin, and skin care.
9. Discuss the preparation and administration of insulin to a child, highlighting any differences between pediatric and adult administration.
10. List three possible causes of insulin shock.
11. Explain the Somogyi phenomenon.
12. Identify a predictable stress that the disease of diabetes mellitus has on children and families during the following periods of life: infancy, toddlerhood, preschool age, elementary school age, puberty, and adolescence.

Key Terms

antidiuretic hormone
dawn phenomenon
diabetes mellitus
glucagon
glycated hemoglobin test ($HgbA_{1c}$) (glī-kā-tĭd HĒ-mō-glō-bĭn tĕst)
glycosuria (glī-kō-SYŪ-rē-ă)
hormones
hyperglycemia (hī-pŭr-glī-SĒ-mē-ă)
hypoglycemia (hī-pō-glī-SĒ-mē-ă)
hypotonia (hī-pō-TŌ-nē-ă)
ketoacidosis (kē-tō-ă-sĭ-DŌ-sĭs)
lipoatrophy (lĭp-ō-ĂT-rō-fē)
polydipsia (pŏl-ē-DĬP-sē-ă)
polyphagia (pŏl-ē-FĀ-jhă)
polyuria (pŏl-ē-YŪ-rē-ă)
Somogyi phenomenon (sō-mō-gēē)
vasopressin (văz-ō-PRĔS-ĭn)

INTEGRATION OF THE NERVOUS AND ENDOCRINE SYSTEMS

The two major control systems that monitor the functions of the body are the nervous system and the endocrine system. These systems are interdependent. The endocrine, or ductless glands regulate the body's metabolic processes. They are primarily responsible for growth, maturation, reproduction, and the response of the body to stress. Fig. 31.1 depicts the organs of the endocrine system and outlines how this system in children differs from that in adults. **Hormones** are chemical substances produced by these ductless glands. As blood flows through an organ of the endocrine system hormonal secretions from the associated gland are secreted into the bloodstream. An organ specifically influenced by a certain hormone is called a *target organ*. Too much or too little of a given hormone may result in a disease state.

Most of the glands and structures of the endocrine system develop during the first trimester of fetal development. Hormonal control is immature until at least 18 months of age, thus infants are more prone to problems related to the functioning of the endocrine system. Maternal endocrine dysfunction may affect the fetus; therefore, an in-depth maternal history is a valuable tool in data collection.

The absence or deficiency of an enzyme that has a role in metabolism causes a defect in the metabolic process, which can result in illness. Most inborn errors of metabolism can be detected by clinical signs or screening tests that can be performed in the newborn. Lethargy, poor feeding, failure to thrive, vomiting, and an enlarged liver may be early signs of an inborn error of metabolism in the newborn. When clinical signs are not manifested in the newborn period, an infection or body stress can precipitate symptoms of a latent defect in the older child. Unexplained intellectual disability, developmental delay, convulsions, an odour from the body or from the urine, or episodes of vomiting may be subtle signs

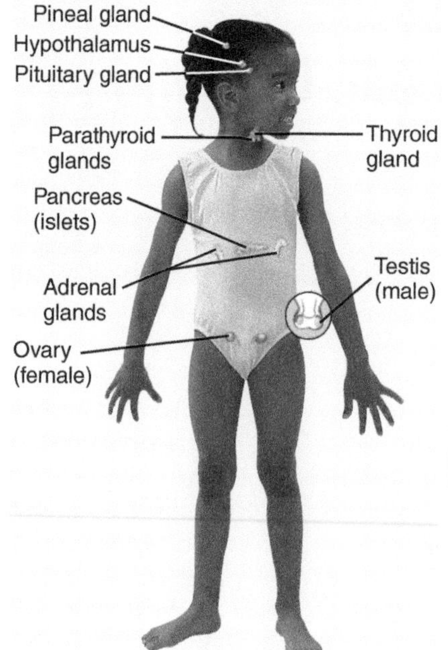

Fig. 31.1 Summary of some endocrine system differences between the child and the adult. The endocrine system consists of the ductless glands that release hormones. It works with the nervous system to regulate metabolic activities. (Art overlay courtesy Observatory Group, Cincinnati, Ohio.)

ENDOCRINE SYSTEM

- The endocrine system of the newborn is supplemented by maternal hormones that cross the placental barrier. In males and females, this may result in swelling of the breasts and genital changes.
- Hormone disturbances during childhood may cause disrupted growth patterns, resulting in short stature or gigantism.
- Congenital hypothyroidism may occur as a result of an absent, nonfunctioning thyroid gland.
- In childhood the pancreas may be deficient in insulin, causing type 1 (insulin-dependent) diabetes.

of a metabolic dysfunction. Phenylketonuria (PKU), galactosemia, and maple syrup urine disease are discussed in Chapter 12. Cystic fibrosis is discussed in Chapter 25.

Many diagnostic tests can be used to diagnose metabolic conditions:

- Radiographic studies are used to determine bone age.
- Serum electrolytes and glucose, hormonal, and calcium level tests may be required.
- Newborn screening is an important device for identifying enzyme deficiencies such as PKU.
- Chromosomal studies and tissue biopsy are used.
- Sexual maturation and skin texture, pigment, and temperature may be indicators of specific disorders.
- Thyroid function tests may be done.
- Ultrasonography is helpful in determining the size and character of adrenal glands, ovaries, and other organs.
- A 24-hour urine specimen is useful.

Genetic counselling can provide parents with information that may help in preventing some disorders.

Most endocrine dysfunctions involve chronic problems and call for long-term nursing care. The nurse must assess the effect of such dysfunctions on growth and development, advocate for early detection and intervention, and promote comprehensive follow-up care that will minimize complications.

DISORDERS AND DYSFUNCTION OF THE ENDOCRINE SYSTEM

Some common metabolic dysfunctions, their manifestations, and their treatments are outlined in Table 31.1.

Nursing Tip

Growth hormone is administered at bedtime to simulate the natural timing of hormone release.

INBORN ERRORS OF METABOLISM

There are hundreds of inherited biochemical disorders that affect body metabolism. The pattern of inheritance is generally autosomal recessive. These conditions range from mild to severe.

Tay-Sachs Disease

Pathophysiology

Tay-Sachs disease involves a deficiency of lysosomal-beta-hexosaminidase, an enzyme necessary for the metabolism of fats. Lipid deposits accumulate on nerve cells, causing both physical and mental deterioration. The incidence of this disease is significantly higher among people of eastern European (Ashkenazi) Jewish descent and non-Jewish French Canadians living near the St. Lawrence River (National Human Genome Research Institute, 2011). It is an autosomal recessive trait carried by 1 in 25 of the Ashkenazi Jewish population (McGovern & Desnick, 2016).

Manifestations

The infant with Tay-Sachs disease has no symptoms until about age 5 to 6 months, when physical development begins to slow. There may be head lag or an inability to sit. The disease progresses, and when cherry-red deposits occur on the optic nerve, blindness may result. Intellectual delay eventually develops because the brain cells become damaged. Most children with

Nutrition Considerations

Diet Therapy in Pediatric Metabolic Disorders

DISORDER	MAJOR SIGNS AND SYMPTOMS	DIETARY REGIMEN
Phenylketonuria (PKU)	Intellectual disability	Low phenylalanine diet, Lofenalac formula for infants
Celiac disease	Chronic diarrhea, irritability, distention, failure to thrive	Eliminate gluten; use corn flour and vitamin B supplements
Cystic fibrosis	Thick mucus causes obstruction of pancreatic enzymes and poor absorption of nutrients, flatulence, and foul-smelling stools	Pancreatic enzyme replacement with normal meals
Lactose intolerance	Abdominal distention, cramps, diarrhea, failure to thrive	Lactose-free diet; use soy formulas; avoid milk and milk products
Galactose intolerance	Jaundice, vomiting, convulsions, lethargy, blindness	No galactose or lactose in diet; use milk substitutes
Fructose intolerance	Vomiting, diarrhea, failure to thrive	Fructose-free diet; avoid honey, fruit, sorbitol, and sucrose; offer vitamin C and vegetables
Maple syrup urine disease	Acidosis, convulsions	Low-leucine and low-valine diet
Urea cycle defect	Lethargy	Low-protein diet
Acidemia	Seizures, elevated ammonia levels	May need to restrict meat proteins
Diabetes insipidus	Inability to concentrate urine, diuresis	Unrestricted water intake
Diabetes mellitus	Inability to produce insulin to metabolize sugar, protein, and fat	Controlled sugar intake regulated with insulin administration; high-fibre, balanced diet

Tay-Sachs disease die before 5 years of age from secondary infection or malnutrition.

Treatment and nursing care

There is no treatment for this devastating disease. The nursing care is mainly palliative. Most care is administered in the home, with periodic hospitalization for complications such as pneumonia. Chapter 22 discusses the care of the dying child.

Carriers can be identified with screening tests, preferably prior to pregnancy. Genetic testing and prenatal counselling have markedly decreased the occurrence of Tay-Sachs disease.

Hypothyroidism

Pathophysiology

Hypothyroidism occurs when there is a deficiency in the secretions of the thyroid gland. It may be congenital or acquired. It is one of the more common disorders of the endocrine system in children. The thyroid gland controls the rate of metabolism in the body by producing thyroxine (T_4) and triiodothyronine (T_3). In *congenital hypothyroidism*, the gland is absent or not functioning. The symptoms of hypothyroidism may not be apparent for several months.

In the noncongenital form, *juvenile hypothyroidism*, the child acquires hypothyroidism when they are older, It may be caused by a number of conditions, the most common being lymphocytic thyroiditis. Often it appears during periods of rapid growth. Predisposing factors include infectious disease, irradiation for cancer, certain medications containing iodine, and a lack of dietary iodine (uncommon in Canada). The symptoms, diagnosis, and treatment are similar to those for congenital hypothyroidism. Intellectual disability and neurological complications are not seen in the older child as brain growth is nearly complete by 2 to 3 years of age.

Manifestations

The infant with hypothyroidism appears very sluggish and sleeps more often than an unaffected same-age child. The tongue becomes enlarged, causing noisy respiration (Fig. 31.2); the skin is dry; hair becomes dry and brittle; there is an absence of perspiration; and the hands and feet are cold. The infant feels floppy when handled. This **hypotonia** also affects the intestinal tract, causing chronic constipation. If hypothyroidism is left untreated, irreversible intellectual delay and physical disabilities result in the young child.

Treatment and nursing care

Early recognition and diagnosis are essential to prevent the developing sequelae. In all Canadian provinces and territories newborn screening for hypothyroidism is conducted shortly after birth (Canadian Organization for Rare Disorders, 2015). This is generally part of an overall screen for other metabolic defects.

Treatment involves the administration of the synthetic hormone levothyroxine sodium (Synthroid, Levothroid). Therapy reverses the symptoms and prevents further intellectual delay but does not reverse existing disability. Hormone levels need to be monitored regularly.

Table 31.1 Metabolic Dysfunctions

GLAND	PROBLEM	INVOLVED HORMONE	MANIFESTATION	THERAPY
Pituitary—anterior	Decreased: hypopituitarism	Growth hormone	Short stature, dwarfism	Synthetic growth hormone replacement
	Increased: hyperpituitarism	Growth hormone	Before epiphyseal closure, gigantism	Cryosurgery, irradiation
			After epiphyseal closure, acromegaly	Radioactive implants
			Sexual precocity (puberty before 8 to 9 years of age)	Monthly hormone injection to control secretions until puberty
Pituitary—posterior	Decreased: hypopituitarism	Decreased antidiuretic hormone	Diabetes insipidus	Vasopressin by injection or nasal spray Provide adequate fluids
	Increased: hyperpituitarism (SIADH)	Increased antidiuretic hormone	SIADH Decreased urine output Edema Fluid overload	Fluid restriction and hormone antagonists
Parathyroid	Decreased: hypoparathyroidism	Decreased parathyroid hormone	Decreased blood calcium and increased phosphorus levels, causing tetany and laryngospasm	Calcium gluconate, vitamin D supplements
	Increased: hyperparathyroidism	Increased parathyroid hormone	Elevated blood calcium and lowered phosphorus levels, causing spontaneous fractures and CNS problems	Restore calcium balance, excise tumour, vitamin D, low-phosphorus diet
Adrenal	Decreased: adrenal cortical insufficiency (Addison disease)	Decreased steroids, sex steroids, epinephrine	Craving for salt, seizures, neurological and circulatory changes, decreased sexual development	Replace cortisol and aldosterone, genetic sexual assessment
	Increased: hyperadrenalism (Cushing syndrome)	Increased cortisol	Cushing syndrome, hyperglycemia, electrolyte problems, pheochromocytoma	Depends on cause, tumour removal, and hormone replacement

CNS, Central nervous system; *SIADH,* syndrome of inappropriate antidiuretic hormone.

The medication is taken at the same time each day, preferably in the morning. Parents are cautioned not to use different brands of the medication. Children may experience reversible hair loss, insomnia, and aggressiveness, and their schoolwork may decline during the first few months of therapy. These effects are temporary. It may take 1 to 3 weeks for the medication to reach the full therapeutic effect. Medication is not to be discontinued, because hormone replacement for hypothyroidism is lifelong. Parents should be taught the signs and symptoms of overdose, which include rapid pulse rate, dyspnea, irritability, weight loss, and sweating. Signs of inadequate dosage or nonadherence are fatigue, sleepiness, and constipation. Parents need to be instructed about these issues and advised to consult their health care provider before giving the child other medications.

Diabetes Insipidus

Pathophysiology

Diabetes insipidus can be hereditary (autosomal dominant) or it can be acquired as the result of a head injury or tumour. It is the consequence of posterior pituitary hypofunction that results in a decreased secretion of **vasopressin**, the **antidiuretic hormone**. A lack of antidiuretic hormone results in uncontrolled diuresis. As a consequence, the kidneys do not concentrate the urine during episodes of dehydration.

Manifestations

Polydipsia and polyuria are the initial signs. The infant cries and prefers water to milk. Weight loss, growth failure, inefficient perspiration, dry skin, and dehydration occur rapidly. As the child grows older, enuresis may be a problem. Excessive thirst and the search for

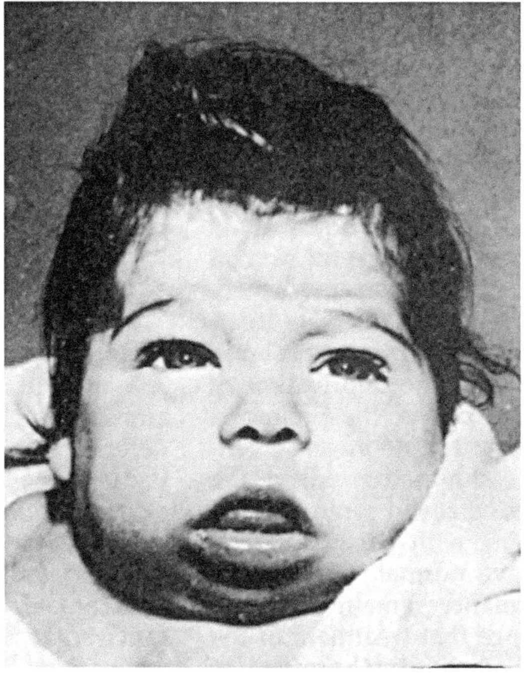

Fig. 31.2 An infant with hypothyroidism. Note the large head and tongue, puffy face, and broad nasal bridge. The infant is not alert and feeds poorly. (From Kliegman, R., Stanton, B., St. Geme, J., et al. (Eds.). [2016]. *Nelson textbook of pediatrics* [20th ed.]. Philadelphia: Saunders.)

water may overshadow the desire to play, explore, eat, learn, or sleep.

Treatment and nursing care

Treatment involves hormone replacement of vasopressin in the form of desmopressin by subcutaneous injection, orally, or DDAVP (desmopressin acetate) nasal spray. Parents should be taught to monitor for signs of overdose, which include symptoms of water intoxication (edema, lethargy, and nausea).

Children with diabetes insipidus who are admitted to the hospital in an unconscious state and are unable to express thirst are at great risk. These children should wear a medical identification bracelet. School personnel should be advised of the child's needs. School protocol often limits children's access to bathrooms and water fountains, but such restrictions could be life-threatening to a child with diabetes insipidus. The child's nurse should contact the school and educate staff concerning the child's care needs and medication. At home, care instructions should include recognizing the signs of water intoxication, dehydration, and hyponatremia.

Diabetes Mellitus

Pathophysiology

Diabetes mellitus (DM) is a chronic metabolic syndrome (group of symptoms) in which the body is unable to use carbohydrates properly, leading to an impairment of glucose transport (sugar cannot pass into the cells). The body is also unable to store and use fats properly and there is a decrease in protein synthesis. When the blood glucose level becomes dangerously high, glucose spills into the urine, and diuresis occurs. Incomplete fat metabolism produces ketone bodies that accumulate in the blood. This condition is termed *ketonemia* and is a serious complication.

Nearly one-third of Canadians have diabetes or prediabetes (Diabetes Canada, 2017). By 2026, it is estimated that 14 million Canadians will be living with DM (Diabetes Canada, 2017).

DM affects the physical and psychological growth and development of children because it requires lifestyle alterations (diet, glucose monitoring, and insulin administration). There are also many long-term complications related to hyperglycemia that can result in blindness, circulatory problems, kidney disease, and neuropathy. Treatment is designed to optimize affected children's growth and development and to minimize complications.

Table 31.2 Classification of Diabetes Mellitus

Type 1	Destruction of beta cells in pancreas results in lack of insulin production Formerly known as insulin-dependent diabetes mellitus (IDDM) or juvenile-onset diabetes mellitus
Type 2	Involves insulin resistance or decreased insulin production Formerly known as non–insulin-dependent diabetes mellitus (NIDDM) or adult-onset diabetes mellitus Associated with obesity and elevated blood lipids
Gestational diabetes	Transient form of diabetes mellitus that is triggered by pregnancy Resolves after birth but may reoccur several years later (see Chapter 5)
Other genetic defects	Defects in chromosomes 6 and 11 and other genetic disorders are associated with diabetes mellitus syndrome

Classification

The major forms of DM have been classified according to whether they are caused by a deficiency of insulin secretion due to pancreatic beta-cell damage (type 1) or are a consequence of insulin resistance (type 2).

The classifications of DM (Table 31.2) pertinent to pediatrics are as follows:

- *Type 1 DM* is an autoimmune condition that occurs when a child with a genetic predisposition is exposed to an environmental factor such as a viral infection that triggers the syndrome by causing destruction of beta cells in the pancreas, resulting in insufficient insulin production. Medications, chemicals, and ionizing radiation may cause beta-cell destruction in some cases (Svoren & Jospe, 2016).
- *Type 2 DM* involves a resistance to insulin. It is often triggered by a sedentary lifestyle and obesity. It also

occurs more frequently in certain ethnic groups, such as Blacks and East Indians, especially those who have hypertension and elevated blood lipid levels. Acanthosis nigricans (a dark pigmentation in the flexor creases of the skin) may be a cutaneous marker for patients with type 2 DM.

Table 31.3 lists the clinical features of types 1 and 2 DM.

Type 1 diabetes mellitus. Type 1 diabetes is the most common metabolic disorder of childhood. Although there is a genetic susceptibility to type 1 diabetes, a large percentage of affected children have no known family history. Genetic studies have implicated chromosome numbers 6 and 11, but other genetic and environmental risk factors have also been identified, such as viruses or stress. Diet, such as the timing of introducing new foods in infancy, may also play a role in autoimmunity, but no conclusive findings have been found. Research is ongoing in this area of practice (Svoren & Jospe, 2016).

Symptoms of type 1 DM may occur at any time in childhood, but the rate of occurrence of new cases is highest among 5- and 7-year-old children and pubescent children 11 to 13 years of age. In the former group, the stress of school and the increased exposure to infectious diseases may be the precipitating events that trigger onset. During puberty, rapid growth, increased emotional stress, and the insulin antagonism of sex hormones may be implicated as contributing to development of diabetes. DM occurs in both sexes with equal frequency.

The disease is more difficult to manage in childhood because the patients are growing, expend a great deal of energy, have varying nutritional needs, and face a lifetime of diabetic management. The initial diagnosis may be determined when the child develops ketoacidosis. Nurses must be particularly astute in their observations during assessment of children in these age groups.

Type 2 diabetes mellitus. Type 2 diabetes is thought to be caused by insulin resistance and decreased insulin secretion. It is precipitated by obesity, low physical activity, and a lipid-rich diet resulting in insulin resistance. In Canada, 9 out of 10 people with diabetes have type 2 diabetes (Government of Canada, 2018).

Risk factors for type 2 DM include the following:

- Family history of type 2 DM
- *Acanthosis nigricans* (a dark pigmentation of the flexure creases of the skin and back of neck)
- Hypertension
- Increased lipids (hyperlipidemia)
- Repeated vaginal monilial *(Candida)* infections resulting from chronic glycosuria
- Obesity (body mass index [BMI] 35 to 39 kg/m^2 or weight and height or greater than the one hundred–twentieth percentile for the ideal weight for height)

Twins who have had intrauterine growth restriction and infants born with low birth weight who gain rapidly in the first few months of life are at increased risk for developing type 2 DM. These infants are more prone to weight gain later in life. However, the combination of obesity, poor diet, lack of adequate exercise, smoking, some psychiatric conditions, and some medications that induce weight gain (such as fluoxetine) also contribute to the risk factors for the development of type 2 diabetes (Svoran & Jospe, 2016).

Diagnosis

A random blood glucose level may be obtained at any time and requires no preparation of the patient. The results should be within the normal limits for both nondiabetic patients and diabetic patients who have good control of their disease. A nonfasting random blood glucose over 11.1 mmol/L and symptomology of unexplained weight loss, polydipsia, and polyuria are diagnostic for DM type 1 (Punthakee, Goldenberg, & Katz, 2018).

- *Fasting blood glucose* level is a standard and reliable test for diabetes. The blood glucose level is measured in the fasting patient, usually immediately on awakening in the morning. The results of the test will not be accurate if the patient is receiving a dextrose intravenous (IV) solution. If a person's fasting blood glucose level is greater than 7.0 mmol/L on two separate occasions and the history is positive, the patient is considered to have DM and requires treatment.
- **Glycated hemoglobin test (HgbA$_{1c}$)** reflects glycemic levels throughout a period of months. Values are found to be elevated in virtually all children with

Table 31.3 Clinical Features of Type 1 and Type 2 Diabetes

FEATURE	TYPE 1	TYPE 2
Onset	Abrupt; patient can often state week of onset	Insidious; often found by screening tests
Body size	Normal or thin	Often obese
Blood glucose level	Fluctuates widely with exercise and infection	Fluctuations are less marked
Ketoacidosis	Common	Infrequent
Sulfonylurea responsiveness	Rare	>50%
Insulin required	Almost all	<25%
Insulin dosage	Increases until glucose control is stable	May remain stable

newly diagnosed diabetes. Glucose in the bloodstream constantly enters red blood cells and links with, or *glycosylates*, molecules of hemoglobin. The more glucose in the blood, the more hemoglobin becomes coated with glucose. The red blood cells carry this glucose until cells with fresh hemoglobin replace them. This process takes about 3 to 4 months. Values vary according to the measurement used (Box 31.1).

Diabetes Canada (Panagiotopoulos, Hadjiyannakis, & Henderson, 2018) recommends using a combination of HgbA1c and fasting or random blood glucose to screen for type 2 diabetes in children and youth with risk factors. The oral glucose tolerance test has little value in diagnosing type 2 DM. Many adolescents remain asymptomatic for years because the hyperglycemia is moderate and signs and symptoms are not dramatic. Asymptomatic adolescents are often not diagnosed until diabetic **ketoacidosis** (DKA) occurs. Lifestyle intervention is the cornerstone of preventing or delaying the onset of type 2 DM in susceptible individuals.

Manifestations

Children with DM present a classic triad of symptoms: **polydipsia** (symptoms of excessive thirst), **polyuria** (excretes large amounts of urine frequently), and **polyphagia** (constantly hungry). The symptoms appear more rapidly in children. An insidious onset with lethargy, weakness, and weight loss is also common. The child who is toilet independent may begin wetting the bed or have frequent "accidents" during play periods, may lose weight, and become irritable. The skin becomes dry. Vaginal yeast infections may be seen in the adolescent girl. There may be a history of recurrent infections. Symptoms can be missed until an infection becomes apparent or coma results.

Laboratory findings indicate glucose in the urine (**glycosuria**). **Hyperglycemia** (*hyper*, "above," *gly*, "sugar," and *emia*, "blood") is also apparent. Hyperglycemia occurs because glucose cannot enter the cells without the help of insulin, and therefore glucose remains in the bloodstream. The cells use protein and fat for energy; therefore, protein stores in the body are depleted. The lack of glucose in the cells triggers the body to develop polyphagia. This intake of glucose further increases glucose levels in the blood. Hyperglycemia is the cause of the many complications associated with uncontrolled DM.

The honeymoon period. When type 1 DM is initially diagnosed and the child is stabilized by insulin dosage, the condition may appear to improve. Insulin requirements decrease and the child feels well. This phenomenon can support the parent's phase of denial in accepting the long-term diagnosis of DM for their child. The "honeymoon period" lasts a short time (a few months), and parents should be encouraged to closely monitor blood glucose levels to prevent complications.

Box 31.1 Recommended Glycated Hemoglobin Levels

Most adolescents and young adults with type 1 diabetes (13 to 18 years old)

- A1c: 7.0% or less

School-age children with type 1 diabetes (6 to 12 years old)

- A1c: 7.5% or less

Toddlers and preschoolers with type 1 diabetes (younger than 6 years old)

- A1c: 8.0% or less

Children, adolescents, and young adults with type 2 diabetes (up to 18 years old)

- A1c: 7.0% or less

Source: Punthakee, Z., Goldenberg, R., & Katz, J. (2018). Definition, classification and diagnosis of diabetes, prediabetes and metabolic syndrome. *Canadian Journal of Diabetes*, 42(Suppl 1), S10-S15. Retrieved from http://guidelines.diabetes.ca/cpg/chapter3.

Nursing Tip

A period of remission, or the "honeymoon" phase of the disease, may occur within a few weeks of beginning insulin administration. There is a decline in insulin need and improved metabolic control. This phase, however, is temporary.

Diabetic ketoacidosis. DKA is also referred to as *diabetic coma*, although a person may have DKA with or without being in a coma. It is manifested by ketonemia and may be precipitated by a secondary infection. It may also occur if the signs and symptoms of DM go unrecognized, which happens fairly often in children. Even minor infections, such as a cold, increase the body's metabolic rate and thereby change the body's demand for insulin and the severity of diabetes. Ketoacidosis is the end result of the effects of insulin deficiency.

Symptoms of ketoacidosis are compared with those of **hypoglycemia** in Table 31.4. Signs and symptoms include a fruity odour to the breath, nausea, decreased level of consciousness, and dehydration. Laboratory values include hyperglycemia, ketonuria, decreased serum bicarbonate concentration (decreased CO_2 levels), low pH, and hypertonic dehydration. Diabetic teaching should include this information. A medical identification bracelet should be worn at all times for anyone with DM. The symptoms range from mild to severe and occur within hours to days. The child with DKA is managed in the hospital setting with close monitoring of fluid, electrolytes, laboratory values, and clinical status.

Treatment and nursing care

The three goals of treatment in DM are:

1. Ensure normal growth and development through metabolic control.
2. Enable the child to live with a chronic illness and have a happy and active childhood.
3. Prevent complications.

Table 31.4 Hyperglycemia and Hypoglycemia

HYPEREGLYCEMIA (KETOACIDOSIS)	HYPOGLYCEMIA
Cause	
Inadequate insulin Excess CHO intake	Excess exercise Too little CHO intake Insulin overdose
Signs and Symptoms	
Blood glucose levels >11 mmol/L Polyuria, polydipsia, polyphagia Fruity odour to breath Fatigue Abdominal pain Red lips, flushed face Dehydration Disorientation Drowsiness progressing to coma Deep, rapid (Kussmaul) respirations	Blood glucose <4 mmol/L Fatigue, hunger Pale, clammy skin Diaphoresis Tremors Lethargy Headache Irritability Tachycardia
Treatment	
Regular insulin	Administer glucagon IM, orange juice, or CHOs orally or IV glucose

CHO, Carbohydrate; *IM*, intramuscularly; *IV*, intravenous.

Maintaining the blood glucose at consistently normal levels can minimize complications.

Ideally, teaching begins when the diagnosis is confirmed. A planned education program is important in order to provide a consistent body of information, which can then be individualized. The patient's age and financial, educational, cultural, and religious background must be considered. Many hospitals hold group clinics for diabetic patients and their families. These sessions are conducted by a multidisciplinary health care team and can include the diabetes nurse educator, dietitian, and pharmacist. Sometimes patients who are living with DM are invited to attend these sessions to share their experiences as well as provide encouragement and support. Health professionals become directly involved with the patient's progress and can offer necessary feedback and education. Continuous follow-up is essential.

Because children with diabetes are growing, additional dimensions of the disorder and its treatment become evident. Growth is not steady but occurs in spurts and plateaus that affect treatment. Infants and toddlers may have hydration problems, especially during illness. Preschool children have irregular activity and eating patterns. School-age children may grieve over the diagnosis and ask, "Why me?" They may use their illness to gain attention or to avoid responsibilities. The onset of puberty may require insulin adjustments as a result of growth and the antagonistic effect of the sex hormones on insulin. Adolescents often resent this condition, which deviates from their concept of the "ideal body." They may have more difficulty in resolving their conflict between dependence and independence, which may lead to rebellion against parents and treatment regimens.

The impact of the disease on the rest of the family must also be considered. Parents may feel guilty for having passed the disease on to their child. Siblings may feel jealous of the attention the patient receives. The sharing of responsibility by parents is ideal but not necessarily a reality. Some may have difficulty accepting the diagnosis and the more regimented lifestyle it imposes. Family members must learn to cope with their individual reactions to the stress of the illness.

Children with diabetes need to assume responsibility for their own care gradually, and with a minimum of pressure. Overprotection can be as detrimental as neglect. Parents who have received satisfaction from their child's dependence on them may need help "letting go."

The nursing care of childhood diabetes requires knowledge of growth and development, pathophysiology, blood glucose self-monitoring, nutritional management, insulin management, insulin shock, exercise, skin and foot care, infections, effects of emotional upsets, and long-term care. Nursing Care Plan 31.1 lists interventions for the child with diabetes.

Teaching plan. The patient and family are instructed about the location of the pancreas and its normal function. The nurse explains the relationship of insulin to the pancreas, differentiating between type 1 and type 2 diabetes. All information should be provided gradually and at the level of understanding of the child and family. Audiovisual aids, pamphlets, and online information can be incorporated into the session. If the patient is newly diagnosed, hospitalization offers opportunities for instruction.

Blood glucose self-monitoring. Patients test their own blood glucose level at home. The patient can make changes in insulin dosage (sliding scale dosage) based on home blood glucose tests, nutritional requirements, and daily exercise. This is of great psychological value to the child, adolescent, and parents because it reduces feelings of helplessness and complete dependence on medical personnel. Home glucose monitoring should be taught to all young patients and their caregivers. The patient not only must be skilled in the techniques but also should understand the results and how to incorporate them into daily regimens. This means involving the entire health care team in ongoing supervision, demonstrations, and support. Although instructions are included with the various products, patients need personalized education.

Glucometer systems can provide readouts and can automatically store data by time and date. Some also keep track of diet and the amount of exercise for the day. They can be connected to a computer, electronic tablet, or smartphone for review or to an insulin pump. Records can be transmitted electronically to the health care provider.

Nursing Care Plan 31.1 The Child With Type 1 Diabetes Mellitus

PATIENT DATA

A 10-year-old boy is admitted with new-onset type 1 diabetes mellitus. An insulin regimen is prescribed. The child states that he wishes to return to a normal life with his peers.

Selected Nursing Diagnosis Risk for hypoglycemia or diabetic ketoacidosis (hyperglycemia) as a result of lack of knowledge about the disease

Goals	Nursing Interventions	Rationales
Child will be able to measure blood glucose level with glucometer, as age appropriate.	Teach child home glucose monitoring.	Self-care increases feelings of control.
	Record vital signs regularly.	Vital signs are used to detect infection and illness, which affect diabetes; in ketoacidosis, Kussmaul respirations may be seen until blood pH and serum bicarbonate levels normalize.
Child will be adequately hydrated as evidenced by good tissue turgor and intake and output records.	Monitor fluid intake and output.	Dehydration may occur as a result of vomiting, polyuria, and hyperglycemia.
	Serve meals and snacks on time.	Serving meals on time prevents hypoglycemia and minimizes hyperglycemia.
	Administer or have patient administer insulin as ordered.	Insulin is individualized to meet the response of patients. It cannot be taken by mouth because stomach juices would destroy it before it could be used.
Child will be asymptomatic of hypoglycemia or hyperglycemia.	Determine level of consciousness. Carefully observe patient for signs of hypoglycemia or hyperglycemia.	Both hypoglycemia and hyperglycemia affect sensorium, depending on stage of reaction.
		Factors such as diet, increased exercise, or illness can contribute to the body's balance of insulin and glucose; changes in hormone levels that accompany menstruation can cause swings of high or low blood glucose levels.

Selected Nursing Diagnosis Need for education about exercise

Goals	Nursing Interventions	Rationales
Child will describe physical exercise program.	Determine child's activity level as age appropriate.	Exercise increases glucose use.
	Explain that exercise lowers the blood glucose level and in this respect acts like more insulin.	Patient may need to adjust insulin dose for days when involved in high-impact exercise.
Child will be prepared for hypoglycemia should it occur.	Teach symptoms of hypoglycemia, such as irritability, shakiness, hunger, headache, and altered levels of consciousness.	Early recognition and prompt treatment will prevent injury.
	Teach child importance of carrying extra sugar when exercising or playing sports.	Taking sugar reverses symptoms of hypoglycemia.
	Teach child the dangers of swimming alone.	Child could drown if symptoms occur.

Selected Nursing Diagnosis Need for education about safety

Goals	Nursing Interventions	Rationales
Child will state understanding of importance of wearing proper identification bracelet.	Child demonstrates proper identification.	Diabetes symptoms may be mistaken for other conditions, such as flu.
Family will acquire medical identification bracelet.	Encourage purchase of means of identification.	Child may be unconscious or too young to inform others of condition.

CRITICAL THINKING QUESTION

1. A child comes to the clinic for follow-up after discharge from the hospital with a diagnosis of diabetic ketoacidosis. He states he is excited about returning to school and rejoining his cross-country team with his friends. His father states he wants his son to stay home and do more sedentary activities to prevent any more health problems. What is the best response of the nurse?

Obtaining blood specimens before meals and at bedtime has been simplified by the use of capillary bloodletting devices. These devices automatically control the depth of penetration of the lancet into the skin. The sides of the fingertips are recommended testing sites because there are fewer nerve endings and more capillary beds in these areas. The best fingers to use are the middle, ring, or little fingers on either hand. The finger will bleed more easily if the child washes the hands in warm water for about 30 seconds. To perform the test, a drop of blood is put on a chemically treated reagent strip. The test strip with a drop of blood is inserted into the glucometer, and the blood glucose reading appears.

Methods of glucose monitoring provide different information. The *finger-stick* method of glucose monitoring shows the glucose level at a moment in time. *Continuous glucose monitoring* measures real-time levels within the interstitial tissues and shows trends in glucose levels but does not completely replace glucometers.

Cost, convenience, and portability are factors to consider when selecting glucometers. Most products can be obtained at the local pharmacy, and cost is generally covered by the provincial health plan and other forms of health insurance. Newer and more precise instruments are being developed constantly.

Continuous glucose monitoring. The continuous glucose monitor consists of a sensor placed under the skin in the abdomen that transmits interstitial blood glucose levels every 10 to 60 seconds to a monitor that can be worn on the patient's clothing or to an electronic device such as a smartphone. This glucose monitoring technique helps identify fluctuation and trends that cannot be picked up by the standard intermittent finger-stick measurements or $HgbA_{1c}$ test. The continuous glucose monitoring system is used to devise an individualized treatment plan for the patient. A continuous glucose monitoring system can usually be used by children age 7 years and older.

Insulin administration. Insulin is a specific medication for the control of DM. When injected into the diabetic patient, it enables the body to burn and store sugar. The dose of insulin is measured in units. U-100 (100-unit) insulin is the standard form. The dosage of insulin is determined by monitoring glucose levels and adjusting the insulin dose to avoid hypo- or hyperglycemia that could result in serious long-term complications. Storage of insulin in extreme temperatures (below [2.2°C, or 36°F] or above [29.4°C, or 85°F]) can destroy insulin. Insulin potency can be decreased if the bottle has been open longer than 1 month.

Intermittent administration of insulin. It is important to teach the parents and child about the administration of insulin. Insulin cannot be taken orally because it is a protein and would be broken down by the gastric juices. The usual method of administration is subcutaneous injection (Fig. 31.3). When injected at a 90-degree angle, the short needle enters the subcutaneous space. This technique may be easier for the child to learn because it takes less coordination to administer than a 45-degree angle technique. Insulin "pens" and injectors for insulin are convenient alternatives from the traditional syringe technique of administering insulin. Administration is as simple as rotating a dial to the intended dose.

The site of the injection is rotated to prevent poor absorption and injury to tissues (Fig. 31.4). One suggested site rotation pattern is to use one area for 1 week. A different site within that area is used for each injection. Injections should be about 2.5 cm apart. In general, a child can be taught to perform self-injection after 7 years of age. The young child and parents can use a doll or a simulator to practice self-injection (Fig. 31.5). Injection models made from construction paper and site rotation patterns are also useful for practice.

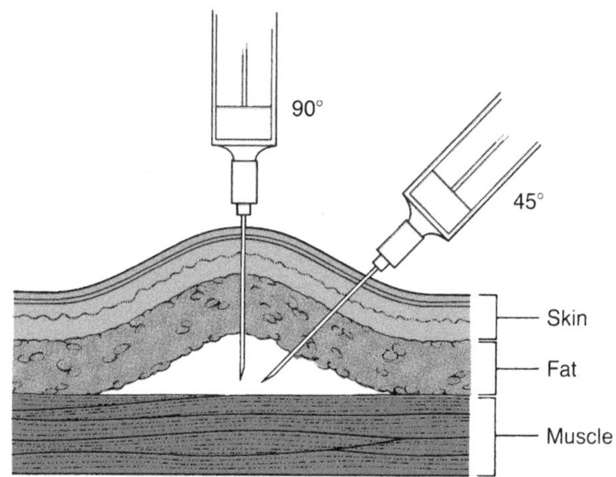

Fig. 31.3 Subcutaneous injection of insulin.

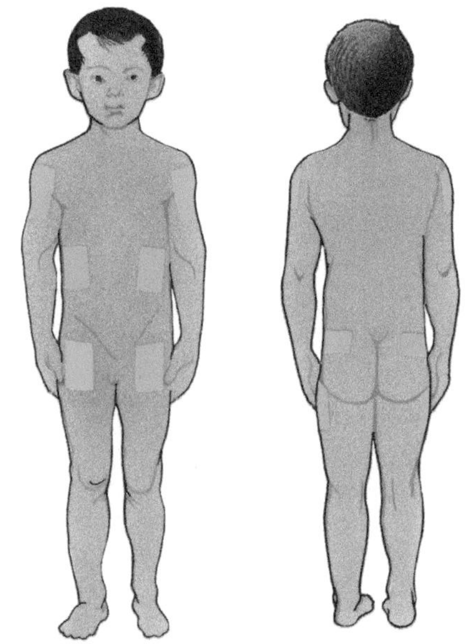

Fig. 31.4 Sites of injection of insulin. (From McKinney, E. S., James, S. R., Murray, S. S., & Ashwill, J. W. [2018]. *Maternal-child nursing* [5th ed.]. Philadelphia: Saunders.)

Insulin should not be injected into an area in which circulation is temporarily increased. In such areas, a more rapid than expected absorption and effect can trigger hypoglycemia. For example, a more rapid circulation to the legs can be expected in a child who is riding a tricycle; therefore, the thigh should not be selected as a site for injection after such activity. If a child has just played tennis, the upper arm is avoided as an injection site for the same reason.

Lipoatrophy (lipo, "fat," and atrophy, "loss of") and *lipohypertrophy* (lipo, "fat," and hypertrophy, "increase of") refer to changes that can occur in the subcutaneous tissue at the injection site. Proper rotation of sites and the availability of the newer purified insulins have helped to eliminate this condition. The child is taught to "feel for lumps" every week and to avoid using any sites that are suspicious.

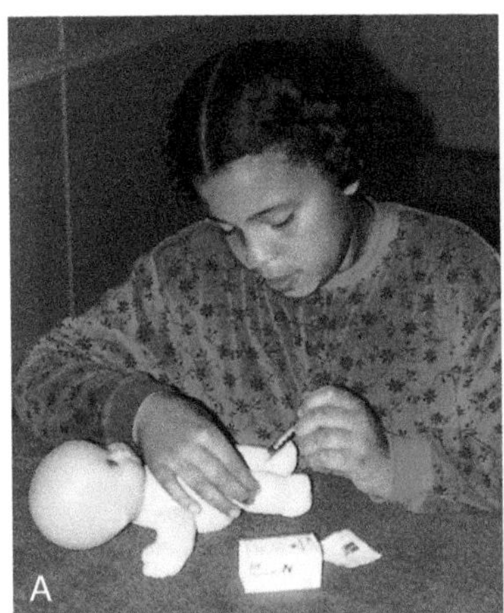
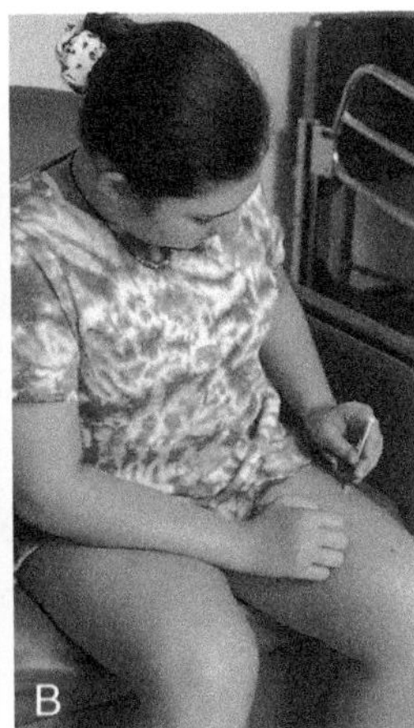

Fig. 31.5 **A,** By giving injections to dolls or puppets, children can be prepared for this procedure and may be less frightened by it. **B,** A child 7 years of age or older can take responsibility for self-injection, with proper supervision. (**A**, courtesy Pat Spier, RN-C; **B**, from McKinney, E. S., James, S. R., Murray, S. S., & Ashwill, J. W. [2018]. *Maternal-child nursing* [5th ed.]. Philadelphia: Saunders.)

The various types of insulin and their action are listed in Table 31.5. The main differences between insulins are the amount of time required for the insulin to take effect, peak action, and duration of the protection provided. The values listed in the table are only *guidelines.* The response of each diabetic child to any given insulin dose is highly individual and depends on many factors, such as stress, site of injection, local destruction of insulin by tissue enzymes, and insulin antibodies.

The health care provider will often order a combination of short-acting and intermediate-acting insulin; for example, "Give 10 units of NPH insulin and 5 units of regular insulin at 0730." This offers the patient immediate and longer-lasting protection. Neutral protamine (NPH) insulin may be administered in the same syringe as regular or crystalline insulin (Fig. 31.6). Stable, premixed insulins are more readily available and tend to be the most common form used. Insulin analogues such as glargine and detemir more closely mimic human insulin.

Current data emphasize the importance of blood glucose control in the prevention of micro- and macrovascular disease. Glucose control is obtained by administering insulin in a basal-dose bolus regimen that involves a combination of slow-onset–long-duration types of insulin with a rapid insulin as necessary for meals or snacks. For example, once a day a basal dose of long-acting insulin may be administered, such as glargine or detemir, and a bolus of shorter-acting insulin, such as Lispro or Aspart, may be administered with meals. An alternate plan may include combining NPH insulin with a rapid-acting bolus at breakfast, a rapid-acting analogue bolus at dinner, and a long-acting glargine at bedtime, which reduces the number of daily injections required. Blood glucose finger-stick monitoring is essential, as activity levels and snacks in young children will affect their needs. Nutritional education is also essential. Illness, infection, and surgery require special modifications in the glucose regimen until the child is healthy again.

Table 31.5 Types of Insulin*

TYPE	ONSET	APPROXIMATE PEAK	APPROXIMATE DURATION
Short-Acting			
Regular	30–60 minutes	2–5 hours	5–8 hours
Rapid-Acting			
Insulin Lispro	15–30 minutes	30–90 minutes	3–5 hours
Aspart	10–20 minutes	40–50 minutes	3–5 hours
Intermediate-Acting			
NPH	1–2 hours	4–12 hours	14+ hours
Long-Acting			
Insulin glargine†	1 hour	Relatively flat	20–24 hours
Detemir†	1 hour	Relatively flat	24 hours

*There are many combined mixtures of insulin available commercially. Synthetic insulin, free of animal impurities, is used for children.
†Do not mix with other insulins.
Lente and Ultra-Lente insulins are no longer used.
From Canadian Pharmacist Association. (2018). *Compendium of pharmaceuticals and specialties*. Ottawa: Author; Clayton, B., & Willihnganz, W. (2016). *Basic pharmacology for nurses* (17th ed.). St. Louis: Elsevier.

1. Perform hand hygiene.
2. Gently rotate the intermediate insulin bottle.
3. Wipe the tops of the insulin vials with an alcohol sponge.
4. Draw back an amount of air into the syringe equal to the total dose.
5. Inject air equal to the NPH dose into the NPH vial. Remove the syringe from the vial.

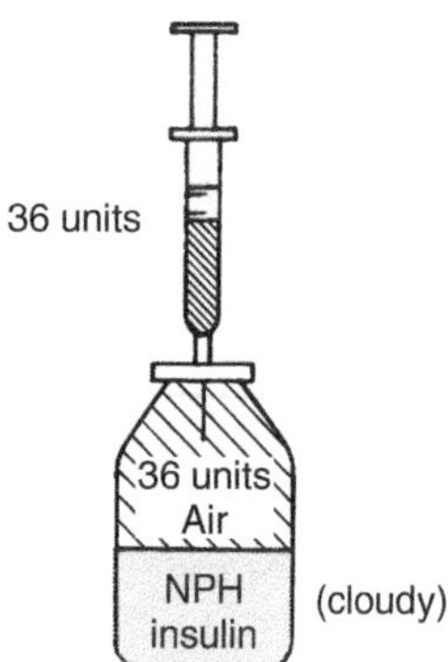

6. Inject air equal to the regular dose into the regular vial.

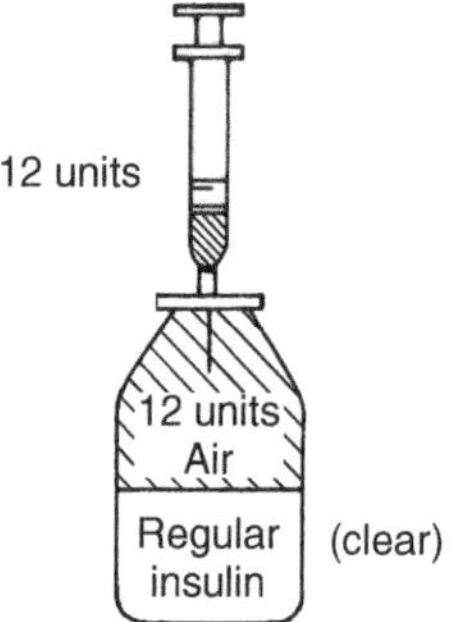

7. Invert the regular insulin bottle and withdraw the regular insulin dose.

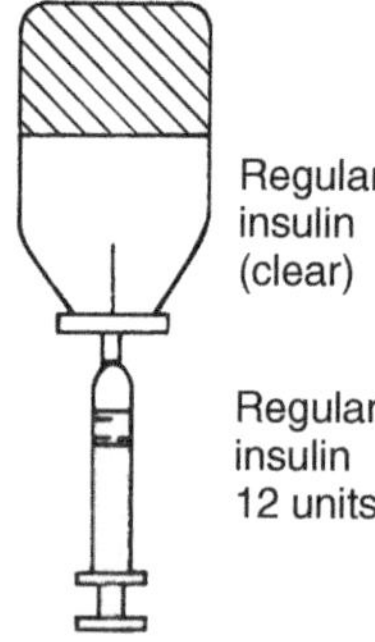

8. Without adding more air to the NPH vial, carefully withdraw the NPH dose.

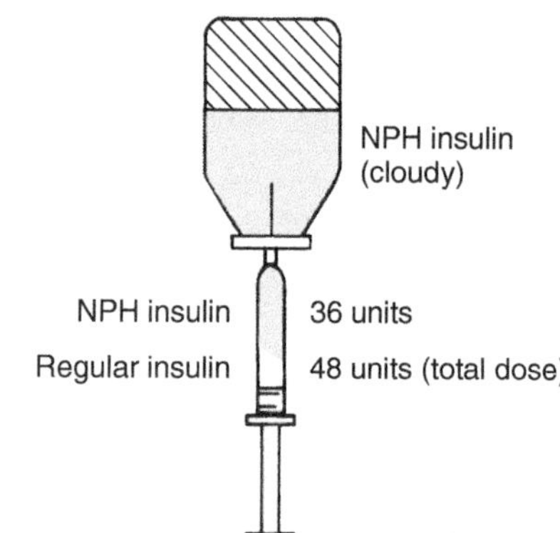

Fig. 31.6 Mixing insulin. This step-order process avoids the problem of contaminating the regular insulin with the intermediate-acting insulin. If contamination of the regular insulin does occur, the rapid-acting effect of this medication is diminished, and it is unreliable as a quick-acting insulin in an acute situation such as diabetic ketoacidosis. (From Bowden, V. R., Dickey, S. B., & Greenberg, S. C. [1998]. *Children and their families: The continuum of care*. Philadelphia: Saunders.)

Medication Alert!

Although not as common a practice today, when mixing insulin, always withdraw the regular insulin first and then add the long-acting insulin into the syringe.

The insulin pump. The insulin pump offers continuous personalized subcutaneous insulin infusion without the need for frequent injections

Closed loop system. A closed loop wireless system provides glycemic control with minimum intervention, by connecting the glucose monitor to an insulin pump that more closely mimics normal physiology. A small, pager-sized, battery-powered, programmable pump holds a cartridge supply of insulin. A catheter attaches to a needle that is inserted into the subcutaneous tissue and is secured with tape. An insulin pump can deliver a personalized 24-hour cycle of insulin plus manual delivery of bolus doses as needed. When connected by wireless technology to a glucose monitor, changes in insulin doses can be programmed and automatic reminders for appropriate actions offered (Fig. 31.7). The closed loop system is designed to alarm and stop insulin delivery when interstitial glucose levels fall below a predetermined level or provide a dose of insulin if the glucose level is above a predetermined level (Svoren & Jospe, 2016). A closed loop system does not completely eliminate the need for blood glucose monitoring checks (which is usually done before meals) to determine the need for a bolus injection based on the food intake.

Some models of closed loop insulin pumps/glucometers have wireless technology with a free smartphone app that shares information with the health care provider. Some models are waterproof. The insulin

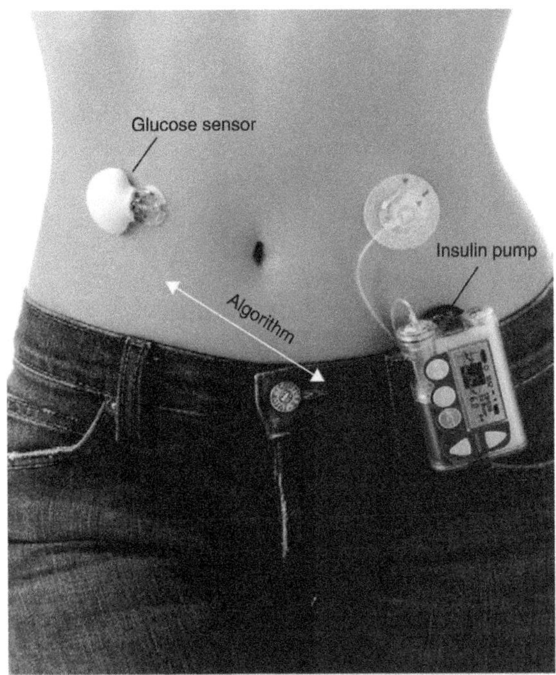

Fig. 31.7 The closed loop system involves both a glucose monitor and insulin delivery catheters attached to needles that are inserted under the skin of the abdomen, secured, and wirelessly communicate with a pager-sized insulin delivery device. This unit provides programmed amounts of insulin around the clock with required changes made by remote control. It can also provide reminders, such as the need to check blood glucose levels and health care provider appointments. (From Atkinson, M. A., Eisenbarth, G. S., & Michels, A. W. [2014]. Type 1 diabetes. *Lancet, 383*, 69–78; Kliegman, R., Stanton, B., St. Geme, J., et al. [Eds.]. [2016]. *Nelson textbook of pediatrics* [20th ed.]. Philadelphia: Saunders.)

pump may need to be disconnected for some procedures, such as magnetic resonance imaging (MRI), and other sources of insulin must be provided.

Inhaled or oral insulin. Inhaled insulin has been under study and appears to be effective. Health Canada has not approved inhaled insulin for marketing in Canada (Canadian Agency for Drugs and Technologies in Health, 2013). More research is needed to determine its long-term effects on the lung tissue before it is released for general use. Oral insulin is not available in Canada. An insulin patch is under development but not approved for use in Canada.

Insulin shock. Insulin shock, also known as *hypoglycemia* (*hypo,* "below," *glyco,* "sugar," and *emia,* "blood"), occurs when the blood glucose level becomes abnormally low. Too much insulin is one cause of this condition. Factors that may contribute to this imbalance include poorly planned exercise, reduced diet, illness, and errors in insulin administration.

Children are more prone to insulin reactions than adults because of the following:

- The condition itself is more unstable in young people.
- Children are growing.
- Children's activities are more irregular.

Unplanned exercise is often the cause of insulin shock during childhood. Hospitalized patients must be observed frequently during naptime and at night. The nurse should become suspicious of problems if there is difficulty in arousing the patient or if the child is perspiring heavily.

The symptoms of an insulin reaction, which range from mild to severe, are generally noticed and treated in the early stages. They appear suddenly in the otherwise well person. Examination of the blood shows a lowered blood glucose level. The child becomes irritable, may behave poorly, is pale and sweaty, and may state feelings of hunger and weakness. Symptoms related to disorders of the nervous system arise because glucose is vital to the proper functioning of nerves. The child may become mentally confused and giddy, and muscular coordination is affected. If insulin shock is left untreated, coma and convulsions can occur.

The immediate treatment consists of administering sugar in some form, such as 125 mL of orange juice, hard candy, a small box of raisins, or a commercial (glucose tablet) product. The patient begins to feel better within a few minutes and at that time may eat a small amount of protein or starch (sandwich, milk, cheese) to prevent another reaction. **Glucagon** is recommended for the treatment of severe hypoglycemia. It quickly restores the child to consciousness in an emergency; the child can then consume some form of sugar or a planned meal.

The **Somogyi phenomenon** (rebound hyperglycemia) occurs when blood glucose levels are lowered to a point at which the body's counterregulatory hormones (epinephrine, cortisol, glucagon) are released. Glucose is released from muscle and liver cells, which precipitates a rapid rise in blood glucose levels. It is generally the result of chronic insulin use, especially in patients who require fairly large doses of insulin to regulate their blood glucose levels. Hypoglycemia during the night and high glucose levels in the morning are suggestive of the phenomenon. The child may awaken at night or have frequent nightmares and experience early morning sweating and headaches. The child actually needs less insulin, not more, to rectify the problem. The Somogyi phenomenon differs from the **dawn phenomenon**, in which early morning elevations of blood glucose occur *in the absence of* preceding hypoglycemia and may be a response to growth hormone secretion that occurs in the early morning hours.

Together, the Somogyi and dawn phenomena are the most common causes of instability in diabetic children. Testing blood glucose levels around 0300 helps to differentiate the two conditions and aids in regulating insulin dosage. Whenever the insulin regime is changed, close monitoring of blood glucose levels is essential to detect the Somogyi and dawn effects that are common in children. Continuous glucose monitoring systems may help prevent either phenomenon (Svoren & Jospe, 2016).

Oral medication. Treatment guidelines for type 2 DM include lifestyle changes to reduce obesity and antidiabetic medication such as metformin, which is the only oral antidiabetic agent approved for children and adolescents. Newer antidiabetic medications have been developed for adult use, but the risks and benefits must be closely evaluated before use in the pediatric setting. A combination therapy of metformin and insulin may be required for adequate glucose control.

When metformin is prescribed, the creatinine level and kidney and liver function should be monitored and metformin should be temporarily discontinued during radiological tests that include IV iodized contrast dyes.

Blood glucose monitoring is essential to ensure the appropriate medication is being prescribed.

Nutrition management. The triad of diabetes management consists of a well-balanced diet, precise medication administration, and regular exercise. Glycemic control is important in decreasing the incidence of symptoms and complications of the disease. The advent of blood glucose self-monitoring has affected patients' food intake in that diets can be fine-tuned and made more flexible while the cornerstone of *consistency* (in amount of food and time of feeding) is maintained.

Contrary to popular belief, there is no scientific evidence indicating that persons with diabetes require special foods. In fact, if it is good for the diabetic patient, it is good for the entire family. The nutritional needs of diabetic children are essentially no different from those of nondiabetic children. The timing of food consumption has to be correlated with the timing and action of the type of insulin or oral hypoglycemic prescribed so that blood glucose levels will not become abnormally high or abnormally low.

The goals of nutrition management in children are to ensure normal growth and development, to distribute food intake so that it aids metabolic control, and to individualize the diet in accordance with the child's ethnic background, age, gender, weight, activity, family economics, and food preferences. Total estimated caloric intake is based on body size or surface area and can be obtained in standard tables. The recommended intake is 55% carbohydrates (mostly complex carbohydrates), 30% fat, and 15% protein (Svoren & Jospe, 2016). Most of the carbohydrate intake should consist of complex carbohydrates that absorb slowly and do not cause sudden and wide elevation of blood glucose level. Dietary fat from animal sources should be limited and replaced with polyunsaturated fats found in vegetables. Occasional excesses for birthdays or special occasions can be accommodated to prevent the child's resistance to dietary restrictions and to promote adherence. Special supplements may be required to accommodate the exercise patterns and growth needs of children.

After a diet prescription is received from the health care provider, a dietitian may assist the family in designing an individualized diet plan. The dietitian should also explain the use of exchange lists (a list of foods that may be substituted with any other food on the same list equal in carbohydrates, calories, protein, and fat).

Carbohydrate counting, in which one carbohydrate choice equals 15 g of carbohydrate, enables flexibility in meal planning. Generally, one unit of insulin covers 15 g of carbohydrate. A general nutrition plan can be created for a child using foods they like, including snacks. The diet prescription usually includes carbohydrate values. Carbohydrate counting offers adolescents in particular control of their diet and involvement in maintaining a positive self-concept and self-esteem, which can promote adherence. An aid in developing food plans is the Government of Canada's (2019) "Eat Well Plate" website, which is aligned with *Canada's Food Guide.*

Education of the child and family regarding diet should be ongoing, without offering too much information at one time, which can overwhelm the parents and discourage the child. For hospitalized patients, ordering of meals can provide an excellent opportunity for teaching. Nurses need to respect cultural patterns and personal preferences when discussing food plans. Nurses can also offer reinforcement and support, for example, by clarifying terms such as *dietetic, sugar free, juice-packed, water-packed,* and *unsweetened.*

The importance of fibre in diets is well documented. In the diabetic patient, soluble fibre has been shown to reduce blood glucose levels, lower serum cholesterol values, and sometimes reduce insulin requirements. Fibre appears to slow the rate of absorption of sugar by the digestive tract. Raw fruits and vegetables, bran cereals, wheat germ, beans, peas, and lentils are good sources of soluble fibre.

! Safety Alert!

Instruct the patient and family to read food labels carefully. The word *dietetic* does not mean *diabetic.* Dietetic merely means something has been changed or replaced; for example, the food may contain less salt or less sugar.

Glycemic index of foods. The glycemic index for selected foods has an impact on the manipulation of dietary needs (Table 31.6). The *glycemic index* is the impact of a portion of food on the blood glucose as compared to the same portion of pure glucose. With intake of foods with a low glycemic index (less than 55), it takes longer to increase the glucose levels in the blood. Foods that have a high glycemic index (more than 70) increase blood glucose levels more rapidly. The glycemic index may be higher for the liquid form (apple juice) than the same carbohydrate in solid form (whole apple). The fibre content of the food can lower the glycemic index. Some chocolate may have a low glycemic index, but the high saturated fat content limits its nutritional and health value.

The *glycemic load* takes into account the amount of glucose in a food combined with the total carbohydrate content of a serving portion. Knowledge of foods' glycemic load enables a person to select optimal foods to eat before, during, and after exercise. The size of portions, the type of processing or cooking, and the combinations of foods have also been shown to have an effect on glucose responses.

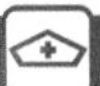 **Nursing Tip**

Patients should be instructed to take snacks seriously—they are an important part of the day's food supply.

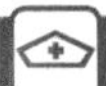 **Nursing Tip**

Avoid the use of sorbitol or xylitol as artificial sweeteners in the diets of children with diabetes (Svoren & Jospe, 2016).

Patient teaching

Exercise. Exercise is important for the patient with diabetes because it causes the body to metabolize sugar and promotes good circulation. It lowers the blood glucose level and, in this respect, it acts like more insulin. The diabetic patient who has planned vigorous exercise should carry extra sugar to avoid insulin reactions. The child or teenager with diabetes should also carry money for candy or a drink and, if possible, carry a cell phone. The diabetic child can participate in almost all active sports, with thoughtful planning and preparation. Exercise that is not well planned, however, can lead to negative consequences, as discussed previously.

For children with type 2 DM, exercise is also very important. Moderate to vigorous physical activity for 1 hour per day and fewer than 2 hours of nonacademic screen time per day are recommended, as many of these children require weight reduction (Svoran & Jospe, 2016).

Skin care. The patient should bathe daily and dry skin well, especially between the toes. Cleansing of the inguinal area, axillae, perineum, and inframammary areas is especially important because yeast and fungal infections tend to occur at these sites. The skin must be inspected for injection site lumps and any cuts, rashes, abrasions, bruises, cysts, or boils. If found, they should be treated promptly. If skin is very dry, an oil such as Alpha Keri may be used in the bath water. Adolescents should be taught to use electric razors. All patients should be urged to avoid exposing the skin to extremes in temperatures.

Foot care. Although circulatory problems of the feet are less common in children, proper habits of foot hygiene must be established. Patients should be instructed to wash and dry their feet well each day. The feet should be inspected for interdigital cracking, and the condition of the toenails needs to be checked. Nails are trimmed straight across. Patients should change socks daily and not wear tight socks or large ones that bunch up. Shoes should be replaced often as the child grows.

Infections. Immunizations against communicable diseases are essential (see Chapter 32). Meticulous skin care and care of needles and insulin equipment can prevent infections.

Emotional upsets. Patients experiencing emotional upset and stress may need food adjustments, insulin adjustments, or both. Table 31.7 lists nursing interventions for stress on the child and family that are related to the child having type 1 diabetes.

Urine checks. Routine urine checks for sugar are being replaced by the more accurate glucose blood monitoring. However, this procedure does not test for acetone level, which the patient may need to determine, particularly during illness and when the blood glucose level is high. When urine checks are advocated for patients, saying urine "check" rather than "test" is less confusing to young children.

Glucose-insulin imbalances. Patients should be taught how to recognize the signs of insulin shock and ketoacidosis (see Table 31.4). Early attention to changes and daily record keeping are stressed. Many excellent teaching films, brochures, and online resources are available. Teachers, athletic coaches, and guidance personnel should be informed about the disease and have the telephone numbers of the patient's parents or guardian.

Travel. With planning, children can enjoy travel with their families, and older adolescents can travel alone. Before leaving on a trip, the child should be seen by the health care provider for a checkup and get prescriptions for supplies. The parents or adolescent should have a written statement and a bracelet identifying the child as having diabetes. Time changes may affect meals. Additional supplies of insulin, sugar, glucagon, and food need to be kept with the child. These are never checked with luggage, especially on an airplane, because they may be lost or damaged.

If foreign travel is planned, parents must become familiar with the food in the area so that dietary requirements can be met. Diabetes Canada has created a thorough and complete resource to assist families in planning to travel with a child with diabetes. Contacting a local chapter of Diabetes Canada is also helpful for on-site support.

Follow-up care. The child with diabetes must see the health care provider regularly. The parents and child should also be taught to visit the dentist regularly for cleaning of teeth and gums. Brushing and flossing daily are essential. Eyes should be examined regularly; blurry vision must not be ignored. There are many brochures, books, websites, and apps that offer excellent suggestions and guidance at an age-appropriate level.

Illness or surgery. When illness occurs, close glucose monitoring and control are essential. Hyperglycemia causes diuresis and dehydration, and ketosis can involve vomiting. Counteracting regulatory hormones that are secreted during periods of stress interfere with the effectiveness of insulin, resulting in increased glucose levels. Modification of insulin doses may be necessary.

The patient with diabetes usually tolerates surgery well. Insulin may be given before, during, or after the operation. If the patient is restricted to nothing by mouth, calories may be supplied by IV glucose. Careful review of the patient's history helps in formulating nursing care plans and provides a basis for teaching.

Long-term complications. The complications of DM include microvascular (mostly referring to kidney, eye, neurological, and circulatory problems) and macrovascular (referring to coronary artery disease, peripheral arterial disease, and stroke) issues. Diabetic retinopathy (pathology of the retina) is the most common eye disease in Canada (Diabetes Canada, 2019). Preventing hyperglycemia is essential in avoiding this complication. Routine eye examinations should be scheduled and are an important part of follow-up care.

Nephropathy (kidney pathology) affects 20 to 30% of diabetic children. Stabilizing glucose levels and preventing the development of hypertension can decrease this risk. The nervous system is also affected by hyperglycemia. Adolescents should be assessed for peripheral neuropathy (decreased sensation). A decline in diabetic complications has been noted since the use

Table 31.6 Glycemic Index of Selected Foods

FOOD	GLYCEMIC INDEX*
All-Bran cereal	44
Apple	36
Baked potato	78
Banana	48
Carrots	39
Corn flakes	81
French baguette bread	95
Cranberry juice cocktail	68
Cola	65 +
Sports beverages	75 +
Peach	43
Peanuts	13
Skim milk	31
Spaghetti	46
Watermelon	72
White bread	70

*Foods with a low glycemic index take a longer time to increase the glucose levels in the blood.

Data from Atkinson, F., Foster-Powell, R., & Brand-Miller, J. (2008). International table of glycemic index and glycemic load values. *Diabetic Care, 31*(12), 2281–2283; Mahan, L., & Escott-Stump, S. (2017). *Krause's food and the nutrition care process* (15th ed.). Philadelphia: Saunders.

Table 31.7 Nursing Interventions for Predictable Types of Stress in a Child With Type 1 Diabetes and in the Family

AGE	ISSUE	NURSING INTERVENTION
Infant	Trust versus mistrust Onset and diagnosis particularly difficult during infancy; anxiety can be transmitted to infant	Stress consistency in fulfilling needs. Involve all appropriate family members in education. Avoid information overload. Instill hope and confidence. Focus on child rather than disease. Review normal growth and development of infancy. Assist in problem solving (e.g., babysitters, difficulty in obtaining specimens, baby food exchange lists).
Toddler	Autonomy versus shame and doubt Is this a temper tantrum or high or low blood glucose?	Prepare child for procedures or separations. Encourage exploration of environment. Stress limit setting as a form of love. Admit it is difficult to distinguish temper tantrums from symptoms. If behaviour worsens or is prolonged or if physical symptoms appear, check blood glucose level. Provide 24-hour telephone number for advice from nurse.
Preschool	Initiative versus guilt May view injections as punishment May view denial of sweets as lack of love "Picky eater"	Foster sense of competence. Educate parents to provide consistent warmth, reassurance, and love. Discuss feelings about child's life and diabetes. Avoid use of words with a negative connotation, such as "bad blood test" or "cheating." Help parents sort out child's fantasies. Plan favourite party dishes on occasion. Invite a playmate for lunch. Suggest alternative nutritious snacks.

Continued

Table 31.7 Nursing Interventions for Predictable Types of Stress in a Child with Type 1 Diabetes and in the Family—cont'd

AGE	ISSUE	NURSING INTERVENTION
Elementary school	Industry versus inferiority Patients may feel they will be cured by hospitalization Grief over lack of cure Rebellion about treatment regimen Rebellion regarding food plan Anxiety about disclosure of condition to friends Embarrassed about reactions in school, missed days Unpredictable effects of exercise	Assist child in how to respond to teasing from peers ("Yecch, needles"). Explain "honeymoon" stage of disease. Accept child's disappointment. Gradually promote self-management of insulin and specimen tests; this increases feelings of mastery and control. Provide lists of fast-food exchanges. Provide group-related education with diabetic peers. Promote open dialogue among health personnel, teachers, and fellow students. Continually reinforce treatment principles with specific regard to hypoglycemia or hyperglycemia and emergencies.
Puberty	"Bouncing" blood glucose levels may make adolescent feel out of control Anger at the disease: "Why must I be different?" More frequent hospitalizations	Explain that growth and sex hormones affect blood glucose levels. Girls in particular experience difficulties during the time of menstruation. Adjustments in insulin and food are common for most diabetic patients at this stage. Assist patient in acceptable ways of expressing anger; discuss anger with parents, because parents are often its target. Provide encouragement and support; be alert to marital stress and sibling deprivation.

Get Ready for the Certification Examination!

Key Points

- The two major systems that control and monitor the functions of the body are the nervous system and the endocrine system.
- The term *inborn error of metabolism* refers to a group of inherited biochemical disorders that affect body metabolism.
- Screening programs for early detection of inborn errors are important because some conditions can cause irreversible neurological damage.
- Growth hormone is administered at bedtime to simulate the natural time of hormone release.
- A deficiency in the secretions of the thyroid gland is termed *hypothyroidism.* It may be congenital or acquired and necessitates lifelong treatment with oral administration of a synthetic thyroid hormone.
- A child with diabetes insipidus requires unlimited access to water.
- Diabetes mellitus type 1 is the most common endocrine disorder of children. The body is unable to use carbohydrates properly because of a deficiency of insulin, which is an internal secretion of the pancreas.
- Insulin resistance causes type 2 diabetes mellitus. It is precipitated by obesity, a lipid-rich diet, and inactivity, and it is becoming more prevalent in children.
- The symptoms of diabetes mellitus appear more rapidly in children. Three symptoms are polydipsia, polyuria, and polyphagia.
- The mainstays of the management of type 1 diabetes mellitus are insulin replacement, diet, and exercise.
- Diabetic ketoacidosis is a serious complication that may become life-threatening.
- The Somogyi phenomenon and the dawn phenomenon are common causes of glucose instability in children.
- Self-management to maintain glucose control and prevent complications is a major goal of education of the child with diabetes mellitus.
- A continuous glucose monitoring system can be programmed to meet individual needs.
- An insulin pump provides subcutaneous doses of insulin that are controlled by a computerized monitor.
- The glycated hemoglobin test (A_{1c}) reflects glucose control over a specific time period.
- Sugar substitutes such as sorbitol and xylitol should not be provided to children.

Additional Learning Resources

evolve Go to your Evolve website (http://evolve.elsevier.com/Canada/Leifer) for the following learning resources:

- Answer Key for Critical Thinking Questions
- Answer Key for Textbook Review Questions
- Audio Glossary
- Interactive Review Questions
- Skills Performance Checklists
- Video clips and more!

Online Resources

- Canadian Inherited Metabolic Diseases Research Network*:* http://www.cimdrn.ca/
- Diabetes Canada: https://www.diabetes.ca/

Review Questions

1. What is an important aspect of a teaching plan for the parent of a child with hypopituitarism?
   a. The child should be enrolled in a special education program at school.
   b. The routine administration of growth hormone should be performed at bedtime.
   c. All family members should have an endocrine workup.
   d. The routine medication should be administered before the school day starts.
2. A child who has diabetes mellitus asks why he cannot take insulin orally instead of by subcutaneous injection. Which is the best response of the nurse?
   a. Pills are only for adults.
   b. Digestive enzymes destroy insulin.
   c. Insulin can cause a stomach ulcer.
   d. Insulin interacts with food in the stomach.
3. What may indicate a need for insulin in a diabetic child?
   a. Diaphoresis and tremors
   b. Red lips and fruity odour to the breath
   c. Confusion and lethargy
   d. Headache and pallor
4. Why would a nurse teach the diabetic child to rotate sites of insulin injection?
   a. Prevent subcutaneous deposit of the medication
   b. Prevent lipoatrophy of subcutaneous fat
   c. Decrease the pain of injection
   d. Increase absorption of insulin
5. While teaching the child with type 1 diabetes mellitus how to prevent hypoglycemia during afternoon volleyball practice, what should a nurse reinforce in the teaching? *(Select all that apply.)*
   a. Eat extra food at lunch time.
   b. Administer a smaller dose of insulin at midday.
   c. Drink a half a cup of orange juice before practice.
   d. Check blood glucose before practice.
6. The family of a child with diabetes insipidus states that the school is planning a field trip and asks the nurse for advice. Which of the following needs for the child should be emphasized by the nurse? *(Select all that apply.)*
   a. Have access to a bathroom
   b. Have free access to water supply
   c. Not eat food containing salt
   d. Have a dose of glucose available during activity

of continuous glucose monitoring devices and insulin pumps (Svoren & Jospe, 2016).

Prospects for the future

Diabetic research is being conducted on many fronts. Pancreas transplantation has been performed in adults. Laser eye surgery has aided the treatment for complicated eye conditions. Such advances hold promise for resolving or eradicating the dilemma of diabetes in children.

REFERENCES

Canadian Agency for Drugs and Technologies in Health. (2013). *Afrezza inhaled insulin for diabetes mellitus. Issues in Emerging Health Technologies*, 120. Retrieved from https://www.cadth.ca/media/pdf/EH0003InhaledInsulin_eh_e_rev.pdf.

Canadian Organization for Rare Disorders. (2015). *Newborn screening in Canada status report*. Retrieved from https://www.raredisorders.ca/content/uploads/Canada-NBS-status-updated-Sept.-3-2015.pdf.

Diabetes Canada. (2017). *Diabetes Canada 2018 pre-budget submission: 90-90-90—Measurable change and improved productivity by 2021. To the House of Commons Standing Committee on Finance, August 4, 2017*. Retrieved from https://www.diabetes.ca/DiabetesCanadaWebsite/media/Advocacy-and-Policy/Submissions%20to%20Government/Federal/2018-Federal-PBS.pdf.

Diabetes Canada. (2019). *What is diabetes?* Retrieved from https://www.diabetes.ca/about-diabetes/prediabetes.

Government of Canada. (2019). *Make healthy meals with the Eat Well Plate*. Retrieved from http://www.healthycanadians.gc.ca/eating-nutrition/healthy-eating-saine-alimentation/tips-conseils/interactive-tools-outils-interactifs/eat-well-bien-manger-eng.php.

Government of Canada. (2018). *Type 2 diabetes*. Retrieved from https://www.canada.ca/en/public-health/services/diseases/type-2-diabetes.html.

McGovern, M., & Desnick, R. (2016). Liposomal storage disorders. In R. Kliegman, B. Stanton, J. St. Geme, et al. (Eds.), *Nelson textbook of pediatrics* (20th ed.). Philadelphia: Saunders.

National Human Genome Research Institute. (2011). *Learning about Tay-Sachs disease*. Retrieved from https://www.genome.gov/10001220/learning-about-taysachs-disease/.

Panagiotopoulos, C., Hadjiyannakis, S., & Henderson, M. I. (2018). Type 2 diabetes in children and adolescents. Clinical Practice Guidelines. *Canadian Journal of Diabetes*, 42(Suppl 1), S247-S254. Retrieved from http://guidelines.diabetes.ca/cpg/chapter35#sec3.

Punthakee, Z., Goldenberg, R., & Katz, J. (2018). Definition, classification and diagnosis of diabetes, prediabetes and metabolic syndrome. *Canadian Journal of Diabetes*, 42(Suppl 1), S10-S15. Retrieved from http://guidelines.diabetes.ca/cpg/chapter3.

Svoren, B., & Jospe, N. (2016). Diabetes mellitus. In R. Kliegman, B. Stanton, J. St. Geme, et al. (Eds.), *Nelson textbook of pediatrics* (20th ed.). Philadelphia: Saunders.

Childhood Communicable Diseases

32

Krystal Buchanan

http://evolve.elsevier.com/Canada/Leifer

Objectives

1. Define each key term listed.
2. Discuss the characteristics of common childhood communicable diseases.
3. Outline the detection and prevention of common childhood communicable diseases.
4. Discuss three principles involved in routine practices and additional precautions used to prevent the transmission of communicable diseases in children.
5. Describe Canadian immunization guidelines.
6. Develop an awareness of worldwide efforts to control the spread of communicable diseases.
7. Describe the nurse's role in the immunization of children.
8. Outline a teaching plan for preventing sexually transmitted infections (STIs) in an adolescent.
9. Formulate a nursing care plan for a child with acquired immunodeficiency syndrome (AIDS).
10. Describe the symptoms of sepsis.

Key Terms

acquired immunity
active immunity
additional precautions
body substance
communicable disease
endemic (ĕn-DĔM-ĭk)
epidemic (ĕp-ĭ-DĔM-ĭk)
erythema (ĕr-ĭ-THĒ-mă)
fomite (FŌ-mīt)
health care–associated infection (HAI)
incubation period
macule (MĂK-yūl,)
natural immunity
opportunistic infections
pandemic (păn-DĔM-ĭk)
papule (PĂP-yūl)
passive immunity
pathogens (PĂTH-ō-jĕnz)
pathognomonic (păth-ŏg-nō-MŎN-ĭk)
portal of entry
portal of exit
prodromal period (prō-DRŌ-mŭl PĒ-rē-ŏd)
pustule (PŬS-tyūl)
reservoir for infection
routine precautions
scab
vector (VĔK-tŭr)
vesicle (VĔS-ĭ-kŭl)

There have been only a few brief periods in history when infectious disease did not dominate the attention of health care professionals. Despite immunization, sanitation, antimicrobial medications, and other controls, the world continues to face infectious agents such as hepatitis, tuberculosis, and sexually transmitted infections (STIs), including human immunodeficiency virus (HIV). Despite our knowledge of immunizations, some children still develop common communicable diseases. Antimicrobial medication-resistant organisms are increasing in number and virulence, and immunocompromised patients are threatened by nonpathogenic organisms. Prevention and control are key factors in managing infectious disease.

COMMON CHILDHOOD COMMUNICABLE DISEASES

The incidence of common childhood communicable diseases has dramatically decreased as immunological agents have been developed. Diseases such as smallpox have declined to a point worldwide that routine immunizations are no longer recommended. Providing all children with the appropriate immunizations is the health care challenge of today. Air travel is commonplace, and rapid transmission of contagious diseases from around the world makes alert assessment by the nurse and all health care workers essential. Most viral infections are contagious for 2 to 3 days before the characteristic symptoms occur. Home care is the preferred care setting for children with communicable diseases.

In many families, both parents work and childcare facilities have become the primary day care setting for preschool children. Intimate contact is a routine part of children's play in childcare settings, so hand hygiene and a clean environment as well as immunization of children and staff are essential to minimize the spread of infection. Policies for excluding children who are ill should be well understood by parents and childcare staff. Staff who serve food should not be assigned to change diapers. See Table 32.1 for selected recommendations concerning excluding children with communicable disease from childcare facilities or school.

REVIEW OF TERMS

A communicable disease is one that can be transmitted, directly or indirectly, from one person to another. Organisms that cause disease are called pathogens.

The incubation period is the time between the invasion by the pathogen and the onset of clinical symptoms. The prodromal period refers to the initial stage of a disease: the interval between the earliest symptoms and the appearance of a typical rash or fever. Children are often contagious during this time, but because the symptoms are not specific they may attend preschool or another group program and spread the disease.

A fomite is any inanimate material that carries and transmits infection. A vector is an insect or animal that carries and spreads a disease.

A pandemic is a worldwide high incidence of a communicable disease. An epidemic is a sudden increase of a communicable disease in a localized area. Endemic refers to a continuous incidence of a communicable disease expected in a localized area.

Body substance refers to moist secretions or parts of the body that can contain microorganisms. Emesis, saliva, sputum, semen, urine, feces, and blood are examples of body substances. Routine precautions indicate the need to wear disposable protective gloves and garments when coming in contact with these body substances.

A portal of entry is a route by which the organisms enter the body (e.g., a cut in the skin). A portal of exit is the route by which the organisms exit the body (e.g., feces or urine). A reservoir for infection is a place that supports the growth of organisms (e.g., standing, stagnant water). The *chain of infection* refers to the way in which organisms spread and infect the individual (see Fig. 32.4). Careful hand hygiene is basic and essential to preventing the spread of infection.

HOST RESISTANCE

Many factors contribute to the virulence of an infectious disease. The age, sex, and genetic makeup of the child have a bearing on the degree of resistance. The nutritional status of the person, as well as physical and emotional health, is also important. The efficiency of the blood-forming organs and of the immune systems affects resistance. Important factors in host resistance to disease include the following:

- *Intact skin and mucous membranes:* A break in the skin can be a portal of entry for an organism that can cause illness.
- *Phagocytes* in the blood attack and destroy organisms.
- The functioning *immune system* in the body responds to fight infection. Some factors in this immune response include interferon, T cells, B cells, and anti-bodies. Vaccinations assist the body in manufacturing antibodies that can help the child to resist infections.

The child who has an underlying chronic illness, such as diabetes, cystic fibrosis, burns, or sickle cell disease, may be more susceptible to certain organisms. Children with HIV or acquired immunodeficiency syndrome (AIDS) or cancer and children receiving steroid or immunosuppressive drugs often have depressed immune systems. This makes them very susceptible to opportunistic infections (an opportunistic infection is caused by organisms *normally* found in the environment that the immune-suppressed individual cannot resist or fight). An infection acquired in a health care facility during hospitalization is termed a health care–associated infection (HAI).

TYPES OF IMMUNITY

Immunity is the natural or acquired resistance to infection. In natural immunity, resistance is inborn. Some races apparently have a greater natural immunity to certain diseases than other races. Immunity also varies from person to person. If two persons are exposed to the same disease, one may become very ill and the other may show no evidence of the disease.

Acquired immunity is not the result of inherited factors but is gained as a result of having the disease or is artificially acquired by receiving vaccines or immune serums. Vaccines contain live attenuated (weakened) or dead organisms that are not strong enough to cause the disease but stimulate the body to develop an immune reaction and antibodies. When the person produces their own immunity, it is called active immunity.

If a person is exposed and needs immediate protection from a specific infectious disease, antibodies can be obtained in immune serums; most are from animals, but some are from humans. For example, tetanus serum (used to prevent lockjaw) is procured from the horse, but gamma globulin, which is rich in antibodies, is obtained from human blood. This type of immunity, known as passive immunity, acts immediately but does not last as long as immunity actively produced by the body. Passive immunity provides the antibody. It does not stimulate the system to produce its own antibodies.

A *carrier* is a person who is capable of spreading a disease but does not show evidence of it. Typhoid fever is an example of a disease spread by a carrier.

TRANSMISSION OF INFECTION

Infection can be transmitted from one person to another by direct or indirect means. *Direct transmission* involves contact with the person who is infected (the body fluids of that person, such as nasal discharge or an open lesion). *Indirect transmission* involves contact with objects that have been contaminated by the infected person. These objects are called *fomites*. Bedrails, intravenous (IV) pumps, bedside tables, door handles, used tissues, countertops, and toys are examples of fomites. For example, the respiratory syncytial virus (RSV) lives on dry soap for several hours. Therefore, picking up soap used by a person infected with RSV transmits the organism. This is one of the reasons why the use of liquid soap is advocated. The chain of

Table 32.1 Communicable Diseases of Childhood

DISEASE	CAUSATIVE ORGANISM	SIGNS AND SYMPTOMS	INCUBATION PERIOD	PREVENTION AND TREATMENT	HOW LONG CONTAGIOUS	NURSING INTERVENTIONS
Rotavirus (RV) (common cause of gastroenteritis)	Reoviridae	Acute onset of fever and vomiting, followed by diarrhea, which can last up to 7 days.	18 hours to 3 days	Vaccine is available, two doses are required. See Fig. 32.6. There is no specific treatment for this virus; prevention of dehydration is important. Clean contaminated areas and perform hand hygiene to prevent spread.	Highly infectious with viral shedding within a few days and up to 21 days after onset	In infants and small children, risk of dehydration and electrolyte imbalance is higher so monitor for signs and symptoms. Additional contact precautions are required. Encourage diet as tolerated.
Norwalk virus (common cause of gastroenteritis)	Norovirus	Nausea, vomiting, diarrhea, and abdominal pain. Usually symptoms arise 1 to 2 days after eating food or water that has been contaminated with Norwalk virus. Sometimes headache and low-grade fever may occur.	12–48 hours	Prevent dehydration. Hand hygiene is the most important measure to prevent transmission.	Contagious for as long as symptoms persist	Monitor for signs and symptoms of dehydration. Additional contact precautions.
Chickenpox (varicella) (Fig. 32.1)	Varicella-zoster virus	Symptoms include flu-like symptoms, fatigue, mild headache, a mild fever, chills, and muscle or joint pain that occurs 1–2 days before the rash appears, then a rash consisting of blisters that are raised (called *vesicles*). All stages of lesions are present on the body at the same time. They dry up and form scabs in 5 to 6 days.	2–3 weeks (10–21 days average)	Vaccine is available; two doses are given at same time as MMR (schedule varies from province to province). See Fig. 32.6. Acyclovir (Zovirax) or immune globulin (VZIG) is given to immuno-suppressed children who are exposed.	Most contagious 1 to 2 days before to shortly after onset of rash	Trim fingernails to prevent scratching. (Removal of scabs may cause scars.) Calamine lotion may reduce itching. Additional airborne precautions required. Monitor acyclovir adverse effects.
German measles (rubella) (Fig. 32.2)	Rubella virus	Mild fever and cold symptoms precede a rose-coloured, maculopapular rash that usually starts on the face and then spreads to the body. Glands at ears and back of neck are enlarged more commonly in older children or adults.	2–3 weeks (14–17 days post-exposure)	Vaccine is available; two doses are given, MMR or MMRV (schedule varies from province to province). See Fig. 32.6.	Until rash fades (5 days) Congenital rubella: use contact precautions, person sheds virus for up to 1 year of age. Exclude from day care until after 3 months of age with two negative cultures obtained at least 1 month apart	Provide symptomatic treatment and comfort measures. Avoid exposure to any woman who might be in early months of pregnancy, because rubella can cause fetal anomalies. Additional droplet precautions are required.

Continued

Table 32.1 Communicable Diseases of Childhood—cont'd

DISEASE	CAUSATIVE ORGANISM	SIGNS AND SYMPTOMS	INCUBATION PERIOD	PREVENTION AND TREATMENT	HOW LONG CONTAGIOUS	NURSING INTERVENTIONS
Measles (rubeola) (Fig. 32.3)	Rubeola virus	Fever, cough, and conjunctivitis are followed by small white (Koplik) spots on inner cheeks (enanthem); maculopapular rash (exanthem) then erupts.	1–2 weeks (10 days average)	Vaccine is available. See Fig. 32.6. Gamma globulin may be given after exposure. Vitamin A is recommended to reduce morbidity in severe cases in some children with certain health concerns, such as a low retinol level.	From 4 days before to 5 days after rash appears	Provide symptomatic care. Use additional airborne precautions and provide quiet activities. Use measures to reduce eyestrain caused by photophobia. Give detailed oral care. Avoid use of soap.
Fifth disease (erythema infectiosum)	Human parvovirus B19	Child has "slapped cheek" appearance. Generalized rash appears, subsides, and reappears if skin is irritated by sun or heat. If developed during pregnancy fetal complications include hemolysis, anemia, and nonimmune hydrops fetalis, and fetal loss occurs in approximately 3% of infected women.	4–14 days	No vaccine is available. Once the rash is present, the child is no longer contagious and can return to day care.	During incubation period	This is a benign condition except in a child who is immunocompromised or a pregnant woman who is <20 weeks' gestation, so exposure should be avoided. Isolation is not required other than routine precautions. Condition may last 1–3 weeks. Use oatmeal baths for itching.
Roseola (sixth disease) (exanthem subitum)	Human herpes-virus 6 or 7 (HHV-6 or HHV-7)	Persistent high fever (39.4° to 40.5°C [103° to 105°F]) is present, then drops rapidly as rash appears. The maculopapular rash is nonpruritic and blanches easily.	2 weeks	There is no vaccine. High fever may precipitate convulsions.	Until rash fades	Rest and quiet should be provided. Teach parents temperature-reducing techniques and prevention of seizures. Use routine precautions. Patients are rarely hospitalized.
Mumps (parotitis)	Para-myxovirus	Fever, headache, glands near ear and toward jawline ache and develop painful swelling. Parotid gland is enlarged. Condition may be bilateral.	14–21 days (18 days average)	Vaccine is available; two doses are given, MMR or MMRV (schedule varies from province to province). See Fig. 32.6.	Until swelling subsides Keep out of day care or school	Encourage fluids, apply ice compresses to neck for comfort. Use additional droplet precautions if patient is hospitalized. Avoid citrus and spices that stimulate salivary flow.

Whooping cough (pertussis)	*Bordetella pertussis*	Fever, cold, and cough are present. Spells of coughing are accompanied by a noisy gasp for air that creates a "whoop."	6–20 days (9–10 days average)	Vaccine is available. See Fig. 32.6. May administer erythromycin to exposed, unvaccinated child. Antibiotics are used for treatment.	Several weeks Exclude from day care for 5 days after antimicrobial treatment has been completed	Use additional droplet precautions until 5 days after antibiotics. Encourage bed rest, provide abdominal support during coughing spell. Observe for airway obstruction and O_2 saturations.
Polio (infantile paralysis; polio-myelitis)	Enterovirus	Fever, headache, stiff neck and stiff back, paralysis.	1–2 weeks	Vaccine is available. See Figure 32.6. May necessitate respirator care.	1 week for throat secretions; 4 weeks for feces	Use routine precautions. Encourage bed rest, observe for respiratory distress. Provide positioning, physiotherapy, and range-of-motion exercises.
Infectious mono-nucleosis (glandular fever)	Epstein-Barr virus (EBV) type 4	Low-grade fever, sore throat, generalized lymphadenopathy malaise, jaundice, enlarged spleen.	2–6 weeks	Limit contact with saliva. Do not share eating utensils.	Spread by direct contact only Return to school when fever and swallowing are normal	Provide rest and supportive treatment. Use routine precautions. Provide school tutoring to maintain schoolwork. Contact sports are avoided until spleen and liver lab tests normal.
Hepatitis A	Enterovirus 72	Children often do not show symptoms, but 10 to 15% may carry the disease for up to 6 months. If symptoms are present, they usually include fever, anorexia, headache, abdominal pain, malaise, jaundice, dark urine, and chalklike stools.	15–45 days	Vaccine is available. See Fig. 32.6. Gamma globulin is provided if child is exposed.	Virus may be shed for up to 6 months in newborns. Hepatitis A–positive infants under 6 months of age should not be in childcare facilities.	Educate family and community about ingestion of contaminated water or shellfish from contaminated water or swimming in contaminated water. Proper hand hygiene is essential. Routine and additional contact precautions are essential.

Continued

Table 32.1 Communicable Diseases of Childhood—cont'd

DISEASE	CAUSATIVE ORGANISM	SIGNS AND SYMPTOMS	INCUBATION PERIOD	PREVENTION AND TREATMENT	HOW LONG CONTAGIOUS	NURSING INTERVENTIONS
Hepatitis B	Hepatitis B virus (HBV)	Symptoms are the same as in type A. Can manifest liver pathology.	30–180 days	Vaccine is available. Immunization schedule varies among provinces. See Fig. 32.6. Interferon or reverse transcriptase inhibitors may be an effective treatment. Immune globulin may be indicated for exposed, susceptible children.	May persist in carrier state	Prevent contact with blood or blood products. Identify high-risk mothers and newborns. Educate concerning need for vaccination.
Lyme disease	*Borrelia burgdorferi*	Skin lesions at site of tick bite. Macule with raised border and clear centre (target or bulls-eye appearance that is 5 cm in diameter). May "burn." Fever, arthralgia. May lead to heart and neurological involvement.	3–30 days after being bitten by an infected tick	Wear protective clothing in wooded areas. Inspect for ticks after play and when camping. Light-coloured clothing makes tick more noticeable. Remove tick with tweezers. Inspect pets for ticks. Treat with amoxicillin or doxycycline. The tick may be sent to Public Health for further testing to confirm if tick is infected.	Spread by infected tick	Educate concerning prevention of exposure. Use routine precautions. Patient should avoid sun if treated with doxycycline. Insect repellant containing 20 to 30% DEET on skin and clothes and camping gear is advised (Onyett & CPS Infectious Diseases and Immunization Committee, 2014/2017).
Tuberculosis	*Mycobacterium tuberculosis*	Low-grade fever, malaise, anorexia, weight loss, cough, night sweats. Children are often asymptomatic. Adenopathy, pneumonia, and positive tuberculin skin test.	2–10 weeks (airborne infection)	Early detection is through routine PPD skin test or serum IGRA. Examine contacts. Exposed children may receive isoniazid, rifampin, and pyrazinamide, administered for several months.	After treatment has been started and written medical clearance to return to day care or school is received from health care provider or local public health authority	Isolate newborn from infected mother if mother has not been treated. Identify contacts. Use additional airborne precautions.

Diphtheria	*Corynebacterium diphtheriae*	Common cold with purulent nasal discharge. Malaise, sore throat. White or grey membrane forms in throat, causing respiratory distress.	2–5 days	Vaccine is available. See Fig. 32.6. Intravenous antibiotics, antitoxin, and tracheotomy are required. Provide oxygen and suction as needed.	Until 4 days after antibiotic therapy	Observe for respiratory, cardiac, and central nervous system involvement. Have emergency airway equipment available. Use additional droplet precautions. Identify contacts for treatment.
Scarlet fever	Group A beta-hemolytic *Streptococcus*	Tachycardia, strawberry tongue, pinpoint rash, circumoral pallor, desquamation	2–5 days	Penicillin therapy is provided for 10 days. Culture for and treat streptococcal infections.	During incubation and clinical illness; may become a carrier	Provide bed rest and quiet activity. Teach regarding prevention of streptococcal infections and culture of sore throats.

DTaP, Diphtheria-tetanus–acellular pertussis vaccine; *IGRA,* interferon-gamma release assay; *MMR,* measles-mumps-rubella vaccine; MMRV, measles-mumps-rubella-varicella vaccine; *PPD,* purified protein derivative; *VZIG,* varicella-zoster immune globulin.
Note: DTaP is administered to infants and children up to age 7 years; Tdap (tetanus-diphtheria–acellular pertussis vaccine) is provided to children age 11 years and older.

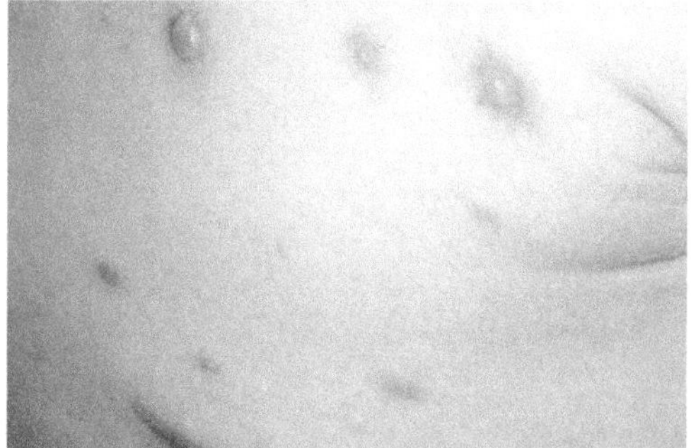

Fig. 32.1 Chickenpox. (From Feigin, R. D., & Cherry, J. D. [1987]. *Textbook of pediatric infectious diseases* [2nd ed.]. Philadelphia: Saunders.)

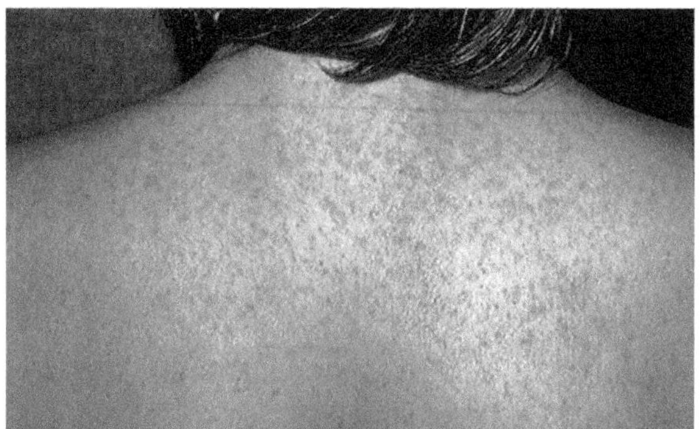

Fig. 32.2 German measles. (From Hurwitz, S. [2016]. *Clinical pediatric dermatology: A textbook of skin disorders of childhood and adolescence* [5th ed.]. Philadelphia: Elsevier.)

infection transmission is shown in Fig. 32.4. Preventing the spread of infection depends on breaking the chain.

Various tests are available to determine whether an individual has been exposed to a particular disease, such as the *Mantoux* intradermal purified protein derivative (PPD) skin test or a blood serum test called the interferon-gamma release assay (IGRA) (more commonly referred to as either QuantiFERON-TB Gold or T spot) that tests for tuberculosis infection. The *Schick test* for diphtheria and the *Dick test* for scarlet fever have been replaced by serum DNA-PCR (DNA polymerase chain reaction) testing.

MEDICAL ASEPSIS, ROUTINE PRECAUTIONS, AND ADDITIONAL PRECAUTIONS

The purpose of medical aseptic techniques used with *all* patients is to prevent the spread of infection from one person to another. A person or object is considered *contaminated* if they or it has touched the infected patient or any equipment or fomite that has come in contact with the patient or their bodily fluids, or ingested or inhaled any infectious agent.

Articles that have come in direct contact with the patient must be disinfected before others can use them. When something is disinfected, the microorganisms in or on it are killed by physical or chemical means. The autoclave, which uses steam under pressure, is considered effective in killing most microbes when the article is adequately exposed and sterilized for the proper length of time.

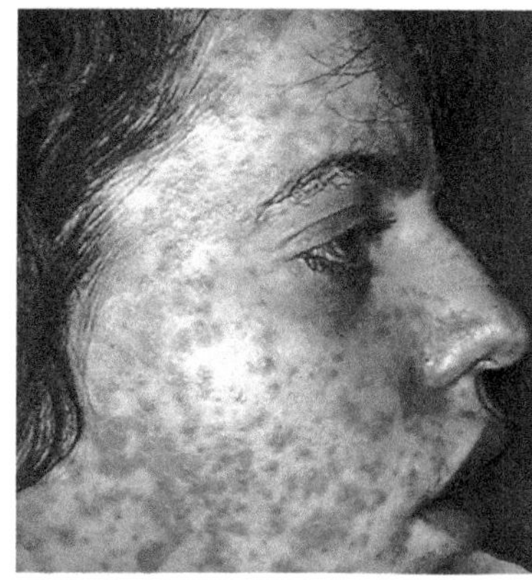

Fig. 32.3 Measles. (From Hurwitz, S. [2016]. *Clinical pediatric dermatology: A textbook of skin disorders of childhood and adolescence* [5th ed.]. Philadelphia: Elsevier.)

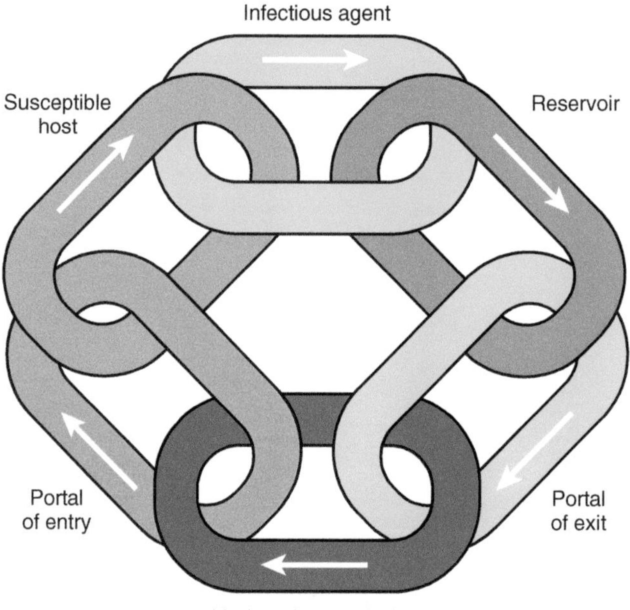

Fig. 32.4 The chain of infection. The series of events through which germs can cause a person to become sick with an infection. If any portion of the chain is broken, the spread of infection may stop. (From Royal College of Nursing. [2016]. *Chain of infection*. Retrieved from https://rcni.com/hosted-content/rcn/first-steps/chain-of-infection.)

All children suspected of having a communicable disease who are admitted to the hospital are placed on both routine and additional precautions until a definite diagnosis is established. A private room or negative-pressure room (prevents air from flowing out of the room when the door is opened) may be assigned.

Disposable items are used, if available, when a child is placed on additional precautions; these include tissues, suction catheters, thermometers, suture sets, bottles, and blood pressure cuffs. They are disposed of according to hospital protocol.

Nurses must understand the importance of protecting themselves and others from a contagious patient. This is accomplished by specific precautions, called **routine precautions**. The Public Health Agency of Canada (PHAC) (2016) recommends that *routine* precautions be used for *all* patients; these involve, at minimum, hand hygiene and the use of personal protective equipment (PPE) when exposure to body substances will occur. In addition to these precautions, **additional precautions** are designed according to the method of spread of infection, such as airborne isolation, contact, droplet, and droplet-contact isolation.

Airborne precautions are used for patients with conditions such as tuberculosis, varicella (chickenpox), and rubeola (measles). Small airborne particles floating in the air can be inhaled any place in the room. The use of negative-pressure rooms and respirator masks (e.g., N95 particulate masks) are required when entering the room. The respirator masks are removed when exiting the room (Nursing Care Plan 32.1).

Nursing Care Plan 32.1 QSEN Interdisciplinary Patient Care Plan for Patient with Tuberculosis

HEALTH HISTORY

A 16-year-old male adolescent is admitted to the unit with pulmonary tuberculosis (TB). During data collection, the nurse discovers he has an autoimmune disorder and that this past summer he travelled with his parents and grandparents to a country that has a high prevalence of TB. His symptoms are unexplained weight loss, night sweats, and a cough with hemoptysis, which began about 3 months after they returned home.

Nursing Diagnosis 1

Need for education concerning additional airborne precautions*

Nursing Diagnosis 2

Need for improved nutrition status as a result of unexplained weight loss*

Competency	Knowledge	Skill	Attitude
Quality improvement	Risk of transmission of TB to staff and visitors is decreased by confirming with Infection Prevention and Control Department that airborne precautions are needed for this patient on this unit.	Provide education and training to patient and family members to minimize their continued spread of and exposure to TB while in the unit and at home.	The patient and family state they understand what must be done to adhere to isolation precautions and treatment plan.
	Medication orders are confirmed with health care provider to ensure accurate information was entered into MAR.	Contact pharmacy to confirm health care provider's medication and dosage orders related to patient's autoimmune disorder and antituberculin medications.	By confirming the orders, the nurse ensures that the right medications are being given at the right time and at the right dose to the right patient.
Safety	Infection Prevention and Control Department contacted to confirm appropriate additional precautions and report admission of patient with TB.	Implement airborne precautions by noting type of isolation protocol instituted in EHR; post appropriate signage on door to patient's room; ensure all necessary supplies are readily available next to door to patient's room.	These actions inform anyone who wants to enter patient's room that they must wear N-95 respirator mask in the room and perform hand hygiene before entering and when leaving room. Ensuring that negative pressure is working properly helps decrease risk of TB mycobacterium spreading in the environment.
	Engineering Department contacted to ensure negative pressure was turned on and working accurately in patient's room.	Note that monitor next to negative pressure room began working within minutes of contacting engineering.	
Teamwork and collaboration	Given patient's need for nutritional adjustments, a dietitian contacted to discuss special dietary needs of patient.	Confirm that correct foods are on patient's meal tray before delivering it to patient.	Ask patient to inform nursing or dietary staff of other foods he would prefer that also meet his cultural preferences and any dietary restrictions he must follow. Ensures that patient will be able to attain and maintain expected weight of a 16-year-old male.
	In handoff report, nurse provides updated status concerning need for continued airborne precautions, which diagnostic labs are still outstanding, and nursing interventions still needing action.	Update charge nurse and other members of nursing team on safety measures that need to be followed to ensure their health and safety while providing nursing care and to help in implementation of patient-specific nursing plan of care.	

(Continued)

Nursing Care Plan 32.1 QSEN Interdisciplinary Patient Care Plan for Patient with Tuberculosis—cont'd

Competency	Knowledge	Skill	Attitude
			Ensure that current and future staff will have airborne precaution supplies stocked and signage posted as required prior to entering room to begin patient care.
Patient-centred care	As indicated by nursing diagnosis related to airborne precautions education, patient and family provided with education and rationales for need to adhere to airborne precaution protocols.	Demonstrate to family and visitors how to don and take off respirator masks and where to dispose of them upon leaving patient's room. Stress importance of performing hand hygiene before going into patient's room and upon removing mask after leaving room.	Patient and family state they understand the required processes.
	Child-life specialist (CLS) contacted and provided with necessary information in order to provide age-appropriate activities while patient is on airborne precautions.	Accompany CLS when visiting patient and provide information regarding patient's needs and environmental limitations.	Confirm with patient later in the shift that CLS was helpful in providing needed materials.
	Patient is a junior in high school and is worried about midterm exams scheduled to take in next few days.	Contact social worker and discuss options for maintaining patient's academic status. Social worker will contact patient's school to make arrangements for obtaining recordings of lectures and schoolwork missed.	Discuss with nursing team and patient's parents how to incorporate study and homework into daily plan of care.
	Lab technician consulted to confirm that enough sputum was collected to perform AFB cultures ordered by health care provider.	Assist lab technician in helping patient provide adequate sputum for collection and reassure patient during process.	Make note of any outstanding sputum cultures that need to be collected.
Evidence-informed practice	Patient teaching materials provided about pulmonary TB, including PHAC website that has more detailed information in many languages.	Assist patient and family in accessing websites on electronic devices. Assist patient in accessing hospital's Wi-Fi system and using electronic devices in the unit that can help him maintain schoolwork assignments so he can maintain his grade level.	Return later in shift to review what patient and family have learned and provide opportunity for them to ask questions and receive answers related to materials provided. Unanswered questions are relayed to charge nurse and health care provider.
Informatics	Admission data collected, isolation precautions implemented, and teaching provided are documented in EHR.	Access Public Health Department's (PHD) communicable disease reporting form and, in collaboration with charge nurse, complete required report notification to PHD.	Family is aware that they will be contacted by local PHD, TB control division, given level of exposure they have had with patient. Patient is also aware that he may be contacted by PHD–TB control nurse.
	MAR reviewed to determine which medications to administer before dinner.	Administer medications and document this in patient's EHR, as well as nursing care and nursing observations made and patient responses noted.	Notations in EHR used in preparing hand-off report to next shift to ensure seamless progression of care.

AFB, Acid-fast bacilli; *EHR*, electronic health record; *MAR*, medication administration record; *PHAC*, Public Health Agency of Canada; *QSEN*, Quality and Safety Education for Nurses (http://QSEN.org).

*Summary of participants in the multidisciplinary team for care given related to this nursing diagnosis: charge nurse, child-life specialist, dietitian, engineering department, family, health care provider, infection prevention and control nurse, lab technician, nursing team members, patient, pharmacist, Public Health Department –TB control nurse, social worker.

QSEN is based on the Institute of Medicine Competencies. (2003). *Health profession education—A bridge to quality*. Washington, DC: National Academy Press; Cronewett, L., Sherwood, G., & Barnsteiner, J. (2007). Quality and safety education for nurses. *Nursing Outlook, 55*(3), 122–131.

Contact precautions are used when the condition causes organisms to be transmitted via skin-to-skin contact or through direct touch of a contaminated fomite. Gloves and a cover gown are worn for close contact with patients with rotavirus, patients with hepatitis A who are incontinent, patients with contagious skin diseases such as impetigo, and patients with wound infections. Some diseases may have more than one mode of spread and therefore necessitate more than one additional precaution technique.

Droplet precautions are used with diseases such as pertussis and pneumonia. When the patient coughs or sneezes, the droplets can contaminate an area 2 metres around the patient. Beyond the 2-metre radius, a mask and gown are not usually necessary.

Droplet-contact precautions are used with diseases such as RSV and influenza. The PHAC (2016) recommends that droplet and contact precautions be used for all patients with suspected or confirmed cases of influenza.

PPE should be worn when anticipating the risk of exposure to blood, body fluids, or other potentially infectious materials.

Safety Alert!

Disposable gloves should be worn whenever there is a risk of contact with another person's body fluids but should not be worn for routine care if there is no risk for exposure e.g., taking vital signs.

PROTECTIVE ENVIRONMENT ISOLATION

Protective environment isolation precautions (previously called *reverse isolation*) are used for patients whose illness is not communicable but who have a lowered resistance, perhaps because of neutropenia, and are highly susceptible to infection. This simple procedure reduces the incidence of health care–associated infections. The patient is placed in a private room with the door closed. It is recommended that all persons wear a gown, a mask, and gloves when attending the child. Both the child and family need adequate explanations concerning the protective environment precautions.

HAND HYGIENE

The nurse must utilize the five moments of hand hygiene, which involve performing hand hygiene at each of the following times (World Health Organization, 2018):

- Before touching a patient
- Before performing clean/aseptic procedures
- After body fluid exposure or risk
- After touching a patient
- After touching patient surroundings

Alcohol-based hand-rub (ABHR) or antibacterial soaps and lotions are used. The use of hot water, instead of warm water, can irritate skin and may promote the development of resistant strains of microorganisms. Self-contained liquid soap dispensers are preferable to bar soap that can harbour organisms. ABHRs should be used as long as the hands are not visibly soiled. Artificial fingernails, including tips, wraps, and nail jewellery, are not permitted in patient care areas. Refer to hospital infection prevention and control protocol. Caregivers with skin lesions on exposed areas of their bodies should not provide direct patient care until the lesions are completely cleared.

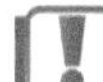

Safety Alert!

Alcohol-based hand rubs should not be used when caring for a patient diagnosed with *Clostridium difficile* diarrhea because this organism is spore forming and resistant to alcohols. Soap and water must be used after every contact.

Nursing Tip

Teaching children and their families to wash their hands before meals and after using the toilet, blowing their nose, sneezing, or handling soiled objects is important in order to minimize the spread of infection and promote healthy living. Making hand hygiene fun for children can motivate them to wash appropriately for a minimum of 15 seconds.

FAMILY EDUCATION

It is essential that family members receive education in ways to prevent communicable disease. Factors to be emphasized include the need to immunize children, proper storage of food (particularly perishables), use of pasteurized milk, proper cooking of meats, cleanliness in food preparation, and proper hand hygiene. The nurse should review the ways in which infectious diseases are spread. Children must be taught to avoid using community hand towels. Other modes of transmission, such as crowded living conditions, insects, rodents, and sandboxes, may also be discussed.

RASHES

Many infectious diseases begin with a rash. Rashes tend to be itchy (pruritic) and uncomfortable. Symptomatic care is provided by the administration of acetaminophen (Tylenol) and diphenhydramine (Benadryl) or topical lotions. Rashes can be described as follows (see Box 30.1):

- **Erythema**: diffused reddened area on the skin
- **Macule**: circular reddened area on the skin
- **Papule**: circular reddened area on the skin that is elevated
- **Vesicle**: circular reddened area on the skin that is elevated and contains fluid
- **Pustule**: circular reddened area on the skin that is elevated and contains pus
- **Scab**: dried pustule that is covered with a crust
- **Pathognomonic**: term used to describe a lesion or symptom that is *characteristic* of a specific illness (e.g., Koplik spots are pathognomonic for measles)

Safety Alert!

Apply lotions to open lesions sparingly to prevent absorption that could lead to medication toxicity.

IMMUNIZATIONS

Federally funded programs to provide vaccines and educate the public are in place in Canada. The efforts of the World Health Organization (WHO) and the United Nations Children's Fund (UNICEF) have resulted in dramatic declines in vaccine-preventable illnesses worldwide, especially in developing countries. New vaccines are developed and assessed for routine use in endemic areas.

At a meeting in Switzerland of the Strategic Advisory Group of Experts (SAGE) in 2018 concerning immunization practices around the world, recommendations and guidelines were endorsed by the WHO. Recommendations included the development of a global vaccine action plan, identification of regional challenges, establishment of a storage stockpile for vaccines, and universal access to vaccines as well as research priorities.

VACCINES

Table 32.2 presents types of immunization agents. Current vaccinations against varicella, hepatitis, influenza (for children 6 months of age and older or high-risk children), and pneumonia (for children greater than 2 months of age) are available. Vaccines for cholera and yellow fever are available for families travelling to endemic areas. The PHAC provides advice concerning vaccinations needed for persons travelling to various parts of the world.

Table 32.2 Types of Immunization Agents

AGENT	DESCRIPTION
Vaccine	A suspension of weakened or inactivated (killed) organisms that stimulate immune bodies to form A form of *active* immunity
Toxoid	A modified toxin that stimulates the production of antitoxin A form of *active* immunity
Immune globulin	A solution containing antibodies extracted from human or animal blood Provides *passive* immunity
Specific immune globulins or antitoxins	Special preparations obtained from blood donors selected for their high antibody level against a specific disease Provides *passive* immunity to the specific disease

In newborn infants, the presence of passively acquired immunity from the mother may inhibit the infant's natural immune response to vaccines. Therefore, most routine immunizations are not started until 2 months of age in Canada, unless a high risk of infection exists.

Most antibodies cannot reach intracellular sites of infection but can prevent spread from the site of entry into the body to a target organ. Thus vaccinations can prevent the disease, but most cannot be used to treat the disease after cellular penetration of the organism has occurred. For some diseases, postexposure immunization is recommended; immune globulins are most often the choice.

Multiple doses of a vaccine at predetermined intervals may be needed to achieve immunity status. The nurse should educate parents about immunization schedules and assess the immunization status of each child at every clinic visit (Fig. 32.5).

Nursing Tip

The earliest age a vaccine should be administered is the youngest age at which the infant can respond by developing antibodies to that illness.

Routes and Timing of Administration

The oral, subcutaneous, and intramuscular (IM) routes are used for various vaccines. The correct route of administration is an important factor in achieving immunization; the recommended route must be used to

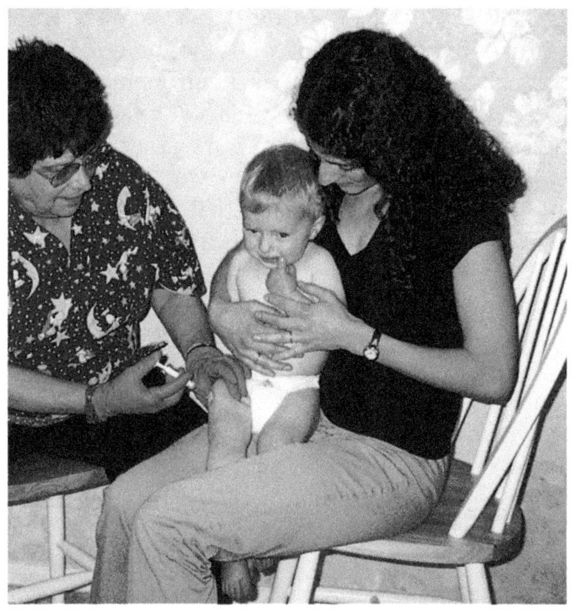

Fig. 32.5 The "hug" restraining position for administration of vaccinations. Note that the mother restrains the arms, and the child's legs are restrained between the mother's knees. The mother comforts the child and may breastfeed during the procedure. The site for intramuscular injections in infants is the thigh. The nurse wears a protective glove. The use of skin-to-skin contact, sucrose solution, aerosol sprays, EMLA cream, or distraction techniques may reduce the pain of multiple injections in infants and children.

obtain optimum response. For example, the administration of hepatitis B vaccine into the buttock will not result in the same optimal level of immunity as administration of the vaccine into the deltoid muscle. The route of administration of a vaccine also influences the response of the infant. Refer to Chapter 20 for principles and techniques of administering IM injections to pediatric patients.

 Safety Alert!

Immune globulin, blood products, and immunosuppressive agents must not be given at the same time as live-virus vaccines.

 Safety Alert!

A period of 2 to 4 weeks should separate the administration of an inactivated vaccine and a live-virus vaccine, and 4 weeks before immunosuppressive therapy.

 Medication Alert!

Varicella vaccine, if not given on the same day as measles, mumps, and rubella (MMR) or in combination as MMRV, must be given *no less* than 28 days later. A tuberculin test should not be administered within 6 weeks of receiving an MMR or varicella immunization because the results will not be accurate.

Storage and Handling

Correct storage of vaccines is essential to ensure their potency. The nurse should check the label or package insert to determine what type of storage or refrigeration is needed. Improper temperature can reduce the potency of the vaccine, and there are often no visible signs of these changes.

Vaccines should not be stored in the doors of refrigerators or freezers, near the cold air vents in the refrigerator, or in storage bins. They must be placed in the centre of shelves to allow the free flow of air around the vaccines. Most vaccines are stored inside the refrigerator at 2° to 8°C (36° to 46°F). The temperature should never fall below 2°C. Vaccines such as Varivax, herpes zoster virus (HZV), measles, mumps, and rubella (MMR), and measles, mumps, rubella, and varicella (MMRV) are very fragile and must be stored in the freezer at −15°C (+5°F) and used within 30 minutes of reconstitution. *The vaccines cannot be refrozen after they have been thawed*. Inactivated vaccines can be harmed if frozen, and live vaccines are harmed by heat and light. This information is especially important to know when participating in outdoor mass immunization programs.

In clinic or office settings, the refrigerator temperatures must be documented at the beginning and the end of each workday, and the records must be kept on file for at least 3 years. Refrigerator-freezers with automatic defrost cycles are not appropriate for vaccine storage because temperatures may not be held stable as required.

Manufacturer-filled syringes should remain in the original package until ready for use, to protect them from exposure to light. Vaccines predrawn from a vile cannot be reinserted into a multidose vial and must be discarded if not used.

Allergies and Thimerosal Content

Parents of children who have a history of allergy should notify the health care provider before the child receives vaccinations. Some multidose containers of vaccines have a latex cover that must be penetrated by the needle and should be used with caution in individuals who may have a latex allergy. Epinephrine should be available in the unit where vaccines are administered, and the child should be observed for a minimum of 20 minutes before they leave the area.

Thimerosal is a mercury-containing preservative used to prevent fungal and bacterial contamination of vaccines that are in multidose containers. The use of thimerosal as a preservative has decreased since the introduction and widespread use of single-dose vials for vaccinations. All vaccines for pregnant women and children under 6 years of age are available in thimerosal-free vials.

Vaccine Hesitancy

The Canadian Paediatric Society (CPS) strongly endorses universal immunization. In order for universal immunization programs to be successful, parents must comply with the recommendations. *Vaccine hesitancy* is defined as the reluctance or refusal to vaccinate despite the availability of vaccines. It threatens to reverse progress made in tackling vaccine-preventable diseases (World Health Organization, 2019). The WHO has identified complacency, inconvenience in accessing vaccines, and lack of confidence as key reasons underlying vaccine hesitancy (WHO, 2019). When a caregiver refuses immunizations for their child, the nurse should listen carefully for the reasons and offer appropriate education. Even after continued discussion and education, some parents may continue to refuse immunizations. Parents may have many reasons for vaccine refusal: some may object to the painful procedure, others believe that the benefits of immunization do not justify the risks associated with immunizations. Many commonly held beliefs about the risks are not supported by enough available data and frequently originate from unsupported claims of organizations or individuals that are critical of immunizations. Children who are not immunized increase the risk of disease transmission in children who cannot be immunized due to age or immunocompromised status.

Some vaccines may contain heavy metals, antibiotics, or animal products. A list of ingredients found in vaccines can be accessed at the Government of Canada site listed in the Additional Learning Resources section at the end of this chapter. Animal products contained in a vaccine may present a problem for parents with specific cultural or religious beliefs. The nurse should be culturally sensitive and offer education concerning the values of the vaccine as well as options.

Parents with doubts about immunizations should still have access to and receive good medical care. Continuing a relationship with parents that fosters trust and respect allows additional opportunities to discuss the refusal of vaccinations over time.

Nursing Care

Nurses must remain alert to signs and symptoms of communicable diseases. Measles is rarely seen in developed countries, although more outbreaks are being seen in developed countries, often related to vaccine hesitancy. The nurse is a vital link in educating parents about the need for immunizations. The CPS and Government of Canada have resources available listing the risk and benefits of immunizations to aid in parent education (see Additional Resources section at the end of the chapter).

The nurse must be aware of when a patient's vaccines are due to be scheduled for administration, the immunization history of the child, the vaccines that can be given together, contraindications, the routes of administration, and the proper equipment needed if a reaction occurs. Before a vaccine is administered to a child, the nurse should provide vaccine-specific information to the caregiver and obtain consent.

The National Advisory Committee on Immunization (NACI), an advisory body to PHAC, makes the recommendations for the use of vaccines in Canada. Following NACI recommendations, provinces and territories determine the best schedule for their specific regions; therefore, publically funded programs vary from province to territory. Routine vaccine practices can vary from province to province; it is important to review the vaccine schedule available within the province.

Serious adverse events occurring within a designated time after vaccination should be reported to the Canadian Adverse Events Following Immunization Surveillance System (CAEFISS). All patients should be directly observed for a minimum of 20 minutes after receiving an immunization, and appropriate equipment for the treatment of anaphylaxis should be immediately available. Epinephrine should be on hand for emergencies.

Reducing pain at the site of injection, especially when multiple injections are required, should be a priority. The use of vapocoolant sprays or EMLA cream is effective. Using the proper technique of injection of vaccines is also important. The *Haemophilus influenzae* type B (Hib) vaccine must be dispensed in a separate syringe from that used for other vaccines administered at the same clinic visit. The varicella vaccine is given subcutaneously, whereas the diphtheria-tetanus–acellular pertussis (DTaP) vaccine causes significant tissue irritation if given subcutaneously and careful IM technique is essential. Combination vaccines have been developed that reduce the number of injections required at each clinic visit.

Alternative methods of vaccine delivery are being developed, including use of the intranasal route and transdermal techniques.

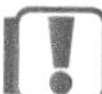

Medication Alert!

There should be a 3- to 11-month interval between the administration of an immune globulin and administration of a live-virus vaccine.

Informed consent concerning the potential risks and the documentation of immunization are essential. Parents should have copies of their child's immunization records. Some provinces have online immunization records that make retrieving information easier. The immunization program for children in Canada is described in Fig. 32.6, which outlines the different provincial guidelines.

Contraindications to live-virus vaccine administration may include the following:

- Immunocompromised state (necessitates individual evaluation by the health care provider)
- Pregnancy
- Bacteremia or meningitis
- Immunocompromised caregiver in the home (necessitates individual evaluation by the health care provider)
- Corticosteroid therapy or immunosuppressive drugs (necessitates individual evaluation)
- History of high fever (40.5° C [105° F]) after previous vaccinations
- Anaphylaxis to contents in the vaccine

A subcutaneous injection should be administered with a 1.5-cm (⅝-inch), 23- to 25-gauge needle; an IM injection should be administered with a 2.5- to 3.2-cm (1- to 1 ¼-inch), 22- to 25-gauge needle; and an intradermal injection should be administered with a 0.6- to 1.3-cm (¼- to ½ inch), 25- to 27-gauge needle with the bevel up and parallel to the volar surface of the forearm.

Children from 4 months to 18 years of age who start the immunization process late or are more than 1 month behind should adhere to the catch-up schedule

Nursing Tip

An interrupted vaccination series can usually continue without restarting the entire series.

THE FUTURE OF IMMUNOTHERAPY

Research concerning the development of new vaccines and the refinement of established vaccines continues

Canada's Provincial and Territorial Routine (and Catch-up) Vaccination Routine Schedule Programs for Infants and Children

This table summarizes the current routine vaccination schedule for infants and children in all provinces and territories across Canada. Changes to this schedule are updated regularly in collaboration with the Canadian Nursing Coalition for Immunization (CNCI) and the Canadian Immunization Committee (CIC) schedules for each province or territory can be found here. Additional information is available on Canada.ca\vaccines (last update: May 2018).

VACCINES		Provincial & Territorial Vaccination Schedules												
Abbreviations	Description	BC	AB	SK	MB	ON	QC	NB	NS	PE	NL	YT	NT	NU
DTaP-IPV-Hib	Diphtheria, Tetanus, acellular Pertussis, Inactivated Polio Virus, *Haemophilus Influenzae* type B vaccine	Age: 18 mos	Age: 18 mos	Age: 2, 4, 6, 18 mos	Age: 2, 4, 6, 18 mos	Age: 2, 4, 6, 18 mos	Age: 6 mos	Age: 2, 4, 6, 18 mos	Age: 2, 4, 6, 18 mos	Age: 18 mos	Age: 2, 4, 6, 18 mos	Age: 18 mos	Age: 2, 4, 6, 18 mos	Age: 2, 4, 6, 18 mos
DTaP-HB-IPV-Hib	Diphtheria, Tetanus, acellular Pertussis, Hepatitis B, Inactivated Polio Virus, *Haemophilus Influenzae* type B vaccine	Age: 2, 4, 6 mos	Age: 2, 4, 6 mos				Age: 2, 4, 18 mos			Age: 2, 4, 6 mos		Age: 2, 4, 6 mos		
Tdap-IPV	Tetanus, diphtheria (reduced toxoid), acellular pertussis (reduced toxoid), Inactivated Polio Virus vaccine	Age: 4–6 yrs	Age: 4–6 yrs	Age: 4–6 yrs	Age: 4–6 yrs	Age: 4–6 yrs	Age: 4–6 yrs	Age: 4 yrs	Age: 4–6 yrs	Age: 4–5 yrs	Age: 4–6 yrs	Age: 4–6 yrs	Age: 4–6 yrs	Age: 4–6 yrs
Tdap	Tetanus, diphtheria (reduced toxoid), acellular pertussis (reduced toxoid) vaccine	Grade 9	Grade 9	Grade 8	Age: 13–15 yrs	Age: 14–16 yrs	3rd year of high school	Grade 7	Grade 7	Grade 9	Grade 9	Grade 9	Grade 7	Grade 6
HB	Hepatitis B vaccine	HB is provided in a 3-dose combination vaccine (DTaP-HB-IPV-Hib) in infancy	(3-dose) Grade 5	(2-dose) Grade 6	(2-dose), Grade 6	(2-dose) Grade 7	HB is provided in a 3-dose combination vaccine (DTaP-HB-IPV-Hib) in infancy Catch-up (2-dose) 2013/14 to 2022/23 Grade 4	Age: At birth, 2,6 mos	(2-doses) Grade 7	HB is provided in a 3-dose combination vaccine (DTaP-HB-IPV-Hib) in infancy	(2-dose) Grade 6	HB is provided in a 3-dose combination vaccine (DTaP-HB-IPV-Hib) in infancy	Age: At birth, 1, 6 mos	Age: At birth, 1, 9 mos
MMR	Measles, Mumps, Rubella vaccine	Age: 12 mos				Age: 12 mos	Age: 12 mos					Age: 12 mos		
Var	Varicella vaccine	Age: 12 mos		Catch- (2nd dose) 2015 to 2021 Grade: 6		Age: 15 mos	Age: 4–6 yrs	Catch-up (2nd dose) 2016/17 to 2022/23 Grade 9				Age: 12 mos		Catch-up Grade 6
MMRV	Measles, Mumps, Rubella, Varicella vaccine	2nd dose Age: 4–6 yrs	Age: 12 mos, 4–6yrs	Age: 12, 18 mos	Age: 12 mos, 4–6yrs	2nd dose Age: 4–6 yrs	Age: 18 mos	Age: 12, 18 mos	Age: 12 mos, 18 mos–6 yrs	Age: 12, 18 mos	Age: 12, 18 mos	2nd dose Age: 4–6 years	Age: 12, 36 mos	Age: 12, 18 mos
Men-C-C	Meningococcal conjugate (Strain C) vaccine	Age: 2, 12 mos	Age: 4, 12 mos	Age: 12 mos	Age: 12 mos[4]	Age: 12 mos	Age: 12 mos, 3rd yr of high school	Age: 12 mos	Age: 12 mos	Age: 12,18 mos	Age: 12 mos	Age: 2, 12 mos	Age: 2,12 mos	Age: 12 mos
Men-C-ACYW-135	Meningococcal conjugate (Strains A, C, Y, W135) vaccine	Grade 9	Grade 9	Grade 6		Grade 7		Grade 9	Grade 7	Grade 9	Grade 4	Grade 9	Grade 12[a]	Grade 9
Pneu-C-13	Pneumococcal conjugate (13-valent) vaccine	Age: 2, 4, 12 mos	Age: 2, 4, 12 mos	Age: 2, 4, 12 mos	Age: 2, 4, 12 mos	Age: 2, 4, 12 mos		Age: 2, 4, 12 mos	Age: 2, 4, 12 mos	Age: 2, 4, 6 if high risk, 12 mos	Age: 2, 4, 6 if high risk 12 mos	Age: 2, 4, 12 mos	Age: 2, 4, 6, 18 mos	Age: 2, 4, 6, 18 mos
Pnue-C-10	Pneumococcal conjugate (10-valent) vaccine						Age: 2, 4, 12 mos							
Rota	Rotavirus vaccine	Age: 2, 4 mos Starting June 2018 age 2, 4, 6 mos	Age: 2, 4 mos	Age: 2, 4, 6 mos	Age: 2, 4, 6 mos	Age: 2, 4, 6 mos	Age: 2, 4 mos	Age: 2, 4, 6 mos		Age: 2, 4, 6 mos	Age 2, 4 mos	Age: 2, 4, 6 mos	Age: 2, 4 mos	Age: 2, 4, 6 mos
HPV	Human Papillomavirus vaccine	(2-dose) Grade: 6[1]	(3-dose) Grade 5[1] Catch-up (3-dose) 2014 to 2018 Grade 9[3]	(2-dose) Grade 6[1]	(2-dose) Grade 6[1]) Catch-up (2-dose) Grade: 8, 9[3]	(2-dose) Grade 7[1] Catch-up (2 or 3 -dose) Grade 8[1], Grades 9 to 12[2]	(2-dose) Grade 4[1]	(2-dose) Grade 7[1])	(2-dose) Grade 7[1]	(2-dose) Grade 6[1]	(2-dose) Grade 6[1]	(2-dose) Grade 6[1]	(9–14 yrs: 2-dose 15 yrs +: 3-dose) Grade 4–6[1]	(2-dose) Grade 6[1]

LEGEND

Abbreviation/footnote	Definition
yrs	Years (age)
mos	Months (age)
a	If attending post-secondary school out-of territory
1	Males and Females
2	Females only
3	Males only
(dark shading)	Vaccine is not publicly funded in this province/territory
(light shading)	A specific catch-up program is currently underway. A catch-up program is defined as a time-limited measure to implement a new vaccine program to a certain age cohort (e.g. an additional dose of a vaccine is recommended and a targeted program is put in place). It can also be used when a vaccine is added at a younger age (e.g. in infancy) and the existing program continues until that infancy age cohort "catches up" to the current age cohort (e.g. hepatitis b vaccine is added to the infancy program, but the school immunization program continues until those infants reach school aged immunization). With that said, a province or territory can still provide catch-up vaccine at the individual level even if there's no specific program in place.

Fig. 32.6 Canada's provincial and territorial routine (and catch-up) vaccination routine schedule programs for infants and children. (From Public Health Agency of Canada. [2018]. Canada's provincial and territorial routine (and catch-up) vaccination routine schedule programs for infants and children. Retrieved from https://www.canada.ca/content/dam/phac-aspc/documents/services/provincial-territorial-immunization-information/childhood_schedule-04-2018.pdf.)

at a rapid pace. The use of transgenic plants for oral administration of bacterial and viral antigens would enable low-cost, effective distribution. Research in the field of transcutaneous immunization involves the application of an antigen with an adjuvant to the intact skin. Recombinant DNA technology and the use of adjuvants are being developed for rheumatic fever and malaria. Alum is an adjuvant currently used in the vaccine against hepatitis B to increase its effectiveness. RNA and DNA viruses are being developed for use as carriers (vectors) of other antigens. Forms of bacterial DNA are also being developed as carriers of antigens.

The most exciting development in immunology is the use of immunotherapy for noncommunicable diseases. An example would be the mucosal administration of myelin in multiple sclerosis and a type 2 collagen for rheumatic arthritis. The possibility of preventing specific types of cancer has been recognized, and the challenge of developing tumour antigens that lyse tumour cells is also a clear possibility. In Alzheimer's disease, the formation of neurotoxic plaques in the brain causes the loss of mental function. Early immunization with amyloid B may prevent or lyse the plaque formation and prevent the devastating problems of this disease.

SEXUALLY TRANSMITTED INFECTIONS

Sexually transmitted infection (STI) is the general name given to infections spread through direct sexual activity. This term replaces the terms *sexually transmitted disease* and *venereal disease*. STIs can be transmitted by a pregnant woman to her unborn child and can cause serious problems in the fetus such as blindness, birth defects, or death (Table 32.3). The occurrence of an STI in a prepubertal patient should always prompt investigation into the possibility of sexual abuse. STIs in adults are discussed in Chapter 2.

To guide Canada's efforts to reduce the health impact of sexually transmitted and blood-borne infections (STBBI), a Pan-Canadian framework has been developed that has been endorsed by federal, provincial, and territorial ministers of health and provides a comprehensive approach to addressing STBBIs (Centre for Communicable Diseases and Infection Control, 2018).

Nursing Tip

The use of condoms to prevent STIs, although recommended, is not considered 100% effective because condoms are apt to slip or break during intercourse and can be damaged by oil-based lubricants. The only method to prevent STIs that is 100% effective is abstinence.

Table 32.3 Nursing Care to Prevent and Treat Sexually Transmitted Infections (STIs)

NURSING GOALS

- To provide anticipatory guidance concerning sexuality at a level that the child or young person can comprehend throughout developmental cycle
- To prevent infection
- To identify early symptoms and provide prompt treatment if infection occurs
- To prevent sequelae

CONCERN	NURSING INTERVENTIONS
Children less than 12 years of age	Provide age-appropriate instruction concerning sexuality; also explore expected patterns that might occur before next visit.
Puberty and adolescence	Review structure and function of reproductive systems; review personal hygiene; discuss values and decision making, possible sexual behaviour and consequences, and prevention of pregnancy and STIs.
Self-concept: anticipate evidence of fear, embarrassment, anger, and decreased self-esteem on suspicion of infection	Create nonjudgemental atmosphere; listen, assess level of knowledge, observe nonverbal behaviour, establish confidentiality; provide privacy when assisting with pelvic or genital examination; provide appropriate draping of patient; realize anger is often a mask for depression or grief—do not take it personally.
Skin and hair	Assess for skin rashes, "crabs" (pubic lice), or scabies (mites).
Sexual partners	Determine sexual preference; investigate and direct to treatment; persons at particular risk are those who have multiple sexual partners, are with new partners, or have a history of previous STI.
Sexual intercourse	Encourage patient to abstain from sex during treatment and to use condoms to prevent reinfection.
Medication	Encourage patient to take all of prescribed medication; if taking tetracycline, advise to take 1 hour before or 2 hours after meals (on empty stomach); avoid intake of dairy products, antacids, and iron and avoid sunlight.
Adherence to treatment	Stress importance of follow-up
Sequelae	Discuss possible complications, such as birth defects and infertility, that can occur with specific STIs.

NURSING CARE

Nurses who wish to help adolescents with STIs must create an environment in which the adolescent feels safe and at ease. Adolescents need emotional support, which the nurse can provide through listening and maintaining a nonjudgemental attitude. The nurse is also responsible for staying up to date on PHAC changes in recommended vaccine protocols.

The nurse needs to approach the patient with sensitivity, recognizing that the adolescent may be embarrassed and in need of privacy, especially during examinations. Girls are often nervous about a pelvic examination. This is true even when their outward manner appears otherwise. Careful explanations are needed. The patient should be draped appropriately, and the nurse may remain in the room during the examination to provide reassurance when required. The findings should be discussed with the patient and questions encouraged. Most adolescents need to be drawn out and do not readily ask questions, even when they do not understand something.

The requirement to report sexual contacts is an emotionally charged topic that often prevents patients from seeking help. The person who is assured of confidentiality and who has been treated in a dignified manner is more apt to work with the health care team. Teenagers who are sexually active must be taught how to take responsibility for their own health. Young people must be made aware of the fact that sex with only one partner does not eliminate the risk, because this partner may have had contact with others; the partner needs to have had only one sexual experience with one infected person to transmit disease.

The nurse should assess the person's level of knowledge and provide information at an understandable level. Many young people have little knowledge of their body and their developing sexuality. They may be involved in relationships they no longer desire and may need help in formulating positive attitudes toward themselves. They also need help understanding their behaviour and that of others.

Prevention of STIs is discussed in Chapter 2.

> **Nursing Tip**
>
> Sex education is not limited to the mechanics of intercourse but rather includes the feelings involved in a sexual experience: expectations, fantasies, fulfillments, and disappointments.

HUMAN PAPILLOMAVIRUS

The most common viral STI in Canada and worldwide is human papillomavirus (HPV). It is contracted via direct sexual contact, and the risk is increased when multiple sexual partners are involved. Many types of HPV are associated with the development of cancer in both males and females. HPV may be a significant cause of cervical cancer in women. HPV is discussed in more detail in Chapter 2.

Prevention

In Canada, there are three vaccines available to help prevent various types of HPV, including ones that are responsible for up to 70% of anal and genital cancer and up to 90% of genital warts. These vaccines have been approved for use in females ages 9 to 45 and in males between the ages of 9 to 26. An initial dose is given, followed by one dose 2 months later and another dose given 6 months after the first dose. These vaccines may also be given according to a two-dose schedule among healthy individuals between the ages of 9 and 14 years of age. All provinces and territories have publicly funded, school-based HPV vaccination programs for girls 9 to 13 years of age (grades 4 to 8), and some programs include vaccination of boys (Canadian Cancer Society, 2019). Parental acceptance of the adolescent vaccine can be increased by emphasizing the values related to cancer prevention for their son or daughter.

Pregnant and lactating women should avoid getting this vaccine (Government of Canada, 2017).

HIV/AIDS IN CHILDREN

Pediatric HIV/AIDS is a worldwide public health problem with a devastating outcome. Children usually acquire the HIV infection through the following:

- Contact with an infected mother at birth (approximately 90% of cases in infants)
- Sexual contact with an infected person
- Use of contaminated needles or contact with infected blood

A challenge for public health authorities is educating the public about the role of unprotected sex and IV drug use in increasing the risk of HIV infection. Nonetheless, the recommended HIV counselling and testing for pregnant women and antiretroviral therapy (ART) have played an important role in preventing perinatal transmission (Money, Tulloch, Boucoiran, et al., 2014).

AIDS is caused by a retrovirus known as HIV-1 that attacks lymphocytes (the white blood cells that protect against disease) and destroys the body's ability to fight infection and increases susceptibility to opportunistic infections that normally would not affect a healthy immune system. AIDS is the advanced stage of HIV infection. Improvements in the treatment of HIV have decreased the incidence of HIV/AIDS in children.

Because passive transmission of antibodies from the mother occurs, infants are born with antibodies that crossed the placenta. Some infants' systems become clear of antibodies in about 15 months, whereas other infants eventually experience the infection. In children with perinatal exposure, virologic assay tests, for example, HIV RNA and HIV DNA nucleic acid tests, are now used to test for HIV infection in children younger than 18 months of age. HIV antibody tests should not be used in infants under 18 months of age (Money et al., 2014).

Treatment and Nursing Care

The goals of care are to slow the growth of the virus, prevent opportunistic infections, and provide adequate nutrition and supportive therapy. The doses of antiretroviral medication for children differ from those for adults because of children's reduced absorption, increased elimination, and immature liver. Monitoring blood levels is essential. Birth control should be encouraged, as most antiviral drugs are teratogenic. Prophylaxis against severe opportunistic infections is available for children. Prognosis has improved and progression to AIDS has diminished.

Psychological support for these children and families is paramount. Sensory stimulation and touching are especially important for infants.

The nurse needs to anticipate interventions related to the care of the child with a life-threatening disease. Efforts to support families in crisis are particularly pertinent. Often assistance from the extended family may be needed. Many families require financial resources and may be exhausted from the child's frequent hospitalizations and physical care. They may need to be introduced to the appropriate community agencies, such as social service, financial aid, HIV/AIDS and grief support groups, home health, nutritional programs, and hospice.

Nursing Tip

Rapid HIV tests are offered to high-risk patients and include a blood sample with results usually available within 1 hour. Traditional tests are used to confirm positive results. Counselling should be available to all patients.

Prevention

Prevention is the core of education related to HIV/AIDS. Education of adolescents should include methods of transmission, hazards of IV and illicit drug use, and the important of using safer sex practices. Nurses should encourage high-risk adolescents to undergo counselling and testing with the hope of modifying risky behaviours. The health education curriculum in elementary school for students and staff should include information concerning STI and HIV/AIDS prevention.

The strict use of routine precautions when caring for all patients is essential, especially when handling blood and other body fluids.

SEPSIS

Sepsis is the systemic response to infection with bacteria and can also result from viral and fungal infections. Sepsis causes a systemic inflammatory response syndrome (SIRS) because of the endotoxin of the bacteria that causes tissue damage. Untreated sepsis results in septic shock, multiorgan dysfunction syndrome (MODS), and death. Children who are immunocompromised, who have neutropenia, or who are in intensive care receiving invasive therapy are at increased risk for developing sepsis.

MANIFESTATIONS

Manifestations of sepsis include fever, chills, tachypnea, tachycardia, and neurological signs such as lethargy. In infants, septic shock is not diagnosed by a decrease in blood pressure, because the infant's body initially compensates for the poor circulation and tissue perfusion by increasing the heart rate and vasoconstriction of peripheral blood vessels.

Get Ready for the Certification Examination!

Key Points

- Routine precautions and additional precautions are techniques recommended by the Public Health Agency of Canada to prevent the transmission of communicable diseases.
- *Body substance* refers to secretions of the body that can contain microorganisms.
- An opportunistic infection is caused by organisms normally found in the environment that the immunosuppressed child cannot fight.
- Koplik spots are white spots on the mucous membrane of the oral cavity that occur before a skin rash and are indicative of measles (rubeola) infection.
- In chickenpox (varicella), all stages of the skin lesions are present on the skin at the same time.
- A woman in the early months of pregnancy should not care for a child with German measles (rubella) because the virus can cause fetal anomalies.
- In children with roseola, a persistently high fever suddenly drops as the rash erupts.
- Immunization programs in Canada provide active immunity for children.
- Proper hand hygiene is the basic essential factor in preventing the transmission of infection.
- Proper storage of vaccines and appropriate routes of administration are essential to ensure the potency of the vaccine.
- Education of parents about the need for immunizations against common childhood communicable diseases is a primary nursing responsibility.
- It is the responsibility of the nurse to know when immunizations are due, the immunization history of the child, contraindications, routes of administration, and which vaccines can be given together. The child should be observed for adverse reactions for at least 20 minutes following immunization.

- Gamma globulin offers passive immunity for exposed children who are immunosuppressed.
- Listening skills and a nonjudgemental attitude are essential when caring for adolescents with sexually transmitted infections.
- Children acquire the HIV infection through contact with an infected mother at birth, sexual contact with an infected person, use of contaminated needles during drug use or through blood transfusions of infected blood.
- The long-term nursing goals in the care of a child with HIV are to promote adherence to long-term medication therapy and provide support to maintain optimum growth and development.
- Sepsis can be the result of an overwhelming infection that affects the entire body.

Additional Learning Resources

evolve Go to your Evolve website (http://evolve.elsevier.com/Canada/Leifer) for the following learning resources:

- Answer Key for Critical Thinking Questions
- Answer Key for Textbook Review Questions
- Audio Glossary
- Interactive Review Questions
- Skills Performance Checklists
- Video clips and more!

Online Resources

- Canadian Paediatric Society (Caring for Kids), *Vaccination and Your Child:* https://www.caringforkids.cps.ca/handouts/vaccination_and_your_child
- CATIE—Canada's source for information on HIV and hepatitis C: http://www.catie.ca/en/home
- Government of Canada, *Canadian Adverse Events Following Immunization Surveillance System (CAEFISS):* https://www.canada.ca/en/public-health/services/immunization/canadian-adverse-events-following-immunization-surveillance-system-caefiss.html
- Government of Canada, *Canadian Immunization Guide:* https://www.canada.ca/en/public-health/services/canadian-immunization-guide.html
- Government of Canada, *National Advisory Committee on Immunization (NACI):* https://www.canada.ca/en/public-health/services/immunization/national-advisory-committee-on-immunization-naci.html#rec
- Government of Canada, *Travel Health and Safety:* https://travel.gc.ca/travelling/health-safety?_ga=2.160068089.517347514.1529895616-440366529.1516216001
- Government of Canada, *Vaccines and Immunizations:* https://www.canada.ca/en/public-health/topics/immunization-vaccines.html

Review Questions

1. The nurse is caring for a newborn with HIV/AIDS. What is the priority goal?
   a. Encourage breastfeeding.
   b. Prevent infections.
   c. Provide initial immunizations.
   d. Notify social services.
2. An adolescent diagnosed with AIDS asks about the mode of transmission for the illness. An accurate response is that it was most likely through which of the following?
   a. Casual contact with a friend who is HIV-positive.
   b. A latent response to an inherited predisposition.
   c. Use of a contaminated toilet seat.
   d. Contact with contaminated body substance through sex or intravenous needle use.
3. When providing play therapy for a child with a communicable disease who is in an isolation room, what would be one priority principle or rationale for toy selection?
   a. The toy should be selected from the hospital playroom.
   b. Most children love books.
   c. It is best to bring the child's favourite toy from home.
   d. The toy should be washable.
4. How is the DTaP immunization administered?
   a. Orally
   b. Subcutaneously
   c. Intramuscularly
   d. Intravenously
5. The nurse is preparing to administer live virus vaccine to a 4-month-old infant. Which observations would indicate that the nurse should contact the health care provider before proceeding? *(Select all that apply.)*
   a. The mother states that the infant cried incessantly for hours after the last immunization
   b. The infant is receiving steroids for a skin problem.
   c. The infant has mild diarrhea.
   d. The infant had a temperature of 37.9°C (100.2°F) this morning.

Hypotension is an ominous sign that may indicate that the body is unable to compensate adequately and cardiorespiratory arrest is about to occur. Laboratory test results may include positive blood cultures, reduced fibrinogen and thrombocyte levels, and the presence of immature white blood cells. Neutropenia (neutrophil count below $1000 \times 10^6/L$) is an ominous sign.

The nursing responsibilities include monitoring neurological status and vital signs; observing for shock; and maintaining strict routine and additional precautions if required. IV antibiotics are prescribed. To prevent sepsis, immunization against Hib and administration of pneumococcal conjugate vaccine (PCV) are recommended for all children between 2 months and 4 years of age. Immunization may prevent some cases of sepsis; however, sepsis may be the result of other bacterial sources.

REFERENCES

Canadian Cancer Society. (2019). *All about HPV vaccines.* Retrieved from http://www.cancer.ca/en/prevention-and-screening/reduce-cancer-risk/make-informed-decisions/get-vaccinated/all-about-hpv-vaccines/?region=on.

Centre for Communicable Diseases and Infection Control. (2018). A summary of the Pan-Canadian framework on sexually-transmitted and blood-borne infections. *Canadian Communicable Disease Report, 44*(7/8), 179–181. Retrieved from https://www.canada.ca/content/dam/phac-aspc/documents/services/reports-publications/canada-communicable-disease-report-ccdr/monthly-issue/2018-44/issue-7-8-july-5-2018/ccdrv44i0708a05-eng.pdf.

Government of Canada. (2017). *Human papillomavirus (HPV) prevention and HPV vaccines: Questions and answers.* Retrieved from https://www.canada.ca/en/public-health/services/infectious-diseases/sexual-health-sexually-transmitted-infections/hpv-prevention-vaccines-questions-answers.html.

Money, D., Tullock, K., Boucoiran, I., et al. (2014). SOGC clinical practice guideline: Guidelines for the care of pregnant women living with HIV and interventions to reduce perinatal transmission. *Journal of Obstetrics and Gynaecology Canada, 36*(8 eSuppl. A), S1–S46.

Onyett, H., & Canadian Paediatric Society (CPS), Infectious Diseases and Immunization Committee. (2014). Lyme disease in Canada: Focus on children. *Paediatrics & Child Health, 19*(7), 379–383. Reaffirmed 2017.

Public Health Agency of Canada (PHAC). (2016). *Routine practices and additional precautions for preventing the transmission of infection in healthcare settings.* Ottawa, ON: Author. Retrieved from https://www.canada.ca/content/dam/phac-aspc/documents/services/publications/diseases-conditions/routine-practices-precautions-healthcare-associated-infections/routine-practices-precautions-healthcare-associated-infections-2016-FINAL-eng.pdf.

World Health Organization (WHO). (2018). *My 5 moments for hand hygiene.* Geneva: Author. Retrieved from http://www.who.int/infection-prevention/campaigns/clean-hands/5moments/en/.

World Health Organization (WHO). (2019). *10 threats to global health in 2019.* Geneva: Author. Retrieved from https://www.who.int/emergencies/ten-threats-to-global-health-in-2019.

The Child With an Emotional or Behavioural Condition

33

Cheryl L.Pollard

http://evolve.elsevier.com/Canada/Leifer

Objectives

1. Define each key term listed.
2. Discuss factors contributing to emotional and behavioural conditions in children and adolescents.
3. List the five service levels within the continuum of care for children and adolescents with emotional and behavioural concerns.
4. Summarize the role of the nurse in supporting children, adolescents, and their families when children or adolescents display symptoms of emotional or behavioural conditions.
5. Describe the emotional and behavioural signs and symptoms of at least three mental disorders that manifest in childhood and adolescence.
6. Describe risk factors and warning signs for suicide.
7. Identify three treatment modalities used in the treatment of children and adolescents with emotional or behavioural symptoms.
8. List three substances that are often misused.
9. Describe the consequences of substance misuse for children and adolescents.

Key Terms

anxiety disorders
attention/-deficit/hyperactivity disorder (ADHD)
autism spectrum disorder (ASD)
clarity
club drugs
cognitive behavioural therapy (CBT)
consistency
continuation
continuum of services
depression
generalized anxiety disorder (GAD)
harm reduction
mood disorders
neurodevelopmental disorders
physical dependence
pica
psychological dependence
psychosocial interventions
separation anxiety
simplicity
social anxiety disorder
street drugs
substance use disorders
supportive and interpersonal therapy
tolerance

Every day, everywhere, children are trying to cope with stress. Many succeed and grow stronger, some do not. Approximately one in five children will experience significant impairments at home, school, with peers, or in the community because of emotional or behavioural symptoms. Many of these problematic symptoms are related to an underlying mental or neurodevelopmental disorder. Children who have been abused or neglected are at greater risk for developing emotional, intellectual, and social problems as a result of their traumatic experiences than children who are not abused (Akresh, Carusp, & Thirumurthy, 2016). A child with a parent with depression is at risk for developing an anxiety disorder, mood disorder, conduct disorder, or substance use disorder. The parent's inability to model effective coping strategies can lead to learned helplessness, the creation of anxiety or apathy, and an inability to master the environment. The most common mental disorders that occur in childhood include mood disorders, anxiety disorders, and neurodevelopmental disorders, such as attention-deficit/hyperactivity disorder (ADHD). Substance use is also a growing concern for caregivers of children and youth. Children will often meet the diagnostic criteria for more than one disorder. One of the most common comorbid disorders is ADHD, which occurs in approximately 90% of individuals with juvenile-onset bipolar disorder, 90% of children with oppositional defiant disorder, and 50% of those with conduct disorder (Gleason, 2016).

THE CONTINUUM OF CARE

To prevent harm, address needs, and ensure that services are delivered with the appropriate intensity and by providers with adequate preparation and training, the goal in treating children with mental disorders is to have a continuum of services available for children, adolescents, and their families (Mental Health Commission of Canada, 2015). Once a decision is made to initiate treatment, there are a variety of individual and family-focused interventions that can be used, including those addressing psychological, social, physical, educational, and spiritual well-being. The decision to initiate treatment is a complicated decision. In addition to considering the severity of symptoms, some health care providers and many caregivers worry that starting treatment will lead to stigmatization and potential marginalization of the child. The fear of stigmatization is a key deterrent to initiation of and engagement in treatment (Kaushik, Kostaki, & Kyriakopoulos, 2016).

The continuum of services begins with health promotion, prevention, and harm reduction. This is the first step in reducing the effect of emotional and behavioural symptoms in child and adolescent populations. The period of childhood and adolescence is the optimal time to target prevention and intervention strategies, as 80% of adults with mental illness experienced their first symptoms in childhood. Should symptoms emerge despite these efforts, then utilizing community-based generalized practitioners is appropriate. Such generalized practitioners may include general practice physicians, pediatric nurse practitioners, or pediatricians. For children with more complex presentations, local mental health and addiction services are required for more detailed assessments, treatment planning, crisis management, system navigation, and delivery of interventions. Children with severe or difficult-to-treat symptoms are usually referred to specialist acute inpatient services with day and mobile treatment teams. Children and adolescents with unremitting symptoms despite multiple attempts at treatment and intervention may require highly specialized treatment within longer-term inpatient or residential settings.

THE ROLE OF THE NURSE

The main goal of nursing care is to assist the family and child in promoting an optimal level of functioning. The significant physical, cognitive, and social changes that occur as children develop also increase the complexity of assessment and treatment of disorders with emotional and behavioural symptoms. A thorough understanding of growth and development, developmental needs, expectations, and abilities is essential. Clinicians and parents may decide to wait to see if the symptoms are a result of a developmental lag or a response to trauma, and hope that the symptoms will resolve on their own. This can result in treatment being delayed and the child and their family experiencing elevated levels of distress.

Children's emotional and behavioural problems necessitate a total family approach to care. Education of the community (school personnel), family (parents and siblings), and child is an essential nursing responsibility during every patient contact. A knowledgeable, caring, understanding, and supportive nature is valuable for any nurse caring for children with behavioural disorders. Patient advocacy with a focus on prevention and long-term management are goals of care. As such, the nurse can support organizations concerned with mental health and become an advocate on issues that are pertinent to the welfare of children in the community.

Meeting the emotional and behavioural needs of youth and their families can be a challenge, as emotional, neurodevelopmental, and behavioural intervention services are often fragmented. Assisting caregivers in navigating a complex system of community, outpatient, and inpatient services can improve the prognosis of emotional and behavioural disorders, enabling children to reach their potential in growth and development. As nurses facilitate optimal family functioning, early bonding and attachment are important goals, as both are essential parts of developing positive mental health. No matter how dysfunctional the parent–child relationship, most children consciously and unconsciously identify with parental values. If the health care provider discredits the parents' values, it threatens the child's security and can create anxiety. The nurse needs to reassure parents and help them regain or maintain confidence in their parenting role. In addition, because children do not seek treatment on their own, the nurse should assist parents in becoming invested in the treatment modality established for their child.

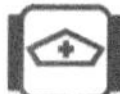 **Nursing Tip**

Parents provide important assessment data about their child that the young child cannot provide. They also bring the child to therapy. Discrediting parents threatens the child and is not therapeutic.

COMMON MENTAL DISORDERS

Children and adolescents with a mental disorder often display behavioural signs and emotional signs and symptoms related to changes in their psychological, social, physical, educational, and spiritual well-being. The most common mental disorders in childhood and adolescence are mood disorders, specifically major depressive disorder; anxiety disorders, specifically generalized anxiety disorder (GAD); and neurodevelopmental disorders, specifically ADHD. There are many other psychiatric disorders that may occur during childhood. For example, children may display symptoms related to pica, avoidant food intake disorder, rumination disorder, anorexia, or bulimia nervosa. It is rare that a child or youth will experience another psychiatric disorder without experiencing a concurrent mood, anxiety, or neurodevelopmental disorder. As a nurse, it is essential to help the patient and their family understand and cope with these complex and often perplexing symptoms. Therefore, the main focus of this chapter will be on the symptoms related to the three most common childhood mental disorders.

MOOD DISORDERS

Mood disorders, sometimes referred to as *affective disorders,* are characterized by pain and suffering, experienced by individuals of all ages. Clinicians and researchers believe that mood disorders remain one of the most underdiagnosed mental health problems. Children and adolescents do not necessarily have or experience the same symptoms as adults. Because of the abstract nature of psychological pain, children may not be able to articulate their emotional experiences. Mood disorders in adolescents also put them at risk of experiencing symptoms of anxiety, behavioural disturbances, and substance misuse that may persist long after the initial episode of the mood disorder is treated.

There are many different mood disorders experienced by children and adolescents (Box 33.1), the most common being major depression. Inheritance factors, organic factors, and environmental factors all contribute to the occurrence of mood disorders in children. Treatment of mood disorders can be on an outpatient basis and may include prescribed medications.

Depression

Depression in a child is not as easy to identify as depression in an adult. Many children have difficulty expressing their feelings and often "act out" their concerns. Depression is an emotion common to childhood. Sadness caused by receiving poor grades, moving to a new community, or losing a pet may trigger a depressive mood that results in either a dependent type or a disruptive type of behaviour. These manifestations are resolved in a short time and are considered perfectly normal.

Box 33.1 Common Mood Disorders

- **Major depression:** a period of a depressed or irritable mood or a noticeable decrease in interest or pleasure in usual activities, along with other signs, lasting at least 2 weeks
- **Persistent depressive disorder (dysthymia):** a chronic, low-grade, depressed, or irritable mood for at least 1 year
- **Bipolar disorder:** manic episodes (period of persistently elevated mood) interspersed with depressed periods or periods of flat or blunted emotional response
- **Disruptive mood dysregulation disorder:** a persistent irritability and extreme inability to control behaviour exhibited in children under the age of 18
- **Premenstrual dysmorphic disorder:** includes depressive symptoms, irritability, and tension before menstruation
- **Mood disorder due to a general medical condition:** many medical illnesses (including cancer, injuries, infections, and chronic medical illnesses) can trigger symptoms of depression
- **Substance-induced mood disorder:** symptoms of depression that are due to effects of medication or other forms of treatment, drug misuse, or exposure to toxins

Manifestations

A major depressive disorder and other mood disorders are usually characterized by a prolonged behavioural change that interferes with school, family life, and age-specific activities. There are many signs and symptoms manifested when a child or adolescent experiences depression (Box 33.2). Individuals who experience thoughts of suicide are often depressed. If left untreated, depressive behaviour can lead to substance misuse, suicide, or both. Suicidal ideation can be a symptom of many psychiatric illnesses. Suicide is discussed later in the chapter.

Treatment and nursing care

Nursing responsibilities include recognizing the signs of depression and initiating appropriate and prompt referral (Nursing Care Plan 33.1). Educating parents and school personnel about the identification of children at risk for depression is an important nursing responsibility. The nurse may choose to use a depression screening questionnaire to help determine the likelihood of an underlying depressive disorder. Common screening tools are the Patient Health Questionnaire (PHQ-9), which is most appropriate for individuals between 12 and 18 years of age. For children between the ages of 7 and 17 years, the Child Depression Inventory 2 (CDI-2) may be used, which is completed by the child, parent, and teacher. See Additional Learning Resources at the end of this chapter for more information about the CDI-2. The Mood and Feelings Questionnaire (MFQ) is a multiversion self-reporting tool. The parents complete one version and the child completes another version. This tool requires that the child is verbal and able to identify if they feel unhappy, sad, or restless; find it hard to think; and believe they are a bad person. All assessment scales are used in an attempt

Box 33.2 Signs and Symptoms of Depression

- Decreased interest in activities or inability to enjoy previously interests
- Hopelessness
- Persistent boredom
- Low energy
- Social isolation
- Poor communication
- Low self-esteem
- Guilt
- Extreme sensitivity to rejection or failure
- Increased irritability, anger, or hostility
- Difficulty with relationships
- Frequent physical illnesses, such as headaches and stomach aches
- Frequent absences from school or poor performance in school
- Poor concentration
- Major change in eating or sleeping patterns, or both
- Thoughts or expressions of suicide or self-destructive behaviour

Nursing Care Plan 33.1 The Depressed Adolescent

PATIENT DATA

An adolescent is admitted with a diagnosis of depression after being treated for injuries that were a result of attempting to die by suicide.

Selected Nursing Diagnosis Possible risk for self-harm as a result of depression and stress

Goals	Nursing Interventions	Rationales
Adolescent will state whether suicide is contemplated.	Ask adolescent if suicidal thoughts are present.	This information is important to know because it will determine intervention; most depressed adolescents are filled with contradictory feelings; talking honestly about feelings helps to clarify them.
	Inquire about precipitating event (e.g., broken romance, poor grades).	Suicidal reactions are associated with feelings of hopelessness, often related to loss of a significant or valued relationship or to a disappointment.
	Determine if adolescent has a specific suicidal plan.	How person plans to take their life is one of the most significant criteria for assessing suicidal potential; more specific plans are a more dangerous threat.
Adolescent does not harm self.	Determine if adolescent has a history of self-harming behaviours.	The situation is considered more critical if the adolescent has made increasing lethal self-harming behaviours.
	Determine if adolescent has a history of emotional instability.	A history of emotional instability is more dangerous.
	Determine if adolescent has the means available to injure self.	If the means to commit suicide are available (e.g., drugs, gun), the threat is imminent and more serious.
	Provide supervision as outlined by health care provider or institution.	Surveillance and support by staff and family are important.
Adolescent will verbalize acceptance of protective measures.	Determine if a "safe contract" has been signed and discussed with adolescent.	This is a written agreement that the adolescent will contact a nurse, counsellor, or crisis line or go to an emergency department before harming self.
	The family will attend team conferences as appropriate.	It is wise to have available as many persons as possible to support one another and to share stress of the situation.
	Administer antidepressants if ordered.	Antidepressants elevate mood of the patient; unfortunately, most antidepressants must be taken for 3 to 4 weeks before a therapeutic response is evident; some require monitoring of blood values.
	Monitor room for potentially dangerous articles.	Belts, glasses, rope, and other materials may be used for self-harm.
	Explain precautions to adolescent and family members.	Explanations will lessen fear and increase compliance.
Family will verbalize seriousness of suicidal threats.	Reinforce to parents the seriousness of adolescent's suicidal ideation.	All suicidal threats need to be taken seriously.

Selected Nursing Diagnosis Poor self-management resulting from poor self-esteem, isolation, and inability to handle painful feelings

Goals	Nursing Interventions	Rationales
Adolescent will make a positive statement about self.	Have adolescent list two positive things about self and reinforce daily.	Determines adolescent's strengths so the nurse can build on them.
Adolescent will accept positive statements from others.	Instruct adolescent to draw "how I see myself" and "how others see me."	Provides valuable information about adolescent's self-esteem. Self-destructive behaviour reflects underlying depression related to low self-esteem and anger directed inward. Drawing offers a release from feelings, helps to clarify emotions, and is a vehicle for discussion between the patient and the nurse.

Nursing Care Plan 33.1 The Depressed Adolescent—cont'd

Goals	Nursing Interventions	Rationales
Adolescent will accept the presence of the nurse, peers, or significant others.	Build extra time into visits so that adolescent does not feel rushed; give your undivided attention.	This indicates that you are truly interested; a ringing telephone and personal interruptions devalue the visit.
Adolescent will gradually cope with painful feelings by sharing and expressing them either verbally or nonverbally.	Instruct adolescent to draw a box and put things that bring happy feelings in the box; then instruct to draw another box and place things that cause sadness in that box. Encourage adolescent to verbalize feelings about drawings; respect adolescent's wish not to talk, should this occur.	Drawings help adolescents distance themselves from the problem and see it more clearly.
Adolescent will speak in future terms.	Review methods of coping.	Discovering how the adolescent coped in the past when less distressed is of importance so that these methods can be reinforced.
Adolescent states two healthy coping measures.	Suggest healthy methods of coping, such as exercise, relaxation recordings or apps, and talking things out with parents or peers.	Many adolescents are not aware of healthy coping methods.

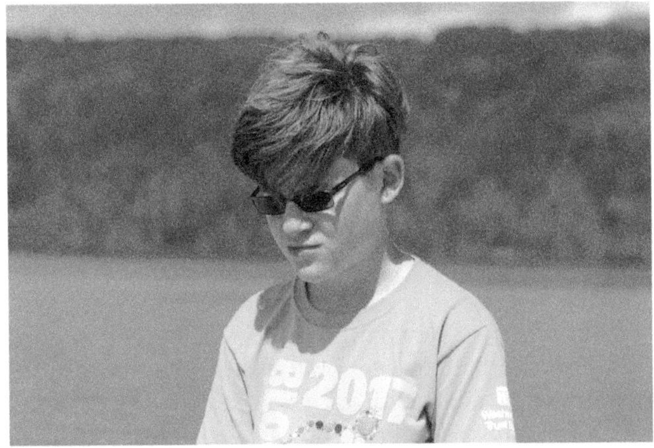

Fig. 33.1 Assessing severity of depressive symptoms. (Photo courtesy of Cheryl L.Pollard.)

to quantify emotional and functional problems in order to determine the level of depressive symptoms (Fig. 33.1).

The treatment of depression typically involves a combination of two treatment modalities, psychosocial and pharmacological. The National Institute for Health and Care Excellence (2017) in the United Kingdom has developed the *Depression in Children and Young People: Identification and Management,* a clinical practice guideline that is recognized by Canadian researchers (Bennet, Duda, Brouwers, et al., 2018) as the best and most trustworthy evidence-informed guideline.

Psychosocial interventions include providing the child or young person and their family with information concerning how to cope with stressful situations. Information regarding strengthening of parent–child relationships may be shared, and **cognitive behavioural therapy (CBT)** may be used. This therapy focuses on skills related to problem solving and management of emotions.

Should the family and child or young person be agreeable to taking medication, a selective serotonin reuptake inhibitor (SSRI) medication is often chosen. When using medication to help treat a depression it should never be used without offering complementary psychosocial interventions. Medications such as paroxetine (Paxil), venlafaxine (Effexor), tricyclic antidepressants, or St. John's wort should not be used concomitantly, because of undesirable medication interactions. As with all interventions, an effective means of evaluating effectiveness must be identified. A recognized assessment scale is often used to evaluate treatment efficacy.

Adverse effects of the medication also require astute monitoring. At highest risk for developing serious adverse effects from medications are adolescents who use alcohol, diet pills, over-the-counter medications, or recreational drugs. SSRI medications are generally well tolerated by adolescents; however, there is the potential for those who take the medication to develop agitation and suicidal thoughts. Close monitoring is essential.

Suicide

Suicide is the second leading cause of death in adolescence (Statistics Canada, 2019a). Death by suicide is more common among boys than in girls, but girls engage more often in nonlethal self-harming behaviours. The spectrum of suicidality ranges from thinking about suicide to death by suicide. To determine the cause of the distress and the risk for violence, the nurse must use active listening when interacting with any young person expressing the wish to hurt self or others. The risk of death by suicide increases when there is a plan of action, a means to carry out the plan, and an absence of obvious resources to turn to for help. The breakdown of family ties, pressure to succeed, or estranged relationships may trigger a low self-esteem or frustration that results in the turning of feelings of hostility or hopelessness inward and further increase the risk of suicide.

In Canada, an Indigenous adolescent has an increased risk of suicide compared to that for non-Indigenous youth. Historical rates indicate that First Nation youth are 5 to 6 times more likely to die by suicide than a non-Indigenous peer, and Inuit children and teenagers are up to 30 times more likely to die by suicide than are their non-Indigenous peers in the rest of Canada (McLoughlin, Gould, & Malone, 2015). Some of the factors that increase risk for suicide among Indigenous teenagers are the high prevalence of mental health disorders, increased substance and alcohol use, and increased social deprivation and stressful life events. Some of this risk is due to the historical undermining and dismantling of cultural processes and structures, due to forced colonial practices such as relocation and placement in residential schools, which have had a profound impact on family functioning (McLoughlin et al., 2015).

Some signs and symptoms of increasing suicidality include deterioration in school performance, isolation from friends and family, changes in physical appearance, giving away of cherished possessions, and talk of death. Some adolescents may exhibit rage behaviours or emotional outbursts that result in impulsive acts causing death that are not directly related to suicidality. Additionally, others may display a chronic type of high-risk behaviour that can lead to serious injury or death.

The nurse's priority is to promote the safety of the child or adolescent, provide education and support to establish healthy mechanisms for coping with their pain and suffering, initiate harm-reduction strategies, identify those children at risk of death by suicide, and facilitate engagement in a more specialized service along the continuum of care. The nurse can also work with school personnel to develop peer support groups and educate families on the available community resources.

Safety Alert!

Every threat of suicide must be taken seriously.

Assessing suicidality in children and youth is complicated by youths' distorted concept of death, underdeveloped ego functioning, and an immature understanding of lethality. The most salient predictor of suicide risk is a past suicide attempt. Additional areas to explore when assessing suicidal risk include the following:

- Existence of a plan, lethality of the plan, and accessibility of any necessities for carrying out the plan
- Feelings of hopelessness
- Changes in level of energy
- Circumstances, state of mind, and motivation
- Viewpoints about suicide and death (e.g., has a family member or friend who attempted suicide)
- Mood or feelings (e.g., anger, guilt, rejection)
- History of impulsivity or poor judgement
- Drug or alcohol use
- Prescribed medications and any recent adherence issues

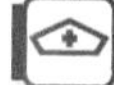

Nursing Tip

When an adolescent feels hopeless and talks about feeling useless or worthless, do not contradict what they are saying. Instead, listen, indicate your understanding, and encourage the expression of feelings. Do not promise not to tell anyone what they tell you. If the adolescent is at imminent risk or if there has been a change in level of risk, other treatment team members will need to be notified.

ANXIETY DISORDERS

Anxious feelings, worries, or fears are common among children. Most children and adolescents will experience apprehension in certain situations, such as during a thunderstorm, being in the dark, being left alone for the first time, receiving grades, or having an argument with a friend (Table 33.1).

Anxiety disorders are caused by a combination of life events, heredity, temperament, and biochemical factors. The physiological, behavioural, and cognitive characteristics of anxiety in children and adolescents are similar to those in adults. This similarity is often helpful when the nurse is teaching family members about "how anxiety feels." When the worries and fears interfere with daily activities like going to school, playing, falling asleep, trying new things, or engaging with friends, this is when further assessment is needed. Children and adolescents can experience many different types of anxiety disorders; see Box 33.3 for common anxiety disorders. The onset of these disorders varies. Phobias and obsessive-compulsive disorder (OCD) arise in early childhood, and panic disorders and social phobias tend to occur in the teen years.

Manifestations

All anxiety disorders share four common features. First, the anxiety or preoccupation interferes with the child's or

Table 33.1 Common Fears of Children

AGE OF CHILD	FEARS
0–1 year	Loss of support, strangers, loud noise
1–3 years	Parental separation, toilet, animals, darkness
3–5 years	Separation, darkness, "bad people"
5–7 years	Being alone, supernatural, harm, dark
7–9 years	School, injury, appearance, death
9–17 years	Personal relations, appearance, school, future, safety, world events, animals

Box 33.3 Common Anxiety Disorders

- **Generalized anxiety disorder (GAD)** is an excessive worry or apprehension about a number of events or activities. These feelings are experienced almost all the time and are not triggered by any one specific issue.
- **Phobias** are highly specific and exclusive of fears. The child or adolescent functions normally until confronted by the specific object, event, or situation.
- **Separation anxiety disorder** is the child's or adolescent's excessive worry and apprehension about being away from their caregivers. Children with separation anxiety disorder often fear that their parents will be harmed in some way or will not return to them as promised.
- **Obsessive-compulsive disorder (OCD)** is a condition involving obsessions and compulsions. Obsessions are recurrent thoughts, impulses, or images that are difficult to control and cause significant distress. Compulsions are behaviours that the child engages in (such as handwashing, checking, redoing) to make the distress feel better.
- **Panic disorder** is characterized by discrete and intense periods of anxiety that occur unexpectedly and without warning and are not always linked to a specific place or situation.
- **Post-traumatic stress disorder (PTSD)** is characterized by re-experiencing the traumatic event. This can occur through intrusive thoughts, dreams, or re-creation through play. As a result, the child can have difficulty sleeping or concentrating, become nervous about their surroundings, act jumpy around loud noises, and withdraw from friends and family.

adolescent's ability to enjoy life or to complete activities of daily living. Second, the reasons behind the development of feelings of anxiety or worries are often unclear. Third, attempts to use logical explanations to reduce the experience of anxiety do not decrease the worries. The last feature is that problems with symptoms of anxiety can be helped with effective treatment strategies. Common symptoms of anxiety are listed in Box 33.4.

A combined treatment approach with CBT, family interventions, and medication based on the needs of the child or adolescent is used to reduce symptoms of anxiety disorders. Medications should not be used without offering at least one other treatment modality.

Generalized Anxiety Disorder

Children with generalized anxiety disorder (GAD) worry more often and more intensely than other children. They tend to be very hard on themselves and strive for perfection. They may worry excessively about their grades, family issues, relationships with peers, performance in sports, personal safety and the safety of family members, or natural disasters and future events. The focus of worry may shift, but the inability to control the worry persists. GAD occurs in over 10% of children and adolescents and has an average age of onset of 8.5 years and is more often reported in girls (Keeton, Kolos, & Walkup, 2009). Common co-occurring conditions include separation anxiety disorder and social phobia.

Box 33.4 Common Symptoms of Anxiety

- Feeling nervous or "on edge"
- Unfounded or unrealistic fears
- Trouble separating from parents
- Sleep disturbance
- Obsessive thoughts or compulsive behaviours
- Trembling, sweating, shortness of breath, stomach aches, headaches, muscle tension, or other physical symptoms

Box 33.5 Potential Complications of Generalized Anxiety Disorder (GAD)

- Insecurity
- Strained family relationships when the child's anxiety contributes to irritability, demanding behaviour, or chronic reassurance seeking
- Withdrawal from other age-appropriate activities
- Decreased school performance or attendance
- "Self-medication" leading to substance misuse by adolescents

Because children with GAD have a hard time "turning off" the worrying, they may have difficulty concentrating, processing information, and engaging successfully in various activities. Potential complications of GAD are listed in Box 33.5. Children with GAD may also seem overly conforming and perfectionistic. They may insist on redoing even fairly insignificant tasks several times to get them "just right." This excessive structuring of one's life is used as a defense against the generalized anxiety related to the quality of their performance.

Nursing Tip

The first step in effective treatment of generalized anxiety disorder is a thorough assessment. This assessment will include the following:

- A review of current symptoms, their duration, and intensity
- A thorough review of the child's development
- Past medical and psychiatric history of the child and family

Separation Anxiety

Separation anxiety is developmentally normal when it occurs between 6 months and 2 years of age and usually involves a response to temporary absence of a parent or primary caregiver. By 3 years of age, the child should be able to accept temporary separations. Separation anxiety is not developmentally normal when it occurs in the school-age child. Fear of harm to self or parent causes the child to resist going to school or even going to sleep without a parent present. Older children refuse to go to school and a panic disorder may develop. When the disorder only involves going to school, it is called *school phobia*.

Social Anxiety Disorder

Social anxiety disorders affect many adolescents; referral is not indicated unless the behaviour significantly interferes with social interactions or academic achievements. Many adolescents are shy, but social anxiety disorders are marked by fear or anxiety in social situations that involve observation and possible criticism by others. The adolescent fears embarrassment or rejection to the extent they may avoid social situations. Basic shyness can be a totally normal characteristic and should not be confused with a social anxiety disorder, which most often involves distress that impairs functioning.

 **Health Promotion**

Emphasizing the strengths of the child rather than their problems is essential to any plan of care for anxiety disorders.

Treatment and Nursing Care

There are a number of types of treatment that can decrease symptoms associated with anxiety. These include supportive and interpersonal therapy; CBT, acceptance and commitment therapy, and pharmacological therapy. All of these therapies help change how individuals relate to their symptoms. Supportive and interpersonal therapy utilizes attachment and communication strategies to help individuals adjust how they see their world. This type of therapy starts with identifying the underlying reasons why the person is having interpersonal difficulties and gauges the amount and depth of the available social support. Interpersonal therapy is most effective in making a person's relationships, transitions, and sense of social isolation more understandable.

CBT specifically target thoughts, physical symptoms, and behaviours, including the over-preparation, planning, and avoidance that characterizes GAD. Through CBT, skills and techniques to reduce anxiety are taught. Individuals learn to recognize their thinking patterns and to replace negative thoughts with more realistic and positive thoughts. Children and adolescents need to be supported when engaged in CBT as they will have "homework" to practice between sessions. For CBT therapy to be successful, the child must be motivated and be capable of following directions. Parent and sibling involvement and support are essential.

Acceptance and commitment therapy involves use of mindfulness strategies to help the individual live in the moment and allow themselves to experience life without judgement.

Medication can be another form of effective treatment for anxiety disorders. The most effective treatment plans have a combination of therapies such as CBT and an SSRI (Rosenberg & Chiriboga, 2016). The nurse's role includes engaging the parent, the mental health therapist, and the school personnel to manage the problem as a team. The nurse also has an important role in assessing the treatment response and the adverse effects of the medication.

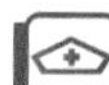 **Nursing Tip**

It is important for nurses who work with youth to also assess for post-traumatic stress disorder (PTSD) and assess the safety of the environment of young people who have been traumatized or have experienced abuse (physical, psychological, or sexual) or a history of other violence. Interventions should focus on teaching coping skills to deal with trauma, supporting efforts to achieve socially appropriate goals, and facilitating integration into healthy social support systems. For example, for those children who have experienced a sexual assault, interventions may focus on developing coping skills to reduce behavioural and emotional changes such as the child becoming withdrawn or very clingy, reverting to younger behaviours such as bed wetting, having outbursts of anger, or becoming unusually secretive.

NEURODEVELOPMENTAL DISORDERS

Neurodevelopmental disorders are those primarily associated with the functioning of the neurological system and brain. Included in this category of disorders are ADHD, autism spectrum disorder (ASD), and learning and intellectual disabilities. The most common neurodevelopmental disorders are ADHD and ASD.

ATTENTION-DEFICIT/HYPERACTIVITY DISORDER

Attention-deficit/hyperactivity disorder (ADHD) refers to a developmentally inappropriate degree of gross motor activity, impulsivity, and inattention in the school and home setting that begins before age 7 years, lasts more than 6 months, and is not related to the existence of any other central nervous system illness. It includes inattention, increased distractibility, poor impulse control, and motor restlessness. The child often underachieves in school, has problems with interpersonal relationships, and has low self-esteem. It often occurs with learning disabilities; however, learning disabilities are not part of ADHD, and the child usually has average or above-average intellectual ability.

An increased risk for ADHD has been associated with brain injury, exposure to environmental toxins, alcohol and tobacco use during pregnancy, premature birth, and low birth weight (Murcia, 2017). Genetic factors have also been identified involving disturbances in the dopamine system, leading to a theory labelled the "dopamine hypothesis," which is the basis for the development of the condition as well as the medications used to treat it (Urion, 2016).

Manifestations

Diagnostic criteria include receptive and expressive language difficulties, memory problems, and motor coordination challenges (American Psychiatric Association [APA], 2013). Many children have trouble focusing or behaving at one time or another. For children with ADHD, these symptoms interfere with their daily functioning and development. There are three different types of ADHD: predominantly inattentive, predominantly hyperactive-impulsive, and combined inattentive and hyperactive-impulsive. Children with ADHD do not "grow out" of these behaviours.

Box 33.6 summarizes common manifestations of ADHD. Not all of these manifestations are present with every child, but when several of these are present, further assessment is appropriate.

> **Nursing Tip**
>
> ADHD is characterized by inattention, hyperactivity, impulsivity, and distractibility.

Treatment and Nursing Care

ADHD is one of the most common neurodevelopmental disorders among children. Early detection, diagnosis, and treatment can prevent long-term consequences of this disorder. As there is no single test to diagnose ADHD, a multidisciplinary approach is needed to confirm a suspected diagnosis. At a minimum, the multidisciplinary team should include the parent, child, physicians, nurses, and teachers. Treatment is individualized for the child and family, with the main focus being on CBT and, depending on the child's needs; a stimulant medication (e.g., methylphenidate, methylphenidate hydrochloride extended-release, amphetamine, dextroamphetamine) may also be prescribed (Findling & Dinh, 2014). Family education to manage a potential knowledge deficit about the condition and counselling to help the family and child cope with the problems encountered are essential. Complementary and alternative health modalities (CAHM) therapy, such as biofeedback, yoga, and dietary interventions, has also been used useful in decreasing the intensity of the symptoms (Farone & Antshel, 2014).

Support groups can aid parents in their coping skills. Parents and other caregivers often find it useful to feel less isolated and to identify the commonalities of their experience. Other important people in the care of a child with ADHD are their teachers. The nurse can help teachers develop strategies for managing children with ADHD in the classroom (see Health Promotion box). Increasing positive interactions, providing tutoring, giving computer assistance, and using behavioural management strategies, under the supervision of a specialized health care provider (e.g., psychologist, advanced practice nurse, social worker), are helpful approaches in the classroom and at home. Some children who are labelled ADHD in school may develop low self-esteem and antisocial behaviour. Engaging these children in a self-esteem group may also lessen the social isolation that often accompanies those who have relational difficulties.

Box 33.6 Common Behavioural Symptoms Associated With ADHD

- Forgetting or losing things frequently
- Squirming or fidgeting
- Lacking in fine-motor control
- Having a hard time following instruction
- Detaching from immediate surroundings
- Having difficulty completing long-term projects
- Talking too much
- Making careless mistakes or taking unnecessary risks
- Having a hard time resisting temptation
- Having trouble taking turns
- Having difficulty getting along with others
- Not contributing to group work and even keeping a group from accomplishing a task

Health Promotion

Strategies for Managing the Child With ADHD in the Classroom

- Seat child in the front of the classroom to minimize distraction.
- Give instructions one at a time and repeat as necessary.
- If possible, work on the most difficult material early in the day.
- Use visuals: charts, pictures, colour coding.
- Create outlines for note-taking that organize the information.
- Create worksheets and tests with fewer items, give frequent, short quizzes rather than long tests, and reduce the number of timed tests.
- Test students with ADHD in the way they do best, such as orally or filling in blanks.
- Divide long-term projects into segments and assign a completion goal for each segment.
- Have student keep a master binder with a separate section for each subject, and make sure everything that goes into the notebook is put in the correct section. Colour-code materials for each subject.
- Make sure student has a system for writing down assignments and important dates and uses it.
- Signal the start of a lesson with an aural cue, such as an egg timer, a cowbell, or a horn. (Subsequent cues can be used to show how much time remains in a lesson.)
- Establish eye contact with any student who has ADHD.
- List activities of the lesson on the board.
- In opening a lesson, tell students what they're going to learn and what the expectations are. Tell students exactly what materials they will need.
- Keep instructions simple and structured. Use props, charts, and other visual aids.
- Vary the pace and include different kinds of activities. Many students with ADHD do well with competitive games or other activities that are rapid and intense.
- Have an unobtrusive cue set up with students who have ADHD, such as a touch on the shoulder or placing a sticky note on their desk, to remind them to stay on task.
- Allow students with ADHD frequent breaks and let them squeeze a rubber ball or tap something that doesn't make noise as a physical outlet.
- Try not to ask a student with ADHD to perform a task or answer a question publicly that might be too difficult.

Box 33.7 Behaviours Associated With Autism Spectrum Disorder

- Tending not to look at or listen to people
- Rarely sharing enjoyment of objects or activities by pointing to or showing things to others
- Having difficulties with the back and forth of conversation
- Often talking at length about a favourite subject without noticing that others are not interested or giving others a chance to respond
- Having facial expressions, movements, and gestures that do not match what is being said
- Having trouble understanding another person's point of view or being unable to predict or understand other people's actions
- Repeating certain behaviours or having unusual behaviours
- Having a lasting intense interest in certain topics, such as numbers, details, or facts
- Having overly focused interests, such as with moving objects or parts of objects
- Getting upset by slight changes in a routine
- Being more or less sensitive than other people to sensory input, such as light, noise, clothing, or temperature

AUTISM SPECTRUM DISORDER

Autism spectrum disorder (ASD) is a group of neurodevelopmental disorders characterized by difficulties in social interaction and communication, repetitive behaviours, and stereotyped interests and activities (Raviola, Trieu, Demaso, et al., 2016). It includes formerly separate conditions such as autism, Asperger syndrome, Rett syndrome, and others (APA, 2013). The cause of this spectrum disorder is thought to be related to factors such as advanced parental age, prematurity, prenatal environment, and multiple genetic factors (Raviola et al., 2016).

Manifestations

People with ASD have difficulty with social communication, relationships, and repetitive behaviours. See Box 33.7 for examples of behaviours that may be displayed by an individual with ASD.

Diagnosis can be made as early as 1 to 2 years of age and is well established by 18 years of age (APA, 2013). In early childhood, there is evidence of little pretend play, the use of rigid rules in play, or preference for solitary play. Often the child shows little empathy for others. Parents need to be educated about normal growth and development so they can recognize deviations and seek early interventions. Red flags to report include the following:

- No babbling or pointing by 12 months
- No two-word spontaneous phrases by 24 months
- Loss of social skills or language previously attained

The Modified Checklist for Autism in Toddlers (M-CHAT) and the Ages and Stages questionnaire are two popular screening tools for ASD. If these preliminary assessments suggest there is a possibility of ASD, a referral to professionals experienced in diagnosing ASD is warranted, such as a developmental pediatrician, child psychologist, child psychiatrist, neuropsychologist, or speech-language pathologist. Their assessment involves evaluation of cognitive thinking skills, language abilities, and age-appropriate skills needed to complete daily activities independently. In Canada, it is recommended that specific screening for ASD occur at 18 to 24 months of age, using the M-CHAT for all children with any of the following: failed items on the social, emotional, or communication skills inquiry; a sibling with autism; or developmental concern expressed by the parent, caregiver, or physician (Ip, Zwaigenbaum, Nicholas, et al., 2015).

Treatment

In many provinces there are provincial funding sources for children with ASD; however, these vary by province (Table 33.2).

Managing behaviours associated with ASD involves a combination of approaches. For example, any underlying medical or psychiatric concerns need to be addressed, and behavioural and educational supports are used to teach replacement skills and self-regulation. There are no medications or any other type of treatment that will "cure" this disorder, but there are several strategies that can help reduce the distress the symptoms cause to the child and to help improve functioning.

Health Promotion

Although people with autism spectrum disorder (ASD) experience many challenges, they may also have many strengths, including:

- Being able to learn things in detail and remember information for long periods of time
- Being strong visual and auditory learners
- Excelling in math, science, music, or art

When a child has several challenging behaviours, it is important to establish priorities. The first priority is the safety of the child. Thus, the plan should focus first on targeting particularly risky or dangerous behaviours. There are four essential components to successful treatment plans: clarity, consistency, simplicity, and continuation. These components are further described in Box 33.8.

Nursing Care

The nurse's role is to identify abnormal behaviour as early as possible, refer for follow-up care, and monitor the adverse effects of prescribed medications used to treat underlying conditions. When the nurse provides services to a child with a neurodevelopmental disorder and their family

Table 33.2 Government Funding and Programs for Autism Spectrum Disorder

PROVINCE OR TERRITORY	WEB LINK TO GOVERNMENT FUNDING AND PROGRAMS
Alberta	https://www.alberta.ca/disability-supports.aspx
British Columbia	http://autisminfo.gov.bc.ca/
Manitoba	http://www.gov.mb.ca/fs/cds/index.html
New Brunswick	http://www2.gnb.ca/content/gnb/en/services/services_renderer.13836.Services_for_Preschool_Children_with_Autism_Spectrum_Disorders.html
Newfoundland/Labrador	http://www.health.gov.nl.ca/health/personsdisabilities/fundingprograms_hcs.html
Northwest Territories	http://services.exec.gov.nt.ca/service/417
Nova Scotia	https://novascotia.ca/dhw/mental-health/autism.asp
Nunavut	https://www.gov.nu.ca/health
Ontario	http://www.children.gov.on.ca/htdocs/English/specialneeds/autism/ontario-autism-program.aspx
Prince Edward Island	https://www.princeedwardisland.ca/en/topic/education-early-learning-and-culture
Quebec	https://www.rrq.gouv.qc.ca/en/enfants/enfant_handicape/Pages/enfant_handicape.aspx
Saskatchewan	https://www.saskatchewan.ca/residents/health/accessing-health-care-services/health-services-for-people-with-disabilities/autism-services
Yukon	http://www.hss.gov.yk.ca/socialservices.php

Box 33.8 Essential Components of Treatment for Autism Spectrum Disorder

- *Clarity*: Information about the plan, expectations, and procedures are clear to the individual, family, staff, and any other team members.
- *Consistency:* Team and family members have the same understanding of interventions and approaches, and strive to apply the same expectations and rewards.
- *Simplicity:* Supports are simple, practical, and accessible so that everyone is on the team, including the family.
- *Continuation:* As behaviour improves, it is important to keep the teaching and positive supports in place to continue to help the child develop good habits and more adaptive skills.

within a hospital or residential clinical setting, the change of setting can be a significant stressor to the child. The stress of the hospitalization and the challenges the child experiences because of the illness can result in an escalation of maladaptive behaviours. The nurse's approach to the child should be slow paced, with few distractions. The child should be allowed to become familiar with the office, room, or equipment. The child should be asked for permission before touching them, and sudden movements or loud noise should be avoided. Safety and family support are priorities.

The development of meaningful language by 5 years of age is a favourable prognosis. Recent clinical trials have shown that the use of intranasal oxytocin aids in increasing positive social interaction and relieving other characteristic symptoms, although research is still ongoing (Raviola et al., 2016).

SUBSTANCE USE DISORDERS

Children and adolescents are exposed to many different types of substances, in the community, at school, and sometimes at home. Commonly misused substances include alcohol, cannabis, and nicotine. Prescription drugs such as analgesics, sedatives, and stimulants can also be misused (Fig. 33.2). Children who have experienced or have been exposed to trauma are at higher risk of misusing substances. The substances will often become a means of "self-medicating" symptoms related to historical trauma, anxiety, psychosis, and emotional and functional problems. A history of colonization, isolation, and poverty has been found to increase the risk of children of northern and remote communities experiencing higher rates of substance use disorders (Canadian Centre on Substance Abuse, 2014).

There are a number of **street drugs** that are sold illegally for the purpose of producing an altered state of consciousness. Substances may be ingested, injected, or inhaled to produce the desired effect. Common street drugs are fentanyl, heroin, cocaine, and methamphetamine. A subgroup of street drugs is referred to as **club drugs**. These substances are commonly found at parties, bars, nightclubs, and concerts. Most forms of the drugs are illegal and can cause serious illness or injury. In some cases, club drug use can lead to death, which can occur from one use, repeated use, or use with other substances, such as alcohol. Examples of club drugs include GHB (liquid ecstasy), MDMA (ecstasy), flunitrazepam (roofies), mephedrone (4-MMC, M-cat, meow-meow), ketamine (special K, K-hole, "date-rape" drug), and LSD (acid). New "legal" psychoactive substances are emerging regularly and are made to mimic the effects of established illegal drugs. Children and

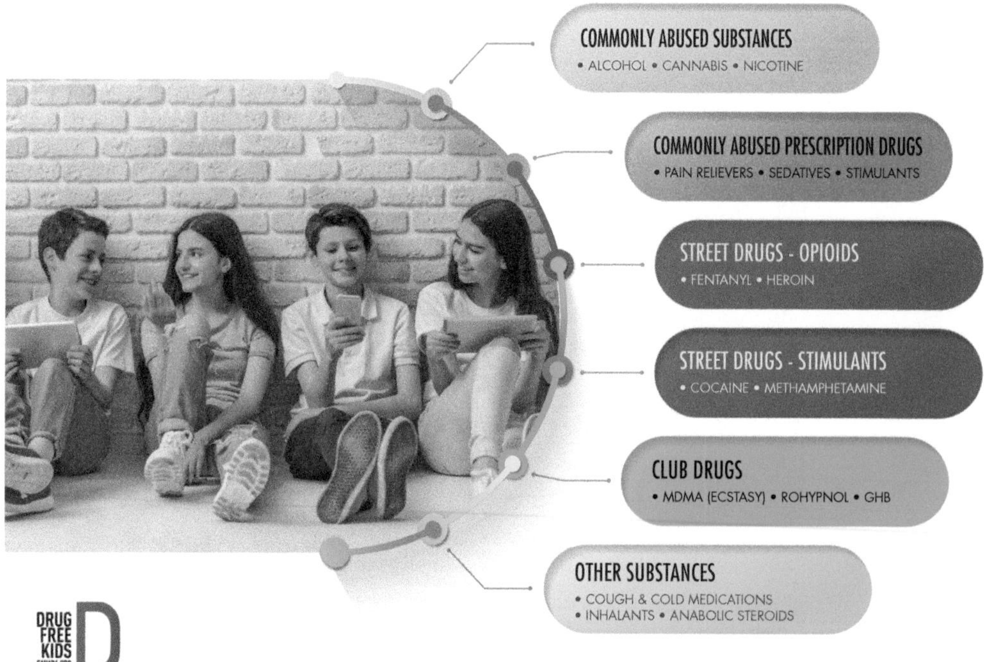
COMMONLY ABUSED SUBSTANCES
• ALCOHOL • CANNABIS • NICOTINE
COMMONLY ABUSED PRESCRIPTION DRUGS
• PAIN RELIEVERS • SEDATIVES • STIMULANTS
STREET DRUGS - OPIOIDS
• FENTANYL • HEROIN
STREET DRUGS - STIMULANTS
• COCAINE • METHAMPHETAMINE
CLUB DRUGS
• MDMA (ECSTASY) • ROHYPNOL • GHB
OTHER SUBSTANCES
• COUGH & COLD MEDICATIONS
• INHALANTS • ANABOLIC STEROIDS
DRUG FREE KIDS CANADA.ORG

Fig. 33.2 Examples of substances that can be misused by children. (From: Drug Free Kids Canada, 2018. *Drug guide for parents: Learn the facts to keep your kids safe*; © CanStock Photo Inc. /GeorgeRudy.)

adolescents may also misuse other substances such as cough and cold medications, inhalants (glue, gas), and anabolic steroids. More information on these types of drugs can be obtained from Drug Free Kids Canada (see Additional Learning Resources at the end of this chapter) (Fig. 33.3).

Substance use disorders are characterized by use, abuse, and physical and psychological dependence as well as by certain patterns of behaviour: (1) loss of control of substance consumption, (2) continued substance use despite associated problems, and (3) cravings and a tendency to relapse after efforts to change behaviour. The main systems that seem to be involved in substance misuse are the endorphin, catecholamine (especially dopamine), serotonin, endocannabinoid, and GABA systems. Substance use disorders develop much more quickly in children and adolescents than in adults (Castellanos-Ryan, O'Leary Barret, & Conrod, 2013). The process of addiction can be experienced by both children and adults. Those who acquire an addiction progress through a process from no contact with the substance; to experimentation; to integrated use, then excessive use, and then addiction. When individuals move from integrated substance use where the use is generally socially and culturally accepted and has few negative consequences to excessive substance use or misuse, they can experience negative social and physical issues because of the effects of the substance. Their relationships may deteriorate and school or vocational performance decrease, and they may start to engage in acts that they would not consider if not under the influence of the substance.

Dependence can be experienced psychologically, physically, or both. **Psychological dependence** includes a mild wish to a craving for a substance or a compulsive emotional need to use it. Dependence occurs when the substance becomes so important to the individual that they believe they cannot manage life without it. In **physical dependence** physiological cellular adaptation occurs and the central nervous system and peripheral nervous system become habituated to the substance such that the person physically needs the drug in order to function or to avoid the physical pain of withdrawal. **Tolerance** develops when a user's body becomes accustomed to certain drugs. The person must then increase the dose each time to maintain its effect.

Health Promotion

It is important to understand why a child or adolescent might turn to substance use. It may be to escape boredom, fit in better with their friends, escape perceived problems, or ease anxiety. Have a conversation with the child or adolescent about what they see as the benefits of using alcohol, cannabis, or other drugs.

From Alcohol to Adderall – The drugs that your child are most likely to come across.

90% of all addictions begin in adolescence. These are common substances that most kids find out about and have relatively easy access to. They are often the drugs that kids will experiment with first. Many kids think that taking someone else's prescription from a doctor is a safe alternative to trying illegal drugs.

CATEGORY		NAME	COMMON NAMES // STREET NAMES	LOOKS LIKE	USE/ABUSE	WHAT TEENS MAY HAVE HEARD	HEALTH RISKS // DANGEROUS BECAUSE	SIGNS OF ABUSE	IMPORTANT TO KNOW
COMMONLY ABUSED SUBSTANCES		ALCOHOL	Liquor, spirits, beer, wine // booze	Liquid	Swallowed	Makes a boring night fun // Everyone is drinking	Increased risk of injuries, violence, fetal damage (in pregnant women); depression; neurologic deficits; hypertension; liver and heart disease; addiction; fatal overdose	Slurred speech, lack of coordination, nausea, vomiting, hangovers	Alcohol is often mixed with other substances such as caffeinated energy drinks increasing the potential health risks // Youth are the biggest consumers of caffeinated alcoholic beverages, drinking at levels up to four times higher than the general public
		CANNABIS	Marijuana // Blunt, dope, ganja, grass, herb, joint, bud, Mary Jane, pot, reefer, green, trees, smoke, sinsemilla, skunk, weed	A green or brown mixture of dried flowers, fruiting tops and leaves of the marijuana plant	Smoked, brewed into tea or mixed into foods	Relaxing, natural, not dangerous and often easier to get than alcohol	Euphoria; relaxation; slowed reaction time; distorted sensory perception; impaired balance and coordination; anxiety; panic attacks; psychosis; frequent respiratory infections; impaired learning memory; possible mental health decline; addiction	Slowed thinking and reaction time, impaired coordination, paranoia	Canadian youth are the top users of cannabis in the developed world // Cannabis is the most commonly used illegal drug among Canadian youth, 15 to 24 years of age.
		NICOTINE	Cigarettes, Electronic Cigarettes // Cancer Sticks, Chew, Snuff, Dip, Fags, Smokes, E-cigs, E-hookahs, vapes, mods	Brown, cut up leaves // A propylene glycol based internal fluid that is combined with other ingredients and flavours and vapourized by battery-operated devices	Smoked, snorted, chewed // Vaped	An oral fixation and appetite suppressant // E-cigarettes are cool and a safer alternative to tobacco because less nicotine	An addictive substance // Smoking harms every organ in the body and causes coronary heart disease, and stroke, as well as many forms of cancer, nonsmoking teens who use E-cigarettes are more likely to start smoking conventional cigarettes	Addictive behaviours, smell on clothes and hair, yellowing of teeth and fingers that hold cigarettes, throat irritation, cough	Smoking tobacco is the leading cause of premature death in Canada // Electronic nicotine delivery systems are growing in popularity.
COMMONLY ABUSED PRESCRIPTION DRUGS		PAIN RELIEVERS	Codeine, Oxycodone, OxyContin, OxyNeo Percocet // Oxy, OC, Percs	Pills, tablets and capsules	Swallowed, injected	A free high from the home medicine cabinet. If it's a prescribed medication, It must be safe	Euphoria, drowsiness //respiratory depression and arrest, nausea, confusion, sedation, unconsciousness, coma, tolerance, addiction	Medicine bottles present without illness, Rx bottles missing, medications missing, disrupted eating and sleeping patterns, addictive behaviours	Problematic use of prescription opioid painkillers can be just as dangerous, addictive and deadly as using illicit heroin
		SEDATIVES	Barbiturates, benzodiazepines Xanax, Valium, Ativan // Benzos, xanies, xani-bars, xani-bombs, and roofies	Multi-colored tablets and capsules; some can be in liquid form	Swallowed, injected	A great release of tension	Sedation, slowed pulse and breathing; lowered blood pressure; poor concentration //confusion, fatigue; impaired coordination, memory, judgment; respiratory depression and arrest, addiction	Slurred speech, shallow breathing, sluggishness, disorientation, lack of coordination	Combining prescription sedatives and/or tranquilizers with alcohol can slow both the heart and respiration and possibly lead to death
		STIMULANTS	Methylphenidate, Amphetamine and Detroamphetamine, Adderall, Dexedrine, Ritalin // Ritz, rippers, dexies, and bennies, smart drug, study drug	Tablets, capsules	Swallowed, injected, snorted	Keeps you attentive and focused	Increased heart rate, blood pressure, metabolism; feelings of exhilaration, energy, increased mental alertness /rapid or irregular heart beat; reduced appetite, weight loss, heart failure	Taking high doses may result in dangerously high body temperatures and an irregular heartbeat. Potential for heart attacks or lethal seizures	Many teens misuse this prescribed medication to help them cram for exams or suppress their appetite.

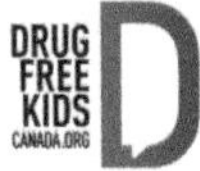

Illegal Street Drugs – Inherently dangerous and potentially fatal.

Highly addictive, these drugs are particularly dangerous for the young because they damage the developing body and the brain. Often laced with toxins like illicit fentanyl analogues and with a high probability of accidental overdose, these drugs can be fatal, even after first time trial.

CATIGORIE		NAME	COMMON NAMES // STREET NAMES	LOOKS LIKE	USE/ABUSE	WHAT TEENS MAY HAVE HEARD	HEALTH RISKS // DANGEROUS BECAUSE	SIGNS OF ABUSE	IMPORTANT TO KNOW
STREET DRUGS - OPIOIDS	Fentanyl $C_{22}H_{28}N_2O$	FENTANYL	Actiq, Duragesic, Sublimaze // Beans, Green Beans, Shady 80s, Apache, China girl, China white, dance fever, friend, goodfella, jackpot, murder 8, TNT, Tango and Cash	White powder, patch, green, pink or white pill, illicit fentanyl is made to look like other medication	Mixed with other drugs, swallowed, snorted, injected	Alternative to opioid // The stronger painkiller // A cheaper high than heroin	Euphoria, drowsiness, respiratory depression and arrest, nausea, confusion, constipation, sedation, tolerance, addiction, unconsciousness, coma, overdose, death	Small pupils; dizziness; suppression of breathing; itching or hives; nausea and vomiting; weight loss; depression; hallucinations; difficulty seeing; sleep problems; sweating; shaking; swollen extremities; addictive behaviours	50 to 100 times more potent than morphine// Overdose is a risk with illicit fentanyl // Can be used to cut other drugs such as cocaine, counterfeit oxycodone or heroin// Dangerous for those with substance use disorders and recreational users
		HEROIN	Diacetylmorphine // Smack, horse, brown sugar, dope, H, junk, skag, skunk, horse, China white	White to dark brown powder or tar-like substance	Injected, smoked, freebased or snorted	Full-on euphoria, but super risky	Euphoria, drowsiness, respiratory depression and arrest, nausea, confusion, constipation, sedation, tolerance,addiction, unconsciousness, coma, overdose, death	Track marks on arms, slowed and slurred speech, vomiting, addictive behaviours	Heroin overdose is a risk on the street, where the purity of the drug cannot be accurately determined
STREET DRUGS - STIMULANTS		COCAINE	Cocaine hydrochloride // Blow, bump, C, candy, Charlie, coke, crack, flake, rock, snow, toot	White crystalline powder, chips, chunks or white rocks	Snorted, smoked, injected	Keeps you amped up // you'll be the life of the party	Weight loss, insomnia; cardiac or cardiovascular complications; stroke; seizures; addiction; nasal damage from snorting	Nervous behavior, restlessness, bloody noses, high energy, addictive behaviours	Cocaine is a highly addictive drug // Increased risk of overdose when injected or smoked (crack cocaine)
		METH-AMPHETAMINE	Desoxyn // Meth, ice, crank, chalk, crystal, fire, glass, go fast, speed	White or slightly yellow crystal-like powder, large rock-like chunks	Swallowed, injected, snorted or smoked	Can keep you going for days	Chronic long-term use, or high dosages, can cause psychotic behavior (including paranoia, delusions, hallucinations, violent behavior, insomnia and strokes) cardiac or cardiovascular complications; stroke; seizures; addiction	Nervous physical activity, scabs and open sores, decreased appetite, Inability to sleep, severe dental problems	Meth has a high potential for abuse and addiction, putting children at risk, increasing crime and causing environmental harm

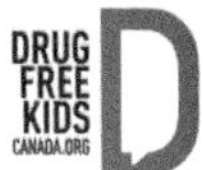

Fig. 33.3 Common street drugs used by children. (From: Drug Free Kids Canada, 2018. *Drug Guide for Parents: Learn the facts to keep your kids safe. Images A. iStock.com/monticelllo; B. iStock.com/digihelion; C. iStock.com/Ary6; D. iStock.com/VladimirSorokin; E. iStock.com/gcsherman1; F. iStock.com/catenarymedia; G. iStock.com/Zerbor; H. iStock.com/FotoMaximum; I. iStock.com/inkit; J. iStock.com/kaarsten)*

Club Drugs and other Substances – A new generation of highs.

Youth culture, performance pressure and getting a quick and cheap fix have given rise to a wide variety of ordinary substances that are used by youth in different ways. Ecstasy at a dance party, sniffing home cleaning products, over the counter medications mixed with grape juice and the date rape drug have all parents concerned about what their kids are doing. Get to know the substances your child is hearing about.

CATIGORIE		NAME	COMMON NAMES // STREET NAMES	LOOKS LIKE	USE/ABUSE	WHAT TEENS MAY HAVE HEARD	HEALTH RISKS // DANGEROUS BECAUSE	SIGNS OF ABUSE	IMPORTANT TO KNOW
CLUB DRUGS		MDMA (ECSTASY)	Methylenedioxy-methamphetamine // Molly, Ecstasy, Adam, clarity, Eve, lover's speed, peace, uppers	Branded tablets (Playboy bunnies, smiley face, stars, hearts, etc.)	Swallowed, snorted, injected	Enhances the senses and you'll love everyone	Can cause severe dehydration, liver and heart failure and even death	Sleep disturbances; depression; impaired memory; teeth clenching, muscle cramping, chills, sweating, dehydration, empathetic feelings; lowered inhibition, anxiety	Can be addictive. A popular club drug because of its stimulant properties, allowing users to dance for long periods of time
		ROHYPNOL	Flunitrazepam // Forget-me pill, R2, roach, Roche, roofies, roofinol, rope, rophies	Clear liquid, white powder, tablets and capsules	Swallowed, snorted	Associated with sexual assault. Known as a "date rape drug"	Sedation; muscle relaxation; confusion; memory loss; dizziness; impaired coordination, addiction	Relaxation, sedation incapacitation, addictive behaviours	Associated with sexual assaults // Rohypnol produces sedative-hypnotic effects including muscle relaxation and amnesia // Can be lethal
		GHB	Gamma-hydroxybutyrate // G, Georgia home boy, grievous bodily harm, liquid ecstasy, soap, scoop, goop, liquid X	Clear liquid, white powder, tablets and capsules	Swallowed	Associated with sexual assault. Known as a "date rape drug"	Sedation; muscle relaxation; confusion; memory loss; dizziness; impaired coordination, seizures, addiction, death	Relaxation, sedation, unconsciouness, seizures, coma, death	Associated with sexual assaults // GHB is odourless and tasteless, it can be slipped into someone's drink without detection
OTHER SUBSTANCES		COUGH & COLD MEDICATIONS	Dextromethorphan (DXM) // Robotripping, Robo, Dex, Red Devils, Triple C, Tussin, Skittles, Syrup, Sizzurp, Purple Drank (promethazine, codeine, sprite, jolly rancher and mountain dew)	Liquid, capsules, pills	Swallowed	Easy to get // Causes a trippy high with various plateaus	Can cause abdominal pain, nausea, seizures, liver damage, panic attacks, psychosis	Slurred speech, loss of coordination, disorientation, vomiting, loss of consciousness, numbness of fingers and toes, abdominal pain, irregular heartbeat, aches, seizures, cold flashes, dizziness, diarrhea	Over the counter medications are relatively easy for teens to purchase // Their use is made popular by several celebrities
		INHALANTS	Solvents (paint thinners, gasoline, glues); gases (butane, propane, aerosol propellants, nitrous oxide); nitrites (isoamyl, isobutyl, cyclohexyl) // Poppers, snappers, whippets, bagging, huffing, dusting	Paint thinners, glues, nail polish remover, whipped cream aerosol, nitrites, air conditioner fluid (Freon) and more	Inhaled through nose or mouth	Easy to get // A cheap, 20-minute high // Enhances sexual experience (Poppers)	These toxins have serious negative effects such as brain damage, respiratory failure and death. Poppers - shortness of breath, blue skin, loss of consciousness, respiratory arrest. Whippets - Euphoria, decreased level of consciousness. Chronic use can cause permanent spinal cord damage.	Missing household products, a drunk, dazed or dizzy appearance	More than 1000 common products are potential inhalants that can kill on the first use or any time thereafter
		ANABOLIC STEROIDS	Juice, Rhoids, Stackers, Pumpers, Gym Candy	Tablet, liquid or skin application	Swallowed, applied to skin or injected	Will guarantee a spot on the starting line-up	Hypertension, blood clotting, cholesterol changes, liver cysts, hostility and aggression, acne, premature stoppage of growth // Boys can develop breasts, girls can develop facial hair and a deepened voice. Can cause heart attacks and strokes	Rapid growth of muscles, opposite sex characteristics and extreme irritability	Teens who abuse steroids before the typical adolescent growth spurt risk staying short and never reaching their full adult height

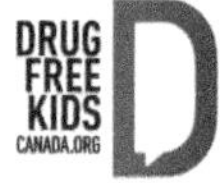

Fig. 33.3, cont'd *K. iStock.com/portokalis; L. iStock.com/Peopleimages; M. iStock.com/VictorZwiers; N. iStock.com/studiocasper; O. iStock.com/Antoine2K; P. iStock.com/Stockernumber2) (Source: Drug Free Kids Canada, 2018. Drug Guide for Parents: Learn the facts to keep your kids safe. Images K. iStock.com/portokalis; L. iStock.com/Peopleimages; M. iStock.com/VictorZwiers; N. iStock.com/studiocasper; O. iStock.com/Antoine2K; P. iStock.com/Stockernumber2)*

ALCOHOL

Alcohol is a central nervous system depressant and, as a result, increases the bioavailability of glutamate, norepinephrine, and dopamine (Csiernik, 2016). Increased levels of glutamate can interfere with memory and learning, whereas dopamine plays a key role in mood, motivation, desire, and pleasure. Likewise, norepinephrine plays a role in concentration, alertness, and how one responds to stressful situations. Alcohol, depending on the extent of use, can have either sedative or excitatory effects. Given the social and cultural acceptance of alcohol use, experimentation with alcohol has traditionally been accepted as a normal part of growing up. Most provinces have legal drinking-age laws that are well defined and enforced.

Nursing Care

Nurses have a significant role in educating the public about the effects of alcohol and addictions more broadly. Education should include discussion about the devastating physical consequences of alcohol misuse as well as the increased risk of accidents and injury. Because it is not uncommon for middle-school-age children to have experimented with beverages containing alcohol, it is appropriate to begin discussions about preventing addiction with children as young as elementary-school age. Public health nurses, parent–teacher associations, school counsellors, and pediatricians can work together to prevent alcohol misuse.

Early identification of behaviours linked with substance use and appropriate referrals for treatment and follow-up care are essential. A common treatment approach is the use of a 12-step program. Groups such as Al-Anon, Alateen, and Alcoholics Anonymous (AA) are 12-step programs that welcome the young adolescent seeking help with an alcohol or substance misuse problem (see Additional Learning Resources).

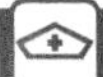 Nursing Tip

Alcoholism is often a family disease. Adults often serve alcohol freely at social events in the home and therefore offer mixed messages about alcohol use to their children.

CANNABIS

Until recently, cannabis sativa, also known as marijuana, was the most commonly used illegal drug used in Canada. Despite the illegality of cannabis, approximately 45% of people between the ages of 15 and 24 have used cannabis (Statistics Canada, 2019b). The Canadian cannabis prohibition began in 1923; however, in 2001, medical cannabis was legalized. Then, in 2018, the *Cannabis Act*, Bill-45, was passed, which legalized the use of cannabis nationwide (Government of Canada, 2018). As with alcohol, provinces have the responsibility to determine the method of sale and distributions, as well as establishing the legal age for cannabis use.

 Health Promotion

The purpose of decriminalizing the possession of cannabis for adults was to protect the health and safety of Canadians, by displacing the illegal market that profits criminals and organized crime. To prevent youth from being persuaded to use cannabis products, advertising restrictions, like those for tobacco products, have been established.

Cannabis is usually smoked, but it can also be baked in foods and ingested orally. Cannabis products are made from the dried flowers and leaves of the cannabis plant. Various strains of cannabis plants give rise to the different varieties of cannabis. When the plants are compressed, a resinous secretion is gathered to create oil, wax, or shatter. Generally, there are higher concentrations of tetrahydrocannabinol (THC) in these products than in the unpressed flower and leaf products. Preliminary evidence suggests that greater health risks are associated with higher levels of THC (Canadian Centre on Substance Abuse, 2016). Cannabis strains with increased cannabidiol (CBD) levels are grown for medicinal consumers.

Cannabis acts on endocannabinoids (Csiernik, 2016). The endocannabinoid neurotransmitters have an effect on sleep, appetite, mood, motor control, pleasure, pain, and memory. Therefore, cannabis can produce relaxation and euphoria and alter the perception of pain. It also changes perception, distorts time, and decreases attention span, and it use can result in deficits in memory, in body tremors, and in impaired motor functioning. Other physical effects of recent cannabis use include increased heart rate and appetite, increased blood pressure, dilated pupils, red eyes, dry mouth and throat, and bronchodilation (Beirness, & Porath-Waller, 2015).

Long-term cannabis use is associated with deficits in memory, attention, psychomotor speed, and executive functioning, particularly among those who started using cannabis during early adolescence. Individuals with respiratory disease are particularly susceptible to symptom aggravation (e.g., asthma). Use of cannabis during pregnancy can affect children's cognitive functioning, behaviour, and future substance use behaviour and increases the risk of mental illness (Cook, Green, de la Ronde, et al., 2017).

 Nursing Tip

Cannabis is not a benign drug. There are risks and harms associated with its use.

OPIOIDS

Recently, there has been a significant rise in the number of deaths related to problematic opioid use. In April 2016, British Columbia declared it a public health crisis. The effects of problematic opioid use are being experienced in many communities across the country, affecting all socioeconomic, gender, and age groups. One factor that may have contributed to the increase in opioid misuse is increased prescription and dispensing rates for opioid medications. Second only to Americans, Canadians are one of the highest per-capita users of opioids in the world (Government of Canada, 2017).

One opioid being misused that is of particular concern is carfentanil, an opioid used by veterinarians. It is 10 000 times more potent than morphine. Veterinarians use this medication only on very large animals. When this substance is obtained illegally, it is used to make "look-alike" pills. There is no smell or taste to this drug, and there is no way to tell if this drug has been added to any illegally obtained drugs. Because of the potency of carfentanil, even a very small amount can result in overdose and death.

 Safety Alert!

Illegally obtained fentanyl, and fentanyl derivatives, are often mixed with other drugs such as heroin or cocaine and made to look like prescription opioids (oxycontin or Percocet pills). There is a high rate of accidental overdose with these "look-alike" pills, as the dosing in the pills is inconsistent and individuals may take these pills while consuming other substances, such as alcohol, benzodiazepines, or stimulants.

MANIFESTATIONS OF SUBSTANCE USE

Drug use rarely begins randomly; generally, there are precursors to individuals' use of substances. These might include increasing intensity or prolonged symptoms of depression or anxiety. General signs that a child or adolescent might be using substances include changes in mood, attitude, hobbies, sleeping habits, or interests or unusual temper outbursts. See Box 33.9 for a list of signs and symptoms that may signal problematic substance use.

Box 33.9 Signs and Symptoms of Potential Substance Use

- Changes in friends
- Negative changes in schoolwork, missing school, or declining grades
- Increased secrecy about possessions or activities
- Use of incense, room deodorant, or perfume to hide smoke or chemical odours
- Subtle changes in conversations with friends, for example, more secretive, using "coded" language
- Change in clothing choices: new fascination with clothes that highlight drug use
- Increase in borrowing money
- Evidence of drug paraphernalia such as pipes and rolling papers
- Evidence of use of inhalant products (such as hairspray, nail polish, correction fluid, common household products); rags and paper bags are sometimes used as accessories
- Bottles of eyedrops, which may be used to mask bloodshot eyes or dilated pupils
- New use of mouthwash or breath mints to cover up smell of alcohol
- Missing prescription medications—especially opioids and mood stabilizers

Source: Drug Free Kids Canada. (2018). *Signs & symptoms of youth drinking and drug use.* Retrieved from https://www.drugfreekidscanada.org/prevention/what-to-look-for-checklist/.

Management and Nursing Care

As with other disorders that have significant emotional and behavioural symptoms, the continuum of services related to youth substance use encompasses health promotion, prevention, and harm reduction. **Harm reduction** is a therapeutic approach used to attempt to reduce the negative consequences associated with substance use. Those who practice from a harm reduction perspective incorporate a number of practical strategies aimed at "meeting people where they are at"; facilitating safer use, managed use, and abstinence; and addressing other concerns related to a variety of determinants of health. The nurse has a significant role in promoting health through education, advocating for public policies that can improve health, and creating supportive environments for the delivery of harm reduction–orientated services as part of a comprehensive approach to protecting youth, particularly with regard to substance misuse and addiction.

The prevention of substance misuse begins by helping expectant parents to develop good parenting skills. It is imperative that children learn to feel good about themselves very early in life. They need a safe environment and adults whom they can trust and who serve as good role models. As development proceeds, the growing child learns to interact with others and develops a sense of identity. A positive self-image and feelings of self-worth help adolescents fine-tune their adaptive coping skills. In time, they learn to rely on their own problem-solving abilities and, ideally, do not need chemicals to manage the complexities of life. Nurses in their various settings can contribute to this process of positive development. They can also educate patients about the seriousness of substance misuse.

Adolescents who have a substance use disorder generally require specialized services. The treatment for this disorder is complicated by the general lack of insight into the social, vocational, and physical consequences of substance misuse. Most adolescents involved in substance misuse do not choose to enter treatment but are coerced by family members or the juvenile justice system. Although the issue is controversial, clinical experience in substance misuse treatment settings has shown that many adolescents become interested in treatment and make behavioural changes after they have been required to enter a treatment program.

Each province has services available for people coping with symptoms of a substance use disorder at the end of the chapter.

Get Ready for the Certification Examination!

Key Points

- Many children and adolescents experience significant impairments at home, in school, with peers, or in the community because of emotional or behavioural symptoms.
- Early childhood experiences are critical to personality formation.
- Treatment of illnesses with significant emotional and behavioural concerns often requires an interdisciplinary approach.
- A continuum of services is utilized to help support and treat children with significant emotional or behavioural concerns and their families.
- Education, prevention, identification, and referral are essential nursing functions in the care of the child with a behavioural disorder.
- The main goal of nursing care is to assist the family in promoting an optimal level of functioning.
- Nurses play an important role in assessing the growth and development, developmental needs, expectations, and abilities of children and their families.
- The child's environment must be safe, and the child must be able to trust caretakers.
- There are emotional and behavioural symptoms associated with childhood mental disorders.
- Depression is characterized by depressed or irritable mood or a noticeable decrease in interest or pleasure in usual activities, along with other signs, lasting at least 2 weeks.
- Talk of suicide must always be taken seriously.
- The risk of suicide increases when there is a definite plan of action, the means are available, and the person has few resources for help and support.
- Anxiety is characterized by worries and fears that interfere with daily activities.
- Attention-deficit/hyperactivity disorder is characterized by a developmentally inappropriate degree of gross motor activity, impulsivity, distractibility, and inattention in school or at home.
- Neurodevelopmental disorders are those primarily associated with the functioning of the neurological system and brain.
- Autism spectrum disorder is characterized by difficulties in social interaction and communication, repetitive behaviours, and stereotyped interests and activities.
- Emphasizing the strengths of the child rather than their weaknesses is essential when caring for a child with a behavioural disorder.
- Substance misuse disorder is a significant problem among Canadian youth.
- The neurotransmitters involved in substance misuse are the endorphins, catecholamines (especially dopamine), serotonin, endocannabinoid, and GABA.
- Substance use disorders involve both physical and psychological dependence.

Additional Learning Resources

evolve Go to your Evolve website (http://evolve.elsevier.com/Canada/Leifer) for the following learning resources:

- Answer Key for Critical Thinking Questions
- Answer Key for Textbook Review Questions
- Audio Glossary
- Fluids & Electrolytes tutorial
- Interactive Review Questions
- Skills Performance Checklists
- Video clips and more!

Online Resources

- Al-Anon Family Groups: https://al-anon.org/
- Anxiety Canada: http://www.anxietycanada.ca
- Autism Canada: https://autismcanada.org
- Canadian ADHD Resource Alliance: https://www.caddra.ca/
- Canadian Association for Suicide Prevention: https://suicideprevention.ca
- Canadian Paediatric Society, *Cannabis and Canada's Children and Youth:* https://www.cps.ca/en/documents/position/cannabis-children-and-youth
- Children's Depression Inventory 2: https://www.mhs.com/MHS-Assessment?prodname=cdi2
- Drug Free Kids Canada: https://www.drugfreekidscanada.org/
- Government of Canada, *Get Help With Problematic Substance Use:* https://www.canada.ca/en/health-canada/services/substance-abuse/get-help/get-help-with-drug-abuse.html
- Mental Health Commission of Canada: https://www.mentalhealthcommission.ca
- Mood Disorders Society of Canada: https://mdsc.ca/

Review Questions

1. What is the first step in addressing illnesses with significant emotional or behavioural symptoms?
   a. Health promotion
   b. Harm reduction
   c. Establishing the treatment team
   d. Ensuring family engagement
2. When will the nurse initiate a discussion about available treatment with a child and family who are displaying emotional or behavioural symptoms of a mental disorder?
   a. At the parents' request
   b. When a referral is made by the teacher
   c. At the next scheduled appointment
   d. When there is impairment in daily functioning

3. Which individual has the highest risk factors for dying by suicide?
   a. A 13-year-old male who plays video war games.
   b. An 8-year-old girl who reports thinking about death.
   c. A 16-year-old girl who recently broke up with her significant other.
   d. A 9-year-old boy who has previously tried to hang himself.
4. When assessing an 8-year-old child who is suspected of misusing substances, what behavioural changes would the nurse expect to find? *(Select all that apply.)*
   a. Depressed mood
   b. Generalized worry
   c. Changes in friends
   d. Secrecy about activities
5. The priorities of nursing care for a child with autism spectrum disorder are which of the following? *(Select all that apply.)*
   a. Safety
   b. Engage in meaningful relationships
   c. Parental support
   d. Strict discipline measures for behaviour problems
6. What disorder is characterized by a loss of pleasure in most activities and feelings of worthlessness?
   a. Autism spectrum disorder
   b. Depression
   c. Conduct disorder
   d. Anxiety

REFERENCES

Akresh, R., Carusp, G. D., & Thirumurthy, H. (2016). *Detailed geographic information, conflict exposure, and health impacts: Discussion paper*. Institute for the Study of Labor (IZA), 1–45. Retrieved from http://ftp.iza.org/dp10330.pdf.

American Psychiatric Association. (2013). In *Diagnostic and statistical manual of mental disorders* (5th ed.). (DSM-5). Washington, DC: Author.

Beirness, D. J., & Porath-Waller, A. J. (2015). *Clearing the smoke on cannabis: Cannabis use and driving—An update*. Ottawa, ON: Canadian Centre on Substance Abuse.

Bennett, K., Duda, S., Brouwers, M., et al. (2018). Towards high-quality, useful practice guidelines for child and youth mental health disorders: Protocol for a systematic review and consensus exercise. *BMJ Open, 8*. https://doi.org/10.1136/ bmjopen-2017-018053.

Canadian Centre on Substance Abuse. (2014). *Competencies for Canada's substance abuse workforce*. Ottawa, ON: Author.

Canadian Centre on Substance Abuse. (2016). *Clearing the smoke on cannabis: Highlights—An update*. Ottawa, ON: Author.

Castellanos-Ryan, N., O'Leary-Barret, M., & Conrod, P. (2013). Substance-use in childhood and adolescence: A brief overview of developmental processes and their clinical implications. *Journal of the Canadian Academy of Child and Adolescent Psychiatry*, 22(1), 41–46.

Cook, J., Green, C., de la Ronde, D., et al. (2017). Epidemiology and effects on substance use in pregnancy. *Journal of Obstetrics and Gynaecology Canada*, 39(10), 906–915. https://doi.org/10.1016/j.jogc.2017.07.005.

Csiernik, R. (2016). *Substance use and abuse: Everything matters* (2nd ed.). Toronto: Canadian Scholars Press.

Farone, S., & Antshel, K. (2014). Toward an evidence based taxonomy of non-pharmacological treatment for ADHD. *Child and Adolescent Psychiatric Clinic of North America*, 23, 965–972.

Findling, R., & Dinh, S. (2014). Transdermal therapy for ADHD with the methylphenidate patch (MTS). *CNS Drugs, 28*, 217–228.

Gleason, M. (2016). Addressing early childhood emotional and behavioral problems. *Pediatrics, 138*(6), e20163025. https://doi.org/10.1542/peds.2016-3025.

Government of Canada. (2017). *Government of Canada actions on opioids: 2016 and 2017*. Ottawa, ON: Author.

Government of Canada. (2018). *Legalization and regulation of cannabis*. Ottawa, ON: Author.

Ip, A., Zwaigenbaum, L., Nicholas, D., et al. (2015). Factors influencing autism spectrum disorder screening by community paediatricians. *Paediatrics & Child Health, 20*(5), e20–e24. https://doi.org/10.1093/pch/20.5.e20.

Kaushik, A., Kostaki, E., & Kyriakopoulos, M. (2016). The stigma of mental illness in children and adolescents: A systematic review. *Psychiatry Research, 243*, 469–494. https://doi.org/10.1016/j.psychres.2016.04.042.

Keeton, C., Kolos, A., & Walkup, J. (2009). Pediatric generalized anxiety disorder. *Pediatric Drugs, 11*(3), 171–183. https://doi.org/10.2165/00148581-200911030-00003.

McLoughlin, A. B., Gould, M. S., & Malone, A. K. (2015). Global trends in teenage suicide: 2003–2014. *QJM: An International Journal of Medicine, 108*(10), 765–780. https://doi.org/10.1093/qjmed/hcv026.

Mental Health Commission of Canada. (2015). *Taking the next step forward: Building a responsive mental health and addictions system for emerging adults*. Ottawa, ON: Mental Health Commission of Canada.

Murcia, C. (2017). Unhealthy prenatal diet linked to ADHD. *Contemporary Pediatrics, 34*(1), 27–30.

National Institute for Health and Care Excellence. (2017). *Depression in children and young people: Identification and management [CG28]*. London, UK: Author.

Raviola, G., Trieu, M., Demaso, D., et al. (2016). Autism spectrum disorders. In R. M. Kliegman, B. F. Stanton, J. W. St. Geme, et al. (Eds.), *Nelson textbook of pediatrics* (20th ed.). Philadelphia: Saunders.

Rosenberg, D., & Chiriboga, J. (2016). Anxiety disorders. In R. M. Kliegman, B. F. Stanton, J. W. St. Geme, et al. (Eds.), *Nelson textbook of pediatrics* (20th ed.). Philadelphia: Saunders.

Statistics Canada. (2019a). *Leading causes of death, total population, by age group*. Table 13-10-0394-01. Retrieved from https://www150.statcan.gc.ca/t1/tbl1/en/tv.action?pid=1310039401#F6.

Statistics Canada. (2019b). *Mental health indicators. Table 13-10-0465-01*. Retrieved from https://www150.statcan.gc.ca/t1/tbl1/en/tv.action?pid=1310046501.

Urion, D. (2016). Attention deficit hyperactivity disorders. In R. M. Kliegman, B. F. Stanton, J. W. St. Geme, et al. (Eds.), *Nelson textbook of pediatrics* (20th ed.). Philadelphia: Saunders.

Normal Vital Signs and Temperature Equivalents of Infants and Children

http://evolve.elsevier.com/Canada/Leifer

Normal Pediatric Vital Signs

AGE	HEART RATE (BEATS/MIN)	RESPIRATORY RATE (BREATHS/MIN)	BLOOD PRESSURE (MM HG)†
Preterm	120–170	40–70‡	55–75/35–45
Newborn	110–160*	30–60	65–85/45–55
1–3 months	100–150	30–55	65–85/45–55
3–6 months	90–120	30–45	70–90/50–65
6–12 months	80–120	25–40	80–100/55–65
1–3 years	70–110	20–30	90–105/55–70
3–6 years	65–110	20–25	95–110/60–75
6–12 years	60–95	14–22	100–120/60–75
>12 years	55–85	12–20	110–135/65–85

*In sleep, infant heart rates may drop significantly lower, but if perfusion is maintained, no intervention is required.
†A blood pressure cuff should cover approximately two thirds of the arm; too small a cuff yields spuriously high pressure readings, and too large a cuff yields spuriously low pressure readings.
‡Many premature infants require mechanical ventilatory support, making their spontaneous respiratory rate less relevant.
Adapted from Kliegman, R. M., Stanton, B., Geme, J., & Schor, N. (2016). *Nelson textbook of pediatrics* (20th ed.). St. Louis: Elsevier.

Normal Temperature Ranges

MEASUREMENT METHOD	NORMAL TEMPERATURE RANGE
Rectal	36.6° to 38°C (97.9° to 100.4°F)
Ear	35.8° to 38°C (96.4° to 100.4°F)
Oral	35.5° to 37.5°C (95.9° to 99.5°F)
Axillary	36.5° to 37.5°C (97.8° to 99.5°F)

Data from Leduc, D., Woods, S., & Canadian Paediatric Society, Community Paediatrics Committee. (2000/2015). *Temperature measurement in paediatrics*. Retrieved from http://www.cps.ca/documents/position/temperature-measurement#ref38.

Centigrade to Fahrenheit Temperature Conversions

°C	°F	°C	°F	°C	°F
35.0	95.0	37.0	98.6	39.0	102.2
35.2	95.4	37.2	99.0	39.2	102.6
35.4	95.7	37.4	99.3	39.4	102.9
35.6	96.1	37.6	99.7	39.6	103.3
35.8	96.4	37.8	100.0	39.8	103.6
36.0	96.8	38.0	100.4	40.0	104.0
36.2	97.2	38.2	100.8	40.2	104.4
36.4	97.5	38.4	101.1	40.4	104.7
36.6	97.9	38.6	101.5	40.6	105.1
36.8	98.2	38.8	101.8	40.8	105.4
				41.0	105.8

Conversion Formulas

°F = (°C × 9/5) + 32 or (°C × 1.8) + 32

°C = (°F − 32) ÷ 5/9 or (°F − 32) ÷ 0.55

Updated Definitions of Blood Pressure (BP) Categories and Stages

FOR CHILDREN AGED 1–13 YEARS	FOR CHILDREN AGED ≥13 YEARS
Normal BP: <90th percentile	Normal BP: <120/<80 mm Hg
Elevated BP: ≥90th percentile to <95th percentile or 120/80 mm Hg to <95th percentile (whichever is lower)	Elevated BP: 120/<80 to 129/<80 mm Hg
Stage 1 hypertension (HTN): ≥95th percentile to <95th percentile + 12 mmHg, or 130/80 to 139/89 mm Hg (whichever is lower)	Stage 1 HTN: 130/80 to 139/89 mm Hg
Stage 2 HTN: ≥95th percentile + 12 mm Hg, or ≥140/90 mm Hg (whichever is lower)	Stage 2 HTN: ≥140/90 mm Hg

Source: Flynn, J. T., Kaelber, D. C., Baker-Smith, C. M., Blowey, D., Carroll, A. E., Daniels, S. R., de Ferranti, S. D., Dionne, J. M., et al. (2017). Clinical practice guideline for screening and management of high blood pressure in children and adolescents. *Pediatrics, 140*(3). Retrieved from http://pediatrics.aappublications.org/content/140/3/e20171904.

Screening Blood Pressure (BP) Values Requiring Further Evaluation, According to Age and Gender

	BP (MM HG)			
	BOYS		GIRLS	
AGE (YEARS)	SYSTOLIC	DIASTOLIC	SYSTOLIC	DIASTOLIC
1	98	52	98	54
2	100	55	101	58
3	101	58	102	60
4	102	60	103	62
5	103	63	104	64
6	105	66	105	67
7	106	68	106	68
8	107	69	107	69
9	107	70	108	71
10	108	72	109	72
11	110	74	111	74
12	113	75	114	75
≥13	120	80	120	80

This simplified table is designed as a screening tool only for the identification of children and adolescents who need further evaluation of their BP starting with repeat BP measurements. It should not be used to diagnose elevated BP or hypertension by itself.
Source: Flynn, J. T., Kaelber, D. C., Baker-Smith, C. M., Blowey, D., Carroll, A. E., Daniels, S. R., de Ferranti, S. D., Dionne, J. M., et al. (2017). Clinical practice guideline for screening and management of high blood pressure in children and adolescents. *Pediatrics, 140*(3). Retrieved from http://pediatrics.aappublications.org/content/140/3/e20171904.

Pediatric Laboratory Values Reference

http://evolve.elsevier.com/Canada/Leifer

Normal Results

TEST	AGES	INTERNATIONAL UNITS (SI)	CONVENTIONAL UNITS
Leukocyte (WBC) count			
	Newborn (0–6 weeks)	9.0–30.0 × 10^9/L	9 000–30 000 cells/mm^3
	Child (<2 years)	6.2–17.0 × 10^9/L	6 200–17 000 cells/mm^3
	Adult/child >2 years)	5.0–10.0 × 10^9/L	5 000–10 000 cells/mm^3
Erythrocyte (RBC) count			
	Newborn	4.8–7.1 × 10^{12}/L	4.8–7.1 × 10^6 mcg/L
	2–6 months	3.5–5.5 × 10^{12}/L	3.5–5.5 × 10^6 mcg/L
	6 months–1 year	3.5–5.2 × 10^{12}/L	3.5–5.2 × 10^6 mcg/L
	1–18 years	4.0–5.5 × 10^{12}/L	4.0–5.5 × 10^6 mcg/L
Hemoglobin (Hgb)	Newborn (0–28 days)	140–240 g/L	14.0–24.0 g/dL
	1–2 months	120–200 g/L	12.0–20.0 g/dL
	2–6 months	100–170 g/L	10.0–17.0 g/dL
	6 months–1 year	95–140 g/L	9.5–14.0 g/dL
	1–6 years	95–140 g/L	9.5–14.0 g/dL
	6–18 years	100–150 g/L	10.0–15.0 g/dL
Hematocrit (Hct)		Volume fraction	
	Newborn	0.37–0.48	37–48%
	2–6 months	0.31–0.39	31–39%
	6 months–18 years	0.31–0.39	31–39%
Mean corpuscular volume (MCV)	Newborn	96–108 fL	96–108 mm^3
	Adult/child	80–95 fL	80–95 mm^3
Mean corpuscular hemoglobin concentration (MCHC)	Newborn	32–33 g/dL	32–33%
	Adult	32–36 g/dL	32–36%
Reticulocyte count		% of total number of RBCs	
	Newborn	2.5–6.5%	
	Infant	0.5–3.1%	
	Adult/child	0.5–2%	
Platelet count	Newborn	150–300 × 10^9/L	150 000–300 000/mm^3
	Infant	200–475 × 10^9/L	200 000–475 000/mm^3
	Adult/child	150–400 × 10^9/L	150 000–400 000/mm^3
Leukocyte differential count	Percentage (%)		Absolute
Myelocytes	0	0	0
Neutrophils	55–70	2.5–8.0 × 10^9/L	2 500–8 000 per mm^3
Lymphocytes	20–40	1.0–4.0 × 10^9/L	1 000–4 000 per mm^3
Monocytes	2–8	0.1–0.7 × 10^9/L	100–700 per mm^3
Eosinophils	1–4	0.0–0.5 × 10^9/L	50–500 per mm^3
Basophils	0.5–1.0	0.02–0.05 × 10^9/L	15–50 per mm^3
Glucose	Cord	2.5–5.3 mmol/L	45–96 mg/dL
	Newborn	1.7–3.3 mmol/L	30–60 mg/dL
	Infant	2.2–5.0 mmol/L	40–90 mg/dL
	Child (<2 years)	3.3–5.5 mmol/L	60–100 mg/dL
	>2 years to adult	<6.1 mmol/L	<110 mg/dL
$HgbA_{1c}$	Nondiabetic adult/child	4.0–5.9% of total Hgb	
	Good diabetic control	<7% of total Hgb	

Normal Results—cont'd

TEST	AGES	INTERNATIONAL UNITS (SI)	CONVENTIONAL UNITS
Antistreptolysin O titre	Infant (0–6 months) 6 months–2 years 2–4 years 5–12 years	Similar to mother's value ≤50 Todd units/mL ≤160 Todd units/mL 170–330 Todd units/mL	
Ammonia nitrogen	Newborn Adult/child	52–88 mcmol/L 6–47 mcmol/L	90–150 mcg/dL 10–80 mcg/dL
Lactate dehydrogenase (LDH)	Newborn Infant Child	160–450 U/L 100–250 U/L 60–170 U/L	
Amylase	Newborn Child/adolescent Adult	<18 U/L <106 U/L 100–300 U/L	 60–120 Somogyi units/dL
Phosphorus	Newborn Child	1.4–3.0 mmol/L 1.45–2.10 mmol/L	4.3–9.3 mg/dL 4.5–6.5 mg/dL
Alkaline phosphatase	1–3 years 4–6 years 7–9 years 10–11 years 12–13 years 14–15 years 16–19 years	185–383 U/L 191–450 U/L 218–499 U/L Male: 174–624 U/L Female: 169–657 U/L Male: 245–584 U/L Female: 141–499 U/L Male: 169–618 U/L Female: 103–283 U/L Male: 98–317 U/L Female: 82–169 U/L	
Total bilirubin	Full term Cord 0–1 day 1–2 days 2–5 days >5 days	 <34 mcmol/L <103 mcmol/L <137 mcmol/L <205 mcmol/L <171 mcmol/L	 <2.0 mg/dL <6.0 mg/dL <8.0 mg/dL <12.0 mg/dL <10.0 mg/dL
Cholesterol	Newborn Infant (7–12 months) 10–11 years	Male: 0.98–4.50 mmol/L Female: 1.45–5.04 mmol/L Male: 2.15–5.30 mmol/L Female: 1.76–5.59 mmol/L Male: 3.10 mmol/L Female: 3.16–6.26 mmol/L	38–174 mg/dL 56–195 mg/dL 83–205 mg/dL 68–216 mg/dL 120–228 mg/dL 122–242 mg/dL
Uric acid	Newborn Child	120–370 mcmol/L 150–320 mcmol/L	2.0–6.2 mg/dL 2.5–5.5 mg/dL
Sodium	Newborn Infant Child Thereafter	134–144 mmol/L 134–150 mmol/L 136–145 mmol/L 136–145 mmol/L	134–144 mEq/L 134–150 mEq/L 136–145 mEq/L 136–145 mEq/L
Chloride	Cord Newborn Thereafter	96–104 mmol/L 96–106 mmol/L 90–110 mmol/L	96–104 mEq/L 96–106 mEq/L 90–110 mEq/L
Potassium	Newborn Infant Child Adult	3.9–5.9 mmol/L 4.1–5.3 mmol/L 3.4–4.7 mmol/L 3.5–5.0 mmol/L	3.9–5.9 mEq/L 4.1–5.3 mEq/L 3.4–4.7 mEq/L 3.5–5.0 mEq/L
Carbon dioxide content (CO_2)	Newborn Infant Child	13–22 mmol/L 20–28 mmol/L 20–28 mmol/L	13–22 mEq/L 20–28 mEq/L 20–28 mEq/L

Normal Results—cont'd

TEST	AGES	INTERNATIONAL UNITS (SI)	CONVENTIONAL UNITS
Calcium (Total)	Cord	1.25–1.50 mmol/L	9.0–11.5 mg/dL
	Newborn (3–24 hours)	2.3–2.65 mmol/L	9.0–10.6 mg/dL
	24–48 hours	1.75–3.0 mmol/L	7.0–12.0 mg/dL
	4–7 days	2.25–2.73 mmol/L	9.0–10.9 mg/dL
	Child	2.2–2.7 mmol/L	8.8–10.8 mg/dL
	Thereafter	2.1–2.55 mmol/L	8.4–10.2 mg/dL
International normalized ratio (INR)		0.8–1.2	
Prothrombin Time (PT)		11.0–12.5 seconds	
Partial thromboplastin time (PTT)		60–70 seconds	
Urea nitrogen (BUN)	Cord	7.5–14.3 mmol/L	21–40 mg/dL
	Newborn	0.7–4.6 mmol/L	2–13 mg/dL
	Infant	1.8–6.0 mmol/L	5–17 mg/dL
	Child	1.8–6.4 mmol/L	5–18 mg/dL
	Adult	3.6–7.1 mmol/L	10–20 mg/dL
Creatinine	Newborn	53–97 mcmol/L	0.6–1.1 mg/dL
	Infant	18–35 mcmol/L	0.2–0.4 mg/dL
	Child/adolescent	18–62 mcmol/L	0.2–0.7 mg/dL
Thyroxine-binding globulin (TBG)	1–5 days	22–42 mg/L	2.2–4.2 mg/dL
	1–11 months	Male: 16–36 mg/L	1.6–3.6 mg/dL
		Female: 17–37 mg/L	1.7–3.7 mg/dL
	1–9 years	Male: 12–28 mg/L	1.2–2.8 mg/dL
		Female: 15–27 mg/L	1.5–2.7 mg/dL
	10–19 years	Male: 14–26 mg/L	1.4–2.6 mg/dL
		Female: 14–30 mg/L	1.4–3.0 mg/dL
Fibrinogen	Newborn	3.68–8.82 mcmol/L	125–300 mg/dL
	Thereafter	5.8–11.8 mcmol/L	200–400 mg/dL
Erythrocyte sedimentation rate (ESR)	Newborn	0–2 mm/hr	
	Child	0–10 mm/hr	
Phenylalanine	Premature	120–450 mcmol/L	2.0–7.5 mg/dL
	Newborn	70–210 mcmol/L	1.2–3.4 mg/dL
	Thereafter	50–110 mcmol/L	0.8–1.8 mg/dL
Lead		<0.48 mcmol/L	<10 mcg/dL
Total protein	Newborn	46–74 g/L	4.6–7.4 g/dL
	Infant	60–67 g/L	6.0–6.7 g/dL
	Child	62–80 g/L	6.2–8.0 g/dL
	Adult	64–83 g/L	6.4–8.3 g/dL
Albumin	Newborn	35–54 g/L	3.5–5.4 g/dL
	Infant	44–54 g/L	4.4–5.4 g/dL
	Child	40–59 g/L	4.9–5.9 g/dL
Blood gas arterial			
pH	Newborn	7.32–7.49	
	2 months–2 years	7.34–7.46	
	Adult/child	7.35–7.45	
Partial pressure of oxygen (PO_2)	Newborn	60–70 mm/Hg	
	Adult/child	80–100 mm/Hg	
Partial pressure of carbon dioxide (PCO_2)	<2 years	26–41 mm/Hg	
	Adult/child	35–45 mm/Hg	
Bicarbonate (HCO_3)	Newborn/Infant	16–24 mmol/L	16–24 mEq/L
	>2 years	21–28 mmol/L	21–28 mEq/L

Note: Results of laboratory tests are method dependent or instrument dependent. Measurements are approximate.

Modified from Kliegman, R. M., et al. (Eds.). (2016). *Nelson textbook of pediatrics* (20th ed.). Philadelphia: Saunders; Lippincott Williams & Wilkins; Pagana, K. D., Pagana, T. J., & Pike-MacDonald, S. A. (2013). *Mosby's Canadian manual of diagnostic and laboratory tests* (1st Canadian ed.). Toronto, ON: Elsevier.)

Appendix

C Canada's Food Guide–2019

http://evolve.elsevier.com/Canada/Leifer

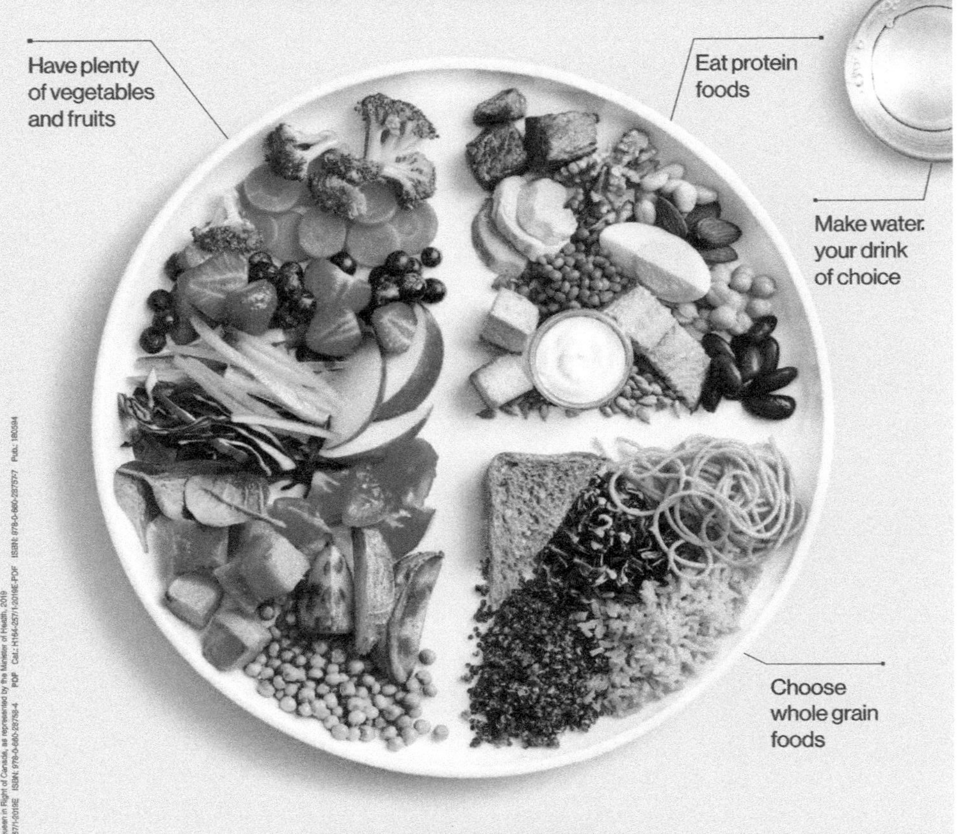
Canada's food guide
Eat well. Live well.
Eat a variety of healthy foods each day
Have plenty of vegetables and fruits
Eat protein foods
Make water your drink of choice
Choose whole grain foods
Discover your food guide at
Canada.ca/FoodGuide
Health Canada Santé Canada
Canada

Canada's food guide

Healthy eating recommendations

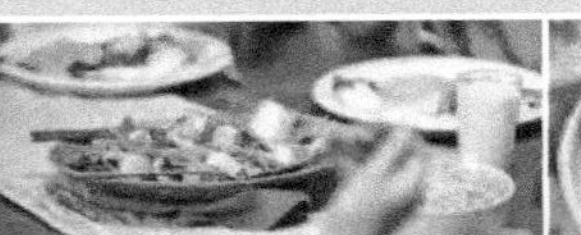
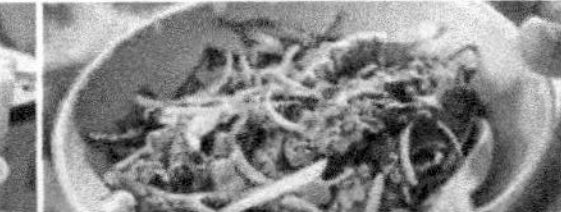
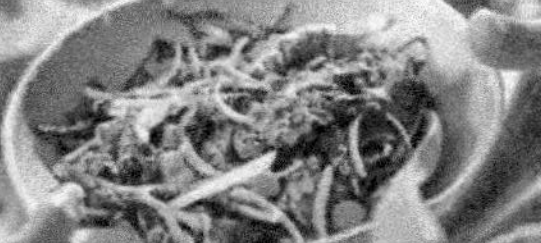
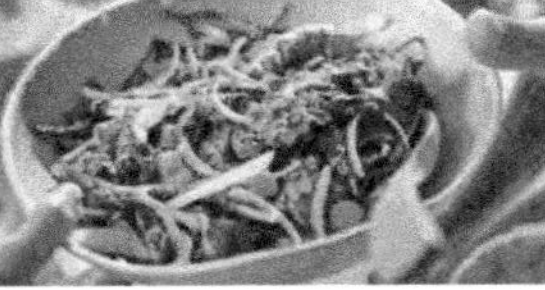
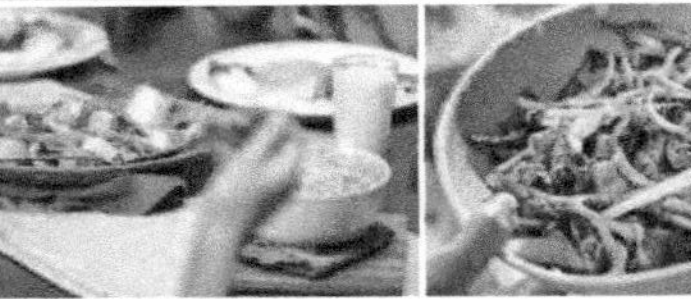
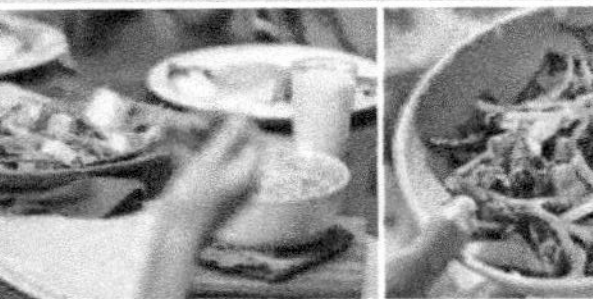
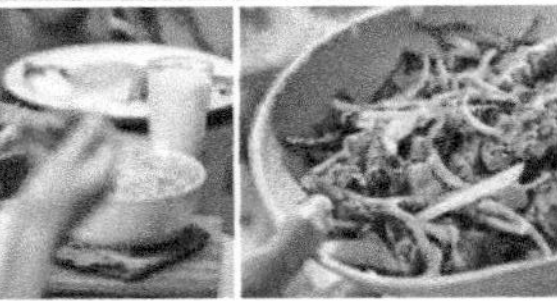
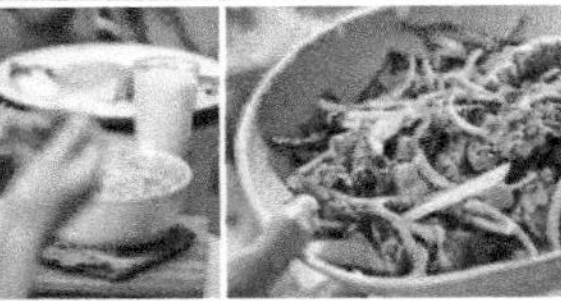
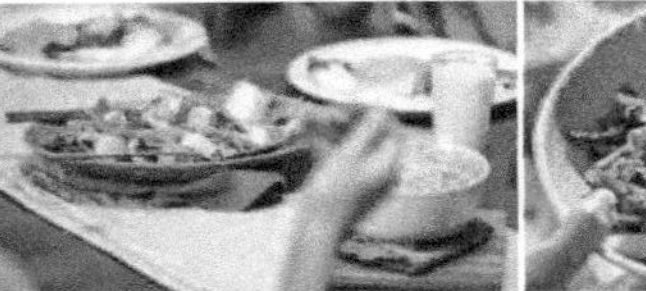
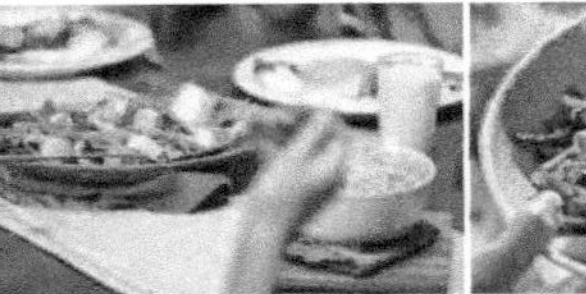
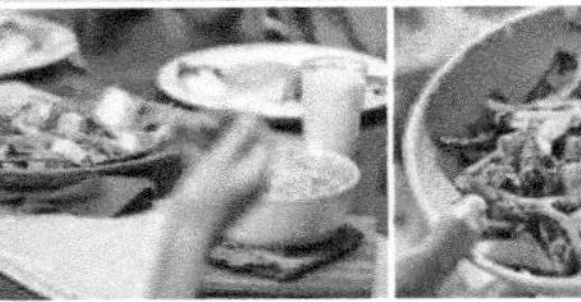
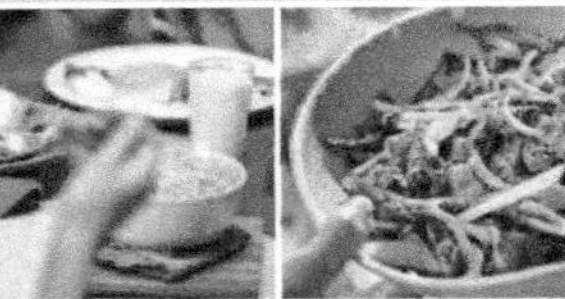
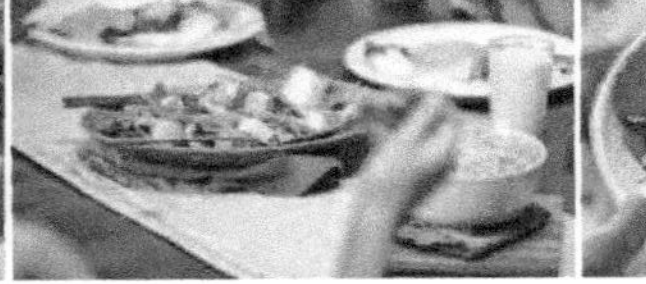
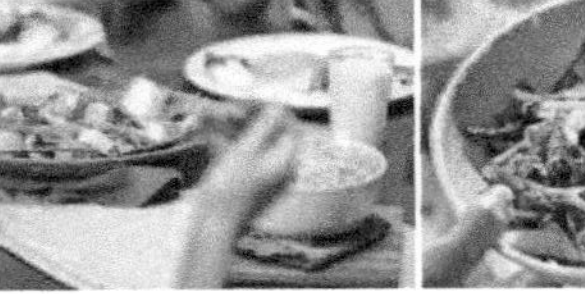
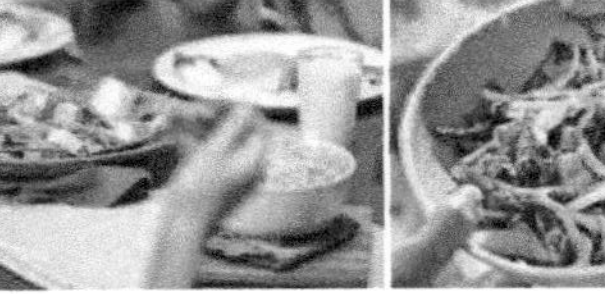
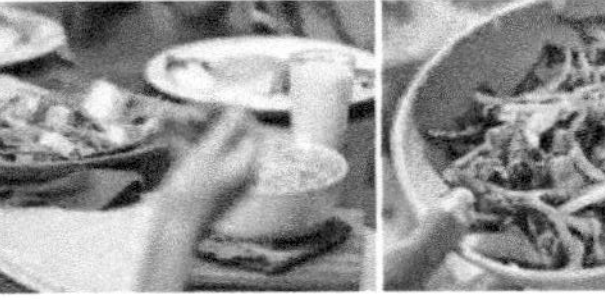
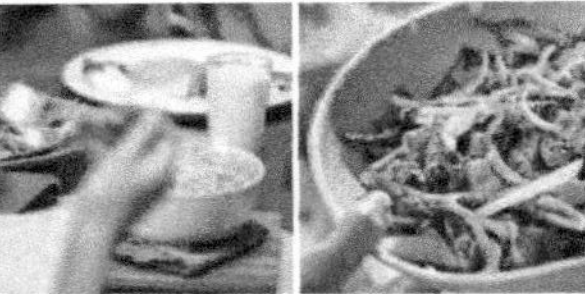
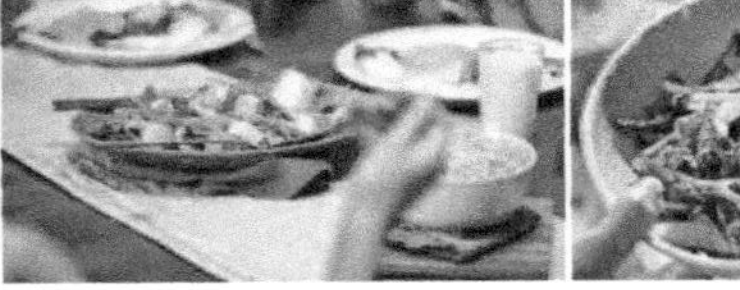
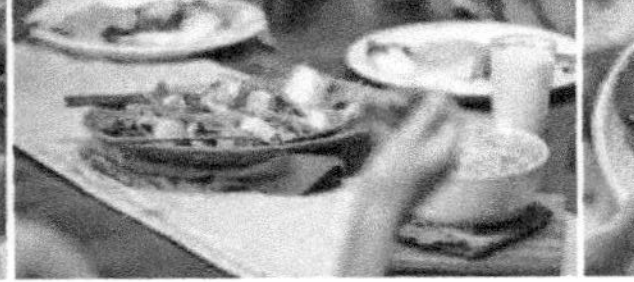
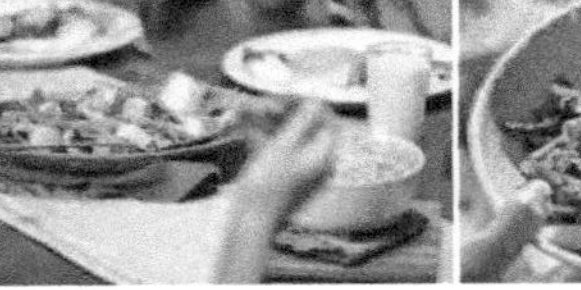
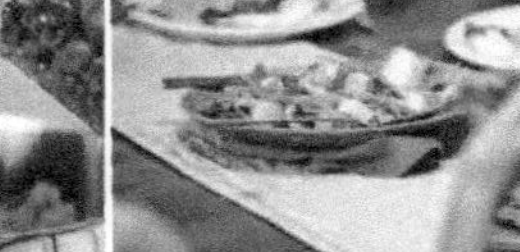
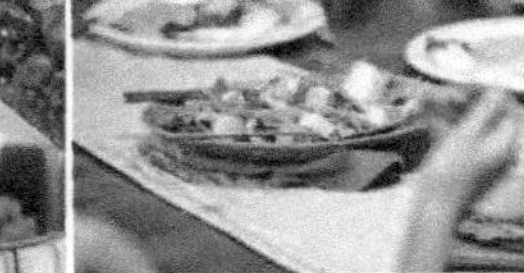
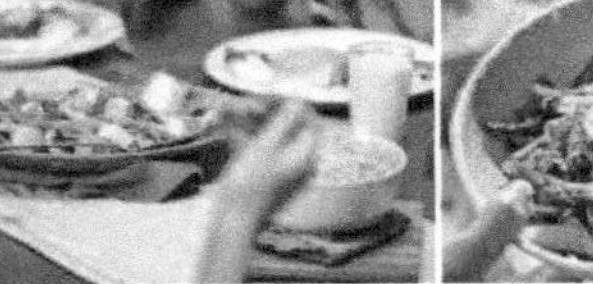

Healthy eating is more than the foods you eat. It is also about where, when, why and how you eat.

Be mindful of your eating habits

- Take time to eat
- Notice when you are hungry and when you are full

Cook more often

- Plan what you eat
- Involve others in planning and preparing meals

Enjoy your food

- Culture and food traditions can be a part of healthy eating

Eat meals with others

Make it a habit to eat a variety of healthy foods each day.

Eat plenty of vegetables and fruits, whole grain foods and protein foods. Choose protein foods that come from plants more often.

- Choose foods with healthy fats instead of saturated fat

Limit highly processed foods. If you choose these foods, eat them less often and in small amounts.

- Prepare meals and snacks using ingredients that have little to no added sodium, sugars or saturated fat
- Choose healthier menu options when eating out

Make water your drink of choice

- Replace sugary drinks with water

Use food labels

Be aware that food marketing can influence your choices

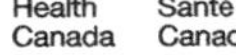

Health Canada
Santé Canada

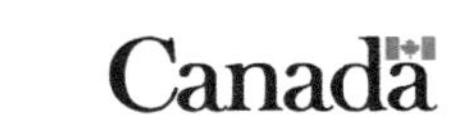
Canada

Fig. C.1 *Canada's Food Guide* recommends daily food intake for people of all ages, as well as serving sizes. Using this guide will help improve overall health. Please note that there Food Guide Snapshots in many languages available at https://www.canada.ca/en/health-canada/services/canada-food-guide/resources/snapshot/languages.html. (© All rights reserved. *Canada's food guide: Eat well. Live well.* Health Canada, 2019. Adapted and reproduced with permission from the Minister of Health, 2019. Retrieved from https://food-guide.canada.ca/en/.)

Appendix

D Pediatric Growth Charts

http://evolve.elsevier.com/Canada/Leifer

WHO GROWTH CHARTS FOR CANADA

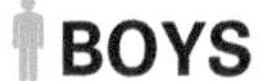

BIRTH TO 24 MONTHS: BOYS

Length-for-age and Weight-for-age percentiles

NAME: ______

DOB: ______ RECORD # ______

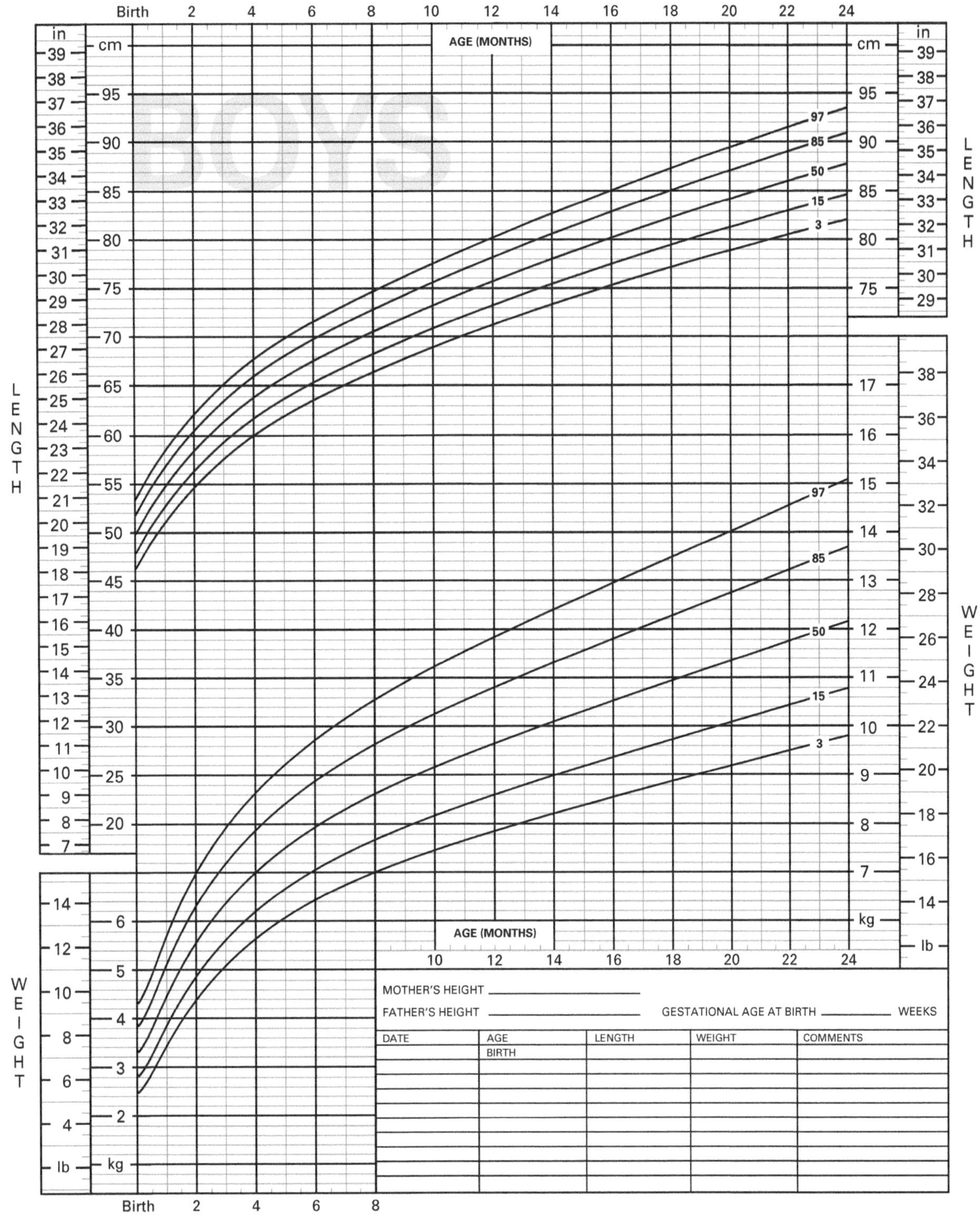

MOTHER'S HEIGHT ______

FATHER'S HEIGHT ______ GESTATIONAL AGE AT BIRTH ______ WEEKS

DATE	AGE	LENGTH	WEIGHT	COMMENTS
	BIRTH			

SOURCE: Based on World Health Organization (WHO) Child Growth Standards (2006) and WHO Reference (2007) and adapted for Canada by Canadian Paediatric Society, Canadian Pediatric Endocrine Group, College of Family Physicians of Canada, Community Health Nurses of Canada and Dietitians of Canada.

WHO GROWTH CHARTS FOR CANADA

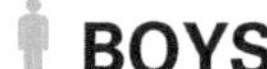
BOYS

2 TO 19 YEARS: BOYS

Height-for-age and Weight-for-age percentiles

NAME: ______________

DOB: ______________ RECORD # ______________

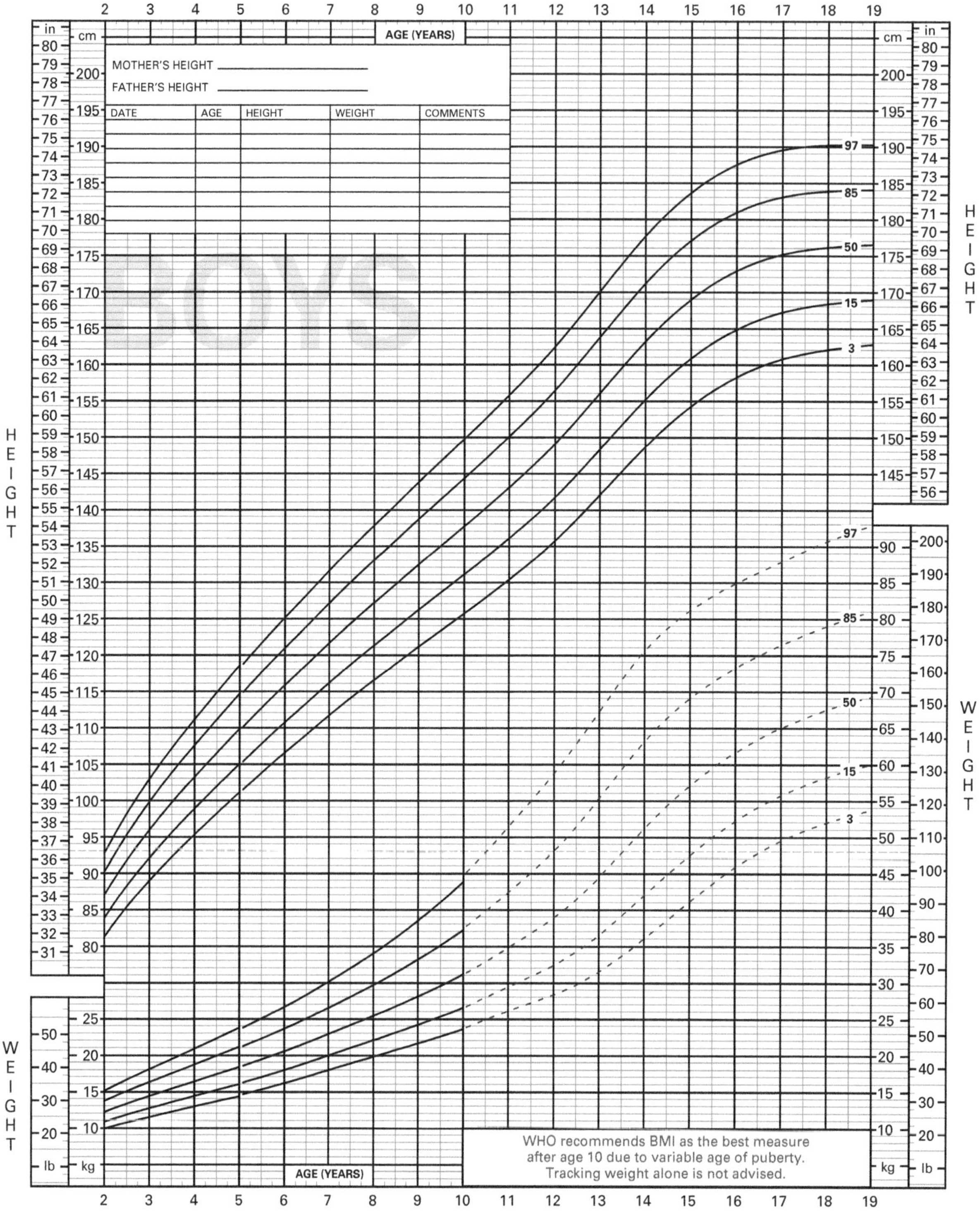

MOTHER'S HEIGHT ______________

FATHER'S HEIGHT ______________

DATE	AGE	HEIGHT	WEIGHT	COMMENTS

AGE (YEARS)
HEIGHT
WEIGHT
cm
in
kg
lb
97
85
50
15
3
BOYS
WHO recommends BMI as the best measure after age 10 due to variable age of puberty. Tracking weight alone is not advised.

SOURCE: The main chart is based on World Health Organization (WHO) Child Growth Standards (2006) and WHO Reference (2007) adapted for Canada by Canadian Paediatric Society, Canadian Pediatric Endocrine Group (CPEG), College of Family Physicians of Canada, Community Health Nurses of Canada and Dietitians of Canada. The weight-for-age 10 to 19 years section was developed by CPEG based on data from the US National Center for Health Statistics using the same procedures as the WHO growth charts.

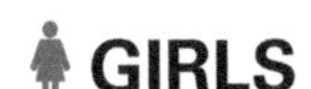

WHO GROWTH CHARTS FOR CANADA

GIRLS

BIRTH TO 24 MONTHS: GIRLS

Length-for-age and Weight-for-age percentiles

NAME: ____________

DOB: ____________ RECORD # ____________

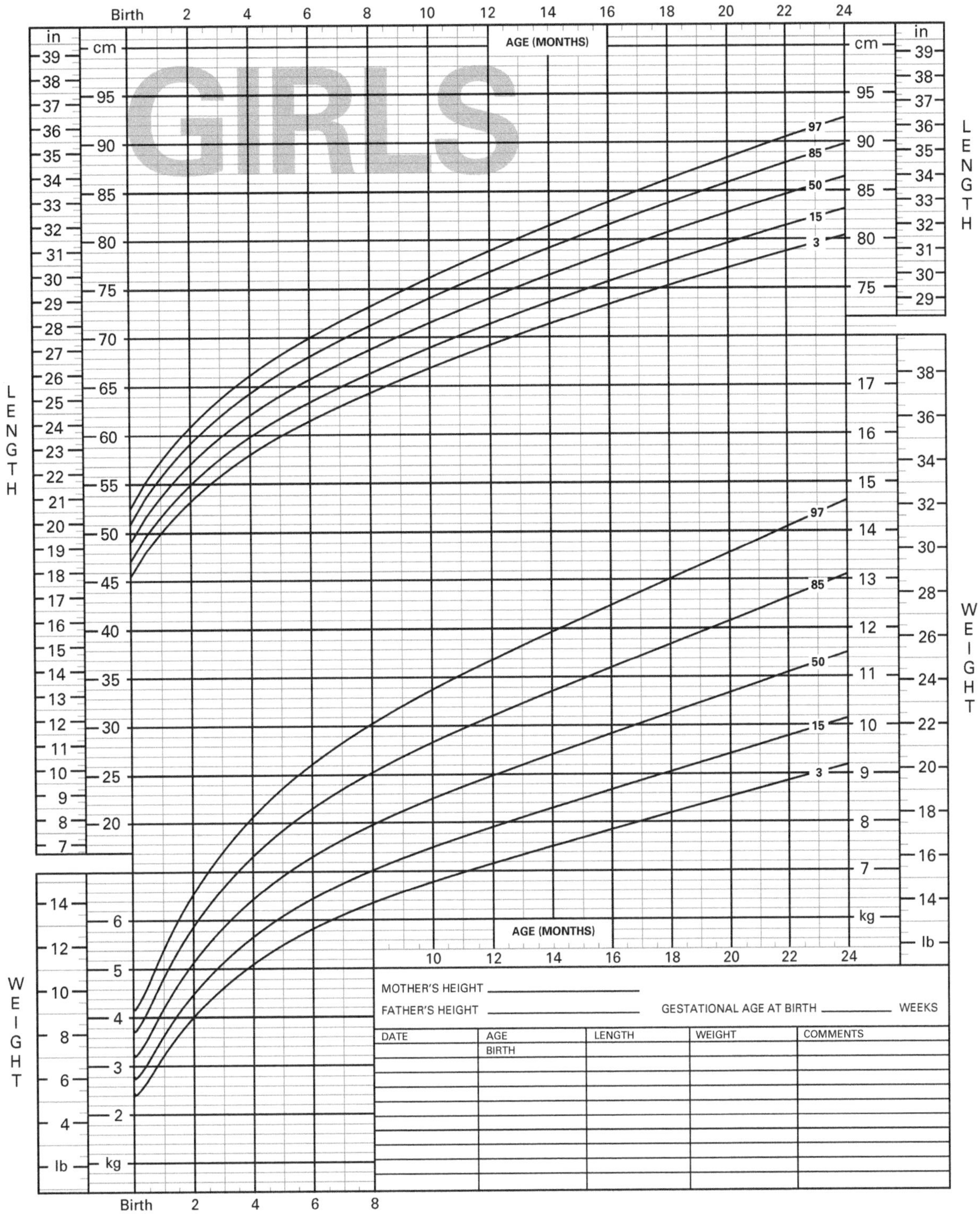

MOTHER'S HEIGHT ____________

FATHER'S HEIGHT ____________ GESTATIONAL AGE AT BIRTH ____________ WEEKS

DATE	AGE	LENGTH	WEIGHT	COMMENTS
	BIRTH			

SOURCE: Based on World Health Organization (WHO) Child Growth Standards (2006) and WHO Reference (2007) and adapted for Canada by Canadian Paediatric Society, Canadian Pediatric Endocrine Group, College of Family Physicians of Canada, Community Health Nurses of Canada and Dietitians of Canada.

WHO GROWTH CHARTS FOR CANADA

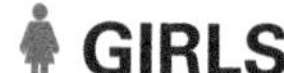

2 TO 19 YEARS: GIRLS

Height-for-age and Weight-for-age percentiles

NAME: ______________________

DOB: ______________ RECORD # __________

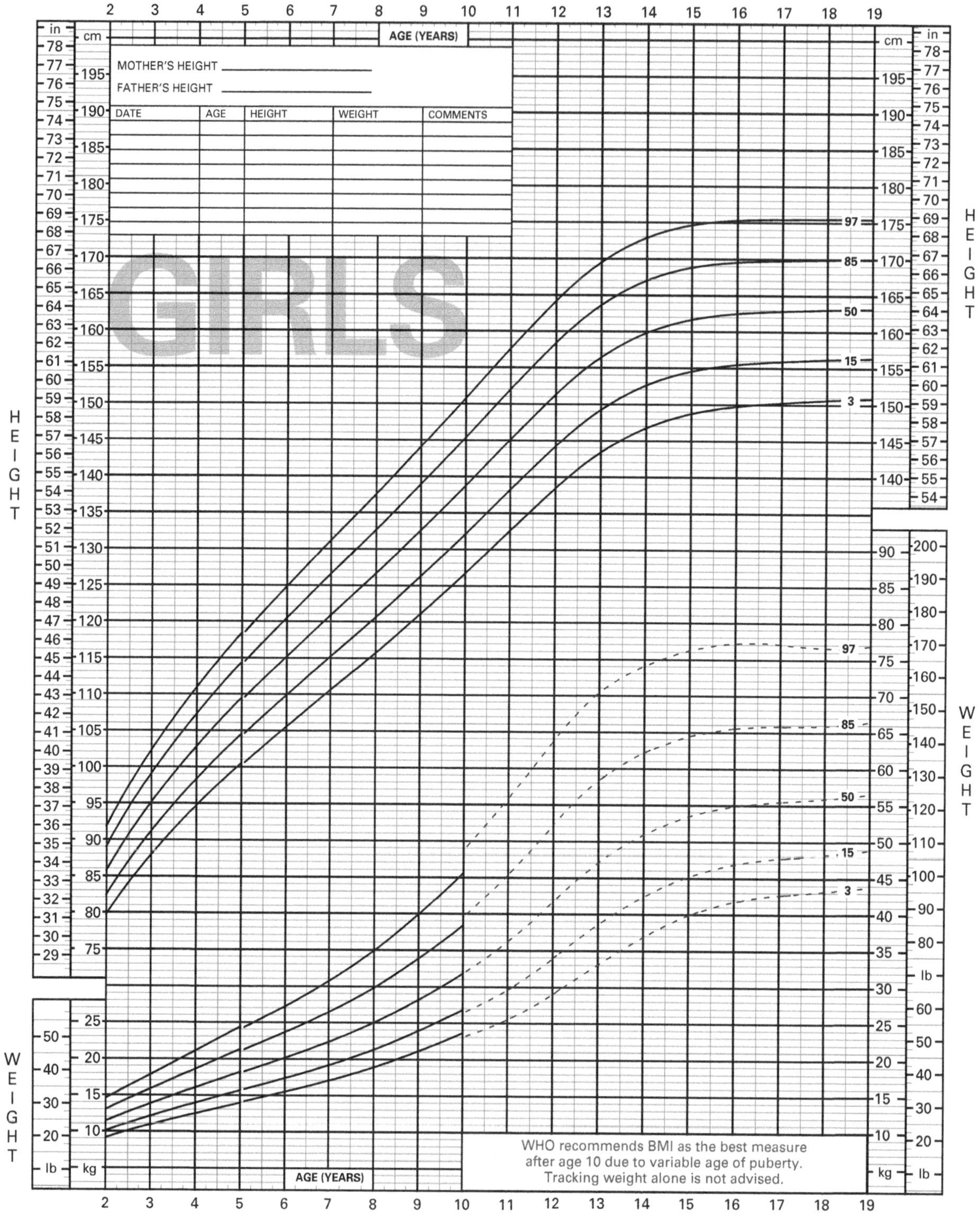

AGE (YEARS)

MOTHER'S HEIGHT ______________

FATHER'S HEIGHT ______________

DATE	AGE	HEIGHT	WEIGHT	COMMENTS

GIRLS

HEIGHT

WEIGHT

WHO recommends BMI as the best measure after age 10 due to variable age of puberty. Tracking weight alone is not advised.

AGE (YEARS)

SOURCE: The main chart is based on World Health Organization (WHO) Child Growth Standards (2006) and WHO Reference (2007) adapted for Canada by Canadian Paediatric Society, Canadian Pediatric Endocrine Group (CPEG), College of Family Physicians of Canada, Community Health Nurses of Canada and Dietitians of Canada. The weight-for-age 10 to 19 years section was developed by CPEG based on data from the US National Center for Health Statistics using the same procedures as the WHO growth charts.

Glossary

A

abortion The end of a pregnancy before the fetus is viable, whether spontaneous or elective.

absent variability Fetal heart rate that is less than 6 beats/minute change from baseline for a 10-minute period; often caused by uteroplacental insufficiency or administration of certain medications.

abstract reasoning A type of logical thought that Jean Piaget used when discussing moral reasoning.

accelerations A temporary increase of the fetal heart rate over the baseline rate of at least 15 beats/minute for at least 15 seconds in a fetus greater than 32 weeks of gestation.

acquired heart disease Heart disease that occurs after birth because of a defect or illness.

acquired immunity Immunity acquired through vaccination or the development of antibodies resulting from exposure to an infectious disease.

acrocyanosis A peripheral blueness of the hands and feet due to reduced peripheral circulation (normal in newborns).

active immunity When a person develops their own immunity.

additional precautions Precautions designed according to the method of spread of infection, such as airborne, contact, droplet, and droplet-contact isolation.

adolescence Period of human development beginning with puberty and ending with young adulthood.

adolescent Ages 12 to 18 years.

advanced practice nurses A term used often to describe the pediatric nurse practitioner (PNP) and the clinical nurse specialist (CNS).

advocate Someone who speaks or acts in support of a person's rights and needs.

afterpains Painful contractions of the uterus that occur for several days after birth; they occur most often in multiparas and are more painful during breastfeeding.

age of viability The time in a pregnancy when the fetus has reached a point in development that it can potentially survive outside of the uterus after birth. Although 22 weeks' gestation is thought to be a baseline age of viability, biomedical and technological advances now influence a fetus's survival; therefore, currently no worldwide specific age of viability can be defined.

alopecia The loss of hair, which can be an adverse effect of chemotherapy.

alternative therapy Forms of therapy that generally replace or substitute for traditionally accepted Western practice of medicine.

alveoli The area in the lungs where the exchange of carbon dioxide and oxygen occurs.

amblyopia The reduction or loss of vision that occurs in children who strongly favour one eye. Also known as "lazy eye."

amenorrhea The absence or suppression of menstruation; normal before puberty, during pregnancy and lactation, and after menopause.

amnioinfusion The infusion of warmed saline into the uterus to relieve cord compression or to wash meconium out of the cavity to prevent aspiration of it at birth.

amniotic fluid embolism Also known as anaphylactoid syndrome, it occurs when there is a massive inflammatory response or maternal immunological response possibly to components of amniotic fluid such as fetal materials.

amniotic sac The sac formed by the amnion and chorion and containing fluid and the fetus; it is commonly known as the "bag of waters."

amniotomy A procedure in which the amniotic sac is ruptured to facilitate labour.

anaphylactoid syndrome An unpredictable, catastrophic condition that occurs during labour or birth, in which an amniotic fluid embolism is released into the mother's circulation and causes cardiogenic shock or respiratory failure. It is a leading cause of maternal mortality.

anasarca Generalized edema.

anemia A decrease in the amount of hemoglobin or red blood cells circulating within the body.

animism A type of thinking characteristic of a period of cognitive development in which the child attributes life to inanimate objects.

antepartum Before the onset of labour.

anthelmintics anti, "against," and helminth, "worms."

antidiuretic hormone A hormone that regulates the balance of water in the body by concentrating the amount of urine excreted by the kidney.

anxiety disorder A disorder caused by a combination of life events, heredity, temperament, and biochemical factors.

aortocaval compression A condition that occurs when a pregnant woman lies in the supine position which allows the heavy uterus to compress her inferior vena cava, reducing the amount of blood returned to her heart. Also known as supine hypotension.

apnea A cessation of respirations.

aromatherapy The absorption of essential oils or their aromas by the lungs or skin for systemic effects.

art therapy A type of therapy that assists children in expressing their feelings and communicate through drawings, clay, and other media.

arthroscopy Using fibre optic cameras this procedure looks inside the joint (knee or shoulder) to determine the extent of the injury.

artificial rupture of membranes (AROM) Artificial rupture of the (amniotic) membranes with a sterile instrument, such as an Amnihook or Allis clamp.

artificialism The idea that people created the world and everything in it.

associative play Playing in loosely associated groups.

asynchrony The lack of concurrence in time. A growing child may look gangling because of asynchrony of growth (i.e., different body parts mature at different rates).

atelectasis An incomplete expansion of the lungs or a collapse of the alveoli after expansion.

athetosis When a child has involuntary, purposeless movements that interfere with normal motion.

atony A lack of muscle tone or strength.

attachment A strong psychological bond of affection between an infant and a caregiver.

attention-deficit hyperactivity disorder (ADHD) A disorder that causes an inappropriate degree of inattention, impulsiveness, and hyperactivity, all of which interfere with functioning or development.

augmentation of labour The enhancement of labour after it has begun but is not progressing at an appropriate rate, through use of medication.

auscultation Listening to the heart rate through a stethoscope (for blood pressure) or a Doppler or fetoscope for fetal heart rate.
autism spectrum disorder (ASD) A group of neurodevelopmental disorders characterized by difficulties in social interaction and communication, repetitive behaviours, and stereotyped interests and activities.
autograft A tissue graft that is healthy tissue obtained from another part of the patient's body. This is a more permanent graft than any other type of graft.
autonomy Independent functioning; self-control.
autosome Any chromosome within the body except the sex chromosomes (X and Y).

B

Ballard scoring system A standardized method used to estimate gestational age within the first 1 to 2 weeks of age, based on the infant's external characteristics and neurological development.
barotrauma A phenomenon that occurs when there is a change in the atmospheric pressure between the internal body systems and the surrounding environment.
baseline fetal heart rate The average fetal heart rate that occurs during a 10-minute period.
baseline variability Fluctuation or constant changes in the baseline fetal heart rate above and below the baseline in a 10-minute window.
birth defects Abnormalities that are apparent at birth.
Bishop score A scoring system that uses cervical dilation, effacement, fetal station, cervical consistency, and position to determine if labour induction will likely be successful.
blepharitis An inflammation of the eyelids that include symptoms such as redness, edema, and itching.
bloody show Appearance of a mixture of blood and mucus from the cervix that often precedes labour.
body substance The moist secretions or parts of the body that can contain microorganisms.
body surface area (BSA) The surface area of the body based on weight and height.
bonding Attachment; the process whereby a unique relationship is established between two people; used in conjunction with parent–newborn attachment.
Bradley method Also called "husband-coached childbirth," and this method of childbirth was the first to include the partner as an integral part of labour. It emphasizes slow abdominal breathing and relaxation techniques.
bradycardia A heart rate slower than the expected rate for age.
Braxton Hicks contractions Intermittent contractions of the uterus; they occur more frequently toward the end of pregnancy and are sometimes mistaken for true labour contractions.
bronchopulmonary dysplasia A complication of artificial oxygen ventilation characterized by scarring of the lung tissue, which inhibits lung ventilation and perfusion.
Bryant traction A type of skin traction apparatus commonly used for toddlers with a fractured femur. Vertical suspension is used.
Buck skin traction A type of skin traction used in fractures of the femur and in hip and knee contractures.

C

CAHM The use of complementary or alternative health modalities for treatment. This therapy is used *with* traditional or conventional therapy. Alternative therapy involves treatments that are used to *replace* conventional or traditional therapy.
caput succedaneum Swelling or edema of the newborn scalp that crosses the suture lines; usually simply called *caput*. It is self-limiting and requires no treatment.
carbon dioxide narcosis Increased levels of oxygen are given, which decreases the drive to breathe and results in increased levels of carbon dioxide (hypercapnia).
carditis An inflammation of the heart; it is a manifestation of rheumatic fever that can be fatal.
centring The tendency to concentrate on a single outstanding characteristic of an object while excluding its other features.
cephalocaudal The orderly development of muscular control, which proceeds from head to toe.
cephalohematoma Subperiosteal swelling containing blood, found on the head of some newborns. The swelling does not cross suture lines and therefore often appears unilateral; it disappears within a few weeks without treatment.
cephalopelvic disproportion (CPD) A condition in which the fetus cannot pass through the maternal pelvis; also called *fetopelvic disproportion*.
cerclage Closing of the cervix with a suture to prevent early dilation and spontaneous abortion.
cerebral palsy (CP) Term used to describe a group of non-progressive motor disorders caused by a lesion in the various motor centres of the developing fetal brain.
Chadwick sign A violet-blue colour of the vaginal mucous membrane caused by increased vascularity; it is a probable sign of pregnancy that is visible about the fourth week of pregnancy.
cheiloplasty Surgical repair for a cleft lip.
chilblain A cold injury with erythema and the formation of vesicles and ulcerative lesions that occur as a result of vasoconstriction.
chloasma A yellow-brown pigmentation over the bridge of the nose and cheeks during pregnancy and in some women who are taking oral contraceptives; also known as the *mask of pregnancy*.
chordee A congenital anomaly in which a fibrous strand of tissue extends from the scrotum to the penis, preventing urination with the penis in the normal elevated position; commonly associated with hypospadias.
chorea A disorder of the central nervous system that is characterized by involuntary, purposeless movements of the muscles.
chorioamnionitis Inflammation of the amniotic sac (fetal membranes), usually caused by bacterial or viral infections.
chorion The fetal membrane closest to the interior uterine wall; it gives rise to the placenta and continues as the outer membrane surrounding the amnion.
Christmas disease A type of hemophilia also called *hemophilia B*. It is due to little or no factor IX.
chronic condition A condition or illness that is long term and either is without cure or has a residual effect that limits activities of daily living.
circumcision The surgical removal of the foreskin of the penis.
clarity Information about the plan, expectations, and procedures are clear to the individual, family, staff, and any other team members.
classic phenylketonuria A genetic disorder caused by the faulty metabolism of phenylalanine; associated with abnormally high blood phenylalanine levels.
cleansing breath A slow, deep breath taken at the beginning and end of each contraction of labour.
cleft lip Congenital separation of one or both sides of the upper lip.
cleft palate Congenital incomplete closure of the roof of the mouth.
climacteric The physiological and psychological alterations that occur around the time of menopause.
clinical nurse specialist (CNS) The CNS provides care in the hospital or community to patients in specific specialty areas, such as cardiac, neurological, or oncological care.
clinical pathways Also known as *critical pathways, care maps*, or *multidisciplinary action plans*, clinical pathways are collaborative guidelines that define multidisciplinary care in terms of outcomes within a timeline.
cliques Small groups of friends that make up an exclusive group with similar interests, values, and tastes.

clonic movement An alternating contraction and relaxation of muscles.
club drugs Substances commonly found at parties, bars, nightclubs, and concerts. See also *street drugs*.
clubbing of the fingers A deformity of the fingers (or toes) often related to lung or cardiovascular disease.
clubfoot A congenital anomaly characterized by a foot that has been twisted inward or outward.
cognition A term referring to intellectual ability.
cognitive behavioural therapy (CBT) A type of therapy that focuses on skills related to problem solving and management of emotions.
coin-rubbing A form of CAHM therapy in which the skin is manipulated; it is thought to help bring the body into healthy alignment.
coitus interruptus Removal of the erect penis from the vagina before ejaculation.
cold stress Environmental chilling that causes increased metabolism and increased oxygen consumption in the body.
colic A condition characterized by periods of unexplained irritability and crying in a healthy, well-fed infant.
colitis An inflammation of the colon.
colostrum A secretion from the breast before the onset of true lactation; it has a high protein content, provides some immune properties, and cleanses the newborn's intestinal tract of mucus and meconium.
colposcopy A procedure in which a special type of scope is used to examine the vagina and cervix for unusual changes or neoplasms.
comedo A skin lesion caused by a plug of keratin, sebum, and bacteria; there are two types: blackheads and whiteheads.
communicable disease A disease that can be transmitted, directly or indirectly, from one person to another.
community A group of people who have a common interest or who live within the same geographic area.
compartment syndrome A progressive loss of tissue perfusion caused by an increase in pressure resulting from edema or swelling that presses on the vessels and tissues; often related to a cast that is too tight.
competitive play Play involving competition with structured rules and highly interactive physical activity.
complementary and alternative health modalities (CAHM) Nontraditional treatment method or methods used to maintain health or treat disease; used in conjunction with traditional medical therapy or treatment.
complementary therapy See *complementary and alternative health modalities (CAHM)*.
compound fracture An injury in which a wound in the skin accompanies the broken bone.
concrete operations A type of thought process that involves logical thinking and an understanding of cause and effect.
concussion A temporary disturbance of the brain that is usually followed by a period of unconsciousness related to a head injury.
congenital Present at birth.
congenital heart disease (CHD) Heart disease that may be caused by genetic or maternal factors or environmental factors.
congenital malformation An anomaly present at birth.
conjunctivitis Inflammation of the mucous membrane lining of the eyelids.
conscious sedation The administration of intravenous (IV) drugs to a patient to impair consciousness.
consistency Team and family members have the same understanding of interventions and approaches and strive to apply the same expectations and rewards.
continuation As a child with Autism spectrum disorder's behaviour improves, it is important to keep the teaching and the positive supports in place to continue to help the child develop good habits and more adaptive skills.
continuum of services Health care services that begin with health promotion, prevention, and harm reduction and follow the patient and their family through treatment and follow-up care.
cooperative play Organized play with group goals.
coping Dealing effectively with stress and problems.
coryza A cold, which is the most common infection of the respiratory tract.
critical congenital heart disease (CCHD) Heart disease with any potentially life-threatening duct-dependent defect in which the infant will die or require surgical repair or intervention within the first 28 days of life to optimize health outcomes.
critical thinking Applying creativity and ingenuity to solve a problem; combining basic standard principles with data specific to the patient.
crowning The appearance of the presenting fetal part (head) at the vaginal orifice during labour.
crust See *scab*.
cryptorchidism When one or both testes fail to lower into the scrotum.
cultural awareness A conscious awareness of one's own cultural values, beliefs, and perceptions and those of others.
cultural competence A quality, attained by cultural awareness and sensitivity, that enables health care providers to adapt practices to meet the needs of patients from various cultures.
cultural humility A process of self-reflection and discovery for building honest and trustworthy relationships.
cultural sensitivity An understanding of and sensitivity to cultural practices and values that differ from one's own.
culture The body of symbols, ideas, values, traditions, and practices shared by a group of people. *Culture* can also mean the growth of organisms in a special medium.
Curling ulcer A stress ulcer; it is common in patients with severe burns.
currant jelly stools Movements of blood and mucus that contain no feces. They are common about 12 hours after the onset of an obstruction.
curettage The scraping or vacuuming of the inner surface of the uterus.
cystometrogram A clinical procedure that evaluates bladder function.

D

DASH diet The Dietary Approach to Stop Hypertension diet: a plant-based diet high in fruits and vegetables, multigrains, and low-fat meats and dairy, as well as low in sodium. Some sugar and sweets are allowed.
dawn phenomenon A phenomenon in which early morning elevations of blood glucose occur *in the absence of* preceding hypoglycemia and may be a response to growth hormone secretion that occurs in the early morning hours.
debridement The removal of dried crusts of necrotic tissue.
deceleration A periodic decrease in baseline fetal heart rate; it can be early, late, or variable.
decidua The part of the decidua that unites with the chorion to form the placenta. It is shed in lochial discharge after birth.
deciduous Baby teeth.
depression A mood disorder characterized by sadness and loss of interest in activities.
dermabrasion A technique used to remove the outer layers of skin to minimize scarring.
dermatomes Areas of the skin that are innervated by the dorsal roots of the spinal cord and affect specific segments of the skin and adjacent structures.
developmental delay A maturational lag; an abnormal, slower rate of development in which a child demonstrates a functioning level below that observed in normal children of the same age.

developmental disability A disability that affects children's intellect or ability to cope or face some unique difficulties.
developmental dysplasia of the hip (DDH) The head of the femur is partly or completely displaced as a result of a shallow hip socket (acetabulum). This is usually diagnosed in a newborn, so treatment can be initiated immediately.
diabetes mellitus A chronic metabolic syndrome in which the body is unable to use carbohydrates properly, leading to an impairment of glucose transport. Nearly one third of Canadians have diabetes or prediabetes.
diastasis rectus Separation of the longitudinal muscles of the abdomen (rectus abdominis) during pregnancy.
diffusion The movement of particles from an area of high concentration to an area of low concentration.
dilate The cervix opens during contractions to allow the fetus to descend the birth canal.
dimensional analysis A method of calculating dosages using basic arithmetic and algebra.
diploid Cell or organism containing a set of maternal and a set of paternal chromosomes. In humans, the diploid number of chromosomes is 46.
disability A physical or intellectual impairment that may affect the life of the person.
disseminated intravascular coagulation (DIC) Coagulation disorder in which clotting factors are consumed and maternal blood does not clot.
dizygotic twins Fetuses that develop from two fertilized ova; fraternal twins.
documentation The written or electronic recording of any action taken by the nurse or other health care provider, including when a medication is given or a treatment performed. This information must be accurately entered on the patient's chart.
doula A person who provides supportive care to the labouring woman.
dysfunctional labour Abnormally painful or prolonged labour.
dysmenorrhea Menstruation that is painful.
dyspareunia Painful sexual intercourse.
dysphagia Difficulty in swallowing.
dystocia Difficult labour due to mechanical factors produced by the fetus or the maternal pelvis or due to inadequate uterine or other muscular activity.
dysuria A urinary dysfunction that makes urinating difficult.

E

early decelerations Gradual fetal heart rate (FHR) decreases during contractions; the FHR always returns to baseline rate by the end of the contraction.
early term infant An infant born between 37 weeks' gestation and 38 weeks, 6 days of gestation.
ecchymosis A bluish-black area on the skin associated with bleeding into that area.
echolalia Repetition of words without comprehension.
eclampsia Gestational hypertension complicated by one or more generalized tonic-clonic seizures.
efface The cervix thins during contractions to allow the fetus to descend the birth canal.
effleurage Using the tips of the fingers to lightly stroke a part of the body in a patterned movement; a relaxation technique used to help cope with the pain of active labour.
egocentric thinking A way of thinking that relates everything back to one's self.
egocentrism A type of thinking in which a child has difficulty seeing anyone else's point of view; this self-centring is normal in young children.
emancipated minor An independent person younger than 18 years who is not supported by their family.
emollient A treatment used to sooth the effect on the skin (sometimes treatments include oatmeal and constarch or baking soda).
empowerment Providing tools and knowledge to a patient and their family to enable informed participation in decision making about health care.
encephalitis Inflammation of the brain.
encopresis Fecal soiling as a result of constipation due to an overflow of stool.
endemic A continuous incidence of a communicable disease expected in a localized area.
endometriosis A medical condition in which endometrial tissue is found in areas of the body other than the uterus.
endometritis An inflammation or infection of the uterine lining, usually from bacterial invasion.
endorphins A natural body substance secreted by the pituitary gland that is similar in action to morphine. Levels of endorphins increase during pregnancy and peak during the labour process.
endoscopy A medical procedure that allows for the direct visualization of the gastrointestinal tract.
enterocolitis An inflammation of the colon and the small intestine.
enucleation The removal of the eye either for treatment of disease or accidentally.
enuresis The abnormal inability to control urine excretion after the age at which control should be established; may be due to organic, allergic, or psychological problems.
epicanthal folds Folds of skin that extend on either side of the bridge of the nose and cover the inner eye canthus; often present in infants with Down syndrome.
epidemic A sudden increase in a communicable disease in a localized area.
epididymis A structure on the posterior border of the testis, where coiled storage ducts provide for maturation and transport of the spermatozoa.
epidural blood patch (EDP) An injection of blood into the epidural space that provides relief from a postdural puncture headache (PDPH).
epiphyseal closure In the long bones when new growth no longer occurs because growing has stopped, the growth plate (or epiphyseal plate) is replaced by growth plate fusion (also known as *epiphyseal closure*)
episiotomy An incision of the perineum that is rarely needed to facilitate birth.
epispadias A congenital anomaly in which the urethral meatus is located on the dorsal surface of the penis.
Epstein pearls The accumulation of yellow-white epithelial cells on the hard palate of a newborn. They usually disappear within a few weeks of birth.
Erikson's stages According to Erikson's theory, the stages of child development that demonstrate the various tasks that must be mastered at each age to achieve optimum maturity.
erythema Diffused reddened area on the skin.
erythropoietin A hormone produced in the kidney that stimulates red blood cell production.
eschar A dry and dark scab that occurs after a burn wound begins to heal.
esophageal atresia (EA) A birth defect caused by a failure of the tissues of the esophagus to separate properly. The upper esophagus and the lower esophagus (leading from the stomach) end in a blind pouch.
estimated date of birth (EDB) This is an *estimated* date; many births occur before or after this date.
evidence-informed practice Taking the best evidence obtained from current, valid, published research and combining that information with the nurse's critical thinking process, experiences, and patient needs to plan safe, effective nursing care for the patient.
exacerbation The increase in severity of symptoms of a condition.
exanthem A skin rash.

extended family Refers to many generations: grandparents, parents, children, and other relatives.
extensor posturing Abnormal extension of the upper extremities with internal rotation of the upper arms and wrists; lower extremities will extend with some internal rotation.
external cephalic version (ECV) A method of changing the fetal presentation, usually from breech or oblique to cephalic.
extrusion reflex Protrusion of the tongue, which pushes food out of the mouth to prevent intake of inappropriate food. Usually present during the first 2–3 months of life.

F

failure to thrive (FTT) When infants and children who, without an obvious cause, fail to gain and often lose weight.
family care plan An expansion of the nursing care plan that includes family members.
fertilization The union of an ovum and sperm.
fetal bradycardia A fetal heart rate that is less than 110 beats/minute for 10 minutes or longer.
fetal fibronectin (fFN) A protein produced by fetal membranes that, when present, may indicate the possibility of preterm labour between 22 and 34 weeks.
fetal tachycardia A baseline fetal heart rate greater than 160 beats/minute that lasts 10 minutes or longer.
fetus A term used for the developing structure from the ninth gestational week until birth.
fever An elevation in body temperature that results in increased metabolic demand on the heart and lungs.
flexor posturing Abnormal flexion of the upper extremities and extension of the lower extremities.
fluorosis A chronic conditions that can occur with excessive use of products containing fluoride.
focal point Concentrating on a specific object or other point.
fomite Any inanimate material that carries and transmits infection.
fontanelles Openings at the point of union of skull bones, often referred to as *soft spots*.
foremilk Milk obtained at the beginning of each breastfeeding session. See also *hindmilk*.
formal operations In Piaget's system of cognitive development this as the ability to think abstractly.
frequency In labour, the period of time from the beginning of one contraction to the beginning of the next.
frostbite The result of the freezing of a body part.
full-term infant An infant born between 39 weeks' gestation and 40 weeks, 6 days' gestation.
fundus The upper portion of the uterus between the fallopian tubes.

G

gait A characteristic manner of walking.
galactogogue An agent that promotes the flow of human breast milk.
galactosemia Disorder in which the body is unable to use the carbohydrates galactose and lactose; can cause cirrhosis of the liver, cataracts, and developmental delays.
gametogenesis The development of a sex cell, such as an ovum or sperm.
gastroenteritis Infectious diarrhea caused by viral, bacterial, or parasitic infection.
gastrostomy A surgically placed tube designed to introduce food directly into the stomach through the abdominal wall.
gay A male person who prefers other males for sexual partners.
gender identity A person's perception of what gender they feel they are, which may be different from their biological sex.
generalized anxiety disorder (GAD) An anxiety reaction characterized by persistent and exaggerated apprehension and tension.
germ layers The three primary germ layers known as ectoderm, mesoderm, and endoderm, each of which develops into a different part of the growing embryo.
gestational age The actual time, from conception to birth, that the fetus remains in the uterus.
gestational diabetes mellitus (GDM) An endocrine disorder that manifests during pregnancy in which the body becomes resistant to insulin.
glomeruli The working units of the kidney that filter the blood and form urine.
glucagon A hormone produced by the alpha cells of the pancreas; counteracts the action of insulin by converting liver stores of glycogen to blood glucose, resulting in an elevation of the blood glucose concentration.
glycosuria Glucose in the urine.
glycated hemoglobin test ($HgbA_{1c}$) A test that reflects glycemic levels throughout a period of months. The more glucose in the blood, the more hemoglobin becomes coated with glucose; this test measures the amount of hemoglobin coated with glucose.
Goodell sign A probable sign of pregnancy occurring during the second month of pregnancy that involves a softening of the cervix.
grasp reflex The newborn's tendency to grasp anything that lightly stimulates the palm; used in determining neurological or muscular maturity of the newborn infant.
gravid Pregnant.
gravida The number of times a woman has been pregnant; a pregnant woman.
greenstick fracture An incomplete fracture in which one side of the bone is broken and the other is bent.
growth An increase in physical size; measured in centimetres and kilograms.
growth spurt Growth to the final, mature height that occurs during adolescence.

H

habilitation A term used to describe the treatment of a patient who has disability from birth and therefore is learning, not relearning, a task.
haploid A single set of chromosomes that are not paired. In the human embryo this number is 23.
harm reduction A range of programs, policies, and interventions designed to reduce or minimize the adverse consequences, such as overdose, infections, and spread of communicable diseases, associated with drug use.
head lag When an infant cannot maintain the neutral position of the head; the head falls back when the infant is lifted from the bed.
health care–associated infection (HAI) An infection acquired in a health care facility.
Hegar sign A probable sign of pregnancy that involves softening of the lower uterine segment found on palpation in the second or third month of pregnancy.
height Standing measurement.
hemarthrosis Bleeding into the joints; a characteristic sign of hemophilia A.
hematoma A collection of clotted blood in a confined space, usually caused by breakage of a blood vessel.
hematopoiesis Production of blood cells; normally occurs in the bone marrow but may occur in extramedullary sites.
hemodynamics The study of blood circulation.
hemolytic disease of the newborn (HDN) When an Rh-negative mother has an Rh-positive fetus there is a possibility that fetal and maternal blood may mix during labour, which causes the mother's body to respond by producing antibodies that cross the placenta and destroy the blood cells of the fetus, causing anemia and possible heart failure.
hemosiderosis The deposits of iron in the organs and tissues.

herbal medicine An alternative or complementary method for treating various ailments by using herbs and plants.
herniorrhaphy A surgical operation in which hernias are repaired.
heterograft A tissue graft that is donated from a different species.
hindmilk The milk an infant obtains after initial minutes of breastfeeding; contains a higher fat content than foremilk and is most hunger relieving.
Hirschsprung disease Occurs when there is an absence of ganglionic innervation to the muscle of a segment of the bowel; also called *congenital aganglionic megacolon*.
hives A general rash that appears abruptly; it is often an allergic or medication reaction.
homeostasis A uniform state.
homografts A tissue graft that is donated from a disease-free cadaver.
hormones A substance produced in an organ or gland and conveyed by the bloodstream to another part of the body to exert an effect.
hydramnios Polyhydramnios; an excess of amniotic fluid, leading to overdistention of the uterus. Often seen in diabetic pregnant women, even if there is no coexisting fetal anomaly.
hydrocele An excessive amount of fluid in the sac that surrounds the testicle; it causes the scrotum to swell.
hydrocephalus An abnormal condition in which there is an excessive amount of cerebral fluid within the brain cavities or surrounding the brain, or both.
hydronephrosis Distension of the renal pelvis as a result of an obstruction.
hyperbaric oxygen therapy (HBOT) Treatment in which an airtight enclosure is used to provide compressed air or oxygen under increased pressure; used to revive children with carbon monoxide poisoning and aid wound healing.
hyperbilirubinemia An excessive amount of bilirubin in the blood; more commonly seen in association with hemolytic disorders of the newborn, infection, and extreme cold stress.
hyperglycemia An excessive amount of glucose in the blood; seen most often in diabetic patients.
hyperkalemia An excess of potassium in the blood.
hyperopia Farsightedness.
hyperthermia is an increase in core body temperature due to a central nervous system impairment. Hyperthermia can result from a medication reaction, trauma, or environmental overheating.
hypertonic More fluids are lost than electrolytes.
hypertrophic pyloric stenosis An obstruction at the lower end of the stomach (pylorus) caused by an overgrowth (hypertrophy) of the circular muscles of the pylorus or by spasms of the sphincter. Projectile vomiting is a common manifestation.
hypoalbuminemia The level of protein in the blood falls.
hypocalcemia Low calcium level in the blood.
hypoglycemia Low glucose level in the blood.
hypospadias A developmental anomaly in which the urethra opens on the lower surface of the penis.
hypothermia Cooling of body temperature to subnormal levels; temperature levels considered dangerous to infants and children are core body temperatures less than 35.6°C.
hypotonia Muscle tone is low and not flexed.
hypotonic A type of dehydration resulting from the loss of more electrolytes than fluids.
hypovolemic shock Acute peripheral circulatory failure caused by loss of circulating blood volume.
hypoxia Inadequate oxygenation of the tissues.

I

icterus Jaundice in the newborn.
ileus Intestinal muscle paralysis.
impairment A physical, cognitive, psychological, or social deficiency that can range from mild to substantial.
imperforate anus The lower end of the gastrointestinal tract and the anus end in blind pouches that do not open.
incarcerated hernia When a hernia cannot be put back in place by gentle pressure.
incompetent cervix A mechanical defect in the cervix, making it unable to remain closed throughout pregnancy and resulting in spontaneous abortion.
incubation period The time between the invasion by the pathogen and the onset of clinical symptoms.
induction of labour Artificial initiation of labour.
infant Age 4 weeks to 1 year.
informed consent Implies that the parent or legal guardian or child is capable of understanding information given to them, including the purpose and risks of the procedure, and that they voluntarily agree to that procedure.
inguinal hernia A protrusion of part of the abdominal contents through the inguinal canal in the groin.
intimacy The development of a close relationship that can be either friendship or sexual.
intracranial hemorrhage Blood vessels within the skull are broken, and bleeding into the brain occurs; most common type of birth injury.
intracranial pressure (ICP) The pressure inside the skull that includes the brain tissue and cerebrospinal fluid.
intramuscular (IM) injection Injection that places medication into the muscle below the subcutaneous tissue.
intrapartum The time of onset of true labour, followed by the birth of the newborn and, finally, the placenta.
intussusception The slipping of one part of the intestine into another part just below it.
involution Reduction in the size of the uterus after birth.
isograft A tissue graft obtained from the patient's identical twin or genotype; this is a more permanent graft.
isoimmunization The phenomenon in which the Rh-negative woman develops antibodies against the Rh-positive fetus she is carrying.
isotonic The patient has lost equal amounts of fluids and electrolytes.

J

Jones criteria Diagnostic criteria used to enable diagnosis of rheumatic fever.

K

kangaroo care The use of skin-to-skin contact between the newborn or infant and the caregiver; used to promote bonding between the caregiver and the infant.
kernicterus A grave form of jaundice in the newborn caused by hyperbilirubinemia and resulting in brain damage.
ketoacidosis Diabetic ketoacidosis (DKA) is also referred to as *diabetic coma* and is associated with hyperglycemia. Symptoms include a fruity odour to the breath, nausea, decreased level of consciousness, and dehydration.
ketogenic diet A diet that is high in fats and low in carbohydrates that produce ketoacidosis in the body. The diet is used to treat epilepsy in some children.
Kohlberg Lawrence Kohlberg is a childhood developmental theorist who suggested that moral development in children is sequential. He describes three levels: *preconventional, conventional*, and *postconventional*.
kwashiorkor A severe deficiency of protein in the diet despite the fact that the number of calories consumed may be nearly adequate; rare in Canada.

L

laceration In obstetrics, a tear in the perineum, vagina, or cervix.
lactation The process of producing and supplying breast milk.

Lamaze method A method taught in childbirth education classes by which women learn ways to decrease their perception of pain during the childbirth experience.
laminaria Type of kelp or seaweed that can be used to help dilate the cervical canal to aid in delivery of the products of conception.
lanugo Fine, downy hair seen on all parts of the fetus, except the palms of the hands and soles of the feet, by the end of 20 weeks of gestation.
last menstrual period (LMP) The first day of the last menstrual period used to determine the estimated date of birth.
latchkey children Children who are left unsupervised after school because parents are away from home or at work and other caregivers are not available to care for them.
late decelerations A decrease in fetal heart rate during a uterine contraction that continues after the contraction ends.
late-term infant Born between 41 weeks and 41 weeks, 6 days.
length The measurement of infants while in the recumbent position.
Leopold manoeuvre A series of four manoeuvres (abdominal palpation) designed to provide a systematic approach to determine fetal presentation and position.
lesbian A female attracted to other females for a sexual relationship.
let-down reflex A pattern of stimulation, hormone release, and muscle contraction that forces milk into the lactiferous ducts, making it available to the infant; milk ejection reflex.
lie The position of the fetus described by the relationship of the long axis of the fetus to the long axis of the mother.
lightening Movement of the fetus and uterus downward into the pelvic cavity and the fundus no longer presses on the diaphragm.
lipoatrophy Loss of fat tissue in subcutaneous tissue that can occur at the injection site of insulin.
lochia The maternal discharge of blood, mucus, and tissue from the uterus; may last for several weeks after birth.
low-flow oxygen A method of oxygen delivery used for children with chronic lung disease.
lumbar puncture A method of obtaining spinal fluid for examination or to reduce pressure within the brain.
lymphadenopathy An enlargement of lymph nodes that is indicative of infection or disease.

M

macrosomia An abnormally large infant, or newborn birth weight above the ninetieth percentile.
macule Circular reddened area on the skin.
marked variability There are more than 25 beats of fluctuation over the fetal heart rate baseline.
Maslow Abraham Maslow developed the hierarchy of needs. The five stages of needs include *physiological, safety, love/belonging, self-esteem*, and *self-actualization*.
mastitis Acute infection of the breast.
maturation The total way in which a person grows and develops, as dictated by genetics.
McDonald sign A probable sign of pregnancy in which the examiner can easily flex the cervix against the body of the uterus.
Meckel's diverticulum During fetal life, the intestine is attached to the yolk sac by the vitelline duct. A small, blind pouch may form if this duct fails to disappear completely.
meconium The first stools of the newborn; a mixture of amniotic fluid and secretions of the intestinal glands.
meconium aspiration syndrome (MAS) Characteristic symptoms that result from aspiration of meconium in utero. The presence of meconium in the trachea or its appearance on a chest X-ray film helps to confirm this diagnosis.
meconium ileus A condition in which the meconium of the fetus becomes excessively sticky and adheres to the intestinal wall, causing obstruction. It is occasionally seen in babies born with cystic fibrosis.
menarche The beginning of menstrual and reproductive functions in girls.
meningitis An inflammation of the meninges that cover the brain and spinal cord.
meningocele A type of spina bifida in which the mass contains portions of the membranes and cerebrospinal fluid.
meningomyelocele A sac-like cyst containing the meninges, spinal cord, and fluid that has herniated through the spinal column, usually via some form of anatomical defect of the bony spinal canal; often associated with paralysis of the legs and poor control of bowel and bladder functions.
menopause The permanent cessation of menses.
menorrhagia Bleeding from the uterus between menstrual cycles.
meridians An imaginary line that encircles the body; used in some forms of complementary or alternative health modalities.
metabolic rate Refers to energy use and oxygen consumption.
methicillin-resistant *Staphylococcus aureus* (MRSA) Infections that are resistant to certain antibiotics and are handled under strict contact isolation precautions.
metrorrhagia Uterine bleeding that is usually normal in amount but occurs at irregular intervals.
microbiota The human body contains a community of microorganisms (pathogenic and nonpathogenic).
microbiome The normal microbes in the individual's own body; they also play a role in maintaining pregnancy, preparation for labour, and establishing a microbiome that is passed on to the newborn.
micturition Emptying the bladder.
midwives The registered midwife (RM) has graduated from an accredited midwifery program and is nationally certified by the Canadian Association of Midwives. The RM provides comprehensive prenatal, intrapartum, and postnatal care for low-risk women.
milestones The growth and development patterns of achievements at various stages of infancy.
milia Very small, white, keratin-filled cysts or papules normally found on a newborn's face. They generally disappear if left alone.
Millennium Development Goals (MDGs) Developed by the member nations of the United Nations that created eight international goals that focused on improving the health and education of the global community.
Milwaukee brace This apparatus exerts pressure on the chin, pelvis, and convex (arched) side of the spine. Occasionally used to treat scoliosis.
minimal variability Fetal heart rate changes of 3 to 6 beats/minute; often due to medications administered to the mother, maternal smoking, or fetal sleep.
mittelschmerz Abdominal pain occurring at the time of ovulation.
modelling Setting a good example for children.
moderate variability Changes of 6 beats/minute to 25 beats/minute from the baseline fetal heart rate.
Mongolian spot A benign, blue-hued pigmentation caused by melanin deposits usually found around the lower back or the buttock. It is seen most often in non-White infants and may fade during childhood.
monozygotic twins Two fetuses that develop from a single divided, fertilized ovum; identical twins.
mood disorders A group of diagnoses related to disturbances in mood.
morbidity Term pertaining to incidence of illness and disease.
Moro reflex The newborn's symmetrical response, when jarred, to extend and abduct the extremities in an embracing motion, including a spreading apart of the fingers with the thumb and forefinger forming a C shape. Presence of the reflex indicates health of the newborn's central nervous system.

mortality Term pertaining to incidence of death.
moulding The shaping of the fetal head to facilitate movement through the birth canal during labour.
multigravida A woman who has been pregnant before, regardless of the duration of the pregnancy.
multipara A woman who has had more than one pregnancy in which the fetus(es) was (were) greater than 20 weeks of gestation.
mummy restraint A short-term restraint that might be necessary for examination or treatments such as a venipuncture or placement of a nasogastric tube.
muscular dystrophies A group of disorders in which progressive muscle degeneration occurs; most common child form is Duchenne muscular dystrophy (DMD).
myopia Nearsightedness.
myringotomy An incision of the ear drum that is used to drain fluid or relieve pressure.

N

Nägele's rule A method of determining the estimated date of birth (EDB); after obtaining the first day of the last menstrual period, add 7 days and count forward 9 months.
narcissistic To be excessively interested in one's own appearance.
natural immunity The body has built the ability to resist infections.
necrotizing enterocolitis (NEC) Acute inflammation of the bowel that leads to necrosis.
negativism The attitude of opposing or resisting the directions of others.
neonatal opioid withdrawal syndrome (NOWS) Occurs when the fetus has prenatal exposure to drugs such as opiates, amphetamines, tranquilizers, or multiple illicit drugs while in utero. Also known as neonatal abstinence syndrome (NAS).
nephron The functional unit of the kidneys.
neurodevelopmental disorders Disorders that manifest in the functioning of the neurological system and brain.
neurological assessment An assessment that is used to detect central nervous system dysfunction or injury. The neurological examination can also be used to detect decline or improvement in neurological status in order to determine the best care for the patient.
neurovascular checks Assessment for capillary refill, signs of poor circulation, pallor, cyanosis, swelling, coldness, numbness, pain, or burning in any distal fingers or toes when there is a cast or an injury.
neutral thermal environment An environment that is neither too hot nor too cold; thus, the body does not need to overwork to deliver oxygen or increase its metabolic rate to maintain a normal body temperature.
nevi A congenital discoloration of an area of the skin, such as a strawberry mark or mole.
newborn Birth to 4 weeks.
nitrazine test A test done to determine if a woman's membranes have ruptured prior to labour. Alkaline amniotic fluid turns pH paper dark blue-green or dark blue.
nocturia A urinary dysfunction that makes one wake up during the night to void.
norms Milestones of growth and development that are achieved at various stages of development which usually occur during certain developmental periods.
nuchal cord A term to describe a situation in which the umbilical cord is wrapped around the fetus's neck.
nuclear family A family unit that consists of one or more parents and one or more of their children.
nursing care plan Developed as a result of the nursing process, the nursing care plan is a written instrument of communication among staff members that focuses on individualized patient care.
nursing caries This condition occurs when the infant is put to bed with a bottle of milk or sweetened juice. Also known as nursing bottle syndrome.
nursing process This term refers to a series of steps describing the systematic problem-solving approach nurses use to identify, prevent, or treat actual or potential health problems. The steps in the nursing process include assessment, analysis, outcome identification, planning, implementation, and evaluation.
nystagmus Constant jerky movements of the eyeball.

O

object permanence The phenomenon of objects existing even if they are out of visual field.
oligohydramnios A decreased amount of amniotic fluid.
oliguria A decrease in urine secretion by the kidney.
oncologists A health care provider who specialize in the treatment of tumours.
oogenesis The process of mitosis in the ovum.
ophthalmia neonatorum Acute conjunctivitis of the newborn, often caused by gonococci or *Chlamydia*.
opioids Natural and synthetic opium derivative used for analgesia.
opisthotonos Extension of the neck with an arched back, associated with central nervous system problems in the newborn.
opportunistic infection An infection caused by bacteria normally found in the environment that become pathogenic to the body owing to a defective immune system; usually seen in immunosuppressed individuals whose CD4 counts have dropped to a critical level, such as patients with cancer or AIDS.
oral stage A personality stage that occurs during infancy that is shown by sucking and is important for the infant's physical and psychological development.
orchiopexy A surgical procedure to move an undescended testicle into the scrotum.
orthopnea A condition in which the patient must sit up to breathe.
Ortolani sign This is when the femoral head slips back into the acetabulum under gentle pressure.
osteomyelitis An infection of the bone.
osteoporosis A decrease in the overall mass of bones due to an increase in the trabeculae of the bone. It can be caused by age, sedentary lifestyle, smoking, diet, and many other factors.
ovarian cycle The changes that the ovarian follicles undergo throughout the menstrual cycle. Days 1 to 14 comprise the follicular phase, and days 15 to 28 comprise the luteal phase.

P

pain threshold The least amount of sensation that a person perceives as painful.
pain tolerance The amount of pain one is willing to endure.
palliative care A method of care that improves the quality of life of children and their families who are facing problems associated with life-threatening illness, including pain management and the relief of suffering.
pandemic A worldwide high incidence of a communicable disease.
papilledema Edema of the optic nerve.
papule Circular reddened area on the skin that is elevated.
parachute reflex A protective arm extension that occurs when an infant is suddenly thrust downward when prone.
parallel play Playing alongside but not with other children.
paraphimosis Impaired circulation of the uncircumcised penis due to improper retraction of the foreskin.
parenteral A medication route other than the gastrointestinal tract; can be intravenous, intramuscular, or another route
parenteral fluids Fluids given by some route other than the digestive tract.
parity The number of pregnancies ending after 20 weeks' gestation.

passive immunity Antibodies to a communicable disease are given to the patient.
pathogens Organisms that cause disease.
pathognomonic A lesion or symptom that is characteristic of a specific illness.
Pavlik harness Used for long-term immobilization (6 to 8 weeks) of a child with developmental dysplasia of the hip.
pediculosis The infestation of lice.
perfusion The distribution of oxygen to body tissues.
perinatal mood disorders Mood disorders affecting women before or after birth; can range from anxiety to depression or psychosis.
periodic changes Brief changes in the fetal heart rate that are associated with uterine contractions.
Personal Information Protection and Electronic Documents Act (PIPEDA) Legislation that sets standards to protect a person's privacy.
personal space An imaginary space that surrounds us and makes us feel secure.
personality A unique organization of characteristics that determine the individual's typical or recurrent pattern of behaviour or the result of interaction between biological and environmental heritages.
petechiae Tiny, flat, purplish red spots on the skin surface resulting from minute hemorrhages within the dermis.
phimosis Tightening of the prepuce of the uncircumcised penis.
phototherapy The treatment of disease by exposure to light; often used to treat hyperbilirubinemia in the newborn.
phototoxicity A skin reaction when exposed to the sun.
physical dependence Physiological cellular adaptation occurs and the central nervous system and peripheral nervous system become habituated to the substance such that the person physically needs the drug in order to function or to avoid the physical pain of withdrawal.
physiological jaundice A condition characterized by a yellow tinge of the skin.
Piaget A psychologist who focused on cognitive development.
pica The eating of substances not ordinarily considered to be edible or to have nutritive value.
pincer grasp The use of the index finger and thumb to grasp an object.
placenta A specialized disk-shaped organ that connects the fetus to the uterine wall for gas, nutrient, and waste exchanges; also called *afterbirth*.
placenta accreta A placenta that is embedded in the uterine muscle, resulting in failure to separate and be expelled during the third stage of labour.
play therapy A technique used for the child under stress where the child can play with any toy they choose.
plumbism Lead poisoning.
polyarthritis Inflammation of many joints, which causes pain and difficulty moving. It usually affects the larger joints.
polycythemia An excess of red blood cells.
polydipsia Symptoms of excessive thirst.
polyhydramnios An excessive amount of amniotic fluid within the placenta.
polyphagia Symptoms of excessive hunger.
polyuria Increased urine output (>3 mL/kg/hr).
portal of entry A route by which organisms enter the body (e.g., a cut in the skin).
portal of exit A route by which organisms exit the body (e.g., feces or urine).
postdural puncture headache (PDPH) Headache that results from spinal fluid leaking from the hole during dural puncture.
postictal A short period of sleep or decreased alertness after a generalized seizure.
postpartum After childbirth.
postpartum blues A normal fluctuation of mood occurring within 2 weeks of birth.
post-term infant A pregnancy that goes beyond 42 weeks.
posturing Abnormal extension and flexion of the limbs usually seen in a person with a brain injury.
preadolescent Age 10 marks the beginning of this stage.
preconceptual stage Developed by Piaget, this stage involves the increasing development of language and symbolic functioning.
pre-eclampsia An increase in blood pressure that occurs during pregnancy, accompanied by proteinuria (protein in the urine). Symptoms may also include thrombocytopenia, renal insufficiency, elevated liver enzymes, or epigastric pain or cerebral symptoms such as a sudden acute headache.
prehension The use of the hands to pick up small objects; grasping.
preoperational phase Developed by Piaget, it consists of the preconceptual stage and the intuitive thought stage.
preschool Ages 3 to 5 years.
preterm infant Premature infant; an infant born before 37 weeks of gestation.
preterm labour The regular contractions of a pregnant uterus resulting in changes in the cervix (dilation and effacement) that start before 37 weeks' gestation.
previability A fetus before the age of when it is able to survive, which is considered 22 weeks' gestation.
primary care nurse practitioner Focuses on prevention of illness and maintenance of health as well as the treatment of illness.
primigravida A woman who is pregnant for the first time.
primipara A woman who has given birth to her first child (past the point of viability), whether or not that child is living or was alive at birth.
prodromal period The initial symptoms indicating an approaching onset of disease.
products of conception (POC) Tissues that are produced during a pregnancy that are passed or removed during a spontaneous or induced abortion.
projectile vomiting Vomiting that occurs with force (vomitus landing 0.5 to 1.5 metres away).
prolonged decelerations Abrupt fetal heart rate decreases of 15 beats/minute from the baseline for longer than 2 minutes but less than 10 minutes.
proptosis A penetrating injury to the eye.
proximodistal Progression from the centre outward or from the midline to the periphery.
pruritus Severe itching of the skin.
pseudoanemia False anemia often due to dilution of the blood.
psychological dependence A mild wish to a craving for or a compulsive emotional need to use a substance.
psychosis Mental state in which a person's ability to recognize reality, communicate, and relate to others is impaired.
psychosocial interventions Providing the child or young person and their family with information concerning how to manage stressful situations.
puberty The period during which the secondary sexual characteristics develop and the ability to reproduce is attained.
puerperal sepsis An infection or septicemia after childbirth.
puerperium The period after birth until involution of the uterus is complete, usually 6 weeks.
pulse oximeter Equipment that uses a sensor placed on the skin to determine the level of blood oxygen saturation.
pulse pressure The difference between the systolic and diastolic blood pressure.
purpura Larger (greater than 3 mm) areas of nonblanching red, blue, or purplish spots that are the result of intradermal hemorrhage (bruising), often a result of a low platelet count.

pursed-lip breathing A technique of breathing often used in children with asthma.
pustule Circular reddened area on the skin that is elevated and contains pus.
pyelonephritis The infection of the kidney and the renal pelvis.

Q

quickening The first fetal movements felt by the pregnant woman, usually occurring between 16 and 18 weeks of gestation for a primigravida.

R

reactive airway disease (RAD) When asthma is suspected but not yet diagnosed. The bronchioles overreact to an irritant.
rebound tenderness Pressing the right lower quadrant with rapid release of pressure causes severe pain in a child with appendicitis.
reflexology Integrative therapy that uses varying degrees of pressure, usually to the hands or the feet, to promote relaxation.
reflux A backward flow of fluid (e.g., vesicoureteral reflux [urine is forced from the bladder into the ureters], gastric reflux [stomach contents flow into the esophagus; it may or may not enter the oral cavity]).
regression Behaviour that is more appropriate to an earlier stage of development; often occurs in children as a response to stress.
remission A period of time in which there is a decrease in the symptoms of a disease.
reservoir for infection A place that supports the growth of organisms (e.g., standing, stagnant water).
respiratory distress syndrome (RDS) Inability of newborn, especially preterm newborn, to maintain adequate respiratory effort, resulting from insufficient surfactant in the lungs.
respite care Trained workers who provide the opportunity for primary caregivers of an ill child to have a break from the responsibility of caring for the child. They may come into the home or work at locations in the community.
retinopathy of prematurity (ROP) Condition in which there is damage to immature retinal blood vessels, which can lead to blindness; thought to be caused by high oxygen levels of arterial blood. Formerly called *retrolental fibroplasia*.
rheumatic fever (RF) A systemic disease involving the joints, heart, central nervous system, skin, and subcutaneous tissues.
ritualism A need to maintain strict structure and routine.
Rolfing Technique of massage that involves fascia pressure, stretching, and manipulation.
rooting reflex The infant's tendency to turn the head and open the lips to suck when that side of the mouth or cheek is touched or stroked.
routine precautions A method of using personal protection equipment (gloves or gown) when in contact with any blood or other body fluids (emesis, saliva, sputum, semen, urine, feces).
rugae Folds of mucous membranes on internal surfaces such as the vagina.
Russell traction A sling that is positioned under the knee, which suspends the distal thigh above the bed.

S

saline lock A long-term peripheral venous access device that is connected to an intravenous line when required for medication or fluid.
satiety When a person's hunger is satisfied.
SBAR A formal method of communicating with other members of the health care team, which includes **s**ituation, **b**ackground, **a**ssessment, and **r**ecommendation.
scab Dried pustule that is covered with a crust.
scarf sign This refers to the full-term infant's resistance to attempts to bring one elbow farther than the midline of the chest.
school-age Ages 5 to 12 years.
scoliosis Lateral curvature of the spine.
sebum An oily secretion of the enlargement of the sebaceous glands.
self-concept How one views one self.
separation anxiety Distress behaviour that occurs when an infant or a young child is separated from the parents; most severe at 18 months of age.
sepsis A generalized infection of the bloodstream.
sexual latency A period Freud referred to regarding when children identify with the parent of the same sex.
sexual maturity ratings (SMRs) A scale used to assess an adolescent's stage of physical development focusing on the development of secondary sexual characteristics.
shaken baby syndrome Roughly shaking an infant can cause the brain to strike the inside of the skull.
shiatsu Finger pressure used with an emphasis on preventing disease rather than treating symptoms.
shoulder dystocia The fetal head is born, but the shoulders become impacted above the mother's symphysis pubis.
shunt A bypass.
sibling rivalry Feelings of jealousy and fear of replacement when a young child must share parental attention with a newborn infant.
sickle cell crises The painful and often fatal manifestations of sickle cell disease caused by the sickling of red blood cells.
sigmoidoscopy A more invasive form of endoscopy that allows direct visualization of the gastrointestinal tract through the insertion of a flexible lighted tube that has a camera at its tip and is inserted through the mouth.
sign language The use of hand signals that correspond to words and assist in communication with a person who is hearing impaired.
simplicity Supports are simple, practical, and accessible so that everyone on the team, including the family, can understand and use them.
social anxiety disorder A disorder that affects many adolescents, but referral is not indicated unless the behaviour significantly interferes with social interactions or academic achievements.
Somogyi phenomenon This occurs when blood glucose levels are lowered to a point at which the body's counter-regulatory hormones (epinephrine, cortisol, glucagon) are released.
spermatogenesis The process by which mature spermatozoa are formed and during which the number of chromosomes is reduced by half.
spermicide An agent that kills sperm.
spica cast Cast used for long-term (several months) treatment of developmental dysplasia of the hips. It keeps the femur in position.
spina bifida A congenital embryonic neural tube defect in which there is an imperfect closure of the spinal vertebrae. There are two types: *occulta* (hidden) and *cystica* (sac or cyst).
spinnbarkeit Elasticity seen in cervical mucus at the time of ovulation.
spiral fracture A complete fracture that occurs from a forceful twisting motion of the bone.
spirometry Measures air flow and volume during a forced exhalation at a maximal effort into a spirometer.
splenomegaly The enlargement of the spleen.
spontaneous rupture of membranes (SROM) When the amniotic sac breaks on its own, either before or during labour. Labour often starts after this occurs.
stage of industry A period Erikson refers to in the school-age child: there is a thirst for knowledge and accomplishment. Children use skills and knowledge they obtain to attempt to master activities.
station The relationship of the presenting fetal part to an imaginary line drawn between the pelvic ischial spines.

statistics The science of gathering and analyzing numerical data.
status epilepticus A prolonged seizure that does not respond to treatment for 30 minutes or more.
stenosis Narrowing of a vessel.
strabismus (cross-eye or squint) A condition in which the child is not able to direct both eyes toward an object at the same time because of a lack of muscle coordination.
street drugs Illegal substances such as fentanyl, heroin, cocaine, and methamphetamine; illegally sold for the purpose of producing an altered state of consciousness.
stridor Emission of a shrill sound during respiration; caused by air passing through a narrowed portion of the respiratory tract.
stroke volume The amount of blood ejected during one contraction.
stye An infection of the sebaceous gland of the eyelash.
subcutaneous (subcut) injection A method of injection into the skin, by which medication or fluid is absorbed slowly, diffusing into the capillaries.
subinvolution A slower-than-expected return of the uterus to its nonpregnant condition. Infection and a retained placenta are the usual causes.
substance use disorders Disorders characterized by the misuse of drugs and the physical and psychological dependence on them.
suckling When the newborn or infant is breastfeeding, it causes the mother's posterior pituitary gland to release oxytocin to help with uterine contractions after birth and stimulates milk production.
supine hypotension The lowering of blood pressure while in a supine position; occurs as a result of pressure or the weight of the pregnant uterus on the inferior vena cava.
supportive and interpersonal therapy Therapy in which attachment and communication strategies are used to help individuals adjust how they see their world.
surfactant A mixture of lipoproteins secreted in the alveoli and air passages that reduces the surface tension within the alveoli and contributes to the expansion of the lungs.
sutures In obstetrics, separation between fetal skull bones that permits moulding during the birth process.
symbolic functioning Seen in the play of children who create a mental image to stand for something that is not there.

T

tachycardia Rapid heart rate (above normal for the age of the child or fetus).
tachypnea Rapid respiration.
tachysystole Uterine contraction frequency more than every 2 minutes; or five or more contractions within 10 minutes with duration longer than 90 seconds; or resting interval between contractions less than 60 seconds.
temper tantrums Uncontrolled anger reactions; often occur during the toddler years.
teratogen A nongenetic factor that can produce malformations of the fetus.
testicular torsion When the spermatic cord that allows blood to flow to the testicle becomes twisted.
"tet" spells Spontaneous cyanosis, respiratory distress, weakness, and syncope occur. They can last a few minutes to a few hours and are followed by lethargy and sleep. They occur during the first 2 years of life in children who have Tetrology of Fallot.
therapeutic play Guided play that helps children deal with concerns or disabilities and helps nurses gain insight into children's needs (e.g., blowing bubbles is postoperative therapeutic play designed to help expand lungs).
thermoregulation Maintenance of body temperature within normal limits.
thoracotomy A chest incision.
time-out Involves removing a child from an activity and not giving the child attention for a short period of time when their behaviour is unacceptable.
tissue turgor The hydration or dehydration of the skin.
tocolytic A medication that inhibits uterine contractions.
toddler Ages 1 to 3 years old.
tolerance This can develop when a user's body becomes accustomed to certain medications and requires more medication to be effective.
tonic-clonic seizures Seizures in which there is facial muscle twitching followed by generalized contraction of all muscles (tonic phase), then alternate contraction and relaxation of the muscles (clonic phase).
tonic movement A stiffening (contraction) of muscles.
tonic neck reflex A postural reflex in which the head is turned to one side, the arm and leg are extended on the same side, and the opposite arm and leg are flexed in a "fencing" position.
total body surface area (TBSA) An assessment of the injury or disease of the skin, such as burns.
total parenteral nutrition (TPN) Provides the total nutritional needs through a parenteral route, for infants and children who cannot use the gastrointestinal tract for nourishment for a prolonged period.
tracheoesophageal fistula (TEF) Caused by a failure of the tissues of the gastrointestinal tract to separate properly from the respiratory tract early in prenatal life. One part of the esophagus is attached to the trachea and the other part of the esophagus ends in a blind pouch.
tracheostomy A surgical procedure in which an opening is made in the trachea to enable the patient to breathe.
transient tachypnea of the newborn (TTN) A condition seen most often in infants born by Caesarean or a rapid vaginal birth, characterized by tachypnea (rapid respirations). It may also include chest retractions, grunting, and mild cyanosis. The condition is often referred to as *wet lung* or *respiratory distress syndrome.*
transitional object An object that promotes security, such as a blanket or a favourite toy.
trial of labour after Caesarean (TOLAC) A labour experience in which the woman attempts to have a vaginal labour and birth after a previous Caesarean birth. The birth is known as a VBAC (vaginal birth after Caesarean).
trimester One third of the gestational time for pregnancy. Pregnancy has three trimesters.

U

ureteritis The infection of the ureters.
urethritis The infection of the urethra.
urgency The immediate need to urinate often with little warning.
uteroplacental insufficiency When not enough oxygen is being delivered to the fetus.
uterus A hollow, muscular organ in which the fertilized ovum is implanted and the developing fetus is nourished until birth.

V

vaginal birth after Caesarean (VBAC) The vaginal birth of an infant following a previous Caesarean birth.
variable decelerations Abrupt decreases of at least 15 beats/minute below baseline, lasting 15 seconds to 2 minutes in the full-term fetus.
vasopressin The antidiuretic hormone that concentrates urine in the kidney.
vector A carrier that transmits an infective agent from one host to another.

ventilation The process of breathing air into and out of the lungs.
vernix caseosa A protective cheeselike, whitish substance made up of sebum and desquamated epithelial cells that is present on fetal skin and the skin of the newborn.
vesicle Circular reddened area on the skin that is elevated and contains fluid.
vesicoureteral reflux The backward flow of urine into the ureters.

W

walking reflex Stepping movements of the legs of an infant.
weaning The process of substituting a cup for a bottle or breastfeeding.
Wharton's jelly Yellow-white gelatinous material that surrounds and protects the vessels of the umbilical cord.
wheal A large, slightly raised, red or blistered area of skin; it may itch.
Wilms tumour One of the most common malignant renal tumours of early life, thought to have a genetic basis. Also called *nephroblastoma*.

X–Z

xenograft A tissue graft that is of a different species.

Index

Note: Page numbers followed by "f" indicate figures, "t" indicate tables and "b" indicate boxes.

N

O

Q

R